Amino Acids in Human Nutrition and Health

———————————

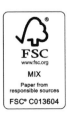

Amino Acids in Human Nutrition and Health

Edited by

J.P.F. D'Mello

Formerly of SAC, University of Edinburgh King's Buildings Campus, Edinburgh, UK

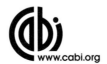

CABI is a trading name of CAB International

CABI Nosworthy Way Wallingford Oxfordshire OX10 8DE UK	CABI 875 Massachusetts Avenue 7th Floor Cambridge, MA 02139 USA
Tel: +44 (0)1491 832111 Fax: +44 (0)1491 833508 E-mail: cabi@cabi.org Website: www.cabi.org	Tel: +1 617 395 4056 Fax: +1 617 354 6875 E-mail: cabi-nao@cabi.org

© CAB International 2012. All rights reserved. No part of this publication may be reproduced in any form or by any means, electronically, mechanically, by photocopying, recording or otherwise, without the prior permission of the copyright owners.

A catalogue record for this book is available from the British Library, London, UK.

Library of Congress Cataloging-in-Publication Data

Amino acids in human nutrition and health / edited by J.P.F. D'Mello.
    p. cm.
  Includes bibliographical references and index.
  ISBN 978-1-84593-798-0 (alk. paper)
1. Amino acids in human nutrition. 2. Amino acids--Metabolism. I. D'Mello, J. P. Felix. II. C.A.B. International.
[DNLM: 1. Amino Acids--metabolism. 2. Amino Acids--therapeutic use. 3. Enzymes--metabolism. 4. Enzymes--therapeutic use. 5. Nutritional Physiological Phenomena. QU 60]

  QP561.A4845 2011
  612'.015756--dc22

                          2011010103

ISBN-13: 978 1 84593 798 0

Commissioning editor: Rachel Cutts
Editorial assistant: Alexandra Lainsbury
Production editor: Fiona Chippendale

Typeset by SPi, Pondicherry, India.
Printed and bound by CPI Group (UK) Ltd, Croydon, CR0 4YY.

Contents

Contributors	xix
Preface	xxiii
Glossary	xxvii

PART I	**ENZYMES AND METABOLISM**	**1**
1	**Glutamate Dehydrogenase**	**3**
	T.J. Smith and C.A. Stanley	
	1.1 Abstract	3
	1.2 Introduction	3
	1.3 GDH in Animals	3
	1.3.1 Structure of animal GDH	4
	1.4 Active Site	5
	1.4.1 GDH dynamics	7
	1.4.2 GTP inhibition site	7
	1.4.3 ADP/second NADH site paradox	8
	1.5 Role of GDH in Insulin Homeostasis	11
	1.5.1 HHS	11
	1.5.2 SIRT4 mutations	13
	1.5.3 SCHAD mutations	13
	1.6 Evolution of GDH Allostery	14
	1.6.1 Possible therapeutics for GDH-mediated insulin disorders	16
	1.6.2 Other novel inhibitors of GDH	17
	1.7 Conclusions	19
	1.8 Acknowledgements	19
2	**Aminotransferases**	**24**
	M.E. Conway	
	2.1 Abstract	24
	2.2 Introduction	24

2.2.1 Transamination	25
2.2.2 Cellular distribution of aminotransferases	25
2.2.2.1 Cellular distribution of the BCAT proteins	27
2.2.2.2 Cellular distribution of the ALT proteins	27
2.2.2.3 Cellular distribution of the AST proteins	28
2.3 The Role of Aminotransferases in Brain Metabolism	28
2.3.1 The role of BCAT in brain metabolism	31
2.4 Alanine Aminotransferases and Glutamate	34
2.5 Aspartate Aminotransferases and their Role in the Malate–Aspartate Shuttle and Glutamate Metabolism	35
2.6 Pathological Conditions Resulting from Impaired Aminotransferase Metabolism	36
2.6.1 Maple syrup urine disease	37
2.6.2 Glutamate toxicity and neurodegeneration	37
2.6.3 Redox sensitivity of BCAT	38
2.7 Aminotransferase Proteins as Biomarkers of Disease	38
2.7.1 Mild elevation of ALT and AST	39
2.7.2 Moderate/marked elevation of ALT and AST	41
2.8 Conclusions and Future Directions	41

3 Arginase
R.W. Caldwell, S. Chandra and R.B. Caldwell

51

3.1 Abstract	51
3.2 Introduction	51
3.3 Isoforms and Distribution	53
3.4 Structure and Location of Arginase	53
3.5 Involvement of Arginase in Health and Disease	54
3.5.1 Arginase in health	54
3.5.1.1 Ammonia detoxification	54
3.5.1.2 Wound healing	54
3.5.1.3 Neuroprotection/regeneration	55
3.5.2 Arginase in disease	55
3.5.2.1 Diabetes	55
3.5.2.2 Hypertension	55
3.5.2.3 Sickle cell disease	56
3.5.2.4 Erectile dysfunction	56
3.5.2.5 Asthma	57
3.5.2.6 Ischaemia/reperfusion injury	57
3.5.2.7 Atherosclerosis	57
3.5.2.8 Nephropathy	58
3.5.2.9 Cancer	58
3.5.2.10 Parasitic infection	59
3.5.2.11 Hyperargininaemia	59
3.5.2.12 Ageing	59
3.5.2.13 Retinopathy	60
3.6 Regulation of Activity	60
3.6.1 Humoral factors	60
3.6.1.1 Reactive oxygen species	60
3.6.1.2 Angiotensin II	61
3.6.2 Elevation of arginase activity and signal transduction mechanisms	61
3.7 Arginase Inhibitors	62
3.8 Conclusions	63

4 Bypassing the Endothelial L-Arginine–Nitric Oxide Pathway: Effects of Dietary Nitrite and Nitrate on Cardiovascular Function — 72
P. Luedike, M. Kelm and T. Rassaf

- 4.1 Abstract — 72
- 4.2 Introduction — 72
- 4.3 L-Arginine: A Semi-Essential Amino Acid in Human Physiology — 73
- 4.4 L-Arginine is the Substrate of the Nitric Oxide Synthases: The L-Arginine–Nitric Oxide Pathway — 73
- 4.5 L-Arginine in Cardiovascular Disease: Perspectives and Limitations — 77
- 4.6 Nitric Oxide Generation without NO-Synthase? Bypassing the L-Arginine Pathway — 78
- 4.7 The Nitrate–Nitrite–Nitric Oxide Pathway — 79
- 4.8 Effects of Nitrite and Nitrate in Human Physiology — 80
- 4.9 Dietary Nitrate and Nitrite — 82
- 4.10 Conclusions — 83
- 4.11 Acknowledgements — 84

5 Histidine Decarboxylase — 89
E. Dere, O. Ambrée and A. Zlomuzica

- 5.1 Abstract — 89
- 5.2 Introduction — 89
- 5.3 Histidine Decarboxylase Enzyme — 91
- 5.4 Histidine Decarboxylase Gene — 91
  - 5.4.1 Gene polymorphism — 92
- 5.5 Pharmacological Inhibition — 92
- 5.6 mRNA Antisense and Gene Knockout — 92
- 5.7 Neurophysiology and Behaviour — 93
  - 5.7.1 Brain neurotransmitters — 93
  - 5.7.2 Nutrition — 93
  - 5.7.3 Sleep, waking and arousal — 94
  - 5.7.4 Reward and drugs — 94
  - 5.7.5 Stress, fear and anxiety — 95
  - 5.7.6 Learning and memory — 96
    - 5.7.6.1 Dementia — 97
- 5.8 Summary and Conclusions — 97
- 5.9 Acknowledgements — 98

6 Glutamate Decarboxylase — 103
H. Ueno, Y. Inoue, S. Matsukawa and Y. Nakamura

- 6.1 Abstract — 103
- 6.2 Introduction — 103
- 6.3 Distribution of GABA — 103
  - 6.3.1 GABA storage, release and uptake — 104
  - 6.3.2 GABA receptors — 104
  - 6.3.3 Metabolism of GABA — 105
  - 6.3.4 Decarboxylation reaction by GAD — 105
  - 6.3.5 Distribution and characterization of GAD — 107
  - 6.3.6 Purification of GAD protein — 110
  - 6.3.7 Gene structure of GAD — 110
- 6.4 GAD 65 in Blood Leucocytes — 110

	6.5 Taste Signalling	113
	6.6 Suggestions for Future Research	115
	6.7 Conclusions	116
	6.8 Acknowledgements	117
7	**Glutaminase**	**122**
	J.M. Matés, J.A. Segura, F.J. Alonso and J. Márquez	
	7.1 Abstract	122
	7.2 Introduction	122
	7.3 Mammalian Glutaminase Genes and Transcripts	123
	7.3.1 *Gls* gene and transcripts	123
	7.3.2 *Gls2* gene and transcripts	124
	7.4 Mammalian Glutaminase Enzymes	125
	7.4.1 Molecular structures and kinetic properties	126
	7.4.2 Subcellular locations	127
	7.5 Glutaminase Expression in Mammalian Brain	127
	7.5.1 Expression of glutaminase L in astrocytes	129
	7.6 State of Art and Perspectives	130
	7.7 Conclusions	131
	7.8 Acknowledgements	132
8	**D-Serine and Serine Racemase in the Retina**	**137**
	S.B. Smith, Y. Ha and V. Ganapathy	
	8.1 Abstract	137
	8.2 Introduction	137
	8.3 NMDA Receptor and D-serine as a Co-agonist	139
	8.4 D-Serine in the Retina	139
	8.5 Mechanisms of D-Serine Uptake in the Retina	140
	8.6 D-Serine and Serine Racemase in Retinal Neurons	142
	8.7 Role of D-Serine in the Retina	144
	8.8 Role of D-Serine and Serine Racemase in Neuronal Cell Death	146
	8.9 Conclusions	147
	8.10 Acknowledgements	148
9	**Tryptophan Hydroxylase**	**150**
	I. Winge, J. McKinney and J. Haavik	
	9.1 Abstract	150
	9.2 Introduction	150
	9.3 General Properties	150
	9.4 Structure and Function of TPH	152
	9.4.1 Domain organization	152
	9.4.2 Ligand binding	154
	9.4.3 Catalytic mechanism	155
	9.5 Enzyme Regulation	156
	9.5.1 Inhibition of TPH	156
	9.5.2 Regulation of TPH	158
	9.5.3 Phosphorylation of TPH	159
	9.5.4 14-3-3 binding to TPH	160
	9.6 TPH Knockout Studies	161
	9.7 Implications of TPH Dysfunction in Human Health	161
	9.8 Concluding Remarks and Future Research	164

| 10 | Methionine Metabolism | 173 |

J.M. Mato, M.L. Martínez-Chantar and S.C. Lu

10.1	Abstract	173
10.2	Introduction	173
10.3	Proliferating Hepatocytes and Liver Cancer Cells Show a Less Efficient Methionine Metabolism than Normal Differentiated Hepatocytes	174
10.4	How Does a Less Efficient Methionine Metabolism Facilitate Hepatocyte Proliferation?	178
10.5	Regulation of Methionine Metabolism is a Crucial Step in Liver Regeneration	180
10.6	How do Both a Defect and an Excess of Liver SAMe Trigger HCC?	182
10.7	Does Changing the Metabolism of Hepatocytes through Manipulation of Methionine Metabolism Hold Promise for Improving HCC Prognosis?	184
10.8	Conclusions	185
10.9	Financial Support	185

PART II   DYNAMICS

| 11 | Amino Acid Transport Across Each Side of the Blood-Brain Barrier | 191 |

R.A. Hawkins, J.R. Viña, D.R. Peterson, R. O'Kane, A. Mokashi and I.A. Simpson

11.1	Abstract	191
11.2	Introduction	192
11.3	A New Approach to Studying the BBB	194
11.4	Facilitative Amino Acid Transporters of the BBB	194
	11.4.1 Facilitative transport of large essential neutral amino acids: system L1	195
	11.4.2 Facilitative transport of cationic amino acids: system y^+	195
	11.4.3 Facilitative transport of glutamine: system n	196
	11.4.4 Facilitative transport of acidic amino acids: system x_G^-	196
11.5	Amino Acid Gradients between Brain and Plasma	197
11.6	Na^+-dependent Transport Systems of the BBB	197
	11.6.1 Na^+-dependent transport of large neutral amino acids: system Na^+-LNAA	199
	11.6.2 Na^+-dependent transport of small non-essential neutral amino acids: system A	199
	11.6.3 Na^+-dependent transport of some large and small neutral amino acids: system ASC	199
	11.6.4 Na^+-dependent transport of nitrogen-rich amino acids: system N	200
	11.6.5 Na^+-dependent transport of acidic amino acids: the EAAT family	200
11.7	Organization of the Various Transport Systems	200
11.8	Branched-chain Amino Acids and Brain Function	201
11.9	Glutamate in Plasma and Brain	201
	11.9.1 Compartmentation of glutamate	202
	11.9.2 Excitotoxicity hypothesis of neuronal death	202
	11.9.3 Glutamate in circulation	202
11.10	Facilitative and Active Transport Systems for Glutamate in the BBB	202
	11.10.1 Facilitative transport of glutamate in the luminal membrane	203
	11.10.2 Active transport systems expel glutamate from the ECF	203
	11.10.3 Current concept of glutamate transport across the BBB	203
11.11	Glutamine and Ammonia Balance	205
	11.11.1 Facilitative transport of glutamine at the luminal membrane	205
	11.11.2 Na^+-dependent transport of glutamine at the abluminal membrane	205
	11.11.3 Ammonia balance	205

11.12 The γ-Glutamyl Cycle and the Role of Pyroglutamate on Na⁺-dependent Carriers	206
11.13 Concluding Comments	208
11.14 Acknowledgements	208

12 Inter-organ Fluxes of Amino Acids — 215
M.C.G. van de Poll and C.H.C. Dejong

12.1 Abstract	215
12.2 Introduction	216
12.3 Glutamine and Ammonia	216
12.3.1 Metabolism	216
12.3.2 Pathophysiology	220
12.3.2.1 Critical illness and trauma	220
12.3.2.2 Hyperammonaemia	221
12.4 Glutamine, Citrulline and Arginine	222
12.4.1 Physiology	222
12.4.1.1 Glutamine and citrulline	222
12.4.1.2 Citrulline and arginine	223
12.4.2 Metabolism after enteral administration	224
12.4.2.1 Glutamine	224
12.4.2.2 Arginine	224
12.4.2.3 Citrulline	225
12.5 Recommendations for Future Research	225
12.6 Conclusions	226

13 Cellular Adaptation to Amino Acid Availability: Mechanisms Involved in the Regulation of Gene Expression — 229
J. Averous, S. Lambert-Langlais, C. Chaveroux, L. Parry, V. Carraro, A.-C. Maurin, C. Jousse, A. Bruhat and P. Fafournoux

13.1 Abstract	229
13.2 Introduction	229
13.3 Regulation of Amino Acid Metabolism and Homeostasis in the Whole Animal	230
13.3.1 Free amino acid pool	230
13.3.2 Specific examples of the role of amino acids in the adaptation to protein deficiency	231
13.3.2.1 Protein undernutrition	231
13.3.2.2 Imbalanced diet	231
13.4 Molecular Mechanisms Involved in the Regulation of Gene Expression by Amino Acid Limitation	232
13.4.1 Transcriptional activation of mammalian genes by amino acid starvation	232
13.4.1.1 Regulation of the human CHOP gene by amino acid starvation	233
13.4.1.2 Regulation of the asparagine synthetase gene by amino acid starvation	233
13.4.1.3 Transcription factors binding the AARE	234
13.4.1.3.1 ATF4	234
13.4.1.3.2 ATF2	234
13.4.1.3.3 Role of ATF4 and ATF2 in the control of the AARE-dependent transcription	235
13.4.2 Signalling pathways regulated by amino acid limitation	235
13.4.2.1 The GCN2/ATF4 pathway (the AAR pathway)	235
13.4.2.2 Signalling pathway leading to ATF2 phosphorylation	236

    13.4.2.3 Other signalling pathways   236
  13.5 Control of Physiological Function by the GCN2/ATF4 Pathway   236
    13.5.1 Amino acid deficiency sensing by GCN2 triggers food aversion   236
    13.5.2 Role of GCN2 in the regulation of neuronal plasticity   237
    13.5.3 Role of GCN2 in the regulation of fatty-acid homeostasis during leucine deprivation   237
    13.5.4 Role of GCN2 in the immune system   238
  13.6 Conclusions   238

PART III NUTRITION   243

14 Endogenous Amino Acids at the Terminal Ileum of the Adult Human   245
P.J. Moughan

  14.1 Abstract   245
  14.2 Introduction   245
  14.3 Endogenous Ileal Amino Acid Losses – How Should They be Determined?   246
    14.3.1 The collection of ileal digesta   246
    14.3.2 Quantification of the endogenous component   247
      14.3.2.1 Protein-free diet   247
      14.3.2.2 Enzyme hydrolysed protein/ultrafiltration method   247
      14.3.2.3 Isotope dilution   248
  14.4 Determined Estimates of Endogenous Ileal Nitrogen and Amino Acid Losses in Humans   248
  14.5 Factors Influencing Endogenous Ileal Amino Acid Losses   249
  14.6 Practical Relevance of Measures of Endogenous Ileal Nitrogen   249
    14.6.1 Metabolic cost   249
    14.6.2 Contribution to amino acid requirement   250
    14.6.3 True ileal amino acid digestibility   251
  14.7 Conclusions   252

15 Metabolic Availability of Amino Acids in Food Proteins: New Methodology   256
C.L. Levesque, R. Elango and R.O. Ball

  15.1 Abstract   256
  15.2 Introduction   256
  15.3 Methods to Estimate Protein Quality   257
  15.4 Metabolic Availability of Amino Acids in Food Protein Sources   258
    15.4.1 Concepts of indicator amino acid oxidation   258
    15.4.2 Application of indicator amino acid oxidation to determine metabolic availability of amino acids in food protein sources   260
    15.4.3 Validation of the metabolic availability method   261
  15.5 Conclusions   263

16 Amino Acid Requirements: Quantitative Estimates   267
R.R. Pillai and A.V. Kurpad

  16.1 Abstract   267
  16.2 Introduction   268
  16.3 Nitrogen Balance   268
  16.4 Isotopic Tracer Methods   271
    16.4.1 Direct amino acid oxidation and balance   272
    16.4.2 Indicator amino acid oxidation and balance   276
    16.4.3 Post-prandial protein utilization   280

16.5 Factorial Prediction of Amino Acid Requirements	281
16.6 Estimates of the Amino Acid Requirement in Potentially Adapted States	282
16.7 Conclusions	283

17 Amino Acid Supplements and Muscular Performance — 291
T.A. Churchward-Venne, D.W.D. West and S.M. Phillips

17.1 Abstract	291
17.2 Introduction	292
17.3 Amino Acids and Protein Turnover	292
17.4 Muscle Protein Synthesis	293
17.5 Enhancing Adaptations to Resistance Exercise with Amino Acid and Protein Supplements	293
17.5.1 Acute studies	294
17.5.2 Chronic studies	295
17.5.3 Dose and distribution considerations to maximize MPS	296
17.6 Enhancing Endurance Exercise Performance and Recovery with Amino Acid and Protein Supplements	296
17.6.1 Amino acids and recovery from endurance exercise	297
17.6.2 Role of protein and amino acids in endurance exercise performance	298
17.7 Cell Signalling Responses to Amino Acids and Resistance Exercise	298
17.7.1 Cell signalling pathways involved in translation initiation and elongation	299
17.7.2 Cell signalling response to amino acids	299
17.7.3 Cell signalling response to amino acids and exercise	299
17.8 Timing Considerations	300
17.8.1 Nutrient timing and acute exercise	300
17.8.2 Nutrient timing and chronic exercise	300
17.9 Amino Acid Source	301
17.9.1 Acute studies	301
17.9.2 Chronic studies	302
17.10 Role of Leucine and Amino Acid Supplements in the Sarcopenia of Ageing	302
17.11 Conclusions and Future Directions	303

18 Amino Acids in Clinical and Nutritional Support: Glutamine in Duchenne Muscular Dystrophy — 312
E. Mok and R. Hankard

18.1 Abstract	312
18.2 Introduction	312
18.3 Duchenne Muscular Dystrophy: the Role of Muscle in Glutamine Metabolism	313
18.4 Glutamine Supplementation in Children with Duchenne Muscular Dystrophy	316
18.4.1 Acute glutamine on protein metabolism	316
18.4.2 Long-term glutamine on clinical outcomes	317
18.5 Conclusions and Future Research	318

19 Adverse Effects — 322
J.P.F. D'Mello

19.1 Abstract	322
19.2 Introduction	323
19.3 Classification	323
19.4 Amino Acid Imbalance	324
19.4.1 Concept	324

19.4.2 Dietary or nutritional amino acid imbalance	324
19.4.2.1 Anorexia	326
19.4.2.2 Dietary preferences	326
19.4.2.3 Mechanisms	326
19.4.2.4 Effects on nutrient utilization	327
19.5 Clinical Amino Acid Imbalance	328
19.5.1 Septic encephalopathy	329
19.5.2 Liver disorders	330
19.5.3 Cancer and other conditions	330
19.5.4 Appetite	330
19.6 Amino Acid Antagonisms	331
19.6.1 Branched-chain amino acid antagonisms	331
19.6.1.1 Leucine and pellagra	332
19.6.2 The lysine–arginine antagonism	332
19.6.2.1 Hyperlysinaemia	332
19.6.3 Antagonisms induced by non-protein amino acids	333
19.6.3.1 Analogues of arginine	333
19.6.3.1.1 Canavanine	333
19.6.3.1.2 Homoarginine	335
19.6.3.1.3 Indospicine	336
19.6.3.2 Analogues of sulphur-containing amino acids	336
19.6.3.2.1 Selenoamino acids	336
19.6.3.2.2 S-Methylcysteine sulphoxide	337
19.6.3.3 Mimosine	337
19.6.3.4 Neurotoxic amino acids	337
19.6.3.4.1 β-N-Oxalylamino-L-alanine	337
19.6.3.4.2 β-Cyanoalanine	337
19.6.3.4.3 α,γ-Diaminobutyric acid	338
19.6.3.4.4 β-N-Methylamino-L-alanine	338
19.6.3.5 Hypoglycin A	338
19.6.3.6 Mechanisms	339
19.6.3.6.1 Arginine analogues	339
19.6.3.6.2 Analogues of the sulphur-containing amino acids	340
19.6.3.6.3 Mimosine	341
19.6.3.6.4 Neurotoxic amino acids	341
19.6.3.6.5 Hypoglycin A	341
19.6.3.6.6 Underlying themes	341
19.7 Amino Acid Toxicity	342
19.7.1 Glutamate	342
19.7.2 Homocysteine	342
19.7.3 Modified lysine residues	342
19.7.4 Phenylalanine	343
19.8 Potential Applications	343
19.8.1 Neuropsychological investigations	343
19.8.2 Therapeutic aspects	343
19.9 Conclusions	345
20 The Umami Taste of Glutamate	**353**
X. Li	
20.1 Abstract	353
20.2 Introduction	353

20.3 The Taste Sensory System	354
20.4 The T1R Family of Taste Receptor	355
20.5 Functional Expression of T1R	356
20.6 T1R Knockout Mice	358
20.7 The Molecular Mechanism of Umami Synergy	358
20.8 Umami Signal Transduction	361
20.9 Functional Neuroimaging of Umami Taste	362
20.10 Conclusions	363

PART IV HEALTH — 367

21 Homocysteine Status: Factors Affecting and Health Risks — 369
L.M. Steffen and B. Steffen

21.1 Abstract	369
21.2 Introduction and Objectives	369
21.3 The Metabolism of Homocysteine	370
21.4 Distribution of Homocysteine Concentrations in the US Population	370
21.5 The Determinants of Serum Total Homocysteine Concentrations	370
21.5.1 Demographic characteristics	370
21.5.2 Diet	370
21.5.3 Smoking	371
21.5.4 Medical conditions and medication use	371
21.5.5 Genetic factors	372
21.6 Homocysteinaemia is a Risk Factor	372
21.6.1 Coronary heart disease, stroke and venous thromboembolism	372
21.6.2 Cognitive function, dementia and Alzheimer's disease	373
21.7 Clinical Efficacy of Folate and Vitamins B_6 and B_{12}	373
21.7.1 Homocysteine, folate, vitamin B_6, vitamin B_{12} and vascular disease	373
21.7.2 Coronary heart disease, stroke and venous thromboembolism	373
21.7.2.1 Observational studies	373
21.7.2.2 Randomized clinical trials	373
21.7.3 Cognitive function, dementia and Alzheimer's disease	373
21.8 Neural Tube Defects	376
21.9 Methodological Issues	376
21.9.1 Differences among studies of homocysteine, B vitamins and vascular disease	376
21.10 Conclusions	377

22 Modified Amino Acid-Based Molecules: Accumulation and Health Implications — 382
S. Bengmark

22.1 Abstract	382
22.2 Introduction	383
22.3 Effects of Heating on Food Quality	383
22.4 AGE/ALE Accumulation in the Body	384
22.5 Modern Molecular Biology: Essential for Understanding the Effects of AGE/ALE	384
22.6 RAGE: a Master Switch and Key to Inflammation	385
22.7 Factors Underlying Enhanced Systemic Inflammation	386
22.8 Dietary Choice	387
22.9 Dairy in Focus	387

22.10 AGE/ALE and Disease	388
22.10.1 Allergy and autoimmune diseases	388
22.10.2 Alzheimer's disease and other neurodegenerative diseases	388
22.10.3 Atherosclerosis and other cardiovascular disorders	389
22.10.4 Cancer	390
22.10.5 Cataract and other eye disorders	390
22.10.6 Diabetes	391
22.10.7 Endocrine disorders	391
22.10.8 Gastrointestinal disorders	392
22.10.9 Liver disorders	392
22.10.10 Lung disorders	392
22.10.11 Rheumatoid arthritis and other skeletomuscular disorders	392
22.10.12 Skin and oral cavity issues	393
22.10.13 Urogenital disorders	394
22.11 Foods Rich in AGE/ALE	394
22.12 Prevention and Treatment of AGE/ALE Accumulation	395
22.12.1 Changing food preparation habits	395
22.12.2 Energy restriction	395
22.12.3 Antioxidants and vitamins	396
22.12.4 Supplementing histidine, taurine, carnitine, or carnosine	396
22.12.5 Pharmaceuticals	396
22.13 Pro- and Synbiotics	396
22.14 Conclusions	397

23 Phenylketonuria: Newborn Identification Through to Adulthood 406
R. Koch and K. Moseley

23.1 Abstract	406
23.2 Introduction	406
23.3 Background	407
23.4 Current Problem: Maternal PKU Therapy	407
23.5 The Role of Tetrahydrobiopterin (BH_4) Treatment for Patients with PKU	408
23.6 Dietary Therapy	409
23.6.1 Large neutral amino acids	412
23.6.2 Glycomacropeptide	412
23.6.3 Tetrahydrobiopterin	412
23.7 Future Research	413
23.8 Conclusions	413

24 Principles of Rapid Tryptophan Depletion and its Use in Research on Neuropsychiatric Disorders 418
F.D. Zepf

24.1 Abstract	418
24.2 Introduction	418
24.3 Basic Principles	419
24.4 RTD Protocol	420
24.4.1 Before administration	421
24.4.2 Administration of amino acids	421
24.5 Effects on Mood	421
24.6 Side Effects and Metabolic Complications	422
24.7 Positron Emission Tomography Studies	422
24.8 Conclusions	423

25 Excitatory Amino Acids in Neurological and Neurodegenerative Disorders   427
G. Flores, J.V. Negrete-Díaz, M. Carrión, Y. Andrade-Talavera, S.A. Bello, T.S. Sihra and A. Rodríguez-Moreno

25.1 Abstract	427
25.2 Introduction	428
25.3 Alzheimer's Disease and Glutamate Receptors	428
25.4 Parkinson's Disease and Glutamate Receptors	429
25.5 Huntington's Disease	430
25.5.1 Animal models	432
25.6 Schizophrenia and Glutamate Receptors	434
25.7 Depression and Glutamate Receptors	435
25.8 Epilepsy and Glutamate Neurotransmission	436
25.8.1 Excitatory amino acids in epilepsy	436
25.8.2 Kainate receptors in epilepsy	437
25.9 Amyotrophic Lateral Sclerosis and Excitatory Amino Acids	440
25.9.1 Glutamate receptors and excitotoxicity in ALS	441
25.9.2 Glutamate metabolism and transport in ALS	442
25.10 Stroke	442
25.10.1 Background	442
25.10.2 Glutamate and glutamate receptors in cerebral ischaemia	443
25.11 Conclusions	445

26 Efficacy of L-DOPA Therapy in Parkinson's Disease   454
G. Sahin and D. Kirik

26.1 Abstract	454
26.2 Introduction	454
26.3 L-DOPA	455
26.4 Dopamine Biosynthesis in Physiological Conditions	456
26.5 Basic Principles of L-DOPA Pharmacotherapy in Parkinson's Disease	456
26.6 Clinical Pharmacokinetics and Pharmacodynamics of L-DOPA Therapy	458
26.7 L-DOPA-induced Dyskinesias	458
26.8 Gene Therapy-mediated Continuous DOPA Delivery in the Parkinsonian Brain	459
26.9 Summary and Concluding Remarks	460

27 Amino Acid Profiles for Diagnostic Applications   464
T. Kimura, M. Takahashi, A. Imaizumi, Y. Noguchi and T. Ando

27.1 Abstract	464
27.2 Introduction	464
27.3 Correlation-based Analysis of Amino Acids	465
27.4 Development of Amino Acid Diagnostics	465
27.4.1 Background	465
27.4.2 Initial studies	466
27.4.3 Measurement of amino acids	468
27.5 Clinical Applications	468
27.5.1 Factors influencing stability of data	468
27.5.2 Application of AminoIndex to liver fibrosis	468
27.5.3 Application of AminoIndex to metabolic syndrome	470
27.5.4 Application of AminoIndex to colorectal and breast cancer	472
27.6 Future Perspectives	472

PART V CONCLUSIONS   477

28 Emergence of a New Momentum   479
J.P.F. D'Mello

28.1 Abstract   479
28.2 Rationale   480
28.3 Objectives and Approach   480
28.4 Key Enzymes and Pathways   481
   28.4.1 Glutamate dehydrogenase   482
   28.4.2 Aminotransferases (transaminases)   483
   28.4.3 Glutamate decarboxylase   484
   28.4.4 Glutamine synthetase   484
   28.4.5 Glutaminase   484
   28.4.6 Ornithine decarboxylase   484
   28.4.7 Urea-cycle enzymes   485
      28.4.7.1 Arginase   485
   28.4.8 Nitric oxide synthase   485
   28.4.9 Histidine decarboxylase   485
   28.4.10 Serine racemase   485
   28.4.11 Hydroxylases   486
   28.4.12 Enzymes of methionine metabolism   486
28.5 Neurotransmitters   487
   28.5.1 Glutamate   487
   28.5.2 Aspartate   488
   28.5.3 Proline   488
   28.5.4 γ-Aminobutyrate and glycine   488
   28.5.5 D-Serine   489
   28.5.6 β-Alanine and taurine   489
   28.5.7 Gases   489
28.6 Molecular Interactions   490
   28.6.1 Transport   490
   28.6.2 Leucine signalling   491
   28.6.3 Hormonal modulation   491
   28.6.4 Umami flavour   492
   28.6.5 Post-translational adducts   492
      28.6.5.1 Advanced glycation end-products 492
      28.6.5.2 Proline-rich proteins   492
28.7 Clinical Support   493
   28.7.1 Biochemical considerations   493
   28.7.2 Supplements   493
28.8 Food Toxicology   496
   28.8.1 Nitrate and nitrite   496
   28.8.2 Plant neurotoxins   496
   28.8.3 Monosodium glutamate   496
   28.8.4 Maillard products   496
   28.8.5 Lysinoalanine   497
28.9 Disorders   497
   28.9.1 Clinical amino acid imbalance   497
   28.9.2 Obesity   497
   28.9.3 Neuropathologies   498
      28.9.3.1 Conditions associated with glutamate excitotoxicity 501
      28.9.3.2 Psychological and cognitive impairments: emerging methodology 502

28.9.4 Cardiovascular disease	503
28.9.5 Diabetes	503
28.9.6 Cancer	504
28.9.7 Genetic defects	505
28.9.8 Risk factors	505
28.9.9 Therapeutics	506
28.9.10 Dietary modulation	506
28.9.11 Non-protein amino acids in cancer prevention	507
28.9.12 Molecular targets	507
28.9.12.1 Enzymes	507
28.9.12.2 Aminoacidergic and monoaminergic receptors	508
28.9.12.3 Transporters	509
28.10 Innovation	509
28.10.1 Modelling	509
28.11 Summary	510
28.11.1 Underlying theme	510
28.11.2 Metabolism	510
28.11.3 Nutrition	510
28.11.4 Food safety	511
28.11.5 Health and disease	511
28.12 Outlook	512
Index	**525**

Contributors

Alonso, F.J., Departamento de Biología Molecular y Bioquímica, Laboratorio de Química de Proteínas, Facultad de Ciencias, Universidad de Málaga, 29071 Málaga, España. E-mail: fcarrion@uma.es

Ambrée, O., Department of Psychiatry, University of Münster, Albert-Schweitzer-Str. 11, 48149 Munster, Germany. E-mail: ambree@uni-muenster.de

Ando, T., AminoIndex Department, Ajinomoto Co., Inc., 1-15-1 Chuo-ku, Tokyo 104-8315, Japan. E-mail: toshihiko_ando@ajinomoto.com

Andrade-Talavera, Y., Laboratorio de Neurociencia Celular y Plasticidad, Universidad Pablo de Olavide, Sevilla, España. E-mail: yandtal@upo.es

Averous, J., Unité de Nutrition Humaine, Institut National de la Recherche Agronomique de Theix, 63122 Saint Genès Champanelle, France. E-mail: julien.averous@clermont.inra.fr

Ball, R.O., Department of Agricultural, Food and Nutritional Sciences, University of Alberta, Edmonton, Alberta, T6G 2P5, Canada, and Department of Nutritional Sciences, University of Toronto, Toronto, ON, M5S 2Z9, Canada. E-mail: ron.ball@ualberta.ca

Bello, S.A., Laboratorio de Neurociencia Celular y Plasticidad, Universidad Pablo de Olavide, Sevilla, España. E-mail: sabina.bello@gmail.com

Bengmark, S., Division of Surgery and Interventional Science, University College London, 4th floor, 74 Huntley Street, London WC1E 6AU, UK. E-mail: stig@bengmark.se

Bruhat, A., Unité de Nutrition Humaine, Institut National de la Recherche Agronomique de Theix, 63122 Saint Genès Champanelle, France. E-mail: alainbruhat@clermont.inra.fr

Caldwell, R.B., Vascular Biology Center, Medical College of Georgia, Augusta, GA 30912, USA. E-mail: rcaldwel@georgiahealth.edu

Caldwell, R.W., Department of Pharmacology and Toxicology, Medical College of Georgia, Augusta, GA 30912, USA. E-mail: wcaldwel@mail.mcg.edu

Carraro, V., Unité de Nutrition Humaine, Institut National de la Recherche Agronomique de Theix, 63122 Saint Genès Champanelle, France. E-mail: valerie.carraro@clermont.inra.fr

Carrión, M., Laboratorio de Neurociencia Celular y Plasticidad, Universidad Pablo de Olavide, Sevilla, España. E-mail: mcarrei@upo.es

Chandra, S., Department of Pharmacology and Toxicology, Medical College of Georgia, Augusta, GA 30912, USA. E-mail: surabhic@email.arizona.edu

Chaveroux, C., Unité de Nutrition Humaine, Institut National de la Recherche Agronomique de Theix, 63122 Saint Genès Champanelle, France. E-mail: cedric.chaveroux@mail.mcgill.ca

Churchward-Venne, T.A., Exercise Metabolism Research Group, Department of Kinesiology, McMaster University, 1280 Main Street West, Hamilton, ON, L8S 4K1, Canada. E-mail: churchta@mcmaster.ca

Conway, M.E., University of the West of England, Coldharbour Lane, Bristol, BS16 1UR, UK. E-mail: Myra.Conway@uwe.ac.uk

Dejong, C.H.C., Department of Surgery, Maastricht University Medical Centre, P.O. Box 6202, AZ Maastricht, the Netherlands. E-mail: chc.dejong@maastrichtuniversity.nl

Dere, E., Université Paris VI: Université Pierre et Marie Curie, UFR des Sciences de la Vie (927), UMR 7102, Neurobiologie des Processus Adaptatifs Bâtiment B (étage 4), Boite 14, 9 quai St Bernard, 75005, Paris, France. E-mail: ekrem.dere@snv.jussieu.fr

D'Mello, J.P.F., Formerly of SAC, University of Edinburgh King's Buildings Campus, West Mains Road, Edinburgh EH9 3JG, UK. E-mail: jpfdmello@hotmail.co.uk

Elango, R., Child & Family Research Institute, BC Children's Hospital, Vancouver, BC, V5Z 4H4, Canada, and Department of Pediatrics, Division of Gastroenterology, Hepatology and Nutrition, University of British Columbia, Vancouver, BC, V5Z 4H4, Canada. E-mail: relango@cfri.ubc.ca

Fafournoux, P., Unité de Nutrition Humaine, Institut National de la Recherche Agronomique de Theix, 63122 Saint Genès Champanelle, France. E-mail: pierre.fafournoux@clermont.inra.fr

Flores, G., Laboratorio de Neuropsiquiatría, Instituto de Fisiología, Universidad Autónoma de Puebla, Puebla, México. E-mail: gonzaloflores56@gmail.com

Ganapathy, V., Vision Discovery Institute, and Department of Biochemistry and Molecular Biology, Medical College of Georgia, 1120 Fifteenth Street, CB 2820, Augusta, GA 30912-2000, USA. E-mail: vganapat@georgiahealth.edu

Ha, Y., Department of Cellular Biology and Anatomy, and Vision Discovery Institute, Medical College of Georgia, 1120 Fifteenth Street, CB 2820, Augusta, GA 30912-2000, USA. E-mail: yha@georgiahealth.edu

Haavik, J., Department of Biomedicine, University of Bergen, Bergen, Norway. E-mail: Jan.Haavik@abm.uib.no

Hankard, R., Pédiatrie Multidisciplinaire-Nutrition de l'Enfant, Centre Hospitalier Universitaire de Poitiers, 2 rue de la Milétrie, 86021 Poitiers Cedex, France. E-mail: regis.hankard@free.fr

Hawkins, R.A., Department of Physiology & Biophysics, The Chicago Medical School, Rosalind Franklin University of Medicine and Science, 3333 Green Bay Road, North Chicago, IL, 60064-3095 USA. E-mail: RAH@post.harvard.edu

Imaizumi, A., Research Institute for Innovation, Ajinomoto Co., Inc., 1-15-1 Chuo-ku, Tokyo 104-8315, Japan. E-mail: akira_imaizumi@ajinomoto.com

Inoue, Y., Laboratory of Applied Microbiology and Biochemistry, Nara Women's University, Nara 630-8506, Japan. E-mail: inoue_1708@yahoo.co.jp

Jousse, C., Unité de Nutrition Humaine, Institut National de la Recherche Agronomique de Theix, 63122 Saint Genès Champanelle, France. E-mail: celine.jousse@clermont.inra.fr

Kelm, M., Division of Cardiology, Pulmonology, and Vascular Medicine, Medical Faculty, University Hospital Düsseldorf, Moorenstrasse 5, D-40225, Düsseldorf, Germany. E-mail: Malte.kelm@med.uni-duesseldorf.de

Kimura, T., R + D Planning Department, Ajinomoto Co., Inc., 1-15-1 Chuo-ku, Tokyo 104-8315, Japan. E-mail: takeshi_kimura@ajinomoto.com

Kirik, D., Brain Repair and Imaging in Neural Systems (BRAINS), Section of Neuroscience, Department of Experimental Medical Science BMC D11, Lund University, 221 84 Lund, Sweden. E-mail: Deniz.Kirik@med.lu.se

Koch, R., Department of Pediatrics, Genetics Division, Keck School of Medicine, University of Southern California, Los Angeles, California 90033, USA. E-mail: drpku@sbcglobal.net

Kurpad, A.V., Division of Nutrition, St. John's Research Institute, St. John's National Academy of Health Sciences, Bangalore 560034, India. E-mail: a.kurpad@sjri.res.in

Lambert-Langlais, S., Unité de Nutrition Humaine, Institut National de la Recherche Agronomique de Theix, 63122 Saint Genès Champanelle, France. E-mail: sarah.langlais@clermont.inra.fr

Levesque, C.L., Department of Animal and Poultry Science, 70 Stone Road, Guelph, ON, N1G 2W1, Canada. E-mail: crystal.levesque@uoguelph.ca

Li, X., GPCR Biology, Senomyx Inc., 4767 Nexus Centre Dr., San Diego, CA 92121, USA. E-mail: xiaodong.li@senomyx.com

Lu, S.C., Division of Gastroenterology and Liver Disease, Keck School of Medicine, USC, Los Angeles, California 90033, USA. E-mail: shellylu@usc.edu

Luedike, P., Division of Cardiology, Pulmonology, and Vascular Medicine, Medical Faculty, University Hospital Düsseldorf, Moorenstrasse 5, D-40225, Düsseldorf, Germany. E-mail: Peter.luedike@med.uni-duesseldorf.de

Márquez, J., Departamento de Biología Molecular y Bioquímica, Laboratorio de Química de Proteínas, Facultad de Ciencias, Universidad de Málaga, 29071 Málaga, España. E-mail: marquez@uma.es

Martínez-Chantar, M.L., CIC bioGUNE, CIBERehd, Technology Park of Bizkaia, 48160 Derio, Bizkaia, España. E-mail: mlmartinez@cicbiogune.es

Matés, J.M., Departamento de Biología Molecular y Bioquímica, Laboratorio de Química de Proteínas, Facultad de Ciencias, Universidad de Málaga, 29071 Málaga, España. E-mail: jmates@uma.es

Mato, J.M., CIC bioGUNE, CIBERehd, Technology Park of Bizkaia, 48160 Derio, Bizkaia, España. E-mail: director@cicbiogune.es

Matsukawa, S., Laboratory of Applied Microbiology and Biochemistry, Nara Women's University, Nara 630-8506, Japan. E-mail: satoko.matsukawa@shionogi.co.jp

Maurin, A-C., Unité de Nutrition Humaine, Institut National de la Recherche Agronomique de Theix, 63122 Saint Genès Champanelle, France. E-mail: anne-catherine.maurin@clermont.inra.fr

McKinney, J., Department of Biomedicine, University of Bergen, Bergen, Norway. E-mail: Jeffrey.Mckinney@biomed.uib.no

Mok, E., Pédiatrie Multidisciplinaire-Nutrition de l'Enfant, Centre Hospitalier Universitaire de Poitiers, 2 rue de la Milétrie, 86021 Poitiers Cedex, France. E-mail: elise.mok@muhc.mcgill.ca

Mokashi, A., Department of Physiology & Biophysics, The Chicago Medical School, Rosalind Franklin University of Medicine and Science, 3333 Green Bay Road, North Chicago, IL, 60064-3095, USA. E-mail: ashwini.mokashi@rosalindfranklin.edu

Moseley, K., Department of Pediatrics, Genetics Division, Keck School of Medicine, University of Southern California, Los Angeles, California 90033, USA. E-mail: kmoseley@usc.edu

Moughan, P.J., Riddet Institute, Massey University, Tennent Drive, Private Bag 11-222, Palmerston North, New Zealand. E-mail: p.j.moughan@massey.ac.nz

Nakamura, Y., Laboratory of Applied Microbiology and Biochemistry, Nara Women's University, Nara 630-8506, Japan. E-mail: nakamuray@missouri.edu

Negrete-Díaz, J.V., Laboratorio de Neuropsiquiatría, Instituto de Fisiología, Universidad Autónoma de Puebla, Puebla, México, and Laboratorio de Neurociencia Celular y Plasticidad, Universidad Pablo de Olavide, Sevilla, España. E-mail: vicentemozart@yahoo.com

Noguchi, Y., Research Institute for Innovation, Ajinomoto Co., Inc., 1-15-1 Chuo-ku, Tokyo 104-8315, Japan. E-mail: yasushi_noguchi@ajinomoto.com

O'Kane, R., Natural and Applied Science Department, La Guardia Community College/CUNY, 31-10 Thomson Ave., Long Island City, NY 11101, USA. E-mail: Robyn.okane@colostate.edu

Parry, L., Unité de Nutrition Humaine, Institut National de la Recherche Agronomique de Theix, 63122 Saint Genès Champanelle, France. E-mail: laurent.parry@clermont.inra.fr

Peterson, D.R., Department of Physiology & Biophysics, The Chicago Medical School, Rosalind Franklin University of Medicine and Science, 3333 Green Bay Road, North Chicago, IL, 60064-3095 USA. E-mail: darryl.peterson@rosalindfranklin.edu

Phillips, S.M., Exercise Metabolism Research Group, Department of Kinesiology, McMaster University, 1280 Main Street West, Hamilton, ON L8S 4K1, Canada. E-mail: phillis@mcmaster.ca

Pillai, R.R., Division of Nutrition, St. John's Research Institute, St. John's National Academy of Health Sciences, Bangalore 560034, India. E-mail: ramaswamy.pillai@gmail.com

Rassaf, T., Division of Cardiology, Pulmonology and Vascular Medicine, Medical Faculty, University Hospital Düsseldorf, Moorenstrasse 5, D-40225, Düsseldorf, Germany. E-mail: Tienush.Rassaf@med.uni-duesseldorf.de

Rodríguez-Moreno, A., Laboratorio de Neurociencia Celular y Plasticidad, Universidad Pablo de Olavide, Sevilla, España. E-mail: arodmor@upo.es

Sahin, G., Brain Repair and Imaging in Neural Systems (BRAINS), Section of Neuroscience, Department of Experimental Medical Science BMC D11, Lund University, 221 84 Lund, Sweden. E-mail: Gurdal.Sahin@med.lu.se

Segura, J.A., Departamento de Biología Molecular y Bioquímica, Laboratorio de Química de Proteínas, Facultad de Ciencias, Universidad de Málaga, 29071 Málaga, España. E-mail: jsegura@uma.es

Sihra, T.S., Department of Neuroscience, Physiology and Pharmacology, University College London, London, UK. E-mail: t.sihra@ucl.ac.uk

Simpson, I.A., Department of Neural and Behavioral Sciences, Milton S. Hershey Medical Center, Pennsylvania State University College of Medicine, Hershey, PA 17033, USA. E-mail: IXS10@psu.edu

Smith, S.B., Department of Cellular Biology and Anatomy, Department of Ophthalmology, and Vision Discovery Institute, Medical College of Georgia, 1120 Fifteenth Street, CB 2820, Augusta, GA 30912-2000, USA. E-mail: sbsmith@georgiahealth.edu

Smith, T.J., Donald Danforth Plant Science Center, 975 North Warson Road, Saint Louis, MO 63132, USA. E-mail: TSmith@danforthcenter.org

Stanley, C.A., Division of Endocrinology, The Children's Hospital of Philadelphia, 34th Street and Civic Center Blvd., Philadelphia, PA 19104, USA. E-mail: stanleyc@email.chop.edu

Steffen, B., Department of Laboratory Medicine and Pathology, University of Minnesota, Minneapolis, MN 55454, USA. E-mail: steff293@umn.edu

Steffen, L.M., Division of Epidemiology and Community Health, University of Minnesota School of Public Health, Minneapolis, MN 55454, USA. E-mail: steffen@umn.edu

Takahashi, M., Research Institute for Innovation, Ajinomoto Co., Inc., 1-15-1 Chuo-ku, Tokyo 104-8315, Japan. E-mail: mitsuo_takahashi@ajinomoto.com

Ueno, H., Laboratory of Applied Microbiology and Biochemistry, Nara Women's University, Nara 630-8506, Japan. E-mail: hueno@cc.nara-wu.ac.jp

van de Poll, M.C.G., Department of Surgery, Maastricht University Medical Centre, P.O. Box 6202, AZ Maastricht, the Netherlands. E-mail: mcg.vandepoll@ah.unimaas.nl

Viña, J.R., Departamento de Bioquímica & Biología Molecular, Facultad de Medicina/ Fundacíon de Investigacíon Hospital Clinico-INCLIVA, Universidad de Valencia, Avenida Blasco Ibañez 17, Valencia, España 46010. E-mail: vinaj@uv.es

West, D.W.D., Exercise Metabolism Research Group, Department of Kinesiology, McMaster University, 1280 Main Street West, Hamilton, ON L8S 4K1, Canada. E-mail: westd3@mcmaster.ca

Winge, I., Department of Biomedicine, University of Bergen, Bergen, Norway. E-mail: ingeborg.winge@biomed.uib.no

Zepf, F.D., Department of Child and Adolescent Psychiatry, Psychosomatics and Psychotherapy, RWTH Aachen University, Aachen, Germany and JARA Translational Brain Medicine, Aachen + Jülich, Germany. E-mail: fzepf@ukaachen.de

Zlomuzica, A., Department of Clinical Psychology, Ruhr-Universität Bochum, Universitaetsstrasse 150, 44780 Bochum, Germany. E-mail: Armin.Zlomuzica@rub.de

Preface

Rationale

Research interest in the biochemistry of amino acids continues apace, generating significant dividends for nutritional support and the elucidation of mechanisms underlying a variety of disorders in humans. The remarkable scale of recent developments has provided the impetus for publication of this first edition of *Amino Acids in Human Nutrition and Health*. It was deemed appropriate to formally acknowledge these advances within a comprehensive volume. The recruitment of authors with exceptional merit constituted an integral part of my strategy.

There appears to be a demand for a book which integrates recent advances relating to amino acids within the two disciplines of nutrition and health. Various symposia have been convened on certain aspects covered in this book, but the published proceedings are distributed in different issues of journals, thereby compromising convenience for consultation by students and research staff. It is an unfortunate reflection of our time that university libraries cannot afford to stock some of the primary journals that have, in the recent past, been judged to be essential reading for advanced students. The publication of *Amino Acids in Human Nutrition and Health* might be viewed as an attempt to rectify this deficiency. Furthermore, the symposia have focused on restricted themes, whereas this volume is designed to address a comprehensive range of issues. The reviews in published proceedings of symposia have also been restricted to a few pages per article, but there is a need for in-depth coverage to more appropriately reflect current developments.

This volume is designed for academic, research, and corporate establishments worldwide, particularly in Europe, the United States, Canada, Japan, and Australia, but generally in all countries where English is a primary medium for education and research. This book should appeal to final year undergraduate and graduate students as well as to research staff. It is anticipated that it will be recommended reading for courses in general and clinical biochemistry, medicine, nursing, human nutrition and food science. The text is also designed with the commercial sector in mind, particularly pharmaceutical companies with extensive R&D laboratories.

Overview

The chapters in *Amino Acids in Human Nutrition and Health* are arranged within a thematic structure as indicated in the sections below. The nature of the subject and the need for interlinking chapters have meant that a limited amount of overlap was inevitable. This is not necessarily a detraction, as individual chapters are now self-contained to ensure continuity for readers, with cross-referencing kept to the minimum. This strategy has also allowed authors increased flexibility in terms of emphasis and interpretation.

Part I Enzymes and metabolism

This section pursues the theme of amino acid metabolism through the driving actions of the principal enzymes, emphasizing recent developments particularly with reference to localization, molecular genetics, biophysical characterization and regulation. Subsequent chapters will also demonstrate the changing facets of amino acid biochemistry. The competing actions of enzymes for critical substrates are also features of relevance in this section. A number of the enzymes under review here catalyse rate-limiting steps in important metabolic pathways, leading to synthesis of physiologically active intermediates and end products. There is scope for elaboration of the important pathways initiated by enzymes under review in this section. Part I has also been developed with the aim of underpinning subsequent chapters in this volume.

Part II Dynamics

This section deals with important issues relating to whole-body amino acid dynamics, with a particular objective of supporting the chapters on nutrition and health that will follow. In this chapter, authors were encouraged to adopt an integrative approach to include their own expertise and that of others in their respective fields. A basic outline of metabolic pathways appears in Part I. The theme in this section centres around kinetics and regulation in broad-spectrum reviews incorporating innovative aspects of the relevant research. In other words, the concept of metabolic networking forms an underlying theme in this series of chapters.

Part III Nutrition

Since the publication of *Mammalian Protein Metabolism* (Munro and Allison, 1964), there has been a steady but perceptible shift in focus towards individual or distinct groups of amino acids, and this change is most clearly seen in nutritional developments. The move away from protein to amino acid considerations is a deliberate theme in the development of the rationale for this section. However, even traditional issues, such as protein-energy malnutrition, are being investigated in the light of kinetics of specific amino acids, with reduced emphasis on whole-body protein dynamics. Against such a background, it was considered appropriate to secure reviews that would reflect a modernizing and progressive agenda in amino acid research.

The chapters cover a number of topical research investigations employing existing technologies to develop novel concepts or to underpin contemporary practices. Methods previously developed and validated with animal models are now being applied to human physiology and nutrition with significant results worthy of publication in this volume.

Part IV Health

The earlier sections have provided the biochemical basis of several of the conditions to be reviewed here. It is now clear that the metabolism of amino acids is associated with or modulated by a diverse array of disorders and, in certain instances, may provide markers for risk assessment. At least four of the chapters in this section will focus on different amino acids associated with neurological issues and cognitive performance measures. The approach here is designed to reflect developments in epidemiology, monitoring, and clinical interventions in the various conditions under consideration in this section.

Part V Conclusions

The final section contains a plenary review designed to summarize the main findings in the foregoing chapters within an integrated account. The main theme centres around the concept of the emergence of a new momentum driving forward a progressive agenda in further elucidating the biochemical and health implications of amino acids.

Acknowledgements

I am indebted to my team of distinguished authors who have made publication of this volume possible despite the constraints imposed by their normal schedules. Their cooperation in submitting manuscripts promptly has ensured that the book remains up-to-date and relevant in an ever-changing scenario. Their lucid chapters have inspired me to enquire further and to challenge existing hypotheses; I trust that my readers will be similarly motivated. I am heartened by responses I have received from a number of my authors. The following words of Professor Deniz Kirik (Chapter 26, with Professor Sahin) encapsulates these sentiments: 'It has been an interesting exercise for us to write this text as it provoked many interesting discussions in areas we thought we knew well but noticed gaps in our knowledge. We will follow on some of these points to inquire more and think that some of them could even become topics for experimentation in the next period. So it has been very valuable and pleasant for us as well.'

Disclaimer

This book necessarily contains references to commercial products. However, authors were asked to refrain from excessive usage of any trade names unless there were compelling reasons for doing so. No endorsement of these products is implied or should be attributed to the editor or to CAB International.

The information set out within *Amino Acids in Human Nutrition and Health* is presented in good faith and in accordance with 'best practice'. Although every effort has been made to verify the facts and figures, neither the editor nor CAB International can accept responsibility for the data presented in individual chapters or for any consequences of their use.

At the time of preparation, I was aware of articles in the popular press extolling the virtues of citrulline and the branched-chain amino acids in the context of health and longevity. However, the publication of this book should not be interpreted as a recommendation for individuals to use these or any other amino acids for whatever purpose. *Amino Acids in Human Nutrition and Health* is intended exclusively for use as a text in education and in R&D establishments.

J.P.F. D'Mello
Editor

Glossary

Introduction

Evaluation of issues underlying the role of amino acids in human nutrition and health inevitably entails an appreciation of specific nomenclature and technical descriptors. Although many of the terms and acronyms used are now in common usage outside scientific circles, it was deemed important to provide as comprehensive a list as possible to assist those readers who are new to this field. Further definitions are available in appropriate scientific dictionaries, for example in the compilations of Hodgson *et al.* (1998), Marcovitch (2005), Parish *et al.* (2006), Martin (2010) and the MedlinePlus (2010) website. Handbooks such as those by D'Mello (1997) and Longmore *et al.* (2010) and current textbooks in medical sciences (Bear *et al.*, 2007; Barker *et al.*, 2008; Baynes and Dominiczak, 2009; Naish *et al.*, 2009) are also recommended as sources of relevant information.

Definition of Terms and Acronyms

The important terms and acronyms are defined in Table 1. This compilation includes standard conventions as well as unique chapter-specific terms. Cross-referencing to individual chapters in this volume is provided in order to permit a greater appreciation of the context of usage of selected terms.

Table 1. Explanation of relevant terms and acronyms used in *Amino Acids in Human Nutrition and Health*.

Abbreviation or Term	Definition
AA	amino acid(s)
AAA	aromatic amino acid(s)
AAAH	aromatic amino acid hydroxylase (Chapter 9)
AADC	aromatic amino acid decarboxylase (Chapters 9 and 26)
AARE	amino acid regulatory element (Chapter 13)
Ac-CoA	acetyl coenzyme A
Acute toxicity	severe adverse effects occurring within a relatively short period of exposure to a potentially harmful substance

Continued

Table 1. Continued.

Abbreviation or Term	Definition
AD	Alzheimer's disease (Chapters 21, 22, 25, and 28)
Adduct	covalent product of a compound or metabolite to large biomolecules such as proteins and DNA (Chapter 28)
ADHD	attention deficit hyperactivity disorder (Chapter 9)
ADI	acceptable daily intake(s)
ADMA	asymmetrical dimethylarginine (Chapter 4)
ADP	adenosine diphosphate (Chapter 1)
AGE	advanced glycation end-product(s) (Chapters 19, 22, and 28)
Agonist	a compound eliciting a biological response by interacting with specific cell receptors, enzymes or metabolites
Akt	protein kinase B (Chapter 17)
ALE	advanced lipoxidation end-product(s) (Chapters 22 and 28)
Allosteric	multi-site enzyme modulation of structure and activity (Chapter 10)
ALP	alkaline phosphatase (Chapter 2)
ALS	amyotrophic lateral sclerosis (Chapter 25)
ALS/PDC	amyotrophic lateral sclerosis/Parkinsonism dementia complex (Chapter 19)
ALT	alanine aminotransferase (Chapter 2)
AMD	age-related macular degeneration (Chapter 22)
Aminoacidergic	relating to amino acids as neurotransmitters (Chapter 28)
AminoIndex	amino acid profiles for diagnostic applications (Chapter 27)
AMP	adenosine monophosphate (Chapter 9)
AMPA	α-amino-3-hydroxy-5-methyl-4-isoxazolepropionic acid (Chapters 8, 25, and 28)
AMPAR	AMPA receptor (Chapter 25)
AMPK	AMP-activated protein kinase (Chapter 10)
ANF	anti-nutritional factor(s) (Chapter 14)
Antagonist	a compound acting as an inhibitor by virtue of structural analogy with nutrients or other intermediates (Chapter 19)
AOAA	aminooxyacetic acid (Chapter 2)
APEX	apurinic/apyrimidinic endonuclease (Chapter 10)
ARA	arachidonic acid (20:4n-6) (Chapter 23)
Arg	arginine
ASNS	asparagine synthetase (Chapter 13)
ASCT	alanine, serine, and cysteine transport system (Chapter 8)
Asn	asparagine
Asp	aspartate
ASS	argininosuccinate synthase (Chapter 3)
AST	aspartate aminotransferase (Chapter 2)
ATA	aurintricarboxylic acid (Chapter 1)
ATF	activating transcription factor (Chapter 13)
ATP	adenosine 5'-triphosphate (Chapters 1, 11, 20, and 28)
AUC	area under the curve (Chapter 27)
BBB	blood–brain barrier (Chapters 9 and 11)
BBMV	brush border membrane vesicles
BCAA	branched-chain amino acids (Chapters 2, 11, 16, 17, 19, and 28)
BCAT	branched-chain aminotransferase (Chapters 2 and 28)
BCH	2-aminobicyclo(2,2,1)-heptane-2-carboxylic acid (Chapter 11)
BCKA	branched-chain keto acids (Chapters 2 and 19)
BCKDH	branched-chain α-keto acid dehydrogenase (Chapter 2)
BH_4	tetrahydrobiopterin (Chapters 4, 9, and 23)
BLMV	basolateral membrane vesicles
BMAA	β-N-methylamino-L-alanine (Chapter 19)
BMI	body mass index (Chapter 23)

Table 1. Continued.

Abbreviation or Term	Definition
BOAA	β-N-oxalylamino-L-alanine (Chapter 19)
CAA	cationic amino acids (Chapter 11)
Carcinogenic	causing cancer
CAT	cationic amino acid transport
CBS	cystathionine β-synthase (Chapter 10)
cDNA	complementary DNA (Chapter 7)
CEL	N^ε-(carboxyethyl) lysine (Chapter 22)
cGMP	cyclic guanosine monophosphate
ChAT	choline acetyltransferase (Chapter 8)
CHD	coronary heart disease (Chapter 21)
CHOP	C/EBP homologous protein (Chapter 13)
Chronic toxicity	adverse effects resulting from prolonged and repeated exposure to relatively small quantities of a potentially harmful substance
Cit	citrulline
CML	N^ε-(carboxymethyl) lysine (Chapters 22 and 28)
cNOS	constitutive nitric oxide synthase (Chapter 28)
CNS	central nervous system (Chapters 1, 7, 8, and 28)
CoA	coenzyme A
COMT	catechol-O-methyltransferase (Chapter 26)
COPD	chronic obstructive pulmonary disease (Chapters 22 and 28)
CPS	carbamoyl phosphate synthase (Chapter 3)
CPu	caudate-putamen (Chapter 25)
CSA	cross-sectional area (of skeletal muscle fibre) (Chapter 17)
CSF	cerebrospinal fluid (Chapter 11)
CVD	cardiovascular disease (Chapter 21)
Cys	cysteine
d	day
DA	dopamine
DAA	dispensable amino acid(s) (see also NEAA) (Chapter 19)
DAAB	direct amino acid balance (Chapter 16)
DAAO	direct measurement of amino acid oxidation (Chapter 16)
DCAM	decarboxylated S-adenosyl-methionine
DDC	DOPA decarboxylase (Chapter 6)
DFMO	α-difluoromethylornithine (Chapter 3)
DHA	docosahexaenoic acid (22:6n-3) (Chapter 23)
DHF	dihydrofolate (Chapter 10)
DMD	Duchenne muscular dystrophy (Chapter 18)
DMI	dry matter intake
$DMPH_4$	6,7-dimethyltetrahydropterin (Chapter 9)
DNA	deoxyribonucleic acid (Chapters 1, 5, 10, 19, and 28)
DOPA	3,4-dihydroxyphenylalanine (Chapters 26 and 28)
DOPAC	3,4-dihydroxyphenylacetate (Chapters 5, 6, and 26)
dUMP	deoxyuridine monophosphate (Chapter 10)
EAA	essential amino acid(s) (see also IAA) (Chapter 17)
EAAT	excitatory amino acid transport (Chapter 11)
EC	epicatechin (Chapter 1)
ECF	extracellular fluid (Chapter 11)
ECG	epicatechin gallate (Chapter 1)
EDTA	ethylendiamine tetraacetic acid (Chapter 27)
EEG	electroencephalogram (Chapter 25)
eEPSC	evoked excitatory postsynaptic current(s) (Chapter 25)
EGC	epigallocatechin (Chapter 1)
EGCG	epigallocatechin gallate (Chapters 1 and 22)

Continued

Table 1. Continued.

Abbreviation or Term	Definition
ELISA	enzyme-linked immunosorbent assay (Chapter 6)
EMG	electromyography (Chapter 25)
EOG	electrooculography (Chapter 25)
EU	European Union
FA	fatty acid(s)
FAD	flavin adenine dinucleotide
FAO	Food and Agriculture Organization (United Nations)
FDA	Food and Drug Administration (USA)
fEPSP	field excitatory postsynaptic potential(s) (Chapter 25)
FMN	flavin mononucleotide (Chapter 4)
fMRI	functional magnetic resonance imaging (Chapter 20)
Fol	folic acid (Chapter 21)
FSR	fractional synthetic rate
GA	glutaminase (Chapter 7)
GAB	glutaminase B (Chapter 7)
GABA	γ-amino butyrate (Chapters 1, 5, 6, 7, 25, and 28)
GABAR	GABA receptor (Chapter 25)
GAC	glutaminase C (Chapter 7)
GAD	glutamic acid decarboxylase (Chapters 6 and 28)
GCH	GTP cyclohydrolase (Chapter 26)
GCN	general control non-derepressive (Chapter 13)
GDH	glutamate dehydrogenase (Chapter 1, 2, and 28)
GDS	gut-derived serotonin (Chapter 9)
GGT	γ-glutamyl transpeptidase (Chapter 11)
GH	growth hormone
Glc-6P	glucose-6 phosphate
Gln	glutamine
Glu	glutamate
Glutamatergic	relating to glutamate neurotransmission (Chapter 28)
Gly	glycine
GMP	guanosine-5′-monophosphate (Chapter 20)
GNMT	glycine N-methyltransferase (Chapter 10)
GPCR	G protein-coupled receptors (Chapter 20)
GS	glutamine synthetase (2 and 28)
GSH	glutathione (Chapter 10)
GTP	guanosine triphosphate (Chapters 1, 4, and 26)
h	hour(s)
HCC	hepatocellular carcinoma (Chapter 10)
HCP	hexachlorophene (Chapter 1)
Hcy	homocysteine (Chapter 21)
HD	Huntington's disease (Chapter 25)
HDC	histidine decarboxylase (Chapters 6 and 28)
HDL	high density lipoproteins (Chapter 22)
Hepatotoxic	toxic to the liver
HHS	hyperinsulinism/hyperammonaemia syndrome (Chapter 1)
His	histidine
HO2	haem-oxygenase-2
HPLC	high-performance liquid chromatography (Chapter 26)
HRI	haem-regulated translational inhibitor (Chapter 13)
5-HT	5-hydroxytryptamine (serotonin) (Chapter 24)
HuR	human antigen R (Chapter 10)
HVA	homovanillic acid (Chapter 26)
hVps34	human vacuolar protein sorting-34 (Chapter 17)
IAA	indispensable amino acid(s) (see also EAA) (Chapters 16 and 19)

Table 1. Continued.

Abbreviation or Term	Definition
IAAB	indicator amino acid balance (Chapter 16)
IAAO	indicator amino acid oxidation (Chapters 15 and 16)
IGF-I	insulin-like growth factor-I (Chapter 13)
IGFBP-1	insulin-like growth factor binding protein-1 (Chapter 13)
ILAE	International League Against Epilepsy (Chapter 25)
Ile	isoleucine
IMP	inosine-5′-monophosphate (inosinate) (Chapter 20)
iNOS	inducible nitric oxide synthase (Chapter 28)
KA	kainate (Chapter 25)
KAR	kainate type glutamate receptor (Chapter 25)
KGA	kidney GA (Chapter 7)
KO	knockout (Chapter 9)
LCMT	leucine carboxyl methyltransferase
LCPUFA	long-chain polyunsaturated fatty acids (Chapter 23)
LDH	lactate dehydrogenase
LDL	low-density lipoprotein(s) (Chapters 3 and 4)
LDR	long-duration response (Chapter 26)
Leu	leucine
LFT	liver function tests (Chapter 2)
LGA	liver GA (Chapter 7)
LKB	liver kinase B (Chapter 10)
LNAA	large neutral amino acid(s) (Chapters 11, 23, and 24)
LTP	long-term potentation (Chapter 25)
Lys	lysine
MA	metabolic availability (Chapters 9 and 15)
MAO	monoamine oxidase (Chapters 9 and 26)
MAP4K3	mitogen activated protein kinase-3 (Chapter 17)
MAT	methionine adenosyltransferase (Chapters 10 and 28)
MDH	malate dehydrogenase (Chapter 2)
ME	malic enzyme (Chapter 2)
MeAIB	N-(methylamino)-isobutyric acid (Chapter 11)
Met	methionine
mGluR	metabotropic G protein-coupled glutamate receptor (Chapter 25)
MMP	mitochondrial membrane potential (Chapter 7)
Monoaminergic	relating to neurotransmission by biogenic amines (Chapter 28)
MPB	muscle protein breakdown (Chapter 17)
MPS	muscle protein synthesis (Chapter 17)
MPTP	1, methyl-4-phenyl-1,2,3,6-tetrahydropyridine (Chapter 26)
M_r	relative molecular mass (Chapter 7)
mRNA	messenger RNA
MSG	monosodium glutamate (Chapters 19, 20, and 28)
MSUD	maple syrup urine disease (Chapter 2)
MT	methyltransferases (Chapter 10)
MTHFR	methylene-tetrahydrofolate reductase (Chapter 21)
mTOR	mammalian target of rapamycin (Chapters 10, 13, 17, and 28)
Mutagenic	causing mutations
N	nitrogen
NAA	neutral amino acids (Chapter 11)
NAcc	nucleus accumbens (Chapter 25)
NAD^+	nicotinamide adenine dinucleotide (oxidized) (Chapter 1)
$NADP^+$	nicotinamide adenine dinucleotide phosphate (oxidized) (Chapter 1)
NADPH	nicotinamide adenine dinucleotide phosphate (reduced) (Chapters 1, 3, and 4)
NAFLD	non-alcoholic fatty liver disease (Chapters 2, 10, and 22)

Continued

Table 1. Continued.

Abbreviation or Term	Definition
NASH	non-alcoholic steatohepatitis (Chapters 10 and 22)
NCHS	National Center for Health Statistics (USA) (Chapter 23)
NDF	neutral detergent fibre (Chapter 14)
NEAA	non-essential amino acid(s)
Nephrotoxic	toxic to the kidney
NIH	National Institutes of Health
NMDA	N-methyl D-aspartate (Chapters 8, 25, and 28)
NMDAR	NMDA receptor(s) (Chapters 8 and 25)
NMMA	N^G-monomethyl arginine (Chapter 4)
NO	nitric oxide (Chapters 3, 4, 11, 12, 19, and 28)
NOHA	N^ω-hydroxy-L-arginine (Chapter 3)
nor-NOHA	N^ω-hydroxy-nor-L-arginine (Chapter 3)
NOS	nitric oxide synthase (Chapters 3, 4, 11, 12, 19, and 28)
NPB	net protein balance (Chapter 17)
NRC	National Research Council (USA)
NSRE	nutrient-sensing response element (Chapter 13)
NTD	neural tube defects (Chapter 21)
OAA	oxaloacetate (Chapters 2 and 7)
OAAL	obligatory amino acid loss (Chapter 16)
OAT	ornithine aminotransferase (Chapter 3)
OCT	ornithine carbamoyltransferase (Chapter 3)
ODC	ornithine decarboxylase (Chapters 3 and 28)
6-OHDA	6-hydroxydopamine (Chapter 26)
3-OMD	3-O-methyl-DOPA (Chapter 26)
Orn	ornithine
Outbreak	two or more incidents of disease attributed to a common cause
PAH	phenylalanine hydroxylase (Chapters 9 and 23)
PCPA	p-chlorophenylalanine (Chapter 9)
PCR	polymerase chain reaction (Chapter 6)
PD	Parkinson's disease (Chapters 25 and 26)
PDCAAS	protein digestibility-corrected amino acid score (Chapters 14 and 15)
PERK	PKR-like endoplasmic reticulum kinase (Chapter 13)
PET	positron emission tomography (Chapter 24)
PFC	prefrontal cortex (Chapter 25)
PHB	prohibitin (Chapter 10)
Phe	phenylalanine
PKR	double-stranded RNA (dsRNA)-dependent protein kinase (Chapter 13)
PKU	phenylketonuria (Chapters 19, 23, and 28)
PLP	pyridoxal phosphate (Chapters 2 and 6)
PMP	pyridoxamine phosphate (Chapter 2)
PPU	post-prandial protein utilization (Chapters 15 and 16)
Pro	proline
Proteomes	total complement of proteins within a cell
PRP	proline-rich proteins (Chapter 28)
PRPP	5-phosphoribosyl-1-pyrophosphate
PRT	protein (Chapter 17)
PTZ	pentylenetetrazole (Chapter 25)
Pyr	pyruvate
rAAV	recombinant-adeno-associated virus (Chapter 26)
R&D	research and development
RAGE	receptor for AGE (Chapter 22)
RBC	red blood cell(s) (Chapter 3)

Table 1. Continued.

Abbreviation or Term	Definition
RCT	randomized clinical trials (Chapter 21)
RDI	recommended daily intake(s) (Chapter 23)
RE	resistance exercise (Chapter 17)
Risk	probability of ill effects
RNA	ribonucleic acid
RNS	reactive nitrogen species (Chapter 3)
ROC	receiver operator characteristic (Chapter 27)
ROS	reactive oxygen species (Chapters 2, 3, 7, and 10)
RTD	rapid tryptophan depletion (Chapter 24)
SAA	sulphur amino acid(s) (Chapter 16)
SAH	S-adenosylhomocysteine (Chapter 10)
SAMe	S-adenosylmethionine (Chapter 10)
SBS	short bowel syndrome (Chapter 18)
SCHAD	short-chain 3-hydroxyacyl-CoA dehydrogenase (Chapter 1)
SD	standard deviation
SDR	short-duration response (Chapter 26)
SDS-PAGE	sodium dodecyl sulphate-polyacrylamide gel electrophoresis (Chapters 6 and 8)
Ser	serine
SERT	serotonin transporter (Chapter 9)
SIRT	silent information regulator (Chapter 1)
SLE	systemic lupus erythematosus (Chapter 19)
SMCO	S-methylcysteine sulphoxide (Chapter 19)
SNc	substantia nigra pars compacta (Chapter 25)
SOD	superoxide dismutase (Chapter 25)
SRI	serotonin reuptake inhibitor(s) (Chapter 9)
STN	subthalamic nucleus (Chapter 25)
STZ	streptozotocin (Chapter 3)
T1R1	one of two class C G protein coupled receptors (Chapter 20)
T1R3	second of two class C G protein coupled receptors (Chapter 20)
Tau	taurine
TCA	tricarboxylic acid (cycle) (Chapters 1, 6, and 7)
TDI	tolerable daily intake
Teratogenic	causing birth defects
TH	tyrosine hydroxylase (Chapter 9)
THF	tetrahydrofolate (Chapter 10)
Thr	threonine
TPH	tryptophan hydroxylase (Chapters 9, 24, and 28)
TRC	taste receptor cells (Chapter 20)
tRNA	transfer RNA
Trp	tryptophan
Tyr	tyrosine
Umami	Japanese for 'delicious'; taste attributed to MSG in foods (Chapter 20)
URL	upper reference limit (Chapter 2)
Val	valine
VFT	Venus flytrap (Chapter 20)
VLDL	very low density lipoproteins (Chapter 10)
VMAT	vesicular monoamine transporter (Chapter 26)
VMH	ventromedial hypothalamus (Chapter 5)
VTE	venous thromboembolism (Chapter 21)
WHO	World Health Organization (United Nations)

References

Barker, R.A., Barasi, S. and Neal, M.J. (2008) *Neuroscience at a Glance*. 3rd ed., Blackwell Publishing, Oxford.

Baynes, J.W. and Dominiczak, M.H. (2009) *Medical Biochemistry*. 3rd ed., Mosby Elsevier, London and New York.

Bear, M.F., Connors, B.W. and Paradiso, M.A. (2007) *Neuroscience: Exploring the Brain*. 3rd ed., Lippincott, Williams and Wilkins, New York.

D'Mello, J.P.F. (1997) *Handbook of Plant and Fungal Toxicants*. 1st ed., CRC Press, Boca Raton, Florida.

Hodgson, E., Mailman, R.B. and Chambers, J.E. (1998) *Dictionary of Toxicology*. 2nd ed., Macmillan Reference Ltd, London.

Longmore, M., Wilkinson, I.B., Davidson, E.H., Foulkes, A. and Mafi, A.R. (2010) *Oxford Handbook of Clinical Medicine*. 8th ed., Oxford University Press, Oxford and New York.

Marcovitch, H. (2005) *Black's Medical Dictionary*. 41st ed., A & C Black, London.

Martin, E.A. (2010) *Oxford Concise Colour Medical Dictionary*. 5th ed., Oxford University Press, Oxford and New York.

MedlinePlus (2010) online: www.nlm.nih.gov/medlineplus/mplusdictionary.html, accessed 15 May 2011.

Munro, H.N. and Allison, J.B. (1964) *Mammalian Protein Metabolism*. Academic Press, New York, 566 pp.

Naish, J., Revest, P. and Court, D.S. (2009) *Medical Sciences*. 1st ed., Saunders Elsevier, London and New York.

Parish, H., Smith, T., Stirling, J. and Vella, F. (2006) *Oxford Dictionary of Biochemistry and Molecular Biology*. 2nd ed., Oxford University Press, Oxford and New York.

Part I

Enzymes and Metabolism

1 Glutamate Dehydrogenase

T.J. Smith[1]* and C.A. Stanley[2]
[1]*Donald Danforth Plant Science Center, Saint Louis, USA;*
[2]*Division of Endocrinology, The Children's Hospital of Philadelphia, Philadelphia, USA*

1.1 Abstract

Glutamate dehydrogenase (GDH) is one of the most extensively studied enzymes, described by hundreds of articles spanning more than five decades of research. The enzyme catalyses the reversible oxidative deamination reaction of L-glutamate to 2-oxoglutarate. All living organisms express this enzyme and key catalytic residues have remained unchanged through the epochs. However, animal GDH exhibits complex allosteric regulation by a wide array of metabolites compared to GDH from the other kingdoms. Recent studies have demonstrated that the loss of some of this allosteric regulation causes hypersecretion of insulin, suggesting that animal GDH is not just important for amino acid oxidation. Discussed here are the atomic details of animal GDH regulation and why these features may have evolved. What is also emerging from these studies is that GDH is a highly dynamic enzyme and regulators act by controlling this movement at key junctions. These details have led to the development of a number of novel inhibitors that may find use in treating a number of GDH-related disorders. It is very clear that we are only beginning to understand the ingenious versatility of this very old enzyme.

1.2 Introduction

GDH is found in all organisms and catalyses the reversible oxidative deamination of L-glutamate to 2-oxoglutarate using NAD^+ and/or $NADP^+$ as coenzyme (Hudson and Daniel, 1993). In nearly all organisms, GDH is a homohexameric enzyme composed of subunits comprised of ~500 residues in animals and ~450 residues in the other kingdoms. While the chemical details of the enzymatic reaction have been tightly conserved through the epochs, the metabolic role of the enzyme has not. Most striking is the fact that GDH from animal sources is allosterically regulated by a wide array of metabolites, while it is mainly regulated at the transcriptional level in the other kingdoms.

1.3 GDH in Animals

In stark contrast to the other kingdoms, animal GDH is regulated by a wide array of metabolites. The two major opposing allosteric regulators, ADP and GTP, appear to exert their effects via abortive complexes. Abortive complexes are where the product is replaced by substrate before the reacted coenzyme has

* E-mail address: TSmith@danforthcenter.org

a chance to dissociate; GDH•glutamate•NAD(P)H in the oxidative deamination reaction and GDH•2-oxoglutarate•NAD(P)$^+$ in the reductive amination reaction. Once these complexes form, coenzyme binds very tightly and there is slow enzymatic turnover. ADP is an activator believed to act, at least in part, by destabilizing the abortive complex (Frieden, 1965; George and Bell, 1980). In contrast, GTP is a potent inhibitor and is thought to act by stabilizing abortive complexes (Iwatsubo and Pantaloni, 1967). GTP binding is antagonized by phosphate (Koberstein and Sund, 1973) and ADP (Dieter et al., 1981), but is proposed to be synergistic with NADH bound in the non-catalytic site (Koberstein and Sund, 1973). Finally, ADP and GTP bind in an antagonistic manner (Dieter et al., 1981) due either to steric competition or to competing effects on abortive complex formation. As discussed below, it is likely that these regulators act by modulating the enzyme dynamics (Smith et al., 2002, Banerjee et al., 2003).

Mammalian GDH is also regulated by several other types of metabolites. Leucine, as well as some other monocarboxylic acids, has been shown to activate mammalian GDH (Yielding and Tomkins, 1961) by increasing the rate-limiting step of coenzyme release in a manner similar to ADP (Prough et al., 1973). However, since ADP and leucine activation were shown to be synergistic, these activators apparently do not bind to the same site (Prough et al., 1973). Since leucine is a weak substrate for GDH, clearly one binding site is the active site. The major question is whether there is a second, allosteric, leucine-binding site. Palmitoyl-CoA (Fahien and Kmiotek, 1981) and diethylstilbestrol (Tomkins et al., 1962) are inhibitors of mammalian GDH, but nothing is known about their binding location.

Mammalian GDH exhibits a number of unusual kinetic properties with unclear physiological roles. Negative cooperativity is observed as 'breaks' in Lineweaver–Burk plots with oxidized coenzyme (NAD$^+$ and NADP$^+$) varied (Engel and Dalziel, 1969). Subsequent studies demonstrated that coenzyme (NAD(P)(H)) binding to the initial subunits weakens the affinity for subsequent subunits (Bell and Dalziel, 1973; Melzi-d'Eril and Dalziel, 1973). This process is dependent upon the substituent at the α-carbon of the substrate backbone (Bell et al., 1985). The physiological role for this behaviour has been suggested to maintain a particular catalytic rate or responsiveness as coenzyme concentrations vary in the mitochondria (Koshland, 1996). However, it is also possible that negative cooperativity is a consequence of inter-subunit communication, necessary for other purposes such as allosteric regulation. This communication has been shown by abrupt and striking changes in the circular dichroism and fluorescence spectra when GDH is half saturated (Bell and Dalziel, 1973), and from chemical modification studies demonstrating that the loss of enzymatic activity is disproportionate to the number of subunits modified (Piszkiewicz and Smith, 1971; Rasool et al., 1976; Syed and Engel, 1984). There is marked substrate inhibition in both reaction directions that is exacerbated by GTP and antagonized by ADP (Bailey et al., 1982). This might be more indicative of product release being the rate-limiting step rather than a form of regulation per se.

1.3.1 Structure of animal GDH

The crystal structures of the bacterial (Baker et al., 1992; Stillman et al., 1993; Yip et al., 1995) and animal forms (Peterson and Smith, 1999; Smith et al., 2002) of GDH have shown that the general architecture and the locations of the catalytically important residues have remained unchanged throughout evolution. The structure of GDH (Fig. 1.1) is essentially two trimers of subunits stacked directly on top of each other with each subunit being composed of at least three domains (Peterson and Smith, 1999; Smith et al., 2001; Smith et al., 2002; Banerjee et al., 2003). The bottom domain makes extensive contacts with a subunit from the other trimer. Resting on top of this domain is the 'NAD binding domain' that has the conserved nucleotide-binding motif. Animal GDH has a long protrusion, an 'antenna' rising above the NAD binding domain, that is not found in bacteria, plants, fungi, and the vast majority of protists. The antenna from each subunit lies immediately behind the adjacent, counter-clockwise neighbour within the trimer. Since these intertwined antennae are only found in the forms of GDH that are

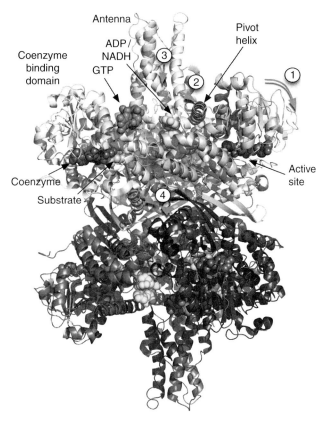

Fig. 1.1. The structure of animal GDH. Shown here is the ribbon diagram of animal GDH with each of the identical subunits represented in different shades of grey. The bound ligands are represented by different space filling objects. The arrows denote the main motions that occur throughout the hexamer as the catalytic cleft closes.

allosterically regulated by numerous ligands, it is reasonable to speculate that they play an important role in regulation.

1.4 Active Site

The first crystal structure of bovine GDH (bGDH) included glutamate, NADH and GTP (Peterson et al., 1998). Initial crystals of the apo form of GDH had been obtained previously, but had an extremely large unit cell and diffracted to modest resolution. Therefore, a substrate-saturated form of the enzyme was crystallized to stabilize the crystal lattice. NADH and glutamate form a tightly bound abortive complex in the active site. In addition, NADH binds to a second site and acts synergistically with the inhibitor GTP (Koberstein and Sund, 1973) to further increase the affinity of glutamate and NADH to the active site (Frieden, 1963a; Iwatsubo and Pantaloni, 1967; Koberstein and Sund, 1973). Therefore, together, it was hoped that high concentrations of these ligands would be sufficient to overcome the negative cooperativity exhibited by GDH with respect to coenzyme binding (Dalziel and Egan, 1972; Bell, 1974; Dalziel, 1975; Bell et al., 1985) so that homogenous and saturated GDH could be crystallized.

From this structure, both the bound NADH and glutamate were clearly visible in the active site (Peterson and Smith, 1999; Smith et al., 2001) (Fig. 1.1). It is important to note that at the time of these structures, only the chemical sequence had been determined for bovine GDH (Smith et al., 1970), and had a number of errors compared to the recently determined DNA sequence (GI:32880220). Figure 1.2 shows the structural details of both NADH and glutamate bound to the active site using the updated and refined bovine GDH structure (Li and Smith, unpublished results). The residues noted by parentheses denote the equivalent amino acids in *Clostridium symbiosum* GDH (csGDH) (Stillman et al., 1993; Maniscalco et al., 1996).

The chemical mechanism of GDH has been extensively studied and well detailed (for a review see Brunhuber and Blanchard, 1994) and the structure of the GDH•NADH•glutamate complex is entirely consistent with this model (Fig. 1.2). In the early 1990s the chemical mechanism was being refined (Singh et al., 1993; Srinivasan and Fisher, 1985; Maniscalco et al., 1996) at the same time that the structure of bacterial glutamate dehydrogenase was being determined (Baker et al., 1992; Dean et al., 1994; Smith et al., 1996;

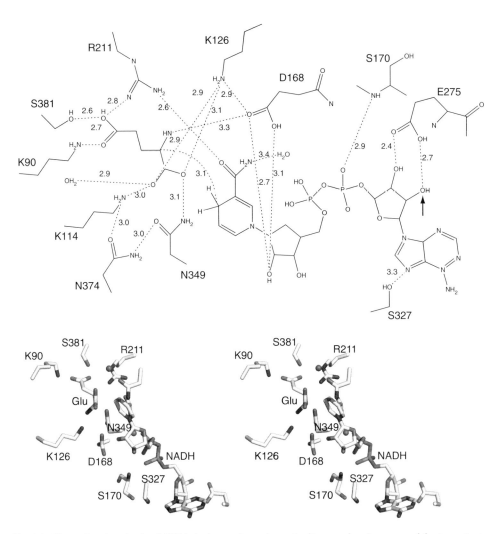

Fig. 1.2. The active site of animal GDH. At the top is a schematic diagram showing some of the important protein/ligand interactions in the active site in the GDH•NADH•glutamate complex. Shown below is a stereo diagram of the substrate and coenzyme bound to the active site.

Stillman et al., 1993). In the proposed mechanism for the reductive amination reaction, the first step is the binding of the γ-carboxyl of 2-oxoglutarate to a protonated lysine. This interaction has been observed in csGDH (Stillman et al., 1993), verified by mutagenesis in csGDH (Wang et al., 1995; Baker et al., 1997), and observed in bGDH (Fig. 1.2). In bGDH, K90, S380, and R211 form hydrogen bonds with the γ-carboxyl of the substrate. These interactions help determine the substrate specificity as has been demonstrated with csGDH, where a mutation of the equivalent to K90 to a leucine decreased the activity with L-glutamate by ~2000 fold, while increasing the activity with monocarboxylic amino acids (norvaline and α-aminobutyrate) by two- to threefold. In the next step of the proposed reaction, ammonium enters the active site and reacts with the α-keto group. A carbinolamine intermediate is then formed when the α-carbonyl oxygen accepts a proton from an active site lysine (K126 in bGDH and K125 in csGDH). The α-carbonyl oxygen then accepts a second proton from an active site carboxyl group (D168 in bGDH and D165 in csGDH) that at the same time accepts a proton from the substrate amine. Water is released as the carbinolamine forms an imine that is, in turn, reduced by NAD(P)H. The product is then protonated by the active site carboxyl group and released by the enzyme. Additional amine groups (K114 and N349) hold the carboxylic acid in place with a network of hydrogen bonds. It was also proposed that a necessary step in this chemical reaction is the closure of the catalytic cleft upon substrate and coenzyme binding (Singh et al., 1993) that expels the bulk water and brings the C-4 atom of the nicotinamide ring into very close contact with the C-α atom of the glutamate. This is clearly the case with only a couple of water molecules found in the closed bGDH•NADH•glutamate complex and the C-4 atom is brought to within ~3.1Å from the C-α atom of glutamate.

1.4.1 GDH dynamics

From the structures of bGDH with and without active site ligands, it is possible to observe the closure of the active site cleft, along with some of the large conformational changes that occur throughout the hexamer during each catalytic cycle (Peterson and Smith, 1999; Smith et al., 2001; Smith et al., 2002; Banerjee et al., 2003). Details of these conformational changes are summarized in Fig. 1.1. Substrate binds to the deep recesses of the cleft between the coenzyme binding domain and the lower domain. Coenzyme binds along the coenzyme binding domain surface of the cleft. Upon binding, the coenzyme binding domain rotates by ~18° to close down firmly upon the substrate and coenzyme (Fig. 1.1; arrow 1). As the catalytic cleft closes, the base of each of the long ascending helices in the antenna appears to rotate out in a counter-clockwise manner to push against the 'pivot' helix of the adjacent subunit (Fig. 1.1; arrow 2). There is a short helix in the descending loop of the antenna that becomes distended and shorter as the mouth closes in a manner akin to an extending spring (Fig. 1.1; arrow 3). The 'pivot helix' rotates in a counter-clockwise manner along the helical axes as well as rotating counter-clockwise around the trimer threefold axis. Finally, the entire hexamer seems to compress as the mouth closes (Fig. 1.1; arrow 4). The three pairs of subunits that sit on top of each other move as rigid units towards each other, compressing the cavity at the core of the hexamer. Therefore, it is quite clear that the bGDH active site cleft does not open and close in isolation, but rather that this motion involves the entire hexamer. As is further detailed in subsequent sections, it is apparent that animal GDH is controlled allosterically via ligand interactions at a number of these flex points.

1.4.2 GTP inhibition site

GTP is a potent inhibitor for the reaction and binds at the base of the antenna, wedged in between the NAD binding domain and the pivot helix (Peterson and Smith, 1999; Smith et al., 2001) (Fig. 1.3). It is important to note that this binding site is only available for GTP binding when the catalytic cleft is closed. Therefore, it is likely that after GTP binds to the 'closed' conformation, it is more difficult for the 'mouth' to open and release

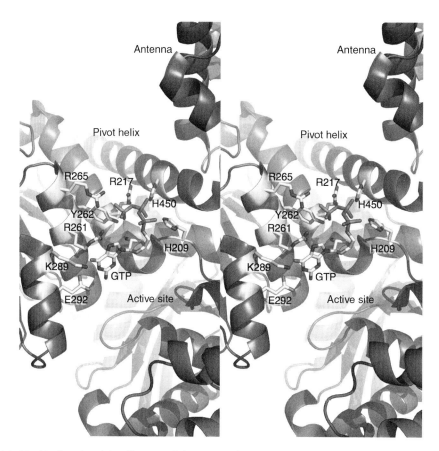

Fig. 1.3. The binding site of the allosteric inhibitor, GTP. This is a stereo diagram of GTP bound to the crevice between the NAD binding domain and the antenna. The highlighted residues are the locations of some of the naturally occurring mutations that cause the loss of GTP inhibition and, in turn, hyperinsulinism/hyperammonaemia.

the product. This is entirely consistent with the finding that GTP inhibits the reaction by slowing down product release and concomitantly increasing the binding affinity of substrate and coenzyme (Frieden, 1963a; Iwatsubo and Pantaloni, 1967; Koberstein and Sund, 1973). The vast majority of the interactions between GTP and bGDH involve the triphosphate moiety with the majority of the salt bridges being made with the γ-phosphate. This explains why, in terms of inhibition, GTP>>GDP>GMP (Frieden, 1965). This site is essentially an energy sensor in that if the mitochondrial energy level is high, then the GTP (and ATP) levels will be elevated and GDH will be inhibited. The environment of the GTP binding site is so favourable for phosphate binding that phosphate buffer was observed to bind in the absence of GTP (Smith et al., 2001). Interestingly, this is consistent with the fact that high phosphate concentrations compete with GTP for binding (Koberstein and Sund, 1973). Further, it is also well known that phosphate buffer stabilizes the enzyme compared to other buffers such as Tris (Frieden, 1963b). Therefore, phosphates binding to this apparently sensitive 'hinge' area somehow protect the enzyme against thermal denaturation.

1.4.3 ADP/second NADH site paradox

Perhaps one of the most confusing regulator sites on animal GDH is the allosteric activator,

ADP, binding site (Fig. 1.4). However, as will be detailed below, NADH also binds to this allosteric site and causes inhibition. In spite of having atomic details as to the interaction of these ligands with the enzyme, it is not at all clear how these regulators can cause opposite effects upon binding to the same site.

The existence of a second NADH binding site per subunit was demonstrated both kinetically and by binding analysis (Frieden, 1959a; Frieden, 1959b; Shafer et al., 1972). It was observed that NADH alone binds with a stoichiometry of 7–8 molecules per hexamer. In the presence of glutamate, NADH binds more tightly and the stoichiometry increases to 12 per hexamer (Shafer et al., 1972). Similarly, GTP also increases the affinity and binding stoichiometry (Koberstein and Sund, 1973). This second coenzyme site strongly favours NADH over NADPH with Kds of 57µM and 700µM, respectively. In the case of oxidized coenzyme, NAD$^+$, two binding sites were also observed. While the recent structures of the various complexes have demonstrated that ADP and NAD(H) bind to the same site (Smith et al., 2001; Banerjee et al., 2003), this was first suggested by ADP binding competition with NAD$^+$ (Limuti, 1983) and NADH (Dieter et al., 1981). Further, these binding studies provided direct evidence that GTP and glutamate enhance binding of NADH to a second site, and ADP blocks binding of both NAD$^+$ and NADH to a second site. A number of chemical reagents affect NADH inhibition by binding to disparate sites of the enzyme: TNBS (Goldin and Frieden, 1971) and FSBA (Pal et al., 1975; Schmidt and Colman, 1984) bind to the antenna; FSBAzA (Dombrowski et al., 1992) and FSBA (Pal et al., 1975; Schmidt and Colman, 1984) modify the core of the hexamer; and 6-BDB-TADP (Batra and Colman, 1986) modifies the outer portion of the NAD binding domain. These results demonstrate that a number of regions distal to the NADH binding site are involved in NADH inhibition. Since, in general terms, NADPH is involved in anabolic reactions in the cell while NADH is important for catabolic processes, it is possible that this regulation offers a feedback mechanism to curtail glutamate oxidation when catabolic reductive potentials (NADH) are high.

In nearly every way, ADP acts in a manner opposite to NADH binding to this site. In the oxidative deamination reaction, ADP activates at high pH, but inhibits at low pH with

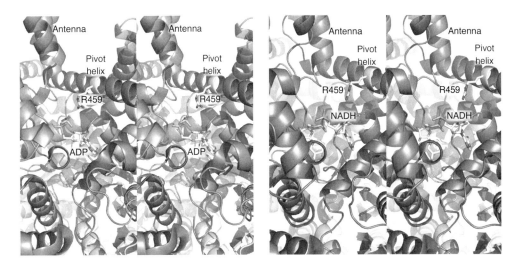

Fig. 1.4. The binding site of the activator, ADP (left), and the second, inhibitory site for NADH (right). This site is behind the NAD binding domain and immediately under the pivot helix. The highlighted residue, R459, was mutated to alanine and caused a loss in ADP activation. Shown on the right is the structure of NADH bound to this site where the adenosine/ribose moiety closely matches that of ADP and the nicotinamide/ribose portion binds into the subunit interface.

either NAD⁺ or NADP⁺ as coenzyme. In the reductive amination reaction, ADP is a potent activator at low pH and low substrate concentration. At pH 6.0, high concentrations of α-KG and NADH, but not NADPH, inhibit the reaction. This substrate inhibition is alleviated by ADP (Bailey et al., 1982). Therefore, while GTP and glutamate bind synergistically with NADH to inhibit GDH, ADP activates the reaction by decreasing the affinity of the enzyme for coenzyme at the active site. Under conditions where substrate inhibition occurs, this activates the enzyme. However, under conditions where the enzyme is not saturated (e.g. low substrate concentrations), this loss in binding affinity causes inhibition. Put another way, under conditions where product release is the rate-limiting step, ADP greatly facilitates the catalytic turnover. It should be noted that the fact that substrate (2-oxoglutarate) inhibition in the reductive amination reaction is only observed using NADH as coenzyme was suggested to be due to NADH (but not NADPH) binding to the second coenzyme site. Further, it was suggested that ADP activation under these conditions was due to ADP displacement of NADH from the second allosteric site (Frieden, 1965).

ADP binds behind the NAD binding domain and immediately under the pivot helix (Banerjee et al., 2003). This location is exactly consistent with chemical modification studies. The ADP analogue, AMPSBDB, reacts with R459 that lies on the pivot helix and is adjacent to the ADP binding site (Wrzeszczynski and Colman, 1994). This modification permanently activates the enzyme by essentially covalently locking an ADP molecule in the activation site. As shown in Fig. 1.4, R459 lies on the pivot helix and interacts with the phosphates of the bound ADP. It was proposed that this interaction might facilitate the rotation of the NAD binding domain and the release of product (Banerjee et al., 2003). To test this, R459 (R463 in human GDH) was mutated to an alanine and this led to a loss in ADP activation. This essentially suggests that ADP activates the reaction by 'pulling' on the back of the NAD binding domain to help open the active site cleft and facilitating product release.

The structures of GDH complexed with NADH, NADPH, and NAD have all been determined (Smith et al., 2001). Because NADH (but not NADPH) has been suggested to be an inhibitor of the reaction, it is somewhat surprising that it binds to the ADP activation site (Banerjee et al., 2003). The adenosine-ribose moiety location exactly matched that of ADP. The electron density of the ribose-nicotinamide moiety was much weaker and was initially built in two alternative conformations. However, the stronger density for this portion of NADH suggests that it points down into the interface between adjacent subunits as shown in Fig. 1.4. As predicted from the binding studies reviewed above, NADPH was found bound to the active site but not the second, allosteric site. From the preferred orientation shown in Fig. 1.4, this is likely due to the fact that there is not enough room to accommodate the additional phosphate on the ribose ring that is buried at the subunit interface.

NAD⁺ was found to bind in a manner essentially identical to NADH (Smith et al., 2001). From steady state kinetic analysis, it was initially thought that NAD⁺ binding to this second site causes activation of the enzyme (Frieden, 1959a), even though NADH causes apparent inhibition. However, subsequent studies demonstrated that this apparent activation was due to negatively cooperative binding with respect to coenzyme (Dalziel and Engel, 1968). Therefore, it is not clear what difference there might be, if any, between NAD⁺ and NADH binding to GDH at this location. It is interesting to note that modification of the ADP site with an ADP analogue did not eliminate NADH inhibition (Wrzeszczynski and Colman, 1994). Perhaps this is due to the nicotinamide moiety still binding to the pocket between the subunits in spite of AMPSBDB being bound to R459. As will be detailed below, recent studies on new GDH inhibitors have shown that compounds binding to subunit interfaces can be potent inhibitors of the enzyme. Perhaps the ribose-nicotinamide moiety is acting in a similar manner.

The physiological role of ADP activation is easily understood: when the energy level of the mitochondria is low and ADP levels are high, the catabolism of glutamate is facilitated for energy production. However, the possible *in vivo* role of NADH inhibition is less clear.

In mammalian mitochondria, assuming a matrix volume of 1 µl mg^{-1} of protein, the concentrations of NAD(H) and NADP(H) are approximate 0.5–2.0 mM (Lenartowicz, 1990). However, activity of the transhydrogenase transfers much of the reductive power of NADH to NADPH. Using metabolite indicators, the mitochondrial NADH/NAD$^+$ ratio was estimated to be ~0.2 and the NADPH/NADP$^+$ ratio was ~200 (Hoek and Rydström, 1988). In experiments on submitochondrial particles, the energy-linked transhydrogenase was found to maintain NADP up to 500 times more reduced than NAD (Rydström *et al.*, 1970). These results suggest that the range of NADH concentration is ~0.083–0.33 mM. NADH inhibition is observed at concentrations above 0.2 mM (e.g. see Batra and Colman, 1986), but only reaches ~50% inhibition at 1mM NADH. Therefore, if NADH inhibition is physiologically relevant, it seems more likely that its purpose is to synergistically enhance GTP inhibition; under conditions of high reductive potential, NADH acts with GTP to keep GDH in a tonic state.

At an atomic level, there is a very clear delineation between ligands binding to the open and closed conformations. NADH alone only binds to the active site. When glutamate is added, the catalytic cleft closes and NADH is able to bind to the second, allosteric site. Further, the GTP binding site collapses when the catalytic cleft opens and therefore GTP also favours the closed conformation. Therefore, the synergism between NADH and GTP is likely due to both ligands binding to, and stabilizing the closed conformation. Again, this supports the contention that NADH inhibition alone may not have a significant physiological role, but rather its main function is the enhancement of GTP inhibition.

1.5 Role of GDH in Insulin Homeostasis

The difference between the allosteric regulation of GDH from animals and the other animal kingdoms has been known for decades, but possible roles for allosteric regulation in animal GDH is only starting to emerge.

Of growing interest is the fact that loss of inhibition of GDH causes inappropriate stimulation of insulin secretion. There have been three GDH-mediated forms of hyperinsulinism identified thus far: hyperinsulinism/hyperammonaemia (HHS) due to mutations that abrogate GTP inhibition, mutations in NAD-dependent deacetylase (SIRT4) and knockout mutations of short-chain 3-hydroxyacyl-CoA dehydrogenase (SCHAD).

1.5.1 HHS

HHS was one of the first diseases that clearly linked GDH regulation to insulin and ammonia homeostasis (Stanley *et al.*, 1998). In brief, the mitochondrion of the pancreatic β-cells plays an integrative role in the fuel stimulation of insulin secretion. The current concept is that mitochondrial oxidation of substrates increases the cellular phosphate potential that is manifested by a rise in the ATP^{4-} MgADP^{2-} ratio. The elevated ATP concentration closes the plasma membrane K$_{ATP}$ channels, resulting in the depolarization of the membrane potential. This voltage change across the membrane opens voltage gated Ca^{2+} channels. The rise of free cytoplasmic Ca^{2+} then leads to insulin granule exocytosis (Fig. 1.5).

The connection between GDH and insulin regulation was initially established using a nonmetabolizable analogue of leucine (Sener and Malaisse, 1980; Sener *et al.*, 1981), BCH (β-2-aminobicycle(2.2.1)-heptane-2-carboxylic acid). These studies demonstrated that activation of GDH was tightly correlated with increased glutaminolysis and release of insulin. In addition, it has also been noted that factors that regulate GDH also affect insulin secretion (Fahien *et al.*, 1988). Subsequently, it was postulated that glutamine could also play a secondary messenger role and that GDH plays a role in its regulation (Stanley, 2000; Li *et al.*, 2003; Li *et al.*, 2004). The *in vivo* importance of GDH in glucose homeostasis was demonstrated by the discovery that a genetic hypoglycaemic disorder, the HHS syndrome, is caused by loss of GTP regulation of GDH (Stanley *et al.*, 1998; Stanley *et al.*, 2000; MacMullen *et al.*, 2001). Children with HHS have increased

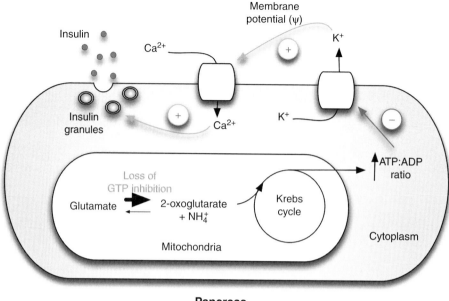

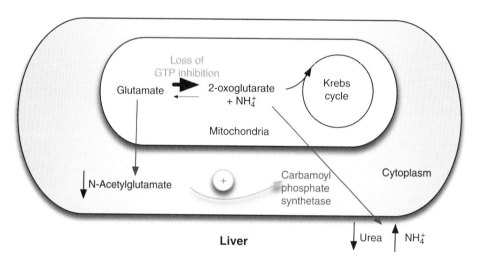

Fig. 1.5. Schematic of how the loss of GTP inhibition can cause the hyperstimulated secretion of insulin (top) and the elevated serum levels of ammonium (bottom). In the pancreas, the loss of GTP inhibition increases the flux of glutamate to the Krebs cycle, leading to elevated ATP levels, and the secretion of insulin. In the liver, not only does accelerated catabolism increase the levels of ammonium, but the lower levels of glutamate also decrease production of N-acetylglutamate, a required activator of ureagenesis that may or may not affect serum ammonium concentrations.

β-cell responsiveness to leucine and susceptibility to hypoglycaemia following high-protein meals (Hsu et al., 2001). This is likely due to uncontrolled catabolism of amino acids yielding high ATP levels that stimulate insulin secretion as well as high serum ammonium levels. The elevation of serum ammonia levels reflects the consequence of altered regulation of GDH, leading to increased ammonia production from glutamate oxidation, and possibly also impaired urea synthesis by carbamoylphosphate synthetase (CPS) due to reduced formation of its activator, *N*-acetyl-glutamate, from glutamate (Fig. 1.5). Essentially, this genetic lesion disrupts the regulator linkage between glycolysis and amino acid catabolism. During glucose-stimulated insulin secretion in normal individuals, it has been proposed that the generation of high energy phosphates inhibits GDH and promotes conversion of glutamate to glutamine, which, alone or combined, might amplify the release of insulin (Li *et al.*, 2003, 2004).

While the glucose and ammonium levels in patients with HHS are alone sufficient to potentially cause damage to the CNS, recent studies have suggested a high correlation between HHS and childhood-onset epilepsy, learning disabilities, and seizures (Bahi-Buisson *et al.*, 2008). Some of these pathologies have been shown to be unrelated to serum glucose and ammonium levels. This is not entirely surprising considering the importance of glutamate and its derivative, γ-aminobutyric acid, as neurotransmitters. The current treatment for HHS is to pharmaceutically control insulin secretion (e.g. diazoxide, a potassium channel activator) but this does not address the serum ammonium and CNS pathologies.

1.5.2 SIRT4 mutations

Sirt2 or sirtuins (silent information regulator two proteins) are found in all organisms and most are NAD-dependent protein deacetylases. The sirtuins have been shown to be implicated in ageing and regulate transcription, involved in stress response, and apoptosis. Recent studies have shown that SIRT4, a mitochondrial enzyme, uses NAD to ADP-ribosylate GDH and inhibit its activity (Herrero-Yraola *et al.*, 2001; Haigis *et al.*, 2006). When SIRT4 knockout mice were generated, the loss of SIRT4 activity led to the activation of GDH and, much like HHS due to the loss of GTP inhibition, up-regulated amino acid-stimulated insulin secretion (Haigis *et al.*, 2006). In addition, they found that, with regard to that ADP-ribosylation,

GDH activity in SIRT4 -/- mice was similar to mice on a calorie restriction diet regime. This suggests that normally SIRT4 in the β cell mitochondria represses GDH activity by ADP-ribosylation and this regulation is removed during times of low caloric intake.

1.5.3 SCHAD mutations

A form of recessively inherited hyperinsulinism has been recently identified to be associated with a deficiency of a mitochondrial fatty acid β-oxidation enzyme, the short-chain 3-hydroxyacyl-CoA dehydrogenase (SCHAD) encoded by the *HADH* gene on 4q (Jackson *et al.*, 1991; Molven *et al.*, 2004; Hussain *et al.*, 2005). Children with this defect have recurrent episodes of hypoglycemia that can be controlled with the K_{ATP} channel agonist diazoxide. These patients also have serum accumulation of fatty acid metabolites such as 3-hydroxybutyryl-carnitine and urinary 3-hydroxyglutaric acid (Molven *et al.*, 2004, Hussain *et al.*, 2005). Similar to HHS, these patients also have severe dietary protein sensitivity (Hussain *et al.*, 2005). However, the loss of SCHAD activity is at odds with increased insulin secretion observed in HHS since it is expected to decrease ATP production. In addition, other genetic disorders of mitochondrial fatty acid oxidation do not lead to hyperinsulinism (Stanley *et al.*, 2006).

Recent studies have now explained this seeming paradox by suggesting that SCHAD regulates GDH activity via protein-protein interactions (Li *et al.*, 2010). From immunoprecipitation and pull-down analysis, it is apparent that GDH and SCHAD interact as had been previously suggested (Filling *et al.*, 2008). This interaction inhibits GDH activity by decreasing GDH affinity for substrate. This effect was found to be limited to the pancreas presumably because of the relatively high levels of SCHAD found in this tissue. Hussain *et al.* (2005) recently demonstrated that SCHAD-deficient children have protein sensitive hypoglycaemia, consistent with an activation of GDH. This would also explain why SCHAD-deficient patients do not have a concomitant increase in serum ammonium levels as observed in HHS. These results are particularly interesting since it strongly suggests that part of GDH regulation comes from associating as a large multienzyme complex in the mitochondria. In addition, this fits in well with the linkage between fatty acid and amino acid oxidation as suggested by the evolution of allostery that came from analysis of ciliate GDH (Allen *et al.*, 2004; Smith and Stanley, 2008) as discussed in the next section.

1.6 Evolution of GDH Allostery

It has been known for some time that animal GDH contain an internal 48-residue insert compared to GDH from the other kingdoms. From the structure of animal GDH, we now know this insert forms the antenna region (Fig. 1.1). Further, kinetic analysis has demonstrated that animal GDH is allosterically regulated by a wide array of metabolites. What was not at all clear was when and why the antenna evolved and whether it was linked to the complex pattern of allostery in animal GDH. With the release of the Tetrahymena Genome Project, it became evident that tetrahymena GDH (tGDH) also has this ~48-residue insert. This possible evolutionary 'missing link' was then further analysed via kinetic and mutagenesis analyses (Allen *et al.*, 2004). Like mammalian GDH,

tGDH is activated by ADP and inhibited by palmatoyl CoA. However, like bacterial GDH, tGDH is coenzyme specific (NAD(H)) and is not regulated by GTP or leucine. Therefore, with regard to allosteric regulation, tGDH is indeed an evolutionary 'missing link' between bacterial and animal GDH.

A major question was how the antenna was linked to allosteric regulation. From structural studies, it was clear that the antenna was not involved in ADP or GTP binding (Peterson and Smith, 1999; Smith *et al.*, 2001; Banerjee *et al.*, 2003). However, when the antenna on human GDH was replaced by the short loop found in bacterial GDH, the enzyme lost GTP, ADP, and palmatoyl-CoA regulation (Allen *et al.*, 2004). When the ciliate antenna was spliced onto human GDH, this hybrid enzyme had a fully functional repertoire of mammalian allostery. This demonstrated that the antenna is essential for exacting allosteric regulation by GTP and ADP while not being directly involved in their binding. Evolutionarily, this also demonstrated that the antenna in ciliate GDH is capable of transmitting the GTP inhibitory signal, but GTP regulation was apparently not needed in the ciliates.

This suggests that GDH allostery evolved in at least a two-step process (Fig. 1.6). The first evolutionary step may have been due to the changing functions of

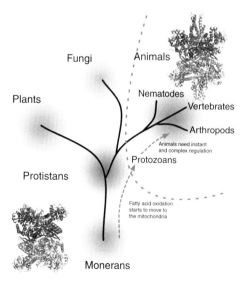

Fig. 1.6. Evolution of glutamate dehydrogenase. The ciliates represent an evolutionary missing link between animals and all of the other kingdoms. In the ciliates, fatty acid oxidation started to move from the peroxisomes to the mitochondria, the location of GDH. Perhaps in response to this, the antenna was created to facilitate allosteric regulation and coordinated control of amino acid and fatty acid oxidation. Using this new architecture, animal GDH added further complexity to allosteric regulation since glutamate has such an important role in insulin homeostasis, neurotransmission and ureagenesis.

the cellular organelles as the ciliates branched off from the other animal kingdoms. In the other eukaryotic organisms, all fatty acid oxidation occurs in the peroxisomes (Gerhardt, 1992; Erdmann *et al.*, 1997). In the ciliates, fatty acid oxidation is shared between the peroxisomes and the mitochondria (Muller *et al.*, 1968; Blum, 1973). Eventually, all medium and long chain fatty oxidation moved into the mitochondria in animals (Reddy and Mannaerts, 1994; Hashimoto, 1999). Therefore, it appears that GDH regulation evolved in response to fatty acid and amino acid oxidation being brought into the same subcellular compartment. Specifically, the pattern of regulation suggests that the catabolism of amino acids is down-regulated when there are sufficient levels of fatty acids. When the mitochondria have run low on fatty acids and their energy state is low (i.e. high ADP levels), only then will amino acids be catabolized. This closely mirrors what was found in the insulin disorders described above; GDH activity is tightly repressed until other energy sources are depleted. Therefore, allostery was necessary to coordinate the growing complexity of mitochondrial metabolism and the antenna feature is needed to exact this regulation.

The second step of evolution was to add leucine and GTP allostery as animals needed even more sophisticated and rapid-response regulation of GDH activity. This is an example of exaptation, where a feature evolves for one reason and is then further refined and used for other functions in subsequent evolution. In animals, GDH is found in high levels in the central nervous system (CNS), pancreas, liver and kidneys. In each organ, the levels of glutamate need to be controlled by very different physiological signals. In the pancreas, GDH needs to coordinate amino acid oxidation with fatty acid and carbohydrate catabolism for an appropriate insulin response. In the liver, glutamate is crucial for ureagenesis. In the CNS, glutamate and its derivative, GABA, are major neurotransmission ligands. These disparate roles for GDH are more than likely why GDH in animals has such sophisticated allosteric regulation compared to all other organisms.

As a likely response to the growing complexity of multi-organ animals, two very important regulators, leucine and GTP, were added to the allosteric regulatory repertoire. In the pancreas, GDH needs to be activated when amino acids (protein) are ingested to promote insulin secretion and appropriate anabolic effects on peripheral tissues. In the glucose-fed state, triphosphate levels are high and GDH needs to be inhibited to redirect amino acids into glutamine synthesis in order to amplify insulin release. In the liver, GDH needs to be suppressed when other fuels, such as fatty acids, are available, but to be increased when surplus amino acids need to be oxidized. To this end, mammals added layers of regulation onto ciliate GDH to include leucine activation and GTP inhibition. The choice of leucine as a regulator is likely not an accident, because leucine is the most abundant amino acid in protein (10%) and provides a good measure of protein abundance. Similarly, the marked sensitivity of GDH for GTP over ATP is also not likely to be accidental. Most of the ATP in the mitochondria is produced from oxidative phosphorylation that is driven by the potential across the mitochondrial membrane created by NADH oxidation. Therefore, the number of ATP molecules generated from one turn of the TCA cycle can vary between 1 and 29. In contrast, one GTP is generated per turn of the TCA cycle and there is a slow mitochondria/cytoplasm exchange rate. Therefore, the GTP/GDP ratio is a much better metric of TCA cycle activity than the ATP/ADP ratio. Indeed, recent results have demonstrated that mitochondrial GTP, but not ATP, regulates glucose-stimulated insulin secretion (Kibbey *et al.*, 2007). This is also consistent with the HHS disorder in that, without GTP inhibition of GDH, glutamate will be catabolized in an uncontrolled manner; the TCA cycle will generate more GTP; and more insulin will be released. Therefore, the addition of GTP and leucine regulation to GDH makes it acutely sensitive to glucose and amino acid catabolism, with obvious implications for insulin homeostasis. It is also likely that this complex network of allostery was also needed to accommodate the differing regulation needed by the CNS and ureagenesis.

1.6.1 Possible therapeutics for GDH-mediated insulin disorders

The current treatment for HHS is to pharmaceutically control insulin secretion (e.g. diazoxide, a potassium channel activator) but this does not address the liver and CNS pathology. One approach to circumvent the extremely high costs of developing therapeutics for diseases with a small patient base is to try to find bioactive compounds commonly found in the food chain. To this end, a broad search led to two bioactive compounds found in green tea.

According to legend, green tea was discovered by the Chinese Emperor Shen-Nung in 2737 BC and for centuries has been used as a folk remedy to treat a number of ailments. Green tea is a significant source of a type of flavonoids called catechins, including epigallocatechin gallate (EGCG); epigallocatechin (EGC); epicatechin gallate (ECG); and epicatechin (EC). One 200 ml cup of green tea supplies 140, 65, 28 and 17 mg of these polyphenols, respectively (Yang and Wang, 1993). Over the past few decades, there has been growing interest in EGCG since it has been suggested to decrease cholesterol levels (Maron et al., 2003), act as an antibiotic (Hamilton-Miller, 1995) and anticarcinogen (Katiyar and Mukhtar, 1996), repress hepatic glucose production (Waltner-Law et al., 2002), and enhance insulin action (Anderson and Polansky, 2002). The exact mechanism of action of EGCG with regard to these various effects is largely unknown and in many cases is assumed to due to its antioxidant activity.

Of the four major catechins found in green tea, only two showed inhibitory activity against GDH: ECG and EGCG (Fig. 1.7). Essentially, activity is dependent upon the presence of the third ring structure, the gallate,

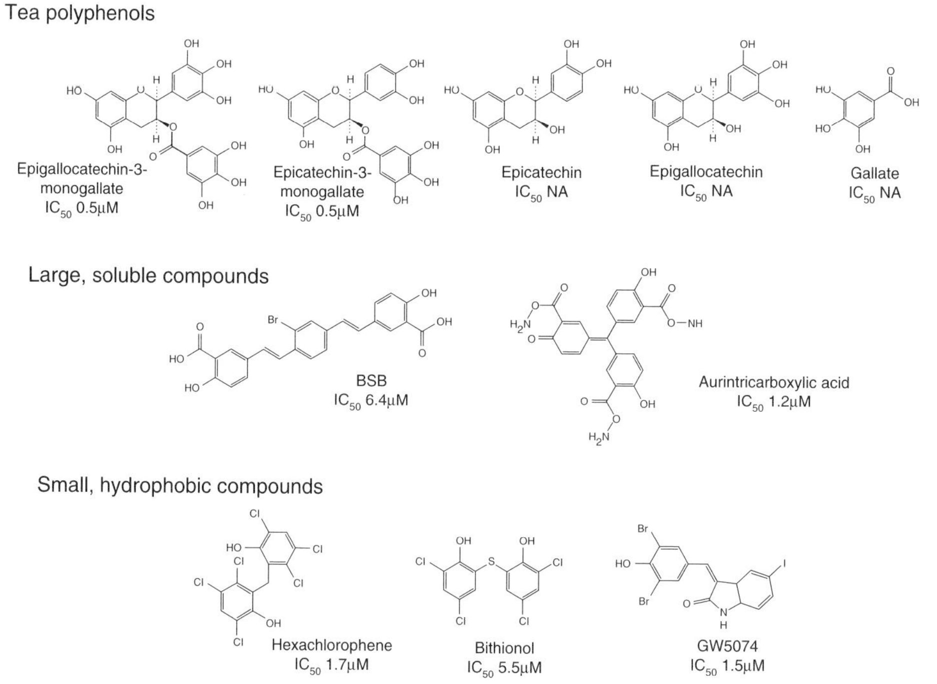

Fig. 1.7. New GDH inhibitors. The top row of compounds shows the various fragments of the polyphenols found in green tea. Note that only ECG and EGCG had any effect on GDH activity. The second row shows other highly soluble compounds uncovered in the high throughput screening. It may very well be that these compounds bind to a site common with the green tea flavonoids. The bottom row shows the bioactive compounds that are smaller, stable and more hydrophobic.

on the flavonoid moiety. EGCG and ECG allosterically inhibit purified animal GDH *in vitro* with a nanomolar ED_{50}. Since EC or EGC were not active against GDH, but have the same antioxidant activity as ECG and EGCG, the antioxidant property of these catechins cannot be relevant to GDH inhibition. EGCG inhibition is non-competitive and, similar to GTP inhibition, is abrogated by leucine, BCH, and ADP. As noted above, the antenna is necessary for GTP inhibition and ADP activation (Allen *et al.*, 2004). Similarly, EGCG does not inhibit the 'antenna-less' form of GDH, thus is further evidence that EGCG is an allosteric inhibitor. Most importantly, EGCG inhibits HHS GDH mutants as effectively as wild type (Li *et al.*, 2006), making it a possible therapeutic lead compound.

The next step was to ascertain whether EGCG was active in tissue. Studies have demonstrated that GDH plays a major role in leucine stimulated insulin secretion (LSIS) by controlling glutaminolysis (Li *et al.*, 2003, 2004). Therefore, EGCG was tested on pancreatic β-cells using the perfusion assay (Li *et al.*, 2006). Importantly, EGCG, but not EGC, blocked the GDH-mediated stimulation of insulin secretion by the β-cells. However, it did not have any effect on insulin secretion, glucose oxidation, or cellular respiration during glucose stimulation where GDH is known to not play a major role in the regulation of insulin secretion. Therefore, EGCG is indeed a specific inhibitor of GDH both *in vitro* and *in situ*, and ongoing studies are evaluating whether it will be similarly active *in vivo*.

More recent studies on glioblastoma cells have demonstrated that EGCG inhibition of GDH might have even broader utility than just with HHS. Increased glucose and glutamine utilization are hallmarks of tumour metabolism (Kim and Dang, 2006; DeBerardinis *et al.*, 2008). The phosphatidylinositol 3'-kinase/Akt pathway is enhanced in many human tumours and up-regulates glucose uptake and utilization (Elstrom *et al.*, 2004; Bauer *et al.*, 2005). c-Myc, on the other hand, up-regulates glutamine utilization by increasing cell surface transporters and enzymes (Wise *et al.*, 2008; Gao *et al.*, 2009). At least *in vitro*, the enhanced utilization of one of these carbon sources also makes the cells sensitive to its withdrawal (Buzzai *et al.*, 2005; Wise *et al.*, 2008). Extending upon all of these results, the DeBerardinis laboratory demonstrated that EGCG sensitizes glioblastoma cells to glucose withdrawal and to inhibitors of Akt signalling and glycolysis (Yang *et al.*, 2009). Indeed, the addition of EGCG mirrored the effects of knocking out GDH in the tissue. Therefore, these results suggest that anti-cancer therapy that combines GDH inhibitors with those that inhibit glucose utilization could be very effective in treating tumours.

1.6.2 Other novel inhibitors of GDH

The results with EGCG/ECG offer proof of concept that it is possible to control GDH activity pharmaceutically. However, it is always important to have more than one lead compound for drug development. Therefore, high throughput screening was used to find additional compounds that might have better efficacy and/or pharmacokinetics (Li *et al.*, 2007; Li *et al.*, 2009).

A search of more than 30,000 compounds yielded a number of interesting active compounds (Fig. 1.7) (Li *et al.*, 2007; Li *et al.*, 2009). First, in agreement with previous studies, the screen identified EGCG as an active compound but EC was found not to be active. With physical properties similar to EGCG, aurintricarboxylic acid (ATA) and 3,3'-[(2-bromo-1,4-phenylene)di(E)ethene-2,1-diyl]bis(6-hydroxybenzoic acid) (BSB) were also found to be efficacious inhibitors of GDH. ATA can interfere with protein-nucleotide interactions such as those found in kinases and phosphatase (Myskiw *et al.*, 2007) and can inhibit influenza virus neuraminidases (Hashem *et al.*, 2009). BSB interacts with amyloid polymers (Skovronsky *et al.*, 2000). The effects of all three of these compounds were strongly abrogated by ADP. Therefore, while not proof evident, it is possible that all three compounds bind to the ADP site. This could be akin to NADH binding to the ADP site and causing inhibition rather than the ADP-mediated activation, and would be consistent with the inhibitory effects that ATA has on kinases/phosphatases. The other group of compounds that were identified in this screen are small, hydrophobic compounds: bithionol, hexachlorophene, GW5074, and diethylstilbestrol. Compared to ATA and EGCG, the inhibition caused by these compounds is not as easily abrogated by ADP. It is likely that these compounds are binding to a site(s) distinct from where the more soluble ATA, EGCG, and BSB compounds are binding.

Subsequent structural studies found that the small, hydrophobic compounds (GW5074, hexachlorophene (HCP), bithionol) bind to subunit interfaces in the enzyme that are critical for conformational transitions (Li et al., 2009). As shown in Fig. 1.8, six molecules of HCP form a ring in the inner cavity of the hexamer, not with sixfold symmetry but rather alternate between two different conformations around the ring. One conformer is relatively flat and tucks into a pocket at the interface between diagonal subunits while the other conformer is more vertically oriented but also interacts with diagonal subunits. Essentially, the symmetrical HCP binds at the interface between twofold related subunits with one ring interacting with one subunit and the other ring interacting with the other. The majority of the interactions between HCP and GDH are hydrophobic, but there is also an almost 'chain link' of aromatic stacking interactions.

Bithionol and GW5074 do not bind to the same site as HCP. While HCP binds to the inner core, these two drugs bind halfway between the core and the exterior of the hexamer (Fig. 1.8). This is in contrast to the binding geometry of HCP where the internal cavity is blocked off from the exterior solvent mainly by the antenna structure. Also unlike HCP, each of the six drug molecules is associated with separate subunits rather than one molecule contacting two symmetrical sites simultaneously. Instead, two drug molecules form pairs that are related by the hexameric twofold axes. The binding environments of the two drugs are nearly identical. Residues 138–155 of the glutamate-binding domain form an α-helix that makes most of the contact between diagonal subunits and draw closer together when the catalytic cleft is closed. These two drugs stack against each other and interact with hydrophobic residues and the aliphatic portions of the polar and charged side chains of

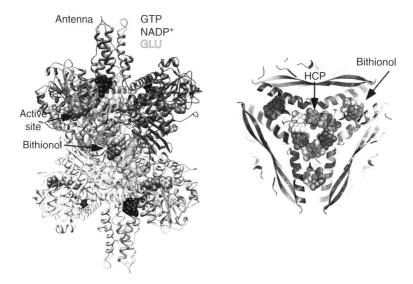

Fig. 1.8. Locations of the binding sites for the new GDH inhibitors. The small, hydrophobic compounds bind to inter-subunit flex points. The left figure is a side view of the entire hexamer showing the location of the bithionol and GW5074. Note that this is the same region that compresses during the closure of the catalytic cleft (Fig. 1.1). On the right is a cutaway view from the top of the hexamer showing that these hydrophobic compounds bind to the subunit interfaces and that HCP forms a ring of aromatic interactions in the core of the enzyme. For clarity, GW5074 is not shown since it binds to the same location as bithionol.

residues K143, R146, R147, and M150. These drugs, therefore, appear to bind directly to the area that compresses during mouth closure.

1.7 Conclusions

It has been suggested that the complex motions within GDH may initially have evolved to improve catalytic efficiency (Smith and Stanley, 2008). The negative cooperativity and extensive subunit communication may have evolved to conserve and transfer the energy involved in substrate binding to one subunit to facilitate product release from adjacent subunits (Smith and Bell, 1982). As is clear in the case of these drugs and the naturally occurring allosteric regulators, this complex ballet of motion creates numerous sites by which ligands can bind and modulate catalytic activity. This has allowed allostery in GDH gradually to evolve in complexity to create new functions and roles, rather than creating entirely new gene products to accommodate the changing needs of the cell (e.g. linkage between amino acid catabolism and insulin secretion). While it seems that GDH regulation is overly complex for an enzyme involved in such a mundane chemical reaction, it is in fact remarkable that this allostery can adequately control a single enzyme that is apparently crucial to regulate central nervous system levels of glutamate, ureagenesis in the liver, and insulin secretion in the pancreas.

1.8 Acknowledgements

This work was supported by National Institutes of Health (NIH) Grant DK072171 (to T.J.S.), NIH Grant DK53012 and American Diabetes Association Research Award 1-05-RA-128 (to C.A.S.) and NIH Grant DK19525 for islet biology and radioimmunoassay cores.

References

Allen, A., Kwagh, J., Fang, J., Stanley, C.A. and Smith, T.J. (2004) Evolution of glutamate dehydrogenase regulation of insulin homeostasis is an example of molecular exaptation. *Biochemistry* 43, 14431–14443.

Anderson, R.A. and Polansky, M.M. (2002) Tea enhances insulin activity. *Journal of Agricultural and Food Chemistry* 50, 7182–7186.

Bahi-Buisson, N., Roze, E., Dionisi, C., Escande, F., Valayannopoulos, V., Feillet, F. and Heinrichs, C. (2008) Neurological aspects of hyperinsulinism-hyperammonaemia syndrome. *Developmental Medicine & Child Neurology* 50, 945–949.

Bailey, J.S., Bell, E.T. and Bell, J.E. (1982) Regulation of bovine glutamate dehydrogenase. *Journal of Biological Chemistry* 257, 5579–5583.

Baker, P.J., Britton, K.L., Engel, P.C., Farrantz, G.W., Lilley, K.S., Rice, D.W. and Stillman, T.J. (1992) Subunit assembly and active site location in the structure of glutamate dehydrogenase. *Proteins: Structure, Function, and Genetics* 12, 75–86.

Baker, P.J., Waugh, M.L., Wang, X.-G., Stillman, T.J., Turnbull, A.P., Engel, P.C. and Rice, D.W. (1997) Determinants of substrate specificity in the superfamily of amino acid dehydrogenases. *Biochemistry* 36, 16109–16115.

Banerjee, S., Schmidt, T., Fang, J., Stanley, C.A. and Smith, T.J. (2003) Structural studies on ADP activation of mammalian glutamate dehydrogenase and the evolution of regulation. *Biochemistry* 42, 3446–3456.

Batra, S.P. and Colman, R.F. (1986) Isolation and identification of cysteinyl peptide labeled by 6-[(4-bromo-2,3-dioxobutyl)thio]-6-deaminoadenosine 5′-diphosphate in the reduced diphosphopyridine nucleotide inhibitory site of glutamate dehydrogenase. *Biochemistry* 25, 3508–3515.

Bauer, D.E., Hatzivassiliou, G., Zhao, F., Andreadis, C. and Thompson, C.B. (2005) ATP citrate lyase is an important component of cell growth and transformation. *Oncogene* 24, 6314–6322.

Bell, E.T., Limuti, C., Renz, C.L. and Bell, J.E. (1985) Negative co-operativity in glutamate dehydrogenase. Involvement of the 2-position in the induction of conformational changes. *Biochemical Journal* 225, 209–217.

Bell, J.E. (1974) Studies on negative cooperativity in glutamate dehydrogenase and glyceraldehyde-3-phosphate dehydrogenase. DPhil thesis, Oxford University, England.

Bell, J.E. and Dalziel, K. (1973) A conformational transition of the oligomer of glutamate dehydrogenase induced by half-saturation with NAD^+ or $NADP^+$. *Biochimica et Biophysica Acta* 309, 237–242.

Blum, J.J. (1973) Localization of some enzymes of β-oxidation of fatty acids in the peroxisomes of *Tetrahymena. Journal of Protozoology* 20, 688–692.

Brunhuber, N.M.W. and Blanchard, J.S. (1994) The biochemistry and enzymology of amino acid dehydrogenases. *Critical Reviews in Biochemistry and Molecular Biology* 29, 415–567.

Buzzai, M., Bauer, D.E., Jones, R.G., DeBerardinis, R.J., Hatzivassiliou, G., Elstrom, R.L. and Thompson, C.B. (2005) The glucose dependence of Akt-transformed cells can be reversed by pharmacologic activation of fatty acid β-oxidation. *Oncogene* 24, 4165–4173.

Dalziel, K. (1975) Kinetics and mechanisms of nicotinamide-nucleotide-linked dehydrogenases. In: Boyer, P.D. (ed.) *The Enzymes.* Academic Press, New York.

Dalziel, K. and Egan, R.R. (1972) The binding of oxidized coenzymes by glutamate dehydrogenase and the effects of glutarate and purine nucleotides. *Biochemical Journal* 126, 975–984.

Dalziel, K. and Engel, P.C. (1968) Antagonistic homotropic interactions as a possible explanation of coenzyme activation of glutamate dehydrogenase. *FEBS Letters* 1, 349–352.

Dean, J.L.E., Wang, X.-G., Teller, J.K., Waugh, M.L., Britton, K.L., Baker, P.J., Stillman, T.J., *et al.* (1994) The catalytic role of aspartate in the active site of glutamate dehydrogenase. *Biochemical Journal* 301, 13–16.

DeBerardinis, R.J., Sayed, N., Ditsworth, D. and Thompson, C.B. (2008) Brick by brick: metabolism and tumor cell growth. *Current Opinion in Genetics & Development* 18, 54–61.

Dieter, H., Koberstein, R. and Sund, H. (1981) Studies of glutamate dehydrogenase. The interaction of ADP, GTP, and NADPH in complexes with glutamate dehydrogenase. *European Journal of Biochemistry* 115, 217–226.

Dombrowski, K.E., Huang, Y.-C. and Colman, R.F. (1992) Identification of amino acids modified by the bifunctional affinity label 5'-(p-fluorosulfonyl)benzoyl)-8-azidoadenosine in the reduced coenzyme regulatory site of bovine liver glutamate dehydrogenase. *Biochemistry* 31, 3785–3793.

Elstrom, R.L., Bauer, D.E., Buzzai, M., Karnauskas, R., Harris, M.H., Plas, D.R., Zhuang, H., *et al.* (2004) Akt stimulates aerobic glycolysis in cancer cells. *Cancer Research* 64, 3892–3899.

Engel, P. and Dalziel, K. (1969) Kinetic studies of glutamate dehydrogenase with glutamate and norvaline as substrates. *Biochemical Journal* 115, 621–631.

Erdmann, R., Veenhuis, M. and Kunau, W.H. (1997) Peroxisomes: organelles at the crossroads. *Trends in Cell Biology* 7, 400–407.

Fahien, L.A. and Kmiotek, E. (1981) Regulation of glutamate dehydrogenase by palmitoyl-coenzyme A. *Archives of Biochemistry and Biophysics* 212, 247–253.

Fahien, L.A., MacDonald, M.J., Kmiotek, E.H., Mertz, R.J. and Fahien, C.M. (1988) Regulation of insulin release by factors that also modify glutamate dehydrogenase. *Journal of Biological Chemistry* 263, 13610–13614.

Filling, C., Kelier, B., Hirschberg, D., Marschall, H.-U., Jörnvall, H., Bennett, M.J. and Oppermann, U. (2008) Role of short-chain hydroxyacyl CoA dehydrogenases in SCHAD deficiency. *Biochemical and Biophysical Research Communications* 368, 6–11.

Frieden, C. (1959a) Glutamic dehydrogenase I. The effect of coenzyme on the sedimentation velocity and kinetic mechanism. *Journal of Biological Chemistry* 234, 809–814.

Frieden, C. (1959b) Glutamic dehydrogenase II. The effect of various nucleotides on the association-disassociation and kinetic properties. *Journal of Biological Chemistry* 234, 815–819.

Frieden, C. (1963a) Different structural forms of reversibly dissociated glutamic dehydrogenase: Relation between enzymatic activity and molecular weight. *Biochemical and Biophysical Research Communications* 10, 410–415.

Frieden, C. (1963b) Glutamate dehydrogenase IV. Studies on enzyme inactivation and coenzyme binding. *Journal of Biological Chemistry* 238, 146–154.

Frieden, C. (1965) Glutamate dehydrogenase VI. Survey of purine nucleotides and other effects on the enzyme from various sources. *Journal of Biological Chemistry* 240, 2028–2037.

Gao, P., Tchernyshyov, I., Chang, T.C., Lee, Y.S., Kita, K., Ochi, T., Zeller, K.I., *et al.* (2009) c-Myc suppression of miR-23a/b enhances mitochondrial glutaminase expression and glutamine metabolism. *Nature* 458, 762–765.

George, S.A. and Bell, J.E. (1980) Effects of adenosine 5'-diphosphate on bovine glutamate dehydrogenase: Diethyl pyrocarbonate modification. *Biochemistry* 19, 6057–6061.

Gerhardt, B. (1992) Fatty acid degradation in plants. *Progress in Lipid Research* 31, 417–446.

Goldin, B.R. and Frieden, C. (1971) Effect of trinitrophenylation of specific lysyl residues on the catalytic, regulatory, and molecular properties of bovine liver glutamate dehydrogenase. *Biochemistry* 10, 3527–3534.

Haigis, M.C., Mostoslavsky, R., Haigis, K.M., Fahie, K., Christodoulou, D.C., Murphy, A.J., Valenzuela, D.M., *et al.* (2006) SIRT4 inhibits glutamate dehydrogenase and opposes the effects of calorie restriction in pancreatic beta cells. *Cell* 126, 941–954.

Hamilton-Miller, J.M. (1995) Antimicrobial properties of tea (Camellia sinensis L.). *Antimicrobial Agents and Chemotherapy* 39, 2375–2377.

Hashem, A.M., Flaman, A.S., Farnsworth, A., Brown, E.G., Van Domselaar, G., He, R. and Li, X. (2009) Aurintricarboxylic acid is a potent inhibitor of influenza A and B virus neuraminidases. *PLoS ONE* 4, e8350.

Hashimoto, T. (1999) Peroxisomal beta-oxidation enzymes. *Neurochemistry Research* 24, 551–563.

Herrero-Yraola, A., Bakhit, S.M., Franke, P., Weise, C., Schweiger, M., Jorcke, D. and Ziegler, M. (2001) Regulation of glutamate dehydrogenase by reversible ADP-ribosylation in mitochondria. *EMBO Journal* 20, 2404–2412.

Hoek, J.B. and Rydström, J. (1988) Physiological roles of nicotinamide nucleotide transhydrogenase. *Biochemical Journal* 254, 1–10.

Hsu, B.Y., Kelly, A., Thornton, P.S., Greenberg, C.R., Dilling, L.A. and Stanley, C.A. (2001) Protein-sensitive and fasting hypoglycemia in children with the hyperinsulinism/hyperammonemia syndrome. *Journal of Pediatrics* 138, 383–389.

Hudson, R.C. and Daniel, R.M. (1993) L-Glutamate dehydrogenases: distribution, properties and mechanism. *Comparative Biochemistry and Physiology* 106B, 767–792.

Hussain, K., Clayton, P.T., Krywawych, S., Chatziandreou, I., Mills, P., Ginbey, D.W., Geboers, A.J., *et al.* (2005) Hyperinsulinism of infancy associated with a novel splice site mutation in the SCHAD gene. *Journal of Pediatrics* 146, 706–708.

Iwatsubo, M. and Pantaloni, D. (1967) Regulation de l'activité de la glutamate dehydrogenase par les effecteurs GTP et ADP: ETUDE par "stopped flow". *Bulletin de la Société de Chimie Biologique* 49, 1563–1572.

Jackson, S., Bartlett, K., Land, J., Moxon, E.R., Pollitt, R.J., Leonard, J.V. and Turnbull, D.M. (1991) Long-chain 3-hydroxyacyl-CoA dehydrogenase deficiency. *Pediatric Research* 29, 406–411.

Katiyar, S.K. and Mukhtar, H. (1996) Tea in chemoprevention of cancer: epidemiologic and experimental studies. *International Journal of Oncology* 8, 221–238.

Kibbey, R.G., Pongratz, R.L., Romanelli, A.J., Wollheim, C.B., Cline, G.W. and Shulman, G.I. (2007) Mitochondrial GTP regulates glucose-stimulated insulin secretion. *Cell Metabolism* 5, 253–264.

Kim, J.W. and Dang, C.V. (2006) Cancer's molecular sweet tooth and the Warburg effect. *Cancer Research* 66, 8927–8930.

Koberstein, R. and Sund, H. (1973) The influence of ADP, GTP and L-glutamate on the binding of the reduced coenzyme to beef-liver glutamate dehydrogenase. *European Journal of Biochemistry* 36, 545–552.

Koshland, D.E.J. (1996) The structural basis of negative cooperativity: receptors and enzymes. *Current Opinion in Structural Biology* 6, 757–761.

Lenartowicz, E. (1990) A complex effect of arsenite on the formation of a-ketoglutarate in rat liver mitochondria. *Archives of Biochemistry and Biophysics* 283, 388–396.

Li, C., Allen, A., Kwagh, K., Doliba, N.M., Qin, W., Najafi, H., Collins, H.W., *et al.* (2006) Green tea polyphenols modulate insulin secretion by inhibiting glutamate dehydrogenase. *Journal of Biological Chemistry* 2006, 10214–10221.

Li, C., Buettger, C., Kwagh, J., Matter, A., Daihkin, Y., Nissiam, I., Collins, H.W., *et al.* (2004) A signaling role of glutamine in insulin secretion. *Journal of Biological Chemistry* 279, 13393–13401.

Li, C., Chen, P., Palladino, A., Narayan, S., Russell, L.K., Sayed, S., Xiong, G., *et al.* (2010) Mechanism of hyperinsulinism in short-chain 3-hydroxyacyl-CoA dehydrogenase deficiency involves activation of glutamate dehydrogenase. *Journal of Biological Chemistry* 285, 31806–31818.

Li, C., Najafi, H., Daikhin, Y., Nissim, I., Collins, H.W., Yudkoff, M., Matschinsky, F.M., *et al.* (2003) Regulation of leucine stimulated insulin secretion and glutamine metabolism in isolated rat islets. *Journal of Biological Chemistry* 278, 2853–2858.

Li, M., Allen, A. and Smith, T.J. (2007) High throughput screening reveals several new classes of glutamate dehydrogenase inhibitors. *Biochemistry* 46, 15089–15102.

Li, M., Smith, C.J., Walker, M.T. and Smith, T.J. (2009) Novel inhibitors complexed with glutamate dehydrogenase: allosteric regulation by control of protein dynamics. *Journal of Biological Chemistry* 284, 22988–23000.

Limuti, C.M. (1983) Glutamate dehydrogenase: equilibrium and kinetic studies. PhD, University of Rochester, New York, USA.

MacMullen, C., Fang, J., Hsu, B.Y.L., Kelly, A., Delonlay-Debeney, P., Saudubray, J.M., Ganguly, A., *et al.* (2001) The Hyperinsulinism/hyperammonemia contributing investigators. Hyperinsulinism/hyperammonemia syndrome in children with regulatory mutations in the inhibitory guanosine triphosphate-binding domain of glutamate dehydrogenase. *Journal of Clinical Endocrinology and Metabolism* 86, 1782–1787.

Maniscalco, S.J., Saha, S.K., Vicedomine, P. and Fisher, H.F. (1996) A difference in the sequence of steps in the reactions catalyzed by two closely homologous forms of glutamate dehydrogenase. *Biochemistry* 35, 89–94.

Maron, D.J., Lu, G.P., Cai, N.S., Wu, Z.G., Li, Y.H., Chen, H., Zhu, J.Q., et al. (2003) Cholesterol-lowering effect of a theaflavin-enriched green tea extract: a randomized controlled trial. *Archives of Internal Medicine* 163, 1448–1453.

Melzi-d'Eril, G. and Dalziel, K. (1973) Negative cooperativity in glutamate dehydrogenase. Coenzyme binding studies. *Biochemical Journal* 130, 3P.

Molven, A., Matre, G.E., Duran, M., Wanders, R.J., Rishaug, U., Njolstad, P.R., Jellum, E., et al. (2004) Familial hyperinsulinemic hypoglycemia caused by a defect in the SCHAD enzyme of mitochondrial fatty acid oxidation. *Diabetes* 53, 221–227.

Muller, M., Hogg, J.F. and De Duve, C. (1968) Distribution of tricarboxylic acid cycle enzymes and glyoxylate cycle enzymes between mitochondria and peroxisomes in *Tetrahymena pyriformis*. *Journal of Biological Chemistry* 243, 5385–5395.

Myskiw, C., Deschambault, Y., Jefferies, K., He, R. and Cao, J. (2007) Aurintricarboxylic acid inhibits the early stage of vaccinia virus replication by targeting both cellular and viral factors. *Journal of Virology* 81, 3027–3032.

Pal, P.K., Wechter, W.J. and Colman, R.F. (1975) Affinity labeling of a regulatory site of bovine liver glutamate dehydrogenase. *Biochemistry* 14, 707–715.

Peterson, P., Pierce, J. and Smith, T.J. (1998) Crystallization and characterization of bovine glutamate dehydrogenase. *Journal of Structural Biology* 120, 73–77.

Peterson, P.E. and Smith, T.J. (1999) The structure of bovine glutamate dehydrogenase provides insights into the mechanism of allostery. *Structure Fold and Design* 7, 769–82.

Piszkiewicz, D. and Smith, E.L. (1971) Bovine liver glutamate dehydrogenase. Equilibria and kinetics of inactivation by pyridoxal. *Biochemistry* 10, 4538–4544.

Prough, R.A., Culver, J.M. and Fisher, H.F. (1973) The mechanism of activation of glutamate dehydrogenase-catalyzed reactions by two different, cooperatively bound activators. *Journal of Biological Chemistry* 248, 8528–8533.

Rasool, C.G., Nicolaidis, S. and Akhtar, M. (1976) The asymmetric distribution of enzymic activity between the six subunits of bovine liver glutamate dehydrogenase. Use of D- and L-glutamyl alpha-chloromethyl ketones (4-amino-6-chloro-5-oxohexanoic acid. *Biochemical Journal* 157, 675–686.

Reddy, J.K. and Mannaerts, G.P. (1994) Peroxisomal lipid metabolism. *Annual Reviews of Nutrition* 14, 343–370.

Rydström, J., Teixeira da Cruz, A. and Ernster, L. (1970) Factors governing the kinetics and steady state of the mitochondrial nicotinamide nucleotide transhydrogenase system. *European Journal of Biochemistry* 17, 56–62.

Schmidt, J.A. and Colman, R.F. (1984) Identification of the lysine and tyrosine peptides labeled by 5'-p-fluorosulfonylbenzoyladenosine in the NADH inhibitory site of glutamate dehydrogenase. *Journal of Biological Chemistry* 259, 14515–14519.

Sener, A. and Malaisse, W.J. (1980) L-leucine and a nonmetabolized analogue activate pancreatic islet glutamate dehydrogenase. *Nature* 288, 187–189.

Sener, A., Malaisse-Lagae, F. and Malaisse, W.J. (1981) Stimulation of pancreatic islet metabolism and insulin release by a nonmetabolizable amino acid. *Proceedings of the National Academy of Sciences USA* 78, 5460–5464.

Shafer, J.A., Chiancone, E., Vittorelli, L.M., Spagnuolo, C., Machler, B. and Antonini, E. (1972) Binding of reduced cofactor to glutamate dehydrogenase. *European Journal of Biochemistry* 31, 166–171.

Singh, N., Maniscalco, S.J. and Fisher, H.F. (1993) The real-time resolution of proton-related transient-state steps in an enzymatic reaction. *Journal of Biological Chemistry* 268, 21–28.

Skovronsky, D.M., Zhang, B., Kung, M.P., Kung, H.F., Trojanowski, J.Q. and Lee, V.M.Y. (2000) In vivo detection of amyloid plaques in a mouse model of Alzheimer's disease. *Proceedings of the National Academy of Sciences USA* 97, 7609–7614.

Smith, C.A., Norris, G.E. and Baker, E.N. (1996) The structure of the thermophilic glutamate dehydrogenase from *Thermococcus* ANI. In: Griffin, J.F. (ed.) *IUCr XVII Congress and General Assembly*. Seattle, WA, AI C 226–227.

Smith, E.J., Landon, M., Piszkiewicz, D., Brattin, W.J., Langley, T.J. and Melamed, M.D. (1970) Bovine liver glutamate dehydrogenase: tentative amino acid sequence; identification of a reactive lysine; nitration of a specific tyrosine and loss of allosteric inhibition by guanosine triphosphate. *Proceedings of the National Academy of Sciences USA* 67, 724–730.

Smith, T.J. and Bell, J.E. (1982) The mechanism of hysteresis in bovine glutamate dehydrogenase: The role of subunit interactions. *Biochemistry* 21, 733–737.

Smith, T.J., Peterson, P.E., Schmidt, T., Fang, J. and Stanley, C. (2001) Structures of bovine glutamate dehydrogenase complexes elucidate the mechanism of purine regulation. *Journal of Molecular Biology* 307, 707–720.

Smith, T.J., Schmidt, T., Fang, J., Wu, J., Siuzdak, G. and Stanley, C.A. (2002) The structure of apo human glutamate dehydrogenase details subunit communication and allostery. *Journal of Molecular Biology* 318, 765–777.

Smith, T.J. and Stanley, C.A. (2008) Untangling the glutamate dehydrogenase allosteric nightmare. *Trends in Biological Chemistry* 33, 557–564.

Srinivasan, R. and Fisher, H.F. (1985) Reversible reduction of an a-amino imino acid to an a-amino acid catalyzed by glutamate dehydrogenase: effect of ionizable functional groups. *Biochemistry* 24, 618–622.

Stanley, C., Bennett, M.J. and Mayatepek, E. (2006) Disorders of mitochondrial fatty acid oxidation and related metabolic pathways. In: Fernandes, J., Saudubray, J.-M., Van den Berg, G. and Walter, J.H. (eds) *Inborn metabolic diseases*. 4th ed., Springer, Heidelberg.

Stanley, C.A. (2000) The hyperinsulinism-hyperammonemia syndrome: gain-of-function mutations of glutamate dehydrogenase. In: O'Rahilly, S. and Dunger, D.B. (eds) *Genetic Insights in Paediatric Endocrinology and Metabolism*. BioScientifica Ltd, Bristol.

Stanley, C.A., Fang, J., Kutyna, K., Hsu, B.Y.L., Ming, J.E., Glaser, B. and Poncz, M. (2000) Molecular basis and characterization of the hyperinsulinism/hyperammonemia syndrome of the glutamate dehydrogenase gene. *Diabetes* 49, 667–673.

Stanley, C.A., Lieu, Y.K., Hsu, B.Y., Burlina, A.B., Greenberg, C.R., Hopwood, N.J., Perlman, K., et al. (1998) Hyperinsulinism and hyperammonemia in infants with regulatory mutations of the glutamate dehydrogenase gene. *New England Journal of Medicine* 338, 1352–1357.

Stillman, T.J., Baker, P.J., Britton, K.L. and Rice, D.W. (1993) Conformational flexibility in glutamate dehydrogenase. Role of water in substrate recognition and catalysis. *Journal of Molecular Biology* 234, 1131–1139.

Syed, S.-E.-H. and Engel, P.C. (1984) Ox liver glutamate dehydrogenase. The use of chemical modification to study the relationship between catalytic sites for different amino acid substrates and the question of kinetic non-equivalence of the subunits. *Biochemical Journal* 222, 621–626.

Tomkins, G.M., Yielding, K.L. and Curran, J.F. (1962) The influence of diethylstilbestrol and adenosine diphosphate on pyridine nucleotide coenzyme binding by glutamic dehydrogenase. *Journal of Biological Chemistry* 237, 1704–1708.

Waltner-Law, M.E., Wang, X.L., Law, B.K., Hall, R.K., Nawano, M. and Granner, D.K. (2002) Epigallocatechin gallate, a constituent of green tea, represses hepatic glucose production. *Journal of Biological Chemistry* 277, 34933–34940.

Wang, X.-G., Britton, K.L., Baker, P.J., Martin, S., Rice, D.W. and Engel, P.C. (1995) Alteration of the amino acid substrate specificity of clostridial glutamate dehydrogenase by site-directed mutagenesis of an active-site lysine residue. *Protein Engineering* 8, 147–152.

Wise, D.R., DeBerardinis, R.J., Mancuso, A., Sayed, N., Zhang, X.Y., Pfeiffer, H.K., Nissim, I., et al. (2008) Myc regulates a transcriptional program that stimulates mitochondrial glutaminolysis and leads to glutamine addiction. *Proceedings of the National Academy of Sciences USA* 105, 18782–18787.

Wrzeszczynski, K.O. and Colman, R.F. (1994) Activation of bovine liver glutamate dehydrogenase by covalent reaction of adenosine 5'-O-[S-(4-bromo-2,3-dioxobutyl)thiophosphate] with arginine-459 at an ADP regulatory site. *Biochemistry* 33, 11544–11553.

Yang, C., Sudderth, J., Dang, T., Bachoo, R.G., McDonald, J.G. and DeBerardinis, R.J. (2009) Glioblastoma cells require glutamate dehydrogenase to survive impairments of glucose metabolism or Akt signaling. *Cancer Research* 69, 7986–7993.

Yang, C.S. and Wang, Z.Y. (1993) Tea and cancer. *Journal of the National Cancer Institute* 85, 1038–1049.

Yielding, K.L. and Tomkins, G.M. (1961) An effect of L-leucine and other essential amino acids on the structure and activity of glutamate dehydrogenase. *Proceedings of the National Academy of Sciences USA* 47, 983.

Yip, K.S.P., Stillman, T.J., Britton, K.L., Artymiuk, P.J., Baker, P.J., Sedelnikova, S.E., Engel, P.C., et al. (1995) The structure of *Pyrococcus furiosus* glutamate dehydrogenase reveals a key role for ion-pair networks in maintaining enzyme stability at extreme temperatures. *Structure* 3, 1147–1158.

2 Aminotransferases

M.E. Conway*
University of the West of England, Bristol, UK

2.1 Abstract

The aminotransferases are PLP-dependent proteins which catalyse the transfer of an amino group from the donor amino acid to α-ketoglutarate, forming glutamate and the respective keto acids. Several key aminotransferase proteins have been identified as playing central roles in whole-body nitrogen metabolism, where they share common functions as nitrogen donors. These pathways play integrated roles within cells and between tissues, shuttling metabolites alluding to distinct pockets of compartmented metabolic activity. These anaplerotic shuttles interface with key metabolic pathways, for example the glutamate/glutamine cycle and TCA cycle, facilitating the regeneration of key metabolites such as the primary neurotransmitter glutamate. Contributions to glutamate levels in the brain from these anaplerotic pathways exceed 30%, illustrating their importance in maintaining the neurotransmitter pool of glutamate in neuronal cells. Knowledge of these pathways is not only important to our understanding of normal physiological mechanisms, but even more to the ways in which they alter and contribute to the pathogenesis of disease. The pathological implications of impaired aminotransferase metabolism is discussed, in particular their potential role in glutamate toxicity, which has been implicated in the pathogenesis of neurodegenerative disease. Finally, because of their tissue distribution these proteins have additional roles as biomarkers of disease, and can be used in the differential diagnosis of acute and chronic hepatic injury.

2.2 Introduction

The compartmentation of metabolic substrates and the subcellular localization of enzymes contribute to a fascinating interplay of highly regulated pathways. Several metabolic pathways, which play central roles in protein metabolism, are governed by the aminotransferases. Although numerous aminotransferase proteins exist, this chapter details the whole-body distribution of several specific aminotransferases, with particular focus on their role in anaplerotic pathways to generate and maintain the pool of brain glutamate through their involvement in metabolic shuttles. Furthermore, their role in disease is discussed with particular reference to the clinical application of serum aminotransferases.

* E-mail address: Myra.Conway@uwe.ac.uk

Transamination reactions are facilitated by pyridoxal phosphate-dependent (PLP) transaminase enzymes (Christen and Metzler, 1985). The key aminotransferase proteins discussed here include the branched chain aminotransferases (BCAT) [E.C. 2.6.1.42], the alanine aminotransferases (ALT) [glutamate pyruvate transaminase or alanine 2-oxo-glutarate E.C. 2.6.1.2], and the aspartate aminotransferase proteins (AST) [glutamic oxaloacetic transaminase or L-aspartate:2-oxo-glutarate aminotransferase, E.C. 2.6.1.1]. These proteins have a mitochondrial and cytosolic isoform with tissue-specific locations. The crystal structures of BCAT and AST have been elucidated, where the catalytically competent structure of these aminotransferases is a homodimer (Jansonius et al., 1984a,b; Yennawar et al., 2002, 2006; Goto et al., 2005). These enzymes belong to a large family of homologous proteins which operate by the same basic mechanism (Jansonius, 1998). PLP-dependent enzymes have been classified into four families with different fold types based on their three-dimensional structures (Jansonius, 1998; Mehta and Christen, 2000; Salzmann et al., 2000; Schneider et al., 2000). With the exception of the BCAT proteins which fall into the fold-type IV class of proteins, most of the PLP aminotransferases have been placed in the fold type I or L-aspartate aminotransferase family. A unique feature of the fold type IV family is that the proton is abstracted from the C4' atom of the coenzyme-imine or external aldimine on the re face instead of the si face of the PLP cofactor (Yoshimura et al., 1996).

2.2.1 Transamination

The mechanism of transamination consists of the coupled half-reaction in which the PLP cofactor transfers between its PLP and pyridoxamine (PMP) form (Fig. 2.1) (Karpeisky and Ivanov, 1966; Ivanov and Karpeisky, 1969; Kirsch et al., 1984). The substrates of the forward reaction are dictated by the specificity of the particular transaminase, whereas L-glutamate features in the reverse reaction for most transaminases. The cofactor PLP is covalently attached to the enzyme via a Schiff base linkage, as a result of the condensation of its aldehyde group with the ε-amino group of a lysine residue. Transamination occurs via a Ping-Pong Bi-Bi mechanism, where each half reaction is divided into three stages. Interaction of the transaminases with their respective substrates involves the nucleophilic attack of the α-amino group of amino acid 1 (e.g. isoleucine) with the enzyme–PLP Schiff base carbon atom to form an amino acid–PLP Schiff base (external aldimine) with release of the enzyme (e.g. BCAT) (Fig. 2.1a). After transamination the second step is keto-enol tautomerism which involves the interconversion between the keto-enol form resulting in the formation of an α-keto acid–PMP Schiff base. This is subsequently hydrolysed to PMP and an α-keto acid, the final step in the first half-reaction (Fig. 2.1b). The second half reaction involves the same three steps but in reverse. In this stage the substrate is a second α-keto acid which reacts with PMP forming a Schiff base. Tautomerization facilitates the conversion from α-keto acid PMP to amino acid 2–PLP Schiff base. Subsequently, an internal aldimine is formed through attack from the ε-amino group of the active site lysine, leading to the release of a new amino acid and the regeneration of the aminotransferase.

The BCAT enzymes catalyse the transfer of the α-amino group from the hydrophobic branched chain amino acids (BCAA) leucine, isoleucine, and valine to α-ketoglutarate, releasing their respective keto acids: ketoisocaproate, keto methyl valerate and keto-isovaline, and glutamate, regenerating the enzyme (Ichihara and Koyama, 1966; Taylor and Jenkins, 1966a,b,c). Both ALT and AST operate by the same basic mechanism generating pyruvate and glutamate, and oxaloacetate and glutamate, respectively (Glinghammar et al., 2009). The transamination reaction of each aminotransferase is summarized in Box 2.1.

2.2.2 Cellular distribution of aminotransferases

Although aminotransferase activity is found in most tissues, each isoform shows tissue specificity with distinct subcellular location, which points to distinct functional roles

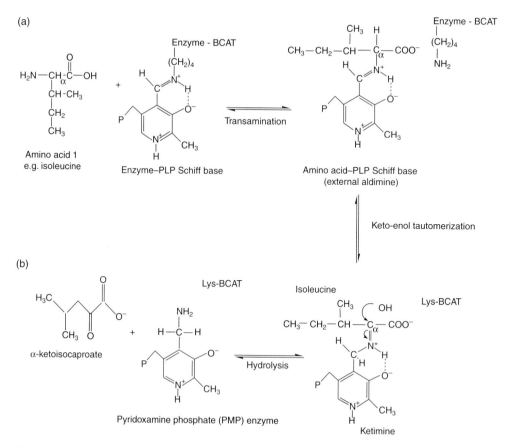

Fig. 2.1. Transamination of the branched chain amino acid isoleucine (first half reaction). (a) The enzyme–PLP Schiff base carbon undergoes a nucleophilic attack by the α-amino group of isoleucine resulting in the formation of an amino acid–PLP Schiff base and the release of BCAT. (b) Following keto-enol tautomerization the resulting ketamine undergoes hydrolysis generating the α-keto acid, α-ketoisocaproate and the PMP form of BCAT.

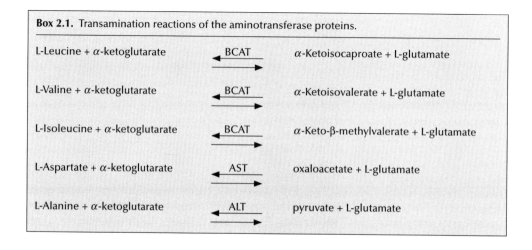

of these proteins in tissues. The cellular distribution of these enzymes was first characterized in murine and rat models and has since progressed to human and cell systems. These models have offered enumerable insights into the compartmentation of many metabolic pathways, and indeed the flow of metabolites between these compartments. Understanding the differential distribution of these proteins and the factors which contribute to their regulation is pivotal to our understanding of the pathogenesis of disease, as many specific enzymes or pathways of metabolism are altered in adverse conditions.

2.2.2.1 Cellular distribution of the BCAT proteins

In mammals there are predominantly two BCAT isoforms, encoded by two different genes, which show both tissue and cellular-specific locations. Although the BCAT isoforms share 58% sequence homology and are structurally very similar, they possess distinct differences in catalytic efficiency and regulation (Davoodi et al., 1998). These enzymes play significant roles in amino acid metabolism and whole-body nitrogen shuttling. The most ubiquitous isoform, $BCAT_m$, is found in mitochondria and is thought to be responsible for the majority of transamination outside the central nervous system with the highest levels of $BCAT_m$ recorded in the pancreas, kidney, stomach, and brain (Suryawan et al., 1998). To date, the cytosolic isoform ($BCAT_c$) has only been isolated from brain, placenta, ovary, and the peripheral nervous system (Hutson, 1988; Hutson et al., 1992, 1998; Hall et al., 1993; Sweatt et al., 2004a,b; Garcia-Espinosa et al., 2007). Although these two isoforms predominate, two other spliced variants have been identified, namely, a novel alternatively spliced PP18b variant found in placental tissue, and a novel co-repressor for thyroid hormone nuclear receptors (P3) (Lin et al., 2001; Than et al., 2001). Both spliced variants are homologous to $BCAT_m$. Although the function of the PP18b variant is unknown, P3 acts as a co-repressor for thyroid hormone nuclear receptors. The biological significance of these variants remains to be determined.

Due to the ease with which the BCAA pass the blood–brain barrier and their role in glutamate metabolism, the subcellular localization of the BCAT proteins in brain has been extensively investigated (Oldendorf, 1973; Cremer et al., 1976, 1979; Bixel et al., 1997, 2001; Bixel and Hamprecht, 2000; Sweatt et al., 2004a,b; Garcia-Espinosa et al., 2007). In brief, $BCAT_c$ was only found in neuronal cells, localized to axons and nerve terminals in glutamatergic neurons, and concentrated in cell bodies in GABAergic neurons (Bixel et al., 2001; Sweatt et al, 2004a,b). Conversely, $BCAT_m$ was the predominant isoform in astrocytic cells. However, low levels of $BCAT_c$ were detected in certain astrocyte populations using a cell culture model, but this was not reported in rat tissue (Bixel et al., 1997, 2001; Bixel and Hamprecht, 2000). To date the BCAT proteins have not been mapped at the subcellular level in the human brain.

2.2.2.2 Cellular distribution of the ALT proteins

Early studies investigating the cellular distribution of ALT in rats suggested that there was only one cytosolic ALT isoform, with the mitochondrial form dismissed as cytosolic contamination of mitochondrial preparations. Subsequent reports have validated that there are two ALT isoforms (ALT1, cytosolic; and ALT2, mitochondrial), encoded by separate genes (ALT1–GTP gene and ALT2-GTP2 gene) (DeRosa and Swick, 1975; Sohocki et al., 1997; Lindblom et al., 2007; Glinghammar et al., 2009). An alternatively spliced isoform of ALT2 (ALT2-2) has been suggested with a predicted sequence of 100 amino acids shorter than ALT2; however this isoform has not been characterized at the protein level and its function is unknown (Lindblom et al., 2007). The ALT proteins play a pivotal role in mediating the passage of intermediates between gluconeogenesis and amino acid metabolism from the muscle to the liver, and more recently have been described as playing a role in the hypothetical alanine–lactate shuttle between neuronal and astrocytic cells (Waagepetersen et al., 2000). Clinically, due to the high expression levels of ALT in liver it is considered to be one of the major biomarkers of liver dysfunction (see below).

Unlike BCAT, both ALT isoforms are widely expressed in rat and murine tissues.

Here high levels of ALT mRNA expression were reported in liver, muscle, and brown/white adipose tissue, with relatively lower ALT expression observed in rat colon, heart, and brain (Jadhao et al., 2004; Yang et al., 2009). With the exception of the kidney, these patterns of mRNA expression largely mapped to those observed in humans (Yang et al., 2002a, 2009). While both ALT isoforms are highly expressed in rat adipose tissue, their expression in human adipose tissue has not been described. Although ALT brain activities have been reported in several rat models there are limited data on the pattern of ALT distribution in the human brain. A study described by Lindblom et al demonstrated that expression of ALT1 was below the detection limit for all brain samples analysed, whereas ALT2 showed low to moderate levels of expression in the cerebral cortex with intense staining in the cerebellum, highlighting the importance for further studies to validate ALT distribution in the brain (Lindblom et al., 2007). These studies would extend our knowledge on the contribution of ALT proteins to glutamate metabolism (see below).

2.2.2.3 Cellular distribution of the AST proteins

Like ALT, the AST proteins are widely distributed with the highest expression found in striated muscle, myocardium and liver tissues. With the exception of the red blood cells which only contain AST_c, all tissues have both isoforms, albeit at varying levels in different cell types. Because of their role in neuronal metabolism the distribution of these isoforms has been extensively studied in various brain preparations with particular focus on the mitochondrial isoform (AST_m). AST_m is not only targeted to mitochondria but also on the cell surface, confirming the role of AST_m as both a mitochondrial and plasma membrane protein (Cechetto et al., 2002). Interestingly AST_m was found to be identical to a fatty acid-binding protein ($FABP_{pm}$), which has a role in permitting the uptake of long chain free fatty acid in cells (Stremmel et al., 1990; Stump et al., 1993; Bradbury and Berk, 2000). For full activity AST must first associate with binding proteins which transfer it to lipids on the inner mitochondrial membrane (Teller et al., 1990). Functionally, AST proteins play a central role in glutamate metabolism and in the malate/aspartate shuttle which transfers reducing equivalents from the mitochondria to the cytosol in the brain. Glutamate dehydrogenase (GDH), like AST, also catalyses the conversion of glutamate to α-ketoglutarate, albeit by a different mechanism (Leong and Clark, 1984). Whereas AST catalyses transamination (Box 2.1), GDH either adds an amino group to α-ketoglutarate utilizing NAD(P)H or removes an amino group from glutamate producing α-ketoglutarate with the reduction of NAD(P). Numerous studies have reported that both these enzymes are co-localized in cells and work in concert with each other to either drive the synthesis or degradation of amino acids (Lai et al., 1977, 1986; Palaiologos et al., 1988).

Immunohistochemical studies on rat brain showed differential staining between glutamatergic or GABAergic neurons. High expression of AST_c was reported in periglomerular cells of the olfactory bulb and basket cells, and in stellate cells of the cerebellum and second layer cells of the neocortex, whereas AST_m was found in mitral cells and glomerular regions of the olfactory bulb and golgi cells of the cerebellum (Kamisaki et al., 1984). Similar reports of isoenzyme compartmentation were also described in the rat retina (Inagaki et al., 1985, 1987). Although high levels of AST activity have been reported in neuronal cells, controversy surrounding the actual activity and indeed its contribution to glutamate metabolism in astrocytes exists, which is in part due to reports of the absence of the malate/asparate carrier (AGC) (see below). Further studies are required to determine the activity of AST relative to GDH in these brain preparations, their localization, and their specific roles in astrocytes.

2.3 The Role of Aminotransferases in Brain Metabolism

The compartmentalization of the aminotransferase isoforms in neuronal or astroglial cells and the observed differences in their catalytic and regulatory mechanisms points to two functionally distinct proteins despite catalysing the same reaction. The aminotransferase proteins and their substrates play a significant role in normal brain function, driving several key metabolic pathways central to energy metabolism and neurotransmitter synthesis (Figs 2.2–2.6). A dysfunction of these pathways can potentially contribute to the pathogenesis of a number of neurodegenerative conditions such as Alzheimer's and Parkinson's disease (Choi, 1988; Esclaire *et al.*, 1997). A key metabolite linking these metabolic pathways is glutamate, the major excitatory neurotransmitter in the mammalian brain as well as the immediate precursor to GABA and glutathione (Attwell and Laughlin, 2001; Danbolt, 2001). Under normal physiological conditions glutamate plays a role in dendrite and synapse formation, but also plays a dominant role in glutamatergic transmission essential for memory and learning (Danbolt, 2001). Activation of excitatory neurotransmission mediated through an increase in calcium, signals the release of glutamate stores within the presynaptic neuron (Fig. 2.2). Excess glutamate not utilized by postsynaptic neurons is taken up by astrocytes, which express high levels of the glutamate-specific transporter (GLAST/EAAT1 and GLT1/EAAT2) facilitating the rapid and efficient removal of glutamate from the extracellular space. In fact transgenic mice that do not express GLT1 are subject to glutamate toxicity (Tanaka *et al.*, 1997). Within the astrocyte, much of the glutamate is converted through

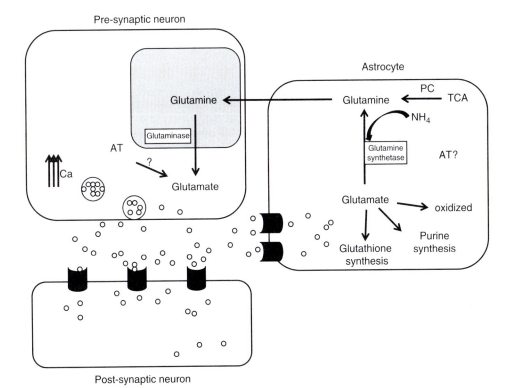

Fig. 2.2. The glutamate–glutamine cycle. Excess glutamate released from pre-synaptic neurons into the synaptic cleft is rapidly taken up by astrocytes through the specific glutamate receptors GLAST/EAA1 and GLT1/EAAT2. Within the astrocyte the majority of glutamate undergoes amidation to glutamine catalysed by glutamine synthetase. Non-neuroactive glutamine is released into the ECF for uptake by pre-synaptic neurons for regeneration of the neuronal glutamate pool. Glutamate may also be oxidized or utilized for the synthesis of glutathione or purines.

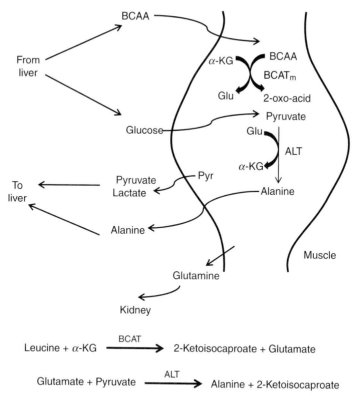

Fig. 2.3. Overview of the glucose–alanine cycle and BCAT in muscle. Both ALT and BCAT are highly concentrated in muscle, playing key roles in energy metabolism, particularly under nutritional stress. The BCAA which are not metabolized by the liver are transported to muscle where they undergo transamination with α-ketoglutarate. The BCAA, in particular leucine, is a major source for the amino group in amino acids such as alanine and glutamine. The alanine generated originates from pyruvate and therefore functions to recycle pyruvate originating from hepatic glucose. This cycle is termed the glucose–alanine cycle, which operates in parallel with the Cori cycle that also generates gluconeogenic substrates (Pyr/lactate) for the liver.

amidation to the non-neuroactive amino acid glutamine, by the microsomal enzyme glutamine synthetase (GS) that is restricted to astrocytes. Glutamine synthetase utilizes the steady supply of ammonia from blood (or brain metabolism) for glutamate synthesis which is then released into the ECF allowing for uptake by the pre-synaptic neuron to recycle the store of glutamate through deamidation of glutamine by mitochondrial phosphate-dependent glutaminase (Fig. 2.2) (Yudkoff et al. 1993, 1994). Thus, astrocytes and neurons play complementary roles in the glutamate–glutamine cycle, maintaining the neuronal glutamate pool at high concentrations, and preventing toxic elevations in the synaptic space. In astrocytes there are several fates for glutamate other than glutamine synthesis, dependent on substrate availability, the differential distribution and regulation of key metabolic enzymes (e.g. glutaminase, GDH, Malate dehydrogenase (MDH), AST, BCAT, ALT, Malic enzyme (ME), and GS), or whether the source of glutamate is exogenous or endogenous (Fig. 2.6). For example, when levels of external glutamate are low, the glial glutamate synthetase pathway is favoured, whereas in glutamate excess, considerable oxidation occurs (McKenna et al., 1996a,b).

Both glutamate and glutamine can be oxidized for energy in astrocytes and neuronal cells (McKenna et al., 1996a,b; Daikhin and Yudkoff, 2000). An estimated 30% of glutamate taken up by astrocytes is metabolized to

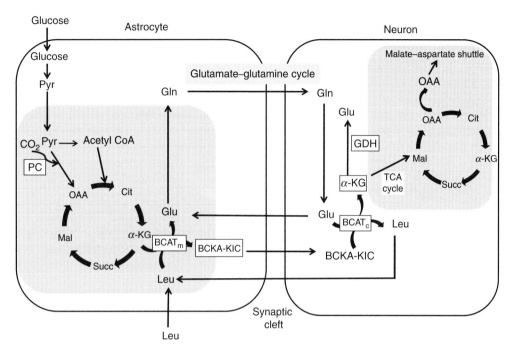

Fig. 2.4. The branched chain aminotransferase-branched chain keto acid shuttle. Leucine is actively taken up by astrocytes where it undergoes transamination via $BCAT_m$ forming glutamate and 2-ketoisocaproate (KIC). The glutamate formed can enter the glutamate–glutamine cycle whereas KIC, which is poorly metabolised by astrocytes, is further metabolized in neuron cells. The keto acid is subsequently transaminated with glutamate to regenerate leucine, which can be subsequently returned to the astrocyte to complete the cycle. These cycles also operate with the TCA cycle and GDH metabolism (Yudkoff et al., 1990; Hutson et al., 2001).

lactate involving TCA cycle intermediates and the pyruvate/malate cycle (Sonnewald et al., 1993; Gamberino et al., 1997). Glutamate in astrocytes is also used in the production of purines and key metabolic amino acids such as glutathione (Fig. 2.2) (Shank and Aprison, 1981; Yudkoff et al., 1988). Therefore, anaplerotic pathways must interface with the glutamate–glutamine cycle to regenerate this 'lost' glutamate necessary to sustain efficient neurotransmission. Pyruvate carboxylase, an enzyme found solely in astrocytes, utilizes brain CO_2 to replenish the carbon required for the TCA cycle, which as a result contributes to the overall concentration of glutamine produced (Oz et al., 2004). A limiting factor in this reaction is the source of nitrogen, where the BCAA, aspartate and more recently alanine serve as potential nitrogen donors (Shank et al., 1985; Bixel and Hamprecht, 1995; Yudkoff et al., 1996a,b; Yudkoff, 1997; Hutson et al., 1998, 2001; Kanamori et al., 1998; Lieth et al., 2001; Magistretti, 2009). The respective roles of the aminotransferase proteins are discussed in the following sections.

2.3.1 The role of BCAT in brain metabolism

The BCAA easily traverse the blood–brain barrier, with leucine more readily accepted than other amino acids (Oldendorf, 1973; Smith et al., 1987). Conversely, glutamate and glutamine are poorly taken up, highlighting the importance of glutamate synthesis in the brain. It has long been established that in peripheral tissues the role of the BCAA, in particular leucine, is to act as a major nitrogen donor for glutamate and glutamine synthesis (Fig. 2.3) (Goldberg and Chang, 1978). Skeletal muscle harbours high concentrations of $BCAT_m$, mediating the formation of glutamate

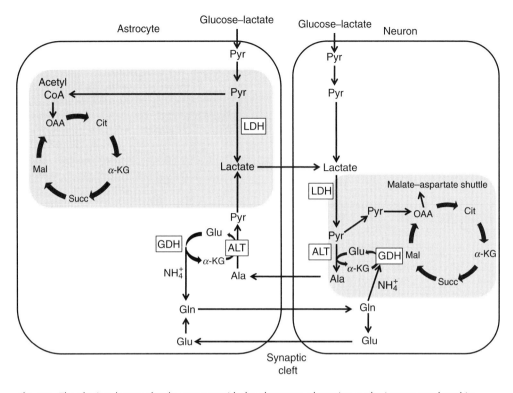

Fig. 2.5. The alanine–lactate shuttle operates with the glutamate–glutamine cycle. Lactate produced in astrocytes can be exchanged in part with alanine from neuronal cells. Lactate is subsequently metabolized to pyruvate which has two fates: i) The TCA cycle, or ii) transamination with glutamate via ALT. The alanine formed through transamination is thought to carry the amino group through GDH metabolism from glutamine deamination to glutamate. The alanine produced acts as a nitrogen donor in astrocytes, ultimately used to regenerate glutamate (adapted from Waagepetersen et al., 2000).

and α-ketoglutarate from BCAA exported from the liver (Fig. 2.2). The role of leucine as a nitrogen donor in brain metabolism has since been extensively studied, where the BCAT proteins are considered to play a key role in the oxidation and synthesis of glutamate owing to both their high expression and subcellular localization.

In rat brain slices the BCAA are metabolized faster than they are incorporated into proteins, supporting the theory that the BCAA serve functions other than just an energy source (Chaplin et al., 1976). In particular, leucine is readily metabolized in astrocytes, where uptake of leucine by glial cells is mediated by a sodium-independent process (Brookes, 1992, 1993). A combination of kinetic and metabolic studies in astrocytes, measuring the incorporation of [^{15}N]leucine into glutamate and glutamine, suggested that the rate of transamination of leucine is greatly favoured over complete oxidation with approximately 30% of the nitrogen of glutamate–glutamine derived from leucine alone (Brand, 1981; Brand and Hauschildt, 1984; Harper and Benjamin, 1984; Yudkoff et al., 1990). These studies, among others, support the hypothesis that although transamination is completely reversible it seems that BCAT transamination in the direction of glutamate and α-keto acid formation is favoured in astrocytes, whereas the reverse holds true for neuronal cells. These produce leucine and α-ketoglutarate, thought to complement the glutamate–glutamine cycle (Yudkoff et al., 1996b; Yudkoff 1997; Daikhin and Yudkoff, 2000). Both in vivo rat brain and ex vivo rat retina models (accepted models of glutamatergic

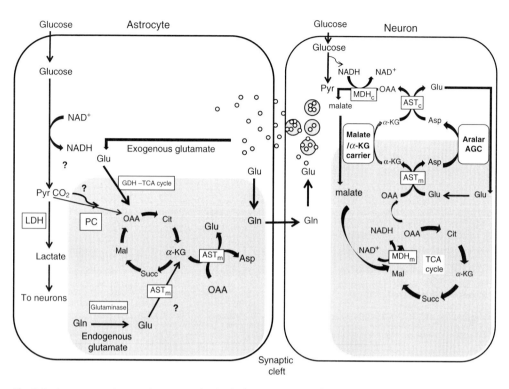

Fig. 2.6. Aspartate aminotransferase proteins in the brain. In neuronal cells AST_m and AST_c operate with the malate/α-KG carrier, the aralar AGC carrier, malate dehydrogenase (MDH), and glutaraldehyde dehydrogenase (GDH), which operate in metabolic complexes to channel NADH-reducing equivalents to the mitochondria for further oxidation. In astrocytes, AST_m is thought to work in synergy with GDH in the metabolism of glutamate. Here, exogenous glutamate is metabolized by GDH, whereas AST_m is thought to process glutamate produced endogenously.

neurons) using gabapentin as an inhibitor of $BCAT_c$ have also supported the *de novo* synthesis of glutamate (LaNoue *et al.*, 2001; Lieth *et al.*, 2001). These studies confirmed that gabapentin inhibited the *de novo* synthesis of glutamate by 30% in retina cells and up to 50–60% of added leucine transamination.

Not only is synthesis affected but so too is oxidation. Both retinal Muller cell (retinal astroglia) and cultured astrocyte models confirmed that transamination was a necessary prerequisite step to glutamate oxidation, where oxidation was blocked by the transaminase inhibitor aminooxyacetic acid (AOAA) (McKenna *et al.*, 1996a,b; Lieth *et al.*, 2001). To fit with the proposed model these results would imply that the supply of branched chain keto-acids (BCKA) would affect the extent of glutamate oxidation. In cultured rat astrocytes, oxidation of [^{14}U]glutamate was stimulated by addition of BCKA (Hutson *et al.*, 1998). In retinal cells the addition of BCKA, gabapentin, and BCKA and gabapentin together, resulted in the stimulation of glutamate oxidation with the latter showing the greatest degree of stimulation. These findings, together with the subcellular localization of $BCAT_m$ to astrocytes and $BCAT_c$ to neuronal cells, led to the development of the BCAA–BCKA shuttle hypothesis between the astrocyte and neuron, which works together with the glutamate–glutamine cycle (Fig. 2.4) (Yudkoff *et al.*, 1996a; Yudkoff, 1997; Hutson *et al.*, 1998, 2001). Here, mitochondrial BCAT catalyses the transamination of the BCAA in astrocytes. The resulting BCKA, which are poorly metabolized by astrocytes, are shuttled to neuronal cells for further metabolism, while glutamate enters the glutamate–glutamine cycle. BCAT$_c$, which is neuronal specific, catalyses transamination of the BCKA with glutamate back to the BCAA, which exit the neuron and return to the astrocyte. α-Ketoglutarate may also undergo reductive amination to glutamate via neuronal GDH but is thought not to be a serious contender, as the flux in this direction is low (Yudkoff et al., 1990; Hutson et al., 2001). Therefore, BCAT proteins in brain metabolism do not only facilitate energy metabolism, but also provide essential nitrogen for the anaplerotic regeneration of glutamate.

2.4 Alanine Aminotransferases and Glutamate

In muscle, BCAA and alanine metabolism are intrinsically linked with glutamate metabolism. During gluconeogenesis both alanine and glutamine are the predominant amino acids which leave the muscle, with alanine preferentially taken up by the liver (Fig. 2.3). Evidently ALT plays a more dominant role in protein metabolism of liver and muscle relative to brain, as the levels of ALT are significantly higher. Alanine released from muscle is derived from pyruvate and glutamate, releasing α-ketoglutarate thought to drive the TCA cycle particularly during exercise; this is known as the glucose–alanine cycle (Fig. 2.3) (Rutten et al., 2005). This is closely linked to the glucose–lactate cycle (Cori cycle), which operates in parallel during gluconeogenesis. Thus, carbohydrate and protein metabolism operate cooperatively, where the direction of metabolism is substrate driven. The role of ALT in brain metabolism has been described in the hypothetical lactate–alanine shuttle between brain cells, with its metabolites potentially linked with glutamate metabolism (Fig. 2.5) (Pellerin and Magistretti, 1994; Peng et al., 1994; Waagepetersen et al., 2000; Schousboe and Waagepetersen, 2005; Bak et al., 2006).

Glucose is considered the main energy source of the brain, where both neuronal and astrocytic cells are capable of its metabolism. Relative to other metabolites glucose is readily taken up by the brain and is available in high concentrations in the blood. Conversely, lactate cannot readily pass the blood–brain barrier (Cremer et al., 1976, 1979) and its levels in the blood fall short in maintaining the energy requirements of the brain, even though neuronal cells express both lactate and glucose transporters (Bergersen et al., 2002). It has been demonstrated that astrocytes have greater glycolytic activity than neuronal cells, with the lactate produced transported to neuronal cells for further oxidation (Schousboe et al., 1997; Waagepetersen et al., 2000; Pellerin, 2003). The lack of metabolic machinery (i.e. the malate–aspartate shuttle) in astrocytes, which would otherwise drive glycolysis through to complete oxidation in the mitochondria, support these findings. In fact, with the proposed lactate–alanine shuttle it was suggested that neuronal cells may actually metabolize lactate as efficiently as glucose, a subject actively debated in the literature (Schurr et al., 1997 a,b,c; Cater et al., 2001; Waagepetersen et al., 2000; Bak et al., 2006, 2007, 2009). Metabolic studies utilizing [U^{13}C]lactate incubated with glutamatergic cerebellar granule cells, astrocytes and co-cultures demonstrated that alanine was preferentially formed or released into the medium in neuronal cells. Incubation of these cells with [U^{13}C]alanine resulted in the preferential enrichment of alanine in astrocytes relative to neuronal cells, suggesting that neurons preferentially synthesize and release alanine, and astrocytes favour uptake supporting a different functional role of alanine metabolism in brain cells. Thus, as described for BCAA in the BCAA–BCKA shuttle, the role of alanine as a carrier for nitrogen between neurons and astrocytes in exchange for lactate was suggested (Fig. 2.5). In this role it was proposed that alanine would serve to transport excess ammonia from neuronal cells to astrocytes, generated from the metabolism of glutamine to glutamate by mitochondrial glutaminase, where it could be utilized by GS for glutamine synthesis from glutamate (Waagepetersen et al., 2000). To establish a link between the alanine–lactate cycle and the glutamate–glutamine cycle, neuronal and astrocyte cells were incubated with [5-^{15}N] glutamine and [^{15}N]alanine, respectively. A minor 3.3% enrichment of alanine in neuronal cells and 22% monolabelling in glutamate and glutamine in astrocytes was reported, offering some evidence in support of the shuttle; however, the actual extent to which it contributes as an anaplerotic pathway is still in dispute.

Production of lactate in astrocytes is thought to correlate with an increase in glycolysis stimulated through glutamate uptake (Pellerin *et al.*, 1998). In brief, it was proposed that lactate generated from astrocytes or through uptake from the peripheral blood is converted to pyruvate by lactate dehydrogenase (LDH), which is further utilized for energy production through the TCA cycle or as a substrate for ALT (Fig. 2.5). In neuronal cells ALT catalyses the transamination of pyruvate to alanine which results in the consumption of glutamate and the generation of α-ketoglutarate. Alanine that is produced is released and taken up by astrocytes to undergo further transamination to pyruvate and α-ketoglutarate, completing the cycle (Fig. 2.5) (Waagepetersen *et al.*, 2000). Here, the role of alanine was proposed to act as a nitrogen carrier from neuronal cells to astrocytes. It was suggested that alanine formed as a result of GDH activity utilizes the excess ammonia formed from the glutaminase reaction, and channels the much-needed source of nitrogen into astrocytes. In retinal Muller cells 60% of glutamate synthesis occurred via AOAA-sensitive transamination (LaNoue *et al.*, 2001). Furthermore, using the inhibitor L-cycloserine, *de novo* synthesis of glutamate was inhibited to a greater degree relative to the specific inhibition of BCAT using gabapentin. This suggests that this alanine shuttle is potentially active in intact neural tissue and that it provides a proportion of nitrogen for glutamate synthesis in the retina (LaNoue *et al.*, 2001). Evidently, ALT does play a role in brain glutamate metabolism; however, the extent to which this contributes to glutamate levels should be considered in the future with the distribution/activity of ALT in neuronal and glial cells.

2.5 Aspartate Aminotransferases and their Role in the Malate–Aspartate Shuttle and Glutamate Metabolism

Functionally, AST proteins play a central role in the malate–aspartate shuttle and in glutamate metabolism. In neuronal cells, the synaptic terminals which are rich in mitochondria have high malate–asparate shuttle activity (Cheeseman and Clark, 1988) and high levels of AST and GDH activity (McKenna *et al.*, 2000a,b), whereas the activity of AST in astrocytes is reported to be considerably lower. Oxidation of glucose to pyruvate yields NADH, a major reducing equivalent which drives the TCA cycle to yield the maximum energy from glucose, which is essential for brain function. The function of the malate–aspartate shuttle is to avoid the build-up of the ratio of $NADH/NAD^+$, which serves to favour metabolism moving in the direction of lactate production, rather than oxidation of pyruvate in the TCA cycle, which would decrease the energy output from glycolysis. Although other shuttle mechanisms may operate, the two most studied shuttles include the malate–aspartate shuttle and the glycerol 3–phosphate shuttle, with the malate–aspartate shuttle considered to be particularly important in neurons and the most important in the brain (Fig. 2.6) (Cheeseman and Clark, 1988). The role of the glycerol 3–phosphate shuttle is disputed, due to conflicting reports of the subcellular localization of this shuttle in various brain cells (Nguyen *et al.*, 2003).

The AST isoforms are central to the operation of this shuttle as they are the rate-limiting enzymes; evidence suggests that this shuttle is more active in neuronal cells relative to astrocytes (McKenna *et al.*, 2006). The AST enzymes work with several other proteins including the aspartate/glutamate carrier (AGC – aralar 1 isoform), the malate/α-ketoglutarate carrier, and GDH and MDH, which have been shown to form metabolomic complexes through physical associations with each other (Ramos *et al.*, 2003; McKenna *et al.*, 2006). These physical interactions between enzymes are thought to facilitate the transfer of substrates between enzymes thus maximizing catalysis. The *in vivo* importance of these interactions is currently unknown. The mitochondrial enzyme AST_m operates in the direction of aspartate synthesis, and the cytosolic in the direction of aspartate conversion to oxaloacetate (OAA). Briefly, the mitochondrial membrane is impermeable to NADH formed during the glycolytic cycle. To facilitate the transfer of reducing equivalents, OAA is reduced to malate in the cytosol, which is exchanged for α-ketoglutarate across the mitochondrial membrane. Malate dehydrogenase catalyses the release of the reducing equivalents from malate with the formation of OAA. Here, mitochondrial AST catalyses the transamination of OAA and glutamate to aspartate and α-ketoglutarate, respectively. Both aspartate and α-ketoglutarate are subsequently transferred to the cytosol where its cytosolic counterpart, AST_c, regenerates glutamate and OAA from cytosolic aspartate and α-ketoglutarate (Fig. 2.6). Over the last few years several groups using immunohistochemistry and *in situ* hybridisation have demonstrated that astrocytes have either no expression or very low levels of AGC, one of the key components of the malate–aspartate shuttle (Ramos *et al.*, 2003; Xu *et al.*, 2007), which suggests that the direction of metabolism results in the production of lactate that must be exported to neuronal cells for further oxidation (Fig. 2.6) (McKenna, 2007; Xu *et al.*, 2007).

In addition to their role in the transfer of reducing equivalents, the AST proteins have been shown to play an important part in glutamate metabolism (Safer and Williamson, 1972; Scholz *et al.*, 1998; Chatziioannou *et al.*, 2003). The rate of oxidation of glutamate differs in neuronal and astrocytic cells. In astrocytes glutamate is oxidized at a rate almost twice that of glutamine, which supports the role of astrocytes in disposing excess glutamate. It has been reported that the role of AST_m in glutamate metabolism is dependent on the origin of glutamate. Using ^{13}C NMR tracer experiments and inhibitors of aminotransferase proteins such as AOA, it was proposed that oxidation of exogenous glutamate is primarily through the action of mitochondrial GDH, whereas glutamate synthesized endogenously from glutamine (oxidized for energy by glutaminase) is metabolized by AST (Fig. 2.6) (McKenna *et al.*, 1993, 1996b). In fact, a congenital deficiency or mutation of GDH can result in neurological disturbances (Plaitakis *et al.*, 1982; Kelly and Stanley, 2001). Irrespective of this, metabolism by either GDH or AST results in the production of key metabolites which enter into the TCA cycle (Sonnewald *et al.*, 1993; McKenna *et al.*, 1996b) and are thought to be particularly important in the disposal of excess glutamate. ^{13}C-NMR studies have shown that the carbon skeleton from [U-^{13}C]glutamate can be traced to lactate, aspartate, or resynthesized glutamate from the TCA cycle (Sonnewald *et al.*, 1993; McKenna *et al.*, 1996a).

As described for astrocytes, both glutamate and glutamine can be oxidized to CO_2 in neuronal cells (McKenna *et al.*, 1993, 1996a); however, here glutamine is metabolized preferentially at a rate five times faster than glutamate. Interestingly, endogenous glutamate is oxidatively deaminated by GDH, which appears to be the opposite to that observed in astrocytes (Tildon *et al.*, 1985; McKenna *et al.*, 1993, 1996a). As both AST and GDH have high activity in the mitochondrial synaptic regions it suggests that the relative importance of these two enzymes in the oxidation of glutamate is substrate driven (Erecinska *et al.*, 1990; McKenna *et al.*, 2000b). Although transamination by AST is freely reversible, the direction or flow of metabolism will be dictated by the concentration of metabolites and possibly how they can influence the metabolomic interactions of AST with other membrane-bound proteins such as glutaminase (Teller *et al.*, 1990; Cooper, 2001). Furthermore, when energy substrates are sufficient, α-ketoglutarate formed in the TCA cycle can be metabolized to glutamate through transamination (Sonnewald *et al.*, 1993). Therefore, taken together these studies suggest both AST and GDH play a central role in glutamate metabolism, favouring catabolism in astrocytes and conservation in neuronal cells.

2.6 Pathological Conditions Resulting from Impaired Aminotransferase Metabolism

To date there are no known mutations of the BCAT, AST, or ALT aminotransferase proteins contributing to a pathological condition. However, a build-up of their substrates or products can lead to disorders leading to neurodegeneration (e.g. glutamate toxicity in Alzheimer's disease). The most accepted consequence of altered BCAA metabolism is a mutation of the BCKDH complex resulting in the accumulation of the BCAA and α-keto acids leading to neuronal dysfunction (see below). Although not discussed in detail in this chapter, the only aminotransferase protein with a known mutation is the alanine:glyoxylate aminotransferase (AGT, EC 2.6.1.44), a PLP-dependent metabolic enzyme which catalyses the transamination of alanine and glyoxylate to pyruvate and glycine. This enzyme is characteristically found in the peroxisomes distributed largely in hepatocytes. In humans, AGT is encoded by the AGXT gene, mutations of which give rise to dysfunctional proteins resulting in the overproduction of oxalate (Coulter-Mackie and Rumsby, 2004; Danpure, 2006). Excess oxalate leads to the progressive accumulation of insoluble calcium oxalate in the kidney and urinary tract leading to urolithiasis, often accompanied by systemic oxalosis, which ultimately results in renal failure.

2.6.1 Maple syrup urine disease

Maple syrup urine disease is a congenital disease characterized by a build-up of both BCAA and their respective keto-acid derivatives. These metabolites are neurotoxic to cells in the cerebrospinal fluid, blood, and tissues resulting in the patient presenting with symptoms such as neurological dysfunction, seizures and infant death (Silberman et al., 1961; Chuang, 1998, 2006). MSUD is an autosomal recessive disorder caused by a deficiency of the multienzyme complex, the branched-chain α-keto acid dehydrogenase complex (BCKDH), the rate-limiting step of transamination (Dancis et al., 1959, 1960; Menkes, 1959, 1962; Dankis 1964). This complex is composed of three catalytic subunits, the E1, E2 and E3 subunits (Harris et al., 2004), where all three units are essential for enzymatic activity (Danner and Doering, 1998). At least 150 mutations in the BCKDH complex genes have been reported, with the most disease-causing mutations seen in E2 (Chuang, 1998; Danner and Doering, 1998, Chuang and Chuang, 2000; Chuang et al., 2006). Five classifications of MSUD have been identified (varying from severe classic forms to mild variant types, and also with a thiamine-responsive form), based on the residual BCKDH activity, the age of onset and the concentration of leucine in serum (Duran and Wadman, 1985; Chuang and Chuang, 2000; Chuang et al., 2006).

Although treatment through restriction of the BCAA in the diet has most value in milder forms of the condition, patients that are not compliant with their diet or those with more severe forms of the disease are still subject to many side effects (Snyderman, 1986, 1988). Investigation into alternative therapies using animal models has been described (Klivenyi et al., 2004; Wu et al., 2004; Homanics et al., 2006). Briefly, the usefulness of these models varies widely, from creating homozygous lethal knockouts, to knockouts that phenotypically resemble BCKDH but on further investigation revealed a $BCAT_m$ mutation (Wu et al., 2004). More useful models include a classical MSUD and intermediate MSUD design (Homanics et al., 2006; Zinnanti et al., 2009). In the homozygous mouse, relative to wild-type (WT), levels of BCAA to alanine were 22-fold higher and 16-fold higher for the cMSUD and iMSUD, respectively. In contrast to the increase in BCAA levels, alanine, glutamate, and glutamine in the blood were all significantly reduced in iMSUD mice compared with WT, with low levels of aspartate and gamma-aminobutyric acid also uniformly reduced. The reduced levels of neurotransmitters are likely to cause encephalopathies such as coma. These models will provide a wealth of knowledge for pathological analysis and metabolic profiling of blood, brain and other tissues (Zinnanti et al., 2009).

2.6.2 Glutamate toxicity and neurodegeneration

Under normal physiological conditions glutamate plays a role in dendrite and synapse formation, and also a dominant role in glutamatergic transmission, essential for memory and learning (Danbolt, 2001). However, high levels of glutamate result in this amino acid becoming a potent neurotoxin (Chapter 25). This has been reported to lead to increased expression of tau protein, neuronal degeneration and cell death (Choi, 1988, 1990; Esclaire et al., 1997). The effect of the excessive synaptic release of glutamate is largely mediated by an increase in the entry of calcium into neurons (Kaplan and Miller, 1997; Sattler and Tymianski, 2000; Mattson, 2003, 2007, 2008), which is the predominant secondary messenger for neurotransmitters and neurotrophins (Choi, 1988; Kaplan and Miller, 1997). An overload of calcium, observed in the brain tissue of patients with AD has been shown to evoke acute degenerative conditions (Mattson and Chan, 2003; Mattson, 2007). Thus, a strong relationship exists between excessive calcium influx and glutamate-triggered neuronal injury. Recently published studies using targeted proteomics in neuronal cells have shown that BCAT proteins have redox-mediated associations with several neuronal proteins involved in G-protein cell signalling, indicating a novel role for BCAT in cellular redox control (Conway et al., 2008). Interestingly, the brain-derived neurotrophin factor, which mediates its action through calcium cell signalling, causes up-regulation of BCAT (Numakawa et al., 2002, 2009; Madeddu et al., 2004). These findings indicate that the BCAT proteins may have fundamental links with calcium-mediated signalling, and because of its primary role in producing glutamate, understanding this mechanism may enhance our knowledge of how glutamate can reach toxic levels in neurodegenerative diseases such as AD, offering potential sites for targeted therapy.

2.6.3 Redox sensitivity of BCAT

Generation of reactive nitrogen and oxygen species (RNS and ROS, respectively) can occur through calcium overload, which as previously mentioned can be generated through glutamate neurotoxicity (Kaplan and Miller, 1997; Sattler and Tymianski, 2000; Mattson, 2003, 2007, 2008). Mitochondrial dysfunction can also generate reactive species, in particular peroxynitrite. Targets of these harmful species include reactive thiols of receptive proteins, resulting in changes to the structure and/or function of a protein, ultimately leading to metabolic imbalances resulting in cell death. The BCAT proteins are unique among the mammalian aminotransferases in that they contain a redox-active CXXC motif subject to reversible mofiication by both ROS and RNS, potentially serving as a biological control point (Conway et al., 2002, 2003, 2004, 2008; Coles et al., 2009; Hutson et al., 2009). Response to cellular stress varies between isoforms, with $BCAT_m$ being completely inactivated by both ROS and RNS, whereas $BCAT_c$ is only partially sensitive to air oxidation and the nitric oxide donor, S-nitrosoglutathione (GSNO). Low concentrations of GSNO caused a reversible time-dependent loss in 50% of $BCAT_c$ activity, characterized predominantly through S-nitrosation (a reaction transferring a NO group to the reactive cysteine of this protein) (Coles et al., 2009). However, increased exposure to GSNO resulted in a shift towards S-glutathionylation (addition of GSH to the reactive thiol), a marker of oxidative stress (Coles et al., 2009). Recent studies have demonstrated that both S-nitrosation and S-glutathionylation of proteins occur in the brains from patients suffering with AD, which is directly correlated to the misfolding of proteins (Yao et al., 2004; Benhar et al., 2006; Uehara et al., 2006; Fang et al., 2007; Lipton et al., 2007; Nakamura and Lipton, 2007, 2008, 2009; Cho et al., 2009). Investigation as to how these mechanisms of S-nitrosation or S-glutathionylation regulate the hBCAT proteins *in vivo*, relative to glutamate toxicity and protein misfolding, may contribute to the understanding of these fundamental pathways involved in the pathogenesis of AD.

2.7 Aminotransferase Proteins as Biomarkers of Disease

Not only do the aminotransferase (AST and ALT) proteins have significant roles in whole-body nitrogen metabolism: they have also been used for decades as biomarkers of disease, most notably liver disease (Panteghini, 1990). The chapter will therefore digress to accommodate their role in clinical biochemistry, detailing how their measurements in serum can assist in the differential diagnosis of hepatic conditions. Biomarkers are used in screening, diagnostics, prognostics, or monitoring of patient outcome. The role of AST and ALT as biomarkers is primarily diagnostic with some prognostic applications. Ideally a diagnostic biomarker should be differentially specific, released in a timely fashion, with rapid robust validated methods of analysis. As both AST and ALT are found in several tissues they fall short as 'ideal' markers of disease. For example, erythrocyte levels of

AST are 10–15 times greater than that measured in serum, so mild elevations could suggest haemolysis rather than hepatic injury. However, to increase their clinical utility and diagnostic relevance, AST and ALT are grouped with other tests of liver function traditionally known as 'liver function tests' (LFT) (Table 2.1). It is relevant to note that although these tests are generically associated as LFT, they do not reflect liver function but rather the structural integrity of liver cells. True liver function tests would include the measurement of albumin, total protein, bilirubin, and/or prothrombin time. As ALT is localized only in the cytosol of liver, and AST is found in both mitochondria and cytosol, the ratio of AST/ALT can be used as an index of the severity of hepatic damage and indeed as a good prognostic indicator. Should the level of AST exceed ALT, damage to the cell is extensive and prognosis is poor.

Abnormal levels of the aminotransferase proteins may reflect both acute and chronic conditions and are interpreted in conjunction with the clinical and biochemical presentation of the patient. Patient history is of utmost importance in this differential diagnosis, as medications (including herbal remedies and over-the-counter preparations), co-morbid conditions, risk factors for viral hepatitis, and age can considerably influence the diagnosis. The reference limits for the aminotransferase proteins can vary among laboratories; however, examples of reference ranges used are summarized in Table 2.1. The use of AST and ALT as biomarkers is normally expressed with respect to the level of magnitude above the reference range, and more so the pattern of alteration often with respect to other LFT markers (Table 2.1). Levels can be defined as mild (≤2×), moderate (3–5×), or a marked increase (≥10–100×) above the upper reference limit (URL), where the rate and nature of change also illustrates the extent of cellular damage. It is important to note that these classifications are broad and may differ among clinicians. Therefore, patient history, the relative degree or elevation, in addition to the pattern of increase of the aminotransferase proteins relative to the other LFT, can differentiate between the causes of both acute and chronic liver disease.

2.7.1 Mild elevation of ALT and AST

The most common causes for a mild elevation of ALT and AST include acute alcoholic-induced or non-alcoholic fatty liver disease (NAFLD), where the activities of AST/ALT are reported as ≤2× the URL (Bayard et al., 2006). Generally, levels of ALT exceed that of AST in acute liver damage, with the exception of toxin-induced or alcoholic hepatitis and Reyes syndrome (Dufour et al., 2000a,b). One explanation for this change in the ratio is due to a deficiency in PLP, common in alcoholics. This has an impact in two ways: ALT is more sensitive to this loss than AST, and alcohol induces the release of AST_m, thus increasing the total amount of serum AST (Dufour et al., 2000a,b). Mildly elevated levels of AST and ALT are also reported for chronic conditions associated with hepatitis B and C, and cirrhosis. A ratio of AST/ALT greater than 1.0 is suggestive of advanced liver disease with a greater risk of advanced fibrosis indicative of a poor prognosis (Williams and Hoofnagle, 1988; Giannini et al., 1999, 2003). An AST/ALT ratio ≥ 1 can be found in 4% of patients with chronic hepatitis C and in 79% of patients who have cirrhosis (Williams and Hoofnagle, 1988; Giannini et al., 1999, 2003). If these conditions are excluded, consideration for more rare causes of mildly elevated AST and ALT must be evaluated, such as haemochromatosis, Wilson's disease (in younger patients), autoimmune liver disease, and α-1-antitrypsin deficiency (Krawitt, 1996; Morrison and Kowdley, 2000; Ferenci et al., 2005). Patients with autoimmune disease, based on elevated levels of hypergammaglobulinaemia, also present with low levels of aminotransferase activity.

Pathologically the first stage of alcoholic liver disease is the appearance of large fatty deposits, without evidence of clinical or biochemical abnormalities. Currently, no biomarker can detect early stage hepatic injury. In stage two, alcoholic hepatitis, increased levels of AST and ALT may be mild or moderate. Because other conditions can also give rise to mild elevations of AST and ALT, γ-glutamyl transferase, a toxin-inducible enzyme often elevated in both alcoholic and drug induced injury and alkaline phosphatase (ALP), may be assessed and taken together with the

Table 2.1. Serum levels of AST and ALT relative to other markers of hepatic injury.

Biomarker	Cellular distribution	Predominant tissue localization	Reference range	Cholestasis	Hepatic ischaemia or toxic injury	Acute viral hepatitis	Acute alcoholic liver disease	Chronic liver disease	Hepatic cirrhosis
Biomarkers of structural integrity									
ALT	Cytoplasm[a]	Liver, muscle and kidney	5–50 IU l^{-1}	Mild or moderate	↑↑↑	↑↑	Mild or moderate	Normal or ↑	Normal or ↑
AST	Cytoplasm and mitochondria	Liver, heart, skeletal muscle, brain, and kidney	AGE RANGE ↑ 5 wks (6–122 IU l^{-1}), 6 wks–1 yr (6–71 IU l^{-1}) 1–4 yrs (6–51 IU l^{-1}) ≥5 yrs (6–35 IU l^{-1})	Mild or moderate	↑↑↑	↑↑	Mild or moderate	Normal or ↑	Normal or ↑
γ-Glutamyl transferase	Cell membrane	Liver, biliary canals, kidney	≤ 55 IU l^{-1}	Mild or moderate	↑↑	↑↑	↑↑	↑↑	↑↑
ALP	Cell membrane	Liver, bone, and kidney	≤ 150 IU l^{-1}	Moderate or marked	↑	↑↑	↑↑	↑↑	↑↑
Functional biomarkers									
Bilirubin		Liver (but also extra hepatic)	≤ 20 μmol l^{-1}	Mild or moderate	Normal or mild	Dependent on the type of infection[b]	Mild or moderate	↑↑	↑↑↑
Albumin[c]		Liver	35–45 g l^{-1}	Normal	Normal	Normal	Normal or ↓	↓	↓
Prothrombin time[d]		Liver	≤ 150 s	Normal	Mild or moderate	Normal or ↑	Normal or ↑	↑↑	↑↑

[a]Only cytosolic form present in the liver; other tissues have both a cytosolic and mitochondrial isoform.
[b]Levels of bilirubin will be elevated relative to infection with hepatitis A, B, C, etc., and the extent of damage.
[c]Albumin levels may also be reduced in patients who are malnourished, have cancer, malabsorption, or immune disorders (therefore it lacks specificity).
[d]The increase in time it takes for the blood to clot will depend on the extent of functional damage, and this can vary greatly within conditions.
↑ mild increase; ↑↑ moderate increase; ↑↑↑ marked increase.

patient history can confirm diagnosis (Rosalki et al., 1971). However, even in the absence of alcohol, γ-glutamyl transferase can be elevated, as seen in patients with NAFLD, and shows a clinical picture similar to chronic hepatitis (Brunt, 2004). If clinical presentation suggests alcoholic-induced liver disease but without evidence of alcohol consumption, other conditions such as diabetes, hyperlipidaemia, and hypertension should be assessed to assist in a diagnosis of NAFLD. Ultimately, a liver biopsy would be required to ascertain the extent of hepatic injury (Dufour et al., 2000a,b).

2.7.2 Moderate/marked elevation of ALT and AST

Acute damage to the liver can also result in a moderate/marked increase in AST and ALT. When levels of AST/ALT reach 100× the URL, it is almost always indicative of ischaemic injury or injury due to toxic ingestion (Dufour et al., 2000a,b). Ischaemic and hypoxic acute liver damage are frequently associated with patients who are clinically challenged, such as those with sepsis (Seeto et al., 2000). Toxin ingestion can captivate prescribed and herbal medications and intended overdose use. Within several hours of an overdose of acetominophen levels of AST can reach in excess of 7000 IU l^{-1}, reflecting the ultimate destruction of liver cells leading to an immediate release of enzymes into the blood stream (Singer et al., 1995). As also seen in ischaemic hepatic injury, the ratio of AST/ALT will be increased and reflect an increase in lactate dehydrogenase, a marker of ischaemic injury. Post insult the levels of AST and ALT can drop dramatically to within the reference range; however, this is not necessarily a good prognosis as it may reflect extensive hepatic necrosis rather than recovery, due to the short circulatory half-life of AST (17 h) and ALT (47 h) (Giannini et al., 2005). In this case the monitoring of true liver function tests such as bilirubin levels or prothrombin time can assess if the patient is at risk from hepatic failure.

It is estimated that over 80% of individuals with acute viral hepatitis are never clinically diagnosed (Giannini et al., 2005; Knight, 2005). This is mostly due to the asymptomatic presentation of those infected and is often passed off as a flu-like illness with non-specific indicators such as fatigue and fever. Although hepatitis A and hepatitis B are on the decrease worldwide due to the introduction of vaccines, hepatitis C is increasing. For those with hepatitis C, 85% develop chronic hepatitis and have a 30% increased risk of developing hepatocellular cancer. Although jaundice is evident in almost 70% of those with acute hepatitis A, it occurs in less than 50% and 33% of cases with acute hepatitis B and C, respectively, and is therefore an insensitive diagnostic indicator (Dufour et al., 2000a,b; Giannini et al., 2005). Levels of the aminotransferases can also be varied dependent on the extent of cellular damage, and can show a moderate or marked increase with or without jaundice. As a result differential diagnosis of acute viral hepatitis can be more challenging for viral hepatitis, in particular hepatitis C. Although biochemically the clinical picture may not be clear, patient history and evidence of high-risk factors such as travel to endemic areas (hepatitis A), intravenous drug use, or transfusions will play a pivotal role in diagnosis. Confirmation of acute viral hepatitis, however, is only obtained when the patient is tested for viral-specific antibodies. Although toxin or viral insult represent the vast majority of acute liver diseases with moderate or marked increases in AST and ALT, other causes such as Epstein–Barr virus, autoimmune, extrahepatic, or congenital disorders must be considered (Giannini et al., 2005).

2.8 Conclusions and Future Directions

Although the intriguing compartmentation of metabolic pathways and the subcellular localization of the aminotransferase isoforms to different brain cells offer enumerable insights into whole-brain metabolism, they also highlight the enormity of what is not understood. Evidently, the cellular distribution of the aminotransferases in brain tissue requires further characterization to substantiate the biochemical findings. Confirmation of the expression and activity of the specific isoforms in brain cells will further assist understanding of the actual extent to which these proteins participate in anaplerotic pathways. The current studies unequivocally support the role that these aminotransferase proteins play in the supply of nitrogen for glutamate synthesis. In particular, studies detailing the role of leucine in glutamate oxidation and synthesis show that it fulfils the criteria as an external nitrogen source:

1. It freely passes the blood–brain barrier.
2. The BCAT proteins are highly expressed in brain cells showing neuronal and astrocytic specificity.
3. Their role in muscle metabolism as a nitrogen donor is substantially characterized.
4. Overwhelming evidence in several model systems support the BCAA–BCKA shuttle with direct evidence of its contribution to the glutamate–glutamine cycle.

However, as with the other aminotransferase proteins, much is still unknown. More sensitive models using inhibitors with greater specificity would further enhance knowledge of these pathways. As these aminotransferase proteins play a key role in facilitating the anaplerotic generation of glutamate it is highly likely that their metabolism will be altered in neurodegenerative disease conditions. Therefore, understanding of how these suggested shuttles are altered in disease will offer possible targets for novel therapeutic treatment to either delay onset or prevent further neuronal destruction. Finally, to date ALT and AST have for decades sustained their role as key biochemical markers of disease, despite their lack of specificity. With the advent of proteomics and the search for the ideal marker of early stage liver disease, new markers are emerging. However, ALT and AST will sustain their prominent role for the foreseeable future and their value may extend if modifications of these proteins are observed at the early stages of disease.

References

Attwell, M., and Laughlin, E. (2001) An energy budget for signalling in grey matter of the brain. *Journal of Cerebral Blood Flow Metabolism* 21, 1133–1145.

Bak, L.K., Schousboe, A., Sonnewald, U. and Waagepetersen, H.S. (2006) Glucose is necessary to maintain neurotransmitter homeostasis during synaptic activity in cultured glutamatergic neurons. *Journal of Cerebral Blood Flow and Metabolism* 26, 1285–1297.

Bak, L.K., Waagepetersen, H.S., Melø, T.M., Schousboe, A. and Sonnewald, U. (2007) Complex glutamate labeling from [U-13C]glucose or [U-13C]lactate in co-cultures of cerebellar neurons and astrocytes. *Neurochemical Research* 32, 671–680.

Bak, L.K., Walls, A.B., Schousboe, A., Ring, A., Sonnewald, U. and Waagepetersen, H.S. (2009) Neuronal glucose but not lactate utilization is positively correlated with NMDA-induced neurotransmission and fluctuations in cytosolic Ca2+ levels. *Journal of Neurochemistry* 109, 87–93.

Bayard, M., Holt, J. and Boroughs, E. (2006) Nonalcoholic fatty liver disease. *American Family Physician* 73, 1961–1968.

Benhar, M., Forrester, M.T. and Stamler, J.S. (2006) Nitrosative stress in the ER: a new role for S-nitrosylation in neurodegenerative diseases. *ACS Chemical Biology* 1, 355–358.

Bergersen, L., Rafiki, A. and Ottersen, O.P. (2002) Immunogold cytochemistry identifies specialized membrane domains for monocarboxylate transport in the central nervous system. *Neurochemical Research* 27, 89–96.

Bixel, M., Shimomura, Y., Hutson, S. and Hamprecht, B. (2001) Distribution of key enzymes of branched-chain amino acid metabolism in glial and neuronal cells in culture. *Journal of Histochemistry and Cytochemistry* 49, 407–418.

Bixel, M.G. and Hamprecht, B. (1995) Generation of ketone bodies from leucine by cultured astroglial cells. *Journal of Neurochemistry* 65, 2450–2461.

Bixel, M.G. and Hamprecht, B. (2000) Immunocytochemical localization of beta-methylcrotonyl-CoA carboxylase in astroglial cells and neurons in culture. *Journal of Neurochemistry* 74, 1059–1067.

Bixel, M.G., Hutson, S.M. and Hamprecht, B. (1997) Cellular distribution of branched-chain amino acid aminotransferase isoenzymes among rat brain glial cells in culture. *Journal of Histochemistry and Cytochemistry* 45, 685–694.

Bradbury, M.W. and Berk, P.D. (2000) Mitochondrial aspartate aminotransferase: direction of a single protein with two distinct functions to two subcellular sites does not require alternative splicing of the mRNA. *Biochemical Journal* 345, 423–427.

Brand, K. (1981) Metabolism of 2-oxoacid analogues of leucine, valine and phenylalanine by heart muscle, brain and kidney of the rat. *Biochimica et Biophysica Acta* 677, 126–132.

Brand, K. and Hauschildt, S. (1984) Metabolism of 2-oxo-acid analogues of leucine and valine in isolated rat hepatocytes. *Hoppe-Seyler's Zeitschrift fur Physiologische Chemie* 365, 463–468.

Brookes, N. (1992) Effect of intracellular glutamine on the uptake of large neutral amino acids in astrocytes: concentrative Na(+)-independent transport exhibits metastability. *Journal of Neurochemistry* 59, 227–235.

Brookes, N. (1993) Interaction between the glutamine cycle and the uptake of large neutral amino acids in astrocytes. *Journal of Neurochemistry* 60, 1923–1928.

Brunt, E.M. (2004) Nonalcoholic steatohepatitis. *Seminars in Liver Disease* 24, 3–20.

Cater, H.L., Chandratheva, A., Benham, C.D., Morrison, B. 3rd and Sundstrom, L.E. (2001) Lactate and glucose as energy substrates during, and after, oxygen deprivation in rat hippocampal acute and cultured slices. *Journal of Neurochemistry* 87, 1381–1390.

Cechetto, J.D., Sadacharan, S.K., Berk, P.D. and Gupta, R.S. (2002) Immunogold localization of mitochondrial aspartate aminotransferase in mitochondria and on the cell surface in normal rat tissues. *Histology and Histopathology* 17, 353–364.

Chaplin, E.R., Goldberg, A.L. and Diamond, I. (1976) Leucine oxidation in brain slices and nerve endings. *Journal of Neurochemistry* 26, 701–707.

Chatziioannou, A., Palaiologos, G. and Kolisis, F.N. (2003) Metabolic flux analysis as a tool for the elucidation of the metabolism of neurotransmitter glutamate. *Metabolic Engineering* 5, 201–210.

Cheesman, A.J., and Clark, J.B. (1988) Influence of the malate-aspartate shuttle on oxidative metabolism in synaptosomes. *Journal of Neurochemistry* 50, 1559–1565.

Cho, D.H., Nakamura, T., Fang, J., Cieplak, P., Godzik, A., Gu, Z. and Lipton, S.A. (2009) S-nitrosylation of Drp1 mediates beta-amyloid-related mitochondrial fission and neuronal injury. *Science* 324, 102–05.

Choi, D.W. (1988) Glutamate neurotoxicity and diseases of the nervous system. *Neuron* 1, 623–634.

Choi, D.W. (1990) Methods for antagonizing glutamate neurotoxicity. *Cerebrovascular and Brain Metabolism Reviews* 2, 105–147.

Chuang, D.T. (1998) Maple syrup urine disease: it has come a long way. *The Journal of Pediatrics* 132, S17–23.

Chuang, D.T., Chuang, J.L. and Wynn, R.M. (2006) Lessons from genetic disorders of branched-chain amino acid metabolism. *Journal of Nutrition* 136, 243S–249S.

Chuang, J.L. and Chuang, D.T. (2000) Diagnosis and mutational analysis of maple syrup urine disease using cell cultures. *Methods in Enzymology* 324, 413–423.

Coles, S.J., Easton, P., Sharrod, H., Hutson, S.M., Hancock, J., Patel, V.B. and Conway, M.E. (2009) S-Nitrosoglutathione inactivation of the mitochondrial and cytosolic BCAT proteins: S-nitrosation and S-thiolation. *Biochemistry* 48, 645–656.

Conway, M.E., Coles, S.J., Islam, M.M. and Hutson, S.M. (2008) Regulatory control of human cytosolic branched-chain aminotransferase by oxidation and S-glutathionylation and its interactions with redox sensitive neuronal proteins. *Biochemistry* 47, 5465–5479.

Conway, M.E., Yennawar, N., Wallin, R., Poole, L.B. and Hutson, S.M. (2002) Identification of a peroxide-sensitive redox switch at the CXXC motif in the human mitochondrial branched chain aminotransferase. *Biochemistry* 41, 9070–9078.

Conway, M.E., Yennawar, N., Wallin, R., Poole, L.B. and Hutson, S.M. (2003) Human mitochondrial branched chain aminotransferase: structural basis for substrate specificity and role of redox active cysteines. *Biochimica et Biophysica Acta* 1647, 61–65.

Conway, M.E., Poole, L.B. and Hutson, S.M. (2004) Roles for cysteine residues in the regulatory CXXC motif of human mitochondrial branched chain aminotransferase enzyme. *Biochemistry* 43, 7356–7364.

Cooper, A.J. (2001) Role of glutamine in cerebral nitrogen metabolism and ammonia neurotoxicity. *Mental Retardation and Developmental Disabilities Research Reviews* 7, 280–286.

Coulter-Mackie, M.B. and Rumsby, G. (2004) Genetic heterogeneity in primary hyperoxaluria type 1: impact on diagnosis. *Molecular Genetics and Metabolism* 83, 38–46.

Cremer, J.E., Braun, L.D. and Oldendorf, W.H. (1976) Changes during development in transport processes of the blood-brain barrier. *Biochimica et Biophysica Acta* 448, 633–637.

Cremer, J.E., Cunningham, V.J., Pardridge, W.M., Braun, L.D. and Oldendorf, W.H. (1979) Kinetics of blood-brain barrier transport of pyruvate, lactate and glucose in suckling, weanling and adult rats. *Journal of Neurochemistry* 33, 439–445.

Daikhin, Y. and Yudkoff, M. (2000) Compartmentation of brain glutamate metabolism in neurons and glia. *Journal of Nutrition* 130, 1026S–1031S.

Danbolt, N.C. (2001) Glutamate uptake. *Progress in Neurobiology* 65, 1–105.

Dancis, J. (1964) Maple syrup urine disease: a manifestation of an unusual metabolic error. *Clinical Pediatrics* 3, 365–367.

Dancis, J., Levitz, M., Miller, S. and Westall, R.G. (1959) Maple syrup urine disease. *British Medical Journal* 1, 91–93.

Dancis, J., Levitz, M. and Westall, R.G. (1960) Maple syrup urine disease: branched-chain keto-aciduria. *Pediatrics* 25, 72–79.

Danner, D.J. and Doering, C.B. (1998) Human mutations affecting branched chain alpha-ketoacid dehydrogenase. *Frontiers in Bioscience* 3, d517–524.

Danpure, C.J. (2006) Primary hyperoxaluria type 1: AGT mistargeting highlights the fundamental differences between the peroxisomal and mitochondrial protein import pathways. *Biochimica et Biophysica Acta* 1763, 1776–1784.

Davoodi, J., Drown, P.M., Bledsoe, R.K., Wallin, R., Reinhart, G.D. and Hutson, S.M. (1998) Overexpression and characterization of the human mitochondrial and cytosolic branched-chain aminotransferases. *Journal of Biological Chemistry* 273, 4982–4989.

DeRosa, G. and Swick, R.W. (1975) Metabolic implications of the distribution of the alanine aminotransferase isoenzymes. *Journal of Biological Chemistry* 250, 7961–7967.

Dufour, D.R., Lott, J.A., Nolte, F.S., Gretch, D.R., Koff, R.S. and Seeff, L.B. (2000a) Diagnosis and monitoring of hepatic injury. I. Performance characteristics of laboratory tests. *Clinical Chemistry* 46, 2027–2049.

Dufour, D.R., Lott, J.A., Nolte, F.S., Gretch, D.R., Koff, R.S. and Seeff, L.B. (2000b) Diagnosis and monitoring of hepatic injury. II. Recommendations for use of laboratory tests in screening, diagnosis, and monitoring. *Clinical Chemistry* 46, 2050–2068.

Duran, M. and Wadman, S.K. (1985) Thiamine-responsive inborn errors of metabolism. *Journal of Inherited Metabolic Disease* 8, 70–75.

Erecińska, M., Zaleska, M.M., Nelson, D., Nissim, I. and Yudkoff, M. (1990) Neuronal glutamine utilization: glutamine/glutamate homeostasis in synaptosomes. *Journal of Neurochemistry* 54, 2057-2069.

Esclaire, F., Lesort, M., Blanchard, C. and Hugon, J. (1997) Glutamate toxicity enhances tau gene expression in neuronal cultures. *Journal of Neuroscience Research* 49, 309–318.

Fang, J., Nakamura, T., Cho, D.H., Gu, Z. and Lipton, S.A. (2007) S-nitrosylation of peroxiredoxin 2 promotes oxidative stress-induced neuronal cell death in Parkinson's disease. *Proceedings of the National Academy of Sciences of the USA* 104, 18742–18747.

Ferenci, P. (2005) Wilson's Disease. *Clinical Gastroenterology and Hepatology* 3, 726–733.

Gamberino, W.C., Berkich, D.A., Lynch, C.J., Xu, B. and LaNoue, K.F. (1997) Role of pyruvate carboxylase in facilitation of synthesis of glutamate and glutamine in cultured astrocytes. *Journal of Neurochemistry* 69, 2312–2325.

Garcia-Espinosa, M.A., Wallin, R., Hutson, S.M. and Sweatt, A.J. (2007) Widespread neuronal expression of branched-chain aminotransferase in the CNS: implications for leucine/glutamate metabolism and for signaling by amino acids. *Journal of Neurochemistry* 100, 1458–1468.

Giannini, E.G., Botta, F., Fasoli, A., Ceppa, P., Risso, D. and Lantieri, P.B. (1999) Progressive liver functional impairment is associated with an increase in AST/ALT ratio. *Digestive Diseases and Sciences* 44, 1249–1253.

Giannini, E.G., Risso, D., Botta, F., Chiarbonello, B., Fasoli, A. and Malfatti, F. (2003) Validity and clinical utility of the aspartate aminotransferase-alanine aminotransferase ratio in assessing disease severity and prognosis in patients with hepatitis C virus-related chronic liver disease. *Archives of Internal Medicine* 163, 218–224.

Giannini, E.G., Testa, R. and Savarino, V. (2005) Liver enzyme alteration: a guide for clinicians. *Canadian Medical Association Journal* 172, 367–379.

Glinghammar, B., Rafter, I., Lindstrom, A.K., Hedberg, J.J., Andersson, H.B., Lindblom, P., Berg, A.L., *et al.* (2009) Detection of the mitochondrial and catalytically active alanine aminotransferase in human tissues and plasma. *International Journal of Molecular Medicine* 23, 621–631.

Goldberg, A.L. and Chang, T.W. (1978) Regulation and significance of amino acid metabolism in skeletal muscle. *Federation Proceedings* 37, 2301–2307.

Goto, M., Miyahara, I., Hirotsu, K., Conway, M., Yennawar, N., Islam, M.M. and Hutson, S.M. (2005) Structural determinants for branched-chain aminotransferase isozyme-specific inhibition by the anticonvulsant drug gabapentin. *Journal of Biological Chemistry* 280, 37246–37256.

Hall, T.R., Wallin, R., Reinhart, G.D. and Hutson, S.M. (1993) Branched chain aminotransferase isoenzymes. Purification and characterization of the rat brain isoenzyme. *Journal of Biological Chemistry* 268, 3092–3098.

Harper, A.E. and Benjamin, E. (1984) Relationship between intake and rate of oxidation of leucine and alpha-ketoisocaproate in vivo in the rat. *Journal of Nutrition* 114, 431–440.

Harris, R.A., Joshi, M. and Jeoung, N.H. (2004) Mechanisms responsible for regulation of branched-chain amino acid catabolism. *Biochemical and Biophysical Research Communications* 313, 391–396.

Homanics, G.E., Skvorak, K., Ferguson, C., Watkins, S. and Paul, H.S. (2006) Production and characterization of murine models of classic and intermediate maple syrup urine disease. *BMC Medical Genetics* 7, 33.

Hutson, S.M. (1988) Subcellular distribution of branched-chain aminotransferase activity in rat tissues. *Journal of Nutrition* 118, 1475–1481.

Hutson, S.M., Berkich, D., Drown, P., Xu, B., Aschner, M. and LaNoue, K.F. (1998) Role of branched-chain aminotransferase isoenzymes and gabapentin in neurotransmitter metabolism. *Journal of Neurochemistry* 71, 863–874.

Hutson, S.M., Lieth, E. and LaNoue, K.F. (2001) Function of leucine in excitatory neurotransmitter metabolism in the central nervous system. *Journal of Nutrition* 131, 846S–850S.

Hutson, S.M., Poole, L.B., Coles, S. and Conway, M.E. (2009) Redox regulation and trapping sulfenic acid in the peroxide-sensitive human mitochondrial branched chain aminotransferase. *Methods in Molecular Biology* 476, 135–148.

Hutson, S.M., Wallin, R. and Hall, T.R. (1992) Identification of mitochondrial branched chain aminotransferase and its isoforms in rat tissues. *Journal of Biological Chemistry* 267, 15681–15686.

Ichihara, A. and Koyama, E. (1966) Transaminase of branched chain amino acids. I. Branched chain amino acids-alpha-ketoglutarate transaminase. *Journal of Biochemistry* 59, 160–169.

Inagaki, N., Kamisaki, Y., Kiyama, H., Horio, Y., Tohyama, M. and Wada, H. (1985) Immunocytochemical localizations of cytosolic and mitochondrial glutamic oxaloacetic transaminase isozymes in rat retina as markers for the glutamate-aspartate neuronal system. *Brain Research* 325, 336–339.

Inagaki, N., Kamisaki, Y., Kiyama, H., Horio, Y., Tohyama, M. and Wada, H. (1987) Immunocytochemical localizations of cytosolic and mitochondrial glutamic oxaloacetic transaminase isozymes in rat primary sensory neurons as a marker for the glutamate neuronal system. *Brain Research* 402, 197–200.

Ivanov, V.I. and Karpeisky, M.Y. (1969) Dynamic three-dimensional model for enzymic transamination. *Advances in Enzymology and Related Areas of Molecular Biology* 32, 21–53.

Jadhao, S.B., Yang, R.Z., Lin, Q., Hu, H., Anania, F.A., Shuldiner, A.R. and Gong, D.W. (2004) Murine alanine aminotransferase: cDNA cloning, functional expression, and differential gene regulation in mouse fatty liver. *Hepatology* 39, 1297–1302.

Jansonius, J.N. (1998) Structure, evolution and action of vitamin B6-dependent enzymes. *Current Opinion in Structural Biology* 8, 759–769.

Jansonius, J.N., Eichele, G., Ford, G.C., Kirsch, J.F., Picot, D., Thaller, C., Vincent, M.G., et al. (1984a) Crystallographic studies on the mechanism of action of mitochondrial aspartate aminotransferase. *Progress in Clinical and Biological Research* 144B, 195–203.

Jansonius, J.N., Eichele, G., Ford, G.C., Kirsch, J.F., Picot, D., Thaller, C., Vincent, M.G., et al. (1984b) Three-dimensional structure of mitochondrial aspartate aminotransferase and some functional derivatives: implications for its mode of action. *Biochemical Society Transactions* 12, 424–427.

Kamisaki, Y., Inagaki, S., Tohyama, M., Horio, Y. and Wada, H. (1984) Immunocytochemical localizations of cytosolic and mitochondrial glutamic oxaloacetic transaminase isozymes in rat brain. *Brain Research* 297, 363–368.

Kanamori, K., Ross, B.D. and Kondrat, R.W. (1998) Rate of glutamate synthesis from leucine in rat brain measured in vivo by 15N NMR. *Journal of Neurochemistry* 70, 1304–1315.

Kaplan, D.R. and Miller, F.D. (1997) Signal transduction by the neurotrophin receptors. *Current Opinion in Cell Biology* 9, 213–221.

Karpeisky, M.Y. and Ivanov, V.I. (1966) A molecular mechanism for enzymatic transamination. *Nature* 210, 493–496.

Kelly, A. and Stanley, C.A. (2001) Disorders of glutamate metabolism. *Mental Retardation and Developmental Disabilities Research Reviews* 7, 287–295.

Kirsch, J.F., Eichele, G., Ford, G.C., Vincent, M.G., Jansonius, J.N., Gehring, H. and Christen, P. (1984) Mechanism of action of aspartate aminotransferase proposed on the basis of its spatial structure. *Journal of Molecular Biology* 174, 497–525.

Klivenyi, P., Starkov, A.A., Calingasan, N.Y., Gardian, G., Browne, S.E., Yang, L., Bubber, P., *et al.* (2004) Mice deficient in dihydrolipoamide dehydrogenase show increased vulnerability to MPTP, malonate and 3-nitropropionic acid neurotoxicity. *Journal of Neurochemistry* 88, 1352–1360.

Knight, J.A. (2005) Liver function tests: their role in the diagnosis of hepatobiliary diseases. *Journal of Infusion Nursing* 28, 108–117.

Krawitt, E.L. (1996) Autoimmune hepatitis. *New England Journal of Medicine* 334, 897–903.

Lai, J.C., Sheu, K.F., Kim, Y.T., Clarke, D.D. and Blass, J.P. (1986) The subcellular localization of glutamate dehydrogenase (GDH): is GDH a marker for mitochondria in brain? *Neurochemical Research* 11, 733–744.

Lai, J.C., Walsh, J.M., Dennis, S.C., and Clarke, J.B. (1977) Synaptic and non-synaptic mitochondrial water as detected by 1H NMR. *Journal of Neurochemistry* 28, 625–631.

LaNoue, K.F., Berkich, D.A., Conway, M., Barber, A.J., Hu, L.Y., Taylor, C. and Hutson, S. (2001) Role of specific aminotransferases in de novo glutamate synthesis and redox shuttling in the retina. *Journal of Neuroscience Research* 66, 914–922.

Leong, S.F. and Clark, J.B. (1984) Regional development of glutamate dehydrogenase in the rat brain. *Journal of Neurochemistry* 43, 106–111.

Lieth, E., LaNoue, K.F., Berkich, D.A., Xu, B., Ratz, M., Taylor, C. and Hutson, S.M. (2001) Nitrogen shuttling between neurons and glial cells during glutamate synthesis. *Journal of Neurochemistry* 76, 1712–1723.

Lin, H.M., Kaneshige, M., Zhao, L., Zhang, X., Hanover, J.A. and Cheng, S.Y. (2001) An isoform of branched-chain aminotransferase is a novel co-repressor for thyroid hormone nuclear receptors. *The Journal of Biological Chemistry* 276, 48196–48205.

Lindblom, P., Rafter, I., Copley, C., Andersson, U., Hedberg, J.J., Berg, A.L., Samuelsson, A., *et al.* (2007) Isoforms of alanine aminotransferases in human tissues and serum–differential tissue expression using novel antibodies. *Archives of Biochemistry and Biophysics* 466, 66–77.

Lipton, S.A., Gu, Z. and Nakamura, T. (2007) Inflammatory mediators leading to protein misfolding and uncompetitive/fast off-rate drug therapy for neurodegenerative disorders. *International Review of Neurobiology* 82, 1–27.

Madeddu, F., Naska, S., Menna, E., Chiellini, C., Sweatt, A.J., Hutson, S.M., Benzi, L., *et al.* (2004) Intraocular delivery of BDNF following visual cortex lesion upregulates cytosolic branched chain aminotransferase (BCATc) in the rat dorsal lateral geniculate nucleus. *European Journal of Neuroscience* 20, 580–586.

Magistretti, P.J. (2009) Role of glutamate in neuron-glia metabolic coupling. *American Journal of Clinical Nutrition* 90, 875S–880S.

Mattson, M.P. (2003) Excitotoxic and excitoprotective mechanisms: abundant targets for the prevention and treatment of neurodegenerative disorders. *Neuromolecular Medicine* 3, 65–94.

Mattson, M.P. (2007) Calcium and neurodegeneration. *Aging Cell* 6, 337–350.

Mattson, M.P. (2008) Glutamate and neurotrophic factors in neuronal plasticity and disease. *Annals of the New York Academy of Sciences* 1144, 97–112.

Mattson, M.P. and Chan, S.L. (2003) Neuronal and glial calcium signaling in Alzheimer's disease. *Cell Calcium* 34, 385–397.

McKenna, M.C. (2007) The glutamate-glutamine cycle is not stoichiometric: fates of glutamate in brain. *Journal of Neuroscience Research* 85, 3347–3358.

McKenna, M.C., Tildon, J.T., Stevenson, J.H., Boatright, R. and Huang, X. (1993) Regulation of energy metabolism in synaptic terminals and cultured rat brain astrocytes: differences revealed using aminooxyacetate. *Developmental Neuroscience* 15, 320–329.

McKenna, M.C., Sonnewald, U., Huang, X., Stevenson, J. and Zielke, H.R. (1996a) Exogenous glutamate concentration regulates the metabolic fate of glutamate in astrocytes. *Journal of Neurochemistry* 66, 386–393.

McKenna, M.C., Tildon, J.T., Stevenson, J.H. and Huang, X. (1996b) New insights into the compartmentation of glutamate and glutamine in cultured rat brain astrocytes. *Developmental Neuroscience* 18, 380–390.

McKenna, M.C., Stevenson, J.H., Huang, X. and Hopkins, I.B. (2000a) Differential distribution of the enzymes glutamate dehydrogenase and aspartate aminotransferase in cortical synaptic mitochondria contributes to metabolic compartmentation in cortical synaptic terminals. *Neurochemistry International* 37, 229–241.

McKenna, M.C., Stevenson, J.H., Huang, X., Tildon, J.T., Zielke, C.L. and Hopkins, I.B. (2000b) Mitochondrial malic enzyme activity is much higher in mitochondria from cortical synaptic terminals compared with mitochondria from primary cultures of cortical neurons or cerebellar granule cells. *Neurochemistry International* 36, 451–459.

McKenna, M.C., Hopkins, I.B., Lindauer, S.L. and Bamford, P. (2006) Aspartate aminotransferase in synaptic and nonsynaptic mitochondria: differential effect of compounds that influence transient hetero-enzyme complex (metabolon) formation. *Neurochemistry International* 48, 629–636.

Mehta, P.K. and Christen, P. (2000) The molecular evolution of pyridoxal-5'-phosphate-dependent enzymes. *Advances in Enzymology and Related Areas of Molecular Biology* 74, 129–184.

Menkes, J.H. (1962) Maple syrup disease and other disorders of keto acid metabolism. *Research Publications – Association for Research in Nervous and Mental Disease* 40, 69–93.

Menkes, J.H. (1959) Maple syrup disease; isolation and identification of organic acids in the urine. *Pediatrics* 23, 348–353.

Morrison, E.D. and Kowdley, K.V. (2000) Genetic liver disease in adults. Early recognition of the three most common causes. *Postgraduate Medicine* 107, 147–152, 155, 158–159.

Nakamura, T. and Lipton, S.A. (2007) Molecular mechanisms of nitrosative stress-mediated protein misfolding in neurodegenerative diseases. *Cellular and Molecular Life Sciences* 13, 1609–1620.

Nakamura, T. and Lipton, S.A. (2008) Emerging roles of S-nitrosylation in protein misfolding and neurodegenerative diseases. *Antioxidants & Redox Signaling* 10, 87–101.

Nakamura, T. and Lipton, S.A. (2009) Cell death: protein misfolding and neurodegenerative diseases. *Apoptosis* 14, 455–468.

Nguyen, N.H., Bråthe, A. and Hassel, B. (2003) Neuronal uptake and metabolism of glycerol and the neuronal expression of mitochondrial glycerol-3-phosphate dehydrogenase. *Journal of Neurochemistry* 85, 831–842.

Numakawa, T., Kumamaru, E., Adachi, N., Yagasaki, Y., Izumi, A. and Kunugi, H. (2009) Glucocorticoid receptor interaction with TrkB promotes BDNF-triggered PLC-gamma signaling for glutamate release via a glutamate transporter. *Proceedings of the National Academy of Sciences of the USA* 106, 647–652.

Numakawa, T., Yamagishi, S., Adachi, N., Matsumoto, T., Yokomaku, D., Yamada, M. and Hatanaka, H. (2002) Brain-derived neurotrophic factor-induced potentiation of Ca(2+) oscillations in developing cortical neurons. *Journal of Biological Chemistry* 277, 6520–6529.

Oldendorf, W.H. (1973) Stereospecificity of blood-brain barrier permeability to amino acids. *American Journal of Physiology* 224, 967–969.

Oz, G., Berkich, D.A., Henry, P.G., Xu, Y., LaNoue, K., Hutson, S.M. and Gruetter, R. (2004) Neuroglial metabolism in the awake rat brain: CO_2 fixation increases with brain activity. *Journal of Neuroscience* 24, 11273–11279.

Palaiologos, G., Hertz, L. and Schousboe, A. (1988) Evidence that aspartate aminotransferase activity and ketodicarboxylate carrier function are essential for biosynthesis of transmitter glutamate. *Journal of Neurochemistry* 51, 317–320.

Panteghini, M. (1990) Aspartate aminotransferase isoenzymes. *Clinical Biochemistry* 23, 311–319.

Pellerin, L. (2003) Lactate as a pivotal element in neuron-glia metabolic cooperation. *Neurochemistry International* 43, 331–338.

Pellerin, L. and Magistretti, P.J. (1994) Glutamate uptake into astrocytes stimulates aerobic glycolysis: a mechanism coupling neuronal activity to glucose utilization. *Proceedings of the National Academy of Sciences of the USA* 91, 10625–10629.

Pellerin, L., Pellegri, G., Bittar, P.G., Charnay, Y., Bouras, C., Martin, J.L., Stella, N. and Magistretti, P.J. (1998) Evidence supporting the existence of an activity-dependent astrocyte-neuron lactate shuttle. *Developmental Neuroscience* 20, 291–299.

Peng, L. Zhang, X. and Hertz, L. (1994) Alteration in oxidative metabolism of alanine in cerebellar granule cell cultures as a consequence of the development of the ability to utilize alanine as an amino group donor for synthesis of transmitter glutamate. *Brain Research Development Research* 79, 128–131.

Plaitakis, A., Berl, S. and Yahr, M.D. (1982) Abnormal glutamate metabolism in an adult-onset degenerative neurological disorder. *Science* 216, 193–196.

Ramos, M., del Arco, A., Pardo, B., Martinez-Serrano, A., Martinez-Morales, J.R., Kobayashi, K., Yasuda, T., et al. (2003) Developmental changes in the Ca2+-regulated mitochondrial aspartate-glutamate carrier aralar1 in brain and prominent expression in the spinal cord. *Brain Research. Developmental Brain Research* 143, 33–46.

Rosalki, S.B., Tarlow, D. and Rau, D. (1971) Plasma gamma-glutamyl transpeptidase elevation in patients receiving enzyme-inducing drugs. *Lancet* 2, 376–377.

Rutten, E.P., Engelen, M.P., Schols, A.M. and Deutz, N.E. (2005) Skeletal muscle glutamate metabolism in health and disease: state of the art. *Current opinion in Clinical Nutrition and Metabolic Care* 8, 41–51.

Safer, H. and Williamson, J.R. (1972) Functional significance of the malate-aspartate shuttle for the oxidation of cytoplasmic reducing equivalents in rat heart. *Recent Advances in Studies on Cardiac Structure and Metabolism* 1, 34–43.

Salzmann, D., Christen, P., Mehta, P.K. and Sandmeier, E. (2000) Rates of evolution of pyridoxal-5'-phosphate-dependent enzymes. *Biochemical and Biophysical Research Communications* 270, 576–580.

Sattler, R. and Tymianski, M. (2000) Molecular mechanisms of calcium-dependent excitotoxicity. *Journal of Molecular Medicine* 78, 3–13.

Schneider, G., Kack, H. and Lindqvist, Y. (2000) The manifold of vitamin B6 dependent enzymes. *Structure* 8, R1–6.

Scholz, T.D., Koppenhafer, S.L., ten Eyck, C.J. and Schutte, B.C. (1998) Ontogeny of malate-aspartate shuttle capacity and gene expression in cardiac mitochondria. *American Journal of Physiology* 274, C780–788.

Schousboe, A. and Waagepetersen, H.S. (2005) Role of astrocytes in glutamate homeostasis: implications for excitotoxicity. *Neurotoxicity Research* 8, 221–225.

Schousboe, A., Westergaard, N., Waagepetersen, H.S., Larsson, O.M., Bakken, I.J. and Sonnewald, U. (1997) Trafficking between glia and neurons of TCA cycle intermediates and related metabolites. *Glia* 21, 99–105.

Schurr, A., Payne, R.S., Miller, J.J. and Rigor, B.M. (1997a) Glia are the main source of lactate utilized by neurons for recovery of function posthypoxia. *Brain Research* 774, 221–224.

Schurr, A., Payne, R.S., Miller, J.J. and Rigor, B.M. (1997b) Brain lactate is an obligatory aerobic energy substrate for functional recovery after hypoxia: further in vitro validation. *Journal of Neurochemistry* 69, 423–266.

Schurr, A., Payne, R.S., Miller, J.J. and Rigor, B.M. (1997c) Brain lactate, not glucose, fuels the recovery of synaptic function from hypoxia upon reoxygenation: an in vitro study. *Brain Research* 744, 105–111.

Seeto, R.K., Fenn, B. and Rockey, D.C. (2000) Ischemic hepatitis: clinical presentation and pathogenesis. *American Journal of Medicine* 109, 109–113.

Shank, R.P. and Aprison, M.H. (1981 Present status and significance of the glutamine cycle in neural tissues. *Life Sciences* 18, 837–842.

Shank, R.P., Bennett, G.S., Freytag, S.O. and Campbell, G.L. (1985) Pyruvate carboxylase: an astrocyte-specific enzyme implicated in the replenishment of amino acid neurotransmitter pools. *Brain Research* 329, 364–367.

Silberman, J., Dancis, J. and Feigin, I. (1961) Neuropathological observations in maple syrup urine disease: branched-chain ketoaciduria. *Archives of Neurology* 5, 351–363.

Singer, A.J., Carracio, T.R. and Mofenson, H.C. (1995) The temporal profile of increased transaminase levels in patients with acetaminophen-induced liver dysfunction. *Annals of Emergency Medicine* 26, 49–53.

Smith, Q.R., Momma, S., Aoyagi, M. and Rapoport, S.I. (1987) Kinetics of neutral amino acid transport across the blood-brain barrier. *Journal of Neurochemistry* 49, 1651–1658.

Snyderman, S.E. (1986) Dietary and genetic therapy of inborn errors of metabolism: a summary. *Annals of the New York Academy of Sciences* 477, 231–236.

Snyderman, S.E. (1988) Treatment outcome of maple syrup urine disease. *Acta Paediatrica Japonica* 30, 417–424.

Sohocki, M.M., Sullivan, L.S., Harrison, W.R., Sodergren, E.J., Elder, F.F., Weinstock, G., Tanase, S., *et al.* (1997) Human glutamate pyruvate transaminase (GPT): localization to 8q24.3, cDNA and genomic sequences, and polymorphic sites. *Genomics* 40, 247–252.

Sonnewald, U., Westergaard, N., Petersen, S.B., Unsgard, G. and Schousboe, A. (1993) Metabolism of [U-13C]glutamate in astrocytes studied by 13C NMR spectroscopy: incorporation of more label into lactate than into glutamine demonstrates the importance of the tricarboxylic acid cycle. *Journal of Neurochemistry* 61, 1179–1182.

Stremmel, W., Diede, H.E., Rodilla-Sala, E., Vyska, K., Schrader, M., Fitscher, B. and Passarella, S. (1990) The membrane fatty acid-binding protein is not identical to mitochondrial glutamic oxaloacetic transaminase (mGOT). *Molecular and Cellular Biochemistry* 98, 191–199.

Stump, D.D., Zhou, S.L. and Berk, P.D. (1993) Comparison of plasma membrane FABP and mitochondrial isoform of aspartate aminotransferase from rat liver. *The American Journal of Physiology* 265, G894–902.

Suryawan, A., Hawes, J.W., Harris, R.A., Shimomura, Y., Jenkins, A.E. and Hutson, S.M. (1998) A molecular model of human branched-chain amino acid metabolism. *American Journal of Clinical Nutrition* 68, 72–81.

Sweatt, A.J., Garcia-Espinosa, M.A., Wallin, R. and Hutson, S.M. (2004a) Branched-chain amino acids and neurotransmitter metabolism: expression of cytosolic branched-chain aminotransferase (BCATc) in the cerebellum and hippocampus. *The Journal of Comparative Neurology* 477, 360–370.

Sweatt, A.J., Wood, M., Suryawan, A., Wallin, R., Willingham, M.C. and Hutson, S.M. (2004b) Branched-chain amino acid catabolism: unique segregation of pathway enzymes in organ systems and peripheral nerves. *American Journal of Physiology Endocrinology and Metabolism* 286, E64–76.

Tanaka, K., Watase, K., Manabe, T., Yamada, K., Wantanabe, M. and Attwell, D. (1997) Epilepsy and exacerbation of brain injury in mice lacking the glutamate transporter GLT-1. *Science* 276, 1699–1702.

Taylor, R.T. and Jenkins, W.T. (1966a) Leucine aminotransferase. 3. Activation by beta-mercaptoethanol. *Journal of Biological Chemistry* 241, 4406–4410.

Taylor, R.T. and Jenkins, W.T. (1966b) Leucine aminotransferase. I. Colorimetric assays. *Journal of Biological Chemistry* 241, 4391–4395.

Taylor, R.T. and Jenkins, W.T. (1966c) Leucine aminotransferase. II. Purification and characterization. *Journal of Biological Chemistry* 241, 4396–4405.

Teller, J.K., Fahien, L.A. and Valdivia, E. (1990) Interactions among mitochondrial aspartate aminotransferase, malate dehydrogenase, and the inner mitochondrial membrane from heart, hepatoma, and liver. *Journal of Biological Chemistry* 265, 19486–19494.

Than, N.G., Sumegi, B., Than, G.N., Bellyei, S. and Bohn, H. (2001) Molecular cloning and characterization of placental tissue protein 18 (PP18a)/human mitochondrial branched-chain aminotransferase (BCATm) and its novel alternatively spliced PP18b variant. *Placenta* 22, 235–243.

Tildon, J.T., Roeder, L.M., and Stevenson, J.H. (1985) Substrate oxidation by isolated rat brain mitochondria and synaptosomes. *Journal of Neuroscience Research* 14, 207–215.

Uehara, T., Nakamura, T., Yao, D., Shi, Z.Q., Gu, Z., Ma, Y., Masliah, E., *et al.* (2006) S-nitrosylated protein-disulphide isomerase links protein misfolding to neurodegeneration. *Nature* 441, 513–517.

Waagepetersen, H.S., Sonnewald, U., Larsson, O.M. and Schousboe, A. (2000) A possible role of alanine for ammonia transfer between astrocytes and glutamatergic neurons. *Journal of Neurochemistry* 75, 471–479.

Williams, A.L. and Hoofnagle, J.H. (1988) Ratio of serum aspartate to alanine aminotransferase in chronic heptatis. Realtionship to cirrhosis. *Gastroenterology* 95, 734–739.

Wu, J.Y., Kao, H.J., Li, S.C., Stevens, R., Hillman, S., Millington, D. and Chen, Y.T. (2004) ENU mutagenesis identifies mice with mitochondrial branched-chain aminotransferase deficiency resembling human maple syrup urine disease. *Journal of Clinical Investigation* 113, 434–440.

Xu, Y., Ola, M.S., Berkich, D.A., Gardner, T.W., Barber, A.J., Palmieri, F., Hutson, S.M. *et al.* (2007) Energy sources for glutamate neurotransmission in the retina: absence of the aspartate/glutamate carrier produces reliance on glycolysis in glia. *Journal of Neurochemistry* 101, 120–131.

Yang, K.S., Kang, S.W., Woo, H.A., Hwang, S.C., Chae, H.Z., Kim, K. and Rhee, S.G. (2002a) Inactivation of human peroxiredoxin I during catalysis as the result of the oxidation of the catalytic site cysteine to cysteine-sulfinic acid. *Journal of Biological Chemistry* 277, 38029–38036.

Yang, R.Z., Blaileanu, G., Hansen, B.C., Shuldiner, A.R. and Gong, D.W. (2002b) cDNA cloning, genomic structure, chromosomal mapping, and functional expression of a novel human alanine aminotransferase. *Genomics* 79, 445–450.

Yang, R.Z., Park, S., Reagan, W.J., Goldstein, R., Zhong, S., Lawton, M., Rajamohan, F., *et al.* (2009) Alanine aminotransferase isoenzymes: molecular cloning and quantitative analysis of tissue expression in rats and serum elevation in liver toxicity. *Hepatology* 49, 598–607.

Yao, D., Gu, Z., Nakamura, T., Shi, Z.Q., Ma, Y., Gaston, B., Palmer, L.A., *et al.* (2004) Nitrosative stress linked to sporadic Parkinson's disease: S-nitrosylation of parkin regulates its E3 ubiquitin ligase activity. *Proceedings of the National Academy of Sciences of the USA* 101, 10810–10814.

Yennawar, N.H., Conway, M.E., Yennawar, H.P., Farber, G.K. and Hutson, S.M. (2002) Crystal structures of human mitochondrial branched chain aminotransferase reaction intermediates: ketimine and pyridoxamine phosphate forms. *Biochemistry* 41, 11592–11601.

Yennawar, N.H., Islam, M.M., Conway, M., Wallin, R. and Hutson, S.M. (2006) Human mitochondrial branched chain aminotransferase isozyme: Structural role of the CXXC center in catalysis. *Journal of Biological Chemistry* 281, 39660–39671.

Yoshimura, T., Jhee, K.H. and Soda, K. (1996) Stereospecificity for the hydrogen transfer and molecular evolution of pyridoxal enzymes. *Bioscience, Biotechnology, and Biochemistry* 60, 181–187.

Yudkoff, M. (1997) Brain metabolism of branched-chain amino acids. *Glia*, 21, 92–98.

Yudkoff, M., Nissim, I. and Pleasure, D. (1988) Astrocyte metabolism of [15N]glutamine: implications for the glutamine-glutamate cycle. Journal of Neurochemistry 51, 843–850.

Yudkoff, M., Nissim, I. and Hertz, L. (1990) Precursors of glutamic acid nitrogen in primary neuronal cultures: studies with 15N. *Neurochemical Research* 15, 1191–1196.

Yudkoff, M., Nissim, I., Daikhin, Y., Lin, Z.P., Nelson, D., Pleasure, D. and Erecinska, M. (1993) Brain glutamate metabolism: neuronal-astroglial relationships. *Developmental Neuroscience* 15, 343–350.

Yudkoff, M., Daikhin, Y., Nissim, I., Pleasure, D., Stern, J. and Nissim, I. (1994) Inhibition of astrocyte glutamine production by alpha-ketoisocaproic acid. *Journal of Neurochemistry* 63, 1508–1515.

Yudkoff, M., Daikhin, Y., Grunstein, L., Nissim, I., Stern, J., Pleasure, D. and Nissim, I. (1996a) Astrocyte leucine metabolism: significance of branched-chain amino acid transamination. *Journal of Neurochemistry* 66, 378–385.

Yudkoff, M., Daikhin, Y., Nelson, D., Nissim, I. and Erecinska, M. (1996b) Neuronal metabolism of branched-chain amino acids: flux through the aminotransferase pathway in synaptosomes. *Journal of Neurochemistry* 66, 2136–2145.

Zinnanti, W.J., Lazovic, J., Griffin, K., Skvorak, K.J., Paul, H.S., Homanics, G.E., Bewley, M.C., *et al.* (2009) Dual mechanism of brain injury and novel treatment strategy in maple syrup urine disease. *Brain* 132, 903–918.

3 Arginase

R.W. Caldwell,[1]* S. Chandra[1] and R.B. Caldwell[2]
[1]*Department of Pharmacology and Toxicology;*
[2]*Vascular Biology Center, Medical College of Georgia, Augusta, USA*

3.1 Abstract

Arginase is one of the several enzymes that metabolize the semi-essential amino acid, L-arginine. The other enzymes which metabolize L-arginine include:

1. Nitric oxide synthase (NO production).
2. Arginyl-tRNA synthetase (protein production).
3. Arginine:glycine aminotransferase (creatine production).
4. Arginine decarboxylase (agmatine production).

Of special note is the competition between arginase and nitric oxide synthase (NOS) for L-arginine. This has been a growing focal point for biomedical research in recent years, because a change in the balance can vastly affect cellular function.

Arginase is distributed in tissue throughout the body in two isoforms and has functions in both health and disease. Arginase converts L-arginine into urea and ornithine – in many tissues ornithine can be further metabolized to polyamines, proline and glutamate. These products have important biological functions. Arginase function in the liver is extremely important. It is part of a cycle which releases urea and produces ornithine, which then accepts hepatic metabolites of NH_3 in the production of citrulline, the precursor of L-arginine. This hepatic urea cycle is essential for ridding the body of toxic NH_3 via the release of urea. Arginase also is beneficial in wound healing and neuroprotection/regeneration. Arginase also has key functions in a number of disease states. These prominently include vascular and endothelial dysfunctions associated with diabetes, hypertension, sickle cell disease, ischaemia/reperfusion injury, atherosclerosis and erectile dysfunction. Other diseases involving elevated arginase activity are asthma, nephropathy, cancer, and parasitic infections.

Stimuli that increase arginase activity/expression include reactive oxygen species, inflammatory cytokines and humoral factors, including angiotensin II and thrombin. Studies of signal transduction mechanisms and development of inhibitors of the activation processes are under way with the goal of limiting arginase function to physiological levels.

3.2 Introduction

Arginase is the hydrolytic enzyme that converts L-arginine to urea and ornithine

* E-mail address: wcaldwel@mail.mcg.edu

(Fig. 3.1). In the liver, this enzyme is a key element of the urea cycle. This cycle removes toxic ammonia, formed through protein catabolism, by processing it along with ornithine via carbamoyl phosphate synthase-1 (CPS-1) and ornithine carbamoyltransferase (OCT) into L-citrulline. L-citrulline can be recycled back to L-arginine by argininosuccinate synthase (ASS) and argininosuccinate lyase (ASL) to complete the urea cycle (Osowska et al., 2004). However, most non-hepatic tissues do not have the complete urea cycle, because they lack OCT or CPS-1 (Fig. 3.2).

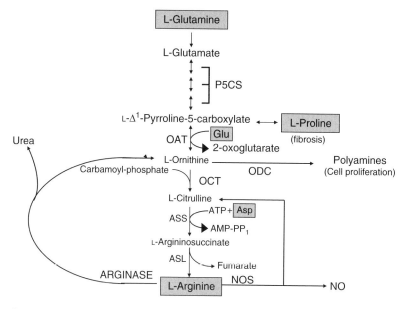

Fig. 3.1. Scheme for synthesis of L-arginine from L-glutamine. Also shown are catabolism of L-arginine to L-ornithine/urea or L-citrulline/NO, production of polyamines, and anabolism and catabolism of proline. ASL, argininosuccinate lyase; ASS, argininosuccinate synthase; Asp, aspartate; NOS, nitric oxide synthase; OAT, ornithine aminotransferase; ODC, ornithine decarboxylase; OCT, orthinine carbamoyltransferase; P5CS, pyrroline-5-carboxylate synthase.

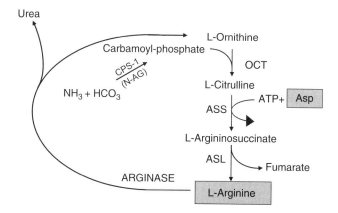

Fig. 3.2. Scheme shows the urea cycle, which is partially included in Fig. 3.1. Note the entry of ammonia (NH_3) into the cycle through the synthesis of carbamoyl-PO4. Abbreviations in addition to those given for Fig. 3.1: CPS-1, carbamoylphosphate synthase-1; N-AG, N-acetylglutamate.

When activated, arginase can compete with NOS for their common substrate, the semi-essential amino acid L-arginine. Decreases in L-arginine availability to NOS can lead to decreased production of NO, and possible NOS uncoupling and increased superoxide formation (White *et al.*, 2006; Romero *et al.*, 2008). These effects and characteristics of arginase can be of pathological importance when its activity and expression are elevated as in disease states such as hypertension and vascular complications of diabetes. In these situations, there is impaired endothelial-dependent vasorelaxation, proliferation of vascular smooth muscle cells, and vascular and perivascular fibrosis (Yang and Ming, 2006). Arginase activity and expression can be enhanced by inflammatory processes and reactive oxygen species associated with disease states.

Ornithine synthesis by arginase in the cytosol leads primarily to the formation of polyamines (putrescine, spermidine, and spermine) via ornithine decarboxylase (ODC) and to the formation of proline via ornithine aminotransferase (OAT). While the actions of polyamines are not completely understood, they are known to be germinally involved in cell cycling and proliferation, but are also implicated in cell death under some conditions (Durante *et al.*, 1998; Li *et al.*, 2001). Proline is essential in collagen synthesis and its organization into fibrous protein structure (Li *et al.*, 2001).

Polyamines are important for processes such as neural development, wound healing and tissue regeneration (Lange *et al.*, 2004) Proline formation and the synthesis of collagen are necessary for wound repair and structural integrity of some tissues (Witte and Barbul, 2003). However, excessive enhancement of these pathways can lead to thickened and stiff blood vessels and airways, hypertrophied and fibrotic hearts and kidneys, growth of cancers and toxicity in some neural cells.

3.3 Isoforms and Distribution

Arginase exists as two isoforms, arginase I and arginase II. Arginase I is a cytosolic enzyme that constitutes a majority of total body arginase activity. It is strongly expressed in the liver and is central to the urea cycle (Morris, 2002). Arginase II is a mitochondrial enzyme expressed primarily in extra-hepatic tissues, especially in the kidney (Miyanaka *et al.*, 1998), but is also found in other tissues. Both arginase I and II have been found in endothelial cells (Romero *et al.*, 2006; Marinova *et al.*, 2008; Romero *et al.*, 2008) while only arginase I has been described in vascular smooth muscle cells (Wei *et al.*, 2000; Topal *et al.*, 2006; White *et al.*, 2006).

Arginase activation provides substrate ornithine for the ornithine decarboxylase (ODC) pathway, producing polyamines which are important in cellular growth and migration and can contribute to cellular hypertrophy and hyperplasia (Liang *et al.*, 2004). In some cases, it is arginase rather than ODC which limits polyamine synthesis (Li *et al.*, 2001; Wei *et al.*, 2001). Arginase II plays a role in the production of proline, a critical component of collagen, through the ornithine aminotransferase (OAT)/pyrroline-5-carboxylate reductase (P5CR) pathway (Durante *et al.*, 2001; Li *et al.*, 2001). Therefore, elevated arginase activity is associated with excess cell growth and collagen accumulation – fibrosis.

3.4 Structure and Location of Arginase

Arginase I and II share 58% homology (Munder, 2009). Human arginase I consists of 322 amino acids and was cloned more than 20 years ago (Dizikes *et al.*, 1986) whereas arginase II was cloned in 1996 and has 354 amino acids (Gotoh *et al.*, 1996). The gene for human arginase I is mapped on chromosome 6q23 (Sparkes *et al.*, 1986) and for arginase II on chromosome 14q24.1–24.3 (Gotoh *et al.*, 1997). High-resolution crystal structures have been determined for arginase I and for arginase II. Each identical subunit of the trimeric enzyme contains an active site at the bottom of a 15 Å deep cleft. Mn(II) ions are located at the bottom of this cleft, separated by approximately 3.3 Å and bridged by oxygen derived from two aspartic acid residues and a solvent-derived hydroxide. This metal bridging is proposed to be the nucleophile that attacks the guanidinium carbon of substrate arginine. Liver arginase is a 105 kDa homotrimer, and each subunit (35 kDa) contains a binuclear Mn(II) centre that is critical for catalytic activity. The overall fold of each subunit belongs to the α/β family, consisting of a parallel, eight-stranded β-sheet flanked on both sides by numerous α-helices (Ash, 2004).

3.5 Involvement of Arginase in Health and Disease

3.5.1 Arginase in health

3.5.1.1 Ammonia detoxification

The urea cycle in liver removes excess ammonia from the body accumulated through dietary sources or due to breakdown of endogenous protein. Various enzymes involved in the urea cycle convert ammonia nitrogen to urea which is non-toxic, more water-soluble, and easily excreted through the kidney in the form of urine. Hyperammonaemia results from deregulation of urea cycle enzymes including N-acetylglutamate synthase (N-AGS), carbamyl phosphate synthetase I (CPS-I), ornithine transcarbamylase (OTC), argininosuccinate synthetase (AS), argininosuccinate lyase (AL) and arginase (Deignan et al., 2008) (see urea cycle in Fig. 3.2). Patients with urea cycle disorder are healthy at birth but develop pathological symptoms progressively. Patients with complete CPS-I or OTC deficiency show symptoms of hyperammonaemia during the first few days of life; patients with AS or AL deficiency develop symptoms during the first month; and patients with ARG deficiency usually present later in childhood (Grody et al., 1993). Deficiency in arginase I, the last enzyme in the urea cycle, causes more severe form of hyperammonaemia. If left untreated, ammonia toxicity manifests as seizures, mental disorders, and early morbidity (Deignan et al., 2008). Arginase deficiency is diagnosed by elevated plasma levels of arginine compared to the lack of any of the other enzymes in the urea cycle, which reduce plasma arginine levels.

Of the two isoforms, arginase I deletion in the mouse model has been associated with hyperammonaemia, decerebrate posture, encephalopathy, tremors in the extremities and death within 10–12 days after birth (Iyer et al., 2002). Arginase II knockout mice do not present any pathological abnormalities. Recently a study showed that arginase II knockout mice displayed hypertension though it was correlated to an up-regulation of sympathetic tone (Huynh et al., 2009a). Treatment of patients with arginase I deficiency involves reduction of protein intake, dietary supplementation with all essential amino acids other than arginine, haemodialysis and in severe cases orthotropic liver transplant and gene replacement therapy (Deignan et al., 2008).

3.5.1.2 Wound healing

The first/acute phase in tissue injury involves oxidative insult through generation of reactive oxygen species (ROS) and reactive nitrogen species (RNS) from the resident macrophages through up-regulation of inducible nitric oxide synthase (iNOS). This helps in eradication of pathogens (Satriano, 2004). Next is the repair phase wherein arginase converts L-arginine to L-ornithine and urea. L-ornithine is further metabolized to form proline via ornithine aminotransferase (OAT) and polyamines via ornithine decarboxylase (ODC). Both of these pathways are essential for wound healing owing to their potential effects on collagen synthesis and cell proliferation. It is reported that arginase activity/expression is strongly induced three to five days post injury (Kampfer et al., 2003). Moreover, supplementation of L-arginine has been shown to enhance wound healing in arginine-depleted animals, as well as in rats with normal dietary intake of arginine (Witte and Barbul, 2003). This response is associated with an accumulation of hydroxyproline, a key constituent of collagen synthesis. Polyamines (putrescine, spermidine and spermine) are required for cell proliferation and homeostasis. Induction or overexpression of arginase I has been shown to cause proliferation of rat aortic smooth muscle cells through increased production of polyamines (Wei et al., 2001). A critical balance between rate of consumption of L-arginine by iNOS

(NO production) and arginase (polyamine and collagen synthesis) determines the course of wound repair.

3.5.1.3 Neuroprotection/regeneration

Arginase has been reported to play important roles in neuroprotection and neural regeneration (Esch *et al.*, 1998; Lange *et al.*, 2004). In a model of enhanced oxidant stress (glutathione depletion) and neuronal cell death, arginase I application was found to be protective, seemingly via depletion of L-arginine and inhibition of protein synthesis. Further, it was protective against several other stimuli which induce apoptosis. Also, a number of studies have shown that up-regulation of arginase I expression can promote axonal regeneration. In one study, acidic fibroblast growth factor along with nerve grafts improved locomotor function after spinal transaction (Kuo *et al.*, 2007). This treatment resulted in a large rise in levels of spermine and arginase I protein in area motor neurons and macrophages. Similar results have been seen by making a small lesion in neuron branches or elevating cAMP levels. This effect seems to be related to elevated levels of cAMP with resultant enhancement of arginase I expression and subsequent blockade of myelin-associated glycol-protein (MAG), a major factor in prohibiting neural regeneration (Deng *et al.*, 2009; Ma *et al.*, 2010). This blockade of MAG through arginase I involves polyamine synthesis, as inhibition of ODC prevents the neural regeneration. In fact, synthesis of spermidine, not putrescine, appears to be necessary for this effect. Polyamines are known to be important in neural growth, development, and regeneration (Filbin, 1996).

However, enhanced arginase activity and polyamine synthesis are not always beneficial to neuronal growth and regeneration. Enhanced arginase activity and polyamine production in the eye can cause retinal ganglion cell death. This appears to be due to excessive activation of the excitotoxic NMDA receptors. Inhibition of arginase and polyamine synthesis is neuroprotective (Pernet *et al.*, 2007). Thus, polyamines appear to promote either cell growth or death, depending on the environment (Wallace *et al.*, 2003).

3.5.2 Arginase in disease

3.5.2.1 Diabetes

Vascular and hepatic arginase activity are increased in diabetic rats, and arginase expression and activity are also increased in aortic and coronary endothelial cells exposed to high glucose (Romero *et al.*, 2006; Romero *et al.*, 2008). Our recent studies show that arginase activity is increased in aortas of diabetic rats and aortic endothelial cells treated with high glucose, and that coronary endothelial-dependent vasorelaxation is reduced in diabetic rats and restored by inhibition of arginase activity (Romero *et al.*, 2006; Tawfik *et al.*, 2006; Romero *et al.*, 2008).

Decreased plasma levels of L-arginine have been reported in diabetic animals and patients (Hagenfeldt *et al.*, 1989; Pieper and Dondlinger, 1997) and in vascular tissue of STZ-diabetic rats (Pieper and Dondlinger, 1997). Increased arginase activity seems to be involved in these conditions. Diabetic rat liver has higher arginase activity than control rats, as well as elevated manganese content, which may stimulate the enzyme (Bond *et al.*, 1983; Spolarics and Bond, 1989). In diabetic patients, arginase activity is also increased in red blood cells (Jiang *et al.*, 2003), and in penile vessels, associated with erectile dysfunction (Bivalacqua *et al.*, 2001). Studies in STZ-diabetic rats show elevated arginase activity and expression in aorta and carotid arteries (Romero *et al.*, 2008).

Diabetes and hyperglycaemic conditions cause production of ROS. These ROS have been shown to increase arginase expression and activity. Several mechanisms are involved in the high glucose-induced elevation of O_2^- and other reactive oxygen species. These are summarized in the Regulation of Activity (see below).

3.5.2.2 Hypertension

Elevated arginase activity in aorta, heart and lung has been reported in adult spontaneously hypertensive rats (SHR) (10 weeks and older), but arginase activity was not altered in kidney, liver and brain (Bagnost *et al.*, 2009). Furthermore, treatment of 25-week-old SHR with the arginase inhibitor N$^\omega$-hydroxy-nor-L-arginine reduced systemic blood pressure, improved vascular function, and reduced cardiac fibrosis (Bagnost et al., 2010). However, arginase II knockout mice display a hypertensive phenotype in adulthood rather than the expected reduction in blood pressure with improved vascular endothelial function. This hypertension appears to be related to an enhanced sympathetic nervous function (Huynh et al., 2009a).

Pulmonary hypertension (PH) is also associated with increased arginase activity. Hypoxia-induced pulmonary hypertension is reported to involve elevated arginase II protein expression and activity (Chen et al., 2009; Jin et al., 2010). This elevation in arginase expression/activity is associated with lower NO production in pulmonary artery endothelial cells and proliferation of these cells (Xu et al., 2004). The enhancement of endothelial cell arginase and cell proliferation with hypoxia can be prevented by blockade of EGF receptor tyrosine kinase (Toby et al., 2010). In addition, lack of MAP kinase phosphatase-1 in mice subjected to hypoxia caused them to suffer a more severe PH and greater lung protein levels of arginase (I and II) (Jin et al., 2010). These data support the involvement of MAP kinase in the increased expression and activity of arginase (Shatanawi et al., 2010).

In secondary pulmonary hypertension (PH) resulting from haemolytic anaemias, such as in sickle cell disease, plasma arginase activity is greatly increased by its release from red cells (see sickle cell disease below). Treatment with arginase inhibitors is projected to be successful in reducing the PH (Morris et al., 2008).

3.5.2.3 Sickle cell disease

In sickle cell disease, haemoglobin S-containing erythrocytes become entrapped in the microcirculation, which leads to repetitive cycles of ischaemia-reperfusion tissue injury and infarction (Bunn, 1997). Primary and secondary inflammation, endothelial activation, oxidant stress and adhesion molecule expression contribute to this process. This disease state is characterized by low tissue levels of NO, sludging of red blood cells (RBC), vaso-occlusive disorders, haemolysis and pulmonary hypertension. Arginase activity and expression are substantially elevated in the plasma, RBCs, and platelets from these patients (Morris et al., 2008). Lysis of the RBCs releases large amounts of both free haemoglobin and arginase. Haemoglobin consumes endothelial NO, while arginase limits L-arginine availability to NOS, further reducing NO levels. Treatment of sickle cell disease patients with supplemental L-arginine and/or L-citrulline has been shown to reduce levels of RBC sludging, vaso-occlusion and pulmonary hypertension (Waugh et al., 2001; Fasipe et al., 2004; Morris et al., 2005). Treatment of sickle cell disease by arginase inhibitors is also a promising therapeutic strategy (Morris, 2006).

3.5.2.4 Erectile dysfunction

Smooth muscle relaxation in the corpus cavernosum is essential for erectile function. The NO/cyclic GMP pathway has been demonstrated to be the principal mediator of cavernous smooth relaxation and penile erection (Masuda et al., 2004). NO is produced from L-arginine by NOS, and both neuronal NOS (nNOS) and endothelial NOS (eNOS) isoforms serve as sources to produce relevant levels of NO in the corpus cavernosum. Recently, both arginase I and II isoforms have been shown to exist in human corpus cavernosum, and the inhibition of arginase resulted in the facilitation of corporal smooth muscle relaxation (Cox et al., 1999; Bivalacqua et al., 2001). It has been reported that basal NO production from the endothelium regulates intrinsic cavernous tone and that endogenous arginase activity in the endothelium modulates tone by inhibiting NO production, presumably through competition with eNOS for the common substrate L-arginine. Both increased arginase activity and reduced NO bioavailability have been strongly associated with erectile dysfunction (ED) in many conditions including obesity (Carneiro et al., 2008), hypercholesterolemia (Xie et al., 2007), ageing (Bivalacqua et al., 2007) and diabetes (Bivalacqua et al., 2001). Angiotensin II-induced elevation of arginase activity and erectile dysfunction can be prevented by inhibition of p38 MAP kinase (Toque et al., 2010a). It also has been recently reported that diabetic mice lacking the gene for ARG II do not exhibit the impaired nitrergic nerve and endothelial dependent relaxations of the corpus cavernosum observed in wild type diabetic mice (Toque et al., 2010b). Thus, arginase is strongly implicated as a regulator of erectile function, and penile arginase is a potential target for the treatment of male sexual dysfunction.

3.5.2.5 Asthma

Allergic asthma is a chronic inflammatory disorder of the airways characterized by allergen-induced bronchoconstriction and inflammation of airways. Lack of available L-arginine for NOS and reduced NO production appears to be centrally involved with the asthmatic state (Maarsingh et al., 2008a). Supplemental L-arginine or treatment with the arginase inhibitor nor-NOHA reduces bronchoconstriction to allergens or other stimulants (de Boer et al., 2001) and enhances nitrergic nerve-mediated airway smooth muscle relaxation (Maarsingh et al., 2006). Both arginase I and II are constitutively expressed in airways tissues, including epithelial and endothelial cells, myofibroblasts, and macrophages (Lindemann and Racke, 2003; Maarsingh et al., 2008b). Arginase activity and expression are elevated in humans with asthma and animal models of asthma (Zimmermann et al., 2003; Kenyon et al., 2008). Asthmatic subjects who are smokers exhibit an even greater elevation of arginase I in airway epithelial cells and myofibroblasts (Bergeron et al., 2007). They also display enhanced levels of ornithine decarboxylase.

Chronic inflammation with asthma also leads to airway remodelling including thickening of basement membranes, fibrosis, and enhanced smooth muscle mass. Structurally, these changes can reduce lung function. Current evidence indicates that this remodelling involves elevated production of polyamines and proline – downstream products of arginase (Meurs et al., 2008). Since several airway functions involve arginase, a key role for arginase in the pathophysiology of asthma is emerging.

3.5.2.6 Ischaemia/reperfusion injury

Reperfusion is aimed to minimize damage in an ischaemic tissue. However, ischaemia/reperfusion (I/R) injury commonly occurs as a result of induction of ROS and pro-inflammatory factors/markers. Endothelial and microvascular dysfunction result from decreased nitric oxide production. As was explained above, arginase competes with NOS for their common substrate L-arginine, thereby reducing NO production. Arginase has been shown to be up-regulated in I/R injury in cardiac tissue (arginase I), and kidney (arginase II), as well as in liver (arginase I) (Hein et al., 2003; Reid et al., 2007; Jeyabalan et al., 2008; Jung et al., 2010). Liver I/R injury releases arginase I from injured hepatocytes leading to hepatic depletion of arginine (Reid et al., 2007; Jeyabalan et al., 2008). The levels of inflammatory cytokines such as tumour necrosis factor-α (TNFα) are shown to be increased in I/R injury and contribute to increased arginase expression and generation of oxidative radicals in endothelial cells leading to endothelial dysfunction (Gao et al., 2007; Zhang et al., 2010). Treatment with the arginase inhibitor, N^{ω} hydroxy-nor-L-arginine (nor-NOHA) has been reported to protect myocardium from I/R injury (Jung et al., 2010). Similarly, infusion with nor-NOHA prevents liver necrosis and increases hepatic arginine and citrulline levels in I/R associated with liver transplant (Reid et al., 2007; Jeyabalan et al., 2008).

3.5.2.7 Atherosclerosis

Pathogenesis of atherosclerosis involves vasoconstriction, inflammation and thrombus formation. Hyperglycaemia contributes significantly to atherosclerosis by increasing pro-inflammatory and pro-thrombotic factors that lead to plaque formation and an increased risk for thromboembolism (Retnakaran and Zinman, 2008). The central mechanism for endothelial dysfunction in atherosclerosis is considered to be due to uncoupling of NOS, reducing NO production, and increasing ROS production (Ozaki et al., 2002; Yang and Ming, 2006). Vascular arginase activity has been shown to be increased with high cholesterol diet in atherogenic-prone mice (ApoE$^{-/-}$) and wild-type mice (Ming et al., 2004). This has been attributed to an increase in the expression of the arginase II isoform as deletion of this gene prevents vascular dysfunction and oxidative stress (Ming et al., 2004; Ryoo et al., 2008). Both isoforms of arginase were expressed in atherosclerotic lesions of hyperlipidaemic rabbits (Hayashi et al., 2006). Arginase II has been reported to increase in endothelial cells of atherosclerotic mice (Zhang et al., 2001) and upon exposure to oxidized LDL in human aortic endothelial cells (Ryoo et al., 2006). Moreover, oxidized LDL induces arginase I expression through PPAR-γ and -α activation in macrophages contributing to atherosclerosis (Gallardo-Soler et al., 2008). Increasing NO bioavailability by citrulline therapy or arginase inhibition improved the prognosis of atherosclerosis in diabetic patients (Hayashi and Iguchi, 2010).

3.5.2.8 Nephropathy

Nitric oxide levels are significantly reduced in chronic kidney disease and end-stage renal disease patients (Zharikov et al., 2008). One of the mechanisms is due to reduced substrate availability, i.e. L-arginine. Although, the liver is the major site of *de novo* L-arginine synthesis, this pool of L-arginine never enters the circulation because of quick consumption by arginase I in the liver to produce urea and ornithine. Moreover, hepatic ornithine is recycled to form citrulline and then arginine. Thus hepatic arginase I activity does not cause significant depletion of the overall arginine supply (Baylis, 2008). Arginase II is the predominant isoform in the kidney, and elevated levels of arginase II can compete with NOS to reduce arginine supply. Indeed there is evidence that inhibition of arginase protects the kidney from structural damage in the renal mass ablation/infarction model of chronic kidney disease (Sabbatini et al., 2003).

In models of nephrotoxic nephritis, it has been shown that both iNOS and arginase are elevated (Waddington et al., 1998a,b). An up-regulation of proline and polyamine production through the arginase II pathway has been considered in the pathology of glomerulonephritis (Waddington et al., 1998b). NO bioavailability is reported to be decreased in renal medulla of diabetic rats due to increased uptake of L-arginine by the CAT-1 transporter in the liver, manifesting in reduced plasma arginine levels (Palm et al., 2008). This is also associated with enhanced arginase activity in the renal cortex of these rats. Early stages in diabetes are characterized by hyperfiltration, postulated to be due to increased glomerular L-arginine uptake and polyamine synthesis (Schwartz et al., 2004). Both arginase I and arginase II were elevated in this 2-week diabetic model, which could affect NO levels as well as increase polyamine levels through the formation of ornithine.

3.5.2.9 Cancer

The level of NO in the tumour milieu determines the rate of cancer progression. Induction of iNOS greatly increases NO generation which can restrict the growth and metastasis of cancer. High expression of iNOS has been reported in the early stages of breast, colon, brain, lung and prostate cancers (Thomsen et al., 1994; Cobbs et al., 1995; Thomsen et al., 1995; Xu et al., 2002). In contrast, moderate levels of NO promote tumour growth. Arginase plays a major role in tumour survival, growth and metastasis. It depletes the substrate, arginine, thereby limiting NO production and increasing ornithine levels which enhance cell replication through polyamine synthesis. Arginase activity and arginase II expression have been shown to be increased in breast, colon and prostate cancers (Buga et al., 1998; Singh et al., 2000; Mumenthaler et al., 2008). A reduction of iNOS and up-regulation of arginase in macrophages causes a phenotypic shift from a tumour-repressive to tumour-supportive microenvironment in which factors that help the tumour grow are released (Mills et al., 1992; Weigert and Brune, 2008). Indeed, elevated arginase I expression has been reported in macrophages isolated from tumours of wild-type mice (Davel et al., 2002; Kusmartsev and Gabrilovich, 2005; Sinha et al., 2005) as well as in tumour cells (Lechner et al., 2005). A recent study showed that knockdown of arginase II causes apoptosis of thyroid cancer cells (de Sousa et al.,

2010). Statin therapy in a breast cancer cell line was found to cause cell death which was attributed to a decrease in arginase II (Kotamraju *et al.*, 2007).

3.5.2.10 Parasitic infection

Several parasites including *Leishmania*, *Trypanosoma*, and *Plasmodium* have been shown to express arginase (Walther *et al.*, 2006; Cuervo *et al.*, 2008; Stempin *et al.*, 2008; Rogers *et al.*, 2009; Dowling *et al.*, 2010). Arginase activity causes ornithine production which promotes proliferation of the pathogen through the polyamine pathway. Macrophages are recruited to the site of infection by factors such as lipopolysaccharide, tumour necrosis factor-α (TNF-α), interleukin-12 (IL-12) and interferon-γ (IFN-γ). During the acute phase of infection, these classically activated macrophages (CAM) induce iNOS to produce NO and peroxynitrite (ONOO$^-$) to control parasitaemia. This has been observed in infections with *Leishmania*, *Trypanosoma*, and *Plasmodium* (Plebanski and Hill, 2000; Peluffo *et al.*, 2004; Walther *et al.*, 2006). Depending on the host genotype, parasite virulence, and stage of the disease (progressed), hosts can produce Type 2 cytokines such as IL-4 and IL-13 which antagonize CAMs and instead up-regulate arginase I to cause collagen synthesis and cell proliferation through the polyamine pathway (Stempin *et al.*, 2010). T helper 1 (Th1) cells generate IFN-γ and induce iNOS, whereas Th2 cells generate IL-4 and IL-10 with resultant induction of arginase I and suppression of iNOS (Munder *et al.*, 1999). Although the polyamine pathway is essential for wound healing, it has been shown to exacerbate parasitic infections by preventing clearance by CAM and promoting parasitic proliferation (Stempin *et al.*, 2010). Further, it has been reported that limiting arginine or inhibiting arginase activation can reduce parasite survival (Wanasen *et al.*, 2007; Rogers *et al.*, 2009).

3.5.2.11 Hyperargininaemia

As was explained above, a deficiency in arginase I leads to accumulation of L-arginine or hyperargininaemia (Dizikes *et al.*, 1986; Vockley *et al.*, 1994; Uchino *et al.*, 1995). It is inherited as an autosomal recessive disease. Patients with this disorder appear normal at birth but start showing symptoms of diminished growth and mental retardation when they are 2–4 years old. They become progressively spastic and develop neurological diseases (Crombez and Cederbaum, 2005). There are sporadic instances of hyperammonaemia and hyperuraemia even though there is an increase in arginine levels by two- to fivefold (Cederbaum *et al.*, 1979; Marescau *et al.*, 1992). This is likely due to compensation by the arginase II isoform in the kidney. Indeed, augmented levels of kidney arginase activity have been reported in arginase-deficient patients whose liver arginase activity is reduced (Spector *et al.*, 1983). Treatment of these patients involves restriction of dietary protein intake, supplementation of essential amino acids, and diversion of ammonia to salvage pathways (Crombez and Cederbaum, 2005).

3.5.2.12 Ageing

Age-related vascular changes have been investigated in humans and in a number of animal species. Arginase plays an important role in regulating vasomotor tone, and its relative contribution varies depending on the vascular bed and the vessel size and type (Santhanam *et al.*, 2008). There is increasing evidence that up-regulation of arginase contributes to impaired endothelial function in ageing (Berkowitz *et al.*, 2003). It has been shown that there is higher arginase activity, lower NO and higher O_2^- production in old rats compared with young rats (Kim *et al.*, 2009). Furthermore, these authors also found that acute inhibition of NOS (with N-nitro-l-arginine methyl ester) and arginase (2S-amino-6-boronohexanoic acid, ABH), can reduce O_2^- production in old rats and prevent uncoupling of the eNOS dimer. Ageing is also associated with endothelial senescence which can contribute to atherosclerosis as well as impairing endothelial function. Indeed, knocking down arginase I (White *et al.*, 2006) or increasing NO bioavailability by citrulline therapy (Hayashi and Iguchi, 2010) restores ageing-related endothelial senescence and improves vascular function. Erectile dysfunction associated with ageing has been found to be improved by inhibiting arginase using ABH or knocking down arginase I (Bivalacqua et al., 2007). Inhibition of arginase also decreases blood pressure and improves vascular function of resistance vessels in hypertensive rats. (Demougeot et al., 2005; Durante et al., 2007; Bagnost et al., 2008). Increased arginase activity can also cause vessel stiffness with age due to collagen deposition and fibrosis through the proline and polyamine pathways.

3.5.2.13 Retinopathy

Ischaemic retinopathies are characterized by a progression of vascular damage, beginning with inflammatory reactions, endothelial cell dysfunction, and reduced blood flow, which can lead to pathological neovascularization and fibrovascular scarring, culminating in retinal detachment and blindness (Friedlander et al., 2007). During the inflammatory stage, excessive arginase activity could enhance cytokine formation by limiting NO production by iNOS. In addition, excessive arginase activity at the level of the retinal endothelial and smooth muscle cells could exacerbate retinal inflammation by reducing NO production by endothelial and neuronal NOS which would decrease blood flow and promote platelet aggregation and leukocyte adhesion to the vessel wall. The ensuing retinal ischaemia would further increase the retinal injury and could contribute to pathological neovascular growth due to the induction of VEGF expression. Excessive arginase activity could also contribute to pathological vascular growth and fibrovascular scarring, by increasing the formation of polyamines and proline, which promote cell growth and collagen formation, respectively.

Arginase I was reported to be increased and localized mainly to Muller cells in rats with endotoxin-induced uveitis (EIU) (Koga et al., 2002). Arginase I is also involved in excitotoxic cell death due to polyamines (Pernet et al., 2007). Studies have shown that arginase activity and arginase I expression are increased in models of EIU and diabetic retinopathy and in cultured retinal endothelial cells, Muller cells, and microglial cells exposed to high glucose or cytokines (Zhang et al., 2009; Caldwell et al., 2010). This was correlated to a concomitant increase in cytokine expression and oxidative stress, reduced NO, vascular dysfunction and pathological angiogenesis. Furthermore, deletion of one copy of the arginase I gene and both copies of arginase II decreases cytokine production in both diabetic retinopathy and EIU (Zhang et al., 2009).

3.6 Regulation of Activity

3.6.1 Humoral factors

3.6.1.1 Reactive oxygen species

Reactive oxygen species (ROS) formation is increased in diabetes. Numerous sources of ROS in diabetes have been described and include advanced glycation end products, flux through the aldose reductase pathway, and activation of PKC (Nishikawa et al., 2000a). ROS play a role in vascular dysfunction in diabetes. Overproduction of O_2^- can lead to scavenging NO and reducing its bioavailability (Yung et al., 2006). Reactive species have been implicated in increased arginase activity and expression. Studies have shown the H_2O_2 causes arginase activation in endothelial cells, leading to decreased NO production which was restored by antioxidant treatment (Thengchaisri et al., 2006). In a model of wound healing, arginase effects in promoting excessive scar formation were mitigated by inhibitors of peroxynitrite actions (Kapoor et al., 2004). Furthermore, treatment with peroxynitrite has been shown to cause increased arginase activity and mRNA and protein expression in coronary and aortic endothelial cells (Romero et al., 2006; Chandra et al., 2010).

High glucose enhances the expression of eNOS and production of O_2^- (Cosentino et al., 1997). The passage of glucose through the polyol pathway generates $O_2^{\cdot -}$ and the toxic reaction product of NO and O_2^-, peroxynitrite (ONOO⁻) (Giugliano et al., 1996). Aldose reductase, the first and rate-limiting enzyme in the polyol pathway, is activated by high glucose and begins the production of sorbitol. In addition to production of ROS, this active pathway consumes NADPH, reducing its supply for many endothelial enzymes, including eNOS. Moreover, large amounts of ATP are consumed, which may compromise the EC energy supply and cell membrane potential. NADH and ATP are also depleted by activation of poly (ADP-ribose) polymerase by ROS (Garcia Soriano et al., 2001). Inhibitors of aldose reductase have been reported to reduce vascular dysfunction in experimental models of diabetes (Cameron and Cotter, 1992). High glucose also stimulates ROS production by mitochondria via actions through the electron transport chain complex II and oxidative phosphorylation (Nishikawa et al., 2000b). The ROS from all sources described above can activate the janus kinases (JAKs) and signal transducers and activators of transcription (STATs) (Marrero et al., 1997; Schieffer et al., 2000), and promote vascular smooth muscle proliferation, collagen deposition and fibrosis. The JAK/STAT pathway has been shown to be involved in up-regulation of arginase (Wei et al., 2000).

3.6.1.2 Angiotensin II

This has been implicated in oxidative stress-induced endothelial dysfunction and vascular remodelling and fibrosis in diabetes. A mechanism of Ang II stimulation of ROS is through stimulation of endothelial NADPH oxidase (Touyz, 2004). In a model of hypertension, inhibitors of the AT1 receptor have been reported to inhibit increased arginase activity and to normalize endothelial function (Kotsiuruba et al., 2002). Studies in our lab have shown that treatment of endothelial cells with Ang II increases both arginase activity and arginase I protein expression (Shatanawi et al., 2011). Cytokines such as IL-4, IL-13, and TNF-α are also activators of arginase activity (Wei et al., 2000; Nelin et al., 2005). Ang II has been shown to play a critical role in inflammatory vascular disease such as arteriosclerosis, and is known to be associated with endothelial nitric oxide synthase (eNOS) dysfunction/uncoupling (Satoh et al., 2008). Inhibitors of the renin angiotensin-aldosterone system (RAAS) have been effective in moderating increased vascular wall thickness clinically and Ang II receptor blockers have inhibited development of atherosclerosis in animal models (Kim and Iwao, 2000).

3.6.2 Elevation of arginase activity and signal transduction mechanisms

Enhanced arginase function can result from increased specific activity/enzyme efficiency or elevated protein levels. The activators of arginase have not been extensively investigated. S-nitrosylation of arginase I through iNOS has been reported to increase its activity by reducing the K_m of arginase (Santhanam et al., 2008). Uric acid also has been reported to activate arginase by reducing its K_m, seemingly for both isoforms (Zharikov et al., 2008).

There is more evidence for mechanisms that increase levels of arginase protein. Protein expression of arginase I is increased in rat smooth muscle in response to interleukins and is apparently mediated through cyclic AMP/protein kinase A and JAK/STAT6 pathways (Wei et al., 2000). In macrophages, it is reported that cAMP mediates activation of arginase I involving protein kinase A type I and histone deacetylase (Haffner et al., 2008). We and others have shown that RhoA and Rho kinase are involved with upregulation of arginase activity/expression in atherosclerosis, inflammatory bowel disease, and diabetes (Ming et al., 2004; Horowitz et al., 2007; Romero et al., 2008). RhoA-GDP is activated by Rho guanosine nucleotide exchange factor (Rho GEF), which promotes exchange of GDP for GTP. The active RhoA-GTP stimulates ROCK to trigger downstream signalling (Loirand et al., 2008). ROS have been shown in several studies to be involved in the enhancement of arginase activity (Ming et al., 2004; Boor et al., 2007; Horowitz et al., 2007; Romero et al., 2008; Zhang et al., 2009). We recently reported that oxidative radicals can increase arginase activity/expression in endothelial cells through a pathway involving protein kinase C-activated p115-Rho GEF and subsequent activation of RhoA/Rho kinase (Chandra et al., 2011). Further, phosphorylation and activation of p115-Rho GEF through protein kinase C alpha (PKCα) is reported to increase endothelial permeability in response to thrombin (Holinstat et al., 2003), a factor which also increases arginase activity (Horowitz et al., 2007).

Active RhoA has also been indicated as an upstream activator of mitogen-activated protein kinase (MAPK) family members such as p38 mitogen-activated protein kinase (MAPK) (Lovett et al., 2006; Guo et al., 2009). Both angiotensin II (Ang II) and high glucose (HG) are reported to activate MAPKs, among which p38 MAPK has been shown to have a central role in cardiovascular dysfunction (Wen et al., 2006; Santhanam et al., 2007). Also, p38 MAPK seems to be involved in increasing arginase I activity and expression in macrophages (Chang et al., 2000; Stempin et al., 2004). Studies also indicate a role for p38 MAPK in increasing arginase activity/expression in endothelial cells upon exposure to Ang II and ROS, which involves intermediate activation of RhoA/ROCK (Chandra et al., 2010; Shatanawi et al., 2010). Activation of p38 MAPK is known to result in activation of transcription factors.

These signal transduction intermediates may be considered targets for the therapeutic limitation of arginase activity. Those intermediate enzymes or processes closest to the enhancement of arginase activity would be expected to be the most specific.

3.7 Arginase Inhibitors

Arginase competes with NOS for their common substrate, L-arginine, thus inhibition of arginase can increase the pool of L-arginine and thereby enhance NO production. Several inhibitors of arginase are available commercially. The first class of inhibitors had non-specific actions and many side effects owing to the high concentrations required (Morris, 2009). For example, norvaline used as an arginase inhibitor is a substrate for amidotransferases (Davoodi et al., 1998). Similarly, N^ω-hydroxy-L-arginine (NOHA) is a potent inhibitor for arginase but is also a precursor for NO synthesis from NOS. α-Difluoromethylornithine (DFMO) is a non-specific weak inhibitor of arginase though it is a potent inhibitor for ornithine decarboxylase (Morris, 2009). Thus the effects of DFMO in increasing NO production are probably due to increased accumulation of ornithine which is known to inhibit arginase. Besides producing urea, arginase is also involved in synthesis of polyamines and amino acids such as ornithine, proline and glutamate. In fact, ornithine, leucine, valine, lysine, isoleucine and nor-valine inhibit arginase with ornithine being the most potent (Huynh et al., 2009b). Also, L-citrulline is an allosteric inhibitor of arginase (Shearer et al., 1997). Recently, competitive inhibitors of arginase with greater specificity for the enzyme have been synthesized. Boronic acid analogues of L-arginine, i.e. S-(2-boronoethyl)-L-cysteine (BEC) and 2(S)-amino-6-boronohexanoic acid (ABH), are highly selective arginase inhibitors that bear N-hydroxyguanidinium or boronic acid heads which bind the manganese cluster in arginase (Berkowitz et al., 2003). Their transition state structures differ significantly from those occurring in NO biosynthesis. Nor-NOHA is also a potent arginase inhibitor and it neither inhibits NOS nor is it an intermediate in NO synthesis. It has a much longer half-life than NOHA. A recent study shows that BEC and NOHA reverse the vascular tolerance to acetylcholine in rat aorta and mesenteric arteries, suggesting an increase in NO bioavailability (Huynh et al., 2009b). It has even been reported that BEC and DFMO could suppress arginase activity and restore NOS activity in the aortic rings from old rats (Berkowitz et al., 2003). L-valine, nor-valine and DFMO have been used to study the relationship or arginase and NOS function by several investigators (Ming et al., 2004; Santhanam et al., 2007; Lewis et al., 2008).

Although several specific arginase inhibitors have been developed and investigated, they are not isoform specific. RNA interference has been used to inhibit expression of specific isoforms. Administration of short hairpin RNA (shRNA) against arginase I greatly reduced IL-13 induced airway hyperresponsiveness, with a concomitant decrease in arginase I mRNA and protein levels in the lungs of mice (Yang et al., 2006). Direct delivery of anti-sense arginase I using adeno-virus vectors in the corpus cavernosum improved

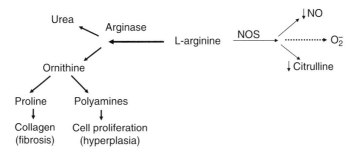

Fig. 3.3. Elevated arginase activity can reduce availability of L-arginine for nitric oxide synthase (NOS) and disrupt its function. Increased production of ornithine can lead to excess collagen formation and cell proliferation.

erectile function in aged mice (Bivalacqua et al., 2007). Anti-sense arginase I also increases NO production in endothelial cells exposed to high glucose (Romero et al., 2008).

3.8 Conclusions

Arginase function/activity is essential for the production of urea in the hepatic urea cycle and the elimination of toxic excess ammonia produced by protein catabolism (Fig. 3.1). Also, wound healing involves enhanced local tissue arginase activity through which ornithine is metabolized to proline (collagen production) and polyamines (cell proliferation). Additionally, arginase activity can be neuroprotective and support regeneration in spinal nerves.

However, elevated arginase activity/expression also occurs and is involved in a variety of disease or pathological states such as diabetes, hypertension, sickle cell disease, asthma, ischaemia/reperfusion injury and atherosclerosis. Activation and excessive function of arginase is closely associated with inflammation and elevated ROS. In these conditions, arginase can compete with NOS and reduce available L-arginine, leading to depressed NO production, and possible NOS uncoupling and increased superoxide (O_2^-) production (Fig. 3.3). Additionally, there is enhanced production of proline and polyamines. In these circumstances, there is impaired endothelial-dependent vasorelaxation (vasoconstriction), proliferation of vascular and other cells, and vascular and tissue fibrosis.

Thus, it is being recognized that arginase plays very important roles in physiological and pathophysiological processes in many cell types and tissues. Its activity and expression are highly regulated. Understanding these signal transduction processes is essential in any efforts to maintain normal arginase function.

References

Ash, D.E. (2004) Structure and function of arginases. *Journal of Nutrition* 134, 2760S–2764S; discussion 2765S–2767S.

Bagnost, T., Berthelot, A., Bouhaddi, M., Laurant, P., Andre, C., Guillaume, Y. and Demougeot, C. (2008) Treatment with the arginase inhibitor N(omega)-hydroxy-nor-L-arginine improves vascular function and lowers blood pressure in adult spontaneously hypertensive rat. *Journal of Hypertension* 26, 1110–1118.

Bagnost, T., Berthelot, A., Alvergnas, M., Miguet-Alfonsi, C., Andre, C., Guillaume, Y. and Demougeot, C. (2009) Misregulation of the arginase pathway in tissues of spontaneously hypertensive rats. *Hypertension Research* 32, 1130–1135.

Bagnost, T., Ma, L., da Silva, R.F., Rezakhaniha, R., Houdayer, C., Stergiopulos, N., Andre, C., *et al.* (2010) Cardiovascular effects of arginase inhibition in spontaneously hypertensive rats with fully developed hypertension. *Cardiovascular Research* 87, 569–577.

Baylis, C. (2008) Nitric oxide deficiency in chronic kidney disease. *American Journal of Physiology Renal Physiology* 294, F1–9.

Bergeron, C., Boulet, L.P., Page, N., Laviolette, M., Zimmermann, N., Rothenberg, M.E. and Hamid, Q. (2007) Influence of cigarette smoke on the arginine pathway in asthmatic airways: increased expression of arginase I. *Journal of Allergy and Clinical Immunology* 119, 391–397.

Berkowitz, D.E., White, R., Li, D., Minhas, K.M., Cernetich, A., Kim, S., Burke, S., et al. (2003) Arginase reciprocally regulates nitric oxide synthase activity and contributes to endothelial dysfunction in aging blood vessels. *Circulation* 108, 2000–2006.

Bivalacqua, T.J., Hellstrom, W.J., Kadowitz, P.J. and Champion, H.C. (2001a) Increased expression of arginase II in human diabetic corpus cavernosum: in diabetic-associated erectile dysfunction. *Biochemical and Biophysical Research Communications* 283, 923–927.

Bivalacqua, T.J., Hellstrom, W.J., Kadowitz, P.J. and Champion, H.C. (2001b) Increased expression of arginase II in human diabetic corpus cavernosum in diabetic-associated erectile dysfunction. *Biochemical and Biophysical Research Communications* 283, 923–927.

Bivalacqua, T.J., Burnett, A.L., Hellstrom, W.J. and Champion, H.C. (2007) Overexpression of arginase in the aged mouse penis impairs erectile function and decreases eNOS activity: influence of in vivo gene therapy of anti-arginase. *American Journal of Physioliology Heart and Circulatory Physiology* 292, H1340–1351.

Bond, J.S., Failla, M.L. and Unger, D.F. (1983) Elevated manganese concentration and arginase activity in livers of streptozotocin-induced diabetic rats. *Journal of Biological Chemistry* 258, 8004–8009.

Boor, P., Sebekova, K., Ostendorf, T. and Floege, J. (2007) Treatment targets in renal fibrosis. *Nephrology Dialysis Transplantation* 22, 3391–3407.

Buga, G.M., Wei, L.H., Bauer, P.M., Fukuto, J.M. and Ignarro, L.J. (1998) NG-hydroxy-L-arginine and nitric oxide inhibit Caco-2 tumor cell proliferation by distinct mechanisms. *American Journal of Physiology Regulatory, Integrative and Comparative Physiology* 275, R1256–1264.

Bunn, H.F. (1997) Pathogenesis and treatment of sickle cell disease. *New England Journal of Medicine* 337, 762–769.

Caldwell, R.B., Zhang, W., Romero, M.J. and Caldwell, R.W. (2010) Vascular dysfunction in retinopathy-an emerging role for arginase. *Brain Research Bulletin* 81, 303–309.

Cameron, N.E. and Cotter, M.A. (1992) Dissociation between biochemical and functional effects of the aldose reductase inhibitor, ponalrestat, on peripheral nerve in diabetic rats. *British Journal of Pharmacology* 107, 939–944.

Carneiro, F.S., Giachini, F.R., Lima, V.V., Carneiro, Z.N., Leite, R., Inscho E.W., Tostes, R.C., et al. (2008) Adenosine actions are preserved in corpus cavernosum from obese and type II diabetic db/db mouse. *Journal of Sexual Medicine* 5, 1156–1166.

Cederbaum, S.D., Shaw, K.N., Spector, E.B., Verity, M.A., Snodgrass, P.J. and Sugarman, G.I. (1979) Hyperargininemia with arginase deficiency. *Pediatric Research* 13, 827–833.

Chandra, S., Romero, M.J., Shatanawi, A., Caldwell, R.B. and Caldwell, R.W. (2011) Oxidative species increase orginase activity in endothelial cells through RhoA/Rho kinase pathway. *British Journal of Pharmacology* July 8, 2011.

Chang, C.I., Zoghi, B., Liao, J.C. and Kuo, L. (2000) The involvement of tyrosine kinases, cyclic AMP/protein kinase A, and p38 mitogen-activated protein kinase in IL-13-mediated arginase I induction in macrophages: its implications in IL-13-inhibited nitric oxide production. *Journal of Immunology* 165, 2134–2141.

Chen, B., Calvert, A.E., Cui, H. and Nelin, L.D. (2009) Hypoxia promotes human pulmonary artery smooth muscle cell proliferation through induction of arginase. *American Journal of Physiology. Lung, Cellular and Molecular Physiology* 297, L1151–1159.

Cobbs, C.S., Brenman, J.E., Aldape, K.D., Bredt, D.S. and Israel, M.A. (1995) Expression of nitric oxide synthase in human central nervous system tumors. *Cancer Research* 55, 727–730.

Cosentino, F., Hishikawa, K., Katusic, Z.S. and Luscher, T.F. (1997) High glucose increases nitric oxide synthase expression and superoxide anion generation in human aortic endothelial cells. *Circulation* 96, 25–28.

Cox, J.D., Kim, N.N., Traish, A.M. and Christianson, D.W. (1999) Arginase-boronic acid complex highlights a physiological role in erectile function. *Nature Structural Biology* 6, 1043–1047.

Crombez, E.A. and Cederbaum, S.D. (2005) Hyperargininemia due to liver arginase deficiency. *Molecular Genetics and Metabolism* 84, 243–251.

Cuervo, H., Pineda, M.A., Aoki, M.P., Gea, S., Fresno, M. and Girones, N. (2008) Inducible nitric oxide synthase and arginase expression in heart tissue during acute Trypanosoma cruzi infection in mice: arginase I is expressed in infiltrating CD68+ macrophages. *Journal of Infectious Diseases* 197, 1772–1782.

Davel, L.E., Jasnis, M.A., de la Torre, E., Gotoh, T., Diament, M., Magenta, G., Sacerdote de Lustig, E., *et al.* (2002) Arginine metabolic pathways involved in the modulation of tumor-induced angiogenesis by macrophages. *Federation of European Biochemical Societies Letters* 532, 216–220.

Davoodi, J., Drown, P.M., Bledsoe, R.K., Wallin, R., Reinhart, G.D. and Hutson, S.M. (1998) Overexpression and characterization of the human mitochondrial and cytosolic branched-chain aminotransferases. *Journal of Biological Chemistry* 273, 4982–4989.

de Boer, J., Meurs, H., Flendrig, L., Koopal, M. and Zaagsma, J. (2001) Role of nitric oxide and superoxide in allergen-induced airway hyperreactivity after the late asthmatic reaction in guinea-pigs. *British Journal of Pharmacology* 133, 1235–1242.

de Sousa, M.S., Latini, F.R., Monteiro, H.P. and Cerutti, J.M. (2010) Arginase 2 and nitric oxide synthase: pathways associated with the pathogenesis of thyroid tumors. *Free Radical Biology and Medicine* 68, 390–394.

Deignan, J.L., Cederbaum, S.D. and Grody, W.W. (2008) Contrasting features of urea cycle disorders in human patients and knockout mouse models. *Molecular Genetics and Metabolism* 93, 7–14.

Demougeot, C., Prigent-Tessier, A., Marie, C. and Berthelot, A. (2005) Arginase inhibition reduces endothelial dysfunction and blood pressure rising in spontaneously hypertensive rats. *Journal of Hypertension* 23, 971–978.

Deng, K., He, H., Qiu, J., Lorber, B., Bryson, J.B. and Filbin, M.T. (2009) Increased synthesis of spermidine as a result of upregulation of arginase I promotes axonal regeneration in culture and in vivo. *Journal of Neuroscience* 29, 9545–9552.

Dizikes, G.J., Grody, W.W., Kern, R.M. and Cederbaum, S.D. (1986) Isolation of human liver arginase cDNA and demonstration of nonhomology between the two human arginase genes. *Biochemical and Biophysical Research Communications* 141, 53–59.

Dowling, D.P., Ilies, M., Olszewski, K.L., Portugal, S., Mota, M.M., Llinas, M. and Christianson, D.W. (2010) Crystal structure of arginase from Plasmodium falciparum and implications for l-arginine depletion in malarial infection. *Biochemistry* 49, 5600–5608.

Durante, W., Liao, L., Peyton, K.J. and Schafer, A.I. (1998) Thrombin stimulates vascular smooth muscle cell polyamine synthesis by inducing cationic amino acid transporter and ornithine decarboxylase gene expression. *Circulation Research* 83, 217–223.

Durante, W., Liao, L., Reyna, S.V., Peyton, K.J. and Schafer, A.I. (2001) Transforming growth factor-beta(1) stimulates L-arginine transport and metabolism in vascular smooth muscle cells: role in polyamine and collagen synthesis. *Circulation* 103, 1121–1127.

Durante, W., Johnson, F.K. and Johnson, R.A. (2007) Arginase: a critical regulator of nitric oxide synthesis and vascular function. *Clinical and Experimental Pharmacology and Physiology* 34, 906–911.

Esch, F., Lin, K.I., Hills, A., Zaman, K., Baraban, J.M., Chatterjee, S., Rubin, L., *et al.* (1998) Purification of a multipotent antideath activity from bovine liver and its identification as arginase: nitric oxide-independent inhibition of neuronal apoptosis. *Journal of Neuroscience* 18, 4083–4095.

Fasipe, F.R., Ubawike, A.E., Eva, R. and Fabry, M.E. (2004) Arginine supplementation improves rotorod performance in sickle transgenic mice. *Hematology* 9, 301–305.

Filbin, M.T. (1996) The Muddle with MAG. *Molecular and Cellular Neurosciences* 8, 84–92.

Friedlander, M., Dorrell, M.I., Ritter, M.R., Marchetti, V., Moreno, S.K., El-Kalay, M., Bird, A.C., *et al.* (2007) Progenitor cells and retinal angiogenesis. *Angiogenesis* 10, 89–101.

Gallardo-Soler, A., Gomez-Nieto, C., Campo, M.L., Marathe, C., Tontonoz, P., Castrillo, A. and Corraliza, I. (2008) Arginase I induction by modified lipoproteins in macrophages: a peroxisome proliferator-activated receptor-gamma/delta-mediated effect that links lipid metabolism and immunity. *Molecular Endocrinology* 22, 1394–1402.

Gao, X., Xu, X., Belmadani, S., Park, Y., Tang, Z., Feldman, A.M., Chilian, W.M. and Zhang, C. (2007) TNF-alpha contributes to endothelial dysfunction by upregulating arginase in ischemia/reperfusion injury. *Arteriosclerosis, Thrombosis and Vascular Biology* 27, 1269–1275.

Garcia Soriano, F., Virag, L., Jagtap, P., Szabo, E., Mabley, J.G., Liaudet, L., Marton, A., *et al.* (2001) Diabetic endothelial dysfunction: the role of poly(ADP-ribose) polymerase activation. *Nature Medicine* 7, 108–113.

Giugliano, D., Ceriello, A. and Paolisso, G. (1996) Oxidative stress and diabetic vascular complications. *Diabetes Care* 19, 257–267.

Gotoh, T., Sonoki, T., Nagasaki, A., Terada, K., Takiguchi, M. and Mori, M. (1996) Molecular cloning of cDNA for nonhepatic mitochondrial arginase (arginase II) and comparison of its induction with nitric oxide synthase in a murine macrophage-like cell line. *Federation of European Biochemical Societies Letters* 395, 119–122.

Gotoh, T., Araki, M. and Mori, M. (1997) Chromosomal localization of the human arginase II gene and tissue distribution of its mRNA. *Biochemical and Biophysical Research Communications* 233, 487–491.

Grody, W.W., Kern, R.M., Klein, D., Dodson, A.E., Wissman, P.B., Barsky, S.H. and Cederbaum, S.D. (1993) Arginase deficiency manifesting delayed clinical sequelae and induction of a kidney arginase isozyme. *Human Genetics* 91, 1–5.

Guo, X., Wang, L., Chen, B., Li, Q., Wang, J., Zhao, M., Wu, W., et al. (2009) ERM protein moesin is phosphorylated by advanced glycation end products and modulates endothelial permeability. *American Journal of Physiology. Heart and Circulatory Physiology* 297, H238–246.

Haffner, I., Teupser, D., Holdt, L.M., Ernst, J., Burkhardt, R. and Thiery, J. (2008) Regulation of arginase-1 expression in macrophages by a protein kinase A type I and histone deacetylase dependent pathway. *Journal of Cellular Biochemistry* 103, 520–527.

Hagenfeldt, L., Dahlquist, G. and Persson, B. (1989) Plasma amino acids in relation to metabolic control in insulin-dependent diabetic children. *Acta Paediatrica Scandinavica* 78, 278–282.

Hayashi, T. and Iguchi, A. (2010) Possibility of the regression of atherosclerosis through the prevention of endothelial senescence by the regulation of nitric oxide and free radical scavengers. *Geriatrics and Gerontology International* 10, 115–130.

Hayashi, T., Esaki, T., Sumi, D., Mukherjee, T., Iguchi, A. and Chaudhuri, G. (2006) Modulating role of estradiol on arginase II expression in hyperlipidemic rabbits as an atheroprotective mechanism. *Proceedings of the National Academy of Sciences of the United States of America* 103, 10485–10490.

Hein, T.W., Zhang, C., Wang, W., Chang, C.I., Thengchaisri, N. and Kuo, L. (2003) Ischemia-reperfusion selectively impairs nitric oxide-mediated dilation in coronary arterioles: counteracting role of arginase. *Federation of American Societies for Experimental Biology Journal* 17, 2328–2330.

Holinstat, M., Mehta, D., Kozasa, T., Minshall, R.D. and Malik, A.B. (2003) Protein kinase Calpha-induced p115RhoGEF phosphorylation signals endothelial cytoskeletal rearrangement. *Journal of Biological Chemistry* 278, 28793–28798.

Horowitz, S., Binion, D.G., Nelson, V.M., Kanaa, Y., Javadi, P., Lazarova, Z., Andrekopoulos, C., et al. (2007) Increased arginase activity and endothelial dysfunction in human inflammatory bowel disease. *American Journal of Physiology. Gastrointestinal and Liver Physiology* 292, G1323–1336.

Huynh, N.N., Andrews, K.L., Head, G.A., Khong, S.M., Mayorov, D.N., Murphy, A.J., Lambert, G., et al. (2009a) Arginase II knockout mouse displays a hypertensive phenotype despite a decreased vasoconstrictory profile. *Hypertension* 54, 294–301.

Huynh, N.N., Harris, E.E., Chin-Dusting, J.F. and Andrews, K.L. (2009b) The vascular effects of different arginase inhibitors in rat isolated aorta and mesenteric arteries. *British Journal of Pharmacology* 156, 84–93.

Iyer, R.K., Yoo, P.K., Kern, R.M., Rozengurt, N., Tsoa, R., O'Brien, W.E., Yu, H., et al. (2002) Mouse model for human arginase deficiency. *Molecular and Cellular Biology* 22, 4491–4498.

Jeyabalan, G., Klune, J.R., Nakao, A., Martik, N., Wu, G., Tsung, A. and Geller, D.A. (2008) Arginase blockade protects against hepatic damage in warm ischemia-reperfusion. *Nitric Oxide* 19, 29–35.

Jiang, M., Jia, L., Jiang, W., Hu, X., Zhou, H., Gao, X., Lu, Z., et al. (2003) Protein disregulation in red blood cell membranes of type 2 diabetic patients. *Biochemical and Biophysical Research Communications* 309, 196–200.

Jin, Y., Calvert, T.J., Chen, B., Chicoine, L.G., Joshi, M., Bauer, J.A., Liu, Y., et al. (2010) Mice deficient in Mkp-1 develop more severe pulmonary hypertension and greater lung protein levels of arginase in response to chronic hypoxia. *American Journal of Physiology. Heart and Circulatory Physiology* 298, H1518–1528.

Jung, C., Gonon, A.T., Sjoquist, P.O., Lundberg, J.O. and Pernow, J. (2010) Arginase inhibition mediates cardioprotection during ischaemia-reperfusion. *Cardiovascular Research* 85, 147–154.

Kampfer, H., Pfeilschifter, J. and Frank, S. (2003) Expression and activity of arginase isoenzymes during normal and diabetes-impaired skin repair. *The Journal of Investigative Dermatology* 121, 1544–1551.

Kapoor, M., Howard, R., Hall, I. and Appleton, I. (2004) Effects of epicatechin gallate on wound healing and scar formation in a full thickness incisional wound healing model in rats. *American Journal of Pathology* 165, 299–307.

Kenyon, N.J., Bratt, J.M., Linderholm, A.L., Last, M.S. and Last, J.A. (2008) Arginases I and II in lungs of ovalbumin-sensitized mice exposed to ovalbumin: sources and consequences. *Toxicology and Applied Pharmacology* 230, 269–275.

Kim, J.H., Bugaj, L.J., Oh, Y.J., Bivalacqua, T.J., Ryoo, S., Soucy, K.G., Santhanam, L., et al. (2009) Arginase inhibition restores NOS coupling and reverses endothelial dysfunction and vascular stiffness in old rats. *Journal of Applied Physiology* 107, 1249–1257.

Kim, S. and Iwao, H. (2000) Molecular and cellular mechanisms of angiotensin II-mediated cardiovascular and renal diseases. *Pharmacological Reviews* 52, 11–34.

Koga, T., Koshiyama, Y., Gotoh, T., Yonemura, N., Hirata, A., Tanihara, H., Negi, A., *et al.* (2002) Coinduction of nitric oxide synthase and arginine metabolic enzymes in endotoxin-induced uveitis rats. *Experimental Eye Research* 75, 659–667.

Kotamraju, S., Williams, C.L. and Kalyanaraman, B. (2007) Statin-induced breast cancer cell death: role of inducible nitric oxide and arginase-dependent pathways. *Cancer Research* 67, 7386–7394.

Kotsiuruba, A.V., Svishchenko, Ie. P., Bukhanevich, O.M., Kosiakova, H.V., Berdyshev, A.H., Radchenko, V.V., Mishchenko, L.A. *et al.* (2002) [Effect of irbesartan, an antagonist of AT-1 receptors for angiotensin II, on L-arginine metabolism in arterial hypertension]. *Fiziolohichnyi Zhurnal* 48, 22–28.

Kuo, H.S., Tsai, M.J., Huang, M.C., Huang, W.C., Lee, M.J., Kuo, W.C., You, L.H., *et al.* (2007) The combination of peripheral nerve grafts and acidic fibroblast growth factor enhances arginase I and polyamine spermine expression in transected rat spinal cords. *Biochemical and Biophysical Research Communications* 357, 1–7.

Kusmartsev, S. and Gabrilovich, D.I. (2005) STAT1 signaling regulates tumor-associated macrophage-mediated T cell deletion. *Journal of Immunology* 174, 4880–4891.

Lange, P.S., Langley, B., Lu, P. and Ratan, R.R. (2004) Novel roles for arginase in cell survival, regeneration, and translation in the central nervous system. *Journal of Nutrition* 134, 2812S-2817S; discussion 2818S–2819S.

Lechner, M., Lirk, P. and Rieder, J. (2005) Inducible nitric oxide synthase (iNOS) in tumor biology: the two sides of the same coin. *Seminars in Cancer Biology* 15, 277–289.

Lewis, C., Zhu, W., Pavkov, M.L., Kinney, C.M., Dicorleto, P.E. and Kashyap, V.S. (2008) Arginase blockade lessens endothelial dysfunction after thrombosis. *Journal of Vascular Surgery* 48, 441–446.

Li, H., Meininger, C.J., Hawker, J.R. Jr, Haynes, T.E., Kepka-Lenhart, D., Mistry, S.K., Morris, S.M. Jr, *et al.* (2001a) Regulatory role of arginase I and II in nitric oxide, polyamine, and proline syntheses in endothelial cells. *American Journal of Physiology. Endocrinology and Metabolism* 280, E75–82.

Li, H., Meininger, C.J., Hawker, J.R. Jr, Haynes, T.E., Kepka-Lenhart, D., Mistry, S.K., Morris, S.M. Jr, *et al.* (2001b) Regulatory role of arginase I and II in nitric oxide, polyamine, and proline syntheses in endothelial cells. *American Journal of Physiology. Endocrinology and Metabolism* 280, E75–82.

Liang, M., Ekblad, E., Hellstrand, P. and Nilsson, B.O. (2004) Polyamine synthesis inhibition attenuates vascular smooth muscle cell migration. *Journal of Vascular Research* 41, 141–147.

Lindemann, D. and Racke, K. (2003) Glucocorticoid inhibition of interleukin-4 (IL-4) and interleukin-13 (IL-13) induced up-regulation of arginase in rat airway fibroblasts. *Naunyn Schmiedeberg's Archive of Pharmacolology* 368, 546–550.

Loirand, G., Scalbert, E., Bril, A. and Pacaud, P. (2008) Rho exchange factors in the cardiovascular system. *Current Opinion in Pharmacology* 8, 174–180.

Lovett, F.A., Gonzalez, I., Salih, D.A., Cobb, L.J., Tripathi, G., Cosgrove, R.A., Murrell, A., *et al.* (2006) Convergence of Igf2 expression and adhesion signalling via RhoA and p38 MAPK enhances myogenic differentiation. *Journal of Cell Science* 119, 4828–4840.

Ma, T.C., Campana, A., Lange, P.S., Lee, H.H., Banerjee, K., Bryson, J.B., Mahishi, L., *et al.* (2010) A large-scale chemical screen for regulators of the arginase 1 promoter identifies the soy isoflavone daidzeinas a clinically approved small molecule that can promote neuronal protection or regeneration via a cAMP-independent pathway. *Journal of Neuroscience* 30, 739–748.

Maarsingh, H., Leusink, J., Bos, I.S., Zaagsma, J. and Meurs, H. (2006) Arginase strongly impairs neuronal nitric oxide-mediated airway smooth muscle relaxation in allergic asthma. *Respiratory Research* 7, 6.

Maarsingh, H., Pera, T. and Meurs, H. (2008a) Arginase and pulmonary diseases. *Naunyn Schmiedeberg's Archives of Pharmacology* 378, 171–184.

Maarsingh, H., Zaagsma, J. and Meurs, H. (2008b) Arginine homeostasis in allergic asthma. *European Journal of Pharmacology* 585, 375–384.

Marescau, B., Deshmukh, D.R., Kockx, M., Possemiers, I., Qureshi, I.A., Wiechert, P. and De Deyn, P.P. (1992) Guanidino compounds in serum, urine, liver, kidney, and brain of man and some ureotelic animals. *Metabolism* 41, 526–532.

Marinova, G.V., Loyaga-Rendon, R.Y., Obayashi, S., Ishibashi, T., Kubota, T., Imamura, M. and Azuma, H. (2008) Possible involvement of altered arginase activity, arginase type I and type II expressions, and nitric oxide production in occurrence of intimal hyperplasia in premenopausal human uterine arteries. *Journal of Pharmacological Sciences* 106, 385–393.

Marrero, M.B., Schieffer, B., Li, B., Sun, J., Harp, J.B. and Ling, B.N. (1997) Role of Janus kinase/signal transducer and activator of transcription and mitogen-activated protein kinase cascades in angiotensin II- and platelet-derived growth factor-induced vascular smooth muscle cell proliferation. *Journal of Biological Chemistry* 272, 24684–24690.

Masuda, H., Yano, M., Sakai, Y., Kihara, K., Yamauchi, Y. and Azuma, H. (2004) Modulation of intrinsic cavernous tone and nitric oxide production by arginase in rabbit corpus cavernosum. *Journal of Urology* 171, 490–494.

Meurs, H., Gosens, R. and Zaagsma, J. (2008) Airway hyperresponsiveness in asthma: lessons from in vitro model systems and animal models. *European Respiratory Journal* 32, 487–502.

Mills, C.D., Shearer, J., Evans, R. and Caldwell, M.D. (1992) Macrophage arginine metabolism and the inhibition or stimulation of cancer. *Journal of Immunology* 149, 2709–2714.

Ming, X.F., Barandier, C., Viswambharan, H., Kwak, B.R., Mach, F., Mazzolai, L., Hayoz, D., et al. (2004) Thrombin stimulates human endothelial arginase enzymatic activity via RhoA/ROCK pathway: implications for atherosclerotic endothelial dysfunction. *Circulation* 110, 3708–3714.

Miyanaka, K., Gotoh, T., Nagasaki, A., Takeya, M., Ozaki, M., Iwase, K., Takiguchi, M., et al. (1998) Immunohistochemical localization of arginase II and other enzymes of arginine metabolism in rat kidney and liver. *Histochemistry Journal* 30, 741–751.

Morris, C.R. (2006) New strategies for the treatment of pulmonary hypertension in sickle cell disease : the rationale for arginine therapy. *Treatments in Respiratory Medicine* 5, 31–45.

Morris, C.R., Kato, G.J., Poljakovic, M., Wang, X., Blackwelder, W.C., Sachdev, V., Hazen, S.L., et al. (2005) Dysregulated arginine metabolism, hemolysis-associated pulmonary hypertension, and mortality in sickle cell disease. *Journal of the American Medical Association* 294, 81–90.

Morris, C.R., Gladwin, M.T. and Kato, G.J. (2008) Nitric oxide and arginine dysregulation: a novel pathway to pulmonary hypertension in hemolytic disorders. *Current Molecular Medicine* 8, 620–632.

Morris, S.M., Jr (2002) Regulation of enzymes of the urea cycle and arginine metabolism. *Annual Review of Nutrition* 22, 87–105.

Morris, S.M., Jr (2009) Recent advances in arginine metabolism: roles and regulation of the arginases. *British Journal of Pharmacology* 157, 922–930.

Mumenthaler, S.M., Yu, H., Tze, S., Cederbaum, S.D., Pegg, A.E., Seligson, D.B. and Grody, W.W. (2008) Expression of arginase II in prostate cancer. *International Journal of Oncology* 32, 357–365.

Munder, M. (2009) Arginase: an emerging key player in the mammalian immune system. *British Journal of Pharmacology* 158, 638–651.

Munder, M., Eichmann, K., Moran, J.M., Centeno, F., Soler, G. and Modolell, M. (1999) Th1/Th2-regulated expression of arginase isoforms in murine macrophages and dendritic cells. *Journal of Immunology* 163, 3771–3777.

Nelin, L.D., Chicoine, L.G., Reber, K.M., English, B.K., Young, T.L. and Liu, Y. (2005) Cytokine-induced endothelial arginase expression is dependent on epidermal growth factor receptor. *American Journal of Respiratory Cell and Molecular Biology* 33, R394–401.

Nishikawa, T., Edelstein, D. and Brownlee, M. (2000a) The missing link: a single unifying mechanism for diabetic complications. *Kidney International. Supplement* 77, S26–30.

Nishikawa, T., Edelstein, D., Du, X.L., Yamagishi, S., Matsumura, T., Kaneda, Y., Yorek, M.A., et al. (2000b) Normalizing mitochondrial superoxide production blocks three pathways of hyperglycaemic damage. *Nature* 404, 787–790.

Osowska, S., Moinard, C., Neveux, N., Loi, C. and Cynober, L. (2004) Citrulline increases arginine pools and restores nitrogen balance after massive intestinal resection. *Gut* 53, 1781–1786.

Ozaki, M., Kawashima, S., Yamashita, T., Hirase, T., Namiki, M., Inoue, N., Hirata, K., et al. (2002) Overexpression of endothelial nitric oxide synthase accelerates atherosclerotic lesion formation in apoE-deficient mice. *Journal of Clinical Investigation* 110, 331–340.

Palm, F., Friederich, M., Carlsson, P.O., Hansell, P., Teerlink, T. and Liss, P. (2008) Reduced nitric oxide in diabetic kidneys due to increased hepatic arginine metabolism: implications for renomedullary oxygen availability. *American Journal of Physiology. Renal Physiology* 294, F30–37.

Peluffo, G., Piacenza, L., Irigoin, F., Alvarez, M.N. and Radi, R. (2004) L-arginine metabolism during interaction of Trypanosoma cruzi with host cells. *Trends in Parasitology* 20, 363–369.

Pernet, V., Bourgeois, P. and Di Polo, A. (2007) A role for polyamines in retinal ganglion cell excitotoxic death. *Journal of Neurochemistry* 103, 1481–1490.

Pieper, G.M. and Dondlinger, L.A. (1997) Plasma and vascular tissue arginine are decreased in diabetes: acute arginine supplementation restores endothelium-dependent relaxation by augmenting cGMP production. *Journal of Pharmacology Experimental Therapeutics* 283, 684–691.

Plebanski, M. and Hill, A.V. (2000) The immunology of malaria infection. *Current Opinion in Immunology* 12, 437–441.

Reid, K.M., Tsung, A., Kaizu, T., Jeyabalan, G., Ikeda, A., Shao, L., Wu, G., et al. (2007) Liver I/R injury is improved by the arginase inhibitor, N(omega)-hydroxy-nor-L-arginine (nor-NOHA). *American Journal of Physiology. Gastrointestinal and Liver Physiology* 292, G512–517.

Retnakaran, R. and Zinman, B. (2008) Type 1 diabetes, hyperglycaemia, and the heart. *Lancet* 371, 1790–1799.

Rogers, M., Kropf, P., Choi, B.S., Dillon, R., Podinovskaia, M., Bates, P. and Muller, I. (2009) Proteophosphoglycans regurgitated by Leishmania-infected sand flies target the L-arginine metabolism of host macrophages to promote parasite survival. *Public Library of Science Pathogens* 5, e1000555.

Romero, M.J., Platt, D.H., El-Remessy, A.B., Tawfik, H.E., Caldwell, R.B. and Caldwell, R.W. (2006) Does Elevated Arginase activity contribute to diabetes-induced endothelial dysfunction. *Circulation* 18, (Supplement 1690):II-328.

Romero, M.J., Platt, D.H., Tawfik, H.E., Labazi, M., El-Remessy, A.B., Bartoli, M., Caldwell, R.B., et al. (2008) Diabetes-induced coronary vascular dysfunction involves increased arginase activity. *Circulation Research* 102, 95–102.

Ryoo, S., Lemmon, C.A., Soucy, K.G., Gupta, G., White, A.R., Nyhan, D., Shoukas, A., et al. (2006) Oxidized low-density lipoprotein-dependent endothelial arginase II activation contributes to impaired nitric oxide signaling. *Circulation Research* 99, 951–960.

Ryoo, S., Gupta, G., Benjo, A., Lim, H.K., Camara, A., Sikka, G., Lim, H.K., et al. (2008) Endothelial arginase II: a novel target for the treatment of atherosclerosis. *Circulation Research* 102, 923–932.

Sabbatini, M., Pisani, A., Uccello, F., Fuiano, G., Alfieri, R., Cesaro, A., Cianciaruso, B., et al. (2003) Arginase inhibition slows the progression of renal failure in rats with renal ablation. *American Journal of Physiology. Renal Physiology* 284, F680–687.

Santhanam, L., Lim, H.K., Lim, H.K., Miriel, V., Brown, T., Patel, M., Balanson, S., et al. (2007) Inducible NO synthase dependent S-nitrosylation and activation of arginase1 contribute to age-related endothelial dysfunction. *Circulation Research* 101, 692–702.

Santhanam, L., Christianson, D.W., Nyhan, D. and Berkowitz, D.E. (2008) Arginase and vascular aging. *Journal of Applied Physiology* 105, 1632–1642.

Satoh, M., Fujimoto, S., Arakawa, S., Yada, T., Namikoshi, T., Haruna, Y., Horike, H., et al. (2008) Angiotensin II type 1 receptor blocker ameliorates uncoupled endothelial nitric oxide synthase in rats with experimental diabetic nephropathy. *Nephrology, Dialysis and Transplantation* 23, 3806–3813.

Satriano, J. (2004) Arginine pathways and the inflammatory response: interregulation of nitric oxide and polyamines: review article. *Amino Acids* 26, 321–329.

Schieffer, B., Luchtefeld, M., Braun, S., Hilfiker, A., Hilfiker-Kleiner, D. and Drexler, H. (2000) Role of NAD(P)H oxidase in angiotensin II-induced JAK/STAT signaling and cytokine induction. *Circulation Research* 87, 1195–1201.

Schwartz, I.F., Iaina, A., Benedict, Y., Wollman, Y., Chernichovski, T., Brasowski, E., Misonzhnik, F., et al. (2004) Augmented arginine uptake, through modulation of cationic amino acid transporter-1, increases GFR in diabetic rats. *Kidney International* 65, 1311–1319.

Shatanawi, A., Romero, M.J., Iddings, J.A., Chandra, S., Umapathy, N.S., Verin, A.D., Caldwell, R.B., et al. (2011) Angiotensin II-induced vascular endothelial dysfunction through RhoA/Rho Kinase/p38 mitogen-activated protein kinase/arginase pathway. *American Journal of Physiology. Cell Physiology* 300, C1183–C1192.

Shearer, J.D., Richards, J.R., Mills, C.D. and Caldwell, M.D. (1997) Differential regulation of macrophage arginine metabolism: a proposed role in wound healing. *American Journal of Physiology* 272, E181–190.

Singh, R., Pervin, S., Karimi, A., Cederbaum, S. and Chaudhuri, G. (2000) Arginase activity in human breast cancer cell lines: N(omega)-hydroxy-L-arginine selectively inhibits cell proliferation and induces apoptosis in MDA-MB-468 cells. *Cancer Research* 60, 3305–3312.

Sinha, P., Clements, V.K. and Ostrand-Rosenberg, S. (2005) Reduction of myeloid-derived suppressor cells and induction of M1 macrophages facilitate the rejection of established metastatic disease. *Journal of Immunology* 174, 636–645.

Sparkes, R.S., Dizikes, G.J., Klisak, I., Grody, W.W., Mohandas, T., Heinzmann, C., Zollman, S., et al. (1986) The gene for human liver arginase (ARG1) is assigned to chromosome band 6q23. *American Journal of Human Genetics* 39, 186–193.

Spector, E.B., Rice, S.C. and Cederbaum, S.D. (1983) Immunologic studies of arginase in tissues of normal human adult and arginase-deficient patients. *Pediatric Research* 17, 941–944.

Spolarics, Z. and Bond, J.S. (1989) Comparison of biochemical properties of liver arginase from streptozocin-induced diabetic and control mice. *Archives of Biochemistry and Biophysics* 274, 426–433.

Stempin, C.C., Tanos, T.B., Coso, O.A. and Cerban, F.M. (2004) Arginase induction promotes Trypanosoma cruzi intracellular replication in Cruzipain-treated J774 cells through the activation of multiple signaling pathways. *European Journal of Immunology* 34, 200–209.

Stempin, C.C., Garrido, V.V., Dulgerian, L.R. and Cerban, F.M. (2008) Cruzipain and SP600125 induce p38 activation, alter NO/arginase balance and favor the survival of Trypanosoma cruzi in macrophages. *Acta Tropica* 106, 119–127.

Stempin, C.C., Dulgerian, L.R., Garrido, V.V. and Cerban, F.M. (2010) Arginase in parasitic infections: macrophage activation, immunosuppression, and intracellular signals. *Journal of Biomedicine and Biotechnology* 2010, 683485.

Tawfik, H.E., El-Remessy, A.B., Matragoon, S., Ma, G., Caldwell, R.B. and Caldwell, R.W. (2006) Simvastatin improves diabetes-induced coronary endothelial dysfunction. *Journal of Pharmacology and Experimental Therapeutics* 319, 386–395.

Thengchaisri, N., Hein, T.W., Wang, W., Xu, X., Li, Z., Fossum, T.W. and Kuo, L. (2006) Upregulation of arginase by H_2O_2 impairs endothelium-dependent nitric oxide-mediated dilation of coronary arterioles. *Arteriosclerosis, Thrombosis and Vascular Biology* 26, 2035–2042.

Thomsen, L.L., Lawton, F.G., Knowles, R.G., Beesley, J.E., Riveros-Moreno, V. and Moncada, S. (1994) Nitric oxide synthase activity in human gynecological cancer. *Cancer Research* 54, 1352–1354.

Thomsen, L.L., Miles, D.W., Happerfield, L., Bobrow, L.G., Knowles, R.G. and Moncada, S. (1995) Nitric oxide synthase activity in human breast cancer. *British Journal of Cancer* 72, 41–44.

Toby, I.T., Chicoine, L.G., Cui, H., Chen, B. and Nelin, L.D. (2010) Hypoxia-induced proliferation of human pulmonary microvascular endothelial cells depends on epidermal growth factor receptor tyrosine kinase activation. *American Journal Physiology. Lung, Cellular and Molecular Physiology* 298, L600–606.

Topal, G., Brunet, A., Walch, L., Boucher, J.L. and David-Dufilho, M. (2006) Mitochondrial arginase II modulates nitric-oxide synthesis through nonfreely exchangeable L-arginine pools in human endothelial cells. *Journal of Pharmacology and Experimental Therapeutics* 318, 1368–1374.

Toque, H.A., Romero, M.J., Tostes, R.C., Shatanawi, A., Chandra, S., Carneiro, Z., Inscho, E., et al. (2010a) p38 Mitogen-activated protein kinase (MAPK) increases arginase activity and contributes to endothelial dysfunction in corpora cavernosa from angiotensin-II treated mice. *Journal of Sexual Medicine* 7(12), 3857–3867.

Toque, H.A., Tostes, R.C., Yao, L., Xu, X., Webb, R.C., Caldwell, R.B. and Caldwell, R.W. (2010b) Arginase II deletion increases corpora cavernosa relaxation in diabetic mice. The Journal of Sexual Medicine [ePub ahead of print]. Nov 3 2010.

Touyz, R.M. (2004) Reactive oxygen species and angiotensin II signaling in vascular cells – implications in cardiovascular disease. *Brazilian Journal of Medical and Biological Research* 37, 1263–1273.

Uchino, T., Snyderman, S.E., Lambert, M., Qureshi, I.A., Shapira, S.K., Sansaricq, C., Smit, L.M., et al. (1995) Molecular basis of phenotypic variation in patients with argininemia. *Human Genetics* 96, 255–260.

Vockley, J.G., Tabor, D.E., Kern, R.M., Goodman, B.K., Wissmann, P.B., Kang, D.S., Grody, W.W., et al. (1994) Identification of mutations (D128G, H141L) in the liver arginase gene of patients with hyperargininemia. *Human Mutation* 4, 150–154.

Waddington, S.N., Mosley, K., Cook, H.T., Tam, F.W. and Cattell, V. (1998a) Arginase AI is upregulated in acute immune complex-induced inflammation. *Biochemical and Biophysical Research Communications* 247, 84–87.

Waddington, S.N., Tam, F.W., Cook, H.T. and Cattell, V. (1998b) Arginase activity is modulated by IL-4 and HOArg in nephritic glomeruli and mesangial cells. *American Journal of Physiology* 274, F473–480.

Wallace, H.M., Fraser, A.V. and Hughes, A. (2003) A perspective of polyamine metabolism. *Biochemical Journal* 376, 1–14.

Walther, M., Woodruff, J., Edele, F., Jeffries, D., Tongren, J.E., King, E., Andrews, L., et al. (2006) Innate immune responses to human malaria: heterogeneous cytokine responses to blood-stage Plasmodium falciparum correlate with parasitological and clinical outcomes. *Journal of Immunology* 177, 5736–5745.

Wanasen, N., MacLeod, C.L., Ellies, L.G. and Soong, L. (2007) L-arginine and cationic amino acid transporter 2B regulate growth and survival of Leishmania amazonensis amastigotes in macrophages. *Infection and Immunity* 75, 2802–2810.

Waugh, W.H., Daeschner, C.W. 3rd, Files, B.A., McConnell, M.E. and Strandjord, S.E. (2001) Oral citrulline as arginine precursor may be beneficial in sickle cell disease: early phase two results. *Journal of the National Medical Association* 93, 363–371.

Wei, L.H., Jacobs, A.T., Morris, S.M., Jr and Ignarro, L.J. (2000) IL-4 and IL-13 upregulate arginase I expression by cAMP and JAK/STAT6 pathways in vascular smooth muscle cells. *American Journal of Physiology Cell Phyisolgy* 279, C248–256.

Wei, L.H., Wu, G., Morris, S.M., Jr and Ignarro, L.J. (2001) Elevated arginase I expression in rat aortic smooth muscle cells increases cell proliferation. *Proceedings of the National Academy of Sciences of the United States of America* 98, 9260–9264.

Weigert, A. and Brune, B. (2008) Nitric oxide, apoptosis and macrophage polarization during tumor progression. *Nitric Oxide* 19, 95–102.

Wen, Y., Gu, J., Li, S.L., Reddy, M.A., Natarajan, R. and Nadler, J.L. (2006) Elevated glucose and diabetes promote interleukin-12 cytokine gene expression in mouse macrophages. *Endocrinology* 147, 2518–2525.

White, A.R., Ryoo, S., Li, D., Champion, H.C., Steppan, J., Wang, D., Nyhan, D., *et al.* (2006) Knockdown of arginase I restores NO signaling in the vasculature of old rats. *Hypertension* 47, 245–251.

Witte, M.B. and Barbul, A. (2003) Arginine physiology and its implication for wound healing. *Wound Repair and Regeneration* 11, 419–423.

Xie, D., Odronic, S.I., Wu, F., Pippen, A.M., Donatucci, C.F. and Annex, B.H. (2007) A mouse model of hypercholesterolemia-induced erectile dysfunction. *Journal of Sexual Medicine* 4, 898–907.

Xu, W., Liu, L.Z., Loizidou, M., Ahmed, M. and Charles, I.G. (2002) The role of nitric oxide in cancer. *Cell Research* 12, 311–320.

Xu, W., Kaneko, F.T., Zheng, S., Comhair, S.A., Janocha, A.J., Goggans, T., Thunnissen, F.B., *et al.* (2004) Increased arginase II and decreased NO synthesis in endothelial cells of patients with pulmonary arterial hypertension. *Federation of American Societies for Experimental Biology Journal* 18, 1746–1748.

Yang, M., Rangasamy, D., Matthaei, K.I., Frew, A.J., Zimmermann, N., Mahalingam, S., Webb, D.C., *et al.* (2006) Inhibition of arginase I activity by RNA interference attenuates IL-13-induced airways hyperresponsiveness. *Journal of Immunology* 177, 5595–5603.

Yang, Z. and Ming, X.F. (2006) Endothelial arginase: a new target in atherosclerosis. *Current Hypertension Reports* 8, 54–59.

Yung, L.M., Leung, F.P., Yao, X., Chen, Z.Y. and Huang, Y. (2006) Reactive oxygen species in vascular wall. *Cardiovascular and Hematological Disorder Drug Targets* 6, 1–19.

Zhang, C., Hein, T.W., Wang, W., Chang, C.I. and Kuo, L. (2001) Constitutive expression of arginase in microvascular endothelial cells counteracts nitric oxide-mediated vasodilatory function. *Federation of American Societies for Experimental Biology Journal* 15, 1264–1266.

Zhang, C., Wu, J., Xu, X., Potter, B.J. and Gao, X. (2010) Direct relationship between levels of TNF-alpha expression and endothelial dysfunction in reperfusion injury. *Basic Research in Cardiology* 105, 453–464.

Zhang, W., Baban, B., Rojas, M., Tofigh, S., Virmani, S.K., Patel, C., Behzadian, M.A., *et al.* (2009) Arginase activity mediates retinal inflammation in endotoxin-induced uveitis. *American Journal of Patholology* 175, 891–902.

Zharikov, S., Krotova, K., Hu, H., Baylis, C., Johnson, R.J., Block, E.R. and Patel, J. (2008) Uric acid decreases NO production and increases arginase activity in cultured pulmonary artery endothelial cells. *American Journal of Physiology. Cell Physiology.* 295, C1183–1190.

Zimmermann, N., King, N.E., Laporte, J., Yang, M., Mishra, A., Pope, S.M., Muntel, E.E., *et al.* (2003) Dissection of experimental asthma with DNA microarray analysis identifies arginase in asthma pathogenesis. *Journal of Clinical Investigation* 111, 1863–1874.

4 Bypassing the Endothelial L-Arginine–Nitric Oxide Pathway: Effects of Dietary Nitrite and Nitrate on Cardiovascular Function

P. Luedike, M. Kelm and T. Rassaf*
Medical Faculty, University Hospital Düsseldorf, Düsseldorf, Germany

4.1 Abstract

L-Arginine (L-Arg) is a semi-essential amino acid that is a natural constituent of most dietary proteins in our daily diet. A fundamental function of this amino acid is its role as the substrate for the synthesis of the signalling molecule nitric oxide (NO). As NO regulates a variety of physiological processes in nearly every organ system of the human organism, L-Arg is a crucial element in mammalian physiology. The family of NO-generating enzymes is called NO synthases (NOS). NOS provide the availability of NO under physiological conditions and depend on an adequate supply of dioxygen (O_2) and several substrates. Under conditions of ischaemia, where O_2 is lacking, the NO production by the NOS shuts down and the generation of the important signalling molecule from L-Arg is disturbed. Until recently it was not known how the organism maintains NO availability under ischaemic conditions. In recent years, biomedical research has demonstrated that along the physiological O_2 gradient NO can be formed independently of its enzymatic synthesis from L-Arg, by reduction of inorganic nitrate and nitrite. Although for a long time both anions have been considered as inert end products of NO metabolism, it has been shown that reduction of nitrate and nitrite could maintain NO homeostasis under hypoxia and ischaemia. It has been demonstrated that low levels of supplemental nitrite and nitrate can influence blood pressure, and that dietary sources of NO metabolites may protect against various cardiovascular disease states. Thus the enzymatic generation of NO from L-Arg under normoxia and the non-enzymatic formation of NO via nitrate and nitrite can be considered as a balance that maintains NO availability along the circulating and metabolic O_2 gradient. Dietary intake of nitrate–nitrite-rich foods such as leafy vegetables may represent an opportunity for disease prevention and health modulation of human physiological functions.

4.2 Introduction

Since the 1998 Nobel Prize in Medicine or Physiology was awarded to Ferid Murad, Louis J. Ignarro, and Robert F. Furchgott for their groundbreaking investigations on the

* E-mail address: Tienush.Rassaf@med.uni-duesseldorf.de

role of NO in human physiology, it is inevitable that one mentions NO when talking about the role of L-arginine (L-Arg) in human nutrition and health (Howlett, 1998). Herein we summarize the role of the amino acid L-Arg as the substrate of human NO synthesis under physiological conditions. Furthermore, we will consider alternative sources of NO under physiological and pathophysiological conditions, with focus on the effects of nitrate and nitrite on cardiovascular function.

4.3 L-Arginine: a Semi-Essential Amino Acid in Human Physiology

L-arginine (2-amino-5-guanidino-pentanoic acid) is a dibasic amino acid that was first discovered over 100 years ago and that is a natural constituent of most dietary proteins (Silk et al., 1985). L-Arg serves as the substrate for the synthesis of the signalling molecule NO and takes part in protein production, endocrine function, wound healing and erectile function (Palmer et al., 1988; Rajfer et al., 1992). L-Arg serves as a precursor for creatine, which plays an essential role in the energy metabolism of muscle, nerve, and testis. As the adult human is able to synthesize L-Arg de novo from the urea cycle, L-Arg is regarded as a non-essential amino acid. However, in infants the amount of synthesized L-Arg is too low to cover the demands of the growing organism, and it becomes essential in this developmental stage. Thus the classification of L-Arg as a semi-essential or conditionally essential amino acid is given. The biosynthesis of L-Arg results from L-citrulline, a by-product of the glutamine metabolism in the gut and in the liver (Hecker et al., 1990). When L-citrulline is excreted into the circulation, it is reabsorbed in the proximal tubule of the kidney where it is converted into L-Arg (Fig. 4.1). Although endogenous synthesis is possible, the dietary intake of L-Arg is the basic determinant of L-Arg plasma levels because the biosynthesis is not able to balance inadequate intake or deficiency. Because of the fact that L-Arg is crucial for ammonia detoxification, dietary deficiency of L-Arg (hypoargininaemia) is a significant nutritional problem in preterm infants. The resulting hyperammonaemia leads to cardiovascular, pulmonary, neurological and intestinal dysfunction, demonstrating the impact of L-Arg on endocrine homeostasis (Wu et al., 2004). The relative amounts of L-Arg in various dietary proteins range from 3% in cereals up to 15% in L-Arg rich protein sources like fish or walnuts. Typical dietary intake of L-Arg is 3.5–5.0 g daily and mainly derives from plant or animal foods (Oomen et al., 2000). Against this background, the different dietary habits between populations and regions may be the underlying reason for differences in L-Arg plasma levels in various parts of the world in recent studies. Ranges from 45–100 µmol l^{-1} in healthy humans as well as in the plasma of patients with vascular disorders (Böger and Bode-Böger, 2001) have been reported. Women show lower levels compared to men, ranging from 72.4 ± 6.7 µmol l^{-1} in the young to 88.0 ± 7.8 µmol l^{-1} in the elderly. This phenomenon is due to the lower muscle mass in women (Moller et al., 1983).

Among the variety of physiological effects of L-Arg, its role as the substrate for the enzyme endothelial NO synthase (eNOS) is one of the most investigated ones and it is supposed to be one of the most important functions of this amino acid. NO exerts various physiological functions in most if not all organ systems throughout the body. To understand the relation between the effects of L-Arg and NO, it is inevitable that one must consider NO synthesis under physiological as well as under pathophysiological conditions.

4.4 L-Arginine is the Substrate of the Nitric Oxide Synthases: The L-Arginine–Nitric Oxide Pathway

The small and relatively unstable free radical NO has become one of the most studied and fascinating molecules in biological chemistry and medicine. It is an important messenger molecule involved in many physiological and

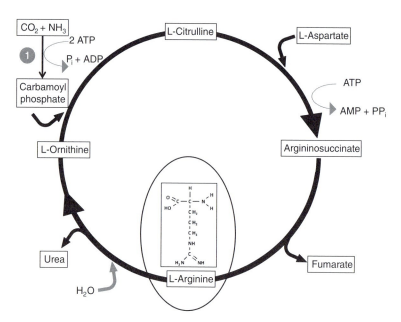

Fig. 4.1. Biosynthesis of L-arginine from citrulline in the urea cycle. ① The primary function of the urea cycle is the detoxification of ammonia (NH_3). The generation of L-arginine is a byproduct of this adenosine triphosphate-dependent (ATP), energy consuming process. Catalysed by cytosolic argininosuccinate synthetase, citrulline and aspartate are condensed to form argininosuccinate. The reaction involves the addition of AMP (from ATP) to the amido carbonyl of citrulline, forming an activated intermediate on the enzyme surface (AMP-citrulline), and the subsequent addition of L-aspartate to form argininosuccinate. L-arginine and fumarate are produced from argininosuccinate by the cytosolic enzyme argininosuccinate lyase (also called argininosuccinase). In the final step of the cycle arginase cleaves urea from arginine, regenerating cytosolic L-ornithine, which can be transported to the mitochondrial matrix for another round of urea synthesis. The fumarate, generated via the action of argininosuccinate lyase, is reconverted to L-aspartate for use in the argininosuccinate synthetase reaction. AMP, adenosine monophosphate; ADP, adenosine diphosphate; P_i, phosphate.

pathophysiological processes within the mammalian body, with both beneficial and detrimental properties (Moncada and Higgs, 1993). NO plays a key role in nearly every organ system within our body and it is primarily known for maintaining normal blood pressure by regulating blood vessel tone, being the major mediator of endothelium-dependent vasodilatation (Furchgott and Zawadzki, 1980, Palmer et al., 1987). NO furthermore regulates the vascular structure by effecting smooth muscle cell proliferation and inhibition of platelet and monocyte adhesion, by maintaining a nonthrombotic endothelial surface (Busse et al., 1987; Ignarro et al., 2001). Risk factors like hypercholesterolaemia, hypertension, diabetes mellitus, or cigarette smoking lead to endothelial dysfunction and thus to the inability of the endothelium to produce NO (Galle et al., 1991; Makimattila et al., 1996; Busse and Fleming, 1999). A decrease of endothelial NO formation is a hallmark of endothelial dysfunction which is a key element in the development of atherosclerosis. This leads to diseases such as hypertension, myocardial infarction, or apoplectic stroke. One of the main consequences of endothelial dysfunction is that the diminishing NO synthesis influences a variety of physiological NO-dependent processes. Beside its impact on cardiovascular function, NO plays a key role in immunomodulatory processes and in the central nervous system (Knowles et al., 1989).

The 'Molecule of the Year' in 1992 is biosynthesized endogenously from the amino acid L-Arg and oxygen by various NOS (Culotta and Koshland, 1992). So far three isoforms of NOS are known, named either according to their distribution within the body

Table 4.1. Isoforms of nitric oxide synthases.

Isoforms	Synonym	K_m^a µmol l^{-1}	Molecular mass, kDa^b	Ca^{2+} – calmodulin dependence
NOS I	neuronal NOS (nNOS)	1.4–2.2	160	+
NOS II	inducible NOS (iNOS)	2.8–32.3	131	−
NOS III	endothelial NOS (eNOS)	2.9	133	+

$^a K_m$, Michaelis–Menten constant, half-saturating L-Arg concentration; ^{b}kDa, Kilo Dalton.

or in the order in which they were first purified and cloned (see Table 4.1) (Forstermann et al., 1994).

All three isoforms function as a homodimer consisting of two identical monomers, which can be functionally divided into a C-terminal reductase-carboxy domain and an N-terminal oxygenase-amino domain (Culotta and Koshland, 1992). Two types are constitutively expressed. They are calcium-calmodulin dependent and release NO for short periods in response to receptor or physical stimulation during signalling processes. The third isoform (iNOS) is inducible upon activation of macrophages, endothelial cells, and a number of other cells by endotoxin and pro-inflammatory cytokines. Once expressed, iNOS synthesizes NO for a prolonged period of time.

NOS produce NO by catalysing a five electron oxidation of guanidino nitrogen of L-Arg. The oxidation of L-Arg into L-citrulline via formation of the intermediate N^Ghydroxy-L-Arg consumes two moles of dioxygen (O_2) and 1.5 moles of nicotinamide adenine dinucleotide (NADPH) per mole of produced NO (Liu and Gross, 1996). Beside O_2 and NADPH, the NOS enzymes require the binding of five cofactors to function properly. These cofactors are: flavin adenine dinucleotide (FAD), flavin mononucleotide (FMN), haem iron, tetrahydrobiopterin (BH$_4$), and calcium-calmodulin (Bredt and Snyder, 1990) (Fig. 4.2). If any of these cofactors becomes limiting, NO production from NOS shuts down, and in many cases NOS then produce superoxide (O_2^-) instead. This mechanism has been termed NOS uncoupling (Landmesser et al., 2003). Consequently a physiological oxygen concentration as well as sufficient substrate supply is necessary for a proper NOS function.

One possible pathway for NO metabolism is the stepwise oxidation to nitrite (NO_2^-) which is rapidly oxidized in whole blood to nitrate (NO_3^-) (Kelm, 1999). For years, both nitrite and nitrate have been considered as inert end products of the NO metabolism. However, we will later illustrate the evolving evidence that the formation of NO from the anions nitrite and nitrate may represent an alternative to the classical L-Arg–NO pathway.

NO derived from the constitutive eNOS mediates vascular smooth muscle relaxation which is the underlying mechanism for the blood pressure regulating effect of this molecule (Ignarro et al., 1986). After entering the target cell, eNOS-derived NO binds to the guanylyl cyclase and activates this enzyme by inducing a conformational change (Ignarro, 1991). Guanylyl cyclase catalyses the formation of cyclic guanylyl monophosphate (cGMP) from guanylyl triphosphate (GTP). cGMP then triggers a cascade of intracellular events that culminate in a reduction of the calcium-dependent vascular smooth muscle tone and vasodilatation (Twort and van Breemen, 1988) (Fig. 4.2).

Under ischaemic conditions the oxidation of L-Arg by NOS is inefficient and NO availability decreases. This is due to the limited O_2 as well as to the lack of substrates and cofactors. If the partial O_2 pressure (pO_2) decreases below 7.6 mmHg, eNOS activity slows down progressively (Abu-Soud et al., 2000). In comparison, a pO_2 of 15 mmHg is considered as normal O_2 level in nonexercised muscle (Marcinek et al., 2003). This limitation of NOS-derived NO is not only of interest under pathological conditions but also under physiological conditions where the O_2 concentration in blood or tissue decreases and the essential NOS cofactor O_2 is lacking, i.e. during physical exercise. Taken together the production of NO from L-Arg can be considered as a critical cellular function in most if not all organ systems throughout the body.

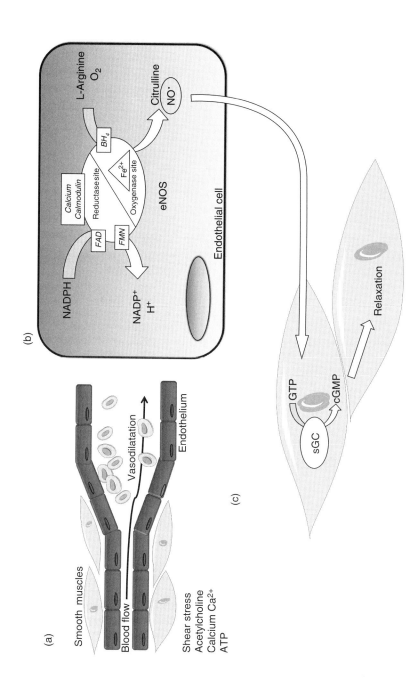

Fig. 4.2. Endothelial NO synthase (eNOS). (a) Upon stimuli such as shear stress via increased blood flow, nitric oxide (NO) is generated in the endothelial cells of blood vessels by the eNOS. (b) The eNOS is a homodimer consisting of two identical monomers, which can be functionally divided into a C-terminal reductase site and an N-terminal oxygenase site. (c) Once released, NO can mediate relaxation of the smooth muscles by activating the soluble guanylate cyclase (sGC). This leads to vasodilatation of the vessel and decreased blood pressure. This reaction requires five bound cofactors beside the substrate L-Arginine (see a). These are: flavin adenine dinucleotide (FAD), flavin mononucleotide (FMN), tetrahydrobiopterin (BH_4), haem iron (Fe^{2+}), and calcium-calmodulin. Nicotinamide adenine dinucleotide (NADPH) and oxygen (O_2) are also required.

4.5 L-Arginine in Cardiovascular Disease: Perspectives and Limitations

NO bioavailability is controlled by its formation through NOS and by its degradation via increased oxidative inactivation by reactive oxygen species (ROS). Considering NO as one of the most important signalling molecules in human physiology, it has been suggested that supplementation of L-Arg might increase NO synthesis in individuals with endothelial dysfunction. The first clinical application of L-Arg, an attempt to improve vascular function in patients with cardiovascular disease, was published by Drexler *et al.* (1991). It was shown that L-Arg enhanced the blood flow response to acetylcholine in the coronary artery of patients with coronary artery disease (CAD), but not in healthy controls. Since then, there have been numerous studies that demonstrated beneficial effects of L-Arg supplementation in both animals and humans under pathophysiological conditions such as hypercholesterolaemia, atherosclerosis and hypertension (Drexler *et al.*, 1991; Rossitch *et al.*, 1991; Hirooka *et al.*, 1992; Böger *et al.*, 1997; Brandes *et al.*, 1997). However, the precise molecular mechanism by which L-Arg improves endothelial function remains unclear.

Increasing the circulating L-Arg concentration by supplementation could not explain the beneficial effects mentioned above, since the intracellular levels of this amino acid are in the mM range (Gold *et al.*, 1989), whereas the enzyme's Michaelis–Menten constant (K_m) for substrate is in the µM (2.9 µmol l^{-1}) range (Bredt and Snyder, 1990). Likewise, circulating L-Arg plasma levels in healthy humans as well as in patients with vascular disorders are up to 15–30-fold higher than the concentration required to saturate the NOS (Böger and Bode-Böger, 2001). Hence, considering enzyme kinetics, eNOS should always be saturated and not depend on extracellular L-Arg supply. This discrepancy is termed the 'arginine paradox' (Tsikas *et al.*, 2000). For this reason, in recent years other possible explanations have been proposed to explain the beneficial effects of supplemental L-Arg:

- McDonald *et al.* demonstrated in 1997 that the eNOS and the L-Arg transporter (CAT1) are co-localized within plasma membrane caveolae. Others proposed that the L-Arg concentration within these caveolae may be lower than in the ambient cytoplasm. It was further hypothesized that eNOS preferentially converts extracellular over intracellular L-Arg. Extracellular L-Arg is taken up into the caveolae via the CAT1 transporter. The intracellular L-Arg concentration could be increased by increasing the extracellular L-Arg concentration. Thus, the co-localization of both eNOS and CAT1 transporter in membrane caveolae may account for the 'arginine paradox', since the high intracellular level of L-Arg may not be utilized for NO synthesis (McDonald *et al.*, 1997).

- Other authors consider the upregulation of the enzyme arginase, which converts L-Arg to ornithine and urea, which may decrease cellular levels of L-Arg and thereby impair NO production (Wei *et al.*, 2000). It has been shown in animal models that upregulation of arginase may contribute to smooth muscle proliferation, resulting in endothelial dysfunction. In vessels of older animals, endothelial arginase activity is elevated and can thus contribute to endothelial dysfunction by reducing the capacity of NO synthesis (Berkowitz *et al.*, 2003). Increasing L-Arg concentrations may override converting activity of arginase and thus contribute to the beneficial effects of L-Arg supplementation.

- Another proposed mechanism by which the 'arginine paradox' could be explained is that oxidized low density lipoproteins (LDL) and lysophosphatidylcholine decrease L-Arg transport into endothelial cells by competing or interfering with transporter systems (Kikuta *et al.*, 1998, Jay *et al.*, 1997). This could be an explanation for the beneficial effects of L-Arg observed in hypercholesterolaemic patients.

- The impact of asymmetrical dimethylarginine (ADMA) on NOS activity and its impact on endothelial dysfunction might serve as another explanation of the way in which L-Arg may affect vascular function.

In 1992, Vallance et al. were the first to describe the presence of endogenous analogues of L-Arg. ADMA and L-N^G-monomethyl-arginine-citrate (L-NMMA) exert biological activity by competing with L-Arg for the active substrate binding site on NO synthase (Vallance et al., 1992). Böger et al. showed that elevation in plasma ADMA occurs in hypercholesterolaemia and correlates with endothelial dysfunction (Böger et al., 1998). Free ADMA as a competitive inhibitor of the NOS is present in the cytoplasm and in the blood plasma. ADMA binds to NOS but could not be used as a substrate through the enzyme. ADMA is eliminated 20% renally, whereas the main excretion route is via metabolism by the enzyme dimethylarginine dimethylaminohydrolase (DDAH) to L-citrulline. DDAH activity is impaired by a variety of factors such as oxidized LDL, hyperglycaemia, or infectious diseases. The resulting increase in plasma ADMA concentrations may contribute to endothelial dysfunction (Stuhlinger et al., 2002). Inhibition of NOS activity might be exceeded by increased extracellular L-Arg/ADMA ratio through excessive substrate and could explain how L-Arg improves endothelial function in patients with vascular disease. The investigators conclude that nutritional supplementation with L-Arg may be able to restore physiological status via this mechanism.

Taken together it has been shown that intravenous or dietary (oral) administration of relatively large doses of L-Arg results in enhanced NO formation in subjects with impaired endothelial function under baseline conditions. According to these findings, long-term administration of L-Arg has been shown to improve the symptoms of cardiovascular disease in several controlled clinical trials. In other trials L-Arg was not beneficial, and in a single study a higher mortality of subjects receiving the amino acid has even been reported (Rector et al., 1996; Bednarz et al., 2005; Schulman et al., 2006). In conclusion more placebo-controlled clinical trials and mechanistic investigations are necessary to resolve the issue of dietary L-Arg as adjunctive therapy for different stages of cardiovascular disease. Furthermore, it will be necessary to assess if individual cofactors such as hypercholesterolaemia or elevated ADMA plasma concentration in patients selectively influence the efficiency of L-Arg supplementation, in comparison to the average population of cardiovascular disease patients.

4.6 Nitric Oxide Generation without NO-Synthase? Bypassing the L-Arginine Pathway

The ability of humans to produce NO from the classical L-Arg pathway is complex and requires undisturbed blood supply, oxygen, and substrate delivery. Under conditions where blood flow is impaired by occlusion or narrowing of vessels, the classical L-Arg pathway is no longer fully functional. A common disease that impairs blood flow by narrowing of the blood vessels and thereby mediating substrate deficiency in tissues is arteriosclerotic vascular disease. Of all diseases, CAD still remains the leading cause of death in the industrialized countries and is the fatal end-stage of endothelial dysfunction. Plaque rupture and the subsequent occlusion of a large epicardial artery cause an acute myocardial infarction. The therapeutic gold standard is the early reperfusion of the ischaemic heart muscle to protect the heart from ischaemia and from the absence of essential substrates. However, when flow through coronary vessels is restored the reperfusion may be an additional source of harm to the myocardium, a phenomenon called ischaemia and reperfusion (I/R) injury (Jennings et al., 1960). This phenomenon is not only limited to the heart but occurs also under all conditions where blood supply is disrupted or deficient over a period and restored afterwards, such as cerebral ischaemia, transplantation surgery, or haemorrhagic shock. In recent years, major advances have been made towards understanding the role of NO in the ischaemic biology of the heart. Numerous studies demonstrate that NO represents one of the most effective protective mechanisms against myocardial I/R injury (Bolli, 2001; Bell et al., 2003; Jones and Bolli, 2006). Although NO offers protective properties, the classical L-Arg–NO pathway is not functional during ischaemia due to insufficient O_2, limited substrate delivery and reduced cofactors. Thus, NOS independent mechanisms must exist to maintain NO homeostasis under hypoxic conditions. The reduction of nitrite, the oxidation product of NO by several 'nitrite-reductases' under hypoxia was identified to be such an alternative pathway (Millar et al., 1998; Cosby et al., 2003; Huang et al., 2005; Rassaf et al., 2007; Shiva et al., 2007). These nitrite reductases operate along the physiological and pathological O_2 gradient and allow a graded nitrite reduction to NO according to the circulating and metabolic need. The reduction of nitrite to NO reflects a major mechanism by which the NO homeostasis is maintained independent of NOS. L-Arg and nitrite maintain the balance of NO sources ensuring NO availability during normoxic as well as hypoxic and ischaemic conditions.

4.7 The Nitrate–Nitrite–Nitric Oxide Pathway

Until recently the inorganic anions nitrate and nitrite were considered inert end products of NO metabolism and unfavourable dietary constituents (Mirvish, 1995). However, a new view is evolving with the accumulating evidence that nitrate and nitrite metabolism occurs in blood and tissues to recycle NO and other bioactive nitrogen oxides. This may represent an alternative to the 'classical' L-Arg-NOS-NO signalling. For the first time in 1994 both Lundberg et al. and Benjamin et al. independently presented evidence for the generation of NO in the stomach resulting from the acidic reduction of inorganic nitrite (Benjamin et al., 1994; Lundberg et al., 1994) (Fig. 4.3). These were the first reports of NO synthase-independent formation of NO in vivo. Further studies identified that commensal bacteria in the crypts of the tongue possess a nitrate reductase enzyme that they utilize for energy metabolism in the absence of oxygen (Duncan et al., 1995; Lundberg et al., 2004). It was known that nitrate is taken up by the salivary glands and concentrated in the saliva. However the reason for this active process could not be explained until the discovery that nitrate serves as substrate for the nitrate reductase enzyme of bacteria in the mouth. These bacteria reduce both plasma-extracted nitrate as well as dietary nitrate, to form nitrite, resulting in salivary nitrite levels that are 1000-fold higher than those found in human plasma (Lundberg and Govoni, 2004). When nitrite-rich saliva meets the acidic gastric juice after swallowing, nitrite is protonated to form nitrous acid (HNO_2) which then decomposes to NO, a process termed acidic disproportionation. Further investigation showed that this gastric NO formation takes part in the human defence against pathogens entering via the alimentary tract. Furthermore it could provide protection against ulcers from drugs or stress (Dykhuizen et al., 1996; Miyoshi et al., 2003; Jansson et al., 2007). Beside the intraluminal formation of NO it has been demonstrated that some of the ingested nitrite survives and reaches the systemic circulation. Thus, ingestion of nitrate increases plasma nitrite by enterosalivary reduction of nitrate and makes it systemically available (Lundberg and Govoni, 2004). It was in 1995, a year after the discovery of gastric-derived NO when Zweier et al. demonstrated that the reduction of nitrite to NO may also occur systemically (Zweier et al., 1995). They discovered that NO was generated in the ischaemic heart from nitrite. In the following years it became clear that nitrite can be reduced in vivo via numerous pathways to form bioactive NO. These include the reduction via deoxygenated myoglobin within the heart muscle, deoxyhaemoglobin, intracellular xanthin oxidoreductase, enzymes of the mitochondrial respiratory chain, cytochrome P-450, and even via the NOS (Millar et al., 1998; Cosby et al., 2003; Kozlov et al., 2003; Castello et al., 2006; Rassaf et al., 2007; Vanin et al., 2007; Hendgen-Cotta et al., 2008). Since then there has been a growing interest in the physiological effects of dietary nitrates and nitrites in human health and disease.

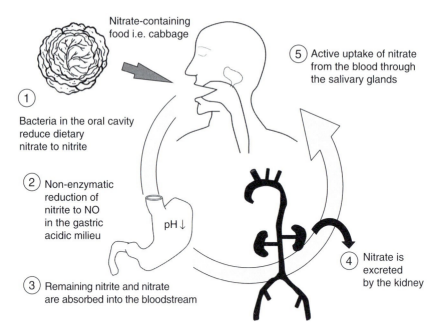

Fig. 4.3. NOS-independent formation of NO in the stomach. Commensial bacteria reduce nitrate to nitrite①. Nitrate is actively extracted from the blood in the salivary glands to concentrate nitrate in the oral cavity⑤. When nitrite-rich saliva is swallowed and meets the acidic gastric juice, nitrite is protonated to form nitrous acid which then decomposes to NO②. Nitrate and remaining nitrite are absorbed from the intestine into the circulation and can convert to bioactive NO in blood and tissue under conditions of hypoxia③. Excess nitrate is excreted by the kidneys④. Nitrite remaining in the blood can be considered as a circulating nitrite source.

4.8 Effects of Nitrite and Nitrate in Human Physiology

To understand the variety of physiological implications of nitrite and nitrate in the human organism it is essential to take a look at the biochemical background of nitrite and nitrate formation. As already outlined above, there are several mechanisms by which NO is generated in the body, including the NO synthase enzymes or the non-enzymatically acidic reduction of nitrite. Once NO is formed, it can be oxidized to nitrite or nitrate through its relatively slow reaction with oxygen. However in most *in vivo* environments like blood or tissue, this autoxidation reaction is not favoured since NO reacts more rapidly with other targets, particularly haem-based proteins. Joshi *et al.* (2002), for example, showed that NO reacts rapidly with oxygenated haemoglobin within the erythrocyte to form nitrate and methaemoglobin. Although it is kinetically unexpected that any NO would be oxidized to nitrite in the blood, it has been shown that the addition of NO to blood does generate significant concentrations of plasma nitrite (Shiva *et al.*, 2006). This nitrite formation was due to the NO-oxidase function of the multi-copper oxidase caeruloplasmin. This was consistent with the finding that caeruloplasmin-deficient mice have lower nitrite levels when NO is added than controls (Shiva *et al.*, 2006). Other sources of nitrite are dietary intake of both nitrite and nitrate, which maintain the plasma nitrite concentration between 300 and 500 nM, whereas the concentration in the tissue is about 1–10 µM (Bryan *et al.*, 2004). The one-electron reduction of nitrite to NO by ferrous haem proteins such as deoxygenated haemoglobin and myoglobin or xanthin oxidoreductase can occur in a much simpler mechanism than the five-electron oxidation that was demonstrated for the synthesis from L-arginine (see Eqn 4.1):

$$NO_2^- + Fe^{(II)} + 2H^+ \leftrightarrow NO + Fe^{(III)} + H_2O \quad (4.1)$$

The outlined reaction occurs in the presence of $Fe^{(II)}$ in haem proteins, a redox state found in deoxygenated haemoglobin in the blood or deoxygenated myoglobin within muscle tissue. Confirming studies for these observations were made by several groups demonstrating that under conditions of low O_2, the nitrite reductase activity of these proteins contributes to NOS independent NO formation (Fig. 4.4). Experiments carried out by our group using wild-type and myoglobin deficient mice (Mb-/-) under moderate hypoxia due to acute coronary artery occlusion established a novel homeostatic mechanism mediated by myoglobin during O_2 deprivation (Rassaf et al., 2007). The imbalance of O_2 supply and demand in the working heart muscle, a consequence of acute hypoxia, results in increased levels of deoxygenated myoglobin, which is able to reduce nitrite to NO. Thus, the decrease in tissue O_2 tension switches the activity of myoglobin from being an NO scavenger under normoxic conditions to an NO producer in hypoxia. Because myoglobin must be at least partially deoxygenated to act as nitrite reductase, the latter reaction pathway can become significant only when the oxygen level falls below the half-loading point (P_{50}) of Mb. The P_{50} of myoglobin is reached when the pO_2 falls below 3.0 mmHg. In comparison the pO_2 of working muscle in humans is 8.0 mmHg (Bylund-Fellenius et al., 1981). During ischaemia the tissue pO_2 can be certainly even lower (Heusch et al., 2005), thereby further augmenting the ability of deoxyMb to form NO from nitrite. This reflects an important O_2 sensing by deoxygenated myoglobin through which NO can regulate muscle function and energetics. The mechanism strongly resembles the characteristics described for acute hibernation (Rassaf et al., 2004). Myocardial short-term hibernation implies an adaptive reduction of energy expenditure through reduced contractile function in response to acute coronary artery inflow reduction. This restores myocardial energy balance over time and maintains myocardial integrity and viability (Heusch, 1998). The protective effects of NO during myocardial I/R are generally accepted (Bolli, 2001, Jones and Bolli, 2006). Our group could provide experimental evidence that the reduction of exogenous nitrite to NO during myocardial I/R leads to a marked decrease of myocardial infarct size which is critically dependent on the presence of myoglobin (Hendgen-Cotta et al., 2008). Concomitantly, ROS formation was attenuated accompanied by lower protein oxidation damage in wild-type mice. These data point out the impact of nitrite reductases under hypoxic conditions. Hence, the observed nitrite mediated cardio-protection was absent in mice lacking myoglobin, supporting the hypothesis that myoglobin serves as an intrinsic nitrite reduction that regulates cellular responses to hypoxia and reoxygenation (Hendgen-Cotta et al., 2008). Other authors report about a nitrite mediated blood flow regulation under conditions of hypoxia (Jia et al., 1996, Cosby et al., 2003). An observation was already made in the "pre-Nitric-Oxide-era" in 1953 from the later Nobel Prize winner Robert Francis Furchgott, who demonstrated that high concentrations of nitrite could mediate vasodilation when applied to isolated aortic rings of rats (Furchgott and Bhadrakom, 1953). Half a century later it was Gladwin et al., who tested

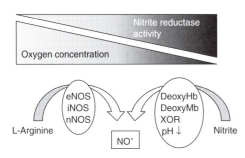

Fig. 4.4. Non-enzymatic NO formation depends on O_2 concentration and is independent of L-arginine (L-Arg). The one-electron reduction of nitrite to NO by ferrous haem proteins such as haemoglobin (Hb), myoglobin (Mb), or xanthin oxidoreductase (XOR) can occur in a much simpler mechanism than the 5-electron oxidation that was demonstrated for the synthesis from L-Arg. Under conditions of low O_2, the nitrite reductase activity of these proteins contributes to NOS-independent NO formation.

whether nitrite could mediate vasodilatation *in vivo* by infusing physiological concentrations of nitrite into the human brachial artery and simultaneously measuring forearm blood flow. They observed that under exercise, at rest and especially in the presence of the NO synthase inhibitor L-N^G-monomethyl Arginine citrate (L-NMMA), nitrite could increase blood flow and hence hypothesized that the observed nitrite reductase activity of haemoglobin can mediate hypoxic vasodilatation and may contribute to blood pressure regulation (Gladwin *et al.*, 2000; Cosby *et al.*, 2003; Gladwin, 2005). One major challenge facing the idea that NO generated from red blood cell deoxyhaemoglobin-nitrite-reaction can mediate vasodilatation is that haemoglobin is a potent scavenger of NO. Hence any NO generated would be scavenged by surrounding haemoglobin before mediating vasodilatation. The oxygen-bound form of nitrite-methaemoglobin shows a degree of ferrous nitrogen dioxide (Fe(II)-$NO_2^\bullet$) character, so it may rapidly react with NO to form dinitrogen trioxide (N_2O_3), a unique species that is not scavenged by haemoglobin and can diffuse out of the red blood cell and homolyse into NO (see Eqn 4.2) (Basu *et al.*, 2007). Briefly, one molecule of nitrite reacts with deoxyhaemoglobin and generates NO and methaemoglobin by the classical nitrite reductase reaction described. Another molecule of nitrite binds to methaemoglobin, and this nitrite bound methaemoglobin has an unusual electron configuration which appears to possess $Fe^{(II)}$-$NO_2^\bullet$ character. The $NO_2^\bullet$ species can react rapidly with a molecule of NO to form N_2O_3. This reaction may allow the NO generated from nitrite to reach distal targets such as the smooth muscle cells, without being scavenged by haemoglobin:

$$\begin{aligned} MetHb+NO_2^- &\leftrightarrow MetHb\text{-}NO_2^- \\ MetHb\text{-}NO_2^- &\leftrightarrow Hb\text{-}NO_2^\bullet \\ Hb\text{-}NO_2^\bullet + NO &\leftrightarrow Hb+N_2O_3 \end{aligned} \quad (4.2)$$

Other nitrite reductases, some much more efficient in generating NO from nitrite, become active at much lower oxygen tensions than haemoglobin (Shiva *et al.*, 2007). The distribution of these proteins in various biological compartments suggests that mechanisms of nitrite reduction may vary by tissue type, and further studies will be necessary to evaluate the physiological function of these proteins. It would go beyond the scope of this chapter to give a complete overview over all nitrite-dependent cytoprotective effects and influences on cellular functions. A comprehensive overview on the role of nitrite as regulator of hypoxic signalling in mammalian physiology is given by van Faassen *et al.* (2009). Furthermore, it is not only the anion nitrite that influences human physiology and serves as a source of NO, but also nitrate. An impressive example was demonstrated by Larsen *et al.* (2006), showing that after three days of oral treatment with inorganic nitrate a reduction of blood pressure occurred in healthy normotonic subjects. These observations could be reproduced with a natural nitrate source. Ingestion of beetroot juice could also decrease blood pressure in healthy volunteers via reduction of nitrate to nitrite (Webb *et al.*, 2008).

However, it becomes clear that nitrate and nitrite are not only the inert end products of NO metabolism, but can be considered as a circulating NO pool that is utilized under conditions where NO synthesis via L-Arg is insufficient.

4.9 Dietary Nitrate and Nitrite

Considering the evidence that nitrite and nitrate mediate cytoprotective effects in human physiology and especially under pathophysiological conditions, it is not unlikely that dietary nitrate and nitrite may positively affect human health and disease. Recognizing that NO is the most important molecule in regulating blood pressure and maintaining vascular homeostasis, food sources rich in NO compounds may provide beneficial effects primarily to the heart and blood vessels. Although there are clear reports on certain foods and diets that have shown a benefit in terms of preventing cancer and cardiovascular disease, the specific nature of the active constituents responsible for the cardioprotective effects of certain foods is still unknown. Viable candidates, promoted not least by TV and food industry campaigns are fibres, minerals, or antioxidants. In order to bring light to this issue several epidemiological studies were carried out. Joshipura *et al.* (1999) found that a high intake of fruits and vegetables was indeed associated with a reduced risk for coronary artery disease and apoplectic stroke. The large study population also allowed for analysis of the protection afforded by specific types of food, and the strongest protection against coronary heart disease was seen with a high intake of green leafy vegetables. According to these findings, Appel *et al.* showed that a dietary supplementation with vegetables lowers blood pressure in subjects with borderline hypertension to the same extent as monotherapy with a standard antihypertensive drug (Appel *et al.*, 1997; Sacks *et al.*, 2001). These observations are concordant with the findings of Larsen and Webb *et al.* who demonstrated the blood pressure-lowering effects of dietary nitrate, and ingestion of beetroot juice, respectively (Larsen *et al.*, 2006; Webb *et al.*, 2008). The investigators of the so-called 'Dietary Approaches to Stop Hypertension study' (DASH) attributed the observed blood pressure-lowering effect to the high calcium, potassium, polyphenols and fibre content, and to the low content of sodium and animal protein (Most, 2004). Bearing in mind that our major dietary sources of nitrate and nitrite are vegetables, these and other findings from the DASH study also point to a less widely acknowledged but highly plausible hypothesis: the observed blood pressure-lowering effect is due to the reduction of nitrate to nitrite and nitric oxide. This hypothesis is encouraged by considering the constituents of the Mediterranean diet, which has been consistently associated with lower incidence of cardiovascular disease and cancer in several studies (Fidanza *et al.*, 1970; Willett *et al.*, 1995; Trichopoulou and Critselis, 2004; Visioli *et al.*, 2004). The main constituent of the Mediterranean diet pyramid is composed of fruits and vegetables, both rich in nitrate and nitrite. The nitrate/nitrite contents of the diet consumed within the DASH study illustrates this coherence. The beneficial, blood pressure-lowering diet results in a consumption of 1222 mg nitrate whereas the unfavourable diet only yields 174 mg nitrate. The latter is comparable with the estimated intake from food in Northern Europe (50–140 mg d^{-1}) (Mensinga *et al.*, 2003). In contrast, the World Health Organization's acceptable daily intake (ADI) for the nitrate ion is set to an exposure limit of 222 mg nitrate and 3.6 mg nitrite for a 60 kg adult.

The hypothesis that dietary nitrate might provide cardiovascular benefit is further encouraged by recent animal models of myocardial infarction, where dietary supplementation of these anions provided beneficial effects on I/R injury (Bryan *et al.*, 2007). But even nowadays it is not possible to talk about the exciting discoveries relating to NO, nitrate, and nitrite without acknowledging the public perception of these anions; for discoveries in the 1960s suggested an increase of cancer incidence from the formation of N-nitrosamines. Despite the early findings of Tannenbaum *et al.* that nitrites and nitrates are formed endogenously in the human intestine, the public perception is still that these anions are harmful food additives that should be avoided (Tannenbaum *et al.*, 1978). Direct evidence for the participation of nitrate and nitrite in human carcinogenesis is lacking, despite extensive epidemiological and animal studies (Powlson *et al.*, 2008). Interestingly, a diet rich in vegetables, such as the Mediterranean and the traditional Japanese diets, contains more nitrate than the recommended acceptable daily intake by the World Health Organization (Katan, 2009). Even a portion of spinach commonly consumed in one serving of salad can exceed the acceptable daily intake for nitrate (Lundberg and Govoni, 2004). Taken together, the current evidence supports the conclusion of the European Food Safety Authority that the benefits of vegetable and fruit consumption outweigh any perceived risk of developing cancer from the consumption of nitrate and nitrite in these foods. The data outlined above, from observational epidemiologic and human clinical studies, support the hypothesis that nitrates and nitrites of plant origin play essential physiologic roles in supporting cardiovascular health.

4.10 Conclusions

Including food rich in nitrite, nitrate and antioxidants combined with L-arginine may provide the optimal combination of substrates to improve NO production and homeostasis. L-arginine alone is not able to restore NO bioavailability under conditions of ischaemia or oxidative stress. The growing field of evidence for the benefit of dietary nitrate and nitrite may provide a rescue or protective pathway for people at risk of cardiovascular disease.

4.11 Acknowledgements

This work was supported by the Deutsche Forschungsgemeinschaft (DFG) and the German Cardiac Society (DGK). Tienush Rassaf is a Heisenberg scholar of the DFG (RA 969/5-1). Malte Kelm is supported by the DFG (Ke405/5-1). Peter Luedike is a scholar of the DGK.

References

Abu-Soud, H.M., Ichimori, K., Presta, A. and Stuehr, D.J. (2000) Electron transfer, oxygen binding, and nitric oxide feedback inhibition in endothelial nitric-oxide synthase. *Journal of Biological Chemistry* 275, 17349–17357.

Appel, L.J., Moore, T.J., Obarzanek, E., Vollmer, W.M., Svetkey, L.P., Sacks, F.M., Bray, G.A., *et al*. (1997) A clinical trial of the effects of dietary patterns on blood pressure. DASH Collaborative Research Group. *The New England Journal of Medicine* 336, 1117–1124.

Basu, S., Grubina, R., Huang, J., Conradie, J., Huang, Z., Jeffers, A., Jiang, A., *et al*. (2007) Catalytic generation of N2O3 by the concerted nitrite reductase and anhydrase activity of hemoglobin. *Nature Chemical Biology* 3, 785–794.

Bednarz, B., Jaxa-Chamiec, T., Maciejewski, P., Szpajer, M., Janik, K., Gniot, J., Kawka-Urbanek, T., *et al*. (2005) Efficacy and safety of oral l-arginine in acute myocardial infarction. Results of the multicenter, randomized, double-blind, placebo-controlled ARAMI pilot trial. *Kardiologia Polska* 62, 421–427.

Bell, R.M., Maddock, H.L. and Yellon, D.M. (2003) The cardioprotective and mitochondrial depolarising properties of exogenous nitric oxide in mouse heart. *Cardiovascular Research* 57, 405–415.

Benjamin, N., O'Driscoll, F., Dougall, H., Duncan, C., Smith, L., Golden, M. and McKenzie, H. (1994) Stomach NO synthesis. *Nature* 368, 502.

Berkowitz, D.E., White, R., Li, D., Minhas, K.M., Cernetich, A., Kim, S., Burke, S., *et al*. (2003) Arginase reciprocally regulates nitric oxide synthase activity and contributes to endothelial dysfunction in aging blood vessels. *Circulation* 108, 2000–2006.

Böger, R.H. and Bode-Böger, S.M. (2001) The clinical pharmacology of L-arginine. *Annual Review of Pharmacology and Toxicology* 41, 79–99.

Böger, R.H., Bode-Böger, S.M., Brandes, R.P., Phivthong-ngam, L., Bohme, M., Nafe, R., Mugge, A., *et al*. (1997) Dietary L-arginine reduces the progression of atherosclerosis in cholesterol-fed rabbits: comparison with lovastatin. *Circulation* 96, 1282–1290.

Böger, R.H., Bode-Böger, S.M., Szuba, A., Tsao, P.S., Chan, J.R., Tangphao, O., Blaschke, T.F., *et al*. (1998) Asymmetric dimethylarginine (ADMA): a novel risk factor for endothelial dysfunction: its role in hypercholesterolemia. *Circulation* 98, 1842–1847.

Bolli, R. (2001) Cardioprotective function of inducible nitric oxide synthase and role of nitric oxide in myocardial ischemia and preconditioning: an overview of a decade of research. *Journal of Molecular and Cellular Cardiology* 33, 1897–1918.

Brandes, R.P., Behra, A., Lebherz, C., Böger, R.H., Bode-Böger, S.M., Phivthong-Ngam, L. and Mugge, A. (1997) N(G)-nitro-L-arginine- and indomethacin-resistant endothelium-dependent relaxation in the rabbit renal artery: effect of hypercholesterolemia. *Atherosclerosis* 135, 49–55.

Bredt, D.S. and Snyder, S.H. (1990) Isolation of nitric oxide synthetase, a calmodulin-requiring enzyme. *Proceedings of the National Academy of Sciences USA* 87, 682–685.

Bryan, N.S., Rassaf, T., Maloney, R.E., Rodriguez, C.M., Saijo, F., Rodriguez, J.R. and Feelisch, M. (2004) Cellular targets and mechanisms of nitros(yl)ation: an insight into their nature and kinetics in vivo. *Proceedings of the National Academy of Sciences USA* 101, 4308–4313.

Bryan, N.S., Calvert, J.W., Elrod, J.W., Gundewar, S., Ji, S.Y. and Lefer, D.J. (2007) Dietary nitrite supplementation protects against myocardial ischemia-reperfusion injury. *Proceedings of the National Academy of Sciences USA* 104, 19144–19149.

Busse, R. and Fleming, I. (1999) Nitric oxide, nitric oxide synthase, and hypertensive vascular disease. *Current Hypertension Reports* 1, 88–95.

Busse, R., Luckhoff, A. and Bassenge, E. (1987) Endothelium-derived relaxant factor inhibits platelet activation. *Naunyn Schmiedebergs Archives of Pharmacology* 336, 566–571.

Bylund-Fellenius, A.C., Walker, P.M., Elander, A., Holm, S., Holm, J. and Schersten, T. (1981) Energy metabolism in relation to oxygen partial pressure in human skeletal muscle during exercise. *Biochemical Journal* 200, 247–255.

Castello, P.R., David, P.S., McClure, T., Crook, Z. and Poyton, R.O. (2006) Mitochondrial cytochrome oxidase produces nitric oxide under hypoxic conditions: implications for oxygen sensing and hypoxic signaling in eukaryotes. *Cell Metabolism* 3, 277–287.

Cosby, K., Partovi, K.S., Crawford, J.H., Patel, R.P., Reiter, C.D., Martyr, S., Yang, B.K., et al. (2003) Nitrite reduction to nitric oxide by deoxyhemoglobin vasodilates the human circulation. *Nature Medicine* 9, 1498–1505.

Culotta, E. and Koshland, D.E., Jr (1992) NO news is good news. *Science* 258, 1862–1865.

Drexler, H., Zeiher, A.M., Meinzer, K. and Just, H. (1991) Correction of endothelial dysfunction in coronary microcirculation of hypercholesterolaemic patients by L-arginine. *Lancet* 338, 8782–8783 and 1546–1550.

Duncan, C., Dougall, H., Johnston, P., Green, S., Brogan, R., Leifert, C., Smith, L., et al. (1995) Chemical generation of nitric oxide in the mouth from the enterosalivary circulation of dietary nitrate. *Nature Medicine* 1, 546–551.

Dykhuizen, R.S., Frazer, R., Duncan, C., Smith, C.C., Golden, M., Benjamin, N. and Leifert, C. (1996) Antimicrobial effect of acidified nitrite on gut pathogens: importance of dietary nitrate in host defense. *Antimicrobial Agents and Chemotherapy* 40, 1422–1425.

Fidanza, F., Puddu, V., Imbimbo, A.B., Menotti, A. and Keys, A. (1970) Coronary heart disease in seven countries. VII. Five-year experience in rural Italy. *Circulation* 41, 163–175.

Forstermann, U., Closs, E.I., Pollock, J.S., Nakane, M., Schwarz, P., Gath, I. and Kleinert, H. (1994) Nitric oxide synthase isozymes. Characterization, purification, molecular cloning, and functions. *Hypertension* 23, 1121–1131.

Furchgott, R.F. and Bhadrakom, S. (1953) Reactions of strips of rabbit aorta to epinephrine, isopropylarterenol, sodium nitrite and other drugs. *Journal of Pharmacology and Experimental Therapeutics* 108, 129–143.

Furchgott, R.F. and Zawadzki, J.V. (1980) The obligatory role of endothelial cells in the relaxation of arterial smooth muscle by acetylcholine. *Nature* 288, 373–376.

Galle, J., Mulsch, A., Busse, R. and Bassenge, E. (1991) Effects of native and oxidized low density lipoproteins on formation and inactivation of endothelium-derived relaxing factor. *Arteriosclerosis, Thrombosis, and Vascular Biology* 11, 198–203.

Gladwin, M.T. (2005) Hemoglobin as a nitrite reductase regulating red cell-dependent hypoxic vasodilation. *American Journal of Respiratory Cell and Molecular Biology* 32, 363–366.

Gladwin, M.T., Shelhamer, J.H., Schechter, A.N., Pease-Fye, M.E., Waclawiw, M.A., Panza, J.A., Ognibene, F.P., et al. (2000) Role of circulating nitrite and S-nitrosohemoglobin in the regulation of regional blood flow in humans. *Proceedings of the National Academy of Sciences USA* 97, 11482–11487.

Gold, M.E., Bush, P.A. and Ignarro, L.J. (1989) Depletion of arterial L-arginine causes reversible tolerance to endothelium-dependent relaxation. *Biochemical and Biophysical Research Communications* 164, 714–721.

Hecker, M., Sessa, W.C., Harris, H.J., Anggard, E.E. and Vane, J.R. (1990) The metabolism of L-arginine and its significance for the biosynthesis of endothelium-derived relaxing factor: cultured endothelial cells recycle L-citrulline to L-arginine. *Proceedings of the National Academy of Sciences USA* 87, 8612–8616.

Hendgen-Cotta, U.B., Merx, M.W., Shiva, S., Schmitz, J., Becher, S., Klare, J.P., Steinhoff, H.J., et al. (2008) Nitrite reductase activity of myoglobin regulates respiration and cellular viability in myocardial ischemia-reperfusion injury. *Proceedings of the National Academy of Sciences USA* 105, 10256–10261.

Heusch, G. (1998) Hibernating myocardium. *Physiological Reviews* 78, 1055–1085.

Heusch, G., Schulz, R. and Rahimtoola, S.H. (2005) Myocardial hibernation: a delicate balance. *American Journal of Physiology - Heart and Circulatory Physiology* 288, H984–999.

Hirooka, Y., Imaizumi, T., Harada, S., Masaki, H., Momohara, M., Tagawa, T. and Takeshita, A. (1992) Endothelium-dependent forearm vasodilation to acetylcholine but not to substance P is impaired in patients with heart failure. *Journal of Cardiovascular Pharmacology* 20, S221–225.

Howlett, R. (1998) Nobel award stirs up debate on nitric oxide breakthrough. *Nature* 39, 625–626.

Huang, Z., Shiva, S., Kim-Shapiro, D.B., Patel, R.P., Ringwood, L.A., Irby, C.E., Huang, K.T., et al. (2005) Enzymatic function of hemoglobin as a nitrite reductase that produces NO under allosteric control. *Journal of Clinical Investigation* 115, 2099–2107.

Ignarro, L.J. (1991) Signal transduction mechanisms involving nitric oxide. *Biochemical Pharmacology* 41, 485–490.

Ignarro, L.J., Adams, J.B., Horwitz, P.M. and Wood, K.S. (1986) Activation of soluble guanylate cyclase by NO-hemoproteins involves NO-heme exchange. Comparison of heme-containing and heme-deficient enzyme forms. *Journal of Biological Chemistry* 261, 4997–5002.

Ignarro, L.J., Buga, G.M., Wei, L.H., Bauer, P.M., Wu, G. and del Soldato, P. (2001) Role of the arginine-nitric oxide pathway in the regulation of vascular smooth muscle cell proliferation. *Proceedings of the National Academy of Sciences USA* 98, 4202–4208.

Jansson, E.A., Petersson, J., Reinders, C., Sobko, T., Bjorne, H., Phillipson, M., Weitzberg, E., et al. (2007) Protection from nonsteroidal anti-inflammatory drug (NSAID)-induced gastric ulcers by dietary nitrate. *Free Radical Biology and Medicine* 42, 510–518.

Jay, M.T., Chirico, S., Siow, R.C., Bruckdorfer, K.R., Jacobs, M., Leake, D.S., Pearson, J.D., et al. (1997) Modulation of vascular tone by low density lipoproteins: effects on L-arginine transport and nitric oxide synthesis. *Experimental Physiology* 82, 349–360.

Jennings, R.B., Sommers, H.M., Smyth, G.A., Flack, H.A. and Linn, H. (1960) Myocardial necrosis induced by temporary occlusion of a coronary artery in the dog. *Archives of Pathology & Laboratory Medicine* 70, 68–78.

Jia, L., Bonaventura, C., Bonaventura, J. and Stamler, J.S. (1996) S-nitrosohaemoglobin: a dynamic activity of blood involved in vascular control. *Nature* 380, 221–226.

Jones, S.P. and Bolli, R. (2006) The ubiquitous role of nitric oxide in cardioprotection. *Journal of Molecular and Cellular Cardiology* 40, 16–23.

Joshi, M.S., Ferguson, T.B. Jr, Han, T.H., Hyduke, D.R., Liao, J.C., Rassaf, T., Bryan, N., et al. (2002) Nitric oxide is consumed, rather than conserved, by reaction with oxyhemoglobin under physiological conditions. *Proceedings of the National Academy of Sciences USA* 99, 10341–10346.

Joshipura, K.J., Ascherio, A., Manson, J.E., Stampfer, M.J., Rimm, E.B., Speizer, F.E., et al. (1999) Fruit and vegetable intake in relation to risk of ischemic stroke. *Journal of the American Medical Association* 282, 1233–1239.

Katan, M.B. (2009) Nitrate in foods: harmful or healthy? *American Journal of Clinical Nutrition* 90, 11–12.

Kelm, M. (1999) Nitric oxide metabolism and breakdown. *Biochimica et Biophysica Acta* 1411, 273–289.

Kikuta, K., Sawamura, T., Miwa, S., Hashimoto, N. and Masaki, T. (1998) High-affinity arginine transport of bovine aortic endothelial cells is impaired by lysophosphatidylcholine. *Circulation Research* 83, 1088–1096.

Knowles, R.G., Palacios, M., Palmer, R.M. and Moncada, S. (1989) Formation of nitric oxide from L-arginine in the central nervous system: a transduction mechanism for stimulation of the soluble guanylate cyclase. *Proceedings of the National Academy of Sciences USA* 86, 5159–5162.

Kozlov, A.V., Dietrich, B. and Nohl, H. (2003) Various intracellular compartments cooperate in the release of nitric oxide from glycerol trinitrate in liver. *British Journal of Pharmacology* 139, 989–997.

Landmesser, U., Dikalov, S., Price, S.R., McCann, L., Fukai, T., Holland, S.M., Mitch, W.E., et al. (2003) Oxidation of tetrahydrobiopterin leads to uncoupling of endothelial cell nitric oxide synthase in hypertension. *Journal of Clinical Investigations* 111, 1201–1209.

Larsen, F.J., Ekblom, B., Sahlin, K., Lundberg, J.O. and Weitzberg, E. (2006) Effects of dietary nitrate on blood pressure in healthy volunteers. *New England Journal of Medicine* 355, 2792–2793.

Liu, Q. and Gross, S.S. (1996) Binding sites of nitric oxide synthases. *Methods Enzymology* 268, 311–324.

Lundberg, J.O. and Govoni, M. (2004) Inorganic nitrate is a possible source for systemic generation of nitric oxide. *Free Radical Biology & Medicine* 37, 395–400.

Lundberg, J.O., Weitzberg, E., Lundberg, J.M. and Alving, K. (1994) Intragastric nitric oxide production in humans: measurements in expelled air. *Gut* 35, 1543–1546.

Lundberg, J.O., Weitzberg, E., Cole, J.A. and Benjamin, N. (2004) Nitrate, bacteria and human health. *Nature Reviews Microbiology* 2, 593–602.

Makimattila, S., Virkamaki, A., Groop, P.H., Cockcroft, J., Utriainen, T., Fagerudd, J. and Yki-Jarvinen, H. (1996) Chronic hyperglycemia impairs endothelial function and insulin sensitivity via different mechanisms in insulin-dependent diabetes mellitus. *Circulation* 94, 1276–1282.

Marcinek, D.J., Ciesielski, W.A., Conley, K.E. and Schenkman, K.A. (2003) Oxygen regulation and limitation to cellular respiration in mouse skeletal muscle in vivo. *American Journal of Physiology - Heart and Circulatory Physiology* 285, H1900–1908.

McDonald, K.K., Zharikov, S., Block, E.R. and Kilberg, M.S. (1997) A caveolar complex between the cationic amino acid transporter 1 and endothelial nitric-oxide synthase may explain the "arginine paradox". *Journal of Biological Chemistry* 272, 31213–31216.

Mensinga, T.T., Speijers, G.J. and Meulenbelt, J. (2003) Health implications of exposure to environmental nitrogenous compounds. *Toxicologic Reviews* 22, 41–51.

Millar, T.M., Stevens, C.R., Benjamin, N., Eisenthal, R., Harrison, R. and Blake, D.R. (1998) Xanthine oxidoreductase catalyses the reduction of nitrates and nitrite to nitric oxide under hypoxic conditions. *FEBS Letters* 427, 225–228.

Mirvish, S.S. (1995) Role of N-nitroso compounds (NOC) and N-nitrosation in etiology of gastric, esophageal, nasopharyngeal and bladder cancer and contribution to cancer of known exposures to NOC. *Cancer Letters* 93, 17–48.

Miyoshi, M., Kasahara, E., Park, A.M., Hiramoto, K., Minamiyama, Y., Takemura, S., Sato, E.F., et al. (2003) Dietary nitrate inhibits stress-induced gastric mucosal injury in the rat. *Free Radical Research* 37, 85–90.

Moller, P., Alvestrand, A., Bergstrom, J., Furst, P. and Hellstrom, K. (1983) Electrolytes and free amino acids in leg skeletal muscle of young and elderly women. *Gerontology* 29, 1–8.

Moncada, S. and Higgs, A. (1993) The L-arginine-nitric oxide pathway. *New England Journal of Medicine* 329, 2002–2012.

Most, M.M. (2004) Estimated phytochemical content of the dietary approaches to stop hypertension (DASH) diet is higher than in the Control Study Diet. *Journal of the American Dietetic Association* 104, 1725–1727.

Oomen, C.M., van Erk, M.J., Feskens, E.J., Kok, F.J. and Kromhout, D. (2000) Arginine intake and risk of coronary heart disease mortality in elderly men. *Arteriosclerosis, Thrombosis, and Vascular Biology* 20, 2134–2139.

Palmer, R.M., Ferrige, A.G. and Moncada, S. (1987) Nitric oxide release accounts for the biological activity of endothelium-derived relaxing factor. *Nature* 327, 524–526.

Palmer, R.M., Ashton, D.S. and Moncada, S. (1988) Vascular endothelial cells synthesize nitric oxide from L-arginine. *Nature* 333, 664–666.

Powlson, D.S., Addiscott, T.M., Benjamin, N., Cassman, K.G., de Kok, T.M., van Grinsven, H., L'Hirondel, J.L., et al. (2008) When does nitrate become a risk for humans? *Journal of Environmental Quality* 37, 291–295.

Rajfer, J., Aronson, W.J., Bush, P.A., Dorey, F.J. and Ignarro, L.J. (1992) Nitric oxide as a mediator of relaxation of the corpus cavernosum in response to nonadrenergic, noncholinergic neurotransmission. *New England Journal of Medicine* 326, 90–94.

Rassaf, T., Feelisch, M. and Kelm, M. (2004) Circulating NO pool: assessment of nitrite and nitroso species in blood and tissues. *Free Radical Biology & Medicine* 36, 413–422.

Rassaf, T., Flogel, U., Drexhage, C., Hendgen-Cotta, U., Kelm, M. and Schrader, J. (2007) Nitrite reductase function of deoxymyoglobin: oxygen sensor and regulator of cardiac energetics and function. *Circulation Research* 100, 1749–1754.

Rector, T.S., Bank, A.J., Mullen, K.A., Tschumperlin, L.K., Sih, R., Pillai, K. and Kubo, S.H. (1996) Randomized, double-blind, placebo-controlled study of supplemental oral L-arginine in patients with heart failure. *Circulation* 93, 2135–2141.

Rossitch, E. Jr, Alexander, E. 3rd, Black, P.M. and Cooke, J.P. (1991) L-arginine normalizes endothelial function in cerebral vessels from hypercholesterolemic rabbits. *Journal of Clinical Investigations* 87, 1295–1299.

Sacks, F.M., Svetkey, L.P., Vollmer, W.M., Appel, L., Bray, G.A., Harsha, D., Obarzanek, E., et al. (2001) Effects on blood pressure of reduced dietary sodium and the Dietary Approaches to Stop Hypertension (DASH) diet. DASH-Sodium Collaborative Research Group. *New England Journal of Medicine* 344, 3–10.

Schulman, S.P., Becker, L.C., Kass, D.A., Champion, H.C., Terrin, M.L., Forman, S., Ernst, K.V., et al. (2006) L-arginine therapy in acute myocardial infarction: the Vascular Interaction With Age in Myocardial Infarction (VINTAGE MI) randomized clinical trial. *Journal of the American Medical Association* 295, 58–64.

Shiva, S., Wang, X., Ringwood, L.A., Xu, X., Yuditskaya, S., Annavajjhala, V., Miyajima, H., et al. (2006) Ceruloplasmin is a NO oxidase and nitrite synthase that determines endocrine NO homeostasis. *Nature Chemical Biology* 2, 486–493.

Shiva, S., Huang, Z., Grubina, R., Sun, J., Ringwood, L.A., MacArthur, P.H., Xu, X., et al. (2007) Deoxymyoglobin is a nitrite reductase that generates nitric oxide and regulates mitochondrial respiration. *Circulation Research* 100, 654–661.

Silk, D.B., Grimble, G.K. and Rees, R.G. (1985) Protein digestion and amino acid and peptide absorption. *Proceedings of the Nutrition Society* 44, 63–72.

Stuhlinger, M.C., Abbasi, F., Chu, J.W., Lamendola, C., McLaughlin, T.L., Cooke, J.P., Reaven, G.M., *et al.* (2002) Relationship between insulin resistance and an endogenous nitric oxide synthase inhibitor. *Journal of the American Medical Association* 287, 1420–1426.

Tannenbaum, S.R., Fett, D., Young, V.R., Land, P.D. and Bruce, W.R. (1978) Nitrite and nitrate are formed by endogenous synthesis in the human intestine. *Science* 200, 1487–1489.

Trichopoulou, A. and Critselis, E. (2004) Mediterranean diet and longevity. *European Journal of Cancer Prevention* 13, 453–456.

Tsikas, D., Böger, R.H., Sandmann, J., Bode-Böger, S.M. and Frolich, J.C. (2000) Endogenous nitric oxide synthase inhibitors are responsible for the L-arginine paradox. *FEBS Letters* 478, 1–3.

Twort, C.H. and van Breemen, C. (1988) Cyclic guanosine monophosphate-enhanced sequestration of Ca2+ by sarcoplasmic reticulum in vascular smooth muscle. *Circulation Research* 62, 961–964.

Vallance, P., Leone, A., Calver, A., Collier, J. and Moncada, S. (1992) Accumulation of an endogenous inhibitor of nitric oxide synthesis in chronic renal failure. *Lancet* 339, 572–575.

van Faassen, E.E., Bahrami, S., Feelisch, M., Hogg, N., Kelm, M., Kim-Shapiro, D.B., Kozlov, A.V., *et al.* (2009) Nitrite as regulator of hypoxic signaling in mammalian physiology. *Medicinal Research Reviews* 29, 683–741.

Vanin, A.F., Bevers, L.M., Slama-Schwok, A. and van Faassen, E.E. (2007) Nitric oxide synthase reduces nitrite to NO under anoxia. *Cellular and Molecular Life Sciences* 64, 96–103.

Visioli, F., Grande, S., Bogani, P. and Galli, C. (2004) The role of antioxidants in the mediterranean diets: focus on cancer. *European Journal of Cancer Prevention* 13, 337–343.

Webb, A.J., Patel, N., Loukogeorgakis, S., Okorie, M., Aboud, Z., Misra, S., Rashid, R., *et al.* (2008) Acute blood pressure lowering, vasoprotective, and antiplatelet properties of dietary nitrate via bioconversion to nitrite. *Hypertension* 51, 784–790.

Wei, L.H., Jacobs, A.T., Morris, S.M. Jr, and Ignarro, L.J. (2000) IL-4 and IL-13 upregulate arginase I expression by cAMP and JAK/STAT6 pathways in vascular smooth muscle cells. *American Journal of Physiology - Cell Physiology* 279, C248–256.

Willett, W.C., Sacks, F., Trichopoulou, A., Drescher, G., Ferro-Luzzi, A., Helsing, E. and Trichopoulos, D. (1995) Mediterranean diet pyramid: a cultural model for healthy eating. *American Journal of Clinical Nutrition* 61, 1402S–1406S.

Wu, G., Jaeger, L.A., Bazer, F.W. and Rhoads, J.M. (2004) Arginine deficiency in preterm infants: biochemical mechanisms and nutritional implications. *Journal of Nutritional Biochemistry* 15, 442–451.

Zweier, J.L., Wang, P., Samouilov, A. and Kuppusamy, P. (1995) Enzyme-independent formation of nitric oxide in biological tissues. *Nature Medicine* 1, 804–809.

5 Histidine Decarboxylase

E. Dere,[1]* O. Ambrée[2] and A. Zlomuzica[3]

[1]Université Paris VI: Université Pierre et Marie Curie, Paris, France;
[2]Department of Psychiatry, University of Münster, Germany;
[3]Department of Clinical Psychology, Ruhr-Universität Bochum, Germany

5.1 Abstract

The mammalian histidine decarboxylase cDNA encodes for a protein with a molecular mass of 74 kDa that is converted into a 53-55 kDa form during post-translational proteolytic processing through the ubiquitin-proteasome system. The resulting enzyme, histidine decarboxylase, converts L-histidine to histamine. In the brain, histamine is an important neurotransmitter and modulator which has been implicated in a wide range of physiological functions and behaviours, such as immune function, gastric acid secretion, nutrition, sleep, anxiety, reward and memory. Furthermore, histamine plays a role in human diseases such as allergy, cancer, epilepsy and autoimmune disorders. The first part of this chapter focuses on the histamine synthesizing enzyme histidine decarboxylase, and summarizes what is known about its molecular structure and catalytic function, its distribution in peripheral and central tissues, its cellular localization, the cell types in which it is expressed, and its gene structure, as well as the regulation of its transcription and translation. The second part of this chapter reviews the literature on neurophysiological and behavioural effects of pharmacological histidine decarboxylase inhibition in the rat, and histidine decarboxylase gene knockout in the mouse. Finally, evidence implicating the brain's histamine system in Alzheimer's disease is discussed.

5.2 Introduction

The imidazolamine histamine is synthesized from its precursor L-histidine by the enzyme histidine decarboxylase and its cofactor pyridoxal phosphate. In the central nervous system, histamine is metabolized to tele-methylhistamine by histamine methyltransferase. Tele-methylhistamine is further degraded to t-methyl-imidazoleacetic acid by monoamine oxidase (Haas *et al.*, 2008; Fig. 5.1a). Histamine plays a role in various physiological functions including nutrition, immune function, cell growth, gastric acid secretion, body temperature, respiration, neurotransmission, sexual behaviour (Rangachari, 1992; Falus, 2003; Ohtsu and Watanabe, 2003), sleep, arousal, anxiety, reward and memory (Dere *et al.*, 2010). It is also involved in several pathological conditions and diseases such as allergic reactions, inflammation, atherosclerosis (Tanimoto *et al.*, 2006), cancer, epilepsy, and autoimmune encephalomyelitis (Watanabe

---

* E-mail address: ekrem.dere@snv.jussieu.fr

and Yanai, 2001; Falus, 2003). The central and peripheral effects of histamine are mediated by the stimulation of four metabotropic G-protein coupled histamine receptors H1-, H2-, H3- and the recently discovered H4-receptors. Histamine receptors differ in terms of pharmacology, central and peripheral localization, and cellular transduction processes (Parson and Ganellin, 2006; Haas et al., 2008).

Although histamine is produced by mast cells in nearly all tissues it is also detected in a variety of other cell and tissue types. The concentration of tissue histamine depends on the status of histidine decarboxylase activity. Expression of histidine decarboxylase in different cell populations and tissues can be investigated, for instance by using quantitative real-time reverse transcription polymerase chain reaction to measure histidine decarboxylase mRNA levels, or by means of immunohistochemical labelling with antibodies raised against histidine decarboxylase. Histidine decarboxylase-positive cells include mast cells, enterochromaffin-like cells in the stomach, basophils, platelets, macrophages, endothelial cells and neurons (Li et al., 2008). In rats, histidine decarboxylase immunoreactive structures were demonstrated in fetal liver and peritoneal mast cells, as well as in skin, stomach and brain tissue (Taguchi et al., 1984). The highest amounts of histidine decarboxylase mRNA expression are measured in the stomach followed by the brain, skin, jejunum, spleen and liver (Kondo et al., 1995).

In the mammalian brain, histidine decarboxylase-positive neurons are clustered in the nucleus tuberomamillaris of the posterior hypothalamus. The tuberomamillary nucleus consists of five subregions known as E1–E5 which are differentiated in terms of cytoarchitecture and projections (Wada et al., 1991). Histamineric projections are diffused widely within the central nervous system, including the septum, hippocampus, amygdala, olfactory bulb, basal ganglia, diagonal band of Broca, thalamus, forebrain, brain stem and spinal cord (Brown et al., 2001; Fig. 5.1b). In the rat brain, the majority of neurons containing histidine decarboxylase mRNA in the nucleus tuberomamillaris are also immunoreactive for glutamate decarboxylase, suggesting that histamine is co-localized with GABA

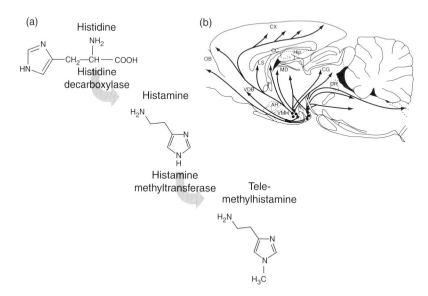

Fig. 5.1. Neuronal histamine. (a) Synthesis and metabolism of histamine in the brain. (b) The histamine system in the rat brain: origins and projections. AH, anterior hypothalamic area; Arc, arcuate nucleus; Cc, corpus callosum; Cer, cerebellum; CG, central grey; CX, cerebral cortex; DR, dorsal raphe nucleus; F, fornix; Hip, hippocampus; LS, lateral septum; MD, mediodorsal thalamus; MMn, medial mammillary nucleus; OB, olfactory bulb; Pn, pontine nuclei; Sol, nucleus of solitary tract; Sox, supraoptic decussation; VDB, Vertical limb of the diagonal band; VMH, ventromedial hypothalamus.

and galanin (Kohler *et al.*, 1986). In the human brain, histidine decarboxylase mRNA only co-localizes with GABA but not with galanin (Trottier *et al.*, 2002).

5.3 Histidine Decarboxylase Enzyme

Mammalian histidine decarboxylase belongs in the fold type I pyridoxal phosphate-dependent enzyme category. It is the only rate-limiting enzyme that catalyses the formation of histamine. Histidine decarboxylase has been purified from various tissues and species including mouse mastocytoma and fetal rat liver. The intracellular localization and post-translational processing of histidine decarboxylase had been investigated in a rat basophilic/mast cell line RBL-2H3 (Tanaka *et al.*, 1998). Histidine decarboxylase mRNA is translated in the cytosol to an endogenous 74 kDa form of the histidine decarboxylase enzyme. This full length 74 kDa form translocates to the endoplasmic reticulum where it undergoes post-translational processing and is truncated into a shorter form by the involvement of the ubiquitin proteasome system (Joseph *et al.*, 1990; Yamamoto *et al.*, 1990; Tanaka *et al.*, 1998). It has been proposed that biologically active histidine decarboxylase is a homodimer consisting of two carboxy-truncated monomers with a molecular mass of 53–55 kDa (Taguchi *et al.*, 1984). However, there is also evidence suggesting that other processed isoforms which are greater in size than 55 kDa might also contribute to histamine biosynthesis *in vivo* (Fleming and Wang, 2003). The histidine decarboxylase enzyme has no amino terminal signal sequence or hydrophobic membrane anchor. COS-7 cell transfection studies with histidine decarboxylase cDNA revealed that the precursor 74 kDa form of L-histidine decarboxylase is tightly associated with the membrane of the endoplasmic reticulum with its carboxyl terminal region exposed on the cytosolic part of the cell (Furuta *et al.*, 2006).

5.4 Histidine Decarboxylase Gene

By means of *in situ* hybridization assays using a rat histidine decarboxylase cDNA probe, the histidine decarboxylase gene has been identified in the 15q21-q22 region of human chromosome number 15 and in the E5-G region of mouse chromosome number 2 (Malzac *et al.*, 1996). The mouse and human histidine decarboxylase genes consist of 12 exons and cover 24 kb of genomic DNA (Suzuki-Ishigaki *et al.*, 2000). In humans, two splicing variants of the histidine decarboxylase gene of 2.4 and 3.4 kb have been detected. In contrast, the mouse homologue does not undergo alternative splicing and generates only a single transcript of 2.4 kb. The exon-intron boundaries of the mouse gene are comparable to those of the human gene and the nucleotide sequences of the exons of the mouse gene show 60–90% homology to their human counterparts (Suzuki-Ishigaki *et al.*, 2000). Research on the regulation mechanism of the histidine decarboxylase gene indicates that in cells that express histidine decarboxylase, the CpG islands in the promoter region of the histidine decarboxylase gene are demethylated, whereas in cells that do not express the histidine decarboxylase gene they are methylated (Watanabe and Ohtsu, 2002). The transcription of the histidine decarboxylase gene is stimulated by various agents, treatments, and physiological conditions. The transcription-initiating factors include gastrin, phorbol ester phorbol 12-myristate 13-acetate, oxidative stress, thrombopointin, tetradecanoylphobol acetate, helicobacter pylori infection and cold-induced stress (Watanabe and Ohtsu, 2002). Gastrin and phorbol ester-induced histidine decarboxylase gene transcription is mediated through protein kinase C- and mitogen-activated protein kinase-dependent pathways (Höcker *et al.*, 1998). In rat tissue, the expression of the histidine decarboxylase protein decreases histidine decarboxylase gene promoter activity in a dose-dependent fashion. Thus, the transcription rate of the histidine decarboxylase gene is controlled by a negative feedback loop. Within the histidine decarboxylase promoter region this negative feedback inhibition is thought to be mediated by gastrin and extracellular signal-related kinase-1 response element recognition sites (Colucci *et al.*, 2001).

5.4.1 Gene polymorphism

Several non-synonymous polymorphisms of the human histidine decarboxylase gene have been detected, including rs17740607 Met31Thr, rs16963486 Leu553Phe, and rs2073440 Asp644Glu (García-Martín et al., 2009). These genetic polymorphisms might be responsible for inter-individual variation in histamine metabolism and possibly some pathological conditions (Zhang et al., 2006).

5.5 Pharmacological Inhibition

α-Fluoromethylhistidine is a specific and irreversible inhibitor of histidine decarboxylase activity (Watanabe et al., 1990). In rats, the intraperitoneal injection of alpha-fluoromethylhistidine at a dose of 200 mg kg^{-1} induced a substantial depletion of neocortical and hippocampal histamine levels three hours after administration of the drug (Servos et al., 1994). Onodera et al. (1992) report that one and three hours after intraperitoneal injection of α-fluoromethylhistidine (200 mg kg^{-1}) to rats the histamine levels were decreased considerably in the hypothalamus, cortex, and thalamus. Histamine levels were moderately reduced in the olfactory bulb, amygdala, pons-medulla oblongata, and midbrain. In contrast to the study by Servos et al. (1994), Onodera et al. (1992) found only minor decreases in histamine levels in the striatum, hippocampus, cerebellum, and pituitary (Onodera et al., 1992). These contradictory results might be due to methodological differences in brain tissue preparation for the measurement of histamine levels. Using a CO_2-trapping enzymatic method it has been found that α-fluoromethylhistidine induced a near-complete inhibition of histidine decarboxylase in the hypothalamus both *in vivo* and *in vitro*, but it failed to do so in the frontal cortex of rats. In the latter, maximal doses of the drug were ineffective in completely inhibiting histidine decarboxylase activity (Skratt et al., 1994). Therefore, it might be possible that a second α-fluoromethylhistidine-resistant form of histidine decarboxylase exists in the mammalian brain. However, there is also evidence that α-fluoromethylhistidine potency to inhibit histidine decarboxylase activity might vary across different brain areas. In this regard it has been suggested that α-fluoromethylhistidine might not necessarily reduce histamine levels in the rat hippocampus because of its scarce innervations by histamine-containing axon terminals (Sakai et al., 1998).

The histamine H3-receptor is an autoreceptor located on histamine-containing cells and regulates histamine synthesis and release at its terminal structures. Intraperitoneal administration of the histamine H3-receptor agonist (R)α-methylhistamine to rats reduces histidine decarboxylase gene expression in the nucleus tuberomamillaris one hour after treatment, and increases histidine decarboxylase gene expression when examined after three hours post treatment (Chotard et al., 2002). The latter might reflect a compensatory or rebound effect required to counteract histamine depletion.

5.6 mRNA Antisense and Gene Knockout

Histidine decarboxylase activity can also be inhibited by molecular genetic techniques including antisense RNAs and gene targeting. The translation of histidine decarboxylase mRNA into the histidine decarboxylase protein can be prevented by a polyclonal histidine decarboxylase-specific antisense oligonucleotide. In melanoma cells, histidine decarboxylase expression is increased by tenfold as compared to normal skin, resulting in high levels of histamine. Histidine decarboxylase-specific antisense oligonucleotides substantially decrease protein levels of histidine decarboxylase and simultaneously inhibit cell proliferation, suggesting that histamine acts as an autocrine growth factor for tumour cell proliferation (Hegyesi et al., 2001).

Histidine decarboxylase knockout mice have been generated by means of homologous gene recombination in embryonic 129/Sv stem cells, and are maintained on a homogenous 129/Sv genetic background. In these mice, the genomic sequence from intron 5 to exon 9 was replaced with an inverted PGK promoter-driven neomycin phosphotransferase gene, resulting in a null mutation (Ohtsu et al., 2001). Exon 8 contains the coding sequence for the binding site of pyridoxal 5´-phosphate which is the essential coenzyme of histidine decarboxylase protein. Therefore it was anticipated that the histidine decarboxylase enzyme produced from this truncated histidine decarboxylase gene would be unable to catalyse the synthesis of histamine from L-histidine. However, histidine decarboxylase gene expression was abolished already at the transcriptional level in these mice. These histidine decarboxylase knockout mice are viable and fertile (although due to their genetic background strain they breed rather poorly as compared to C57BL/6J mice). As expected, the targeted disruption of mouse histidine decarboxylase gene in these mice resulted in the near complete absence of endogenous synthesis of histamine. Furthermore, a decreased number of mast cells have been observed in these mouse mutants. Moreover, the remaining mast cells of histidine decarboxylase knockout mice were characterized by morphological aberrations, reduced levels of granular proteases and generally reduced granular content (Ohtsu et al., 2001). However, it should be noted that although the histidine decarboxylase protein expression was blocked at the transcriptional level, nevertheless some residual minor histamine content was found in the brains of histidine decarboxylase knockout mice, even under low-histamine diet conditions. It therefore remains to be determined whether there is a yet unknown brain enzyme different from histidine decarboxylase which is capable of catalysing the synthesis of histamine.

5.7 Neurophysiology and Behaviour

In the following, some of the behavioural and associated neurophysiological effects of histidine decarboxylase inhibition in rats and mice will be reviewed. The behavioural effects of pharmacological blockade of single histamine receptors, as well as studies with histamine receptor knockout mice, has been reviewed recently elsewhere (Esbenshade et al., 2008; Alvarez, 2009; Dere et al., 2010) and will not be discussed here. Nevertheless the reader should be aware that pharmacological blockade of single histamine receptors can have distinct and sometimes opposed effects on behavioural and neurophysiological measures when compared to pharmacological histidine decarboxylase blockade. For a discussion of these divergent results see Alvarez (2009) and Dere et al. (2010).

5.7.1 Brain neurotransmitters

In the central nervous system histamine interacts with other neurotransmitters including dopamine, serotonin, and acetylcholine, and influences their metabolism, content, and release. Post-mortem neurochemical assessments revealed that the histidine decarboxylase knockout mice exhibited changes in dopamine metabolism in the neo- and ventral striata. In the ventral striatum, the DOPAC/dopamine and 3-MT/dopamine ratios were higher in histidine decarboxylase knockout mice as compared to the controls (Dere et al., 2003). Furthermore, the histidine decarboxylase knockout mice had higher acetylcholine concentrations and a significantly higher serotonin turnover in the frontal cortex, but reduced acetylcholine levels in the neostriatum (Dere et al., 2004). These findings suggest that inhibition of endogenous histamine synthesis modulates the metabolism, content, and release of dopamine, serotonin and acetylcholine in the mouse brain.

5.7.2 Nutrition

Histamine has been implicated in the control of appetite, is a mediator of the anorexigenic action of leptin, and plays an important role in the pathogenesis of age-related obesity in mice. α-Fluoromethylhistidine has been reported to increase food intake in rats via depletion of neuronal histamine (Tuomisto et al., 1994; Sakai et al., 1995). Intracerebroventricular infusion of α-fluoromethylhistidine into the third ventricle of rats induced feeding in the early light phase when the histamine synthesis usually is high (Ookuma et al., 1993).

Chronic administration of α-fluoromethylhistidine to rats via osmotic minipumps over a period of two weeks increased feeding throughout the test period and increased body weights towards the end of the test period (Orthen-Gambill and Salomon, 1992). Furthermore, intraperitoneal administration of α-fluoromethylhistidine abolished leptin-induced suppression of food intake in C57BL/6 mice (Morimoto et al., 1999).

It is well known that the hypothalamus located in the diencephalon mediates the release of nutrition-related hormones, and that the dorsomedial hypothalamic nucleus is involved in the control of feeding and drinking behaviour, as well as in the regulation of body weight (Bellinger and Bernardis, 2002). Furthermore it has been proposed that histamine stimulates the satiety centre located in the ventromedial part of the hypothalamus (Sakata et al., 2003). Given that α-fluoromethylhistidine led to histamine depletion in the hypothalamus, without affecting concentrations of catecholamines (Ookuma et al., 1993), it is likely that α-fluoromethylhistidine increases food intake via histamine depletion in the hypothalamus.

In rats, the intraperitoneal application of the histamine precursor L-histidine decreased both drinking and food ingestion. This effect was reversed in part by the co-administration of α-fluoromethylhistidine (Vaziri et al., 1997). Histidine decarboxylase knockout mice exhibited an enhanced susceptibility to high-fat diet-induced obesity (Jørgensen et al., 2006). In sum, it appears that central histamine depletion increases food and water intake, while it is decreased by the stimulation of histamine synthesis. It remains to be determined whether the brain's histamine system might be a potential pharmacological molecular target for the treatment of eating disorders such as anorexia and obesity (Masaki and Yoshimatsu, 2007).

5.7.3 Sleep, waking and arousal

Animal research using rodents and cats has established a central role of the histaminergic system in the regulation of sleep and wakefulness. Histidine decarboxylase-positive neurons increase their firing frequency during waking and arousal but are silent during sleep (Lin, 2000). In cats, the functional inactivation of the nucleus tuberomamillaris by the microinfusion of muscimol caused hypersomnia associated with reduced arousal and attention (Lin et al., 1989). Similar effects have been observed after microinjections of α-fluoromethylhistidine into the ventrolateral posterior hypothalamus of cats which is innervated by histaminergic fibres. Here, α-fluoromethylhistidine decreased wakefulness and increased slow-wave sleep (Lin et al., 1986). In rats, the intraperitoneal application of the histidine decarboxylase inhibitor α-fluoromethylhistidine prevented the increase in wakefulness induced by intracerebroventricular administration of the hypocretin orexin, a recently discovered wake-promoting agent, suggesting that the sleep–wake regulation by orexin neurons recruits the histaminergic system (Yasuko et al., 2010). Furthermore, histidine decarboxylase knockout mice displayed diminished wakefulness during the dark period of the light–dark cycle and in an unfamiliar environment (Parmentier et al., 2002). Furthermore, they also exhibited an abnormal electroencephalogram, sleep fragmentation and increased paradoxical sleep during the light period (Anaclet et al., 2009). The pharmacological modulation of histamine neurotransmission in the brain has been utilized as a treatment for sleep disorders. For example, histamine H1 receptor antagonists known as 'antihistamines' as well as various psychotropic drugs with antihistamine properties are currently used to ameliorate insomnia (Stahl, 2008).

5.7.4 Reward and drugs

The dopamine hypothesis of reward holds that activation of the mesocorticolimbic and nigrostriatal dopamine system is a common pathway through which both drugs of abuse and natural rewards can reinforce behaviour and/or initiate memory formation (Wise, 2008). There is substantial evidence indicating that neuronal histamine counteracts reward and reinforcement processes, mediated by the dopamine system in the brain (Hasenöhrl and Huston, 2004). Accordingly, it has been hypothesized that the blockade of histamine synthesis should enhance the rewarding or hedonic aspects of addictive drugs. In line with these assumptions it was found that subcutaneous injections of α-fluoromethylhistidine potentiated the conditioned place preference induced by a sub-effective low dose of morphine (Suzuki *et al.*, 1995). Similarly, histidine decarboxylase knockout mice showed stronger morphine-induced conditioned place preference but decreased naloxone-precipitated withdrawal jumping as compared to their wild-type controls (Gong *et al.*, 2010). They also displayed a weaker stimulatory response to acute ethanol but showed stronger ethanol-induced conditioned place preference compared to their wild-type litter mates (Nuutinen *et al.*, 2010). Receptor binding studies suggested that these effects are not related to changes in the expression of the $GABA_A$ receptor in the brain of histidine decarboxylase knockout mice, but rather reflect increases in the rewarding or reinforcing properties of ethanol (Nuutinen *et al.*, 2010). In rodents, the chronic intraperitoneal administration of methamphetamine induces a progressive and long-lasting increase in locomotor and stereotyped behaviour. The behavioural effects of methamphetamine are potentiated by pre-treatment with α-fluoromethylhistidine administered intraperitoneally (Ito *et al.*, 1996). Histidine decarboxylase knockout mice showed increased methamphetamine-induced locomotor hyperactivity and accelerated behavioural sensitization to methamphetamine as compared to the wild-type controls (Iwabuchi *et al.*, 2004). However, the psychostimulant effects of cocaine were lower in histidine decarboxylase knockout mice relative to their wild-type littermates. Furthermore, cocaine-induced conditioned place preference of histidine decarboxylase knockout mice was not significantly different from the controls (Brabant *et al.*, 2007). In conclusion, the majority of findings reviewed above are in accordance with the assumption that central histamine depletion has a disinhibitory effect on the dopamine system of the brain. The meso-cortico-limbic dopamine system is thought to mediate the rewarding and reinforcing effects of natural rewards and drugs of abuse.

5.7.5 Stress, fear and anxiety

Histamine has been implicated in the regulation of the stress response mediated by the hypothalamo-pituitary-adrenocortical axis. In mice, different types of stress including water bathing, cold, body restraint, foot shock, and prolonged walking increase histidine decarboxylase activity in peripheral tissues such as skeletal muscles and the stomach (Taylor and Synder, 1971; Yoshitomi *et al.*, 1986; Ayada *et al.*, 2000). In rats, the application of unavoidable electrical shocks or a chronic restraint of their bodies increased histamine turnover rates in the diencephalon, nucleus accumbens and striatum (Ito, 2000; Westerink *et al.*, 2002). Incomplete lesions of the nucleus tuberomamillaris induced anxiolytic effects in rats (Frisch *et al.*, 1998). The amygdala is a central part of the brain's defence system, modulating fear and anxiety-related behaviours including conditioned and genetically predetermined unconditioned fear responses. Microinfusion of histamine into the amygdala of rats increased anxiety-related behaviours in the elevated plus maze test (Zarrindast *et al.*, 2005). From these findings one would predict an anxiolytic effect of brain histamine depletion. However, the behavioural phenotyping of histidine decarboxylase knockout mice revealed an opposite relationship. These mouse mutants exhibited increased behavioural measures of anxiety in a variety of tasks measuring experimental fear and anxiety including the open field test of anxiety, light–dark box, elevated plus maze and elevated zero maze (Acevedo *et al.*, 2006). Furthermore, histidine decarboxylase knockout mice showed an increase in anxiety-related behaviours in the height–fear task and the graded anxiety test, a modified elevated plus maze based on a combination of the light–dark box and elevated plus maze (Dere *et al.*, 2004). The role of brain histamine in fear and anxiety-related behaviour has been investigated by means of pharmacological, lesion, and genetic approaches. However, to date no clear-cut picture on the question of whether central histamine has anxiolytic or anxiogenic effects has emerged.

5.7.6 Learning and memory

It is well known that histamine plays an important role in various forms of learning and memory, both under physiological as well as pathological conditions (Dere et al., 2010). Histamine has also been implicated in synaptic long-term potentiation and depotentiation, which are assumed to represent electrophysiological correlates of learning and memory formation (Dringenberg and Kuo, 2006; Haas et al., 2008). In rats, the working and reference memory impairment that is induced by the infusion of the muscarinergic acetylcholine receptor blocker scopolamine into the dorsal hippocampus is ameliorated by the co-administration of histamine or its precursor L-histidine (Xu et al., 2009). Moreover, intracerebroventricular injection of histamine or the intraperitoneal injection of L-histidine to rats with hippocampal lesions both ameliorated active avoidance performance (Kamei et al., 1997). Intracerebroventricular injection of the histidine decarboxylase-blocker α-fluoromethylhistidine to rats impaired spatial memory in a radial maze task (Chen et al., 1999) and prolonged the response latency after intracerebroventricular and intraperitoneal injection in an active avoidance paradigm (Kamei et al., 1993). Interestingly, the senescence-accelerated mice-prone strain, which already exhibits learning and memory deficits at the age of 12 months as compared to an age-matched normal-rate ageing strain, also exhibited lower histidine decarboxylase activity in the forebrain including the cortex, hippocampus and striatum (Meguro et al., 1995). These studies suggest that the stimulation of histamine neurotransmission can counteract amnestic manipulations such as acetylcholine receptor blockade or hippocampal lesions, and that the reduction of histamine synthesis has detrimental effects on learning and memory performance in rodents. However, there is also evidence available suggesting the opposite relationship. For example, repeated administration of α-fluoromethylhistidine decreased histamine levels in the hippocampus and cerebral cortex, but concomitantly improved spatial memory in a working-memory version of the eight-arm radial maze (Sakai et al., 1998). Furthermore, histidine decarboxylase knockout mice showed improved cued and contextual fear-conditioning (Liu et al., 2007); and electrophysiological measurements revealed that hippocampal CA1 long-term potentiation was greater in the histidine decarboxylase knockout mice immediately after its induction, but smaller one day after. Additionally, hippocampal glutamate levels were increased in histidine decarboxylase knockout mice up to four days after the induction of long-term potentiation (Liu et al., 2007). In the Morris water maze, histidine decarboxylase knockout mice showed superior performance in the hidden and cued platform versions of the task and on the retention test of the passive avoidance task (Dere et al., 2003; Acevedo et al., 2006). However, the histidine decarboxylase knockout mice were impaired in their learning of a temporal sequence whereby novel objects were successively introduced into a familiar environment (Dere et al., 2003).

These contradictory effects of various forms of brain histamine depletion might be the result of concomitant effects on emotional and reward-mediating systems and their interactions with specific experimental conditions and technical parameters of the different learning and memory tasks used. It is well known that both too low, and excess levels of stress/arousal during testing, can counteract learning and memory performance. In aversively motivated tasks, such as the Morris water maze or the one-trial inhibitory avoidance task, the level of stress/arousal induced to motivate learning and memory formation has to be adjusted to an optimal intermediate range that enables the detection of impaired and improved performance. Interestingly, it has been found that a slight reduction in the brain histamine concentration by α-fluoromethylhistidine enhances attention and accuracy in solving a visuospatial task under stressful conditions (Cacabelos and Alvarez, 1991). In positively motivated learning and memory paradigms, such as the eight-arm radial maze, conditioned place preference or the novelty preference object recognition paradigm, the amount of reward given to reinforce correct responses can likewise modulate learning and memory performance. When the amount of reward given is at the lower end of the spectrum that is sufficient to reinforce correct responses and maintain responding, brain histamine depletion might increase learning motivation by enhancing the rewarding value of natural rewards and drugs (Dere et al., 2010).

5.7.6.1 Dementia

The severe memory impairments of patients suffering from Alzheimer's disease was originally attributed to the degeneration of cholinergic neurons, especially those located in the basal forebrain, due to extracellular amyloid plaque deposits and the intracellular accumulation of neurofibrillary tangles. However, there is substantial evidence suggesting that other neurotransmitter systems, including the brain's histamine system, also contribute to the cognitive impairments of these patients (Musiał et al., 2007; Yanai and Tashiro, 2007; Dere et al., 2010). Individuals suffering from Alzheimer's disease displayed changes in brain histamine levels (Panula et al., 1998) concomitant with a degeneration of histamine-containing neurons in the nucleus tuberomamillaris (Airaksinen et al., 1991; Nakamura et al., 1993; Ishunina et al., 2003). A coupled radioenzymatic assay has been used to determine the activity of histidine decarboxylase in the frontal cortex of ageing Downs's syndrome patients, Alzheimer's patients and healthy control individuals. It was found that histidine decarboxylase activity was reduced in brains of both Downs's syndrome and Alzheimer's patients (Schneider et al., 1997). Tacrine is an anti-Alzheimer's drug (a cholinesterase inhibitor) which increases the availability of acetylcholine, and is widely prescribed during the early stages of the disease. The catabolic activity of histamine-N-methyltransferase, which normally degrades histamine to tele-methylhistamine, is blocked by tacrine. Tacrine has been reported to increase histamine levels in the hippocampus (Nishibori et al., 1991; Morisset et al., 1996). In contrast to tacrine, physostigmine, another anti-Alzheimer's drug, is less effective in ameliorating cognitive symptoms in Alzheimer's disease and has a lower affinity to histamine-N-methyltransferase (Nishibori et al., 1991). Thus, it is possible that the procognitive effects of cholinesterase in early-stage Alzheimer's disease are due at least in part to increases in histamine neurotransmission, e.g. in the hippocampus. Given the growing need for effective cognitive enhancers with minor adverse effects, histamine H3 receptor antagonists which stimulate histamine synthesis and release are currently being evaluated for their potential use in Alzheimer's disease (Medhurst et al., 2009).

5.8 Summary and Conclusions

Mammalian histidine decarboxylase is the rate-limiting enzyme that catalyses the formation of the indolamine histamine from histidine in a one-step oxidative decarboxylating process. Biologically active histidine decarboxylase takes the form of a homodimer consisting of two carboxy-truncated monomers with a molecular mass of 53–55 kDa. Within the cell, histidine decarboxylase is coupled to the membrane of the endoplasmic reticulum with its carboxyl terminal region exposed on the cytosolic part of the cell. Histidine decarboxylase-positive cells include mast cells, enterochromaffin-like cells, macrophages, endothelial cells and neurons. In the brain histidine, decarboxylase-positive neurons are exclusively located in the nucleus tuberomamillaris of the posterior hypothalamus, from where projections to wide parts of the brain arise. The mouse and human histidine decarboxylase gene consists of 12 exons and covers 24 kb of genomic DNA. Histidine decarboxylase gene expression is initiated by several agents, treatments and physiological conditions.

The depletion of brain histamine by means of systemic or intracerebral application of the histidine decarboxylase blocker α-fluoromethylhistidine to rats, or the genetic inactivation of histidine decarboxylase expression in the mouse, modulates a wide range of behavioural and physiological processes. The effects of histamine depletion in rodents include increases in nutritive behaviour; decreased waking and arousal; potentiation of the psychostimulant, rewarding, and reinforcing effects of addictive drugs; modulation of behavioural correlates of stress, fear, and anxiety; changes in brain acetylcholine and monoamine levels; and the modulation of hippocampal synaptic plasticity and learning and memory performance. In terms of learning and memory performance the findings are inconsistent, with both improvements and impairments observed after pharmacological or genetic inhibition of histidine decarboxylase activity. These effects might be explained by simultaneous effects on emotional- and reward-mediating systems, and their interactions with specific experimental conditions and task parameters (Dere *et al.*, 2010).

Pathological changes in the histamine system have been measured in brains of Alzheimer's disease patients. These changes involve neurodegeneration of histamine-positive neurons in the nucleus tuberomamillaris, decreased activity of histidine decarboxylase and changes in the levels of central histamine. It remains to be determined whether some of the cognitive symptoms of patients with Alzheimer's disease might be ameliorated after treatment with histamine-related drugs.

5.9 Acknowledgements

This work was supported by the German Science Foundation through grant DE1149/5-1 to E.D.

References

Acevedo, S.F., Ohtsu, H., Benice, T.S., Rizk-Jackson, A. and Raber, J. (2006) Age-dependent measures of anxiety and cognition in male histidine decarboxylase knockout (Hdc-/-) mice. *Brain Research* 1071, 113–123.

Airaksinen, M.S., Paetau, A., Paljärvi, L., Reinikainen, K., Riekkinen, P., Suomalainen, R. and Panula, P. (1991) Histamine neurons in human hypothalamus: anatomy in normal and Alzheimer diseased brains. *Neuroscience* 44, 465–481.

Alvarez, E.O. (2009) The role of histamine on cognition. *Behavioural Brain Research* 199, 183–189.

Anaclet, C., Parmentier, R., Ouk, K., Guidon, G., Buda, C., Sastre, J.P., Akaoka, H., *et al.* (2009) Orexin/hypocretin and histamine: distinct roles in the control of wakefulness demonstrated using knock-out mouse models. *Journal of Neuroscience* 29, 14423–14438.

Ayada, K., Watanabe, M. and Endo, Y. (2000) Elevation of histidine decarboxylase activity in skeletal muscles and stomach in mice by stress and exercise. American journal of physiology. *American Journal of Physiology. Regulatory, Integrative and Comparative Physiology* 279, R2042–2047.

Bellinger, L.L. and Bernardis, L.L. (2002) The dorsomedial hypothalamic nucleus and its role in ingestive behavior and body weight regulation: lessons learned from lesioning studies. *Physiology and Behavior* 76, 431–442.

Brabant, C., Quertemont, E., Anaclet, C., Lin, J.S., Ohtsu, H. and Tirelli, E. (2007) The psychostimulant and rewarding effects of cocaine in histidine decarboxylase knockout mice do not support the hypothesis of an inhibitory function of histamine on reward. *Psychopharmacology* 190, 251–263.

Brown, R.E., Stevens, D.R. and Haas, H.L. (2001) The physiology of brain histamine. *Progress in Neurobiology* 63, 637–672.

Cacabelos, R. and Alvarez, X.A. (1991) Histidine decarboxylase inhibition induced by alpha-fluoromethylhistidine provokes learning-related hypokinetic activity. *Agents Actions* 33, 131–134.

Chen, Z., Sugimoto, Y. and Kamei, C. (1999) Effects of intracerebroventricular injection of alpha-fluoromethylhistidine on radial maze performance in rats. *Pharmacology, Biochemistry and Behavior* 64, 513–518.

Chotard, C., Ouimet, T., Morisset, S., Sahm, U., Schwartz, J.C. and Trottier, S. (2002) Effects of histamine H3 receptor agonist and antagonist on histamine co-transmitter expression in rat brain. *Journal of Neural Transmission* 109, 293–306.

Colucci, R., Fleming, J.V., Xavier, R. and Wang, T.C. (2001) Histidine decarboxylase decreases its own transcription through downregulation of ERK activity. *American Journal of Physiology. Gastrointestinal and Liver Physiology* 281, G1081–1091.

Dere, E., De Souza Silva, M.A., Topic, B., Spieler, R.E., Haas, H.L. and Huston, J.P. (2003) Histidine-decarboxylase knockout mice show deficient nonreinforced episodic object memory, improved negatively reinforced water-maze performance, and increased neo- and ventro-striatal dopamine turnover. *Learning and Memory* 10, 510–519.

Dere, E., De Souza Silva, M.A., Spieler, R.E., Lin, J.S., Ohtsu, H., Haas, H.L. and Huston, J.P. (2004) Changes in motoric, exploratory and emotional behaviours and neuronal acetylcholine content and 5-HT turnover in histidine decarboxylase-KO mice. *European Journal of Neuroscience* 20, 1051–1058.

Dere, E., Zlomuzica, A., De Souza Silva, M.A., Rocco, L.A., Sadile, A.G. and Huston, J.P. (2010) Neuronal histamine and the interplay of memory, reinforcement and emotions. *Behavioural Brain Research* 215, 209–220.

Dringenberg, H.C. and Kuo, M.C. (2006) Cholinergic, histaminergic, and noradrenergic regulation of LTP stability and induction threshold: cognitive implications. *Neurotransmitter Interactions and Cognitive Function Experientia Supplementum* 98, 165–183.

Esbenshade, T.A., Browman, K.E., Bitner, R.S., Strakhova, M., Cowart, M.D. and Brioni, J.D. (2008) The histamine H3 receptor: an attractive target for the treatment of cognitive disorders. *British Journal of Pharmacology* 154, 1166–1181.

Falus, A. (2003) Histamine, part of the metabolome. *Acta Biologica Hungarica* 54, 27–34.

Fleming, J.V. and Wang, T.C. (2003) The production of 53-55-kDa isoforms is not required for rat histidine decarboxylase activity. *Journal of Biological Chemistry* 278, 686–694.

Frisch, C., Hasenöhrl, R.U., Krauth, J. and Huston, J.P. (1998) Anxiolytic-like behavior after lesion of the tuberomammillary nucleus E2-region. *Experimental Brain Research* 119, 260–264.

Furuta, K., Ichikawa, A., Nakayama, K. and Tanaka, S. (2006) Membrane orientation of the precursor 74-kDa form of Histidine decarboxylase. *Inflammation Research* 55, 185–191.

García-Martín, E., Ayuso, P., Martínez, C., Blanca, M. and Agúndez, J.A. (2009) Histamine pharmacogenomics. *Pharmacogenomics* 10, 867–883.

Gong, Y.X., Zhang, W.P., Shou, W.T., Zhong, K. and Chen, Z. (2010) Morphine induces conditioned place preference behavior in histidine decarboxylase knockout mice. *Neuroscience Letters* 468, 115–119.

Haas, H.L., Sergeeva, O.A. and Selbach, O. (2008) Histamine in the nervous system. *Physiological Reviews* 88, 1183–1241.

Hasenöhrl, R.U. and Huston, J.P. (2004) Histamine. In: Riedel, G. and Platt, B. (eds), *Memories are Made of These: From Messengers to Molecules*. Landes Bioscience, Austin, Texas.

Hegyesi, H., Somlai, B., Varga, V.L., Toth, G., Kovacs, P., Molnar, E.L., Laszlo, V., *et al.* (2001) Suppression of melanoma cell proliferation by histidine decarboxylase specific antisense oligonucleotides. *Journal of Investigative Dermatology* 117, 151–153.

Höcker, M., Rosenberg, I., Xavier, R., Henihan, R.J., Wiedenmann, B., Rosewicz, S., Podolsky, D.K., *et al.* (1998) Oxidative stress activates the human histidine decarboxylase promoter in AGS gastric cancer cells. *Journal of Biological Chemistry* 273, 23046–23054.

Ishunina, T.A., van Heerikhuize, J.J., Ravid, R. and Swaab, D.F. (2003) Estrogen receptors and metabolic activity in the human tuberomamillary nucleus: changes in relation to sex, aging and Alzheimer's disease. *Brain Research* 988, 84–96.

Ito, C. (2000) The role of brain histamine in acute and chronic stresses. *Biomedicine and Pharmacotherapy* 54, 263–267.

Ito, C., Sato, M., Onodera, K. and Watanabe, T. (1996) The role of the brain histaminergic neuron system in methamphetamine-induced behavioral sensitization in rats. *Annals of the New York Academy of Sciences* 801, 353–360.

Iwabuchi, K., Kubota, Y., Ito, C., Watanabe, T., Watanabe, T. and Yanai, K. (2004) Methamphetamine and brain histamine: a study using histamine-related gene knockout mice. *Annals of the New York Academy of Sciences* 1025, 129–134.

Jørgensen, E.A., Vogelsang, T.W., Knigge, U., Watanabe, T., Warberg, J. and Kjaer, A. (2006) Increased susceptibility to diet-induced obesity in histamine-deficient mice. *Neuroendocrinology* 83, 289–294.

Joseph, D.R., Sullivan, P.M., Wang, Y.M., Kozak, C., Fenstermacher, D.A., Behrendsen, M.E. and Zahnow, C.A. (1990) Characterization and expression of the complementary DNA encoding rat histidine decarboxylase. *Proceedings of the National Academy of Sciences of the USA* 87, 733–737.

Kamei, C., Okumura, Y. and Tasaka, K. (1993) Influence of histamine depletion on learning and memory recollection in rats. *Psychopharmacology* 111, 376–382.

Kamei, C., Chen, Z., Nakamura, S. and Sugimoto, Y. (1997) Effects of intracerebroventricular injection of histamine on memory deficits induced by hippocampal lesions in rats. *Methods and Findings in Experimental and Clinical Pharmacology* 19, 253–259.

Kohler, C., Ericson, H., Watanabe, T., Polak, J., Palay, S.L., Palay, V. and Chan-Palay, V. (1986) Galanin immunoreactivity in hypothalamic neurons: further evidence for multiple chemical messengers in the tuberomammillary nucleus. *Journal of Comparative Neurology* 250, 58–64.

Kondo, S., Imamura, I., Shinomura, Y., Matsuzawa, Y. and Fukui, H. (1995) Determination of histidine decarboxylase mRNA in various rat tissues by the polymerase chain reaction. *Inflammation Research* 44, 111–115.

Li, Z., Liu, J., Tang, F., Liu, Y., Waldum, H.L. and Cui, G. (2008) Expression of non-mast cell histidine decarboxylase in tumor-associated microvessels in human esophageal squamous cell carcinomas. *APMIS* 116, 1034–1042.

Lin, J.S. (2000) Brain structures and mechanisms involved in the control of cortical activation and wakefulness, with emphasis on the posterior hypothalamus and histaminergic neurons. *Sleep Medicine Reviews* 4, 471–503.

Lin, J.S., Sakai, K. and Jouvet, M. (1986) Role of hypothalamic histaminergic systems in the regulation of vigilance states in cats. *Comptes rendus de l'Académie des sciences. Série III, Sciences de la vie* 303, 469–474.

Lin, J.S., Sakai, K., Vanni-Mercier, G. and Jouvet, M. (1989) A critical role of the posterior hypothalamus in the mechanisms of wakefulness determined by microinjection of muscimol in freely moving cats. *Brain Research* 479, 225–240.

Liu, L., Zhang, S., Zhu, Y., Fu, Q., Zhu, Y., Gong, Y., Ohtsu, H., et al. (2007) Improved learning and memory of contextual fear conditioning and hippocampal CA1 long-term potentiation in histidine decarboxylase knock out mice. *Hippocampus* 17, 634–641.

Malzac, P., Mattei, M.G., Thibault, J. and Bruneau, G. (1996) Chromosomal localization of the human and mouse histidine decarboxylase genes by in situ hybridization. Exclusion of the HDC gene from the Prader-Willi syndrome region. *Human Genetics* 97, 359–361.

Masaki, T. and Yoshimatsu, H. (2007) Neuronal histamine and its receptors in obesity and diabetes. *Current Diabetes Reviews* 3, 212–216.

Medhurst, A.D., Roberts, J.C., Lee, J., Chen, C.P., Brown, S.H., Roman, S. and Lai, M.K. (2009) Characterization of histamine H3 receptors in Alzheimer's Disease brain and amyloid over-expressing TASTPM mice. *British Journal of Pharmacology* 157, 130–138.

Meguro, K., Yanai, K., Sakai, N., Sakurai, E., Maeyama, K., Sasaki, H. and Watanabe, T. (1995) Effects of thioperamide, a histamine H3 antagonist, on the step-through passive avoidance response and histidine decarboxylase activity in senescence-accelerated mice. *Pharmacology, Biochemistry and Behavior* 50, 321–325.

Morimoto, T., Yamamoto, Y., Mobarakeh, J.I., Yanai, K., Watanabe, T., Watanabe, T. and Yamatodani, A. (1999) Involvement of the histaminergic system in leptin-induced suppression of food intake. *Physiology and Behavior* 67, 679–683.

Morisset, S., Traiffort, E. and Schwartz, J.C. (1996) Inhibition of histamine versus acetylcholine metabolism as a mechanism of tacrine activity. *European Journal of Pharmacology* 315, R1–2.

Musiał, A., Bajda, M. and Malawska, B. (2007) Recent developments in cholinesterases inhibitors for Alzheimer's disease treatment. *Current Medicinal Chemistry* 14, 2654–2679.

Nakamura, S., Takemura, M., Ohnishi, K., Suenaga, T., Nishimura, M., Akiguchi, I., Kimura, J., et al. (1993) Loss of large neurons and occurrence of neurofibrillary tangles in the tuberomammillary nucleus of patients with Alzheimer's disease. *Neuroscience Letters* 151, 196–199.

Nishibori, M., Oishi, R., Itoh, Y. and Saeki, K. (1991) 9-Amino-1,2,3,4-tetrahydroacridine is a potent inhibitor of histamine N-methyltransferase. *Japanese Journal of Pharmacology* 55, 539–546.

Nuutinen, S., Karlstedt, K., Aitta-Aho, T., Korpi, E.R. and Panula, P. (2010) Histamine and H3 receptor-dependent mechanisms regulate ethanol stimulation and conditioned place preference in mice. *Psychopharmacology* 208, 75–86.

Ohtsu, H. and Watanabe, T. (2003) New functions of histamine found in histidine decarboxylase gene knockout mice. *Biochemical and Biophysical Research Communications* 305, 443–447.

Ohtsu, H., Tanaka, S., Terui, T., Hori, Y., Makabe-Kobayashi, Y., Pejler, G., Tchougounova, E., et al. (2001) Mice lacking histidine decarboxylase exhibit abnormal mast cells. *FEBS Letters* 502, 53–56.

Onodera, K., Yamatodani, A. and Watanabe, T. (1992) Effects of alpha-fluoromethylhistidine on locomotor activity, brain histamine and catecholamine contents in rats. *Methods and Findings in Experimental and Clinical Pharmacology* 14, 97–105.

Ookuma, K., Sakata, T., Fukagawa, K., Yoshimatsu, H., Kurokawa, M., Machidori, H. and Fujimoto, K. (1993) Neuronal histamine in the hypothalamus suppresses food intake in rats. *Brain Research* 628, 235–242.

Orthen-Gambill, N. and Salomon, M. (1992) FMH-induced decrease in central histamine levels produces increased feeding and body weight in rats. *Physiology and Behavior* 51, 891–893.

Panula, P., Rinne, J., Kuokkanen, K., Eriksson, K.S., Sallmen, T., Kalimo, H. and Relja, M. (1998) Neuronal histamine deficit in Alzheimer's disease. *Neuroscience* 82, 993–997.

Parmentier, R., Ohtsu, H., Djebbara-Hannas, Z., Valatx, J.L., Watanabe, T. and Lin, J.S. (2002) Anatomical, physiological, and pharmacological characteristics of histidine decarboxylase knock-out mice: evidence for the role of brain histamine in behavioral and sleep-wake control. *Journal of Neuroscience* 22, 7695–7711.

Parson, M.E. and Ganellin, C.R. (2006) Histamine and its receptors. *British Journal of Pharmacology* 147, S127–S135.

Rangachari, P.K. (1992) Histamine: mercurial messenger in the gut. *American Journal of Physiology* 262, G1–G13.

Sakai, N., Sakurai, E., Onodera, K., Sakurai, E., Asada, H., Miura, Y. and Watanabe, T. (1995) Long-term depletion of brain histamine induced by alpha-fluoromethylhistidine increases feeding-associated locomotor activity in mice with a modulation of brain amino acid levels. *Behavioural Brain Research* 72, 83–88.

Sakai, N., Sakurai, E., Sakurai, E., Yanai, K., Mirua, Y. and Watanabe, T. (1998) Depletion of brain histamine induced by alpha-fluoromethylhistidine enhances radial maze performance in rats with modulation of brain amino acid levels. *Life Sciences* 62, 989–994.

Sakata, T., Yoshimatsu, H., Masaki, T. and Tsuda, K. (2003) Anti-obesity actions of mastication driven by histamine neurons in rats. *Experimental Biology and Medicine* 228, 1106–1110.

Schneider, C., Risser, D., Kirchner, L., Kitzmüller, E., Cairns, N., Prast, H., Singewald, N., et al. (1997) Similar deficits of central histaminergic system in patients with Down syndrome and Alzheimer disease. *Neuroscience Letters* 222, 183–186.

Servos, P., Barke, K.E., Hough, L.B. and Vanderwolf, C.H. (1994) Histamine does not play an essential role in electrocortical activation during waking behavior. *Brain Research* 636, 98–102.

Skratt, J.J., Hough, L.B., Nalwalk, J.W. and Barke, K.E. (1994) Alpha-Fluoromethylhistidine-induced inhibition of brain histidine decarboxylase. Implications for the CO_2-trapping enzymatic method. *Biochemical Pharmacology* 47, 397–402.

Stahl, S.M. (2008) Selective histamine H1 antagonism: novel hypnotic and pharmacologic actions challenge classical notions of antihistamines. *CNS Spectrums* 13, 1027–1038.

Suzuki, T., Takamori, K., Misawa, M. and Onodera, K. (1995) Effects of the histaminergic system on the morphine-induced conditioned place preference in mice. *Brain Research* 675, 195–202.

Suzuki-Ishigaki, S., Numayama-Tsuruta, K., Kuramasu, A., Sakurai, E., Makabe, Y., Shimura, S., Shirato, K., et al. (2000) The mouse histidine decarboxylase gene: structure and transcriptional regulation by CpG methylation in the promoter region. *Nucleic Acids Research* 28, 2627–2633.

Taguchi, Y., Watanabe, T., Kubota, H., Hayashi, H. and Wada, H. (1984) Purification of histidine decarboxylase from the liver of fetal rats and its immunochemical and immunohistochemical characterization. *Journal of Biological Chemistry* 259, 5214–5221.

Tanaka, S., Nemoto, K., Yamamura, E. and Ichikawa, A. (1998) Intracellular localization of the 74- and 53-kDa forms of histidine decarboxylase in a rat basophilic/mast cell line, RBL-2H3. *Journal of Biological Chemistry* 273, 8177–8182.

Tanimoto, A., Sasaguri, Y. and Ohtsu, H. (2006) Histamine network in atherosclerosis. *Trends in Cardiovascular Medicine* 16, 280–284.

Taylor, K.M. and Synder, S.H. (1971) Brain histamine: rapid apparent turnover altered by restraint and cold stress. *Science* 172, 1037–1039.

Trottier, S., Chotard, C., Traiffort, E., Unmehopa, U., Fisser, B., Swaab, D.F. and Schwartz, J.C. (2002) Co-localization of histamine with GABA but not with galanin in the human tuberomamillary nucleus. *Brain Research* 939, 52–64.

Tuomisto, L., Yamatodani, A., Jolkkonen, J., Sainio, E.L. and Airaksinen, M.M. (1994) Inhibition of brain histamine synthesis increases food intake and attenuates vasopressin response to salt loading in rats. *Methods and Findings in Experimental and Clinical Pharmacology* 16, 355–359.

Vaziri, P., Dang, K. and Anderson, G.H. (1997) Evidence for histamine involvement in the effect of histidine loads on food and water intake in rats. *Journal of Nutrition* 127, 1519–2156.

Wada, H., Inagaki, N., Itowi, N. and Yamatodani, A. (1991) Histaminergic neuron system in the brain: distribution and possible functions. *Brain Research Bulletin* 27, 367–370.

Watanabe, T. and Yanai, K. (2001) Studies on functional roles of the histaminergic neuron system by using pharmacological agents, knockout mice and positron emission tomography. *Tohoku Journal of Experimental Medicine* 195, 197–217.

Watanabe, T. and Ohtsu, H. (2002) Histidine decarboxylase as a probe in studies on histamine. *Chemical Record* 2, 369–376.

Watanabe, T., Yamatodani, A., Maeyama, K. and Wada, H. (1990) Pharmacology of alpha-fluoromethylhistidine, a specific inhibitor of histidine decarboxylase. *Trends in Pharmacological Sciences* 11, 363–367.

Westerink, B.H., Cremers, T.I., De Vries, J.B., Liefers, H., Tran, N. and De Boer, P. (2002) Evidence for activation of histamine H3 autoreceptors during handling stress in the prefrontal cortex of the rat. *Synapse* 43, 238–243.

Wise, R.A. (2008) Dopamine and reward: the anhedonia hypothesis 30 years on. *Neurotoxicity Research* 14, 169–183.

Xu, L.S., Fan, Y.Y., He, P., Zhang, W.P., Hu, W.W. and Chen, Z. (2009) Ameliorative effects of histamine on spatial memory deficits induced by scopolamine infusion into bilateral dorsal or ventral hippocampus as evaluated by the radial arm maze task. *Clinical and Experimental Pharmacology and Physiology* 36, 816–821.

Yamamoto, J., Yatsunami, K., Ohmori, E., Sugimoto, Y., Fukui, T., Katayama, T. and Ichikawa, A. (1990) cDNA-derived amino acid sequence of histidine decarboxylase from mouse mastocytoma P-815 cells. *FEBS Letters* 276, 214–218.

Yanai, K. and Tashiro, M. (2007) The physiological and pathophysiological roles of neuronal histamine: an insight from human positron emission tomography studies. *Pharmacology and Therapeutics* 113, 1–15.

Yasuko, S., Atanda, A.M., Masato, M., Kazuhiko, Y. and Kazuki, H. (2010) Alpha-fluoromethylhistidine, a histamine synthesis inhibitor, inhibits orexin-induced wakefulness in rats. *Behavioural Brain Research* 207, 151–154.

Yoshitomi, I., Itoh, Y., Oishi, R. and Saeki, K. (1986) Brain histamine turnover enhanced by foot shock. *Brain Research* 362, 195–198.

Zarrindast, M.R., Moghadam, A.H., Rostami, P. and Roohbakhsh, A. (2005) The effects of histaminergic agents in the central amygdala of rats in the elevated plus-maze test of anxiety. *Behavioural Pharmacology* 16, 643–649.

Zhang, F., Xiong, D.H., Wang, W., Shen, H., Xiao, P., Yang, F., Recker, R.R., *et al.* (2006) HDC gene polymorphisms are associated with age at natural menopause in Caucasian women. *Biochemical and Biophysical Research Communications* 348, 1378–1382.

6 Glutamate Decarboxylase

H. Ueno,* Y. Inoue, S. Matsukawa and Y. Nakamura
Laboratory of Applied Microbiology and Biochemistry, Nara Women's University, Nara, Japan

6.1 Abstract

Glutamate decarboxylase (GAD) catalyses the synthesis of γ-aminobutyric acid (GABA), an inhibitory neurotransmitter, from glutamate. Glutamate is an excitatory neurotransmitter and is also known as an umami compound. GAD was known for its localization in the central nervous system, testes and pancreas; however, recent findings suggest wide distribution including skin and digestive system, i.e. stomach, intestine and tongue. This chapter updates some of the findings of GAD in the taste signalling system. It also covers the area of GAD gene structure and reports an unusual form of GAD protein expression, probably evidence for multiple splicing. The role of GAD in diabetes is another emerging issue worthy of further investigation in relation to diagnostic and therapeutic potential.

role as an inhibitory neurotransmitter in the central nervous system (CNS) of higher animals (Ueno, 2000). Since both substrate and product are neurotransmitters but with opposite roles, GAD is a unique enzyme.

Characterization of GAD has been carried out widely and described elsewhere; however, it is important to point out that there was controversy in the properties that were published prior to early 1990, before genes for GAD had been cloned. Molecular analysis made it clear that there are two distinct gene products for GAD, namely GAD 65 and GAD 67. Since then, genetic investigations including knockout mouse studies and immunological analysis for tissue-specific GAD expression have been carried out. Furthermore, GAD 65 involvement in diabetes is also now well recognized. In the following sections, each topic on GAD-related issues is briefly reviewed.

6.2 Introduction

This chapter describes recent advances relating to glutamate decarboxylase (GAD), involving two amino acids: L-glutamate as a substrate and γ-aminobutyrate (GABA) as a product. GABA was first recognized for its

6.3 Distribution of GABA

The role of GABA as an inhibitory neurotransmitter defines its distribution in the mammalian system, mainly at the GABAergic neuron that is estimated at around 25–45% of the total neurons. GABA concentration is estimated at

---

* E-mail address: hueno@cc.nara-wu.ac.jp

mM level, significantly high, but its distribution is uneven (Iversen and Snyder, 1968). On the other hand, there is little GABA present at the peripheral nerves. In the nerve cells, GABA is localized at the synaptic terminals and cell bodies (Ribak et al., 1979a,b) (Fig. 6.1). In vertebrates, GABA occurs at relatively high levels in Purkinje cells in the cerebellum (Obata, 1969; Saito et al., 1974; Storm-Mathisen, 1975); hippocampus (Mihailobic et al., 1965; Delgado et al., 1971; Storm-Mathisen, 1975); substantia nigra (McGeer et al., 1974; Storm-Mathisen, 1975); posterior spinal cord (Henry, 1979); hypothalamus (Storm-Mathisen, 1975; Marczynski, 1998); and at low levels in medulla oblongata (Siemers et al., 1982); cerebral cortex (Thangnipon et al., 1983); and cerebellar cortex (Ikenaga et al., 2005). Outside of the nervous system, GABA was found in pancreatic β-cells (Smismans et al., 1997), ovary (Schaeffer and Hsueh, 1982), heart (Yessaian et al., 1969), and intestine (Taniyama et al., 1982). Crustaceans show significant amount of GABA at the connective part of neurons.

6.3.1 GABA storage, release and uptake

GABA is stored in synaptic vesicles by vesicular GABA transporter (VGAT). Ligand specificity of VGAT is low: i.e., glycine can sometimes be transported (Dumoulin et al., 1999). Nerve impulses release GABA into the synaptic space, where the process depends upon Ca^{2+}. Released GABA molecules are taken up to the nerve ending and/or glia cells. The process depends upon energy and is associated with Na^+ and Cl^-. Currently, four subtypes are known to be GABA transporters; these actions may be inhibited by β-alanine or L-2, 3-diaminobutyrate (Guimbal et al., 1995).

6.3.2 GABA receptors

GABA binds to the GABA receptor to raise Cl^- permeation that leads to hyperpolarization of the membrane in inhibiting nerve excitation. There are three subtypes of GABA receptor, namely $GABA_A$, $GABA_B$ and $GABA_C$. $GABA_A$ and $GABA_C$ are Cl^- ion channel hetero-pentameric subunits. $GABA_A$ is mainly found in the central nervous system (CNS), particularly around synapses, and its subunit construction is quite diverse: five subunits, with four transmembrane domains selected from eight groups of polypeptide chains classified into 19 isoforms. The exact location of $GABA_A$ receptor with one specific combination of subunits defines the role of the particular $GABA_A$ receptor. $GABA_A$ receptor has two GABA binding sites and several allosteric sites; thus, it exhibits complex pharmacological characteristics.

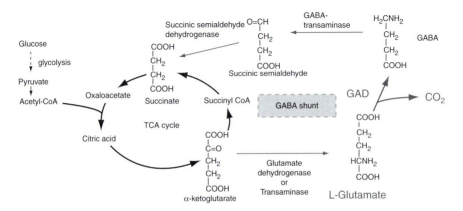

Fig. 6.1. Metabolic pathway of GABA.

GABA$_B$ receptor is a typical G-protein coupled type with seven transmembrane domains and constructed with dimeric subunits. GABA$_B$ is located at the peripheral nerves, pre- and post-synaptic terminals.

GABA$_C$ receptors are ligand-gated Cl⁻ ion channel type receptors constructed with 5ρ family subunits (Qian *et al.*, 1997, 1998). GABA$_C$ receptors mediate slow and sustained responses in contrast to GABA$_A$ receptors. GABA$_C$ receptors are expressed in many brain regions, including retinal neurons. Affinity towards the GABA molecule is tenfold higher than that of GABA$_A$ receptors (Table 6.1).

6.3.3 Metabolism of GABA

In the metabolic network, GABA locates at the GABA shunt (Fig. 6.1), adjacent to the TCA cycle (Erecinska *et al.*, 1996). L-glutamate can be synthesized from α-ketoglutarate by aminotransferase(s), and is decarboxylated by an enzyme, glutamate decarboxylase (GAD, EC: 4.1.1.15) to produce GABA (Martin *et al.*, 1991; Zhang *et al.*, 1999). GABA is then converted to succinic semialdehyde by GABA transaminase, and to succinate by succinic semialdehyde dehydrogenase. Succinate is now returned to the TCA cycle (Bouche *et al.*, 2003). GABA lowers high blood pressure (Daniels and Pettigrew, 1975), and also has diuretic (Krantis and Kerr, 1981) and antitumour activity (Fukushima and Toyoshima, 1975; Lin *et al.*, 1996). These physiological activities might act upon non-neuronal systems. Recently many food products such as chocolate, having GABA as a main ingredient, have been developed commercially for their relaxation effect. However, it is still unclear how GABA acts on non-neuronal systems. GABA is not transported into the brain since it is unable to cross the blood–brain barrier (Purpura and Carmichael, 1960).

6.3.4 Decarboxylation reaction by GAD

Decarboxylation of L-glutamate is a one-step and irreversible reaction catalysed by GAD. GAD requires a coenzyme, pyridoxal 5′-phosphate (PLP) that binds to the active site lysine residue to form an internal Schiff base (Choi and Churchich, 1986), where PLP is an active form of vitamin B$_6$. GAD takes L-glutamate as a substrate and cleaves the α-carboxyl group to form CO$_2$ and GABA. During the catalytic cycle, GAD also utilizes one H⁺.

GAD belongs to a family of PLP-dependent amino acid decarboxylases that includes histidine decarboxylase (HDC) and aromatic amino acid decarboxylase (AroDC), also called DOPA decarboxylase (DDC). The three decarboxylases have a common function that cleaves α-carboxyl group of the substrate amino acids to form CO$_2$ and the corresponding amines. Comparison of the amino acid sequences should show that, if common amino acid residues are found, these should participate in the recognition and cleavage of the α-carboxyl group. When amino acid sequences were compared, it was of interest to note that AroDC is the shortest among the three: mammalian GAD isoforms have a long extra complement of residues, about 100 amino acids, at the N-terminal side, and HDC shows about 150 extra amino acid residues at

Table 6.1. Characteristics of GABA receptors.

	GABA$_A$ receptor	GABA$_B$ receptor	GABA$_C$ receptor
Category	Ligand-gated channel	G-protein coupled receptor	Ligand-gated channel
Subunits	α, β, γ, δ, ε, π	GBR1, GBR2	ρ
Agonists	Muscimol, THIP	Baclofen	
Antagonists	Bicuculline, picrotoxin	Phaclofen	TPMPA, picrotoxin
Desensitization	Yes	No	No
Modulator	Benzodiazepines, barbiturates		Zinc

the C-terminal side (Fig. 6.2). The roles of these extra parts on decarboxylation reactions have not been uncovered; however, some have speculated on the effects of physiological function and/or cellular localization. Further studies are needed on substrate-recognition mechanisms of these three decarboxylases. Those residues with amino acid similarity being highly heterologous should be candidates for substrate

```
                   10         20         30         40         50         60         70         80
Rat GAD67    1 MASSTPSPAT SSNAGADPNT TNLRPTTYDT WCGVAHGCTR KLGLKICGFL QRTNSLEEKS RLVSAFRERQ ASKNLLSCEN   80
Rat GAD65    1 MAS--PGSGF WSFGSEDGSG DPENPGTARA WCQVAQKFTG GIGNKLCALL YGDS--EKPA ESGGSVTSRA ATR-KVACTC   75
Human HDC    0 ---------- ---------- ---------- ---------- ---------- ---------- ---------- ----------    0
Rat ADC      0 ---------- ---------- ---------- ---------- ---------- ---------- ---------- ----------    0
                   90        100        110        120        130        140        150        160
Rat GAD67   81 SDPGARFRRT ETDFSNLFAQ DLLPAKNGEE QTVQFLLEVV DILLNYVRKT FDRSTKVLDF HHPHQLLEGM EGFNLELSDH  160
Rat GAD65   76 DQKPCSCPKG DVNYALLHAT DLLPACEGER PTLAFLQDVM NILLQYVVKS FDRSTKVIDF HYPNELLQ-- -EYNWELADQ  152
Human HDC    1 ---------- --------MM EPEEYRERGR EMVDYICQYL STVRE----- -RRVTPDVGP GYLRACLP-- ----ESAPED   50
Rat ADC      1 ---------- --------M DSREFRRRGK EMVDYIADYL DGIEG----- -RPVYPDVEP GYLRALIP-- ----TTAPQE   49
                  170        180        190        200        210        220        230        240
Rat GAD67  161 PESLEQILVD CRDTLKYGVR TGH-PRFFNQ LSTGLDIIGL AGEWLTSTAN TNMFTYEIAP VFVLMEQITL KKMREIIGWS  240
Rat GAD65  153 PONLEEILTH COTTLKYAIK TGH-PRYFNQ LSTGLDMVGL AADWLTSTAN TNMFTYEIAP VFVLLEYVTL KKMREIIGVP  231
Human HDC   51 PDSWDSIFGD IERIIMPGVV HWQSPHMHAY YPALTSWPSL LGDMLADAIN CLGFTWASSP ACTELEMNVM DWLAKMLGLP  130
Rat ADC     50 PETYEDIIRD IEKIIMPGVT HWHSPYFFAY FPTASSYPAM LADMLCGAIG CIGFSWAASP ACTELETVMM DWLGKMLELP  129
                  250        260        270        280        290        300        310        320
Rat GAD67  240 N-------K DGDGIFSPGG AISNMYSIMA ARYKYFPEVK TKG-----MA AVPKLVLFTS EHSHYSIKKA GAALGFGTDN  306
Rat GAD65  232 G-------G SGDGIFSPGG AISNMYAMLI ARYKMFPEVK EKG-----MA AVPRLIAFTS EHSHFSLKKG AAALGIGTDS  298
Human HDC  131 EHFLHHHPSS QGGGVLQSTV SESTLIALLA ARKNKILEMK TSEPDADESC LNARLVAYAS DQAHSSVEKA G---LISLVK  207
Rat ADC    130 EAFLAGR-AG EGGGVIQGSA SEATLVALLA ARTKMIRQLQ AASPELTQAA LMEKLVAYTS DQAHSSVERA G---LIGGVK  205
                  330        340        350        360        370        380        390        400
Rat GAD67  307 VILIKCNERG KIIPADLEAK ILDAKQKGFV PLYVNATAGT TVYGAFDPIQ EIADICEKYN LWLHVDAAWG GGLLMSRKHR  386
Rat GAD65  299 VILIKCDERG KMIPSDLERR ILEVKQKGFV PFLVSATAGT TVYGAFDPLL AVADICKKYK IWMHVDAAWG GGLLMSRKHK  378
Human HDC  208 MKFLPVDDNF CLRGEALQKA ICEDKQRCLV PVFVCATLCT TCVCAFDCLS ELCPICAREG LWLHIDAAYA GTAFLCPEFR  287
Rat ADC    206 IKATPSDGNY SMRAAALREA LERDKAAGLI PFFVVVTLGT TSCCSFDNLL EVGPICNQEG VWLHIDAAYA GSAFICPEFR  285
                  410        420        430        440        450        460        470        480
Rat GAD67  387 HKLSGIERAN SVTWNPHKMM GVLLQCSAIL VKEKGILQGC NQMCAGYLFQ PDKQYDVSYD TGDKAIQCGR HVDIFKFWLM  466
Rat GAD65  379 WKLNGVERAN SVTWNPHKMM GVPLQCSALL VREEGLMQSC NQMHASYLFQ QDKHYDLSYD TGDKALQCGR HVDVFKLWLM  458
Human HDC  288 GFLKGIEYAD SFTFNPSKWM MVHFDCTGFW VKDKYKLQGT FSVNPIYLRH AN--SGVATD FMHWQIPLSR RFRSVKLWFV  365
Rat ADC    286 YLLNGVEFAD SFNFNPHKWL LVNFDCSAMW VKKRTDLTEA FNMDPVYLRH SHODSGLITD YRHWQIPLGR RFRSLKMWFV  365
                  490        500        510        520        530        540        550        560
Rat GAD67  467 WKAKGTVGFE NQINKCLELA EYLYAKIKNR EEFEMVFNGE PEHTNVCFWY IPQSLRGVPD SPERREKLHR VAPKIKALMM  546
Rat GAD65  459 WRAKGTTGFE AHIDKCLELA EYLYNIIKNR EGYEMVFDGK POHTNVCFWF VPPSLRVLED NEERMSRLSK VAPVIKARMM  538
Human HDC  366 IRSFGVKNLQ AHVRHGTEMA KYFESLVRND PSFEIPAKRH LGLVVFRLKG PNCLTENVLK EIAKAGRLFL IPATIQDKLI  445
Rat ADC    366 FRMYGVKGLQ AVIRKHVKLS HEFESLVRQD PRFEICTEVI LGLVCFRLKG SNQLNETLLQ RINSAKKIHL VPCRLRDKFV  445
                  570        580        590        600        610        620        630        640
Rat GAD67  547 ESGTTIMVGYQ PQGDKANFFR MVISNPAATQ SDIDFLIEEI ERLGQDL--- ---------- ---------- ----------  593
Rat GAD65  539 EYGTTMVSYQ PLGDKVNFFR MVISNPAATH QDIDFLIEEI ERLGQDL--- ---------- ---------- ----------  585
Human HDC  446 IR-FTVTSQF TTRDDILRDW NLIRDAATLI LSQHCTSOPS PRVGNLISQI RGARAWACGT SLQSVSGAGD DPVQARKIIK  524
Rat ADC    446 LR-FAVCSRT VESAHVQLAW EHIRDLASSV LRAEKE---- ---------- ---------- ---------- ----------  480
                  650        660        670        680        690        700        710        720
Rat GAD67  593 ---------- ---------- ---------- ---------- ---------- ---------- ---------- ----------  593
Rat GAD65  585 ---------- ---------- ---------- ---------- ---------- ---------- ---------- ----------  585
Human HDC  525 QPQRVGAGPM KRENGLHLET LLDPVDDCFS EEAPDATKHK LSSFLFSYLS VQTKKKTVRS LSCNSVPVSA QKPLPTEASV  604
Rat ADC    480 ---------- ---------- ---------- ---------- ---------- ---------- ---------- ----------  480
                  730        740        750        760        770        780        790        800
Rat GAD67  593 ---------- ---------- ---------- ---------- ---------- ---------- ..........  ..........  593
Rat GAD65  585 ---------- ---------- ---------- ---------- ---------- ---------- ..........  ..........  585
Human HDC  605 KNGGSSRVRI FSRFPEDMMM LKKSAFKKLI KFYSVPSFPE CSSQCGLQLP CCPLQAMV.. ..........  662
Rat ADC    480 ---------- ---------- ---------- ---------- ---------- ---------- ..........  ..........  480
```

Fig. 6.2. Amino acid sequence alignment of amino acid decarboxylases. Amino acid sequences of rat GAD 67, rat GAD 65, human HDC, and rat ADC were compared by using the homology program (DNASIS®, Hitachi). Protein weight matrix of Gonnet 250 was employed with gap open penalty of 10, and gap extension penalty of 0.1. Amino acid sequences were obtained from public database (Swiss-Prot).

recognition sites for the distal carboxyl group, the aromatic group, and the imidazole group for GAD, AroDC, and HDC, respectively. The answer to this may emerge from the completion of X-ray crystal structure studies.

6.3.5 Distribution and characterization of GAD

GAD is distributed widely, from microbes to mammals (Miyashita and Good, 2008; Ueno, 2000). In higher mammals, GAD is found in the brain, particularly in Purkinje cells in the cerebellum, neuronal cells (Saito *et al.*, 1974; Ogoshi and Weiss, 2003; Sueiro *et al.*, 2004; Castaneda *et al.*, 2005), pancreas (Faulkner-Jones *et al.*, 1993), liver (Wu *et al.*, 1978), kidney (Tursky and Bandzuchova, 1999), and sexual organs, including testis and ovary (Medina-Kauwe *et al.*, 1994).

While attempting to clone a gene for GAD, it was found that there are two separate genes for GAD (Erlander *et al.*, 1991; Erlander and Tobin, 1991; Kaufman *et al.*, 1991; Bu *et al.*, 1992; Soghomonian and Martin, 1998). Due to the difference in the expected molecular mass for the protein products, now called isoforms, those gene products were named GAD 65 and GAD 67. Localization of each isoform was extensively studied and it was found that GAD 65 is localized at the nerve ending, particularly at the vesicular membrane region, whereas GAD 67 is localized in the cytosolic space. Knockout studies showed that mice in which individual genes were depleted showed different morphological behaviour (Asada *et al.*, 1996, 1997). Results suggested each isoform has separate biological functions. GAD 67 knockout induced developmental defects in newborn mice, resulting in immediate death after birth, whereas GAD 65 knockout caused development of seizures but allowed survival (Asada *et al.*, 1996, 1997; Choi *et al.*, 2002). Distribution of GAD isoforms in mammalian tissues and organs has not been totally clear. The GAD/GFP transgenic (knock-in) mouse might be a useful tool for the purpose (Tamamaki *et al.*, 2003; Obata, 2004). The GAD 67/GFP knock-in mouse was used successfully to show that GAD 67 is expressed in the stomach, jejunum, and type III taste buds (Akamatsu *et al.*, 2007; Nakamura *et al.*, 2007). The specific expression of GAD in the non-neuronal system is of great interest and could be a target for future research.

Figure 6.3 shows amino acid homology between two isoforms from the same animal species; also shown is homology among various species. There is about 60% sequence homology between the isoforms from the same species; however, homology reduces to 30% if only N-terminal 100 amino acid sequences are compared. Sequence homology between the isoforms from the same species is lower than that of one of the isoforms from difference species; for example, GAD 65 from human versus GAD 65 from rat, or GAD 67 from human versus GAD 67 from rat.

Different properties for GAD isoforms were reported. PLP affinity appeared to be different: GAD 67 has high affinity to PLP, or in other words, both subunits of GAD 67 bind to PLP with the same affinity. GAD 65 may be asymmetrically constructed; one subunit is bound to PLP but another subunit has no PLP, and this is known as the half-apo form. Therefore, the specific activity of GAD 67 is obviously higher than that of GAD 65. The reason why one subunit of GAD 65 has low affinity for PLP is still unclear.

GAD 65 was reported to be a target antigen for autoantibody found in patients of type 1 diabetes (Baekkeskov *et al.*, 1987, 1990, 2000). Similar autoantibody was found in patients of Stiff-person syndrome (Bjork *et al.*, 1994; Daw *et al.*, 1996). A part of GAD 65 protein, showing sequence homology with a virus coat protein commonly found in type 1 diabetes patients, may be the target site that activates B-cells for antibody production (Von Boehmer and Sarukhan, 1999; Yoon *et al.*, 1999). In an extension of this finding, GAD 65 protein has become a target protein for developing an early diagnostic tool of type 1 diabetes, since autoantibody against 63-64 kDa protein circulates as early as 15–18 years prior to onset of the diabetic symptoms. For this reason, extensive attempts have been made for large-scale preparation of GAD 65 protein, stability tests on GAD 65, immunogenicity examination of GAD 65, and other studies to develop a suitable ELISA system (Daw et al., 1996; Law et al., 1998; Papakonstantinou et al., 2000; Kono et al., 2001).

Besides PLP binding, post-translational modification has been observed with GAD. Palmitoylation of cysteine residue(s) at the N-terminal region of GAD 65 (Christgau et al., 1992; Shi et al., 1994; Solimena et al., 1994; Dirkx et al., 1995; Wei and Wu, 2008), and phosphorylation were reported (Bao et al., 1994, 1995; Namchuk et al., 1997; Hsu et al., 1999; Wei et al., 2004; Wei and Wu, 2008).

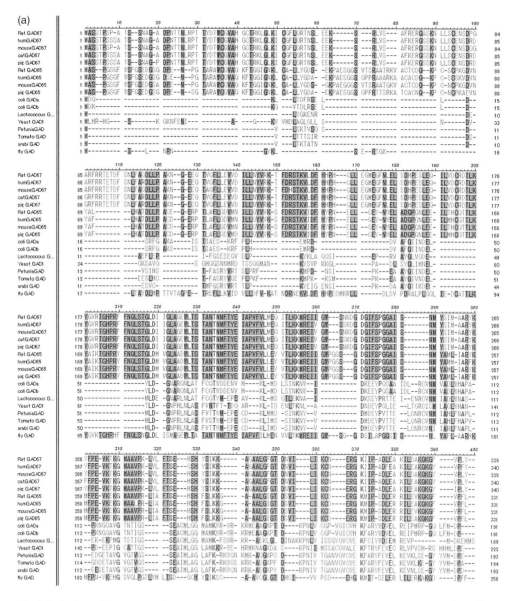

Fig. 6.3. Amino acid sequence alignment of GAD from different species. GAD protein sequences from the following species were compared for the amino acid homology: rat GAD 67, human GAD 67, mouse GAD 67, feline GAD 67, pig GAD 67, rat GAD 65, human GAD 65, mouse GAD 65, pig GAD 65, *Escherichia coli* GAD$_A$, *E. coli* GAD$_B$, *Lactococcus* GAD, baker's yeast GAD1, petunia GAD, tomato GAD, *Arabidopsis* GAD, and fruit fly GAD. Computational condition was as described in Fig. 6.2.

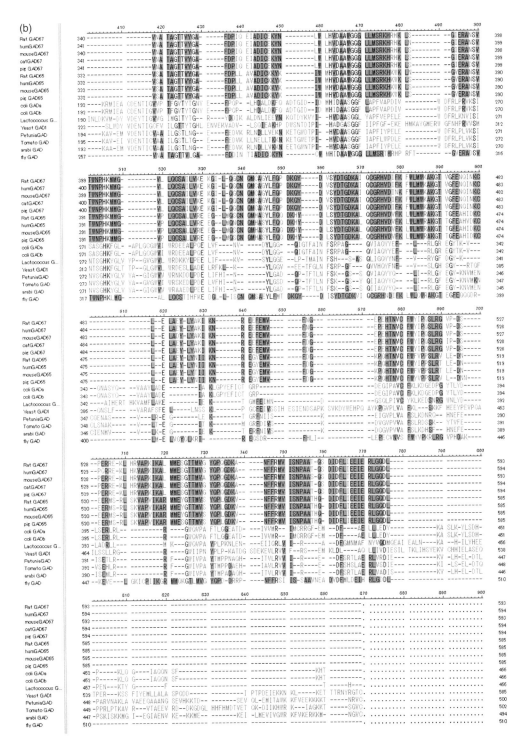

Fig. 6.3. Continued.

The significance of palmitoylation is not clear but it is postulated to show increased membrane affinity of GAD 65. Phosphorylation and dephosphorylation on GAD were reported. It is quite rare that both palmitoylation and phosphorylation are observed on PLP-dependent enzymes.

A typical GAD protein from mammalian sources comprises a dimer, each subunit has one PLP (Denner et al., 1987). Studies on the mechanism of action of GAD, as well as biochemical characterization were extensively carried out on the *Escherichia coli* enzyme; however, mammalian GAD was not fully understood, because until two separate GAD genes were identified, investigators assumed there was only one GAD gene for mammals. Ever since multiple GAD genes became evident, two separate gene products, exhibiting about 60% amino acid sequence homology, are characterized to have separate biological roles. Nevertheless, the difference or similarity between the two GAD protein properties is not fully characterized. Hence it is prudent to be cautious about references to enzymatic studies on GAD that were conducted prior to the discovery of two independent genes.

6.3.6 Purification of GAD protein

Rat (Wu et al., 1985) and mouse sources (Wu et al., 1973) have been used for GAD protein purification. Other attempts to purify brain GAD have been made on rabbit (Brandon, 1986), pig (Nathan et al., 1994), monkey (Inoue et al., 2008) and human tissues (Davis et al., 2000), for example. Soon after the identification of the GAD genes, attempts were made to clone and express GAD isoforms in *E. coli* (Kaufman et al., 1986; Chu and Metzler, 1994), yeast (Kanai et al., 1996), and other host cells (Mauch et al., 1993). More recently, the use of tag, i.e. His-tag and GST, attached at either end of the proteins expressed, has made the purification step easier. By using recombinant GAD proteins, X-ray crystal structures of both isoforms of GAD have been determined, although N-terminal 100 amino acid residues were missing from both preparations (Fenalti et al., 2007). N-terminal region of GAD exhibits low sequence homology and is highly susceptible to proteolysis (Chu and Metzler, 1994). It is desirable to construct the *in vitro* expression system for GAD proteins with full length.

6.3.7 Gene structure of GAD

Human GAD 67 gene is located on chromosome 2 constructed with 16 exons (Erlander et al., 1991; Karlsen et al., 1991; Bu and Tobin, 1994). It encodes a 594 amino acid residue protein with PLP attached at K405. Two truncated isoforms of GAD 67 have been reported: one has not been fully characterized and the other, known as GAD 25, has no enzymatic activity (Chessler and Lernmark, 2000). Rat, mouse, and chicken GAD 67 genomes contain 17 exons, where the 5' untranslated region of GAD 67 mRNA is found within an additional exon, exon 0, together with a part of exon 1. The exon 16 of GAD 67 covers the entire 3' untranslated region of GAD 67 mRNA. Human GAD 65 gene is located on chromosome 10, also constructed with 16 exons. It encodes a 585 amino acid residue protein with PLP attached at K396. Like GAD 67 genomes, gene structure of GAD 65 exhibits high resemblance among animals. Particularly interesting are the locations of exon/intron boundaries, nearly identical for all mammalian GAD genomes.

6.4 GAD 65 in Blood Leucocytes

GAD 65 was found as a target antigenic protein of autoantibody produced by type 1 diabetic patients (Baekkeskov et al., 1990; Richter et al., 1992; Kaufman and Tobin, 1993). It is noteworthy that the autoantibody appears many years before onset of the diabetic symptoms (Atkinson et al., 1994; Hou et al., 1994; Richter et al., 1994; Schloot et al., 1997; Tong et al., 2002; Kawashima et al., 2004). It is thought that a part of GAD 65 amino acid sequence is homologous with a part of the coat protein of Coxsackie virus, a virus suspected for its infection in type 1 diabetes (Fairweather and Rose, 2002). Since GAD 65 is suspected of causing diabetes by inducing antibody production, we have investigated its expression profile in peripheral blood leucocytes (Matsukawa and Ueno, 2007).

Human blood cells were collected and divided into polynuclear and mononuclear leucocyte fractions. After cellular proteins were solubilized, SDS-PAGE was performed and GAD protein was visualized by Western blot analysis. We used two antibodies specific to C-terminal region of GAD 65: one, G4913, is specific to GAD 65 and the other, G5163, recognizes a common sequence in GAD 65 and 67.

G5163 antibody was raised against peptide having a sequence of KDIDFLIEEIERLGQDL that corresponds to residues 570–585 locating at the end of C-terminal region of human GAD 65, and also to residues 579–594 of GAD 67. Those two sequences of GAD 65 and 67 are highly conserved among mammalian species; thus, G5163 should bind to both mammalian GAD 65 and GAD 67. When Western blot analysis was carried out on the leucocyte fractions, no bands appeared, although the control brain sample exhibited two bands at 67 and 65 kDa (Fig. 6.4). The results suggested that both mono- and polynuclear leucocytes may not express GAD proteins.

G4913 antibody was raised against KRTLEDNEERMSRLSKVA that corresponds to residues 514–530 of GAD 65, slightly away from the C-terminal. This sequence is common between human and rat; thus, rat brain homogenate was used as a control. Western blot analysis with G4913 showed positive bands at 80 and 30 kDa for mononuclear leucocyte but only 30 kDa for polynuclear leucocyte extracts, whereas the rat brain extract gave bands at 65 and 30 kDa (Fig. 6.4). Results were unexpected; although there was no 65 kDa band for both mono- and polynuclear leucocytes, an 80 kDa band that is larger than expected GAD 65 was observed, and polynuclear leucocyte extract

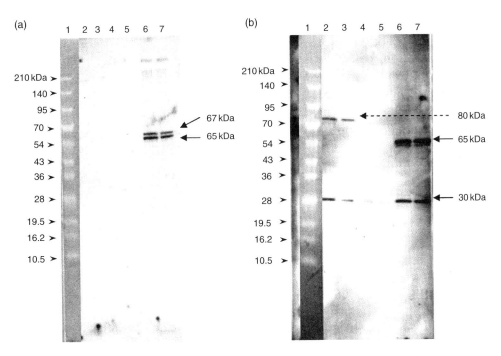

Fig. 6.4. Detection of anti-GAD antibody reactive protein by Western blotting. Lysate from human mononuclear leucocytes or rat brain were separated on polyacrylamide gel, then blotted to PVDF membrane and probed by G5163 anti-GAD 65/67 antibody (a) or G4913 anti-GAD 65 antibody (b). Lane 1, molecular ladder marker; lanes 2–3, mononuclear leucocyte fraction; lanes 4–5, polynuclear leucocyte fraction; lanes 6–7, rat brain extract.

showed a band at 30 kDa. The results suggest, first, that both mono- and polynuclear leucocytes do not express a functional 65 kDa protein; and second, that the 80 kDa band may be the result of multi-splicing specific to mononuclear leucocyte or a fault positive. The small 30 kDa band may be a GAD isoform reported earlier that could be a result of early termination in the biosynthesis of GAD 65.

In addition to Western blot analysis, further study was carried out by using RT-PCR, targeting the antibody recognition region for G5163 and G4913. mRNA isolated from mononuclear leucocytes was converted to cDNA and used as a template for RT-PCR. Two sets of primer pair were designed: primer set 1 was designed to produce a 154 bp fragment that covers G4913 epitope and extends toward 3' (C-terminal region) just prior to the G5163 epitope. Primer set 2 was designed to produce a 58 bp fragment that includes the G4913 epitope. As a positive control, a primer set for GAPDH was employed. When PCR products were analysed by the Agilent Bioanalyzer, a positive band was observed for the cDNA obtained from mononuclear leucocytes with the primer 2 set only (Fig. 6.5). Both GAPDH and brain samples showed positive bands. The results support the Western blot analysis that GAD 65 is expressed in mononuclear leucocytes, but the C terminal region may be missing or truncated. In order to confirm the finding, PCR was carried out by using primer set 2 as primers and mononuclear leucocyte cDNA as a template (Fig. 6.5). After the PCR product was integrated into pGEM®-Teasy, the inserted region was confirmed after DNA sequencing as a valid sequence (data not shown).

The location of G4913 epitopes on the gene sequence of GAD 65 was further examined. The exon/intron interface at the end of exon 15 happens to be correlated with the end of epitope for G4913 (Fig. 6.6). This result

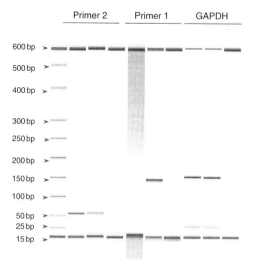

Fig. 6.5. Electrophoresis of PCR products. PCR products were separated on the Agilent Bioanalyzer. Lanes should read from left to right as lane 1 to 10. Lane 1 is a molecular ladder marker. Lanes 2, 5, and 8 are products when cDNA from mononuclear leucocytes is being used as a template. Lanes 3, 6 and 9 are products when cDNA from rat brain is being used as a template. Lanes 4, 7 and 10 are control when no template is added. Primers 1 and 2 are described in Figure 6.6.

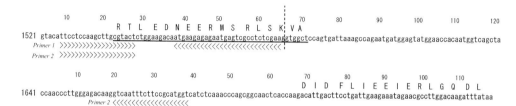

Fig. 6.6. Correlation between PCR primers and epitopes for G5163 and G4913 antibodies. cDNA sequence at the C-terminal of human GAD 65 is shown with PCR primers and epitopes. The epitope for G4913 or G5163 with amino acid above is shown with underline or highlight, respectively. Left primer (>) and right primer (<) are represented for primer set 1 (upper) and set 2 (lower), respectively. The border of exon 15 and 16 is shown by a dotted line.

supports the idea that exon 16 may be omitted during the RNA splicing process. There are two bands with 80 and 30 kDa for mononuclear leucocyte extracts on SDS-PAGE and Western blot analysis. At the present time, there is no evidence whether or not the mRNA isolated corresponds to particular protein bands. Also unknown is the size problem for 80 kDa species: deletion would produce a smaller size protein than the native one, but 80 kDa is larger. There are two possibilities: either some duplication of exons might occur during the splicing process, or post-translational modification might occur. Both possibilities should be considered in the future.

6.5 Taste Signalling

GAD protein has long been known for its localization in few specific organs, including brain, nerves, pancreas and testes. Recently, other localization sites for GAD have been demonstrated in various tissues related to the digestion of food: the stomach, intestine (Fig. 6.7), salivary gland, skin and taste buds (Kuno *et al.*, 2001; Iwahori *et al.*, 2002; Watanabe *et al.*, 2002; Wang *et al.*, 2006; Akamatsu *et al.*, 2007; Ito *et al.*, 2007; Nakamura *et al.*, 2007). Localization is specific, and conventional methods of solubilizing the tissues and by detecting the activity or Western blot analysis might not be sensitive enough to detect the minute amounts of GAD proteins expressed. Recent advancements in RT-PCR and transgenic mouse studies have made the following findings possible.

Mammals have taste buds on their tongue to sense five distinct tastes: sweet, bitter, umami, salt, and sour, where umami is recognized most recently as sodium monoglutamate (MSG) isolated from kelp in 1908 by Kikunae Ikeda (Ajinomoto, 2009; Kurihara, 2009). Taste buds are mainly distributed in papillae, and these are classified into four groups: circumvallate, fungiform, foliate, and filiform. The latter lack taste buds (Fig. 6.8). The first three types of papillae contain about 100 or more taste buds. Taste buds are divided into four types, I–IV, where type I is the connecting cell, type II serves to express taste receptors, type III is for linkage to the nerve, and type IV is the stem cell (Fig. 6.9). There are dedicated receptor proteins for each of the five tastes. For example, sweet materials are considered to bind to sweet-specific receptors, sour materials to sour-specific receptors, and so on to convey the respective taste signals to the brain. It is of interest to understand whether or not each of the type II taste buds express all three receptor types for sweet, bitter, and umami; and whether or not each of the type III taste buds expresses both receptor types for salt and sour tastes. In addition,

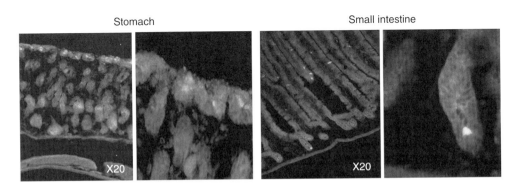

Fig. 6.7. Immunohistochemistry for GAD 65 on mouse stomach and small intestine. GAD 65 immunostaining is shown as a white spot, where propidium iodide staining is used to identify the location of cells. Photos cover a general region to illustrate the principal cells in the stomach, the surface of its mucosa and endocrine cells and crypts in the small intestine.

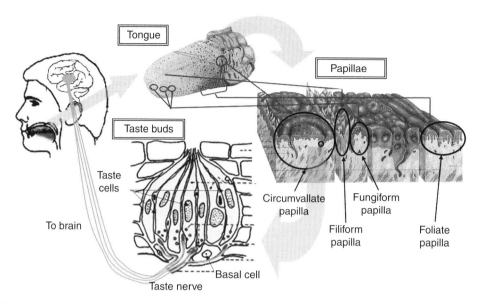

Fig. 6.8. Image of how taste signals are transmitted from tongue to brain.

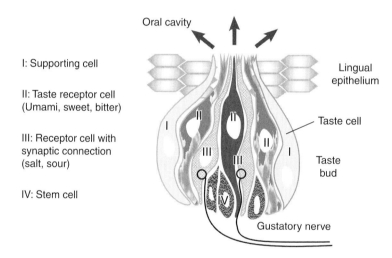

Fig. 6.9. Schematic diagram of circumvallate papilla with four types of taste bud cells.

the nerve from the brain ends up at the tongue, where the nerve connects only with type III taste buds: thus, a question has been raised as to how the signal from type II travels to the nerve.

Expression of GAD protein was examined on the mouse tongue. Thin sections of mouse tongue were subjected to immunohistochemical study with antibodies specific to GAD, as explained in the previous section. There was positive staining at the area where papillae are located (data not shown). More precise evidence was obtained when GAD 67/GFP transgenic mouse was used: under fluorescent light, there was a single spot having green fluorescence on the tongue where the circumvallate papilla locates (Fig. 6.10). Thin sections with the fluorescent spot showed GAD 67 and GABA positive for antibody reactions, and positive

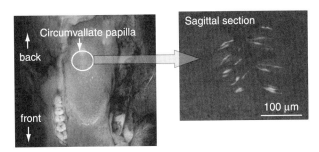

Fig. 6.10. Photos of GAD 67/GFP knock-in mouse tongue and thin section of circumvallate papilla.

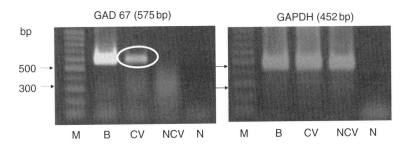

M, marker (100 bp ladder); B, brain; CV, circumvallate papilla; NCV, near circumvallate papilla; N, negative control (water)

Fig. 6.11. Electrophoresis of RT-PCR products. PCR products were separated on agarose gel electrophoresis. For GAD 67, primer specific to GAD 67 was chosen to produce 575 bp product. GAPDH producing 452 bp product was used as a control.

results for RT-PCR probing for GAD 67. The finding supports the notion that GAD 67 is expressed in mouse taste buds, particularly at circumvallate papilla. RT-PCR studies on the sample taken from the fluorescent spot supports the immunohistochemical results (Fig. 6.11). In the next step, taste cell type that may express GAD 67 was determined. Antibodies specific to cell markers for type II and type III were used. The number of cells reacting with antibodies and those having fluorescence were counted. Results suggested that PGP9.5 and serotonin-positive cell populations overlap the most: it indicates that type III cells express GAD 67 protein (Fig. 6.12) (Nakamura *et al.*, 2005; Nakamura *et al.*, 2007). The results suggest a scheme (Fig. 6.13) as to how the salt (or acid) signal is transmitted via GABA in type III cells.

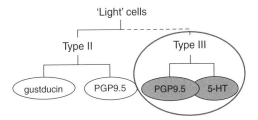

Fig. 6.12. Schematic view of taste bud cell type determination. GFP positive cells were subjected for immunostaining with the use of antibodies specific to cell markers. GFP positive cells were stained with 5-HT and PGP9.5 specific antibodies; thus, they are type III cells.

6.6 Suggestions for Future Research

Studies on the chemistry of glutamate have been relatively subdued recently, partly because of

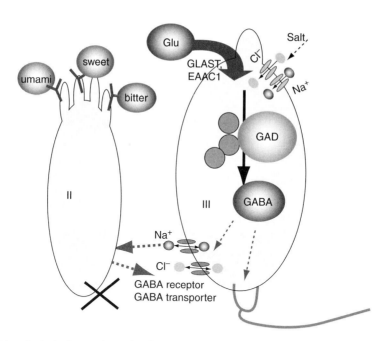

Fig. 6.13. Hypothetical scheme of signal pathway. Left cell is type II and right cell is type III. Nerve is directly connected to type III cell but not to type II cell. GAD is found in type III cell where GABA production is expected. GABA may activate the Cl⁻ ion channel that allows the transport of salt or perhaps acid; hence, GABA may act as a taste signal mediator.

the lack of high-sensitivity analytical tools for amino acids. Recent advancements in chromatography have made it possible to analyse just above femtomol amounts of amino acids within 8 min. This is the most significant breakthrough for amino acid analysis since Moore–Stein's original instrument and the Pico-tag® system developed later by Waters. Enzymological studies on GAD should benefit from this analytical technique as more precise assays should now be possible. Researchers are now more optimistic about the ability to conduct single-cell enzymology for GAD expression and characterization.

6.7 Conclusions

The glutamate-metabolizing enzyme GAD produces GABA, an amino acid credited with the role of inhibitory neurotransmitter in the CNS of higher animals. Mammals have two isoforms of GAD, with a slightly different molecular mass encoded in two independent genes. Differences in subcellular localization and characteristics probably reside in the heterogeneity of their N-terminal amino acid residues. Blood cell analyses have shown that mononuclear leucocytes exhibit a GAD-like protein apparently having a truncated C-terminal region that corresponds to exon 16. The finding implicates a possible multi-splicing phenomenon that may explain the diverse expression pattern of GAD. Recent studies also show that GAD 67 is expressed at the taste bud cells, specifically in the type III cells that contain salt and acid receptors, and also have a physical connection with taste nerve terminals. Since GABA acts as a ligand for $GABA_A$ receptor, also known as a chloride-ion channel, the possibility is strongly suggested that GABA is a mediator for taste signal transduction. In other words, if GAD activity could be altered by external factors, an altered taste signal might result that may lead, for example, to the salt-enhancement effect. The role of GAD in diabetes is another emerging field for potential exploitation in the development of novel diagnostics and therapeutics for this disease.

6.8 Acknowledgements

We appreciate the long-term collaboration with Dr Kenichi Ito of Ichimaru Pharcos Co.; with Professors Masahito Watanabe and Yoshinori Otsuki of Osaka Medical College; with Professor Kunihiko Obata of Riken; and with Professor Yuchio Yanagawa of Gunma University Graduate School of Medicine. We are also grateful for funds provided by Urakami Food and Food Culture Foundation, Nakano Research Foundation, and the Society for Research on Umami Taste.

References

Ajinomoto (2009) Proceedings of the 100th Anniversary Symposium of Umami Discovery: the roles of glutamate in taste, gastrointestinal function, metabolism, and physiology. Tokyo, Japan. September 11–13, 2008. *American Journal of Clinical Nutrition* 90, 705S–885S.

Akamatsu, K., Nakamura, Y., Hayasaki, H., Kanabara, K., Maemura, K., Yanagawa, Y., Obata, K., et al. (2007) Cells expressing GABA synthetic enzyme, glutamate decarboxylase, in stomach and intestine: RT-PCR and immunohistochemistry studies. *Journal of Biological Macromolecules* 7, 55–62.

Asada, H., Kawamura, Y., Maruyama, K., Kume, H., Ding, R.-G., Ji, F.Y., Kanbara, N., et al. (1996) Mice lacking the 65 kDa isoform of glutamic acid decarboxylase (GAD65) maintain normal levels of GAD67 and GABA in their brains but are susceptible to seizures. *Biochemical and Biophysical Research Communications* 229, 891–895.

Asada, H., Kawamura, Y., Maruyama, K., Kume, H., Ding, R.-G., Kanbara, N., Kuzume, H., et al. (1997) Cleft palate and decreased brain γ-aminobutyric acid in mice lacking the 67-kDa isoform of glutamic acid decarboxylase. *Proceedings of the National Academy of Sciences USA* 94, 6496–6499.

Atkinson, M.A., Bowman, M.A., Campbell, L., Darrow, B.L., Kaufman, D.L. and Maclaren, N.K. (1994) Cellular immunity to a determinant common to glutamate decarboxylase and coxsackie virus in insulin-dependent diabetes. *Journal of Clinical Investigation* 94, 2125–2129.

Baekkeskov, S., Landin, M., Kristensen, J.K., Srikanta, S., Bruining, G.J., Mandrup-Poulsen, T., de Beaufort, C., et al. (1987) Antibodies to a 64,000 Mr human islet cell antigen precede the clinical onset of insulin-dependent diabetes. *Journal of Clinical Investigation* 79, 926–934.

Baekkeskov, S., Aanstoot, H.J., Christgau, S., Reetz, A., Solimena, M., Cascalho, M., Folli, F., et al. (1990) Identification of the 64K autoantigen in insulin-dependent diabetes as the GABA-synthesizing enzyme glutamic acid decarboxylase. *Nature* 347, 151–156.

Baekkeskov, S., Kanaani, J., Jaume, J.C. and Kash, S. (2000) Does GAD have a unique role in triggering IDDM? *Journal of Autoimmunity* 15, 279–286.

Bao, J., Nathan, B., Hsu, C.C., Zhang, Y., Wu, R. and Wu, J.Y. (1994) Role of protein phosphorylation in regulation of brain L-glutamate decarboxylase activity. *Journal of Biomedical Sciences* 1, 237–244.

Bao, J., Cheung, W.Y. and Wu, J.-Y. (1995) Brain L-glutamate decarboxylase. Inhibition by phosphorylation and activation by dephosphorylation. *Journal of Biological Chemistry* 270, 6464–6467.

Bjork, E., Velloso, L.A., Kampe, O. and Karlsson, F.A. (1994) GAD autoantibodies in IDDM, stiff-man syndrome, and autoimmune polyendocrine syndrome type I recognize different epitopes. *Diabetes* 43, 161–165.

Bouche, N., Fait, A., Bouchez, D., Moller, S.G. and Fromm, H. (2003) Mitochondrial succinic-semialdehyde dehydrogenase of the gamma-aminobutyrate shunt is required to restrict levels of reactive oxygen intermediates in plants. *Proceedings of the National Academy of Sciences USA* 100, 6843–6848.

Brandon, C. (1986) Purification of L-glutamate decarboxylase from rabbit brain and preparation of a monospecific antiserum. *Journal of Neuroscience Research* 15, 367–381.

Bu, D.F., Erlander, M.G., Hintz, B.C., Tillakaratne, N.J.K., Kaufman, D.L., Wagner-McPherson, C.B., Evans, G.A. et al. (1992) Two human glutamate decarboxylases, 65-kDa GAD and 67-kDa GAD, are each encoded by a single gene. *Proceedings of the National Academy of Sciences USA* 89, 2115–2119.

Bu, D.F. and Tobin, A.J. (1994) The exon-intron organization of the genes (GAD1 and GAD2) encoding two human glutamate decarboxylases (GAD67 and GAD65) suggests that they derive from a common ancestral GAD. *Genomics* 21, 222–228.

Castaneda, M.T., Sanabria, E.R., Hernandez, S., Ayala, A., Reyna, T.A., Wu, J.Y. and Colom, L.V. (2005) Glutamic acid decarboxylase isoforms are differentially distributed in the septal region of the rat. *Neuroscience Research* 52, 107–119.

Chessler, S.D. and Lernmark, A. (2000) Alternative splicing of GAD67 results in the synthesis of a third form of glutamic-acid decarboxylase in human islets and other non-neural tissues. *Journal of Biological Chemistry* 275, 5188–5192.

Choi, S.Y. and Churchich, J.E. (1986) Glutamate decarboxylase side reactions catalyzed by the enzyme. *European Journal of Biochemistry* 160, 515–520.

Choi, S.Y., Morales, B., Lee, H.K. and Kirkwood, A. (2002) Absence of long-term depression in the visual cortex of glutamic acid decarboxylase-65 knock-out mice. *Journal of Neuroscience* 22, 5271–5276.

Christgau, S., Aanstoot, H.-J., Schierbeck, H., Begley, K., Tullin, S., Hejnaes, K. and Baekkeskov, S. (1992) Membrane anchoring of the autoantigen GAD65 to microvesicles in pancreatic β-cells by palmitoylation in the NH_2-terminal domain. *Journal of Cell Biology* 118, 309–320.

Chu, W.C. and Metzler, D.E. (1994) Enzymatically active truncated cat brain glutamate decarboxylase: expression, purification, and absorption spectrum. *Archives of Biochemistry and Biophysics* 313, 287–295.

Daniels, J.D. and Pettigrew, J.D. (1975) A study of inhibitory antagonism in cat visual cortex. *Brain Research* 93, 41–62.

Davis, K.M., Foos, T., Bates, C.S., Tucker, E., Hsu, C.C., Chen, W., Jin, H., *et al.* (2000) A novel method for expression and large-scale production of human brain L-glutamate decarboxylase. *Biochemical and Biophysical Research Communications* 267, 777–782.

Daw, K., Ujihara, N., Atkinson, M. and Powers, A.C. (1996) Glutamic acid decarboxylase autoantibodies in stiff-man syndrome and insulin-dependent diabetes mellitus exhibit similarities and differences in epitope recognition. *Journal of Immunology* 156, 818–825.

Delgado, J.M., DeFeudis, F.V. and Bellido, I. (1971) Injections of GABA and glutamate into the amygdalae of awake monkeys. *Communications in Behavioral Biology* 5, 347–357.

Denner, L.A., Wei, S.C., Lin, H.S., Lin, C.T. and Wu, J.Y. (1987) Brain L-glutamate decarboxylase: purification and subunit structure. *Proceedings of National Academy of Sciences USA* 84, 668–672.

Dirkx, R., Jr, Thomas, A., Li, L., Lernmark, A., Sherwin, R.S., De Camilli, P. and Solimena, M. (1995) Targeting of the 67-kDa isoform of glutamic acid decarboxylase to intracellular organelles is mediated by its interaction with the NH_2-terminal region of the 65-kDa isoform of glutamic acid decarboxylase. *Journal of Biological Chemistry* 270, 2241–2246.

Dumoulin, A., Rostaing, P., Bedet, C., Levi, S., Isambert, M.F., Henry, J.P., Triller, A. *et al.* (1999) Presence of the vesicular inhibitory amino acid transporter in GABAergic and glycinergic synaptic terminal boutons. *Journal of Cell Sciences* 112, 811–823.

Erecinska, M., Nelson, D., Daikhin, Y. and Yudkoff, M. (1996) Regulation of GABA level in rat brain synaptosomes: fluxes through enzymes of the GABA shunt and effects of glutamate, calcium, and ketone bodies. *Journal of Neurochemistry* 67, 2325–2334.

Erlander, M.G., Tillakaratne, N.J., Feldblum, S., Patel, N. and Tobin, A.J. (1991) Two genes encode distinct glutamate decarboxylases. *Neuron* 7, 91–100.

Erlander, M.G. and Tobin, A.J. (1991) The structural and functional heterogeneity of glutamic acid decarboxylase: A review. *Neurochemical Research* 16, 215–226.

Fairweather, D. and Rose, N.R. (2002) Type 1 diabetes: virus infection or autoimmune disease? *Nature Immunology* 3, 338–340.

Faulkner-Jones, B.E., Cram, D.S., Kun, J. and Harrison, L.C. (1993) Localization and quantitation of expression of two glutamate decarboxylase genes in pancreatic beta-cells and other peripheral tissues of mouse and rat. *Endocrinology* 133, 2962–2972.

Fenalti, G., Law, R.H., Buckle, A.M., Langendorf, C., Tuck, K., Rosado, C.J., Faux, N.G., *et al.* (2007) GABA production by glutamic acid decarboxylase is regulated by a dynamic catalytic loop. *Nature Structural and Molecular Biology* 14, 280–286.

Fukushima, K. and Toyoshima, S. (1975) Antitumor activity of amino acid derivatives in the primary screening. *Gann* 66, 29–36.

Guimbal, C., Klostermann, A. and Kilimann, M.W. (1995) Phylogenetic conservation of 4-aminobutyric acid (GABA) transporter isoforms. Cloning and pharmacological characterization of a GABA/beta-alanine transporter from Torpedo. *European Journal of Biochemistry* 234, 794–800.

Henry, J.L. (1979) Naloxone excites nociceptive units in the lumbar dorsal horn of the spinal cat. *Neuroscience* 4, 1485–1491.

Hou, J., Said, C., Franchi, D., Dockstader, P. and Chatterjee, N.K. (1994) Antibodies to glutamic acid decarboxylase and P2-C peptides in sera from coxsackie virus B4-infected mice and IDDM patients. *Diabetes* 43, 1260–1266.

Hsu, C.-C., Thomas, C., Chen, W., Davis, K.M., Foos, T., Chen, J.L., Wu, E., et al. (1999) Role of synaptic vesicle proton gradient and protein phosphorylation on ATP-mediated activation of membrane-associated brain glutamate decarboxylase. *Journal of Biological Chemistry* 274, 24366–24371.

Ikenaga, T., Yoshida, M. and Uematsu, K. (2005) Morphology and immunohistochemistry of efferent neurons of the goldfish corpus cerebelli. *Journal of Comparative Neurology* 487, 300–311.

Inoue, Y., Ishii, K., Miyazaki, M. and Ueno, H. (2008) Purification of L-glutamate decarboxylase from monkey brain. *Bioscience, Biotechnology and Biochemistry* 72, 2269–2276.

Ito, K., Tanaka, K., Nishibe, Y., Hasegawa, J. and Ueno, H. (2007) GABA-synthesizing enzyme, GAD67, from dermal fibroblasts: evidence for a new skin function. *Biochimica et Biophysica Acta* 1770, 291–296.

Iversen, L.L. and Snyder, S.H. (1968) Synaptosomes: different populations storing catecholamines and gamma-aminobutyric acid in homogenates of rat brain. *Nature* 220, 796–798.

Iwahori, M., Akamatsu, K., Kurohara, S., Yokoigawa, K., Ueno, H., Ogawa, H., Ozawa, H., et al. (2002) Immunohistochemical study of the localization of glutamate decarboxylase in rodent's submandibular gland. *Journal of Biological Macromolecules* 2, 76–77.

Kanai, T., Atomi, H., Umemura, K., Ueno, H., Teranishi, Y., Ueda, M. and Tanaka, A. (1996) A novel heterologous gene expression system in *Saccharomyces cerevisiae* using the isocitrate lyase promoter from *Candida tropicalis*. *Applied Microbiology and Biotechnology* 44, 759–765.

Karlsen, A.E., Hagopian, W.A., Grubin, C.E., Dube, S., Disteche, C.M., Adler, D.A., Barmeier, H., et al. (1991) Cloning and primary structure of a human islet isoform of glutamic acid decarboxylase from chromosome 10. *Proceedings of the National Academy of Sciences USA* 88, 8337–8341.

Kaufman, D.L. and Tobin, A.J. (1993) Glutamade decarboxylases and autoimmunity in insulin-dependent diabetes. *Trends in Pharmacological Sciences* 14, 107–109.

Kaufman, D.L., McGinnis, J.F., Krieger, N.R. and Tobin, A.J. (1986) Brain glutamate decarboxylase cloned in lamda.gt-11: Fusion protein produces γ-aminobutyric acid. *Science* 232, 1138–1140.

Kaufman, D.L., Houser, C.R. and Tobin, A.J. (1991) Two forms of the gamma-aminobutyric acid synthetic enzyme glutamate decarboxylase have distinct intraneuronal distributions and cofactor interactions. *Journal of Neurochemistry* 56, 720–723.

Kawashima, H., Ihara, T., Ioi, H., Oana, S., Sato, S., Kato, N., Takami, T., et al. (2004) Enterovirus-related type 1 diabetes mellitus and antibodies to glutamic acid decarboxylase in Japan. *Journal of Infection* 49, 147–151.

Kono, T., Nishimura, F., Sugimoto, H., Sikata, K., Makino, H. and Murayama, Y. (2001) Human fibroblasts ubiquitously express glutamic acid decarboxylase 65 (GAD 65): possible effects of connective tissue inflammation on GAD antibody titer. *Journal of Periodontology* 72, 598–604.

Krantis, A. and Kerr, D.I. (1981) Gaba induced excitatory responses in the guinea-pig small intestine are antagonized by bicuculline, picrotoxinin and chloride ion blockers. *Naunyn-Schmiedeberg's Archives of Pharmacology* 317, 257–261.

Kuno, M., Wang, F.-Y., Maemura, K. and Watanabe, M. (2001) Expression and characterization of γ-aminobutyrate and glutamate decarboxylase in rat jejunum: Implication for the proliferation and differentiation of epithelial cells. *Bulletin of Osaka Medical College* 47, 27–35.

Kurihara, K. (2009) Glutamate: from discovery as a food flavor to role as a basic taste (umami). *American Journal of Clinical Nutrition* 90, 719S–722S.

Law, R.H., Rowley, M.J., Mackay, I.R. and Corner, B. (1998) Expression in Saccharomyces cerevisiae of antigenically and enzymatically active recombinant glutamic acid decarboxylase. *Journal of Biotechnology* 61, 57–68.

Lin, P., Kusano, K., Zhang, Q., Felder, C.C., Geiger, P.M. and Mahan, L.C. (1996) GABAA receptors modulate early spontaneous excitatory activity in differentiating P19 neurons. *Journal of Neurochemistry* 66, 233–242.

Marczynski, T.J. (1998) GABAergic deafferentation hypothesis of brain aging and Alzheimer's disease revisited. *Brain Research Bulletin* 45, 341–379.

Martin, D.L., Martin, S.B., Wu, S.J. and Espina, N. (1991) Cofactor interactions and the regulation of glutamate decarboxylase activity. *Neurochemical Research* 16, 243–249.

Matsukawa, S. and Ueno, H. (2007) Expression of glutamate decarboxylase isoform, GAD65, in human mononuclear leucocytes: a possible implication of C-terminal end deletion by Western blot and RT-PCR study. *Journal of Biochemistry* 142, 633–638.

Mauch, L., Seiffer, J., Haubruck, H., Cook, N.J., Abney, C.C., Berthold, H., Wirbelauer, C., et al. (1993) Baculovirus-mediated expression of human 65 kDa and 67 kDa glutamic acid decarboxylases in SF9 insect cells and their relevance in diagnosis of insulin-dependent diabetes mellitus. *Journal of Biochemistry* 113, 699–704.

McGeer, P.L., Fibiger, H.C., Maler, L., Hattori, T. and McGeer, E.G. (1974) Evidence for descending pallido-nigral GABA-containing neurons. *Advanced Neurology* 5, 153–160.

Medina-Kauwe, L.K., Tillakaratne, N.J., Wu, J.Y. and Tobin, A.J. (1994) A rat brain cDNA encodes enzymatically active GABA transaminase and provides a molecular probe for GABA-catabolizing cells. *Journal of Neurochemistry* 62, 1267–1275.

Mihailobic, L.T., Krzalic, L. and Cupic, D. (1965) Changes of glutamine, glutamic acid and GABA in cortical and subcortical brain structures of hibernating and fully aroused ground squirrels (Citellus citellus). *Experientia* 21, 709–710.

Miyashita, Y. and Good, A.G. (2008) Contribution of the GABA shunt to hypoxia-induced alanine accumulation in roots of Arabidopsis thaliana. *Plant Cell Physiology* 49, 92–102.

Nakamura, Y., Akamatsu, K., Yanagawa, Y., Obata, K., Ueno, H. and Watanabe, M. (2005) GABAergic cells in the mouse taste bud. In: *International Interdisciplinary Conference on Vitamins, Coenzymes, and Biofactors 2005*, Awaji, Japan.

Nakamura, Y., Yanagawa, Y., Obata, K., Watanabe, M. and Ueno, H. (2007) GABA is produced in taste bud. *Chemical Senses* 32, J19.

Namchuk, M., Lindsay, L., Turck, C.W., Kanaani, J. and Baekkeskov, S. (1997) Phosphorylation of serine residues 3, 6, 10, and 13 distinguishes membrane anchored from soluble glutamic acid decarboxylase 65 and is restricted to glutamic acid decarboxylase 65α. *Journal of Biological Chemistry* 272, 1548–1557.

Nathan, B., Bao, J., Hsu, C.C., Aguilar, P., Wu, R., Yarom, M., Kuo, C.Y., *et al.* (1994) A membrane form of brain L-glutamate decarboxylase: identification, isolation, and its relation to insulin-dependent mellitus. *Proceedings of the National Academy of Sciences USA* 91, 242–246.

Obata, K. (1969) Gamma-aminobutyric acid in Purkinje cells and motoneurones. *Experientia* 25, 1283.

Obata, K. (2004) GABAergic neurons revealed in the gene knock-out and knock-in mice. *Protein, Nucleic Acid, and Enzyme* 49, 295–300.

Ogoshi, F. and Weiss, J.H. (2003) Heterogeneity of Ca^{2+}-permeable AMPA/kainate channel expression in hippocampal pyramidal neurons: fluorescence imaging and immunocytochemical assessment. *Journal of Neuroscience* 23, 10521–10530.

Papakonstantinou, T., Law, R.H., Gardiner, P., Rowley, M.J. and Mackay, I.R. (2000) Comparative expression and purification of human glutamic acid decarboxylase from *Saccharomyces cerevisiae* and *Pichia pastoris*. *Enzyme and Microbial Technology* 26, 645–652.

Purpura, D.P. and Carmichael, M.W. (1960) Characteristics of blood-brain barrier to gamma-aminobutyric acid in neonatal cat. *Science* 131, 410–412.

Qian, H., Hyatt, G., Schanzer, A., Hazra, R., Hackam, A.S., Cutting, G.R. and Dowling, J.E. (1997) A comparison of $GABA_C$ and rho subunit receptors from the white perch retina. *Visual Neuroscience* 14, 843–851.

Qian, H., Dowling, J.E. and Ripps, H. (1998) Molecular and pharmacological properties of GABA-rho subunits from white perch retina. *Journal of Neurobiology* 37, 305–320.

Ribak, C.E., Harris, A.B., Vaughn, J.E. and Roberts, E. (1979a) Inhibitory, GABAergic nerve terminals decrease at sites of focal epilepsy. *Science* 205, 211–214.

Ribak, C.E., Vaughn, J.E. and Roberts, E. (1979b) The GABA neurons and their axon terminals in rat corpus striatum as demonstrated by GAD immunocytochemistry. *Journal of Comparative Neurology* 187, 261–283.

Richter, W., Endl, J., Eiermann, T.H., Brandt, M., Kientsch-Engel, R., Thivolet, C., Jungfer, H. and Scherbaum, W.A. (1992) Human monoclonal islet cell antibodies from a patient with insulin-dependent diabetes mellitus reveal glutamate decarboxylase as the target antigen. *Proceedings of the National Academy of Sciences USA* 89, 8467–8471.

Richter, W., Mertens, T., Schoel, B., Muir, P., Ritzkowsky, A., Scherbaum, W.A. and Boehm, B.O. (1994) Sequence homology of the diabetes-associated autoantigen glutamate decarboxylase with coxsackie B4-2C protein and heat shock protein 60 mediates no molecular mimicry of autoantibodies. *Journal of Experimental Medicine* 180, 721–726.

Saito, K., Barber, R., Wu, J., Matsuda, T., Roberts, E. and Vaughn, J.E. (1974) Immunohistochemical localization of glutamate decarboxylase in rat cerebellum. *Proceedings of the National Academy of Sciences USA* 71, 269–273.

Schaeffer, J.M. and Hsueh, A.J. (1982) Identification of gamma-aminobutyric acid and its binding sites in the rat ovary. *Life Science* 30, 1599–1604.

Schloot, N.C., Roep, B.O., Wegmann, D.R., Yu, L., Wang, T.B. and Eisenbarth, G.S. (1997) T-cell reactivity to GAD65 peptide sequences shared with coxsackie virus protein in recent-onset IDDM, post-onset IDDM patients and control subjects. *Diabetologia* 40, 332–338.

Shi, Y., Veit, B. and Baekkeskov, S. (1994) Amino acid residues 24-31 but not palmitoylation of cysteines 30 and 45 are required for membrane anchoring of glutamic acid decarboxylase, GAD_{65}. *Journal of Cell Biology* 124, 927–934.

Siemers, E.R., Rea, M.A., Felten, D.L. and Aprison, M.H. (1982) Distribution and uptake of glycine, glutamate and gamma-aminobutyric acid in the vagal nuclei and eight other regions of the rat medulla oblongata. *Neurochemcal Research* 7, 455–468.

Smismans, A., Schuit, F. and Pipeleers, D. (1997) Nutrient regulation of gamma-aminobutyric acid release from islet beta cells. *Diabetologia* 40, 1411–1415.

Soghomonian, J.J. and Martin, D.L. (1998) Two isoforms of glutamate decarboxylase: why? *Trends in Pharmacological Sciences* 19, 500–505.

Solimena, M., Dirkx, R., Jr, Radzynski, M., Mundigl, O. and De Camilli, P. (1994) A signal located within amino acids 1-27 of GAD65 is required for its targeting to the Golgi complex region. *Journal of Cell Biology* 126, 331–341.

Storm-Mathisen, J. (1975) High affinity uptake of GABA in presumed GABA-ERGIC nerve endings in rat brain. *Brain Research* 84, 409–427.

Sueiro, C., Carrera, I., Molist, P., Rodriguez-Moldes, I. and Anadon, R. (2004) Distribution and development of glutamic acid decarboxylase immunoreactivity in the spinal cord of the dogfish Scyliorhinus canicula (elasmobranchs). *Journal of Comparative Neurology* 478, 189–206.

Tamamaki, N., Yanagawa, Y., Tomioka, R., Miyazaki, J., Obata, K. and Kaneko, T. (2003) Green fluorescent protein expression and colocalization with calretinin, parvalbumin, and somatostatin in the GAD67-GFP knock-in mouse. *Journal of Comparative Neurology* 467, 60–79.

Taniyama, K., Miki, Y. and Tanaka, C. (1982) Presence of gamma-aminobutyric acid and glutamic acid decarboxylase in Auerbach's plexus of cat colon. *Neuroscience Letters* 29, 53–56.

Thangnipon, W., Taxt, T., Brodal, P. and Storm-Mathisen, J. (1983) The corticopontine projection: axotomy-induced loss of high affinity L-glutamate and D-aspartate uptake, but not of gamma-aminobutyrate uptake, glutamate decarboxylase or choline acetyltransferase, in the pontine nuclei. *Neuroscience* 8, 449–457.

Tong, J.C., Myers, M.A., Mackay, I.R., Zimmet, P.Z. and Rowley, M.J. (2002) The PEVKEK region of the pyridoxal phosphate binding domain of GAD65 expresses a dominant B cell epitope for type 1 diabetes sera. *Annals of New York Academy of Sciences* 958, 182–189.

Tursky, T. and Bandzuchova, E. (1999) An endogenous activator of renal glutamic acid decarboxylase effects of adenosine triphosphate, phosphate and chloride on the activity of this enzyme. *European Journal of Biochemistry* 262, 696–703.

Ueno, H. (2000) Enzymatic and structural aspects on glutamate decarboxylase. *Journal of Molecular Catalysis B: Enzymatic* 10, 67–79.

von Boehmer, H. and Sarukhan, A. (1999) GAD, a single autoantigen for diabetes. *Science* 284, 1135–1136.

Wang, F.Y., Zhu, R.M., Maemura, K., Hirata, I., Katsu, K. and Watanabe, M. (2006) Expression of gamma-aminobutyric acid and glutamic acid decarboxylases in rat descending colon and their relation to epithelial differentiation. *Chinese Journal of Digestive Disease* 7, 103–108.

Watanabe, M., Maemura, K., Kanbara, K., Tamayama, T. and Hayasaki, H. (2002) GABA and GABA receptors in the central nervous system and other organs. *International Review of Cytology* 213, 1–47.

Wei, J. and Wu, J.Y. (2008) Post-translational regulation of L-glutamic acid decarboxylase in the brain. *Neurochemical Research* 33, 1459–1465.

Wei, J., Davis, K.M., Wu, H. and Wu, J.Y. (2004) Protein phosphorylation of human brain glutamic acid decarboxylase (GAD)65 and GAD67 and its physiological implications. *Biochemistry* 43, 6182–6189.

Wu, J.Y., Matsuda, T. and Roberts, E. (1973) Purification and characterization of glutamate decarboxylase from mouse brain. *Journal of Biological Chemistry* 248, 3029–3034.

Wu, J.Y., Chude, O., Wein, J., Roberts, E., Saito, K. and Wong, E. (1978) Distribution and tissue specificity of glutamate decarboxylase (EC 4.1.1.15). *Journal of Neurochemistry* 30, 849–857.

Wu, J.Y., Denner, L., Lin, C.T. and Song, G.X. (1985) L-Glutamate decarboxylase from brain. *Methods in Enzymology* 113, 3–10.

Yessaian, N.H., Armenian, A.R. and Buniatian, H.C. (1969) Effect of gamma-aminobutyric acid on brain serotonin and catecholamines. *Journal of Neurochemistry* 16, 1425–1433.

Yoon, J.-W., Yoon, C.-S., Lim, H.-W., Huang, Q.Q., Kang, Y., Pyun, K.H., Hirasawa, K., *et al.* (1999) Control of autoimmune diabetes in NOD mice by GAD expression or suppression in β cells. *Science* 284, 1183–1187.

Zhang, F., Thottananiyil, M., Martin, D.L. and Chen, C.H. (1999) Conformational alteration in serum albumin as a carrier for pyridoxal phosphate: a distinction from pyridoxal phosphate-dependent glutamate decarboxylase. *Archives of Biochemistry and Biophysics* 364, 195–202.

7 Glutaminase

J.M. Matés,* J.A. Segura, F.J. Alonso and J. Márquez
Departamento de Biología Molecular y Bioquímica, Laboratorio de Química de Proteínas, Facultad de Ciencias, Universidad de Málaga, España

7.1 Abstract

A key role for phosphate-activated glutaminase has been proposed for the synthesis of neurotransmitter glutamate and γ-aminobutyric acid (GABA) in the brain. This synthesis must be exquisitely regulated because of its potential harmful effects giving rise to excitotoxic damage. It is noteworthy that two glutaminase isozymes coded by different genes are expressed in the brains of mammals. The need for two genes and two isozymes to support the single process of glutamate synthesis is unexplained, and identifying the role of each glutaminase is an important factor in understanding glutamate-mediated neurotransmission. Furthermore, simultaneous expression of glutaminase isoforms has been reported in other mammalian tissues and cells. Validation of glutaminase expression and regulation as therapeutic tools for brain lesions will be considered here.

7.2 Introduction

Phosphate-activated glutaminase (EC 3.5.1.2; GA) is a glutamine (Gln) amidohydrolase, a true hydrolytic enzyme because the acyl chain and ammonium acceptor is water and not another molecule. Some of the main physiological functions of GA include renal ammoniagenesis, nitrogen supply for urea biosynthesis in the liver, synthesis of the excitatory neurotransmitter glutamate (Glu) in the brain and energy supply for the bioenergetics of many normal and transformed cell types (Kovacevic and McGivan, 1983; Curthoys and Watford, 1995). In brain, although several different precursors have been proposed for the synthesis of transmitter Glu, Gln is considered the most important source through GA reaction (Kvamme, 1984). Besides being the major excitatory neurotransmitter in the central nervous system (CNS) (Fonnum, 1984), Glu fulfils many other crucial roles in synaptogenesis, synaptic plasticity, pathogenesis of neuropsychiatric diseases (Conti and Weinberg, 1999), synthesis of GABA and brain energy metabolism (Erecińska and Silver, 1990).

On the other hand, the role of two key genes of Gln metabolism, glutamine synthetase (GS, EC 6.3.1.2) and GA, has also attracted considerable attention in tumour biology, because Gln behaves as a central metabolite for growth and proliferation (Matés *et al.*, 2002). The high rate of glutaminolysis observed in a wide variety of tumours may be essential to maintain their proliferative capacity (Souba, 1993).

* E-mail address: jmates@uma.es

7.3 Mammalian Glutaminase Genes and Transcripts

In humans, the GA family consists of two main members which are encoded by separate genes in different chromosomes (Table 7.1): the *Gls* gene, located in chromosome 2, encodes isoforms known as kidney (K-type) glutaminases; and the *Gls2* gene, located on chromosome 12, codes for liver (L-type) isozymes (Aledo *et al.*, 2000). Orthologous genes have been described in other mammalian species, such as mouse and rat, for *Gls* (Mock *et al.*, 1989) and *Gls2* (Chung-Bok *et al.*, 1997).

7.3.1 *Gls* gene and transcripts

The human *Gls* gene spans 82 kb. By comparison with available human cDNAs, the gene was split into 19 exons (Porter *et al.*, 2002). At least two different transcripts arise from this gene: the KGA mRNA formed by joining exons 1–14 and 16–19, and the alternative spliced transcript named glutaminase C (GAC) mRNA which uses only the first 15 exons, omitting exons 16–19 (Porter *et al.*, 2002). The K-type cDNA named GAC was originally isolated from an HT-29 human colon cDNA library (Elgadi *et al.*, 1999) but it has also been reported to be present in rat kidney and porcine kidney cell line (Porter *et al.*, 2002). In human tissues, GAC mRNA is expressed predominantly in cardiac muscle and pancreas, appreciably in placenta, kidney and lung, but not in liver and brain (Elgadi *et al.*, 1999).

KGA mRNA was found to be ubiquitous in most non-hepatic human tissues (Aledo *et al.*, 2000). K-type cDNAs have been cloned from different mammalian tissues including kidney (Shapiro *et al.*, 1991), brain (Nagase *et al.*, 1998) and colon cancer cells (Elgadi *et al.*, 1999). Differential expression of multiple K-type mRNAs have been detected in LLC-PK$_1$-FBPase$^+$ porcine proximal tubule-like cells (Porter *et al.*, 1995), rat lymphocytes (Sarantos *et al.*, 1993), mouse splenocytes (Aledo *et al.*, 1998), Ehrlich ascites tumour cells (Aledo *et al.*, 1994) and human kidney (Elgadi *et al.*, 1999). The length of these transcripts is in the range of 3.0–6.0 kb and can be produced by use of alternative polyadenylation sites (Porter *et al.*, 2002) or by alternative splicing (Elgadi *et al.*, 1999).

In kidney, the KGA enzyme is strongly induced by metabolic acidosis. The presence of a pH-response element (AU-rich sequences) in the 3'-UTR region of the KGA mRNA is responsible for its selective stabilization through binding of the protein ξ-crystallin/NADPH-quinone reductase (Tang and Curthoys, 2001). However, in tissues other than kidney, expression of the *Gls* gene is likely to be regulated at the level of transcription. For example, in small intestinal mucosal cells, dexamethasone increased KGA mRNA and specific activity. The increase in message preceded the increase in activity, consistent with *de novo* RNA synthesis followed by protein synthesis. Glucocorticoids may accelerate intestinal Gln utilization by increasing glutaminase expression, an adaptive response that could provide more energy for mucosal cells in stress states (Sarantos *et al.*, 1992). The primary role of glutaminase in the intestine is

Table 7.1. Mammalian glutaminase genes and transcripts. Data are for human glutaminases except for the LGA isoform (rat). The expression data have been collected from different mammalian glutaminases.

	KGA	GAC	LGA	GAB
Gene	*Gls*	*Gls*	*Gls2*	*Gls2*
Chromosome	2	2	12	12
Transcript (nt)	4348	3183	2257	2408
Number of exons	18	15	17	18
Expression	Ubiquitous in most non-hepatic mammalian tissues	Breast cancer cells, colon, heart, kidney, lung, pancreas, placenta	Liver	Brain, breast cancer cells, pancreas

to regulate enterocyte metabolism. This is because Gln is the main respiratory fuel of enterocytes and GA catalyses the rate-limiting step of Gln degradation (Kong et al., 2000).

In proliferative cells and tumours transcriptional regulation of the *Gls* gene seems to be operative and associated with cell growth and proliferation. Glutamine is the principal fuel used by lymphocytes, and a fast rise of KGA mRNA levels was observed after mitogenic challenge with endotoxin (Sarantos et al. 1993). Cytokines such as interleukin-1, interleukin-6, tumour necrosis factor-α, and γ-interferon decreased KGA activity, protein content and mRNA levels in cultured human fibroblast (Sarantos et al., 1994). In Ehrlich ascites tumour cells, a long-term regulation for tumour KGA expression during tumour development was deduced, in such a way that maximum activity and mRNA levels were found in mitochondria isolated from cells in the exponential phase of growth, when compared with the stationary phase of growth (Aledo et al., 1994).

With regard to mammalian brain regulation, it is noteworthy that both rat KGA and human KGA and GAC cDNAs contain variable CAG trinucleotide repeats in their 5' ends (Shapiro et al., 1991). However, the CAG repeats are located in the 5'-nontranslated region of the human K-type mRNAs, while in the rat they are located within the coding region. CAG repeat-length polymorphisms are shown to be the cause of various neurodegenerative diseases, including Huntington's disease, spinocerebellar ataxias and myotonic dystrophy (Singer, 1998).

7.3.2 *Gls*2 gene and transcripts

The human *Gls*2 gene has a length greater than 18 kb and is split into 18 exons (Aledo et al., 2000). Exon 1 shares 62.5% similarity, but it codes for 129 amino acids in KGA and only for 61 amino acids in human glutaminase L, accounting for the 67 extra amino acids of KGA protein at the N-terminal. The sequences encoded by exon 1 contain the signals involved in mitochondrial targeting and translocation processes (Shapiro et al., 1991). Interestingly, exon 1 also contains an LXXLL signature motif for human glutaminase L, which might explain the nuclear localization recently demonstrated for glutaminase L in mammalian brain (Olalla et al., 2002). Likewise, exon 18, which codes for the C-terminal region of both proteins, shows the lowest sequence similarity (29.4%). This region of the human L-type GA protein has been demonstrated recently to be involved in the recognition of PDZ (PSD95/Dlg/ZO1 domains)-interaction modules (Márquez et al., 2009). Therefore, the most significant differences between human *Gls* and *Gls*2 exons are located in regions involved with organelle targeting and protein–protein interactions, which may help to explain their differential function and regulation. L-type transcripts derived from the *Gls*2 gene were originally thought to be present in adult liver tissue and absent in extra-hepatic tissues (Smith and Watford, 1990; Curthoys and Watford, 1995). This restricted pattern of expression was generally accepted until quite recently, when results showed clear evidence that expression also occurs in extra-hepatic tissues like brain, pancreas and breast cancer cells (Gómez-Fabre et al., 2000).

Two different L-type GA transcripts of the mammalian *Gls*2 gene have been characterized so far: a long transcript, named GAB, was isolated as a cDNA clone from ZR75 breast cancer cells, having an ORF of 1806 nucleotides encoding a protein of 602 amino acids (Gómez-Fabre et al., 2000; de la Rosa et al., 2009). A short transcript termed LGA was isolated from rat liver (Smith and Watford, 1990; Chung-Bok et al., 1997). Sequence comparisons showed that human GAB cDNA was very similar (89% identity) to the rat liver LGA cDNA. With regard to the deduced amino acid sequence, human L-type GAB shares a considerable degree of identity (94%) with the rat liver LGA enzyme, but the human enzyme extends over 67 residues at the N-terminal end (Gómez-Fabre et al., 2000). In contrast, the human L-type GAB showed only 68.5% identity with the rat kidney KGA cDNA, a percentage similar to that found between rat liver and kidney GA cDNA species (Chung-Bok et al., 1997).

Glutamine is a major substrate for hepatic gluconeogenesis and urea synthesis (Watford,

1993). In contrast to KGA, hepatic GA is not affected by changes in acid–base status. Analysis of the rat hepatic GA promoter revealed a cAMP-responsive element (CRE) that may explain the gene's responsiveness to low insulin and/or high glucagon levels (Chung-Bok et al., 1997). The proximal promoter of the rat Gls2 gene lacks a functional TATA box, but contains hepatocyte nuclear factor recognition elements (HNF-1 and HNF-5), and CAAT-enhancer binding protein (C/EBP) that may be important for its basal expression in liver (Chung-Bok et al., 1997).

The core promoter regions of both the human and rat Gls2 genes do not contain canonical TATA boxes, but do have G+C-rich domains (Pérez-Gómez et al., 2003). This characteristic is also found in the human KGA promoter (Porter et al., 2002). Unlike rat LGA, human Gls2 has a canonical CAAT box and Ras-responsive element-binding transcription factors (RREBs), though it lacks the HNF-5 site present in rat Gls2. Mutagenesis and transient transfections clearly demonstrated that two CAAT boxes play crucial roles in the transcriptional regulation of the human Gls2 gene, both in cells of liver origin (HepG2), and in MCF-7 breast cancer cells (Pérez-Gómez et al., 2003). C/EBPs control cell growth and differentiation, causing growth arrest and inducing cellular differentiation in several adipocyte, granulocyte, and keratinocyte lineages (Darlington et al., 1998). Furthermore, HepG2 hepatoma cells express significantly lower levels of C/EBPα and C/EBPβ than those found in normal terminally differentiated hepatocytes (Friedman et al., 1989). Thus conversion of hepatocytes into proliferating hepatoma cells might require strong down-regulation of C/EBPα and C/EBPβ expression.

The GAB enzyme from ZR75 human breast cancer cells also showed a long-term regulation depending on the cell proliferation state: maximal activities were found at the beginning of the exponential growth phase, with a remarkable decrease at the stationary phase of growth when cell confluence was achieved. These results agree with those previously reported for Ehrlich ascites tumour cells, and indicate a long-term regulation of GA in tumours by differential gene expression (de la Rosa et al., 2009).

7.4 Mammalian Glutaminase Enzymes

Besides differences in molecular structures, the distinct kinetic behaviour has been a hallmark frequently used to distinguish between GA isoforms (Table 7.2). These enzymes are intricately regulated by a number of low-molecular mass effectors. The main kinetic differences have been observed in the dependence of the activator inorganic phosphate (Pi) (low for L-type, high for K-type); the relative affinity for the substrate Gln (higher in K- than in L-types); and the inhibitory effect of Glu, a unique characteristic reported only for K-type isozymes (Kovacevic and McGivan, 1983; Curthoys and Watford, 1995).

Table 7.2. Mammalian glutaminase proteins. The kinetic data have been collected from different mammalian glutaminases.

	KGA	LGA	GAB
Purification source	Cow, mouse, pig, rat	Rat	Human
Tissues/cells	Brain, EATC[a], kidney	Liver	Recombinant protein expressed in Sf9 insect cells
Length (aas)	669	535	602
Native molecular mass (kDa)	90–137	162–170	Not determined
Glutamine affinity	High	Low	Low
Pi dependence	High	Low	Low
Glutamate inhibition	Yes	No	Moderate
Ammonia activation	No	Strong	Very low

[a]EATC, Ehrlich ascites tumour cells.

7.4.1 Molecular structures and kinetics properties

KGA protein has been purified from pig kidney (Kvamme et al., 1991); pig brain (Svenneby et al., 1973; Nimmo and Tipton, 1980), rat kidney (Curthoys et al., 1976a), rat brain (Haser et al., 1985; Kaneko et al., 1987), cow brain (Chiu and Boeker, 1979) and from Ehrlich ascites tumour cells (Quesada et al., 1988; Segura et al., 1995). These enzymes are not activated by ammonia but inhibited by Glu, have a relatively low $K_{0.5}$ for Gln, a high $K_{0.5}$ for Pi, and their antibodies showed crossed reactions, but not with the LGA isoenzyme (Curthoys et al., 1976b). Purified native KGA in the absence of polyvalent anions is an inactive protomer with an apparent relative molecular mass ranging from 90,000 to 137,000.

Rat renal and brain KGA contain two different peptides of M_r 66,000 and 68,000 that are present in the ratio 3:1 and are produced *in vivo* from a common precursor (Haser et al., 1985; Perera et al., 1990). In rat kidney, the two mature KGA subunits forming the tetramer are produced by mitochondrial processing of a common 74 kDa precursor (Srinivasan et al., 1995). In contrast, KGA from pig brain has been reported to contain a single polypeptide of M_r 64,000 (Svenneby et al., 1973) or 73,000 (Nimmo and Tipton, 1980). These discrepancies can be ascribed to species-specific differences or, alternatively, they could be explained by proteolytic degradation and the use of different molecular mass standards for calibration of the SDS gels (Quesada et al., 1988; Segura et al., 1995).

In contrast to KGA, the liver LGA enzyme is not inhibited by Glu, has a higher K_m for Gln, is fully activated at lower concentrations of Pi, and shows activation by ammonia. Rat liver LGA possesses a unique subunit with an M_r of 58,000, but a great variability has been reported for the molecular mass of the native protein, with values ranging from 162,000 to 170,500 Da (Heini et al., 1987; Smith and Watford, 1988), to more than 300,000 Da (Patel and McGivan, 1984; Smith and Watford, 1988). The molecular data obtained suggest that rat liver glutaminase is a trimer composed of three identical subunits. In contrast to KGA, no signs for a similar aggregation of the liver LGA enzyme were found even at high Pi concentrations (Heini et al., 1987). The human GAB mRNA has been heterologously expressed in prokaryotic (Campos et al., 2003) and baculovirus (Campos-Sandoval et al., 2007) systems. This was the first direct demonstration that the cDNA of human GAB, originally cloned from ZR75 breast cancer cells (Gómez-Fabre et al., 2000), encodes an active GA enzyme.

In particulate preparations from brain, stimulatory effectors include Pi, sulphate, chloride, carboxylic acids, nucleotide triphosphates and riboflavin phosphate, all active in mM concentrations (Erecińska and Silver, 1990). Other compounds such as CoA, short- and long-chain acyl-CoA, and the dye bromothymol blue activate GA at µM concentrations but become inhibitors in mM concentrations (Kvamme et al., 2000). Ca^{2+} activates GA in mitochondria, brain synaptosomes, brain slices and homogenates, but does not act on purified enzyme, indicating that its effect is indirect (Erecińska and Silver, 1990; Kvamme et al., 2000). Phosphate is the most prominent stimulator of GA (Kvamme et al., 1970). Main inhibitors of brain GA include Glu, ammonium ions, protons, and cAMP and cGMP at mM concentrations (Erecińska and Silver, 1990; Kvamme et al., 2000). Other non-specific inhibitors are compounds that react with thiol groups as well as Gln analogues like 6-diazo-5-oxo-norleucine (DON) (Curthoys and Watford, 1995; Campos et al., 1998). A recently discovered KGA-specific inhibitor is BPTES [bis-2-(5-phenylacetamido-1,2,4-thiadiazol-2-yl)ethyl sulphide] which prevents the formation of large phosphate-induced oligomers (Robinson et al., 2007).

Glutamate is a competitive inhibitor and the relative concentrations of Gln and Glu in glutamatergic terminals (Kvamme et al., 2000) suggest that GA can be strongly inhibited in nerve cells. GAB and LGA enzymes differ markedly in their molecular mass, kinetic characteristics, regulatory properties, tissue distribution and subcellular localization (de la Rosa et al., 2009). Human GAB is 67 amino acids longer than rat liver LGA protein. Nuclear GA exhibited a kinetic behaviour that resembles that of the LGA enzyme with regard to the low Pi concentration requirement; however, nuclear GA showed a strong and unexpected inhibition by Glu, a property that is absent in the LGA enzyme (Olalla et al., 2002). Purified human GAB is an allosteric enzyme: measurements of the Gln binding kinetics yielded a sigmoidal curve with a Hill index of 2.7, and $S_{0.5}$ values of 32 and 64 mM for high and low Pi concentrations, respectively (de la Rosa et al., 2009). Whereas the protein showed a low Pi dependence typical for L-type GA, the enzyme was unexpectedly inhibited by Glu, a kinetic characteristic exclusive of K-type isozymes. At low Pi concentration (5 mM) and suboptimal Gln concentration (20 mM) the IC_{50} for Glu was 50mM. These data are in the range of Ki values reported for Glu competitive inhibition of K-type enzymes at high Pi concentrations (de la Rosa et al., 2009).

7.4.2 Subcellular locations

It is now accepted that at least two GA isoforms, with different kinetic and regulatory properties, are expressed in mammalian brain (Olalla et al., 2002). The regional distribution of both GA transcripts in human brain showed a similar pattern of expression: they were ubiquitously expressed in all regions of the brain examined, with the strongest signal in the cerebral cortex. Furthermore, expression of K- and L-type transcripts in brain was also demonstrated in other mammalian species such as cow, mouse, rabbit and rat. Simultaneous expression of both K- and L-type GA isozymes in the same cell type is more frequent than previously thought: apart from neurons, it has been found in human colorectal tumour cells (Turner and McGivan, 2003), human hepatoma HepG2 cells, medullar blood mononuclear cells from patients suffering from leukaemia, KU812F human myeloid cells and human breast cancer cells MCF7 and ZR-75-1 (Pérez-Gómez et al., 2005).

A crucial difference between GAB and the rest of the GA isoforms so far described is that GAB has been found in extra-mitochondrial localizations, while KGA and LGA have always been exclusively confined to mitochondria (Erecińska and Silver, 1990; Curthoys and Watford, 1995). In the cerebral cortex, hippocampus, cerebellum and striatum the immunolocalization revealed an L-type GA immunostaining concentrated in the neuronal nuclei (Olalla et al., 2002). The staining was seen in rat and monkey brains. The nuclear role of this L-type GA has yet to be determined, but this novel location has been linked to a potential function as a transcriptional coregulator (Márquez et al., 2006; Szeliga et al., 2009).

Whereas GAB seems to have structural determinants needed for mitochondrial targeting (Gómez-Fabre et al., 2000), it does not possess a discernible classical nuclear localization signal. However, human GAB has other sequence motifs and conserved modules that may be essential for its nuclear import (Márquez et al., 2006). For example, a PDZ-recognition motif would be implicated in GAB specific targeting to selective cellular locations (Olalla et al., 2008; Márquez et al., 2009). A second extra-mitochondrial localization of GAB, apart from cell nuclei, has been found in human polymorphonuclear neutrophils (PMN) (Castell et al., 2004). The presence of L-type GA in these leukocytes was related to their bactericidal action through a Gln-dependent mechanism of superoxide production. These results point towards a cell-specific subcellular location of GAB, increasing the number of potential roles this protein may fulfil (de la Rosa et al., 2009).

7.5 Glutaminase Expression in Mammalian Brain

Glutamate is the principal excitatory neurotransmitter in the CNS (Fonnum, 1984; Chapter 25). Glutamate homeostasis is achieved by multiple interactions in the tripartite synapse where this amino acid is utilized as a releasable transmitter or for general metabolism (Erecińska and Silver, 1990). Considerable attention has been dedicated to study the regulation of Glu release and inactivation, leading to an exhaustive characterization of Glu receptors, which are among the most studied and best understood molecules of the nervous system (Watkins and Jane, 2006). However, understanding the mechanisms by which Glu plays its role in diverse processes requires not only the detailed knowledge of the implicated postsynaptic receptors but also of the enzymes involved in the production of Glu in the presynaptic neurons (Márquez et al., 2009).

Despite extensive investigations, the source of neurotransmitter Glu has not been completely resolved. Although there is more than one pathway for Glu synthesis in cells, the vesicular Glu pool in neurons is derived primarily from glutamine through GA. Furthermore, neurotransmitter Glu synthesis has also been shown to be dependent on transamination of α-ketoglutarate involving tricarboxylic acid cycle reactions (Palaiologos et al., 1988; Waagepetersen et al., 2005). Most of the released Glu is taken up by the glial compartment and converted to Gln. A Glu–Gln shuttle between neurons and glial cells has been postulated for neurotransmitter recycling (Hertz, 2004). This cycle assumes that Gln, in turn, is released from the glial cells, taken up by neurons, and converted back to Glu. The model nicely explains the neuronal input of a suitable precursor for Glu synthesis, taking into account the lack of quantitatively important anaplerotic enzymes in neurons (Fig. 7.1). The Glu–Gln cycle was also based on the exclusive localization of glutamine synthetase in astrocytes and GA in neurons (Norenberg and Martínez-Hernández, 1979; Aoki et al., 1991; Laake et al., 1995).

Key issues will be to answer the main question of why two GA isoenzymes are needed in mammalian brain, and also to elucidate the functions that glutaminase L fulfils in nuclei. Potential nuclear functions for glutaminase L include the regulation of Gln/Glu levels or its role as a transcriptional coregulator. In this regard, a recent study has revealed that over-expression of human L-type GA gene in the T98 glioblastoma cell line induced a marked change in the cells' transcriptome correlated with a reversion of their transformed phenotype (Szeliga et al., 2009). Human malignant gliomas have been

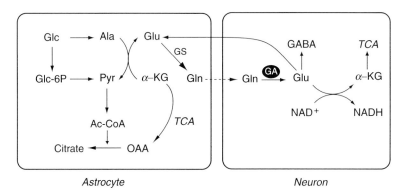

Fig. 7.1. Glutaminase in the glutamate–glutamine cycle between astrocytes and neurons, including pathways followed in energy metabolism. Astrocytes transform Glc to Glc-6P, which is further metabolized to substrates for subsequent transformation into the TCA cycle. The main routes of carbon are from Glc to pyruvate through glycolysis, the anaplerotic pathway at astrocytic oxaloacetate, astrocytic, and neuronal TCA cycles, and the Glu–Gln cycle. Glu is converted to Gln by GS in the astrocytes. Glu can also be degraded in astrocytes, via formation of α-KG. Ac-CoA can also be formed from acetate, but only in astrocytes. Gln is released by the astrocytes, transported into the neurons, and converted to Glu by GA. Ac-CoA, Acetyl coenzyme A; α-KG, alpha-ketoglutarate; GA, glutaminase; GABA, γ-aminobutyric acid; Glc, glucose; Glc-6P, glucose-6Phosphate; GS, Gln synthetase; OAA, oxaloacetate; Pyr, pyruvate; TCA, Tri-carboxylic acid cycle.

shown to express K-type GAs (KGA and GAC isoforms) but with a negligible expression of L-type GA (Szeliga et al., 2005). Taking into account its presence in the nuclei of the cells, it has been speculated that glutaminase L over-expression may contribute to alter the transcriptional programme of glioma cells yielding a less-malignant and more differentiated phenotype, but the concrete molecular mechanisms underpinning this phenotypical change are unknown (Márquez et al., 2009).

The other main neurotransmitter in the CNS – GABA – is produced by L-glutamic acid decarboxylase (EC 4.1.1.15; GAD (Chapter 6)). Interestingly, two GAD isoforms, encoded by different independently regulated genes, are also expressed in brain (Bu et al., 1992). Both forms can synthesize transmitter GABA, but have different roles in the coding of information by GABA-containing neurones and different subcellular localizations (Soghomonian and Martin, 1998). Although it is not fully clear why two GAD enzymes are needed in the brain, recent structural studies are revealing the molecular basis for selective isoform activation and its implication in the regulation of GABA homeostasis (Fenalti et al., 2007). Thus, each of the two main neurotransmitters in the CNS (Glu and GABA) can be synthesized by two isozymes coded by distinct genes, a unique situation to the other neurotransmitters. Production of glutamate and GABA must be a process exquisitely regulated to ensure a proper Glu function (Márquez et al., 2009).

7.5.1 Expression of glutaminase L in astrocytes

The presence of functional GA in astrocytes is a phenomenon which is hard to reconcile with the current model of Glu recycling. This does not consider that any GA activity takes place in astrocytes; rather, astrocytes take up most of the neurotransmitter Glu by specific carriers and convert it into Gln through the Gln synthetase enzyme, exclusively expressed in these cells. We have found L-type GA label in rat brain astrocytes from the cerebral cortex by immunocytochemical analyses (Olalla et al., 2008). Although primary cultures of astrocytes displayed GA activity (Yudkoff et al., 1988), immunohistochemical studies have shown KGA immunoreactivity in rat brain astrocytes (Aoki et al., 1991). Recently, KGA, GAC, and LGA mRNAs have been detected in cultured rat astrocytes (Szeliga et al., 2008). However, no GA signal was found in astrocytes from rat cerebellum via post-embedding immunocytochemistry with colloidal gold (Laake et al., 1999). While an in-depth study of GA isoform expression in glial cells is still lacking (further work is in progress), these findings complement early studies describing GA expression in glial cells (Márquez et al., 2009).

The concept of GAs as exclusive neuron-specific enzymes has been challenged by recent findings reporting expression of GA in astrocytes. These novel findings open a new avenue of research on how Glu and Gln may affect the synapse. As the interactome of brain glutaminases is being investigated, they can be envisioned as multifunctional proteins having additional tasks that seem to be operative in different processes relating to Glu homeostasis, besides their roles in glutamatergic transmission. Some of these novel roles for brain glutaminases may include transcriptional control, neuronal growth and differentiation, and cerebrovascular regulation (Márquez et al., 2009).

On the other hand, the Glu–Gln cycle proposes that astrocytes transform Glu to Gln, which fuels the neuron (Fig. 7.1). The carbon skeletons of oxaloacetate and other intermediates of the tri-carboxylic acid cycle (TCA) can be derived from Gln and Glu as well as glucose (Chambers et al., 2010). The conversion of Gln to Glu occurs in both the extracellular and intracellular compartments in many cell types and organs (Welbourne et al., 2001). Fluxes of nitrogen to and from alanine have been reported to be high in both cultured astrocytes and neurons (Fig. 7.1).

In addition to a role in neuronal Glu synthesis, transamination reactions are critical for Glu utilization by neurons (Erecińska et al., 1994). The expansion of the available pool of oxaloacetate can reflect an increased oxidation of Glu and Gln through a portion of the TCA cycle and enhanced production of oxaloacetate from Glu and Gln carbon (Yudkoff et al., 2000). Interestingly, cerebral Glu and Gln are predominantly localized in glutamatergic neurons and astroglia, respectively (Shen, 2006). Independent studies using *in vivo* microdialysis and mass spectrometry to determine the labelling of extracellular Glu and Gln have shown that neuronal Glu (through Glu–Gln cycling) is the precursor for 80–90% of glial Gln synthesis. In fact, the reported values of the Glu–Gln neurotransmitter cycle flux in humans and the relationship between Glu–Gln cycle flux and neuronal TCA cycle flux are in relatively good agreement (Shen et al., 2009). In addition to its interaction with the predominantly neuronal Glu, the astroglial Gln is also in exchange with blood, allowing for unlabelled Gln from blood to be transported into brain, and the glial compartment, effectively diluting the astroglial Gln pool (Bröer and Brookes, 2001).

Astrocytes play a critical role in the regulation of brain metabolic responses to activity. Astrocytes prepared from different brain regions all gave rise to the same capacity to enhance glycolysis upon Glu stimulation. Thus, this property appears to be an intrinsic feature of astrocytes and is not specifically linked either to culture conditions or cell origin (Pellerin et al., 2007). Interestingly, neuronal consumption of glucose to maintain their antioxidant status may take priority over the use of glucose to fulfil their bioenergetic requirements, which can be met by other sources. Increasing evidence indicates that neurons can use lactate generated by astrocytes to produce energy and that this is not a uniform process but varies as a result of glutamatergic activation. It is likely that the increased use of lactate by neurons is coupled to an increase in their regeneration of reduced glutathione from glucose (Herrero-Méndez et al., 2009). Moreover, incubation of neurons with a plasma membrane-permeable form of glutathione (glutathione ethyl ester) prevented apoptosis. These results indicate that production of reactive oxygen species (ROS) in neurons might be consequent to the diversion of glucose-6-phosphate from the pentose–phosphate pathway to glycolysis (Bolaños et al., 2008).

7.6 State of Art and Perspectives

In most tested experimental models the Gln-responsive genes and the transcription factors involved correspond tightly to the specific effects of Gln in cell proliferation, differentiation and survival, and metabolic functions. Indeed, in addition to the major role played by nuclear factor-kappaB in the anti-inflammatory action of Gln, the stimulatory role of activating protein-1 and the inhibitory role of C/EBP homology binding protein in growth promotion, and the role of c-Myc in cell survival, many other transcription factors are also involved in the action of Gln to regulate apoptosis and intermediary metabolism in different cell types and tissues (Brasse-Lagnel et al., 2009). The influence of Gln on intestinal proteome expression in apoptotic conditions has been studied and evaluated in the human epithelial intestinal cell line HCT-8 (Deniel et al., 2007). By comparing the mitochondrial proteomes of tetracycline-treated and untreated cells with high Myc expression, it has been found that GA expression was increased tenfold in response to Myc. GA levels diminish with decreased Myc expression, and recover on Myc re-induction (Gao et al., 2009). Gln is converted by GA to Glu for further catabolism by the TCA cycle, and previous studies indicate that overexpression of Myc sensitizes human cells to Gln-withdrawal-induced apoptosis (Yuneva et al., 2007).

In both a murine microglia model and the microglial cell line BV-2, inhibition of GA suppresses chromatin condensation and annexin-V labelling. Gln and ammonium enhanced production of ROS. Apoptosis, induced by Gln, was inhibited either by the radical scavenger α-tocopherol or by a nitric oxide synthase blocker. Furthermore, blockade of caspase-9 activity also prevented apoptosis. Taken together, these results indicate that hydrolysis of Gln and, accordingly, accumulation of ammonium in mitochondria can induce the intrinsic pathway of apoptosis (Svoboda and Kerschbaum, 2009).

Glutaminase catabolizes Gln for ATP and glutathione synthesis; its reduction affects proliferation and cell death, presumably through depletion of ATP and augmentation of ROS, respectively (Gao et al., 2009). The predominant neurotoxic factor released from both activated microglia and macrophages is Glu. They synthesize Glu via GA from extracellular Gln, and release it through hemichannels of gap junctions, not through Glu transporters. Inhibiting GA and/or gap junctions with specific antagonists effectively suppresses neuronal dysfunction caused by both macrophages and activated microglia. Both the glutaminase inhibitor DON, and the gap junction inhibitor carbenoxolone (CBX), effectively suppressed Glu production and subsequent neurotoxicity. Therefore, these drugs may be clinically valuable as components of a therapeutic strategy to limit the severity or progression of neurological disorders that promote neurodegeneration (Yawata et al., 2008).

Glucose metabolism via pyruvate dehydrogenation provides energy in both neurons and astrocytes and may include gap junction-mediated lactate transport into astrocytes. The importance of glycogen reflects that it selectively supports *de novo* synthesis of transmitter Glu by combined pyruvate dehydrogenation and carboxylation in astrocytes (Hertz and Gibbs, 2009). Because *de novo* synthesis from α-ketoglutarate is minimal in neurons, metabolic studies have suggested that most neurotransmitter Glu is recycled via the Gln–Glu neuron–astrocyte shuttle, involving GA (Fig. 7.1).

The critical role of GA has been supported further by pharmacological experiments in which a near-complete depletion of neuronal Glu was observed after inhibition of Glu synthesis. Mice *Gls* null mutants failed to feed because of deficits in goal-directed behaviour and died within the first postnatal day with a phenotype of altered respiration (Masson et al., 2006). *Gls* knockout perturbed glutamatergic neural networks such as brainstem respiratory circuits that depend on robust summation of synaptic inputs, and thus could account for the altered respiration phenotype. Despite the conclusions of many previous studies that GA is the principal source of neurotransmitter Glu, knocking out the *Gls* gene had a surprisingly subtle effect on glutamatergic synaptic transmission (Masson et al., 2006). This finding implies that other Glu-synthetic pathways are operative but, surprisingly, glutaminase L was not considered as a plausible compensatory source of transmitter (Masson et al., 2006). Besides Glu synthesis by LGA/GAB, the persistence of glutamatergic synaptic transmission in GA null mutants could be accounted for by other Glu-synthetic pathways such as transamination of α-ketoglutarate with alanine, branched-chain amino acids, or lysine (Hertz, 2004), or by direct reuptake of Glu into neurons (Waagepetersen et al., 2005). In spite of alternative synthetic pathways allowing temporary postnatal survival, the mice breathe poorly and die, indicating that KGA/GAC function is essential for survival (Masson et al., 2006).

7.7 Conclusions

Glutaminase converts Gln to Glu, which is further catabolized through the TCA cycle for the production of ATP, or serves as a substrate for glutathione synthesis. Under pathological conditions, Gln and ammonium are elevated globally in the brain. The Trojan horse hypothesis of L-Gln toxicity assumes that intramitochondrial hydrolysis of L-Gln enhances ammonium locally and leads to mitochondrial dysfunction (Albrecht and Norenberg, 2006). Exposure of brain cells to L-Gln can promote apoptosis (Fig. 7.2). Gln catabolism through GA is critical for cell proliferation induced by Myc, and protection against ROS generated by enhanced mitochondrial function in response to c-Myc (Lora et al., 2004). Intriguingly, elevated levels of c-Myc protein in human cancer

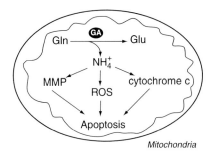

Fig. 7.2. Glutaminase and ammonium are involved in glutamine-dependent apoptosis in brain cells. Gln is accumulated in mitochondria and metabolized to Glu and ammonium. Ammonium contributes to the generation of reactive oxygen species (ROS) by blocking respiratory chain in mitochondria. The Trojan horse hypothesis of Gln toxicity assumes that accumulation and hydrolysis of Gln in mitochondria lead to toxic concentrations of ammonium. Because of the small volume of mitochondria, ammonium interacts rapidly with mitochondrial enzymes involved in energy metabolism leading to production of ROS and mitochondrial membrane depolarization. The efflux of cytochrome c contributes to the induction of caspase-3 and triggers apoptosis. GA, glutaminase; Gln, glutamine; Glu, glutamate; MMP, mitochondrial membrane potential; ROS, reactive oxygen species.

correspond to levels of GA, which are not increased in the accompanying normal tissue from the same patients (Gao et al., 2009). Taken together, the data indicate that GA is a promising pharmacotherapeutic target. The fact that both GA activity and Glu levels are reduced in adulthood suggests that a reduction in GA, and the ensuing decrease in Glu levels, are plausible explanations for the phenotypes observed in heterozygous *Gls* gene knockout mice, and argues against the possibility that these effects are due to neurodevelopmental alterations unrelated to GA or to Glu neurotransmission (Gaisler-Salomon et al., 2009).

7.8 Acknowledgements

This work was supported by Excellence Grant CVI-1543 from the regional Andalusian government (Junta de Andalucía), Grant SAF2007-61953 from the Ministry of Education and Science of Spain, and Grant RD06/1012 of the RTA RETICS network from the Spanish Health Institute Carlos III.

References

Albrecht, J. and Norenberg, M.D. (2006) Glutamine: a Trojan horse in ammonia neurotoxicity. *Hepatology* 44, 788–794.
Aledo, J.C., Segura, J.A., Medina, M.A., Alonso, F.J., Nuñez de Castro, I. and Márquez, J. (1994) Phosphate-activated glutaminase expression during tumor development. *FEBS Letters* 341, 39–42.
Aledo, J.C., Segura, J.A., Barbero, L.G. and Márquez, J. (1998) Early differential expression of two glutaminase mRNAs in mouse spleen after tumor implantation. *Cancer Letters* 133, 95–99.
Aledo, J.C., Gómez-Fabre, P.M., Olalla, L. and Márquez, J. (2000) Identification of two human glutaminase loci and tissue-specific expression of the two related genes. *Mammalian Genome* 11, 1107–1110.
Aoki, C., Kaneko, T., Starr, A. and Pickel, V.M. (1991) Identification of mitochondrial and non-mitochondrial glutaminase within select neurons and glia of rat forebrain by electron microscopic immunocytochemistry. *Journal of Neuroscience Research* 28, 531–548.
Bolaños, J.P., Delgado-Esteban, M., Herrero-Méndez, A., Fernández-Fernández, S. and Almeida, A. (2008) Regulation of glycolysis and pentose-phosphate pathway by nitric oxide: impact on neuronal survival. *Biochimica et Biophysica Acta* 1777, 789–793.
Brasse-Lagnel, C., Lavoinne, A. and Husson, A. (2009) Control of mammalian gene expression by amino acids, especially glutamine. *FEBS Journal* 276, 1826–1844.
Bröer, S. and Brookes, N. (2001) Transfer of glutamine between astrocytes and neurons. *Journal of Neurochemistry* 77, 705–719.
Bu, D.F., Erlander, M.G., Hitz, B.C., Tillakaratne, N.J., Kaufman, D.L., Wagner-McPherson, C.B., Evans, G.A., et al. (1992) Two human glutamate decarboxylases, 65-kDa GAD and 67-kDa GAD, are each encoded by a single gene. *Proceedings of the National Academy of Sciences USA* 89, 2115–2119.

Campos, J.A., Aledo, J.C., del Castillo-Olivares, A., del Valle, A.E., Núñez de Castro, I. and Márquez, J. (1998) Involvement of essential cysteine and histidine residues in the activity of isolated glutaminase from tumour cells. *Biochimica et Biophysica Acta* 1429, 275–283.

Campos, J.A., Aledo, J.C., Segura, J.A., Alonso, F.J., Gómez-Fabre, P.M., Núñez de Castro, I. and Márquez, J. (2003) Expression of recombinant human L-glutaminase in *Escherichia coli*: Polyclonal antibodies production and immunological analysis of mouse tissues. *Biochimica et Biophysica Acta* 1648, 17–23.

Campos-Sandoval, J.A., López de la Oliva, A.R., Lobo, C., Segura, J.A., Matés, J.M., Alonso, F.J. and Márquez, J. (2007) Expression of functional human glutaminase in baculovirus system: affinity purification, kinetic and molecular characterization. *International Journal of Biochemistry & Cell Biology* 39, 765–773.

Castell, L., Vance, C., Abbott, R., Márquez, J. and Eggleton, P. (2004) Granule localization of glutaminase in human neutrophils and the consequence of glutamine utilization for neutrophil activity. *Journal of Biological Chemistry* 279, 13305–13310.

Chambers, J.W., Maguirre, T.G. and Alwine, J.C. (2010) Glutamine metabolism is essential for human cytomegalovirus infection. *Journal of Virology* 84, 1867–1873.

Conti, F. and Weinberg, R.J. (1999) Shaping excitation at glutamatergic synapses. *Trends in Neurosciences* 22, 451–458.

Curthoys, N.P. and Watford, M. (1995) Regulation of glutaminase activity and glutamine metabolism. *Annual Review of Nutrition* 15, 133–159.

Curthoys, N.P., Kuhlenschmidt, T. and Godfrey, S.S. (1976a) Regulation of renal ammoniagenesis. purification and characterization of phosphate-dependent glutaminase from rat kidney. *Archives of Biochemistry and Biophysics* 174, 82–89.

Curthoys, N.P., Kuhlenschmidt, T., Godfrey, S.S. and Weiss, R.F. (1976b) Phosphate-dependent glutaminase from rat kidney. Cause of increased activity in response to acidosis and identity with glutaminase from other tissues. *Archives of Biochemistry and Biophysics* 172, 162–167.

Chiu, J.F. and Boeker, E.A. (1979) Cow brain glutaminase: partial purification and mechanism of action. *Archives of Biochemistry and Biophysics* 196, 493–500.

Chung-Bok, M.-I., Vincent, N., Jhala, U. and Watford, M. (1997) Rat hepatic glutaminase: identification of the full coding sequence and characterization of a functional promoter. *Biochemical Journal* 324, 193–200.

Darlington, G.J., Ross, S.E. and MacDougald, O.A. (1998) The role of C/EBP genes in adipocyte differentiation. *Journal of Biological Chemistry* 273, 30057–30060.

Deniel, N., Marion-Letellier, R., Charlionet, R., Tron, F., Leprince, J., Vaudry, H., Ducrotté, P., *et al.* (2007) Glutamine regulates the human epithelial intestinal HCT-8 cell proteome under apoptotic conditions. *Molecular & Cellular Proteomics* 6, 1671–1679.

Elgadi, K.M., Meguid, R.A., Qian, M., Souba, W.W. and Abcouwer, S.F. (1999) Cloning and analysis of unique human glutaminase isoforms generated by tissue-specific alternative splicing. *Physiological Genomics* 1, 51–62.

Erecińska, M. and Silver, I.A. (1990) Metabolism and role of glutamate in mammalian brain. *Progress in Neurobiology* 35, 245–296.

Erecińska, M., Nelson, D., Nissim, I., Daikhin, Y. and Yudkoff, M. (1994) Cerebral alanine transport and alanine aminotransferase reaction: alanine as a source of neuronal glutamate. *Journal of Neurochemistry* 62, 1953–1964.

Fenalti, G., Law, R.H., Buckle, A.M., Langendorf, C., Tuck, K., Rosado, C.J., Faux, N.G., *et al.* (2007) GABA production by glutamic acid decarboxylase is regulated by a dynamic catalytic loop. *Nature Structural & Molecular Biology* 14, 280–286.

Fonnum, F. (1984) Glutamate: a neurotransmitter in mammalian brain. *Journal of Neurochemistry* 42, 1–11.

Friedman, A.D., Landschulz, W.H. and McKnight, S.L. (1989) CCAAT/enhancer binding protein activates the promoter of the serum albumin gene in cultured hepatoma cells. *Genes & Development* 3, 1314–1322.

Gaisler-Salomon, I., Miller, G.M., Chuhma, N., Lee, S., Zhang, H., Ghoddoussi, F., Lewandowski, N., *et al.* (2009) Glutaminase-deficient mice display hippocampal hypoactivity, insensitivity to pro-psychotic drugs and potentiated latent inhibition: relevance to schizophrenia. *Neuropsychopharmacology*, 34, 2305–2322.

Gao, P., Tchernyshyov, I., Chang, T.C., Lee, Y.S., Kita, K., Ochi, T., Zeller, K.I., *et al.* (2009) c-Myc suppression of miR-23a/b enhances mitochondrial glutaminase expression and glutamine metabolism. *Nature* 458, 762–765.

Gómez-Fabre, P.M., Aledo, J.C., del Castillo-Olivares, A., Alonso, F.J., Núñez de Castro, I., Campos, J.A. and Márquez, J. (2000) Molecular cloning, sequencing and expression studies of the human breast cancer cell glutaminase. *Biochemical Journal* 345, 365–375.

Haser, W.G., Shapiro, R.A. and Curthoys, N.P. (1985) Comparison of the phosphate-dependent glutaminase obtained from rat brain and kidney. *Biochemical Journal* 229, 399–408.

Heini, H.G., Gebhardt, R. and Mecke, D. (1987) Purification and characterization of rat liver glutaminase. *European Journal of Biochemistry* 162, 541–546.

Herrero-Méndez, A., Almeida, A., Fernández, E., Maestre, C., Moncada, S. and Bolaños J.P. (2009) The bioenergetic and antioxidant status of neurons is controlled by continuous degradation of a key glycolytic enzyme by APC/C-Cdh1. *Nature Cell Biology* 11, 747–752.

Hertz, L. (2004) Intercellular metabolic compartmentation in the brain: past, present and future. *Neurochemistry International* 45, 285–296.

Hertz, L. and Gibbs, M.E. (2009) What learning in day-old chickens can teach a neurochemist: focus on astrocyte metabolism. *Journal of Neurochemistry* 109, 10–16.

Kaneko, T., Urade, Y., Watanabe, Y. and Mizuno, N. (1987) Production, characterization, and immunohistochemical application of monoclonal antibodies to glutaminase purified from rat brain. *Journal of Neuroscience* 7, 302–309.

Kong, S.E., Hall, J.C., Cooper, D. and McCauley, R.D. (2000) Glutamine-enriched parenteral nutrition regulates the activity and expression of intestinal glutaminase. *Biochimica et Biophysica Acta* 1475, 67–75.

Kovacevic, Z. and McGivan, J.D. (1983) Mitochondrial metabolism of Glutamine and glutamate and its physiological significance. *Physiological Reviews* 63, 547–605.

Kvamme, E. (1984) Enzymes of cerebral glutamine metabolism. In: Häussinger, D. and Sies, H. (eds) *Glutamine Metabolism in Mammalian Tissues*. Springer Verlag, Berlin, pp. 32–48.

Kvamme, E., Tveit, B. and Svenneby, G. (1970) Glutaminase from pig renal cortex. I. Purification and general properties. *Journal of Biological Chemistry* 245, 1871–187.

Kvamme, E., Torgner, I.A. and Roberg, B. (1991) Evidence indicating that pig renal phosphate-activated glutaminase has a functionally predominant external localization in the inner mitochondrial membrane. *Journal of Biological Chemistry*, 266, 13185–13192.

Kvamme, E., Roberg, B. and Torgner, I. (2000) Phosphate activated glutaminase and mitochondrial Glutamine transport in the brain. *Neurochemistry Research* 25, 1407–1419.

Laake, J.H., Slyngstad, T.A., Haug, F.M. and Ottersen, O.P. (1995) Glutamine from glial cells is essential for the maintenance of the nerve terminal pool of glutamate: immunogold evidence from hippocampal slice cultures. *Journal of Neurochemistry* 65, 871–881.

Laake, J.H., Takumi, Y., Eidet, J., Torgner, I.A., Roberg, B., Kvamme, E. and Ottersen, O.P. (1999) Postembedding immunogold labelling reveals subcellular localization and pathway-specific enrichment of phosphate activated glutaminase in rat cerebellum. *Neuroscience* 88, 1137–1151.

Lora, J., Alonso, F.J., Segura, J.A., Lobo, C., Márquez, J. and Matés, J.M. (2004) Antisense glutaminase inhibition decreases glutathione antioxidant capacity and increases apoptosis in Ehrlich ascitic tumour cells. *European Journal of Biochemistry* 271, 4298–4306.

Márquez, J., López de la Oliva, A.R., Matés, J.M., Segura, J.A. and Alonso, F.J. (2006) Glutaminase: A multifaceted protein not only involved in generating glutamate. *Neurochemistry International* 48, 465–471.

Márquez, J., Tosina, M., de la Rosa, V., Segura, J.A., Alonso, F.J., Matés, J.M. and Campos-Sandoval, J.A. (2009) New insights into brain glutaminases: beyond their role on glutamatergic transmission. *Neurochemistry International* 55, 64–70.

Masson, J., Darmon, M., Conjard, A., Chuhma, N., Ropert, N., Thoby-Brisson, M., Foutz, A.S., et al. (2006) Mice lacking brain/kidney phosphate-activated glutaminase have impaired glutamatergic synaptic transmission, altered breathing, disorganized goal-directed behavior and die shortly after birth. *Journal of Neuroscience* 26, 4660–4671.

Matés, J.M., Pérez-Gómez, C., Núñez de Castro, I., Asenjo, M. and Márquez, J. (2002) Glutamine and its relationship with intracellular redox status, oxidative stress and cell proliferation/death. *International Journal of Biochemistry & Cell Biology* 34, 439–458.

Mock, B., Kozak, C., Seldin, M.F., Ruff, N., D'Hoostelaere, L., Szpirer, C., Levan, G., et al. (1989) A glutaminase (gls) gene maps to mouse chromosome 1, rat chromosome 9, and human chromosome 2. *Genomics* 5, 291–297.

Nagase, T., Ishikawa, K., Suyama, M., Kikuno, R., Hirosawa, M., Miyajima, N., Tanaka, A., et al. (1998) Prediction of the coding sequences of unidentified human genes. XII. The complete sequences of 100 new cDNA clones from brain which code for large proteins in vitro. *DNA Research* 5, 355–364.

Nimmo, G.A. and Tipton, K.F. (1980) Purification of soluble glutaminase from pig brain. *Biochemical Pharmacology* 29, 359–367.

Norenberg, M.D. and Martínez-Hernández, A. (1979) Fine structural localization of Glutamine synthetase in astrocytes of rat brain. *Brain Research* 161, 303–310.

Olalla, L., Gutiérrez, A., Campos, J.A., Khan, Z.U., Alonso, F., Segura, J.A., Márquez, J., et al. (2002) Nuclear localization of L-glutaminase in mammalian brain. *Journal of Biological Chemistry* 277, 38939–38944.

Olalla, L., Gutiérrez, A., Jiménez, A.J., López-Téllez, J.F., Khan, Z.U., Pérez, J., Alonso, F.J., et al. (2008) Expression of scaffolding PDZ protein GIP (glutaminase-interacting-protein) in mammalian brain. *Journal of Neuroscience Research* 86, 281–292.

Palaiologos, G., Hertz, L. and Schousboe, A. (1988) Evidence that aspartate aminotransferase activity and ketodicarboxylate carrier function are essential for biosynthesis of transmitter glutamate. *Journal of Neurochemistry* 51, 317–320.

Patel, M. and McGivan, J.D. (1984) Partial purification and properties of rat liver glutaminase. *Biochemical Journal* 220, 583–590.

Pellerin, L., Bouzier-Sore, A.K., Aubert, A., Serres, S., Merle, M., Costalat, R. and Magistretti, P.J. (2007) Activity-dependent regulation of energy metabolism by astrocytes: an update. *Glia* 55, 1251–1262.

Perera, S.Y., Chen, T.C. and Curthoys, N.P. (1990) Biosynthesis and processing of renal mitochondrial glutaminase in cultured proximal tubular epithelial cells and in isolated mitochondria. *Journal of Biological Chemistry* 265, 17764–11770.

Pérez-Gómez, C., Matés, J.M., Gómez-Fabre, P.M., del Castillo-Olivares, A., Alonso, F.J. and Márquez, J. (2003) Genomic organization and transcriptional analysis of the human L-glutaminase gene. *Biochemical Journal* 370, 771–784.

Pérez-Gómez, C., Campos-Sandoval, J.A., Alonso, F.J., Segura, J.A., Manzanares, E., Ruiz-Sánchez, P., González, M.E., et al. (2005) Co-expression of glutaminase K and L isoenzymes in human tumour cells. *Biochemical Journal* 386, 535–542.

Porter, D., Hansen, W.R., Taylor, L. and Curthoys, N.P. (1995) Differential expression of multiple glutaminase mRNAs in LLC-PK$_1$-F$^+$ cells. *American Journal of Physiology* 269, F363–373.

Porter, L.D., Ibrahim, H., Taylor, L. and Curthoys, N.P. (2002) Complexity and species variation of the kidney-type glutaminase gene. *Physiological Genomics* 9, 57–66.

Quesada, A.R., Sánchez-Jiménez, F., Pérez-Rodríguez, J., Márquez, J., Medina, M.A. and Núñez de Castro, I. (1988) Purification of phosphate-dependent glutaminase from isolated mitochondria of Ehrlich ascites-tumour cells. *Biochemical Journal* 255, 1031–1036.

Robinson, M.M., McBryant, S.J., Tsukamoto, T., Rojas, C., Ferraris, D.V., Hamilton, S.K., Hansen, J.C., et al. (2007) Novel mechanism of inhibition of rat kidney-type glutaminase by bis-2-(5-phenylacetamido-1,2,4-thiadiazol-2-yl)ethyl sulfide (BPTES). *Biochemical Journal* 406, 407–414.

de la Rosa, V., Campos-Sandoval, J.A., Martín-Rufián, M., Cardona, C., Matés, J.M., Segura, J.A., Alonso, F.J. and Márquez, J. (2009) A novel glutaminase isoform in mammalian tissues. *Neurochemistry International* 55, 76–84.

Sarantos, P., Abouhamze, A. and Souba, W.W. (1992) Glucocorticoids regulate intestinal glutaminase expression. *Surgery* 112, 278–283.

Sarantos, P., Ockert, K. and Souba, W.W. (1993) Endotoxin stimulates lymphocyte glutaminase expression. *Archives of Surgery* 128, 920–924.

Sarantos, P., Abouhamze, A., Abcouwer, S., Chakrabarti, R., Copeland, E.M. and Souba W.W. (1994) Cytokines decrease glutaminase expression in human fibroblasts. *Surgery* 116, 276–283.

Segura, J.A., Aledo, J.C., Gómez-Biedma, S., Núñez de Castro, I. and Márquez, J. (1995) Tumor glutaminase purification. *Protein Expression & Purification* 6, 343–351.

Shapiro, R.A., Farrell, L., Srinivasan, M. and Curthoys, N.P. (1991) Isolation, characterization and in vitro expression of a cDNA that encodes the kidney isoenzyme of the mitochondrial glutaminase. *Journal of Biological Chemistry* 266, 18792–18796.

Shen, J. (2006) ^{13}C magnetic resonance spectroscopy studies of alterations in glutamate neurotransmission. *Biological Psychiatry* 59, 883–887.

Shen, J., Rothman, D.L., Behar, K.L. and Xu, S. (2009) Determination of the glutamate-Glutamine cycling flux using two-compartment dynamic metabolic modeling is sensitive to astroglial dilution. *Journal of Cerebral Blood Flow and Metabolism* 29, 108–118.

Singer, R.H. 1998. Triplet-repeat transcripts: a role for DNA in disease. *Science* 280, 696–697.

Smith, E.M. and Watford, M. (1988) Rat hepatic glutaminase: purification and immunochemical characterization. *Archives of Biochemistry and Biophysics* 260, 740–751.

Smith, E.M. and Watford, M. (1990) Molecular cloning of a cDNA for rat hepatic glutaminase. Sequence similarity to kidney-type glutaminase. *Journal of Biological Chemistry* 265, 10631–10636.

Soghomonian, J.-J. and Martin, D.L. (1998) Two isoforms of glutamate decarboxylase: why? *Trends in Pharmacological Sciences* 19, 500–505.

Souba, W.W. (1993) Glutamine and cancer. *Annals of Surgery* 218, 715–728.

Srinivasan, M., Kalousek, F. and Curthoys, N.P. (1995) In vitro characterization of the mitochondrial processing and the potential function of the 68-kDa subunit of renal glutaminase. *Journal of Biological Chemistry*, 270, 1185–1190.

Svenneby, G., Torgner, I. and Kvamme, E. (1973) Purification of phosphate-dependent pig brain glutaminase. *Journal of Neurochemistry* 20, 1217–1224.

Svoboda, N. and Kerschbaum, H.H. (2009) L-Glutamine-induced apoptosis in microglia is mediated by mitochondrial dysfunction. *European Journal of Neuroscience* 30, 196–206.

Szeliga, M., Sidoryk, M., Matyja, E., Kowalczyk, P. and Albrecht, J. (2005) Lack of expression of the liver-type glutaminase (LGA) mRNA in human malignant gliomas. *Neuroscience Letters* 374, 171–173.

Szeliga, M., Matyja, E., Obara, M., Grajkowska, W., Czernicki, T. and Albrecht, J. (2008) Relative expression of mRNAs coding for glutaminase isoforms in CNS tissues and CNS tumors. *Neurochemistry Research* 33, 808–813.

Szeliga, M., Obara-Michlewska, M., Matyja, E., Lazarczyk, M., Lobo, C., Hilgier, W., Alonso, F., *et al.* (2009) Transfection with liver-type glutaminase cDNA alteres gene expression and reduces viability, migration and proliferation of T98G glioma cells. *Glia* 57, 1014–1023.

Tang, A. and Curthoys, N.P. (2001) Identification of zeta-crystallin/NADPH:quinone reductase as a renal glutaminase mRNA pH response element-binding protein. *Journal of Biological Chemistry* 276, 21375–21380.

Turner, A. and McGivan, J.D. (2003) Glutaminase isoform expression in cell lines derived from human colorectal adenomas and carcinomas. *Biochemical Journal* 370, 403–408.

Waagepetersen, H.S., Qu, H., Sonnewald, U., Shimamoto, K. and Schousboe, A. (2005) Role of glutamine and neuronal glutamate uptake in glutamate homeostasis and synthesis during vesicular release in cultured glutamatergic neurons. *Neurochemistry International* 47, 92–102.

Watford, M. (1993) Hepatic glutaminase expression: Relationship to kidney-type glutaminase and to the urea cycle. *FASEB Journal* 7, 1468–1474.

Watkins, J.C. and Jane, D.E. (2006) The glutamate story. *British Journal of Pharmacology* 147, S100–S108.

Welbourne, T., Routh, R., Yudkoff, M. and Nissim, I. (2001) The glutamine/glutamate couplet and cellular function. *News in Physiological Sciences* 16, 157–160.

Yawata, I., Takeuchi, H., Doi, Y., Liang, J., Mizuno, T. and Suzumura, A. (2008) Macrophage-induced neurotoxicity is mediated by glutamate and attenuated by glutaminase inhibitors and gap junction inhibitors. *Life Sciences* 82, 1111–1116.

Yudkoff, M., Nissim, I. and Pleasure, D. (1988) Astrocyte metabolism of [15N]glutamine: implications for the glutamine-glutamate cycle. *Journal of Neurochemistry* 51, 843–850.

Yudkoff, M., Daikhin, Y., Nissim, I. and Nissim, I. (2000) Acidosis and astrocyte amino acid metabolism. *Neurochemistry International* 36, 329–339.

Yuneva, M., Zamboni, N., Oefner, P., Sachidanandam, R. and Lazebnik, Y. (2007) Deficiency in glutamine but not glucose induces MYC-dependent apoptosis in human cells. *Journal of Cell Biology* 178, 93–105.

8 D-Serine and Serine Racemase in the Retina

S.B. Smith,[1,2,3*] **Y. Ha**[1,3] **and V. Ganapathy**[3,4]

[1]*Department of Cellular Biology and Anatomy;* [2]*Department of Ophthalmology;* [3]*Vision Discovery Institute;* [4]*Department of Biochemistry and Molecular Biology, Medical College of Georgia, Augusta, Georgia, USA*

8.1 Abstract

Recent data suggest that D-serine is the endogenous ligand for the 'glycine' binding site of the N-methyl-D-aspartate (NMDA) subtype of glutamate receptor. This chapter reviews evidence that this is the case, not only in brain, but also in the retina. Information is provided documenting the location of D-serine and serine racemase, in retinal Müller glial cells. The transport of D-serine by these cells is discussed. New evidence demonstrating that D-serine and serine racemase are present in retinal neurons is provided, along with data evaluating the effects of excess D-serine on retinal neuronal viability.

8.2 Introduction

The retina is the light-sensitive tissue of the eyeball. It develops from two layers of the invaginated optic vesicle. Figure 8.1 provides a photomicrograph of the mammalian retina. The outermost lamina becomes a single layer of epithelial cells, termed the retinal pigment epithelial cell layer. It is sandwiched between a vascular bed, the choriocapillaris, and the inner retina, frequently referred to as the neural retina. The neural retina is stratified into nuclear layers, which harbour cell bodies and plexiform layers that represent synapses between cells. There are five broad classes of neuronal cells and at least three types of glial cells. The cell bodies of retinal photoreceptors (rods and cones), specialized to capture photons of light, occupy the outer nuclear layer and their processes comprise the inner and outer segments. In the outer plexiform layer, photoreceptor cells synapse with first-order neurons of the visual system, the bipolar cells whose cell bodies are found in the inner nuclear layer. Other neurons in the inner nuclear layer include horizontal cells that modulate the activity of bipolar cells and amacrine cells that modulate the synaptic transmission from bipolar cells to ganglion cells. Synaptic connections to ganglion cells are present in the inner plexiform layer. Ganglion cells are the second-order neurons of the visual pathway and their cell bodies occupy the innermost cellular layer (ganglion cell layer) of the retina. Their axons form the optic nerve and are visualized as the nerve fibre layer in retinal histological sections. The cell bodies of some amacrine cells can also be found in the ganglion cell layer. The major glial cell of the retina,

---

* E-mail address: sbsmith@georgiahealth.edu

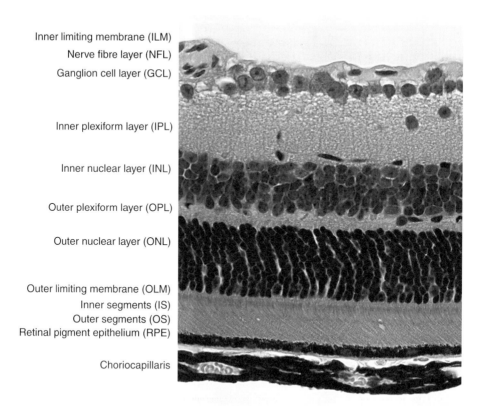

Fig. 8.1. Haematoxylin and eosin-stained JB-4 plastic embedded section of C57Bl/6 adult mouse retina. Note the well-organized, laminar appearance of the retina, distinguished by its orderly nuclear and plexiform (synaptic) layers. Light passes through the thickness of the retina to strike the outer segments of photoreceptor cells initiating a conversion of the photic stimulus into a neuronal stimulus. The impulse travels from the photoreceptor to bipolar cells of the inner nuclear layer, and then to ganglion cells whose axons form the nerve fibre layer that gives rise to the optic nerve.

the Müller cell, is radially oriented and its endfeet form the inner and outer retinal limiting membranes. Müller cells subserve many of the metabolic, ionic, and extracellular buffering requirements of adjacent neurons. Müller cells play a key role in transporting substances from the extracellular milieu into the cell and *vice versa*. Other glial cell types in the retina are astrocytes and microglia.

In the retina, L-glutamate serves as the major excitatory transmitter; it is used in the retinal forward transmission of visual signals by photoreceptors, bipolar, and ganglion cells (Massey and Miller, 1987; Massey and Miller, 1990). Receptors for glutamate are broadly divided into the two categories ionotropic and metabotropic, depending upon whether the channel is gated directly or indirectly. The ionotropic glutamate receptors are further subdivided into three classes, NMDA, AMPA, and kainate, based upon the synthetic agonists that activate them (N-methyl-D-aspartate, alpha-amino-3-hydroxy-5-methyl-isoxazole-4-propionic acid, and kainate).

The focus of this review, the NMDA subtype of glutamate receptor, is arguably one of the most important synaptic receptors in the CNS. This chapter reviews recent evidence that D-serine is an endogenous ligand for the NMDA receptor in the retina. It provides an overview of data showing that both retinal glial cells and retinal neurons express D-serine and serine racemase, the enzyme that converts L-serine to D-serine. Mechanisms by which cells take up D-serine are discussed, as well as the possible effects of excessive levels of D-serine on retinal neuronal viability.

8.3 NMDA Receptor and D-Serine as a Co-agonist

NMDA receptors are heterotetrameric protein complexes, typically comprising two NR1 and two glutamate-binding NR2 subunits. NMDA receptor variety is provided in large part by the four different NR2 subunits (NR2A-D) (Monyer et al., 1994). In addition to the binding of glutamate, NMDA receptors require the binding of a co-agonist on the NR1 subunit to exert physiological actions. The obligatory co-agonist was identified originally as glycine (Johnson and Ascher, 1987). Indeed, this 'glycine binding' site must be occupied to allow glutamate to open the ion channel of the NMDA receptor. Subsequent studies revealed that other compounds could serve as a glutamate co-agonist; indeed some were more effective than glycine. Included among these compounds was D-serine (Kemp and Leeson, 1993; Czepita et al., 1996).

The observation that D-serine could serve as a co-agonist of the NMDA receptor *in vitro* was intriguing. While it was well known that bacteria and many invertebrate species use both D- and L-enantiomers of amino acids for cellular functions, it was generally believed that higher organisms had a more restricted stereospecificity and were confined to the use of L-amino acids. D-Amino acids detected in vertebrates were presumed to arise from intestinal flora or ingested material (Corrigan, 1969). Hashimoto et al. (1992) asked whether D-serine was present in the brain, and found that nearly 25% of the total brain serum was the D-enantiomer. These investigators were the first to suggest that D-serine may be an endogenous, co-agonist for the NMDA receptor. McBain et al., (1989) reported that D-serine was much more effective than L-serine as a co-agonist of the binding site.

An important additional indicator that D-serine might play a key role in NMDA receptor activation came in the form of discovery of the enzyme that catalyses the conversion of L-serine to D-serine (Wolosker et al., 1999a,b). This enzyme, serine racemase, is a 37 kDa protein and was isolated from rat brain. In addition, the enzyme D-amino acid oxidase (D-AAOX) is also present in the brain and represents the principal pathway of serine degradation. D-serine has been studied in other regions of the brain including spinal cord and cerebellum. Levels of D-serine are relatively high in the neonatal rat cerebellum, though levels decrease as the animals develop (Rabacchi et al.,1992).

8.4 D-Serine in the Retina

For almost a decade, studies related to D-serine centred on its presence and role in the brain. In 2003, however, Stevens and colleagues investigated D-serine and serine racemase in the retina for the first time. Their findings implicate D-serine as an NMDA receptor co-agonist in the mammalian and non-mammalian retina (Stevens et al., 2003). D-serine and serine racemase were analysed comprehensively in rats and larval tiger salamanders using immunohistochemistry, immunoblotting, analytical chemistry (HPLC), and electrophysiology. D-serine and serine racemase were localized to Müller glial cells and astrocytes. Exogenous D-serine enhanced NMDA receptor responses and modulated light-evoked activity in retinal ganglion cells. It is noteworthy that several years prior to the report by Stevens, Harsanyi and colleagues (1996) were experimenting with NMDA receptor activation in a fish model and used D-serine in their superfusate. They detected horizontal cell activity in the presence of D-serine, but did not explore this as an NMDA receptor co-agonist. Elegant analytical studies of D-serine levels in the tiger salamander retina complemented the findings of Stevens. O'Brien et al. (2003) used microdialysis-capillary electrophoresis with laser-induced fluorescence detection in a sheath flow detection cell to analyse D-serine levels in their model system. Levels of D-serine in retinal homogenates of larval tiger salamander retinas averaged 11.9 $nmol\,mg^{-1}$ protein. The investigators were also able to study the amount of D-serine released from the isolated retinal preparations (O'Brien et al., 2004). These early studies of D-serine in the retina have been reviewed by Miller (2004). In addition to analyses in rat and salamander, D-serine has been detected in human (fetal) retina (Diaz et al., 2007) and in mouse retina (Dun et al., 2008).

8.5 Mechanisms of D-Serine Uptake in the Retina

The initial studies of mechanisms used by cells to transport D-serine were performed in the brain and investigated the potential role of a variety of neutral amino acid transporters (ASCT1, ASCT2, system A, system L). Studies by Hayashi et al. (1997) and by Ribeiro et al. (2002) provided functional evidence that D-serine uptake is mediated by the ASC type of transporters. No functional experiments were performed to distinguish between ASCT1 and ASCT2 transporters, nor were molecular analyses performed to determine which transporter mediated D-serine transport.

Using whole-retina preparations from the larval tiger salamander, O'Brien et al. (2005) examined whether neutral amino acid transporters mediate D-serine uptake. They argued that an amino acid exchanger that can take up and release D-serine would offer a mechanism for regulation of D-serine levels in the retina. In experiments using capillary electrophoresis, D-serine uptake was shown to be dependent upon Na$^+$, thus ruling out the Na$^+$-independent asc-1 transporter (SLC7A10, a transporter system for small neutral L- and D-amino acids), as a transporter for D-serine in retina. The observation that Na$^+$-dependent uptake of D-serine was inhibited by L-alanine, L-serine, and L-cysteine was consistent with transport mediated by the ASC types of neutral amino acid transporters. The ASCT1 (SLC1A4, alias: SATT) and ASCT2 (SLC1A5, alias: ATB^0) transport systems are Na$^+$-dependent and have high affinity for alanine, serine, and cysteine. They exhibit distinct substrate selectivity: in addition to the common substrates of ASCT transporters, ASCT2 also accepts glutamine and asparagine as high affinity substrates, whereas ASCT1 does not (Kanai and Hediger, 2003).

The studies by O'Brien et al. (2005) did not distinguish between the ASCT1 and the ASCT2 transporters, nor did they rule out transport by a unique amino acid transporter ATB$^{0,+}$, which is energized by Na$^+$- and Cl$^-$-gradients and membrane potential. ATB$^{0,+}$ (SLC6A14) has broad substrate specificity and concentrative ability and recognizes neutral as well as cationic amino acids. Both ASCT2 and ATB$^{0,+}$ have been shown to mediate D-serine uptake (Hatanaka et al., 2002; Thongsong et al., 2005). Immunohistochemical analysis of ocular tissues, using an antibody specific for ATB$^{0,+}$, provided evidence that this transporter is present in the mammalian retina (Hatanaka et al., 2004). Given our familiarity with analysis of transporter systems and our interest in retinal Müller cells, we analysed the mechanism(s) of D-serine uptake in a rat Müller cell line and in primary cultures of Müller cells isolated from mouse retina (Dun et al., 2007a). We used functional methods to distinguish among the three likely transporter candidates (ASCT1, ASCT2, ATB$^{0,+}$), and used molecular methods to establish the identity of the transporter likely to be responsible for the uptake and/or efflux of D-serine in Müller cells. We detected serine racemase mRNA and protein in rMC-1 and primary mouse Müller cells. We examined the uptake of D-serine uptake in the cell line and in the primary Müller cells. We found that D-serine uptake in rMC-1 cells is absolutely dependent on Na$^+$ and that Cl$^-$ is not obligatory for the process (Fig. 8.2a). The Na$^+$-activation kinetics were analysed to determine the Na$^+$: D-serine stoichiometry. The dependence of D-serine uptake on Na$^+$ concentration displayed a hyperbolic relationship and the analysis of the data by the Hill equation yielded a value of 0.8 ± 0.03 for the Hill coefficient, indicating an Na$^+$: D-serine stoichiometry of 1:1 (Fig. 8.2b). We confirmed the ion dependence of D-serine uptake in primary Müller cells. The uptake in these cells exhibited ion dependence that was similar to that observed in rMC-1 cells (Fig. 8.2c).

We examined the substrate specificity of the transport system responsible for D-serine uptake in retinal Müller cells and found that uptake of D-serine was inhibited markedly by L-alanine, L-serine, L-cysteine, L-asparagine, and L-glutamine. The anionic amino acids (L-aspartate and L-glutamate), and cationic amino acids (L-lysine and L-arginine) failed to inhibit the uptake of D-serine, showing

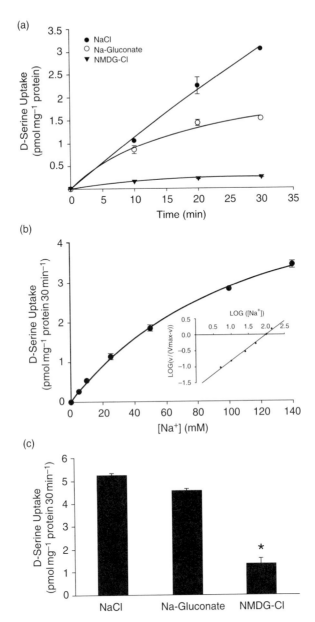

Fig. 8.2. Ion dependence of D-serine uptake in retinal Müller cells. (a) Time course and ion dependence of D-serine uptake in rMC-1 cells. Uptake of [^{3}H] D-serine (0.1 µM) in rMC-1 cells incubated at various times in NaCl-, Na-gluconate-, and NMDG-Cl-containing uptake buffers. (b) Na$^+$-activation kinetics of D-serine uptake in rMC-1 cells. Uptake of [^{3}H] D-serine (0.1 µM) was determined following a 30 min incubation in uptake medium containing increasing concentrations of Na$^+$ (0–140 mM). The concentration of Cl$^-$ was kept constant at 140 mM (inset, Hill plot). (c) Ion dependence of D-serine uptake in primary Müller cells; uptake of [^{3}H] D-serine (0.1 µM) was determined following a 30 min incubation in NaCl-, Na-gluconate- and NMDG-Cl-containing uptake medium. Values are means ± SE for three determinations from two independent experiments. (*Significantly different from NaCl value, $p < 0.05$.) (Adapted from Dun et al., 2007a, and used with permission.)

that the transport process that mediates the uptake of D-serine in Müller cells is specific for neutral amino acids and excludes anionic and cationic amino acids. Our studies ruled out the participation of ATB$^{0,+}$ in the uptake process, leaving two family members of the ASC transporter group as likely mediators of D-serine uptake in Müller cells. The mRNAs encoding ASCT1 and ASCT2 were both expressed in the rMC-1 and primary Müller cells. To distinguish between the two isoforms, we used a battery of known substrates for ASCT1 and ASCT2. Owing to the finding that uptake of D-serine was inhibited by not only alanine, serine, and cysteine, but also by asparagine and glutamine, substrates specific for ASCT2, ASCT2 emerged as the mediator of D-serine transport in Müller cells. Our immunodetection analyses confirmed the presence of ASCT2 in neural retinal and in primary Müller cells. Our studies with the *Xenopus laevis* oocyte heterologous expression system and the cloned human ASCT2 showed that ASCT2 was able to mediate not only the uptake, but also the efflux, of D-serine, a distinct characteristic of ASC-type transporters. Thus, these findings provided definitive evidence that ASCT2 is the transporter for D-serine in retinal Müller cells.

8.6 D-Serine and Serine Racemase in Retinal Neurons

The early analyses of D-serine and serine racemase were performed in the brain, and immunohistochemical studies localized D-serine exclusively to type II astrocytes in the brain (Schell *et al.*, 1995). Shortly thereafter, serine racemase was shown to be enriched in cortical astrocytes (Wolosker *et al.*, 1999a,b). These findings were supportive of the proposed dynamic role of glial cells in influencing neuronal activity, particularly as a third element of the chemical synapse. In the retina, the initial reports of D-serine localized it and serine racemase to Müller glial cells. This location fit well with postulated mechanisms of glial to neuron signalling. Newman speculated that release of D-serine by Müller cells could facilitate NMDA synaptic transmission by binding to the NMDA co-agonist site (Newman, 2004).

Interestingly, two years after the discovery of serine racemase, Yasuda and colleagues published a brief report that D-serine was present not only in glial cells, but also in some neurons of the rat brain (Yasuda *et al.*, 2001). Using highly sensitive immunohistochemical methods, they detected D-serine at low levels in pyramidal neurons of the cerebral cortex and in neurons of the nucleus of trapezoid body. A few years later, other groups examined the notion that D-serine is localized exclusively to glial cells more comprehensively. Investigators from Wolosker's lab provided unambiguous evidence for the presence of D-serine and serine racemase in neurons as well as in glia (Kartvelishvily *et al.*, 2006). Using neurons purified from the embryonic cerebral cortex, they found that virtually all of these cells were immunoreactive for serine racemase. They also detected D-serine in their neuronal cell cultures. At about the same time, studies from Hashimoto's lab were published, reporting the expression of serine racemase in primary cultures of neurons from rat brain (Yoshikawa *et al.*, 2006). High levels of D-serine were reported also during the first three weeks of postnatal development in glial cells of rat vestibular nuclei (Puyal *et al.*, 2006). This time period corresponds to an intense period of plasticity and synaptogenesis. Interestingly, upon maturation, D-serine levels were low and mainly localized in neuronal cell bodies and dendrites.

The reports that D-serine and serine racemase are present in neurons isolated from the brain, coupled with the finding that the expression of D-serine may be developmentally regulated, led us to investigate the neuronal expression of D-serine and its synthesizing enzyme in the retina, specifically focusing on expression in retinal ganglion cells (Dun *et al.*, 2008). It is well established that the processes of Müller cells span much of the retinal thickness and ensheath the neurons of the retina, including the ganglion cells. Our studies demonstrated robust serine racemase expression and appreciable D-serine content in the ganglion cell layer, as well as in other neurons of the intact retina and in the purified cultures of ganglion cells.

As shown in Fig. 8.3, serine racemase was detected in abundance in the ganglion cell layer of mouse retina. Serine racemase also localized to the inner segments of photoreceptor

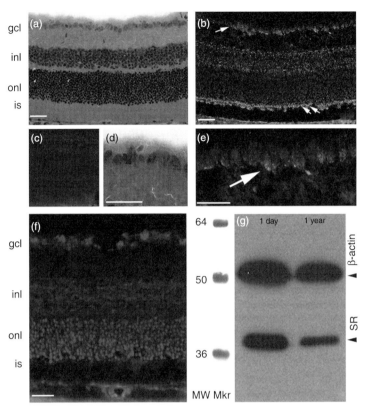

Fig. 8.3. Immunodetection of serine racemase in intact mouse retina. Cryosections of retinas were prepared from animals at 3 and 18 weeks of age. (a) Haematoxylin- and eosin-stained section of three-week-old mouse retina. (gcl, ganglion cell layer; inl, inner nuclear layer; onl, outer nuclear layer; is, inner segment). (b) Three-week-old mouse retina immunostained with an antibody against serine racemase followed by Alexa Fluor® 555 secondary antibody. Bright fluorescence indicates positive immunoreactivity. Immunopositive signals specific for serine racemase are present in the ganglion cell layer (single arrow), inner nuclear layer, and the inner limiting membrane/inner segment region (double arrows). (c) Incubation of cryosections with antibody pre-incubated with blocking peptide yielded no immunopositive reaction. (d) Higher magnification of H&E-stained retina showing the ganglion cells. (e) Higher magnification of immunopositive reaction for serine racemase in ganglion cells. Arrow points to intense immunopositive reaction. (f) Cryosection of retina from adult mouse (18 weeks) subjected to immunohistochemistry with the antibody against serine racemase. The immunodetection procedure and image capturing was identical to that for the 3-week-old retina shown in panel (b). Note the marked decrease in immunopositive reaction in the adult retina compared with the 3-week-old retina (b and e). (g) Immunoblotting of neural retina for serine racemase. Proteins were isolated from neural retinas of 1-day- and 1-year-old mice, subjected to sodium dodecyl sulphate–polyacrylamide gel electrophoresis (SDS-PAGE), transferred to membranes, and incubated with a commercially available antibody against serine racemase. Serine racemase (SR; M_r = 38 kDa) was detected in both preparations, but was more abundant in younger mouse retinas versus the 1-year old. β-Actin (M_r = 50 kDa) served as the loading control. [MW Mkr = pre-stained markers of known molecular weights (kDa), magnification bar = 50 μm]. (Adapted from Dun et al., 2008, and used with permission; original figure shows panels in colour.)

cells and the inner limiting membrane (Fig. 8.3b). It was detected in some of the cells of the inner nuclear layer. Incubation of sections with the antibody that had been pre-incubated with the serine racemase blocking peptide (Santa Cruz Corp.) yielded minimal staining. Our data were acquired in retinas harvested from three-week-old mice. When the pattern of immunostaining for serine racemase was examined in adult mouse retina (18-week-old), the expression levels were considerably less. Figure 8.4f shows a photomicrograph of an adult retina in which the immunodetection procedure was performed exactly as for the retinas of the young mice shown in Figs 8.3b, c, and e panels (including exposure time in capturing the image). There was minimal labelling in the ganglion cell layer of the adult retina. There was a very faint immunopositive reaction associated with some of the cells in the inner nuclear layer, but it was reduced dramatically compared with that observed in the three-week-old retinas. These data suggested that there is a developmental regulation of serine racemase expression in retina such that the protein levels are much higher in neonatal and young mice compared with mature animals. This was investigated further using a more quantitative method (Western blotting, Fig. 8.3g). For these experiments, we isolated retinal proteins from very young (1 day) and very old (1 year) mouse retinas and subjected them to sodium dodecyl sulphate–polyacrylamide gel electrophoresis (SDS-PAGE). After transfer to nitrocellulose membranes and incubation with the antibody against serine racemase, the protein was detected at robust levels in the neural retina from 1-day-old mice, but the level of detection was reduced in the 1-year-old mouse. When data were normalized using β-actin as a loading control and quantified by densitometry, the ratio of serine racemase to β-actin at 1 day was 0.7 and at 1 year was 0.4 (Fig. 8.3g). Thus our studies suggested that serine racemase levels are also developmentally regulated in the retina, with high levels detected during the early postnatal period, but diminishing considerably as the retina matures.

In performing these studies, we recognized that the close proximity of glial processes with neuronal processes complicates the interpretation of immunohistochemical data. Therefore, in addition to studying D-serine and serine racemase gene and protein expression in intact tissue, we used an immunopanning procedure to isolate ganglion cells from the neonatal mouse retina and investigated serine racemase expression and D-serine content in these neuronal cells.

Proteins were isolated from these immunopanned ganglion cells, subjected to SDS-PAGE, transferred to membranes, and incubated with commercially available monoclonal or polyclonal antibodies against serine racemase (Figs 8.4a and 8.4b, respectively.) Primary Müller cells known to express serine racemase served as a positive control. A band of ~38 kDa, consistent with the published size of the monomeric form of serine racemase, was detected in both Müller cells and RGCs using both antibodies. We confirmed the neuronal phenotype of the isolated cells immunocytochemically using NF-L (Fig. 8.4c, note the intense fluorescence of the cell body and the axon (arrowhead)). These cells were immunopositive for serine racemase using two different antibodies (Figs 8.4d, 8.4e). Figure 8.4f depicts immunocytochemical analysis of serine racemase in the neuronal processes, which can be better visualized if the exposure time of the camera is increased; the cell body labelling is saturated (extremely intense fluorescence), axon is more visible (arrowhead). These primary ganglion cells are positive for the ganglion cell marker Thy 1.2 (Fig. 8.4g), but are negative for the amacrine cell marker ChAT (choline acetyltransferase, Fig. 8.4h).

This was the first report of neuronal expression of D-serine and serine racemase in the vertebrate retina and suggested an important contribution of neuronal D-serine during retinal development. Others have confirmed our findings. Takayasu *et al.* (2008) used the rat retina as a model system and employed *in situ* hybridization techniques to detect serine racemase mRNA. They found expression in ganglion cells, amacrine cells, bipolar cells, horizontal cells, and Müller cells of the retina as well as in the astrocytes of the optic nerve head and the lamina cribrosa. They interpreted their findings to suggest that both neuron- and glia-derived D-serine could modulate neurotransmission via the glycine site of the N-methyl-D-aspartate receptors in the retina.

8.7 Role of D-Serine in the Retina

Recent elegant studies have provided compelling evidence that endogenous D-serine plays an essential role as a co-agonist for NMDA receptors, allowing it to contribute to light-evoked responses of retinal ganglion cells (Gustafson *et al.*, 2007). In subsequent studies analysing the retina of the tiger salamander

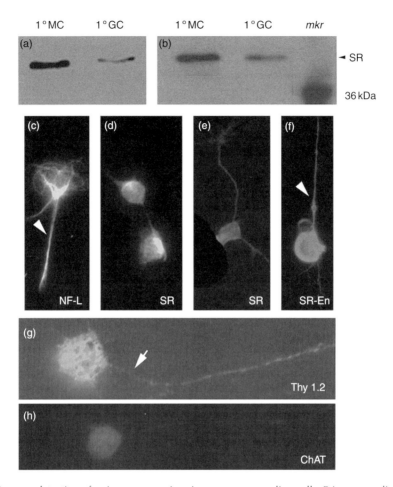

Fig. 8.4. Immunodetection of serine racemase in primary mouse ganglion cells. Primary ganglion cells (1°GC) were isolated by immunopanning from 1–3-day-old mouse retinas and were used for immunoblotting (a, b) or immunocytochemistry (c–h). Proteins were isolated, subjected to SDS-PAGE, transferred to membranes, and incubated with commercially available monoclonal (a) or polyclonal (b) antibodies against serine racemase (SR). Primary Müller cells (1°MC) known to express serine racemase were used as positive controls. A band of ~38 kDa, consistent with the published size of the monomeric form of serine racemase, was detected in both Müller cells and ganglion cells using the two antibodies. (c) Immunocytochemical detection of NF-L, a marker for neurons, in the cultured ganglion cells. Note the intense fluorescence of the cell body and the axon (arrowhead). (d) Immunocytochemical detection of serine racemase in ganglion cells using the Alexa Fluor® 488 secondary antibody. The intense fluorescence reflects the positive reaction in the cell bodies. (e) Immunocytochemical detection of serine racemase in ganglion cells using the Alexa Fluor® 555 for serine racemase; labelling of processes is minimal. (f) Neuronal processes of ganglion cells can be visualized well if the exposure time of the camera is increased; the cell body labelling is saturated (extremely intense fluorescence), axon is more visible (arrowhead). (g) Primary ganglion cells are positive for Thy 1.2 as indicated by fluorescence; arrow points to the axon. (h) Incubation of the cells with an antibody to detect choline acetyltransferase (ChAT), an amacrine cell marker, revealed no positive labelling (which would fluoresce if present). 1°, primary; MC, Müller cell; GC, ganglion cell; arrow heads point to axons; NF-L, neurofilament light polypeptide; SR, serine racemase, SR-En, serine racemase immunofluorescence with increased exposure time. (Adapted from Dun et al., 2008, with permission; original figure shows fluorescent images in colour.)

(*Ambystoma tigrinum*), this same team of investigators blocked the synthesis of D-serine by exposing the retina to phenazine ethosulphate and validated the changes in the tissue levels of D-serine using capillary electrophoresis methods. They found that phenazine ethosulphate exposure decreased D-serine levels in the retina by about 50% and significantly reduced the NMDA receptor contribution to light responses of the inner retina. Theirs was the first report of a linkage between D-serine synthesis and NMDA receptor activity in the vertebrate retina (Stevens *et al.*, 2010). Daniels and Baldridge (2010) have shown that D-serine enhances glutamate-induced calcium responses in immmunopanned retinal ganglion cells. Endogenous D-serine degradation by treatment with D-amino acid oxidase caused ~45% decrease in NMDA-induced responses, which were reversible by co-application of D-serine. Interestingly, in their *in vitro* model, D-serine and glycine were equally effective in enhancing glutamatergic calcium responses. Endogenous D-serine contributes to NMDAR activation in retinal wholemounts and some but not all retinal ganglion cells may experience saturating levels of D-serine or glycine.

8.8 Role of D-Serine and Serine Racemase in Neuronal Cell Death

It is well documented that glutamate, under certain circumstances, can contribute to disease. Excessive amounts of glutamate are highly toxic to neurons. Brief exposure to high concentrations of glutamate to cells in tissue culture can kill many neurons by an action called glutamate excitotoxicity. In many cell types, glutamate excitotoxicity is thought to result predominately from excessive inflow of Ca^{2+} through NMDA-type channels. High concentrations of intracellular Ca^{2+} may activate Ca^{2+}-dependent proteases and phospholipases and may produce free radicals that are toxic to cells. Excessive glutamate has been implicated in various diseases such as stroke and Huntington's disease, and where the retina is involved, diabetic retinopathy. The possible role of glutamate (and other excitotoxic amino acids such as homocysteine) in neuronal cell death associated with diabetic retinopathy has prompted a number of studies in our laboratory, including investigation of D-serine in the retina. Sasabe *et al.* (2007) published data showing that D-serine plays a key role in the glutamate toxicity associated with amyotrophic lateral sclerosis.

We were interested in determining whether D-serine would augment glutamate-induced toxicity in primary ganglion cells. To examine this, we isolated ganglion cells using our published method (Dun *et al.*, 2007b) and exposed the cells to varying concentrations of D-serine [1, 25, or 50 μM] in the presence/absence of glutamate [10 or 20 μM]. Cells were treated for 18 h and then analysed *in situ* by detection of DNA Fragmentation (TUNEL assay). The TUNEL assay was performed using the ApopTAG® Fluorescein *In Situ* Apoptosis Detection Kit (Chemicon, Temecula, California, USA) following our published method (Dun *et al.*, 2007b). Cells were viewed by epifluorescence using a Zeiss Axioplan–2 microscope, equipped with the axiovision programme, and an HRM camera. Cells in five randomly chosen fields for each coverslip were counted for positive fluorescent indicating apoptosis. Three coverslips were examined for each treatment group. The data from these experiments are shown in Fig. 8.5. We found that exposure of ganglion cells to D-serine decreased their viability, especially at 25 and 50 μM concentrations. Exposing ganglion cells to higher levels of glutamate [20 μM] induced significant death of primary ganglion cells. Given that ganglion cell death is a feature of diabetic retinopathy, we investigated the levels of serine racemase in retinas of the diabetic *Ins2^{Akita}*/- mouse. We found that the levels of this enzyme were similar in mice 8 and 18 weeks post-onset of diabetes (unpublished observations) to those levels determined for non-diabetic control animals. Whether alterations in serine racemase are detectable in other models of retinal degeneration remains to be investigated.

Earlier studies from the Akaike laboratory examined the contribution of endogenous glycine site NMDA agonists in the cell death of retinal neurons (Hama *et al.*, 2006) and neurons of the brain (Katsuki *et al.*, 2004). In studies of the retina, the investigators quantified surviving retinal ganglion cells following injections into the superior colliculus of a

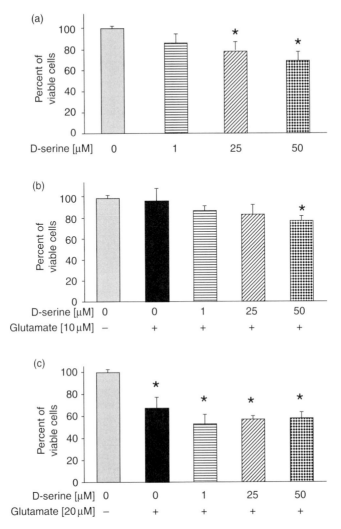

Fig. 8.5. Effects of D-serine on retinal ganglion cell viability. Retinal ganglion cells were isolated from neonatal mice by immunopanning. The primary neuronal cultures were maintained for several days in neurobasal media and then exposed to varying concentrations of D-serine, or D-serine and L-glutamate. Cell viability was determined using the TUNEL assay and the data were expressed as the percentage of cells that were alive compared to all cells in the field. For each experiment, at least five fields were examined and the experiments were performed three times. (*Significantly different from control, $p < 0.05$.)

competitive antagonist of the glycine-binding site following administration of 200 nM NMDA. They showed that blocking the glycine site rescued ganglion cells from excitotoxic death. In addition, they found that retinas exposed to 20 nM NMDA in the presence of 10 nM glycine or 10 nM D-serine increased the death of ganglion cells. They concluded that ganglion cell death under excitotoxic conditions depended upon the levels of glycine and D-serine.

8.9 Conclusions

The NDMA sub-type of glutamate receptor plays a key role in neurotransmission in the retina as well as in the brain. Though for years it was thought that glycine was the endogenous agonist required for activation of the receptor, evidence over the past decade indicates that D-serine is at least as potent an activator of this site as glycine. Indeed, recent work on the retina suggests that D-serine is the endogenous co-agonist of the receptor. While originally thought to be limited to glial cells of the retina, it appears as if D-serine and its synthesizing enzyme serine racemase are present in retinal neurons also, including the ganglion cells. Future analyses of D-serine are likely to uncover the contributions of this NMDA receptor ligand to retinal disease.

8.10 Acknowledgements

This work was supported by NIH R01 EY014560 to S.B.S.

References

Corrigan, J.J. (1969) D-amino acids in animals. *Science* 164,142–149.

Czepita, D., Daw, N.W. and Reid, S.N. (1996) Glycine at the NMDA receptor in cat visual cortex: saturation and changes with age. *Journal of Neurophysiology* 75, 311–317

Daniels, B.A. and Baldridge, W.H. (2010) d-Serine enhancement of NMDA receptor-mediated calcium increases in rat retinal ganglion cells. *Journal of Neurochemistry* 112, 1180–1189.

Diaz, C.M., Macnab, L.T., Williams, S.M., Sullivan, R.K. and Pow, D.V. (2007) EAAT1 and D-serine expression are early features of human retinal development. *Experimental Eye Research* 84, 876–885.

Dun, Y., Mysona, B., Itagaki, S., Martin-Studdard, A., Ganapathy, V. and Smith S.B. (2007a) Functional and molecular analysis of D-serine transport in retinal Müller cells. *Experimental Eye Research* 84, 191–199.

Dun, Y., Thangaraju, M., Prasad, P., Ganapathy, V. and Smith S.B. (2007b) Prevention of excitotoxicity in primary retinal ganglion cells by (+)-pentazocine, a sigma receptor-1 specific ligand. *Investigative Ophthalmology and Visual Science* 48, 4785–4794.

Dun, Y., Duplantier, J., Roon, P., Martin, P.M., Ganapathy, V. and Smith S.B. (2008) Serine racemase expression and D-serine content are developmentally regulated in neuronal ganglion cells of the retina. *Journal of Neurochemistry* 104, 970–978.

Gustafson, E.C., Stevens, E.R., Wolosker, H. and Miller, R.F. (2007) Endogenous D-serine contributes to NMDA-receptor-mediated light-evoked responses in the vertebrate retina. *Journal of Neurophysiology* 98, 122–130.

Hama, Y., Katsuki, H., Tochikawa, Y., Suminaka, C., Kume, T., Akaike, A. (2006) Contribution of endogenous glycine site NMDA agonists to excitotoxic retinal damage in vivo. *Neuroscience Research* 56, 279–285.

Harsanyi, K., Wang, Y. and Mangel, S.C. (1996) Activation of NMDA receptors produces dopamine-mediated changes in fish retinal horizontal cell light responses. *Journal of Neurophysiology* 75, 629–647

Hashimoto, A., Nishikawa, T., Hayashi, T., Fujii, N., Harada, K., Oka, T. and Takahashi, K. (1992). The presence of free D-serine in rat brain. *FEBS Letters* 296, 33–36.

Hatanaka, T., Huang, W., Nakanishi, T., Bridges, C.C., Smith, S.B., Prasad, P.D., Ganapathy, M.E. *et al.* (2002) Transport of d-serine via the amino acid transporter ATB(0,+) expressed in the colon. *Biochemical and Biophysical Research Communications* 291, 291–295.

Hatanaka, T., Haramura, M., Fei, Y.J., Miyauchi, S., Bridges, C.C., Ganapathy, P.S., Smith, S.B., *et al.* (2004) Transport of amino acid-based prodrugs by the Na$^+$- and Cl$^-$-coupled amino acid transporter ATB0,+ and expression of the transporter in tissues amenable for drug delivery. *Journal of Pharmacology and Experimental Therapeutics* 308, 1138–1147.

Hayashi, F., Takahashi, K. and Nishikawa, T. (1997) Uptake of d- and l-serine in C6 glioma cells. *Neuroscience Letters* 239, 85–88.

Johnson, J.W. and Ascher, P. (1987) Glycine potentiates the NMDA response in cultured mouse brain neurons. *Nature* 325, 529–531.

Kanai, Y. and Hediger, M.A. (2003). The glutamate and neutral amino acid transporter family: physiological and pharmacological implications. *European Journal of Pharmacology* 479, 237–247.

Kartvelishvily, E., Shleper, M., Balan, L., Dumin, E. and Wolosker, H. (2006) Neuron-derived d-serine release provides a novel means to activate n-methyl-d-aspartate receptors. *Journal of Biological Chemistry* 281, 14151–14162.

Katsuki, H., Nonaka, M., Shirakawa, H., Kume, T. and Akaike A. (2004) Endogenous D-serine is involved in induction of neuronal death by N-methyl-D-aspartate and simulated ischemia in rat cerebrocortical slices. *Journal of Pharmacology and Experimental Therapeutics* 311, 836–844.

Kemp, J.A. and Leeson, P.D. (1993) The glycine site of the NMDA receptor - five years on. *Trends in Pharmacological Science* 14, 20–25.

Massey, S.C. and Miller, R.F. (1987) Excitatory amino acid receptors of rod- and cone-driven horizontal cells in the rabbit retina. *Journal of Neurophysiology* 57, 645–659.

Massey, S.C. and Miller, R.F. (1990) N-methyl-D-aspartate receptors of ganglion cells in rabbit retina. *Journal of Neurophysiology* 63, 16–30.

McBain, C.J., Kleckner, N.W., Wyrick, S. and Dingledine, R. (1989). Structural requirements for activation of the glycine coagonist site of N-methyl-D-aspartate receptors expressed in Xenopus oocytes. *Molecular Pharmacology* 36, 556–565.

Miller, R.F. (2004) D-Serine as a glial modulator of nerve cells. *Glia* 47, 275–283.

Monyer, H., Burnashev, N., Laurie, D.J., Sakmann, B. and Seeburg, P.H. (1994) Developmental and regional expression in the rat brain and functional properties of four NMDA receptors. *Neuron* 12, 529–540.

Newman, E.A. (2004) A dialogue between glia and neurons in the retina: modulation of neuronal excitability. *Neuron Glia Biology* 1, 245–252.

O'Brien, K.B., Esguerra, M., Klug, C.T., Miller, R.F. and Bowser, M.T. (2003) A high-throughput on-line microdialysis-capillary assay for D-serine. *Electrophoresis* 24, 1227–1235.

O'Brien, K.B., Esguerra, M., Miller, R.F. and Bowser, M.T. (2004) Monitoring neurotransmitter release from isolated retinas using online microdialysis-capillary electrophoresis. *Analytical Chemistry* 76, 5069–5074.

O'Brien, K.B., Miller, R.F. and Bowser, M.T. (2005) D-Serine uptake by isolated retinas is consistent with ASCT-mediated transport. *Neuroscience Letters* 385, 58–63.

Puyal, J., Martineau, M., Mothet, J.P., Nicolas, M.T. and Raymond, J. (2006) Changes in D-serine levels and localization during postnatal development of the rat vestibular nuclei. *Journal of Comparative Neurology* 497, 610–621.

Rabacchi, S., Bailly, Y., Delhaye-Bouchaud, N. and Mariani J. (1992). Involvement of the N-methyl D-aspartate (NMDA) receptor in synapse elimination during cerebellar development. *Science* 256, 1823–1825.

Ribeiro, C.S., Reis, M., Panizzutti, R., de Miranda, J. and Wolosker, H. (2002). Glial transport of the neuromodulator d-serine. *Brain Research* 929, 202–209.

Sasabe, J., Chiba, T., Yamada, M., Okamoto, K., Nishimoto, I., Matsuoka, M. and Aiso, S. (2007) D-serine is a key determinant of glutamate toxicity in amyotrophic lateral sclerosis. *EMBO Journal* 26, 4149–4159.

Schell, M.J., Molliver, M.E. and Snyder, S.H. (1995) D-serine, an endogenous synaptic modulator: localization to astrocytes and glutamate-stimulated release. *Proceedings of the National Academy of Sciences USA* 92, 3948–3952.

Stevens, E.R., Esguerra, M., Kim, P.M., Newman, E.A., Snyder, S.H., Zahs, K.R. and Miller, R.F. (2003) D-serine and serine racemase are present in the vertebrate retina and contribute to the physiological activation of NMDA receptors. *Proceedings of the National Academy of Sciences USA* 100, 6789–6794.

Stevens, E.R., Gustafson, E.C., Sullivan, S.J., Esguerra, M. and Miller, R.F. (2010) Light-evoked NMDA receptor-mediated currents are reduced by blocking D-serine synthesis in the salamander retina. *Neuroreport* 21, 239–244.

Takayasu, N., Yoshikawa, M., Watanabe, M., Tsukamoto, H., Suzuki, T., Kobayashi, H. and Noda, S. (2008) The serine racemase mRNA is expressed in both neurons and glial cells of the rat retina. *Archives of Histology and Cytology* 71, 123–129.

Thongsong, B., Subramanian, R.K., Ganapathy V. and Prasad, P.D. (2005) Inhibition of amino acid transport system a by interleukin-1beta in trophoblasts. *Journal of the Society of Gynecological Investigation* 12, 495–503.

Wolosker, H., Blackshaw, S. and Snyder, S.H. (1999a) Serine racemase: a glial enzyme synthesizing D-serine to regulate glutamate-N-methyl-D-aspartate neurotransmission. *Proceedings of the National Academy of Sciences USA* 96, 13409–13414.

Wolosker, H., Sheth, K.N., Takahashi, M., Mothet, J.P., Brady, R.O. Jr, Ferris, C.D. and Snyder, S.H. (1999b) Purification of serine racemase: biosynthesis of the neuromodulator D-serine. *Proceedings of the National Academy of Sciences USA* 96, 721–725.

Yasuda, E., Ma, N. and Semba, R. (2001) Immunohistochemical evidences for localization and production of d-serine in some neurons in the rat brain. *Neuroscience Letters* 299, 162–164.

Yoshikawa, M., Nakajima, K., Takayasu, N., Noda, S., Sato, Y., Kawaguchi, M., Oka, T., et al. (2006) Expression of the mRNA and protein of serine racemase in primary cultures of rat neurons. *European Journal of Pharmacology* 548, 74–76.

9 Tryptophan Hydroxylase

I. Winge,* J. McKinney and J. Haavik

Department of Biomedicine, University of Bergen, Norway

9.1 Abstract

Tryptophan hydroxylases (TPH1 and TPH2) are the rate-limiting enzymes in the serotonin biosynthesis and have the most restricted tissue distribution of the aromatic amino acid hydroxylases. TPH1 is mainly found in the pineal gland and enterochromaffin cells of the gut, whereas TPH2 is the main TPH in the brain. Here we summarize the structure, reaction mechanism, and physiological effect of both TPHs. Since much of the research was performed before the identification of TPH2, it has been difficult to distinguish what is known for each of the different TPH enzymes. In this review we try to clarify this aspect. In addition we discuss the regulation of the enzymes, both *in vitro* and *in vivo*, and how to use this information in drug treatment. Finally we discuss the implications of TPH dysfunction in human health, based on studies both in patient groups and knockout mice.

9.2 Introduction

The basic processes involved in serotonin biosynthesis, degradation, storage, uptake and release have been well characterized and are schematically shown in Fig. 9.1. In brief, serotonergic neurotransmission depends on three major steps:

1. Synthesis and degradation of serotonin, where the main enzymes are tryptophan hydroxylase (TPH) and monoamine oxidase A (MAO A).
2. Serotonin reuptake from the synaptic cleft, mediated by the monoamine transporters.
3. Activity of serotonin receptors. In the pineal glands, serotonin is further processed to melatonin. This chapter will focus on TPH, the rate-limiting enzyme in the synthesis of serotonin, with emphasis on its role in the mammalian nervous system.

9.3 General Properties

TPH [E.C.1.14.16.4] is a member of the aromatic amino acid hydroxylase enzyme superfamily (AAAH), together with phenylalanine hydroxylase (PAH) [E.C. 1.14.16.1] and tyrosine hydroxylase (TH) [E.C.1.14.16.2], which hydroxylate their respective amino acid substrates in the presence of tetrahydrobiopterin (BH_4), molecular oxygen (O_2) and iron (Fig. 9.2). They are all closely related, i.e. having approximately 60% overall DNA sequence

* E-mail address: ingeborg.winge@biomed.uib.no

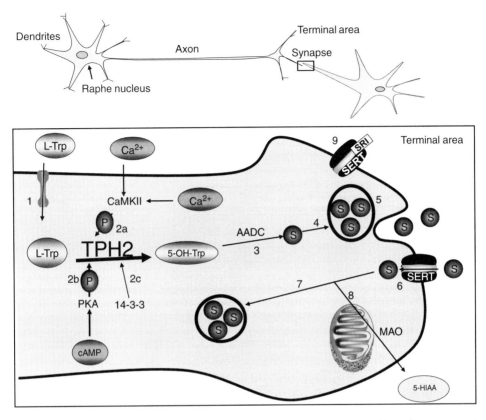

Fig. 9.1. The serotonin pathway. 1. Transport of L-tryptophan (L-Trp) through the blood–brain barrier (BBB) via a transporter (only last step into the neuron is shown). 2a and 2b. Phosphorylation of TPH2 by the putative kinases CaMKII (a) or PKA (b). 2c. Binding of 14-3-3 to the phosphorylated TPH2. TPH2 catalyses the conversion of L-Trp to 5-hydroxy tryptophan (5-OH-Trp). 3. Aromatic amino acid decarboxylase (AADC) catalyses the conversion of 5-OH-Trp to serotonin (S). 4. Serotonin is taken up into storage vesicles. 5. Serotonin is secreted from the vesicles into the synaptic space. 6. Serotonin is taken up into the presynaptic serotonin terminals by serotonin transporter (SERT). 7 and 8. Within these terminals, serotonin will either be taken up by the storage vesicles or be degraded by either monoamine oxidase (MAO) type A, which is in the outer mitochondrial membranes in synapses some distance from the serotonergic terminal, or by MAO type B in the serotonergic neurons. 9. Serotonin reuptake inhibitors (SRI). Figure modified from Wong et al. (2005).

identity and 85% amino acid sequence identity in their catalytic domains, and it has been speculated that they have arisen from a common ancestor gene (Grenett et al., 1987). The two hydroxylases PAH and TH have been studied more at the molecular level, and therefore it is natural to compare characteristics of TPH with the other AAAH throughout this review.

Two distinct *TPH* genes code for their respective enzymes, TPH1 and TPH2. It was only in 2003 that the latter gene was reported (Walther et al., 2003), although many researchers had already distinguished between brain and peripheral TPH (Fig. 9.3) (Kim et al., 1991; Cash, 1998). TPH1 is found in the enterochromaffin cells in the gut, pineal gland, spleen, thymus, skin, and retina, whereas TPH2 is predominantly distributed in the serotonergic neurons of the raphe nuclei in the brain stem and in the gut (Cote et al., 2003; Hornung, 2003; Slominski et al., 2003; Liang et al., 2004; Zill et al., 2004). TPH2 appears to be the major TPH protein in the brain, although TPH1 mRNA levels

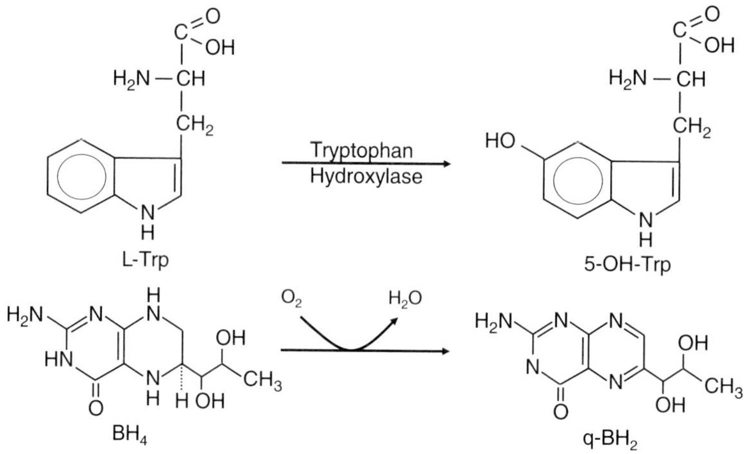

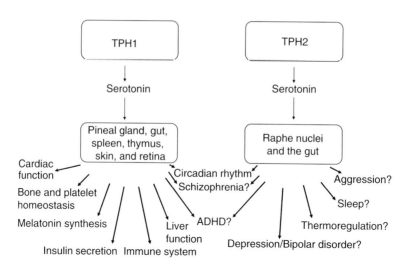

Fig. 9.2. Hydroxylation of L-tryptophan (L-Trp) using tetrahydrobiopterin (BH_4) as cofactor. 5-OH-Trp, 5-hydroxy tryptophan; q-BH_2, quinonoid dihydrobiopterin.

Fig. 9.3. Functions and implications of the peripheral (TPH1) and neuronal (TPH2) tryptophan hydroxylases. (Figure modified from Matthes et al., 2010, with permission from S. Karger AG, Basel.)

(around one-third of TPH2 levels) have also been detected in the anterior and posterior pituitary and in the hypothalamus in addition to the pineal gland (Sugden et al., 2009; Zill et al., 2009). When analysing total brain lysates, these findings will have to be taken into consideration. The possible role of TPH1 in brain function is still being debated since TPH1 appears to be important in the early development of the brain (Nakamura et al., 2006b; Cote et al., 2007; Abumaria et al., 2008; Halmoy et al., 2010).

9.4 Structure and Function of TPH

9.4.1 Domain organization

The two TPH enzymes have a subunit and domain organization that is similar to the other AAAH enzymes. Limited proteolysis, deletion mutagenesis, and crystallographic studies have demonstrated that they are organized in three domains:

1. An amino (N)-terminal regulatory domain of variable length with one or more serine phosphorylation sites, which mediate 14-3-3 binding in the case of TPH and TH.
2. A catalytic core with substrate and cofactor binding sites.
3. A short carboxy (C)-terminal oligomerization domain (Mockus et al., 1998) (Fig. 9.4).

TPH has been shown to exist as homotetramers, similar to TH (Nakata and Fujisawa, 1982; Okuno and Fujisawa, 1982), whereas PAH has been shown to exist in a state of equilibrium between dimeric and tetrameric forms (Iwaki et al., 1986; Kappock et al., 1995; Kleppe et al., 1999). 'Molecular dissection' of TPH has shown that the final 17 C-terminal residues comprise the tetramerization domain, which forms a leucine zipper motif and is conserved in TH (Mockus et al., 1997; Carkaci-Salli et al., 2006; Tenner et al., 2007). However, it has also been suggested that some N-terminal residues may contribute to subunit assembly in TPH1 (Yohrling et al., 1999). X-ray crystal structures of N- and C-terminally truncated forms of rat TH and human PAH have shown that the tetrameric form is held together by a long helix, which forms an antiparallel coiled-coil, and that C-terminal residues contribute to oligomerization via two antiparallel β-strands that contribute to subunit contacts (Erlandsen et al., 1997; Goodwill et al., 1997; Fusetti et al., 1998). A pentapeptide (Val-Pro-Trp-Phe-Pro, 105–109 in TPH1 and 151–155 in TPH2) is conserved in all of the hydroxylase enzymes, and demarcates a border between the catalytic domain and the end of the regulatory region. Removal of the regulatory region dramatically improves the solubility while enzyme activity is retained (Mockus et al., 1998; Carkaci-Salli et al., 2006). Both TPH1 and TPH2 have a tendency to form aggregates when purified, which is attributed to residues in the N-terminus. In TPH2, the N-terminal region is 46 aa longer than in TPH1 and contains several aromatic and basic residues (theoretical pI = 8.69) as well as an important PKA/CaMKII phosphorylation site, Ser19, which modulates 14-3-3 binding in TPH2 (Winge et al., 2008). The TPH2 deletion mutants NΔ41 and NΔ44 show that it exerts a negative effect on enzyme activity *in vitro* and *in vivo*, i.e. they have a higher V_{max}, without affecting the K_m for Trp, higher expression levels and decreased half-life (Murphy et al., 2008; Tenner et al., 2008). Recently a TPH2 isoform (TPH2b) was identified, the product of alternative mRNA splicing, which has two extra amino acids in the N-terminal region, (Gly146-Lys147) (Grohmann et al., 2010), which interrupts a

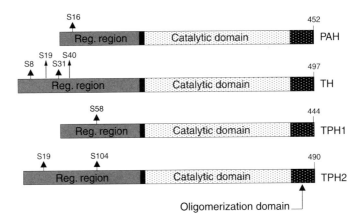

Fig. 9.4. The domain organization of the hAAAHs (PAH, TH1, TPH1, and TPH2); an N-terminal region containing one or more serine (S) phosphorylation sites, the catalytic domain, and the oligomerization domain.

highly acidic sequence in TPH2a, i.e. Glu144-Asp150 where 6 of 7 residues are acidic (theoretical pI = 3.3).

Both TPH1 and TPH2 contain putative ACT domains in the N-terminal regulatory region, based on the consensus sequence and homology with PAH, which correspond to amino acids 18–94 in TPH1 and 66–142 in TPH2 (Liberles *et al.*, 2005). Proteins containing the ACT domain are often involved in amino acid metabolism, and it was originally hypothesized that binding of regulatory ligands was its common function (Chipman and Shaanan, 2001). Several proteins that contain the ACT domain motif βαββαβ have been crystallized, including PAH (PDB: 1PHZ) (Grant, 2006). There is no evidence that phenylalanine binds to the ACT domain in PAH nor tryptophan in TPH, and it has been hypothesized that the ACT domain has adopted other functions in the AAAH enzymes (Siltberg-Liberles and Martinez, 2009).

9.4.2 Ligand binding

The catalytic core domain has been crystallized for TPH1, PAH, and TH and demonstrates that a 2-His-1-carboxylate facial triad is a conserved motif that anchors the catalytic mononuclear non-haem iron at the active site (Erlandsen *et al.*, 1997; Goodwill *et al.*, 1997; Hegg and Que, 1997; Wang *et al.*, 2002; Windahl *et al.*, 2008). They correspond to residues His272, His277 and Glu317 in TPH1; and to His318, His323 and Glu363 in TPH2. A variety of different investigations including rational site directed mutagenesis, naturally occurring missense variants, and computational studies of crystal structures in complex with ligands and ligand analogues demonstrate important ligand selectivity determinants (Daubner *et al.*, 2006; Teigen *et al.*, 2007; Windahl *et al.*, 2008). Both L-Trp and L-Phe are excellent substrates for TPH, which is similar to PAH, whereas TH has the most stringent substrate specificity (Fitzpatrick, 2003). Experiments with substrate analogues showed that nitrogen in position 1 of the indole ring, which could be expected to form a hydrogen bond with the enzyme, is probably important for proper positioning of the indole moiety, but that variations in steric bulk (methyl substituents) and atomic charge (additional ring nitrogens) retain the ability to be hydroxylated at the 5 position (Moran *et al.*, 1999). Several crystal structures of the catalytic domain of TPH1 in complex with substrate, substrate inhibitors and cofactor analogue have been reported (Wang *et al.*, 2002; Windahl *et al.*, 2008; Cianchetta *et al.*, 2010). They provide structural explanations for non-conserved substrate orienting residues that were first identified by use of sequence alignment, homology modelling and mutagenesis, i.e. Tyr236, Phe314 and Ile366 in TPH1; and Tyr281, Phe359 and Ile412 in TPH2 (Teigen *et al.*, 1999; Daubner *et al.*, 2000; Jiang *et al.*, 2000; McKinney *et al.*, 2001). Electrostatic interactions that are important for amino acid substrate orientation are conserved across the hydroxylase enzymes, i.e. between the carboxyl group in tryptophan and phenylalanine with the guanidium group of the Arg257 side chain, the hydroxyl group of the Ser336 side chain, and the nitrogen backbone of Thr265. They were first identified in NMR/modelling studies (Teigen *et al.*, 1999; McKinney *et al.*, 2001) and in crystal structures with substrate analogues in a ternary complex with PAH and BH_4 (Andersen *et al.*, 2001). The importance of those studies was later demonstrated for a naturally occurring Arg303Trp missense variant in TPH2 (McKinney *et al.*, 2008), which had no detectable activity, probably due to loss of the charged Arg residue (McKinney *et al.*, 2001). In the chicken TPH1 structure, tryptophan stacks against Pro268, which is different from both the docked structure and the substrate analogue, which stacked against the imidazole group of His272 (Windahl *et al.*, 2008).

A conformational change is inferred from a comparison of the crystal structure for human TPH1 catalytic domain in complex with cofactor analogue (Wang *et al.*, 2002) and a recent crystal structure of chicken catalytic domain in complex with substrate (Windahl *et al.*, 2008). It was reported that the substrate-bound chicken TPH1 structure is more similar to the PAH structure with bound substrate analogue (PDB: 1MMK) than to the TPH1 structure without substrate: rmsd 0.9 versus 1.47 Å respectively for the Cα atoms. Two loops that are located on either side of the active site channel form a more closed active site in the substrate bound structure; that is, the Cα atoms of Leu130 and Thr368 are 7.1 Å apart with tryptophan bound, which is 10 Å less than in the structure in complex with the cofactor analogue (Windahl et al., 2008). Those loop residues are conserved in human TPH1 and TPH2: Leu124-Asp139 and Ile367-Thr369, Leu123-Asp140 and Ile366-Thre368 in TPH1 and Leu169-Asp184 and Ile412-Thr414 TPH2, respectively. Thus, the crystal structures provide an explanation for the substrate inhibition seen for L-Trp both for the catalytic domain and the full-length enzyme (Wang et al., 2002; McKinney et al., 2005).

There has been a keen interest in the regulation of BH_4-dependent enzymes, the pharmacological effects of BH_4 administration, and the development of selective inhibitors of BH_4-dependent enzymes (Werner-Felmayer et al., 2002). The first TPH crystal structure was of the catalytic domain, aa 102–402, in complex with ferric iron and 7,8-dihydrobiopterin (Wang et al., 2002), which is similar to the binding mode for all the AAAH enzymes as was shown for PAH (Teigen et al., 2004) and TH (Martinez et al., 1993). The BH_4 binding site is similar in the hydroxylase enzymes and comprises aa Tyr235-Pro238 and Phe241 in TPH1 which are also conserved in TPH2. The pterin ring pi-stacks with Phe241 and is hydrogen bonded to Glu273. The binding pocket for the BH_4 dihydroxypropyl side chain is different for each enzyme due to non-conserved residues there, i.e. Pro in TPH1 and TPH2, Ser in PAH, and Ala in TH. Thus, the pterin binding site has important differences that may be exploited for designing hydroxylase-specific inhibitors, which has been demonstrated for TPH using 8-methyl-6,7-dimethyl-5,6,7,8-tetrahydropterin (Teigen et al., 2007).

Besides its function as an essential cofactor for substrate hydroxylation in the AAAH enzymes, BH_4 has also been shown to play a stabilizing effect on PAH and TH (Perez et al., 2005; Takazawa et al., 2008). A subset of persons with phenylketonuria have their phenylalanine levels normalized by oral BH_4 therapy, which is attributed to stabilization of PAH protein variants. In mice that lack BH_4 synthesizing enzymes, oral BH_4 has also been shown to enhance both PAH levels and activity and TH levels in the brain, especially at nerve terminals, whereas TPH does not appear to be affected (Sumi-Ichinose et al., 2001; Takazawa et al., 2008; Thony et al., 2008). Thus, an interest in the identification of ligands that might affect AAAH enzyme stability differently also led to discovery of a compound in a commercially available chemical library that dramatically increased the thermostability of the TPH2, as well as PAH and TH (Pey et al., 2008; Calvo et al., 2010).

9.4.3 Catalytic mechanism

Due to structural and functional similarities, TPH and the other AAAH enzymes are assumed to share a common catalytic mechanism; however, studies on the catalytic mechanism are mainly reported for TH and PAH due to their greater stability *in vitro*. According to enzyme nomenclature, they are categorized as oxidoreductases, i.e. they transfer electrons from a reductant to an oxidant. AAAH enzymes employ a paired electron donor (BH_4), with incorporation or reduction of molecular oxygen, i.e. into tryptophan and transiently to BH_4 (IUPAC-IUB, 1984). Catalysis requires a ferrous iron atom, one molecule of reduced pterin per catalytic site, which is oxidized to a dihydropterin. One molecule of O_2 is consumed in the reaction; one atom of oxygen is incorporated into the amino acid substrate, whereas the other is ultimately reduced to water (Fitzpatrick, 2003). Although a variety of data suggests that BH_4 is the physiological substrate (Frantom et al., 2006), many different synthetic tetrahydropterins, e.g. 6-methyltetrahydropterin (6-MPH_4) and 6,7-dimethyltetrahydropterin ($DMPH_4$), are sufficient for catalysis and have been used in experiments that have generated important data about the catalytic mechanism (Eser et al., 2007; Chow et al., 2009).

Upon purification, the enzymes are typically isolated with ferric iron, whereas the reaction cycle starts and stops with iron in the ferrous state (Fitzpatrick, 2003). Thus, the mechanism for iron reduction has been somewhat controversial due to the stoichiometric incompatibility between the two-electron reductant BH$_4$ and the one-electron oxidant ferric iron (Nieter Burgmayer, 1998). The reaction mechanism is typically described as two partial reactions: formation of the hydroxylating intermediate and oxygen transfer to the aromatic amino acid (Fitzpatrick et al., 2003; Haahr et al., 2010). From kinetic data this mechanism, as shown for PAH and TH, appears to be sequential (Hosoda, 1975; Fitzpatrick et al., 2003). The Fitzpatrick laboratory has made many important findings regarding the nature of the reaction. It has shown evidence for an electrophilic aromatic substitution reaction mechanism with a cationic amino acid intermediate, where a ferryloxy species is responsible for generating the 4a-OH-pterin intermediate. The 4a-OH-pterin intermediate has been demonstrated for all of the hydroxylases including TPH (Haavik and Flatmark, 1987; Moran et al., 2000).

The binding order of amino acid substrate and cofactor is deemed to be somewhat random; however, kinetic data and crystal structures of enzyme–ligand complexes show that binding of the cofactor before substrate enhances enzymatic activity and that catalysis only occurs when both substrate and pterin are bound (Fitzpatrick, 2003). This hypothesis is supported by crystallographic and kinetic data for TPH1 (Windahl et al., 2009). The enzyme exhibits substrate inhibition for L-Trp, i.e. K_{si} 385 µM for the full-length enzyme (McKinney et al., 2004) and 71.7 µM for double-truncated catalytic domain (Windahl et al., 2009) and is in a more closed conformation when in complex with substrate (Windahl et al., 2008) than with cofactor analogue (Wang et al., 2002). For TPH2, no crystal structure has been reported yet, but the kinetic data show that it is less susceptible to substrate inhibition, i.e. K_{si} 970 µM for the full length enzyme (McKinney et al., 2004), and no substrate inhibition up to 100 µM for the isolated catalytic domain (Windahl et al., 2009).

Many researchers have reported that TPH (both TPH1 and TPH2) easily aggregate and are difficult to purify. Kinetic values are also critically dependent on reaction conditions, such as pH and buffer compositions. Together, this can probably explain some of the diverging kinetic values shown in Table 9.1. With plasma and brain levels of L-Trp of about 30 µM (for rats) (Grahame-Smith, 1964; Fernstrom and Wurtman, 1971), and diverging K_m results, as for BH$_4$, it is difficult to conclude whether the substrate availability is limiting in the cells.

9.5 Enzyme Regulation

9.5.1 Inhibition of TPH

The regulation of TPH activity has been studied extensively. One way of regulating enzymes is by substrate or product inhibition. All AAAHs seem to be rather insensitive to product inhibition, whereas they are more sensitive towards their substrate. TPH appears to be regulated by substrate inhibition, by high concentrations of L-Trp or L-Phe, although the inhibition by L-Trp is more pronounced than by L-Phe (Friedman et al., 1972; Tong and Kaufman, 1975). For a long time it was unclear if this had an effect *in vivo*, but it has been shown that patients with phenylketonuria (PKU) have decreased platelet (Friedman et al., 1972; Tong and Kaufman, 1975), cerebrospinal fluid (CSF) (Schulpis et al., 2002), and brain (Burlina et al., 2000) serotonin levels. When treated with BH$_4$, these levels increased in almost all patients, although the L-Trp and L-Phe levels remained the same, suggesting that this is a direct effect of BH$_4$ on TPH, compensating for the inhibition by high L-Phe levels (Ormazabal et al., 2005).

The sensitivity of TPH towards inhibition is also dependent on its cofactor. Substrate inhibition of brain TPH is more pronounced in the presence of BH$_4$ than DMPH$_4$. However, it is debated whether this inhibition is significant *in vivo*, as inhibition in the presence of BH$_4$ has only been seen at concentrations of 100 µM (Ormazabal et al., 2005), exceeding normal tissue levels of BH$_4$.

As for both PAH and TH, TPH has been shown to be very sensitive towards inhibition by catecholamines (Kaufman, 1974), although catecholamines do not seem to be synthesized in TPH1- and TPH2-containing cells. Nevertheless, dopamine and serotonin appear to have a similar distribution in the paraventricular organ, most probably due to uptake of dopamine in the serotonergic cells

Table 9.1. Kinetic parameters (K_m values) of TPH1 and TPH2.

Ligand	TPH1	TPH2	Species	Reference
L-Trp (µM)		50	Native rabbit hind brain	Friedman et al. (1972)
		32	Rabbit hind brain	Tong and Kaufman (1975)
	8		Rabbit (cloned)	Tipper et al. (1994)
		71.2	Mouse (cloned)	Sakowski et al. (2006)
	12		Human (cloned)	Tipper et al. (1994)
	26		Human (cloned)	Yang and Kaufman (1994)
	20		Human (cloned)	Kowlessur and Kaufman (1999)
	22.8	40.3	Human (cloned)	McKinney et al. (2005)
		24.26	Human (cloned)	Carkaci-Salli et al. (2006)
		41.3	Human (cloned)	Winge et al. (2007)
	28		Human (cloned), 92–444	Yang and Kaufman (1994)
	33		Human (cloned), NΔ91	McKinney et al. (2001)
	7.8		Human (cloned), ΔN102–ΔC402	Wang et al. (2002)
	22.8	15	Human TPH1:100–413 TPH2: 146–459 (recombinant)	Windahl et al. (2009)
BH$_4$ (µM)		31	Rabbit hind brain	Friedman et al. (1972)
	39		Rabbit hind brain, 92–444	Yang and Kaufman (1994)
	66		Rabbit (cloned)	Tipper et al. (1994)
		26.8	Mouse (cloned)	Sakowski et al. (2006)
	66		Human (cloned)	Tipper et al. (1994)
	48		Human (cloned)	Yang and Kaufman (1994)
	45		Human (cloned)	Kowlessur and Kaufman (1999)
	39	20.2	Human (cloned)	McKinney et al. (2005)
		17.9	Human (cloned)	Carkaci-Salli et al. (2006)
		68.4	Human (cloned)	Winge et al. (2007)
	39		Human (cloned), 92–444	Yang and Kaufman (1994)
	50.8		Human (cloned), NΔ91	McKinney et al. (2001)
	26.5		Human (cloned), ΔN102–ΔC402	Wang et al. (2002)
	315	26.5	Human (cloned), NΔCΔ 146–459	Windahl et al. (2009)
O$_2$		2.5%		Friedman et al. (1972)
	109	273		Windahl et al. (2009)

Only mammalian forms of the enzyme (preferentially human) are listed. For the measurements of K_m values for the amino acid substrate L-Trp only the data with the natural cofactor BH$_4$ are selected.

(Martinez et al., 2001). This allows for dopamine to have a potential physical contact with neuronal TPH. It has been shown that when studying the inhibition of brain TPH, dopamine is competitive with respect to the pterin cofactor DMPH$_4$ with a K_{si} reported to be 50 µM (Batten et al., 1993), whereas when using BH$_4$ the K_{si} is lower, i.e. 10–50 µM for TPH1 and 10–34 µM for TPH2, respectively (Johansen et al., 1991; Kuhn and Arthur, 1998; Sakowski et al., 2006; Winge et al., 2007). However, as for inhibition by pterins, the significance in vivo is difficult to predict, as it depends on the availability of the catecholamines in the tissue.

As TPH may be involved in many different disorders, there is an increased interest in finding specific inhibitors of TPH1 and TPH2. High concentrations of L-Trp and L-Phe inhibit TPH1 and TPH2. In addition, derivatives of L-Trp and L-Phe such as p-chlorophenylalanine (PCPA), 6-fluorotryptophan and 6-chlorotryptophan are also potent TPH-inhibitors (McGeer et al., 1968; Nicholson and Wright, 1981; Pandey et al., 1983; Nakamura et al., 2006a). PCPA was first introduced as an agent for depleting brain serotonin (McGeer et al., 1968; Nicholson and Wright, 1981; Pandey et al., 1983; Nakamura et al., 2006a), and inhibition of TPH was reported as the main cause of serotonin depletion (Koe and Weissman, 1966). It was shown that *in vivo* the drug would lead to an irreversible inhibition of the enzyme. Pineal TPH (now known as TPH1) has been reported to be less sensitive to inhibition by PCPA (Jequier et al., 1967) than TPH2. The effect of TPH-inhibition has been shown to be dependent on the pterin used, i.e. the inhibition of PCPA is stronger in the presence of BH_4 than in the presence of $DMPH_4$ (Deguchi and Barchas, 1972). Although PCPA is a strong inhibitor, 6-fluorotryptophan appears to be more potent *in vivo* (Tipper et al., 1994). More recently, *p*-ethynylphenylalanine has been found to be an even more selective, reversible, and potent inhibitor than PCPA (Stokes et al., 2000).

Tetrahydroisoquinolines (TIQs) have been proposed to be neurotoxic *in vitro* and constitute another class of TPH inhibitors (Stokes et al., 2000). TIQs such as salsolinol and tetrahydropapaveroline have been identified in the urine of parkinsonian patients receiving L-DOPA therapy. They inhibit the dopamine biosynthesis by a direct binding of TH (Shin et al., 1999; Kim et al., 2001; Scholz et al., 2008). In addition to inhibiting TH, the rate-limiting enzyme in the catecholamine biosynthesis, these TIQs have also been found to inhibit TPH at a similar concentration range (Ota et al., 1992; Kim et al., 2003; Kim et al., 2004).

Recently, Cianchetta and co-workers published their work on TPH1 crystalstructures with the novel inhibitors LP533401, LP521834, and LP534193 (Ota et al., 1992; Kim et al., 2003; Kim et al., 2004). They appear to fill the tryptophan-binding pocket of TPH1 without reaching into the binding site of the cofactor and induces a major conformational change of the enzyme. Since all three inhibitors share a phenylalanine moiety, they are competitive with L-Trp and assume a compact complex that is similar to the TPH1-Trp complex. Apart from the phenylalanine moiety, LP521834 contains a 2-amino-triazine, LP521834 a 2-amino-pyrimidine, and LP-534193 contains a pyrazine as the second component of the molecule (Cianchetta et al., 2010).

LP533401 has also been tested in a group of patients with osteoporosis (Yadav et al., 2010). Gut-derived serotonin (GDS) has been described to be a powerful inhibitor of osteoblast proliferation and bone formation (Yadav et al., 2010). Oral administration of this TPH1-inhibitor decreased the GDS synthesis and may therefore be a potential treatment for osteoporosis (Yadav et al., 2010). Armed with such enzyme-specific inhibitors, it will be easier to explore the biology and pathophysiology of TPH1 and TPH2.

9.5.2 Regulation of TPH

In contrast to the growing numbers of genetic association and functional studies of TPH1 and TPH2, little is known about the normal regulation of TPH expression. In 1997, it was reported that glucocorticoids are involved in the tissue-specific regulation of TPH mRNA levels. Treatments of adrenalectomized rats with the synthetic glucocorticoid dexamethasone led to an increase in TPH mRNA in the pineal gland, whereas in the raphe nuclei it was decreased (Yadav et al., 2010). The identification of TPH2, and the knowledge that the promoters of TPH1 and TPH2 lack sequence homologies, suggests that the main reason for the apparently different regulation was different mRNA species, and not different tissue localization.

Both TPH1 and TPH2 have been shown to exhibit a diurnal rhythm of gene expression, although TPH2 to a lesser extent than TPH1 (Liang et al., 2004; Malek et al., 2004; Malek et al., 2007). The nocturnal increase in TPH1 appears to be dependent on a cyclic adenosine monophosphate (cAMP) increase that both increases mRNA production (Liang et al., 2004; Malek et al., 2004; Malek et al., 2007) and phosphorylation of TPH1 by the cAMP-dependent protein kinase (PKA) (Huang et al., 2008). Phosphorylation appears to stabilize the protein, which may explain the increase in TPH1 at night-time (Huang et al., 2008). The increase in TPH2 mRNA, however, has been found to be stimulated by an increase in corticosterone (Malek et al., 2004; Malek et al., 2007). In addition to being regulated by the diurnal rhythm, expression of both TPH1 and TPH2 mRNA have been shown to be regulated by various hormones and stressors, such as haemorrhaging shock, glucocorticoids, oestrogen and ovarian steroids (Clark et al., 2005; Malek et al., 2005, 2007; Sanchez et al., 2005; Brown et al., 2006; Hiroi et al., 2006).

Recently, a truncated isoform without a catalytic domain (ENST00000266669, g.22879A>G) (Haghighi et al., 2008) and an alternatively spliced variant of *TPH2* with six extra nucleotides between exons 3 and 4 (Haghighi et al., 2008) have been described. This supports the suggestion that alternative splicing and RNA editing may be an additional way of regulating TPH activity. It has also been shown that the N-terminal domain of TPH2 is involved in regulation of enzyme expression, and this might partially explain the different expression levels and stability of TPH1 and TPH2 *in vivo* (Grohmann et al., 2010).

9.5.3 Phosphorylation of TPH

Many enzymes are regulated by reversible phosphorylation at Ser, Thr, or Tyr residues. Multiprotein serine/threonine specific protein kinases such as PKA and the Ca^{2+}/calmodulin-dependent protein kinase (CaMKII) have been reported to phosphorylate and activate the AAAHs. Particularly, regulation of TH by phosphorylation has been thoroughly studied (Kumer and Vrana, 1996; Toska et al., 2002; Dunkley et al., 2004; Fujisawa and Okuno, 2005). Compared to TH, less is known about the phosphorylation of TPH1 and TPH2, and it is sometimes difficult to know whether the findings involve TPH1 or TPH2, as most experiments were performed before the knowledge about TPH2. The pineal gland is, however, known to express mainly TPH1. Phosphorylation of TPH has been reported in both chick pineal cells and rat pineal glands and was increased by addition of cAMP or calcium (Ehret et al., 1991; Florez et al., 1996). Phosphorylation of recombinant forms of TPH1 by bovine PKA has been thoroughly reported (Vrana et al., 1994; Johansen et al., 1996). In mast cells that express TPH1, inhibition of phosphorylation by the CaMKII-specific inhibitor KN-62 indicated that TPH1 could also be phosphorylated by CaMKII. This was confirmed by adding exogenous CaMKII to mast cell lysates in the presence of Ca^{2+} and calmodulin (Iida et al., 2002).

The phosphorylation site on Ser58 in TPH1 was later confirmed by site-directed mutagenesis (Kuhn et al., 1997; Kumer et al., 1997), and although Ser260 has been suggested as an additional phosphorylation site (Jiang et al., 2000), this has not been verified by other groups. Recently, it has been shown that phosphorylation on Ser58 in TPH1 increases during the night, and this may play a regulatory role on the TPH1-levels in the pineal gland, as phosphorylation also appears to stabilize TPH1 (Huang et al., 2008).

Although phosphorylation of TPH2 was not explicitly studied before 2003, it was early shown that addition of ATP and Mg^{2+} in rat brain stem lysates, containing mainly TPH2, increases TPH activity by 40–50%, and that addition of Ca^{2+} increased the activity even more (70–200%). Removing Ca^{2+} by adding EDTA had the opposite effect (Knapp et al., 1975; Hamon et al., 1977). Similar results were also reported using total rat brain lysates (Boadle-Biber, 1978; Boadle-Biber, 1979; Boadle-Biber, 1982). In the presence of Ca^{2+}, calmodulin was reported to be an activator of TPH activity (Boadle-Biber, 1978; Boadle-Biber, 1979; Boadle-Biber, 1982), and it was demonstrated that TPH from rat brain stem (most likely TPH2) is phosphorylated by CaMKII (Yamauchi and Fujisawa, 1979a,b, 1981; Ehret et al., 1989). However, it was not until 2007 that the phosphorylation site for CaMKII in TPH2 was identified as Ser19, using mass spectrometry (MS) and site directed mutagenesis (Kuhn et al., 2007; Winge et al., 2008).

The evidence for activation of TPH by adding cAMP to brain stem extracts is not as clear as for addition of Ca^{2+}. Several investigators state that addition of cAMP activates rat brain stem TPH (TPH2) up to twofold (Kuhn et al., 2007; Winge et al., 2008), whereas others have not observed this increase in enzyme activation (Hamon et al., 1978; Kuhn et al., 1978; Yamauchi and Fujisawa, 1979b; Boadle-Biber, 1982; Johansen et al., 1995). However, these reports are based on findings using brain lysate that may already contain cAMP, so there is no extra activation effect when it is added. Some groups Johansen et al. (1995) and Makita et al. (1990) found that TPH2 was indeed phosphorylated by exogenous PKA. In 2005 the first PKA-phosphorylation site in TPH2 was identified, i.e. Ser19 (McKinney et al., 2005), and later a second phosphorylation site, Ser104, corresponding to Ser58 in TPH1, was identified (Winge et al., 2008). Phosphorylation on Ser19 by PKA appears to increase the stability of TPH2 (Murphy et al., 2008; Winge et al., 2008); however, this may be related to the binding of 14-3-3 proteins (Winge et al., 2008).

So far, little is known about the functional effects of phosphorylation of TPH. However, there appears to be a consensus that phosphorylation activates TPH, although it is still unclear whether the activation is direct, as suggested for TPH1 (Banik et al., 1997; Kuhn et al., 1997), or due to increased stability of the protein, as proposed for TPH1 and TPH2 (Huang et al., 2008; Murphy et al., 2008; Winge et al., 2008). To make any further conclusions about the regulatory effect of phosphorylation, more studies on both enzymes are needed.

9.5.4 14-3-3 binding to TPH

The mammalian 14-3-3 protein family consists of seven different structurally related acidic proteins that are widely distributed and involved in many physiological processes. Activation of TPH and TH by 14-3-3 were the first biological functions associated with binding of 14-3-3 proteins (Ichimura et al., 1987). Most research has been done on 14-3-3 binding to TH, but there are also some findings for TPH. Most of the findings were reported prior to the discovery of TPH and there is no clear distinction between the effects on TPH1 and TPH2. Yamauchi and coworkers reported as early as in 1981 that rat brain stem TPH (mainly TPH2) phosphorylated by CaMKII was activated in the presence of an activator protein that later turned out to be a 14-3-3 (Ichimura et al., 1987). Later, a similar activation was observed for TPH in brain stem phosphorylated by endogenous or exogenous PKA in the presence of 14-3-3 (Ichimura et al., 1987). However, other studies showed no enzyme activation when incubating either rat brain stem TPH or recombinant TPH2 with 14-3-3 (Johansen et al., 1995; McKinney et al., 2005). Binding of 14-3-3 to TPH1 has also been shown to maintain the enzyme in a phosphorylated state, and thereby prolong the phosphorylation-dependent increase in activity (Johansen et al., 1995; McKinney et al., 2005) (Fig. 9.5). This stabilizing effect on the protein activity was also reported for TPH2 (Winge et al., 2008).

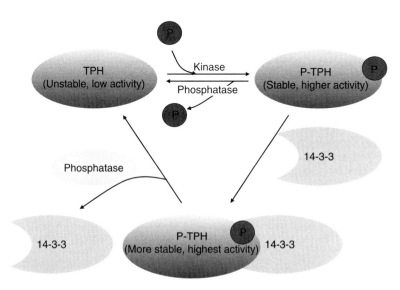

Fig. 9.5. Schematic representation of the interaction of TPH with 14-3-3 proteins. Figure adapted from Winge et al. (2008).

Phosphorylation studies and site-directed mutagenesis have revealed that phosphorylation is necessary for the binding of 14-3-3 to TPH2 (McKinney *et al.*, 2005; Winge *et al.*, 2008), and an interesting finding is that there appears to be a different binding site for TPH2 compared to TPH1. Specific binding sequences of 14-3-3 in TPH1 and TPH2 are yet to be confirmed, but it has been suggested that Ser58 is involved in the binding of 14-3-3 (McKinney *et al.*, 2005; Winge *et al.*, 2008), whereas mutation studies indicate that phosphorylation on Ser19 and not Ser104 (corresponding to Ser58 in TPH1) is essential for binding of 14-3-3 to TPH2 (Winge *et al.*, 2008). This may indicate a different regulation of the enzymes with the 14-3-3 proteins.

9.6 TPH Knockout Studies

Recently, several reports have been published regarding TPH knockout (KO) studies in mice. The first TPH1 KO report was particularly important as it revealed the existence of a second TPH gene (*TPH2*). In these TPH1 KO mice serotonin was found in normal levels in the brain, but was not present in the periphery (Walther *et al.*, 2003). The earliest reports of TPH1 -/- mice showed no morphological or behavioural changes, except for a cardiac dysfunction due to an increased heart size, compared with the wild type (WT) (Cote *et al.*, 2003). The first TPH2 KO reports were also negative with respect to changes in the visible or behavioural features. The phenotypic features that were reported were decreased body size during the first 2 months of life, reduced body fat, and the TPH1/TPH2 double KO mice had also decreased immobility (Gutknecht *et al.*, 2008; Savelieva *et al.*, 2008). However, a recent report showed that TPH2 KO also led to 50% lethality during the first 4 weeks of postnatal life. In addition, the pups had altered regulation of sleep, breathing, thermoregulation, heart rate and blood pressure. As adults, the mice were more aggressive and showed maternal neglect (Alenina *et al.*, 2009). This is also reflected in another report showing that maternal serotonin is crucial for murine embryonic development, as pups born to TPH1 KO mice showed dramatic abnormalities in the development of the brain and other organs (Alenina *et al.*, 2009). In addition to these KO mice, a mutant form (P449R) of TPH2 has also been found in Balb/c mice. These mice had reduced serotonin levels and behaved aggressively (Zhang *et al.*, 2004). All these results indicate that although TPH1 and TPH2 are not essential for adult life, they are involved in both behaviour and autonomic pathways. However, further studies of KO organisms are needed to establish the full effect of TPH-deletion and serotonin depletion.

9.7 Implications of TPH Dysfunction in Human Health

Serotonin is an important neurotransmitter in the CNS, and serotonin-containing diffuse projections from the raphe nuclei in the brainstem are found in many brain regions. Thus, although constituting less than 1% of the total transmitters in the human brain, serotonin may be considered to be one of the most widely distributed neurotransmitters (Hensler *et al.*, 1994) and it has been linked to a variety of CNS functions such as temperature control, attention, pain, and memory (Mochizucki, 2004; Maurer-Spurej, 2005; Mendelsohn *et al.*, 2009). In recent years there has been a dramatic increase in clinical evidence associating dysregulation in central serotonin activity with symptoms such as aggression, impulsivity and hyperactivity, in addition to human disorders such as depression, anxiety, obsessive-compulsive disorder, schizophrenia and attention deficit hyperactivity disorder (ADHD) (reviewed in Arango *et al.*, 2003; Haavik *et al.*, 2008; Matthes *et al.*, 2010).

Although TPH2 is found mainly in neurons, it has been reported that TPH1 is predominantly expressed during the late developmental stage of the brain (Nakamura *et al.*, 2006b). Therefore, both *TPH1* and *TPH2* have been regarded as potential susceptibility genes for psychiatric disorders. The coding regions of *TPH1* and *TPH2* are small compared to the total gene sequence, so most of the single nucleotide polymorphisms (SNPs) that have been reported have been located in the introns and promoter regions (Nakamura *et al.*, 2006b).

TPH1 markers have been reported to be associated with suicidal behaviour (reviewed in Haavik *et al.*, 2008), depression (Sun *et al.*, 2004; Jokela *et al.*, 2007), bipolar disorder (Bellivier *et al.*, 1998; Zaboli *et al.*, 2006; Chen *et al.*, 2008) schizophrenia (Bellivier *et al.*, 1998; Zaboli *et al.*, 2006; Chen *et al.*, 2008) and ADHD (Allen *et al.*, 2008). Since the characterization of the neuronal *TPH2* (McKinney *et al.*, 2005), the focus has mainly been shifted towards this enzyme. Since then, variants of *TPH2* have been reported to be associated with different psychiatric disorders as well, such as major depression, bipolar disorder, suicidal behaviour, personality disorders and ADHD (reviewed in Haavik *et al.*, 2008; Matthes *et al.*, 2010).

One of the first variants reported was in intron 7 of the *TPH1*-gene (Haavik *et al.*, 2008; Matthes *et al.*, 2010), whereas the first coding polymorphism, p.TPH1 V177I, was found in a patient exhibiting motor- and neurodevelopmental problems (Ramaekers *et al.*, 2001). Recently, six other coding polymorphisms have been found in patients with ADHD (Ramaekers *et al.*, 2001): p.TPH1 K54Q, R142C, R145X, L274I, A300T, and I410N. These polymorphisms have been linked to impaired maternal serotonin production that may have long-term effects on brain development and increase the risk of ADHD-related symptoms and behaviour in offspring (Halmoy *et al.*, 2010) (Fig. 9.6 a and b). So far, for TPH1, there are hundreds of variants identified across

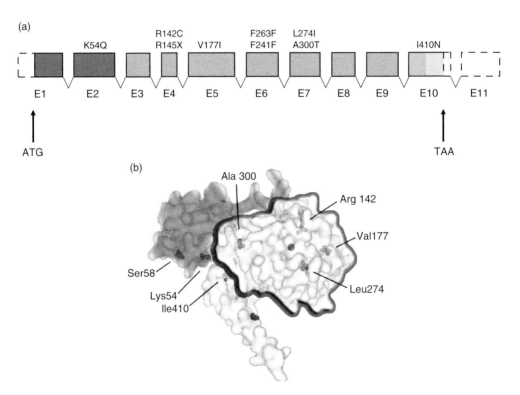

Fig. 9.6. Genomic structure and location of variants in human *TPH1* (a and b) and *TPH2* (c and d). (a and c) Exons encoding the regulatory domain are shown in dark grey (p.Met1-Thr104 (TPH1) and p.Met1-Asp150 (TPH2)), the catalytic domain in lighter grey (p.Val105-Asn402 (TPH1) and Val151-Asn448 (TPH2)), and the oligomerization domain in light grey (p.Pro403-Ile444 (TPH1) and Pro449-Ile490 (TPH2)). Modified from Yadav *et al.*, 2010. (b and d) Molecular model of a full-length subunit of TPH1 (b) and TPH2 (d) WT, illustrating the position of missense mutations and phosphorylation sites. A dark grey ball represents the active site iron atom. Arbitrarily determined domain boundaries are as shown in Fig. 9.6a.
Figure adapted from Haavik *et al.* (2008) with permission from John Wiley and Sons.

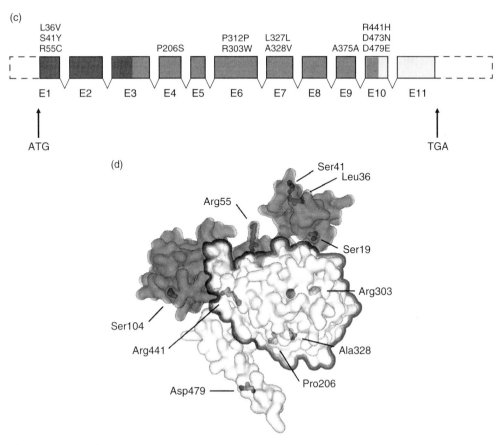

Fig. 9.6. Continued.

different species including the human gene (www.ncbi.nlm.nih.gov/snp?term=TPH1).

The polymorphisms A218C (rs1800532) and A779C (rs1799913) in the introns of TPH1 are the two most studied SNPs in *TPH1* and have been reported to be associated with several disorders such as schizophrenia (Allen *et al.*, 2008), bipolar disorder, suicidality, and depression. However, other groups have not been able to replicate these findings. In a recent large multicentre study, common variants in either TPH1 or TPH2 were not significantly associated with persistent ADHD (Johansson *et al.*, 2010).

So far, almost 2000 SNPs have been identified for *TPH2* across all species, and more than 700 of these are found in the human gene (www.ncbi.nlm.nih.gov/snp?term=TPH2). Among these, eight non-synonymous variants are in the coding region, ten in humans and one in mouse: human p.TPH2 L36V, L36P, S41Y, R55C, P206S, R303W, A328V, R441H, D473N, and D479E; and mouse p.TPH2 P447R (Winge *et al.*, 2005; Zhang *et al.*, 2005; Cichon *et al.*, 2008; McKinney *et al.*, 2009; Halmoy *et al.*, 2010) (Fig. 9.6c and d). There are also five synonymous coding SNPs (Y212Y, P312P, L327L, A375A, and C406C) and many non-coding SNPs reported (470 in humans, June 2010) (www.ncbi.nlm.nih.gov/snp?term=TPH2).

In addition to exerting an impact on psychiatric disorders, TPH2 has been suggested to be involved in sudden infant death syndrome (SIDS) by the observation of decreased protein levels in the SIDS cases compared with controls (Duncan *et al.*, 2010), and to be involved in coronary artery lesions in children with Kawasaki disease (Park *et al.*, 2010). TPH1, as a peripheral enzyme, has been reported to be involved in gastrointestinal disorders such as irritable bowel syndrome (Park *et al.*, 2010) and colonic inflammation (Ghia *et al.*, 2009), in both of which decreased mRNA levels have been observed. In addition, the inhibition of TPH1 by synthetic inhibitors increases bone formation and could potentially be important in the treatment of osteoporosis (Yadav *et al.*, 2010).

Further implications of the reduced serotonin levels on brain function and neuropsychological disorders are discussed in Chapter 24 of this volume.

9.8 Concluding Remarks and Future Research

Studies on TPH have been carried out for several decades, although it was only recently that TPH2 was identified. Most of the early studies were done in cell lysates, but during the last two decades the purified recombinant proteins have also been studied. The mechanism of hydroxylation by both TPH1 and TPH2 appears to be similar to that of the other two AAAHs, with a sequential order of substrate binding and formation of an activated oxygen intermediate. Knowledge of the ligand-binding and catalytic mechanism is also increasing with the aid of crystal structures, spectroscopy, and binding assays. However, the detailed mechanism of hydroxylation is still not known, and more investigation is needed.

Another question that is yet to be answered is why the TPHs are so difficult to purify, and why they aggregate rapidly *in vitro*. TPH2 has been reported to be somewhat less stable than TPH2, and the N-terminal has been suggested to be involved in the susceptibility of the protein to aggregation. Phosphorylation, in contrast, has been suggested to stabilize the protein, and also to label it for degradation. There are still some controversies regarding the different phosphorylation sites in TPH1 and TPH2, and which enzymes truly phosphorylate TPH1 and TPH2 *in vivo*. The effects of TPH phosphorylation on enzyme kinetics and turnover also need further studies.

TPH1 and TPH2 have been reported to be associated with psychiatric disorders, SIDS, and disorders in the gut. However, these aspects need to be clarified as there are contradictory results in the literature, in particular for the different psychiatric disorders. As a consequence of the growing amount of articles concerning TPH and disorders there is increased interest in finding new enzyme inhibitors that can be used as drugs. Some of the naturally occurring mutations reported in TPH1 and TPH2 have been reported to destabilize the enzyme in a way that is compatible with a role in brain disorders. The discovery of pharmacological chaperones that can stabilize these enzymes may therefore be an important finding that should be studied further.

Inhibitors of TPH1 have been suggested as a possible treatment in different diseases such as osteoporosis. However, one should keep in mind that TPH1 has been found to be important for early development of the brain, and pregnant women should probably not be treated with these inhibitors. These findings show the complexity of the serotonin pathway, how important it is to consider all aspects of the enzymes, and the importance of TPH1 and TPH2 in the normal development of the brain and other organs.

References

Abumaria, N., Ribic, A., Anacker, C., Fuchs, E. and Flugge, G. (2008). Stress upregulates TPH1 but not TPH2 mRNA in the rat dorsal raphe nucleus: identification of two TPH2 mRNA splice variants. *Cellular and Molecular Neurobiology* 28, 331–342.

Alenina, N., Kikic, D., Todiras, M., Mosienko, V., Qadri, F., Plehm, R., Boye, P., *et al.* (2009) Growth retardation and altered autonomic control in mice lacking brain serotonin. *Proceedings of the National Academy of Sciences USA* 106, 10332–10337.

Allen, N.C., Bagade, S., Mcqueen, M.B., Ioannidis, J.P., Kavvoura, F.K., Khoury, M.J., Tanzi, R.E., *et al.* (2008) Systematic meta-analyses and field synopsis of genetic association studies in schizophrenia: the SzGene database. *Nature Genetics* 40, 827–834.

Andersen, O.A., Flatmark, T. and Hough, E. (2001) High resolution crystal structures of the catalytic domain of human phenylalanine hydroxylase in its catalytically active Fe(II) form and binary complex with tetrahydrobiopterin. *Journal of Molecular Biology* 314, 279–291.

Arango, V., Huang, Y.Y., Underwood, M.D. and Mann, J.J. (2003) Genetics of the serotonergic system in suicidal behavior. *Journal of Psychiatric Research* 37, 375–386.

Banik, U., Wang, G.A., Wagner, P.D. and Kaufman, S. (1997) Interaction of phosphorylated tryptophan hydroxylase with 14-3-3 proteins. *Journal of Biological Chemistry* 272, 26219–26225.

Batten, T.F., Berry, P.A., Maqbool, A., Moons, L. and Vandesande, F. (1993) Immunolocalization of catecholamine enzymes, serotonin, dopamine and L-dopa in the brain of Dicentrarchus labrax (Teleostei). *Brain Research Bulletin* 31, 233–252.

Bellivier, F., Leboyer, M., Courtet, P., Buresi, C., Beaufils, B., Samolyk, D., Allilaire, J.F., *et al.* (1998) Association between the tryptophan hydroxylase gene and manic-depressive illness. *Archives of General Psychiatry* 55, 33–37.

Boadle-Biber, M.C. (1978) Activation of tryptophan hydroxylase from central serotonergic neurons by calcium and depolarization. *Biochemical Pharmacology* 27, 1069–1079.

Boadle-Biber, M.C. (1979) Decrease in the activity of tryptophan hydroxylase from slices of rat brain stem incubated in a low calcium or a calcium-free manganese-substituted medium. *Biochemical Pharmacology* 28, 3487–3490.

Boadle-Biber, M.C. (1982) Further studies on the role of calcium in the depolarization-induced activation of tryptophan hydroxylase. Effect of verapamil, Tetracaine, haloperidol and fluphenazine. *Biochemical Pharmacology* 31, 2495–2503.

Brown, H.J., Henderson, L.A. and Keay, K.A. (2006) Hypotensive but not normotensive haemorrhage increases tryptophan hydroxylase-2 mRNA in caudal midline medulla. *Neuroscience Letter*, 398, 314–318.

Burlina, A.B., Bonafe, L., Ferrari, V., Suppiej, A., Zacchello, F. and Burlina, A.P. (2000) Measurement of neurotransmitter metabolites in the cerebrospinal fluid of phenylketonuric patients under dietary treatment. *Journal of Inherited Metabolic Disease* 23, 313–316.

Calvo, A.C., Scherer, T., Pey, A.L., Ying, M., Winge, I., McKinney, J., Haavik, J., *et al.* (2010) Effect of pharmacological chaperones on brain tyrosine hydroxylase and tryptophan hydrolylase 2. *Journal of Neurochemistry* 114, 853–863.

Carkaci-Salli, N., Flanagan, J.M., Martz, M.K., Salli, U., Walther, D.J., Bader, M. and Vrana, K.E. (2006) Functional domains of human tryptophan hydroxylase 2 (hTPH2). *Journal of Biological Chemistry* 281, 28105–28112.

Cash, C.D. (1998) Why tryptophan hydroxylase is difficult to purify: a reactive oxygen-derived species-mediated phenomenon that may be implicated in human pathology. *General Pharmacology* 30, 569–574.

Chen, C., Glatt, S.J. and Tsuang, M.T. (2008) The tryptophan hydroxylase gene influences risk for bipolar disorder but not major depressive disorder: results of meta-analyses. *Bipolar Disorder* 10, 816–821.

Chipman, D.M. and Shaanan, B. (2001) The ACT domain family. *Current Opinion in Structural Biology* 11, 694–700.

Chow, M.S., Eser, B.E., Wilson, S.A., Hodgson, K.O., Hedman, B., Fitzpatrick, P.F. and Solomon, E.I. (2009) Spectroscopy and kinetics of wild-type and mutant tyrosine hydroxylase: mechanistic insight into O2 activation. *Journal of the American Chemical Society* 131, 7685–7698.

Cianchetta, G., Stouch, T., Wangsheng, Y., Zhi-Cai, S., Leslie, W.T., Swansson, R.V., Hunter, M.J., *et al.* (2010) Mechanism of inhibition of novel tryptophan hydroxylase inhibitors revealed by co-crystal structures and kinetic analysis. *Current Chemical Genomics* 4, 19–26.

Cichon, S., Winge, I., Mattheisen, M., Georgi, A., Karpushova, A., Freudenberg, J., Freudenberg-Hua, Y., *et al.* (2008) Brain-specific tryptophan hydroxylase 2 (TPH2): a functional Pro206Ser substitution and variation in the 5′-region are associated with bipolar affective disorder. *Human Molecular Genetics* 17, 87–97.

Clark, J.A., Pai, L.Y., Flick, R.B. and Rohrer, S.P. (2005) Differential hormonal regulation of tryptophan hydroxylase-2 mRNA in the murine dorsal raphe nucleus. *Biological Psychiatry* 57, 943–946.

Cote, F., Thevenot, E., Fligny, C., Fromes, Y., Darmon, M., Ripoche, M.A., Bayard, E., *et al.* (2003) Disruption of the nonneuronal tph1 gene demonstrates the importance of peripheral serotonin in cardiac function. *Proceedings of the National Academy of Sciences USA* 100, 13525–13530.

Cote, F., Fligny, C., Bayard, E., Launay, J.M., Gershon, M.D., Mallet, J. and Vodjdani, G. (2007) Maternal serotonin is crucial for murine embryonic development. *Proceedings of the National Academy of Sciences USA* 104, 329–334.

Daubner, S.C., Melendez, J. and Fitzpatrick, P.F. (2000) Reversing the substrate specificities of phenylalanine and tyrosine hydroxylase: aspartate 425 of tyrosine hydroxylase is essential for L-DOPA formation. *Biochemistry* 39, 9652–9661.

Daubner, S.C., McGinnis, J.T., Gardner, M., Kroboth, S.L., Morris, A.R. and Fitzpatrick, P.F. (2006) A flexible loop in tyrosine hydroxylase controls coupling of amino acid hydroxylation to tetrahydropterin oxidation. *Journal of Molecular Biology* 359, 299–307.

Deguchi, T. and Barchas, J. (1972) Effect of p-chlorophenylalanine on tryptophan hydroxylase in rat pineal. *Nature - New Biology* 235, 92–93.

Duncan, J.R., Paterson, D.S., Hoffman, J.M., Mokler, D.J., Borenstein, N.S., Belliveau, R.A., Krous, H.F., *et al.* (2010) Brainstem serotonergic deficiency in sudden infant death syndrome. *Journal of the American Medical Association* 303, 430–437.

Dunkley, P.R., Bobrovskaya, L., Graham, M.E., Von Nagy-Felsobuki, E.I. and Dickson, P.W. (2004) Tyrosine hydroxylase phosphorylation: regulation and consequences. *Journal of Neurochemistry* 91, 1025–1043.

Ehret, M., Cash, C.D., Hamon, M. and Maitre, M. (1989) Formal demonstration of the phosphorylation of rat brain tryptophan hydroxylase by Ca2+/calmodulin-dependent protein kinase. *Journal of Neurochemistry* 52, 1886–1891.

Ehret, M., Pevet, P. and Maitre, M. (1991) Tryptophan hydroxylase synthesis is induced by 3',5'-cyclic adenosine monophosphate during circadian rhythm in the rat pineal gland. *Journal of Neurochemistry* 57, 1516–1521.

Erlandsen, H., Fusetti, F., Martinez, A., Hough, E., Flatmark, T. and Stevens, R.C. (1997) Crystal structure of the catalytic domain of human phenylalanine hydroxylase reveals the structural basis for phenylketonuria. *Nature Structural & Molecular Biology* 4, 995–1000.

Eser, B.E., Barr, E.W., Frantom, P.A., Saleh, L., Bollinger, J.M., Jr, Krebs, C. and Fitzpatrick, P.F. (2007) Direct spectroscopic evidence for a high-spin Fe(IV) intermediate in tyrosine hydroxylase. *Journal of the American Chemical Society* 129, 11334–11335.

Fernstrom, J.D. and Wurtman, R.J. (1971) Brain serotonin content: physiological dependence on plasma tryptophan levels. *Science* 173, 149–152.

Fitzpatrick, P.F. (2003) Mechanism of aromatic amino acid hydroxylation. *Biochemistry* 42, 14083–14091.

Fitzpatrick, P.F., Ralph, E.C., Ellis, H.R., Willmon, O.J. and Daubner, S.C. (2003) Characterization of metal ligand mutants of tyrosine hydroxylase: insights into the plasticity of a 2-histidine-1-carboxylate triad. *Biochemistry* 42, 2081–2088.

Florez, J.C., Seidenman, K.J., Barrett, R.K., Sangoram, A.M. and Takahashi, J.S. (1996) Molecular cloning of chick pineal tryptophan hydroxylase and circadian oscillation of its mRNA levels. *Brain Research. Molecular Brain Research* 42, 25–30.

Frantom, P.A., Seravalli, J., Ragsdale, S.W. and Fitzpatrick, P.F. (2006) Reduction and oxidation of the active site iron in tyrosine hydroxylase: kinetics and specificity. *Biochemistry* 45, 2372–2379.

Friedman, P.A., Kappelman, A.H. and Kaufman, S. (1972) Partial purification and characterization of tryptophan hydroxylase from rabbit hindbrain. *Journal of Biological Chemistry* 247, 4165–4173.

Fujisawa, H. and Okuno, S. (2005) Regulatory mechanism of tyrosine hydroxylase activity. *Biochemical and Biophysical Research Communications* 338, 271–276.

Fusetti, F., Erlandsen, H., Flatmark, T. and Stevens, R.C. (1998) Structure of tetrameric human phenylalanine hydroxylase and its implications for phenylketonuria. *Journal of Biological Chemistry* 273, 16962–16967.

Ghia, J.E., Li, N., Wang, H., Collins, M., Deng, Y., El-Sharkawy, R.T., Cote, F., *et al.* (2009) Serotonin has a key role in pathogenesis of experimental colitis. *Gastroenterology* 137, 1649–1660.

Goodwill, K.E., Sabatier, C., Marks, C., Raag, R., Fitzpatrick, P.F. and Stevens, R.C. (1997) Crystal structure of tyrosine hydroxylase at 2.3 A and its implications for inherited neurodegenerative diseases. *Nature Structural & Molecular Biology* 4, 578–585.

Grahame-Smith, D.G. (1964) Tryptophan hydroxylation in brain. *Biochemical and Biophysical Research Communications* 16, 586–592.

Grant, G.A. (2006) The ACT domain: a small molecule binding domain and its role as a common regulatory element. *Journal of Biological Chemistry* 281, 33825–33829.

Grenett, H.E., Ledley, F.D., Reed, L.L. and Woo, S.L. (1987) Full-length cDNA for rabbit tryptophan hydroxylase: functional domains and evolution of aromatic amino acid hydroxylases. *Proceedings of the National Academy of Sciences USA* 84, 5530–5534.

Grohmann, M., Hammer, P., Walther, M., Paulmann, N., Buttner, A., Eisenmenger, W., Baghai, T.C., *et al.* (2010) Alternative splicing and extensive RNA editing of human TPH2 transcripts. *PLoS ONE* 5, e8956.

Gutknecht, L., Waider, J., Kraft, S., Kriegebaum, C., Holtmann, B., Reif, A., Schmitt, A., et al. (2008) Deficiency of brain 5-HT synthesis but serotonergic neuron formation in Tph2 knockout mice. *Journal of Neural Transmission* 115, 1127–1132.

Haghighi, F., Bach-Mizrachi, H., Huang, Y.Y., Arango, V., Shi, S., Dwork, A.J., Rosoklija, G., et al. (2008) Genetic architecture of the human tryptophan hydroxylase 2 Gene: existence of neural isoforms and relevance for major depression. *Molecular Psychiatry* 13, 813–820.

Halmoy, A., Johansson, S., Winge, I., McKinney, J.A., Knappskog, P. and Haavik, J. (2010) ADHD symptoms in offspring of mothers with impaired serotonin production. *Archives of General Psychiatry* 67, 1033–1043.

Hamon, M., Bourgoin, S., Artaud, F. and Hery, F. (1977) Rat brain stem tryptophan hydroxylase: mechanism of activation by calcium. *Journal of Neurochemistry* 28, 811–818.

Hamon, M., Bourgoin, S., Hery, F. and Simonnet, G. (1978) Activation of tryptophan hydroxylase by adenosine triphosphate, magnesium, and calcium. *Molecular Pharmacology* 14, 99–110.

Hegg, E.L. and Que, L., Jr (1997) The 2-His-1-carboxylate facial triad–an emerging structural motif in mononuclear non-heme iron(II) enzymes. *European Journal of Biochemistry* 250, 625–629.

Hensler, J.G., Ferry, R.C., Labow, D.M., Kovachich, G.B. and Frazer, A. (1994) Quantitative autoradiography of the serotonin transporter to assess the distribution of serotonergic projections from the dorsal raphe nucleus. *Synapse* 17, 1–15.

Hiroi, R., Mcdevitt, R.A. and Neumaier, J.F. (2006) Estrogen selectively increases tryptophan hydroxylase-2 mRNA expression in distinct subregions of rat midbrain raphe nucleus: association between gene expression and anxiety behavior in the open field. *Biological Psychiatry* 60, 288–295.

Hornung, J.P. (2003) The human raphe nuclei and the serotonergic system. *Journal of Chemical Neuroanatomy* 26, 331–343.

Hosoda, S. (1975) Further studies on tryptophan hydroxylase from neoplastic murine mast cells. *Biochimica et Biophysica Acta* 397, 58–68.

Huang, Z., Liu, T., Chattoraj, A., Ahmed, S., Wang, M.M., Deng, J., Sun, X. and Borjigin, J. (2008) Posttranslational regulation of TPH1 is responsible for the nightly surge of 5-HT output in the rat pineal gland. *Journal of Pineal Research* 45, 506–514.

Haahr, L.T., Jensen, K.P., Boesen, J. and Christensen, H.E. (2010) Experimentally calibrated computational chemistry of tryptophan hydroxylase: trans influence, hydrogen-bonding, and 18-electron rule govern O2-activation. *Journal of Inorganic Biochemistry*, 104, 136–145.

Haavik, J. and Flatmark, T. (1987) Isolation and characterization of tetrahydropterin oxidation products generated in the tyrosine 3-monooxygenase (tyrosine hydroxylase) reaction. *European Journal of Biochemistry* 168, 21–26.

Haavik, J., Blau, N. and Thony, B. (2008) Mutations in human monoamine-related neurotransmitter pathway genes. *Human Mutation* 29, 891–902.

Ichimura, T., Isobe, T., Okuyama, T., Yamauchi, T. and Fujisawa, H. (1987). Brain 14-3-3 protein is an activator protein that activates tryptophan 5-monooxygenase and tyrosine 3-monooxygenase in the presence of Ca2+,calmodulin-dependent protein kinase II. *FEBS Letters* 219, 79–82.

Iida, Y., Sawabe, K., Kojima, M., Oguro, K., Nakanishi, N. and Hasegawa, H. (2002) Proteasome-driven turnover of tryptophan hydroxylase is triggered by phosphorylation in RBL2H3 cells, a serotonin producing mast cell line. *European Journal of Biochemistry* 269, 4780–4788.

IUPAC-IUB (1984) IUPAC-IUB Joint Commission on Biochemical Nomenclature (JCBN). Nomenclature and symbolism for amino acids and peptides. Recommendations 1983. *Biochemical Journal* 219, 345–373.

Iwaki, M., Phillips, R.S. and Kaufman, S. (1986) Proteolytic modification of the amino-terminal and carboxyl-terminal regions of rat hepatic phenylalanine hydroxylase. *Journal of Biological Chemistry* 261, 2051–2056.

Jequier, E., Lovenberg, W. and Sjoerdsma, A. (1967) Tryptophan hydroxylase inhibition: the mechanism by which p-chlorophenylalanine depletes rat brain serotonin. *Molecular Pharmacology* 3, 274–278.

Jiang, G.C., Yohrling, G.J.T., Schmitt, J.D. and Vrana, K.E. (2000) Identification of substrate orienting and phosphorylation sites within tryptophan hydroxylase using homology-based molecular modeling. *Journal of Molecular Biology* 302, 1005–1017.

Johansen, P.A., Wolf, W.A. and Kuhn, D.M. (1991) Inhibition of tryptophan hydroxylase by benserazide and other catechols. *Biochemical Pharmacology* 41, 625–628.

Johansen, P.A., Jennings, I., Cotton, R.G. and Kuhn, D.M. (1995) Tryptophan hydroxylase is phosphorylated by protein kinase A. *Journal of Neurochemistry* 65, 882–888.

Johansen, P.A., Jennings, I., Cotton, R.G. and Kuhn, D.M. (1996) Phosphorylation and activation of tryptophan hydroxylase by exogenous protein kinase A. *Journal of Neurochemistry* 66, 817–823.

Johansson, S., Halmoy, A., Mavroconstanti, T., Jacobsen, K.K., Landaas, E.T., Reif, A., Jacob, C., *et al*. (2010) Common variants in the TPH1 and TPH2 regions are not associated with persistent ADHD in a combined sample of 1,636 adult cases and 1,923 controls from four European populations. *American Journal of Medical Genetics Part B: Neuropsychiatric Genetics* 153B, 1008–1015.

Jokela, M., Raikkonen, K., Lehtimaki, T., Rontu, R. and Keltikangas-Jarvinen, L. (2007) Tryptophan hydroxylase 1 gene (TPH1) moderates the influence of social support on depressive symptoms in adults. *Journal of Affective Disorders* 100, 191–197.

Kappock, T.J., Harkins, P.C., Friedenberg, S. and Caradonna, J.P. (1995) Spectroscopic and kinetic properties of unphosphorylated rat hepatic phenylalanine hydroxylase expressed in Escherichia coli. Comparison of resting and activated states. *Journal of Biological Chemistry* 270, 30532–30544.

Kaufman, S. (1974) Properties of the pterin-dependent aromatic amino acid hydroxylases. In: Wolstenholme, G.E.W. and Fitzsimons, D.W. (eds) *Aromatic Amino Acids in the Brain*. Novartis Foundation Symposia, pp. 85–115.

Kim, E.I., Yin, S., Kang, M.H., Hong, J.T., Oh, K.W. and Lee, M.K. (2003) Reduction of serotonin content by tetrahydropapaveroline in murine mastocytoma P815 cells. *Neuroscience Letters* 339, 131–134.

Kim, E.I., Kang, M.H. and Lee, M.K. (2004) Inhibitory effects of tetrahydropapaverine on serotonin biosynthesis in murine mastocytoma P815 cells. *Life Science* 75, 1949–1957.

Kim, K.S., Wessel, T.C., Stone, D.M., Carver, C.H., Joh, T.H. and Park, D.H. (1991) Molecular cloning and characterization of cDNA encoding tryptophan hydroxylase from rat central serotonergic neurons. *Brain Research. Molecular Brain Research* 9, 277–283.

Kim, S.H., Shin, J.S., Lee, J.J., Yin, S.Y., Kai, M. and Lee, M.K. (2001) Effects of hydrastine derivatives on dopamine biosynthesis in PC12 cells. *Planta Medica* 67, 609–613.

Kleppe, R., Uhlemann, K., Knappskog, P.M. and Haavik, J. (1999) Urea-induced denaturation of human phenylalanine hydroxylase. *Journal of Biological Chemistry* 274, 33251–33258.

Knapp, S., Mandell, A.J. and Bullard, W.P. (1975) Calcium activation of brain tryptophan hydroxylase. *Life Science* 16, 1583–1593.

Koe, B.K. and Weissman, A. (1966) p-Chlorophenylalanine: a specific depletor of brain serotonin. *Journal of Pharmacology and Experimental Therapeutics* 154, 499–516.

Kowlessur, D. and Kaufman, S. (1999) Cloning and expression of recombinant human pineal tryptophan hydroxylase in Escherichia coli: purification and characterization of the cloned enzyme. *Biochimica et Biophysica Acta* 1434, 317–330.

Kuhn, D.M. and Arthur, R., Jr (1998) Dopamine inactivates tryptophan hydroxylase and forms a redox-cycling quinoprotein: possible endogenous toxin to serotonin neurons. *Journal of Neuroscience* 18, 7111–7117.

Kuhn, D.M., Vogel, R.L. and Lovenberg, W. (1978) Calcium-dependent activation of tryptophan hydroxylase by ATP and magnesium. *Biochemical and Biophysical Research Communications* 82, 759–766.

Kuhn, D.M., Arthur, R., Jr and States, J.C. (1997) Phosphorylation and activation of brain tryptophan hydroxylase: identification of serine-58 as a substrate site for protein kinase A. *Journal of Neurochemistry* 68, 2220–2223.

Kuhn, D.M., Sakowski, S.A., Geddes, T.J., Wilkerson, C. and Haycock, J.W. (2007) Phosphorylation and activation of tryptophan hydroxylase 2: identification of serine-19 as the substrate site for calcium, calmodulin-dependent protein kinase II. *Journal of Neurochemistry* 103, 1567–1573.

Kumer, S.C. and Vrana, K.E. (1996) Intricate regulation of tyrosine hydroxylase activity and gene expression. *Journal of Neurochemistry* 67, 443–462.

Kumer, S.C., Mockus, S.M., Rucker, P.J. and Vrana, K.E. (1997) Amino-terminal analysis of tryptophan hydroxylase: protein kinase phosphorylation occurs at serine-58. *Journal of Neurochemistry* 69, 1738–1745.

Liang, J., Wessel, J.H. 3rd, Iuvone, P.M., Tosini, G. and Fukuhara, C. (2004) Diurnal rhythms of tryptophan hydroxylase 1 and 2 mRNA expression in the rat retina. *Neuroreport* 15, 1497–1500.

Liberles, J.S., Thorolfsson, M. and Martinez, A. (2005) Allosteric mechanisms in ACT domain containing enzymes involved in amino acid metabolism. *Amino Acids* 28, 1–12.

Makita, Y., Okuno, S. and Fujisawa, H. (1990) Involvement of activator protein in the activation of tryptophan hydroxylase by cAMP-dependent protein kinase. *FEBS Letters* 268, 185–188.

Malek, Z.S., Pevet, P. and Raison, S. (2004) Circadian change in tryptophan hydroxylase protein levels within the rat intergeniculate leaflets and raphe nuclei. *Neuroscience* 125, 749–758.

Malek, Z.S., Dardente, H., Pevet, P. and Raison, S. (2005) Tissue-specific expression of tryptophan hydroxylase mRNAs in the rat midbrain: anatomical evidence and daily profiles. *European Journal of Neuroscience* 22, 895–901.

Malek, Z.S., Sage, D., Pevet, P. and Raison, S. (2007) Daily rhythm of tryptophan hydroxylase-2 messenger ribonucleic acid within raphe neurons is induced by corticoid daily surge and modulated by enhanced locomotor activity. *Endocrinology* 148, 5165–5172.

Martinez, A., Abeygunawardana, C., Haavik, J., Flatmark, T. and Mildvan, A.S. (1993) Interaction of substrate and pterin cofactor with the metal of human tyrosine hydroxylase as determined by 1H-NMR. *Advances in Experimental Medicine and Biology* 338, 77–80.

Martinez, A., Knappskog, P.M. and Haavik, J. (2001) A structural approach into human tryptophan hydroxylase and its implications for the regulation of serotonin biosynthesis. *Current Medicinal Chemistry* 8, 1077–1091.

Matthes, S., Mosienko, V., Bashammakh, S., Alenina, N. and Bader, M. (2010) Tryptophan hydroxylase as novel target for the treatment of depressive disorders. *Pharmacology* 85, 95–109.

Maurer-Spurej, E. (2005) Circulating serotonin in vertebrates. *Cellular and Molecular Life Sciences,* 62, 1881–1889.

McGeer, E.G., Peters, D.A. and McGeer, P.L. (1968) Inhibition of rat brain tryptophan hydroxylase by 6-halotryptophans. *Life Science* 7, 605–615.

McKinney, J., Teigen, K., Froystein, N.A., Salaun, C., Knappskog, P.M., Haavik, J. and Martinez, A. (2001) Conformation of the substrate and pterin cofactor bound to human tryptophan hydroxylase. Important role of Phe313 in substrate specificity. *Biochemistry* 40, 15591–15601.

McKinney, J., Knappskog, P.M., Pereira, J., Ekern, T., Toska, K., Kuitert, B.B., Levine, D., et al. (2004) Expression and purification of human tryptophan hydroxylase from Escherichia coli and Pichia pastoris. *Protein Expression and Purification* 33, 185–194.

McKinney, J., Knappskog, P.M. and Haavik, J. (2005) Different properties of the central and peripheral forms of human tryptophan hydroxylase. *Journal of Neurochemistry* 92, 311–320.

McKinney, J., Johansson, S., Halmoy, A., Dramsdahl, M., Winge, I., Knappskog, P.M. and Haavik, J. (2008) A loss-of-function mutation in tryptophan hydroxylase 2 segregating with attention-deficit/hyperactivity disorder. *Molecular Psychiatry* 13, 365–367.

McKinney, J.A., Turel, B., Winge, I., Knappskog, P.M. and Haavik, J. (2009) Functional properties of missense variants of human tryptophan hydroxylase 2. *Human Mutation* DOI 10.1002/humu.20956.

Mendelsohn, D., Riedel, W.J. and Sambeth, A. (2009) Effects of acute tryptophan depletion on memory, attention and executive functions: a systematic review. *Neuroscience & Biobehavioral Reviews* 33, 926–952.

Mochizuki, D. (2004) Serotonin and noradrenaline reuptake inhibitors in animal models of pain. *Human Psychopharmacology* 19, S15–19.

Mockus, S.M., Kumer, S.C. and Vrana, K.E. (1997) Carboxyl terminal deletion analysis of tryptophan hydroxylase. *Biochimica et Biophysica Acta* 1342, 132–140.

Mockus, S.M., Yohrling, G.J.T. and Vrana, K.E. (1998) Tyrosine hydroxylase and tryptophan hydroxylase do not form heterotetramers. *Journal of Molecular Neuroscience* 10, 45–51.

Moran, G.R., Phillips, R.S. and Fitzpatrick, P.F. (1999) Influence of steric bulk and electrostatics on the hydroxylation regiospecificity of tryptophan hydroxylase: characterization of methyltryptophans and azatryptophans as substrates. *Biochemistry* 38, 16283–16289.

Moran, G.R., Derecskei-Kovacs, A., Hillas, P.J. and Fitzpatrick, P.F. (2000) On the catalytic mechanism of tryptophan hydroxylase. *Journal of the American Chemical Society* 122, 4535–4541.

Murphy, K.L., Zhang, X., Gainetdinov, R.R., Beaulieu, J.M. and Caron, M.G. (2008) A regulatory domain in the N-terminus of tryptophan hydroxylase 2 controls enzyme expression. *Journal of Biological Chemistry* 283, 13216–13224.

Nakamura, K., Koyama, Y., Takahashi, K., Tsurui, H., Xiu, Y., Ohtsuji, M., Lin, Q.S., et al. (2006a) Requirement of tryptophan hydroxylase during development for maturation of sensorimotor gating. *Journal of Molecular Biology* 363, 345–354.

Nakamura, K., Sugawara, Y., Sawabe, K., Ohashi, A., Tsurui, H., Xiu, Y., Ohtsuji, M., et al. (2006b) Late developmental stage-specific role of tryptophan hydroxylase 1 in brain serotonin levels. *Journal of Neuroscience* 26, 530–534.

Nakata, H. and Fujisawa, H. (1982) Purification and properties of tryptophan 5-monooxygenase from rat brain-stem. *European Journal of Biochemistry* 122, 41–47.

Nicholson, A.N. and Wright, C.M. (1981) (+)-6-fluorotryptophan, an inhibitor of tryptophan hydroxylase: sleep and wakefulness in the rat. *Neuropharmacology* 20, 335–339.

Nieter Burgmayer, S.J. (1998) Electron transfer in transition metal-pteridine systems In: Clarke, M.J. (ed.) *Structure and Bonding*. Springer, Berlin/Heidelberg.

Okuno, S. and Fujisawa, H. (1982) Purification and some properties of tyrosine 3-monooxygenase from rat adrenal. *European Journal of Biochemistry* 122, 49–55.

Ormazabal, A., Vilaseca, M.A., Perez-Duenas, B., Lambruschini, N., Gomez, L., Campistol, J. and Artuch, R. (2005) Platelet serotonin concentrations in PKU patients under dietary control and tetrahydrobiopterin treatment. *Journal of Inherited Metabolic Disease* 28, 863–870.

Ota, M., Dostert, P., Hamanaka, T., Nagatsu, T. and Naoi, M. (1992) Inhibition of tryptophan hydroxylase by (R)- and (S)-1-methyl-6,7-dihydroxy-1,2,3,4-tetrahydroisoquinolines (salsolinols). *Neuropharmacology* 31, 337–341.

Pandey, A., Habibulla, M. and Singh, R. (1983) Tryptophan hydroxylase and 5-HTP-decarboxylase activity in cockroach brain and the effects of p-chlorophenylalanine and 3-hydroxybenzylhydrazine (NSD-1015). *Brain Research* 273, 67–70.

Park, S.W., Ban, J.Y., Yoon, K.L., Kim, H.J., Chung, J.Y., Yi, J.W., Lee, B.J., et al. (2010) Involvement of tryptophan hydroxylase 2 (TPH2) gene polymorphisms in susceptibility to coronary artery lesions in Korean children with Kawasaki disease. *European Journal of Pediatrics* 169, 457–461.

Perez, B., Desviat, L.R., Gomez-Puertas, P., Martinez, A., Stevens, R.C. and Ugarte, M. (2005) Kinetic and stability analysis of PKU mutations identified in BH4-responsive patients. *Molecular Genetics and Metabolism* 86, S11–16.

Pey, A.L., Ying, M., Cremades, N., Velazquez-Campoy, A., Scherer, T., Thony, B., Sancho, J., et al. (2008) Identification of pharmacological chaperones as potential therapeutic agents to treat phenylketonuria. *Journal of Clinical Investigation* 118, 2858–2867.

Ramaekers, V.T., Senderek, J., Hausler, M., Haring, M., Abeling, N., Zerres, K., Bergmann, C., et al. (2001) A novel neurodevelopmental syndrome responsive to 5-hydroxytryptophan and carbidopa. *Molecular Genetics and Metabolism* 73, 179–187.

Sakowski, S.A., Geddes, T.J. and Kuhn, D.M. (2006) Mouse tryptophan hydroxylase isoform 2 and the role of proline 447 in enzyme function. *Journal of Neurochemistry* 96, 758–765.

Sanchez, R.L., Reddy, A.P., Centeno, M.L., Henderson, J.A. and Bethea, C.L. (2005) A second tryptophan hydroxylase isoform, TPH 2 mRNA, is increased by ovarian steroids in the raphe region of macaques. *Brain Research. Molecular Brain Research* 135, 194–203.

Savelieva, K.V., Zhao, S., Pogorelov, V.M., Rajan, I., Yang, Q., Cullinan, E. and Lanthorn, T.H. (2008) Genetic disruption of both tryptophan hydroxylase genes dramatically reduces serotonin and affects behavior in models sensitive to antidepressants. *PLoS ONE* 3, e3301.

Scholz, J., Toska, K., Luborzewski, A., Maass, A., Schunemann, V., Haavik, J. and Moser, A. (2008) Endogenous tetrahydroisoquinolines associated with Parkinson's disease mimic the feedback inhibition of tyrosine hydroxylase by catecholamines. *FEBS Journal* 275, 2109–2121.

Schulpis, K.H., Tjamouranis, J., Karikas, G.A., Michelakakis, H. and Tsakiris, S. (2002) In vivo effects of high phenylalanine blood levels on Na+,K+-ATPase, Mg2+-ATPase activities and biogenic amine concentrations in phenylketonuria. *Clinical Biochemistry* 35, 281–285.

Shin, J.S., Yun-Choi, H.S., Kim, E.I. and Lee, M.K. (1999) Inhibitory effects of higenamine on dopamine content in PC12 cells. *Planta Medica* 65, 452–455.

Siltberg-Liberles, J. and Martinez, A. (2009) Searching distant homologs of the regulatory ACT domain in phenylalanine hydroxylase. *Amino Acids* 36, 235–249.

Slominski, A., Pisarchik, A., Johansson, O., Jing, C., Semak, I., Slugocki, G. and Wortsman, J. (2003) Tryptophan hydroxylase expression in human skin cells. *Biochimica et Biophysica Acta* 1639, 80–86.

Stokes, A.H., Xu, Y., Daunais, J.A., Tamir, H., Gershon, M.D., Butkerait, P., Kayser, B., et al. (2000) p-ethynylphenylalanine: a potent inhibitor of tryptophan hydroxylase. *Journal of Neurochemistry* 74, 2067–2073.

Sugden, K., Tichopad, A., Khan, N., Craig, I.W. and D'souza, U.M. (2009) Genes within the serotonergic system are differentially expressed in human brain. *BMC Neuroscience* 10, 50.

Sumi-Ichinose, C., Urano, F., Kuroda, R., Ohye, T., Kojima, M., Tazawa, M., Shiraishi, H., et al. (2001) Catecholamines and serotonin are differently regulated by tetrahydrobiopterin - A study from 6-pyruvoyltetrahydropterin synthase knockout mice. *Journal of Biological Chemistry* 276, 41150–41160.

Sun, H.S., Tsai, H.W., Ko, H.C., Chang, F.M. and Yeh, T.L. (2004) Association of tryptophan hydroxylase gene polymorphism with depression, anxiety and comorbid depression and anxiety in a population-based sample of postpartum Taiwanese women. *Genes Brain Behavior* 3, 328–336.

Takazawa, C., Fujimoto, K., Homma, D., Sumi-Ichinose, C., Nomura, T., Ichmose, H. and Katoh, S. (2008) A brain-specific decrease of the tyrosine hydroxylase protein in sepiapterin reductase-null mice as a mouse model for Parkinson's disease. *Biochemical and Biophysical Research Communications* 367, 787–792.

Teigen, K., Froystein, N.A. and Martinez, A. (1999) The structural basis of the recognition of phenylalanine and pterin cofactors by phenylalanine hydroxylase: implications for the catalytic mechanism. *Journal of Molecular Biology* 294, 807–823.

Teigen, K., Dao, K.K., McKinney, J.A., Gorren, A.C., Mayer, B., Froystein, N.A., Haavik, J., et al. (2004) Tetrahydrobiopterin binding to aromatic amino acid hydroxylases. Ligand recognition and specificity. *Journal of Medicinal Chemistry* 47, 5962–5971.

Teigen, K., McKinney, J.A., Haavik, J. and Martinez, A. (2007) Selectivity and affinity determinants for ligand binding to the aromatic amino acid hydroxylases. *Current Medicinal Chemistry* 14, 455–467.

Tenner, K., Walther, D. and Bader, M. (2007) Influence of human tryptophan hydroxylase 2 N- and C-terminus on enzymatic activity and oligomerization. *Journal of Neurochemistry* 102, 1887–1894.

Tenner, K., Qadri, F., Bert, B., Voigt, J.P. and Bader, M. (2008) The mTPH2 C1473G single nucleotide polymorphism is not responsible for behavioural differences between mouse strains. *Neuroscience Letters* 431, 21–25.

Thony, B., Calvo, A.C., Scherer, T., Svebak, R.M., Haavik, J., Blau, N. and Martinez, A. (2008) Tetrahydrobiopterin shows chaperone activity for tyrosine hydroxylase. *Journal of Neurochemistry* 106, 672–681.

Tipper, J.P., Citron, B.A., Ribeiro, P. and Kaufman, S. (1994) Cloning and expression of rabbit and human brain tryptophan hydroxylase cDNA in Escherichia coli. *Archives of Biochemistry and Biophysics* 315, 445–453.

Tong, J.H. and Kaufman, S. (1975) Tryptophan hydroxylase. Purification and some properties of the enzyme from rabbit hindbrain. *Journal of Biological Chemistry* 250, 4152–4158.

Toska, K., Kleppe, R., Cohen, P. and Haavik, J. (2002) Phosphorylation of tyrosine hydroxylase in isolated mice adrenal glands. *Annals of the New York Academy of Sciences* 971, 66–68.

Vrana, K.E., Rucker, P.J. and Kumer, S.C. (1994) Recombinant rabbit tryptophan hydroxylase is a substrate for cAMP-dependent protein kinase. *Life Science* 55, 1045–1052.

Walther, D.J., Peter, J.U., Bashammakh, S., Hortnagl, H., Voits, M., Fink, H. and Bader, M. (2003) Synthesis of serotonin by a second tryptophan hydroxylase isoform. *Science* 299, 76.

Wang, L., Erlandsen, H., Haavik, J., Knappskog, P.M. and Stevens, R.C. (2002) Three-dimensional structure of human tryptophan hydroxylase and its implications for the biosynthesis of the neurotransmitters serotonin and melatonin. *Biochemistry* 41, 12569–12574.

Werner-Felmayer, G., Golderer, G. and Werner, E.R. (2002) Tetrahydrobiopterin biosynthesis, utilization and pharmacological effects. *Current Drug Metabolism* 3, 159–173.

Windahl, M.S., Petersen, C.R., Christensen, H.E. and Harris, P. (2008) Crystal structure of tryptophan hydroxylase with bound amino acid substrate. *Biochemistry* 47, 12087–12094.

Windahl, M.S., Boesen, J., Karlsen, P.E. and Christensen, H.E. (2009) Expression, purification and enzymatic characterization of the catalytic domains of human tryptophan hydroxylase isoforms. *Protein Journal*, 28, 400–406.

Winge, I., McKinney, J.A., Knappskog, P.M. and Haavik, J. (2005) Effects of mutations in human tryptophan hydroxylase associated with behavioural differences. *Journal of Neurochemistry* 94, suppl.2 172.

Winge, I., McKinney, J.A., Knappskog, P.M. and Haavik, J. (2007) Characterization of wild-type and mutant forms of human tryptophan hydroxylase 2. *Journal of Neurochemistry* 100, 1648–57.

Winge, I., McKinney, J.A., Ying, M., D'santos, C.S., Kleppe, R., Knappskog, P.M. and Haavik, J. (2008) Activation and stabilization of human tryptophan hydroxylase 2 by phosphorylation and 14-3-3 binding. *Biochemical Journal* 410, 195–204.

Wong, D.T., Perry, K.W. and Bymaster, F.P. (2005) Case history: the discovery of fluoxetine hydrochloride (Prozac). *Nature Reviews Drug Discovery* 4, 764–774.

Yadav, V.K., Balaji, S., Suresh, P.S., Liu, X.S., Lu, X., Li, Z., Guo, X.E., et al. (2010) Pharmacological inhibition of gut-derived serotonin synthesis is a potential bone anabolic treatment for osteoporosis. *Nature Medicine* 16, 308–312.

Yamauchi, T. and Fujisawa, H. (1979a) Activation of tryptophan 5-monooxygenase by calcium-dependent regulator protein. *Biochemical and Biophysical Research Communications* 90, 28–35.

Yamauchi, T. and Fujisawa, H. (1979b) Regulation of rat brainstem tryptophan 5-monooxygenase. Calcium-dependent reversible activation by ATP and magnesium. *Archives of Biochemistry and Biophysics* 198, 219–226.

Yamauchi, T. and Fujisawa, H. (1981) A calmodulin-dependent protein kinase that is involved in the activation of tryptophan 5-monooxygenase is specifically distributed in brain tissues. *FEBS Letters* 129, 117–119.

Yang, X.J. and Kaufman, S. (1994) High-level expression and deletion mutagenesis of human tryptophan hydroxylase. *Proceedings of the National Academy of Sciences USA* 91, 6659–6663.

Yohrling, G.J.T., Mockus, S.M. and Vrana, K.E. (1999) Identification of amino-terminal sequences contributing to tryptophan hydroxylase tetramer formation. *Journal of Molecular Neuroscience* 12, 23–34.

Zaboli, G., Gizatullin, R., Nilsonne, A., Wilczek, A., Jonsson, E.G., Ahnemark, E., Asberg, M. and Leopardi, R. (2006) Tryptophan hydroxylase-1 gene variants associate with a group of suicidal borderline women. *Neuropsychopharmacology* 31, 1982–1990.

Zhang, X., Beaulieu, J.M., Sotnikova, T.D., Gainetdinov, R.R. and Caron, M.G. (2004) Tryptophan hydroxylase-2 controls brain serotonin synthesis. *Science* 305, 217.

Zhang, X., Gainetdinov, R.R., Beaulieu, J.M., Sotnikova, T.D., Burch, L.H., Williams, R.B., Schwartz, D.A., *et al.* (2005) Loss-of-function mutation in tryptophan hydroxylase-2 identified in unipolar major depression. *Neuron* 45, 11–16.

Zill, P., Buttner, A., Eisenmenger, W., Bondy, B. and Ackenheil, M. (2004) Regional mRNA expression of a second tryptophan hydroxylase isoform in postmortem tissue samples of two human brains. *European Neuropsychopharmacology* 14, 282–284.

Zill, P., Buttner, A., Eisenmenger, W., Muller, J., Moller, H.J. and Bondy, B. (2009) Predominant expression of tryptophan hydroxylase 1 mRNA in the pituitary: a postmortem study in human brain. *Neuroscience* 159, 1274–1282.

10 Methionine Metabolism

J.M. Mato,[1]* M.L. Martínez-Chantar[1] and S.C. Lu[2]

[1]*CIC bioGUNE, CIBERehd, Technology Park of Bizkaia, Bizkaia, Spain;* [2]*Division of Gastroenterology and Liver Disease, Keck School of Medicine, USC, Los Angeles, USA*

10.1 Abstract

The steatosic and hepatocarcinogenic effect of diets deficient in methyl groups (methionine and choline) has been known for decades. Knockout mice with either a deficiency or excess in hepatic *S*-adenosylmethionine (SAMe, the first step in methionine metabolism and the main biological methyl donor) spontaneously develop steatosis (fatty liver) and hepatocellular carcinoma (HCC). Thus, a model has emerged in which changes in cellular pools of hepatic SAMe, fluctuating in response to a variety of conditions such as hepatocyte growth and differentiation, could provide the rheostat by which the methylation status and consequently the activity of critical proteins can be modulated. The relevance of this observation to human health is obvious since SAMe synthesis is impaired in humans with liver cirrhosis and HCC, and SAMe treatment increases survival in patients with alcoholic liver cirrhosis. Several molecular mechanisms have emerged to explain how abnormal fluctuations in hepatic SAMe content lead to the development of non-alcoholic fatty liver disease and HCC. This review analyses the methionine requirement of resting and proliferating hepatocytes as well as of liver cancer cells, in an attempt to understand why abnormal methionine metabolism can lead to liver injury and HCC. It is concluded that a less efficient methionine metabolism facilitates hepatocyte proliferation, and that manipulation of methionine metabolism holds promise for improving HCC prognosis.

10.2 Introduction

The body of a normal, adult, lean individual has an energy reserve of about 138,000 kcal, the majority of them (about 135,000 kcal) stored in the white adipose tissue as triglycerides (TGL). In addition, a small amount of TGL (about 450 kcal) playing a critical role in maintaining metabolic homeostasis for the whole body is stored in the liver (Cahill, 1976). Current estimates indicate that about 20–40% of the general adult population living in Western countries has non-alcoholic fatty liver disease (NAFLD, defined as more than 5% of fat by weight) (Adams and Lindor, 2007). In these individuals, the liver loses its characteristic reddish colour and turns a yellowish tint, due to the excessive accumulation of TGL. NAFLD is mainly associated with obesity although it is also frequent in individuals

* E-mail address: director@cicbiogune.es

suffering from essential nutrient deficiency. NAFLD is a progressive disease that moves from the simple accumulation of fat in the liver (steatosis) to steatosis with inflammation, necrosis, and fibrosis (non-alcoholic steatohepatitis, NASH). In turn, NASH may progress to cirrhosis and hepatocellular carcinoma (HCC), indicating that metabolic imbalance may be at the origin of the association of cancer with NAFLD (Reid, 2001).

While our current knowledge of the existence of this synchronization of nutrient metabolism and cell growth is principally based on studies on glucose consumption (Vander Heiden *et al.*, 2009), the hepatocarcinogenic activity of diets deficient in methyl groups (methionine and choline) (Mikol *et al.*, 1983) indicates that the metabolism of methionine may also be adapted to meet the needs of proliferating cells. This realization has brought renewed attention to Charles Best's observation in 1932 that choline prevented the deposition of fat in the liver, a phenomenon known as 'lipotropism' (Fig. 10.1) (Best, 1956). Best also realized that the rate of oxygen uptake by the slices of livers from rats on a diet low in choline was appreciably less than that of the normal liver slices, indicating a synchronization of the metabolism of choline and mitochondrial oxidative phosphorylation. In a subsequent study carried out in 1937, Tucker and Eckstein discovered the lipotropic action of methionine (Best, 1956). Then in 1940 du Vigneaud and his colleagues administered deuterium-labelled methionine to rats fed a diet low in methionine and choline, finding a massive accumulation of the isotope in choline (Best, 1956). This process, referred as 'transmethylation', undoubtedly established the synthesis of choline from methionine. Later work by Stetten established that ethanolamine (we know now that in the form of phosphatidylethanolamine) receives methyl groups from methionine to form choline (Best, 1956). In 1953 Cantoni showed that, in order to transfer its methyl group, methionine needs first to be converted to an active sulphonium ion by reacting with ATP and forming S-adenosylmethionine (SAMe) (Best, 1956). In 1983, Poirier observed that a severe deficiency in methyl groups causes liver cancer (Mikol *et al.*, 1983). More recently, Lu and Mato (2008) demonstrated that knockout mice deficient in hepatic SAMe synthesis fed a normal diet spontaneously develop fatty liver (Lu *et al.*, 2001) and HCC (Martínez-Chantar *et al.*, 2002). An explanation for these observations has remained elusive, since the connection of methionine metabolism with carbohydrate and lipid utilization as well as with hepatocyte proliferation is, at first glance, not obvious (Fig. 10.2).

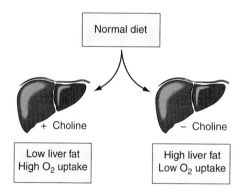

Fig. 10.1. Schematic representation of the lipotropic effect of choline: Best's effect. In 1932, Charles Best discovered that choline prevented the deposition of fat in the liver, a phenomenon known as 'lipotropism'. Best also realized that the rate of oxygen consumption by the slices of livers from rats on a diet low in choline was appreciably lower than that of the normal liver slices. In a subsequent study carried out in 1937, Tucker and Eckstein discovered the lipotropic effect of methionine.

10.3 Proliferating Hepatocytes and Liver Cancer Cells Show a Less Efficient Methionine Metabolism than Normal Differentiated Hepatocytes

SAMe is synthesized by methionine adenosyltransferase (MAT), an enzyme extremely well conserved through evolution, with 59% sequence homology between the human and *Escherichia coli* isoenzymes (Markham and Pajares, 2009). MAT is one of the minimal set of about 300 proteins that sustain independent life (Fraser *et al.*, 1995) because it catalyses the only reaction that generates SAMe, the main biological methyl donor (Mato and Lu, 2007; Mato *et al.*, 2008). In mammals there are three isoforms of MAT (MATI, MATII, and MATIII)

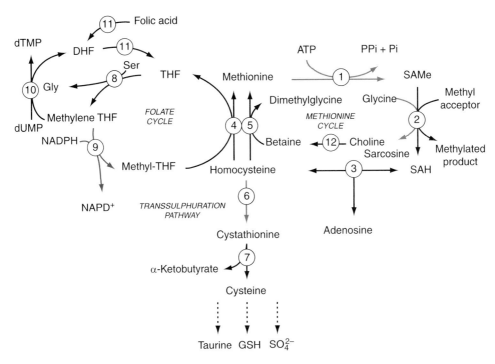

Fig. 10.2. Liver methionine metabolism comprises the methionine cycle, the folate cycle, and the transsulphuration pathway. SAMe (S-adenosylmethionine) is synthesized by methionine adenosyltransferase (1), an enzyme extremely well conserved through evolution. SAMe synthesized by the liver is utilized in hundreds of transmethylation reactions (2) to maintain the methylated status of DNA, histones, and numerous other proteins and small molecules. Excess SAMe is eliminated by glycine N-methyltransferase, the main enzyme involved in hepatic SAMe catabolism that converts glycine into sarcosine (methyl glycine). Transmethylation reactions convert SAMe into homocysteine via S-adenosylhomocysteine (SAH) (3). Once formed, homocysteine is used for the synthesis of cysteine and α-ketobutyrate as result of its transsulphuration. The transsulphuration pathway involves two enzymes: cystathionine β-synthase (6) and cystathionase (7). Cysteine is then utilized for the synthesis of glutathione (GSH) as well as other sulphur-containing molecules such as taurine, while α-ketobutyrate penetrates the mitochondria where it is decarboxylated to carbon dioxide and propionyl CoA. Homocysteine may also be used to regenerate methionine via two reactions: methionine synthase (4) and betaine-homocysteine methyltransferase (5). Methionine synthase links the methionine cycle with the folate cycle. The folate cycle also comprises the conversion of tetrahydrofolate (THF) into methylene-THF (8), and the synthesis of methyl-THF by the action of the enzyme methylenetetrahydrofolate reductase (9). Methylene-THF is also used for the synthesis of deoxy-TMP (thymidylic acid) (10), a reaction catalysed by the enzyme thymidylate synthase, a crucial step in DNA synthesis. Dietary folic acid may be converted into THF (11) through the intermediary dihydrofolate (DHF). dUMP, deoxyuridine monophosphate.

that are encoded by two genes (*MAT1A* and *MAT2A*). MATI and MATIII are tetrameric and dimeric forms, respectively, of the same subunit (α1) encoded by *MAT1A*, whereas the MATII isoform is a tetramer of a different subunit (α2) encoded by *MAT2A*. A third gene, *MAT2β*, encodes for a β subunit that regulates the activity of MATII (lowering the K_m and K_i, for methionine and SAMe, respectively) but not of MATI or MATIII (Halim *et al.*, 1999; Yang *et al.*, 2008). Adult differentiated liver expresses mainly *MAT1A*, whereas extrahepatic tissues, fetal liver, and HCC express *MAT2A* and *MAT2β* (Halim *et al.*, 1999; Yang *et al.*, 2008). The question why there are three different MAT isoforms in the liver is intriguing.

The predominant liver form, MATIII, has lower affinity for its substrates, a hysteretic response to methionine (a hysteretic behaviour, defined as a slow response to changes in substrate binding, has been described for many important enzymes in metabolic regulation), and higher V_{max}, contrasting with the other two enzymes (del Pino et al., 2000). Based on the differential properties of hepatic MAT isoforms, it has been postulated that MATIII is the truly liver-specific enzyme.

In a quiescent differentiated liver, when the levels of methionine are low, MATI would, as MATII outside the liver, synthesize most SAMe required by the hepatic cells to maintain the methylated status of DNA, histones, etc., and the homocysteine thus generated is mainly used for methionine regeneration (Fig. 10.3). However, after an increase in methionine concentration, i.e. after a protein-rich meal, conversion to the high activity MATIII would occur and methionine excess will be eliminated (del Pino et al., 2000). This will lead to an accumulation of SAMe and to the activation of glycine N-methyltransferase (GNMT), the main enzyme involved in hepatic SAMe catabolism (Luka et al., 2009). Consequently, the excess of SAMe will be eliminated and converted to homocysteine via S-adenosylhomocysteine (SAH). Once formed, the excess of homocysteine will be used mainly for the synthesis of cysteine and α-ketobutyrate as result of its transsulphuration (oxidative methionine metabolism) (Fig. 10.3).

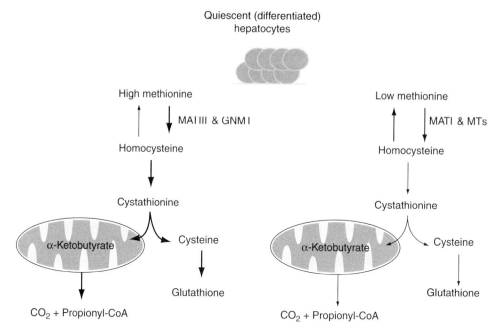

Fig. 10.3. Methionine metabolism in hepatocytes. In quiescent differentiated hepatocytes, when the levels of methionine are low, MATI (methionine adenosyltransferase I) synthesizes most SAMe required by the hepatic cells which is used by hundreds of methyltransferases (MTs) to maintain the methylated status of DNA, histones, and numerous other proteins and small molecules. The homocysteine thus generated is mainly used for methionine regeneration and only a small part is channelled through the transsulphuration pathway to be converted into cysteine and α-ketobutyrate (aerobic methionine metabolism). On the contrary, when the levels of methionine are high (i.e. after a protein-rich meal), the excess of this amino acid will be eliminated by the concerted action of MATIII (methionine adenosyltransferase III) and GNMT (glycine N-methyltransferase), and the resulting homocysteine is mainly channelled into the transsulphuration pathway to be converted into cysteine and α-ketobutyrate. Cysteine is then utilized for the synthesis of glutathione, while α-ketobutyrate penetrates the mitochondria and is decarboxylated to carbon dioxide and propionyl CoA (oxidative methionine metabolism). See text for details.

This pathway involves two enzymes: cystathionine β-synthase (CBS), which is activated by SAMe, and cystathionase. Cysteine is then utilized for the synthesis of glutathione as well as other sulphur-containing molecules such as taurine, while α-ketobutyrate penetrates the mitochondria where it is decarboxylated to carbon dioxide and propionyl CoA. Since SAMe is an inhibitor of methylene-THF reductase (MTHFR), this will prevent the regeneration of methionine after an oral load of this amino acid. At the mRNA level, SAMe maintains *MAT1A* expression while inhibiting *MAT2A* expression (Mato *et al.*, 2002). This modulation by SAMe of both the flux of methionine into the transsulphuration pathway and the regeneration of methionine maximizes the production of cysteine and α-ketobutyrate after a methionine load and minimizes the regeneration of this amino acid (Fig. 10.3).

In contrast to normal non-proliferating hepatocytes, which rely primarily on MATI/III to generate SAMe and maintain methionine homeostasis, embryonic and proliferating adult hepatocytes – as well as liver cancer cells – instead rely on MATII to synthesize SAMe (Fig. 10.4) (Cai *et al.*, 1996; Gil *et al.*, 1996; Huang *et al.*, 1998; García-Trevijano *et al.*, 2002). Moreover, liver cancer cells often have very low levels of *GNMT* and *CBS* expression and increased expression of *MAT2β*, which as mentioned above lowers the K_m for methionine and the K_i for SAMe of MATII (Huang *et al.*, 1998; Martínez-Chantar *et al.*, 2003). Consequently, *MAT2A/MAT2β*-expressing hepatoma cells have lower SAMe levels than cells expressing *MAT1A* favouring the regeneration of methionine and THF. This mechanism maximizes the incorporation of methionine into biomass, which in turn facilitates hepatocyte and hepatoma growth regardless of whether methionine is present in high or low amounts. By analogy with the 'Warburg effect', a well-known phenomenon that maximizes the conversion of glucose into biomass (facilitating rapid cell division even in the presence of enough oxygen to support mitochondrial oxidative phosphorylation) (Vander Heiden *et al.*, 2009), we designate this process as aerobic methionine metabolism.

The finding that MAT1A, GNMT, and CBS knockout mice spontaneously develop steatosis (Lu *et al.*, 2001; Robert *et al.*, 2005; Martínez-Chantar *et al.*, 2008; Varela-Rey *et al.*, 2009a) and, in the case of MAT1A- and GNMT-deficient animals, also HCC (Martínez-Chantar *et al.*, 2002, 2008; Liao *et al.*, 2009) additionally

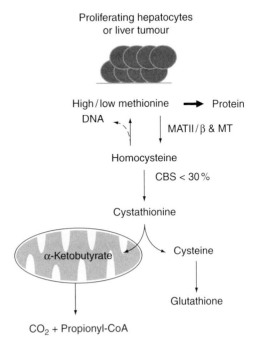

Fig. 10.4. Methionine metabolism in proliferating hepatocytes and liver tumour cells. In contrast to normal non-proliferating hepatocytes, which rely primarily on MATI/III (methionine adenosyltransferase I/III) to generate SAMe and maintain methionine homeostasis, embryonic and proliferating adult hepatocytes as well as liver cancer cells, rely instead on MATII and its regulatory subunit MAT2β to synthesize SAMe. Consequently, proliferating hepatocytes and hepatoma cells consume less methionine and maintain lower SAMe levels than non-proliferating hepatocytes. Moreover, liver cancer cells have very low levels of CBS (cystathionine β-synthase). This mechanism maximizes the regeneration of methionine and the incorporation of this amino acid into biomass, which in turn facilitates hepatocyte and hepatoma growth regardless of whether methionine is present in high or low amounts. This minimizes the channelling of homocysteine into the transsulphuration pathway. By analogy with the 'Warburg effect', we designate this process aerobic methionine metabolism. Methionine metabolism is coupled to the synthesis of dTMP, and consequently of DNA, through the folate cycle. MT, methyltransferases. See text for details.

demonstrates the synchronization of methionine metabolism with lipid metabolism and hepatocyte growth. It has been observed that genetic polymorphisms that associate with reduced MTHFR activity and increased thymidylate synthase (TYMS) activity, both of which are essential in minimizing uracyl misincorporation into DNA (Fig. 10.2), may protect against the development of HCC in humans (Yuang et al., 2007). This further supports the view that this synchronization may be an adaptive mechanism that is programmed to fit the specific needs of hepatocytes, and that alterations in the appropriate balance between methionine metabolism and proliferation may be at the origin of the association of cancer with fatty liver disease.

10.4 How Does a Less Efficient Methionine Metabolism Facilitate Hepatocyte Proliferation?

From these results it becomes evident that proliferating hepatocytes and hepatoma cells are not very tolerant of high SAMe levels or converting methionine via the transsulphuration pathway to cysteine and α-ketobutyrate. The underlying question is whether a less efficient methionine metabolism is simply an adaptation to the 'Warburg effect', allowing the conservation of this amino acid to optimize its utilization for protein and DNA synthesis (methionine metabolism is coupled to the synthesis of dTMP, and consequently of DNA, through the folate cycle), or if is also a primordial factor in the hepatocyte proliferation process and hepatocarcinogenesis. There is increasing evidence that SAMe works as a rheostat that regulates hepatocyte and liver cancer cell growth. As a rule, low SAMe levels facilitate hepatocyte and hepatoma cell growth, and elevated SAMe prevents cell growth. Thus, whereas in hepatoma cells over-expression of *MAT2β* reduces SAMe content and increases DNA synthesis, down-regulation of *MAT2β* expression increases SAMe content and reduces DNA synthesis (Halim et al., 1999; Martínez-Chantar et al., 2003; Yang et al., 2008). Similarly, hepatoma cells transfected with *MAT1A* grow more slowly than control tumour cells (Li et al., 2010), and the addition of SAMe to hepatoma cells, but not to normal hepatocytes, induces apoptosis (Ansorena et al., 2002; Lu et al., 2009). *In vivo*, SAMe treatment is also effective in preventing the establishment of HCC, although in a rodent model it is ineffective as a treatment for existing liver tumours (possibly due to the adaptation of the surrounding normal liver tissue to eliminate excess exogenous SAMe) (Lu et al., 2009). The mitogenic effect of HGF (hepatocyte growth factor) in hepatocytes requires the induction of both *MAT2A* and *MAT2β* expression, and is blocked by exogenous SAMe administration (Latasa et al., 2001; Martínez-Chantar et al., 2002; Luka et al., 2009; Vázquez-Chantada et al., 2009). Moreover, the administration of SAMe preceding partial hepatectomy (PH) in mice prevents the fall in SAMe concentration and impairs liver regeneration (Vázquez-Chantada et al., 2009). Intriguingly, although in hepatoma cells the mitogenic effect of leptin (an adipose tissue-derived hormone that plays a pivotal role in the progression of liver fibrogenesis and carcinogenesis) is blocked by SAMe administration, inducing apoptosis, this adipokine increases hepatic SAMe levels by about 45% despite inducing both *MAT2A* and *MAT2β* expression (Ramani et al., 2008). Our hypothesis is that for hepatoma cells, like non-hepatocytes that express only *MAT2A* and have low levels of SAMe, an increase in this molecule may be beneficial in supporting polyamine synthesis and growth. However, at higher doses SAMe inhibits growth and induces apoptosis. With regards to MAT2β, this protein may have other activities independent of the modulation of MATII, including the regulation of the activity of several mitogen-activated protein kinases by mechanisms that we do not know yet (Ramani et al., 2008; Yang et al., 2008). These results demonstrate that the effect of SAMe can vary drastically in normal versus malignant hepatocytes.

A signalling pathway that senses the cellular SAMe content and that involves AMPK (adenosine 5'-monophosphate (AMP) activated protein kinase) has been recently identified in hepatocytes (Fig. 10.5) (Martínez-Chantar et al., 2006; Vázquez-Chantada et al., 2009). AMPK is a serine/threonine protein kinase that plays a key role

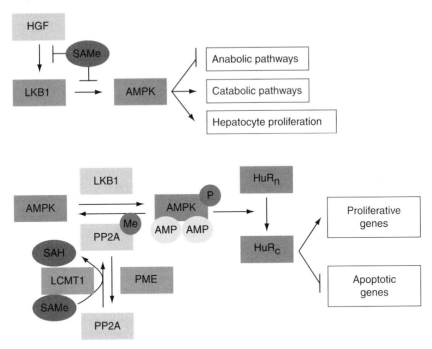

Fig. 10.5. A signalling pathway that senses the cellular SAMe content. AMPK (AMP-activated protein kinase) is a protein kinase that plays a key role in the regulation of energy homeostasis. AMPK is activated by an increase in the AMP/ATP ratio. This activation is dependent of LKB1, a protein kinase that phosphorylates AMPK. Binding of AMP is thought to be responsible for allosteric regulation of AMPK by making the enzyme less accessible to phosphoprotein phosphatase inactivation and facilitating phosphorylation by LKB1. Once activated, AMPK shuts down anabolic pathways that mediate the synthesis of proteins, lipids, and glycogen and stimulates catabolic pathways such as lipid oxidation and glucose uptake. This coordinated action of AMPK on metabolism restores ATP levels, keeping the cellular energy balance. In hepatocytes, LKB1 and AMPK are phosphorylated in response to HGF. SAMe blocks this activation by HGF of LKB1 and AMPK phosphorylation, through a mechanism possibly involving increased dephosphorylation of the enzymes, by making them more accessible to PP2A (phosphoprotein phosphatase 2A). PP2A enzymes exist as heterotrimeric complexes consisting of catalytic (PP2A$_C$), structural (PP2A$_A$), and regulatory (PP2A$_B$) subunits. Different PP2A$_B$ subunits have been described that determine the substrate specificity of the enzyme. PP2A$_C$ subunit is methylated by LCMT1 (leucine carboxyl methyltransferase-1) and demethylated by PME1, a specific phosphoprotein phosphatase methylesterase. PP2A$_C$ methylation has no effect on PP2A activity but has a crucial role in the recruitment of specific PP2A$_B$ subunits to the PP2A$_{A,C}$ complex and therefore on PP2A substrate specificity. AMPK activation leads to the mobilization of HuR from the nucleus (HuR$_n$) to the cytoplasm (HuR$_c$). HuR is a RNA-binding protein that increases the stability and translation of numerous target mRNAs involved in cell proliferation and apoptosis under conditions of stress. SAH, S-adenosylhomocysteine.

in the regulation of energy homeostasis (Viollet *et al.*, 2009). AMPK is activated by an increase in the AMP/ATP ratio. This activation is dependent on LKB1, a serine/threonine protein kinase that phosphorylates AMPK. Binding of AMP is thought to be responsible for allosteric regulation of AMPK by making the enzyme less accessible to phosphoprotein phosphatase inactivation, and facilitating phosphorylation by LKB1. Once activated, AMPK shuts down anabolic pathways that mediate the synthesis of proteins, fatty acids (FA), cholesterol and glycogen, and stimulates catabolic pathways such as lipid oxidation and glucose uptake. This coordinated action of AMPK on metabolism restores ATP levels, keeping the cellular energy balance. In hepatocytes, LKB1 and

AMPK are phosphorylated in response to HGF (Fig. 10.5) (Martínez-Chantar et al., 2006; Vázquez-Chantada et al., 2009). SAMe blocks this activation by HGF of LKB1 and AMPK phosphorylation through a mechanism that may involve increased dephosphorylation of the enzymes by making them more accessible to PP2A (phosphoprotein phosphatase 2A) (Martínez-Chantar et al., 2006). PP2A enzymes exist as heterotrimeric complexes consisting of catalytic ($PP2A_C$), structural ($PP2A_A$), and regulatory ($PP2A_B$) subunits (Sontag et al., 2008). Different $PP2A_B$ subunits have been described, that determine the substrate specificity of the enzyme. $PP2A_C$ subunit is methylated by SAMe-dependent leucine carboxyl methyltransferase-1 (LCMT1), and demethylated by a specific phosphoprotein phosphatase methylesterase (PME1). $PP2A_C$ methylation has no effect on PP2A activity but has a crucial role in the recruitment of specific $PP2A_B$ subunits to the $PP2A_{A,C}$ complex, and therefore on PP2A substrate specificity. In hepatocytes, AMPK interacts with PP2A through a process stimulated by SAMe (Martínez-Chantar et al., 2006) and which is associated with increased PP2A methylation (MLMC, SCL, JMM, unpublished). In the brain, alterations in methionine metabolism that lead to a decrease in the ratio of SAMe/SAH (SAH is a potent competitive inhibitor of LCMT1) associate with down-regulation of LCMT1, PP2A methylation, and $PP2A_B$ expression, and enhanced Tau phosphorylation (Sontag et al., 2008). It is however unknown whether physiologically induced changes in hepatic SAMe content lead to changes in PP2A methylation and its association with AMPK.

Down-regulation of LKB1 or AMPK with specific RNA interference (RNAi) inhibits the mitogenic effect of HGF in hepatocytes, through a mechanism that involves HuR mobilization from the nucleus to the cytoplasm and that is inhibited by SAMe (Fig. 10.5) (Vázquez-Chantada et al., 2009). HuR is an RNA-binding protein that increases the stability and translation of numerous target mRNAs involved in cell proliferation and apoptosis under conditions of stress (Doller et al., 2008). HuR can regulate both cell proliferation (by varying the levels of proteins that control cell-cycle progression such as cyclins D1 and A2) and apoptosis (by changing the expression of pro- and anti-apoptotic proteins such as p53 and Bcl-2) (Doller et al., 2008). As a rule, elevated cytoplasmic HuR associates with cell survival and proliferation, whereas reduced cytoplasmic HuR associates with apoptosis. In *MAT1A* knockout (KO) mice, a reduction in hepatic SAMe content is associated with LKB1- and AMPK-hyperphosphorylation, HuR mobilization to the cytoplasm, increased expression of proliferative genes and mitogenesis (Martínez-Chantar et al., 2006; Vázquez-Chantada et al., 2009). In contrast, in *GNMT*-KO animals the large increase in hepatic SAMe associates with LKB1- and AMPK-hypophosphorylation, reduced cytoplasmic HuR, increased expression of apoptotic genes and cell death (Varela-Rey et al., 2009a). From this perspective, it seems that increased SAMe content is a problem when hepatocytes have to grow. This explains, at least in part, the selective advantage provided to proliferating hepatocytes by the switch from *MAT1A* to *MAT2A* expression. Uncontrolled liver proliferation is prevented because hepatocytes do not normally express MATII unless forced to do so by growth factors. Cancer cells overcome this growth factor dependence by silencing *MAT1A* expression (Gil et al., 1996; Avila et al., 2000).

10.5 Regulation of Methionine Metabolism is a Crucial Step in Liver Regeneration

Hepatocyte proliferation is infrequent in normal adult liver, since these cells are arrested in the G0 phase of the cell cycle (Taub, 2004). However, after PH the majority of the hepatic cells re-enter the cell cycle within hours of surgery, achieving liver mass restoration in several days. Re-entering the cell cycle after PH is preceded by a decrease in *MAT1A* expression and inhibition of MATI/III activity, possibly mediated by the nitric oxide and reactive oxygen substances (ROS) generated in response to the stress imposed by the loss of liver mass (Corrales et al., 1990), an increase in the expression of *MAT2A*, and a reduction of SAMe content (Huang *et al.*, 1998; Ramani *et al.*, 2008). This reduction in hepatic SAMe content releases the inhibition that this molecule exerts on HGF-mediated phosphorylation of LKB1 and AMPK, HuR mobilization, and the expression of mitogenic genes such as cyclin D1 (Fig. 10.5) (Vázquez-Chantada *et al.*, 2009). These results suggest that switching to a less efficient methionine metabolism with the concomitant reduction in SAMe content is a crucial step in liver regeneration. Accordingly, SAMe administration preceding PH to prevent the fall in hepatic SAMe content during liver regeneration inhibited LKB1- and AMPK-phosphorylation, HuR mobilization, and the activation of cyclin D1, thereby blocking progression through G1 and entry into the DNA-synthesis phase of the cell cycle (Vázquez-Chantada *et al.*, 2009). Similarly, *in vivo* down-regulation of *GNMT* with specific RNAi to prevent the fall in SAMe content following PH also induced a marked reduction in the expression of cyclin D1 (Varela-Rey *et al.*, 2009a); and *MAT1A*- and *GNMT*-KO mice show impaired liver regeneration after PH (Chen *et al.*, 2004;Varela-Rey *et al.*, 2009a).

As mentioned above, a switch accompanies cell growth from complete catabolism of glucose, using mitochondrial oxidative phosphorylation to maximize the generation of ATP required for cellular processes, to aerobic glycolysis (conversion of glucose into lactate, the Warburg effect). Hepatocytes are the exception to this rule. Unlike most growing cells, after PH regenerating hepatocytes not only need to proliferate rapidly but also continue functioning to maintain metabolic homeostasis for the whole organism (Taub, 2004). This fundamental difference between proliferating hepatocytes and other growing cells is reflected in their metabolic needs. Hepatic regeneration results in a rapid mobilization of FA from the white adipose tissue to the liver, causing a transient accumulation of fat in hepatocytes. These FA are then oxidized, mainly in the mitochondria, providing the necessary ATP to support the metabolic demands of rapid proliferation (catabolic metabolism), a process that is activated by AMPK. In parallel, liver regeneration induces the expression of gluconeogenic genes (anabolic metabolism), a critical function to maintain the serum glucose level and compensate for the hypoglycaemic effect of AMPK activation (Taub, 2004). Hepatic regeneration also induces the activation of the protein kinase complex mTOR, another key energy sensor controlling gluconeogenesis and directing amino acids into protein synthesis (Taub, 2004).

Steatosis occurs when the rate of hepatic FA uptake from blood and lipogenesis is greater than the rate of FA oxidation and secretion (as TGL forming very low density lipoproteins, VLDL). Isotope-labelling experiments have shown that adipose tissue-derived FA account for up to 60% of the liver TGL in steatosis, whereas hepatic lipogenesis accounts for about 25%, and other pathways, such as impaired lipid oxidation or secretion, are less important (Parks and Hellerstein, 2006). In *MAT1A*-KO mice, chronic deficiency in hepatic SAMe induces hepatocyte proliferation which possibly stimulates a constant flux of FA from the adipose tissue to the liver and steatosis (Fig. 10.6). Similarly, in *GNMT*-KO mice the excess of hepatic SAMe triggers activation of the Ras and JAK/STAT pathways, inducing hepatocyte proliferation and possibly leading to an increased flux of FA from the adipose tissue to the liver, and to steatosis (Fig. 10.6). Additionally, altered SAMe metabolism may impair the flux of VLDL from hepatocytes to other parts of the body, as suggested by the finding that phosphatidylethanolamine methyltransferase (PEMT) KO mice are defective in VLDL secretion and develop liver steatosis (Zhao *et al.*, 2009). Interestingly, patients with liver cirrhosis have impaired SAMe synthesis and reduced PEMT activity (Duce *et al.*, 1988).

Hepatic steatosis has been proposed as an essential precursor of steatohepatitis, but the simple accumulation of fat in the liver is not sufficient to induce the necroinflammatory lesions associated with steatohepatitis, as seen in models of chronically obesity such as in obese (*ob/ob*) mice (Koteish and Diehl, 2002; Varela-Rey *et al.*, 2009b). One of the factors associated with the progression of steatosis to steatohepatitis is the oxidative stress originated by toxic lipid peroxidation catalysed by

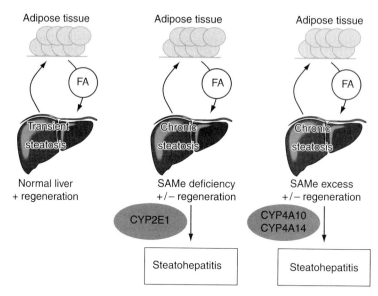

Fig. 10.6. Schematic representation of fatty acid mobilization in normal regenerative liver and in the liver of animals with altered SAMe metabolism. Liver regeneration after partial hepatectomy induces the mobilization of fatty acids (FA) from the white adipose tissue to the liver causing a transient accumulation of triglycerides (steatosis). These FA are then oxidized, mainly in the mitochondria, providing the necessary ATP to support the metabolic demands of rapid proliferation. In *MAT1A*-KO and *GNMT*-KO mice, regardless of whether the liver is regenerating or not, abnormal hepatic SAMe content induces hepatocyte proliferation, which stimulates a constant flux of FA from the adipose tissue to the liver causing chronic steatosis. The increased FA flux to the liver and decreased FA oxidation results in toxic lipid peroxidation catalysed by CYP2E1 in the case of *MAT1A*-KO mice, and CYP4A10 and CYP4A14 in the case of *GNMT*-KO animals, leading to steatohepatitis (steatosis with inflammation, necrosis and fibrosis).

cytochrome P4502E1 (CYP2E1), the main enzyme involved in NADPH-dependent reduction of oxygen leading to lipid peroxidation (Lieber, 1997). The CYPs constitute a superfamily of haem-containing microsomal mono-oxygenases that play a central role in the detoxification of xenobiotics, as well as in the metabolism of endogenous compounds including FA. *CYP2E1* expression is up-regulated in *MAT1A*-KO mouse liver (Martínez-Chantar *et al.*, 2002). In contrast, *CYP2E1* expression in *GNMT*-KO mouse liver is reduced, but the expression of two alternative FA-hydroxylases (*CYP4A10* and *CYP4A14*, the two major *CYP4A* genes) is markedly induced (Latasa *et al.*, 2001). It has been demonstrated that CYP4A enzymes are key intermediates of an adaptive response to perturbation of hepatic lipid metabolism. Thus, in *CYP2E1*-KO mice, lipid peroxidation induced by the accumulation of hepatic FA in response to a methyl-deficient diet is mediated by the up-regulation of *CYP4A10* and *CYP4A14* expression (Leclerq *et al.*, 2000). Alterations in the appropriate balance of CYPs that deal with FA oxidation may underline the predisposition to develop steatohepatitis and HCC associated with methionine deficient metabolism. A better understanding of how hepatic SAMe levels differentially interact with *CYP2E1*, *CYP4A10*, and *CYP4A14* expression, and with lipid metabolism, may help to identify points for therapeutic intervention.

10.6 How do Both a Defect and an Excess of Liver SAMe Trigger HCC?

Through its regulation of the LKB1/AMPK signalling pathway, SAMe is linked to both growth control and metabolism, and through the methylation of DNA and histones, SAMe regulates gene expression. In addition, there is evidence indicating that SAMe also regulates proteolysis, widening its spectrum of action (Fig. 10.7). In hepatocytes, the protein levels of both prohibitin 1 (PHB1) and the apurinic/apyrimidinic endonuclease (APEX1) are stabilized by SAMe (Santamaria et al., 2003; Tomasi et al., 2009). PHB1 is a chaperone-like protein involved in mitochondrial function and APEX1 is a key protein involved in DNA repair. Proteasomal chymotrypsin- and caspase-like activities are increased in MAT1A-KO livers and cultured hepatocytes, but were blocked by SAMe treatment (Tomasi et al., 2010). Moreover, SAMe inhibits chymotrypsin- and caspase-like activities in 20S proteasomes and causes rapid degradation of some of the 26S proteasomal subunits (Tomasi et al., 2010). Recently, methylated proteins have been identified in mammalian 20S proteasome complex (Zong et al., 2008), suggesting that this may be a key regulatory mechanism of proteasome function.

Under normal conditions, liver SAMe content is low enough not to induce aberrant DNA and histone hypermethylation, which would result in epigenetic modulation of specifics and critical carcinogenic pathways, such as the Ras and JAK/STAT signalling pathways. Nevertheless it is sufficiently elevated to avoid the spontaneous activation of the LKB1/AMPK signalling pathway resulting in uncontrolled hepatocyte growth and, possibly, undesired proteolysis. In MAT1A-KO mice, liver SAMe content is reduced chronically about threefold, resulting in the continuous activation of the LKB1/AMPK signalling pathway, abnormal proteasomal activity, and inefficient DNA repair. This leads to uncontrolled hepatocyte growth and HCC formation (Lu et al., 2001; Martínez-Chantar et al., 2002). Tumorigenic progenitor oval cells (OC), capable of forming epithelial tumours, have been isolated from MAT1A-KO mouse liver (Rontree et al., 2008; Ding et al., 2009), indicating that liver cancer stem cells contribute to carcinoma formation in this mouse model of SAMe deficiency. OC are liver stem cells found in the nonparenchimal fraction of the liver, and reside near the terminal bile ducts, at the hepatocyte–cholangiocyte interface. In normal adult liver, OC are quiescent and few in number, and proliferate only during severe, prolonged liver injury and in various models of experimental carcinogenesis (Lee et al., 2009). OC-derived carcinomas tend to have a more aggressive phenotype, with as many as 50% of HCC defined as having a progenitor cell phenotype. Related to this is a recent

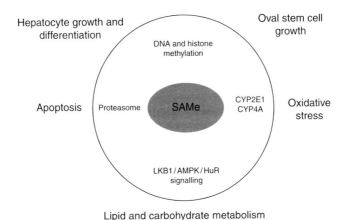

Fig. 10.7. Schematic representation of the spectrum of SAMe action in the liver. The modulation of the activity of critical genes and proteins by modification of their methylation status supports a model in which changes in cellular pools of hepatic SAMe, fluctuating in response to a variety of conditions, regulates key cellular functions such as hepatocyte growth and differentiation, oval cell proliferation, apoptosis, proteasomal activity, oxidative stress and lipid and carbohydrate metabolism.

report finding that patients with HCC where MAT1A expression was silenced had more aggressive tumours and shorter survival (Calvisi *et al.*, 2007).

In *GNMT*-KO mice, hepatic SAMe content is chronically increased about 50-fold, resulting in the inhibition of the LKB1/AMPK signalling pathway and increased apoptosis (Martínez-Chantar *et al.*, 2008; Varela-Rey *et al.*, 2010). These supra-physiological levels of hepatic SAMe also induce loss of expression of the Ras and JAK/STAT inhibitors *RASSF1*, *RASSF4*, *SOCS1*, *SOCS2*, *SOCS3*, and *CIS*, resulting in uncontrolled growth and HCC (Martínez-Chantar *et al.*, 2008). These inhibitors of the Ras and JAK/STAT signalling pathways, which are frequently inactivated by promoter methylation, have been involved in carcinogenesis, including HCC formation (Calvisi *et al.*, 2006). In *GNMT*-KO mouse liver the methylation of *RASSF1* and *SOCS2* promoters has been demonstrated, as well as the hypermethylation of H3K27 (lysine 27 in histone 3) (Martínez-Chantar *et al.*, 2008), which is also linked to gene repression and carcinogenesis (Calvisi *et al.*, 2006). Tumorigenic OC have also been identified in *GNMT*-KO mouse liver (Martínez-Chantar *et al.*, 2010).

This effect of *GNMT* silencing on HCC formation is possibly related to the more common phenomenon of methionine auxotrophy in cancer cells. Methionine auxotrophy (or methionine stress) is defined as the inability of a cell to grow in a medium devoid of methionine but containing instead homocysteine together with folic acid and vitamin B_{12} (Kokkinakis *et al.*, 2006). Most cancer cells, but not normal cells, are methionine dependent (Kokkinakis *et al.*, 2006). The biochemical basis of methionine dependency of tumour cells is not totally clear. Normal cells grow slowly and possibly have lower needs of methionine for protein synthesis than cancer cells, being able to cover their need for this amino acid by regenerating methionine from homocysteine. In contrast, an imbalance may exist in tumour cells between the needs of methionine and the capacity of the cells to regenerate this amino acid from homocysteine. As a consequence, tumour cells cannot compensate for a relative deficiency in methionine and therefore cease growing. From this perspective, silencing *MAT1A*, *GNMT*, and *CBS* (a most efficient pathway to remove methionine from protein synthesis and convert it to cysteine and α-ketobutyrate) will facilitate liver tumour cell growth.

GNMT is also present in large amounts in the prostate (Mato *et al.*, 2008; Luka *et al.*, 2009). *GNMT*-KO mice, however, do not develop prostate pathology, indicating that the function of GNMT in this organ is different than that in the liver. Interestingly, down-regulation of GNMT with RNAi results in a significant reduction in cell invasion in DU145 prostate cancer cells (Sreekumar *et al.*, 2009), demonstrating that when it comes to methionine metabolism and cancer, generalization is very difficult.

10.7 Does Changing the Metabolism of Hepatocytes through Manipulation of Methionine Metabolism Hold Promise for Improving HCC Prognosis?

An explanation of Best's effect is that where the cellular levels of SAMe and the activity of the transsulphuration pathway are maintained low, a less efficient methionine metabolism enhances the capacity of hepatocytes and hepatoma cells to utilize nutrients for anabolic processes, and supports growth. In principle, this dependency of HCC on methionine metabolism may be utilized for cancer treatment. Understanding how *MAT1A*, *GNMT*, and *CBS* are silenced and how *MAT2A* and *MAT2β* are activated in hepatoma cells may identify potential points for therapeutic intervention. Recently, we have provided some mechanistic insight into how this switch between *MAT1A* and *MAT2A* occurs (Vázquez-Chantada *et al.*, 2010). It was first observed that under a variety of conditions (embryonic liver development, hepatocyte growth, and liver regeneration), the timely switch from *MAT1A* to *MAT2A* coincides with an increase in the expression of the mRNA binding proteins HuR and AUF1. We also observed that HuR associates with *MAT2A* increasing its stability, while AUF1 associates with *MAT1A* mRNA decreasing its stability. Understanding how HuR and AUF1 expression is regulated during NAFLD progression and hepatocarcinogenesis may identify potential points for therapeutic intervention. Additionally, understanding how SAMe interacts with HGF-stimulated LKB1/AMPK/HuR signalling may better define how alterations in methionine metabolism lead to fatty liver, abnormal growth, and increased cancer predisposition. Furthermore, a better understanding of how liver regeneration mobilizes FA from the adipose tissue to the liver and of how SAMe interacts with *CYP2E1*, *CYP4A10*, and *CYP4A14* expression and, perhaps, with VLDL secretion, may help to prevent the progression of fatty liver disease from steatosis to steatohepatitis. The finding that SAMe regulates proteolysis in the liver has widened its spectrum of action, opening new and unexpected areas of clinical interest. From this perspective, maintaining a tight control of hepatic SAMe and methionine metabolism is likely to have a major impact in the development and progression of fatty liver disease and on the predisposition to cancer in these patients. Both patients with alcoholic and non-alcoholic liver cirrhosis have low *MAT1A* expression and MATI/III activity (Cabrero *et al.*, 1988; Duce *et al.*, 1988; Corrales *et al.*, 1990), and SAMe treatment has been shown to increase survival in patients with alcoholic liver cirrhosis (Mato *et al.*, 1999). Additionally, patients with HCC where *MAT1A* expression is silenced have more aggressive tumours and shorter survival (Calvisi *et al.*, 2007). Treatment of *GNMT*-KO mice with nicotinamide, a substrate of nicotinamide *N*-methyltransferase – an enzyme mainly expressed in the liver (Cantoni, 1951) – leads to the normalization of hepatic SAMe content and prevents liver injury. The clinical importance of this finding is obvious, since children with mutations that lead to a drastic reduction of GNMT develop liver injury (Mudd *et al.*, 2001; Augoustides-Savvopoulou *et al.*, 2003).

10.8 Conclusions

Mammalian cells metabolize methionine by converting it into SAMe, the main biological methyl donor. Widespread methylation of DNA and proteins indicates methylation is important in controlling cell function. Changes in the availability of methionine could directly affect the methylation status, and hence the activity of critical substrates. The issue then is how, after an increase in dietary methionine, mammals metabolize it and, at the same time, control SAMe content intracellularly. This is crucial for the liver, where methionine is mainly metabolized. Two genes, *MAT1A* and *GNMT*, play critical roles in controlling methionine metabolism and hepatic SAMe content. *MAT1A*- and *GNMT*-KO mice spontaneously develop NAFLD and HCC. SAMe-regulation of AMPK, and proteasomal activity, as well as that of DNA and histone methylation, have been causally implicated in these animal models and in human studies. Changing the metabolism of methionine in hepatocytes through manipulation of methionine metabolism provides potential for improving NAFLD and HCC prognosis.

10.9 Financial Support

This work is supported by grants from NIH AT-1576 (to S.C.L., M.L.M-C. and J.M.M.); SAF 2008-04800, HEPADIP-EULSHM-CT-205, and ETORTEK-2008 (to J.M.M. and M.L.M.-C); and from Sanidad Gobierno Vasco 2008111015 (to M.L.M.-C). CIBERehd is funded by the Instituto de Salud Carlos III.

References

Adams, L.A. and Lindor, K.D. (2007) Nonalcoholic fatty liver disease. *Annals of Epidemiology* 17, 863–869.
Ansorena, E., García-Trevijano, E.R., Martínez Chantar, M.L., Huang, Z.Z., Chen, L., Mato, J.M., Iraburu, M., *et al.* (2002) S-Adenosylmethionine and methylthioadenosine are antiapoptotic in cultured rat hepatocytes but proapoptotic in human hepatoma cells. *Hepatology* 35, 274–280.

Augoustides-Savvopoulou, P., Luka Z., Karyda, S., Stabler, S.P., Allen, R.H., Patsiaoura, K., Wagner, C., *et al*. (2003) Glycine N-methyltransferase deficiency: a new patient with a novel mutation. *Journal of Inherited Metabolic Disease* 26, 745–759.

Avila, M.A., Berasain, C., Torres, L., Martín-Duce, A., Corrales, F.J., Yang, H., Prieto, J., *et al*. (2000) Reduced mRNA abundance of the main enzymes involved in methionine metabolism in human liver cirrhosis and hepatocellular carcinoma. *Journal of Hepatology* 33, 907–914.

Best, C.H. (1956) The lipotropic agents in the protection of liver, kidney, heart and other organs of experimental animals. *Proceedings of the Royal Society of London. Series B, Biological Sciences* 145, 151–169.

Cabrero, C., Duce, A.M., Ortiz, P., Alemany, S. and Mato, J.M. (1988) Specific loss of the high-molecular-weight form of S-adenosyl-L-methionine synthetase in human liver cirrhosis. *Hepatology* 8, 1530–1534.

Cahill, G.F. (1976) Starvation in man. *Journal of Clinical Endocrinology & Metabolism* 5, 397–415.

Cai, J., Sum, W.M., Hwang, J.J., Stain, S.C. and Lu, S.C. (1996) Changes in S-adenosylmethionine synthase in human liver cancer: molecular characterization and significance. *Hepatology* 24, 876–881.

Calvisi, D.F., Ladu, S., Gorden, A., Farina, M., Conner, E.A., Lee, J.S., Factor, V.M., *et al*. (2006) Ubiquitous activation of Ras and Jak/Stat pathways in human HCC. *Gastroenterology* 130, 1117–1128.

Calvisi, D.F., Simile, M.M., Ladu, S., Pellegrino, R., DeMurtas, V., Pinna, F., Tomasi, M.L., *et al*. (2007) Altered methionine metabolism and global DNA methylation in liver cancer: relationship with genomic instability and prognosis. *International Journal of Cancer* 121, 2410–2420.

Cantoni, G.L. (1951) Methylation of nicotinamide with soluble enzyme system from rat liver. *Journal of Biological Chemistry* 189, 203–216.

Chen, L., Zeng, Y., Yang, H., Lee, T.D., French, S.W., Corrales, F.J., García-Trevijano, E.R., *et al*. (2004) Impaired liver regeneration in mice lacking methionine adenosyltransferase 1A. *FASEB Journal* 18, 914–916.

Corrales, F.J., Cabrero, C., Pajares, M.A., Ortiz, P., Martín–Duce, A. and Mato, J.M. (1990) Inactivation and dissociation of S–adenosylmethionine synthetase by modification of sulfhydryl groups and its possible occurrence in cirrhosis. *Hepatology* 11, 216–222.

del Pino, M.M., Corrales, F.J. and Mato, J.M. (2000) Hysteretic behavior of methionine adenosyltransferase III. Methionine switches between two conformations of the enzyme with different specific activities. *Journal of Biological Chemistry* 275, 23476–23482.

Ding, W., Mouzaki, M., You, H., Laird, J.C., Mato, J.M., Lu, S.C. and Rountree, C.B. (2009) CD133+ liver cancer stem cells from methionine adenosyltransferase 1A-deficient mice demonstrate resistance to transforming growth factor (TGF)-beta-induced apoptosis. *Hepatology* 49, 1277–1286.

Doller, A., Pfeilschifter, J. and Eberhardt, W. (2008) Signalling pathways regulating nucleo-cytoplasmic shuttling of the mRNA-binding protein HuR. *Cell Signaling* 20, 2165–2173.

Duce, A.M., Ortiz, P., Cabrero, C. and Mato, J.M. (1988) S-adenosyl-L-methionine synthetase and phospholipid methyltransferase are inhibited in human cirrhosis. *Hepatology* 8, 65–68.

Fraser, C.M., Gocayne, J.D., White, O., Adams, M.D., Clayton, R.A., Fleischmann, R.D., Bult, C.J., *et al*. (1995) The minimal gene complement of Mycoplasma genitalium. *Science* 270, 397–403.

García-Trevijano, E.R., Martínez-Chantar, M.L., Latasa, M.U., Mato, J.M. and Avila, M.A. (2002) NO sensitizes rat hepatocytes to proliferation by modifying S-adenosylmethionine levels. *Gastroenterology* 122, 1355–1363.

Gil, B., Casado, M., Pajares, M., Boscá, L., Mato, J.M., Martín-Sanz, P. and Alvarez, L. (1996) Differential expression pattern of S-adenosylmethionine synthetase isoenzymes during rat liver development. *Hepatology* 24, 876–881.

Halim, A., LeGros, L., Geller, G. and Kotb, M. (1999) Expression and functional interaction of the catalytic and regulatory subunits of human methionine adenosyltransferase mammalian cells. *Journal of Biological Chemistry* 274, 29720–29725.

Huang, Z.Z., Mao, Z., Cai, J. and Lu, S.C. (1998) Changes in methionine adenosyltransferase during liver regeneration in the rat. *American Journal of Physiology* 275, G14–G21.

Kokkinakis, D.M. (2006) Methionine-stress: a pleiotropic approach in enhancing the efficacy of chemotherapy. *Cancer Letters* 233, 195–207.

Koteish, A. and Diehl, A.M. (2002) Animal models of steatohepatitis. *Best Practice & Research: Clinical Gastroenterology* 16, 679–690.

Latasa, M.U., Boukaba, A., García-Trevijano, E.R., Torres, L., Rodríguez, J.L., Caballería, J., Lu, S.C., *et al*. (2001) Hepatocyte growth factor induces MAT2A expression and histone acetylation in rat hepatocytes: role in liver regeneration. *FASEB Journal* 15, 1248–1250.

Leclerq, I.A., Farrell, G.C., Field, J., Bell, D.R., Gonzalez, F.J. and Robertson, G.R. (2000) CYP2E1 and CYP4A as microsomal catalysts of lipid peroxides in murine nonalcoholic steatohepatitis. *Journal of Clinical Investigation* 105, 1067–1075.

Lee, T.K., Castilho, A., Ma, S. and Ng, I.D. (2009) Liver cancer stem cells: implications for a new therapeutic target. *Liver International* 29, 955–965.

Li, J., Ramani, K., Sun, Z., Zee, C., Grant, E.G., Yang, H., Xia, M., et al. (2010) Forced expression of methionine adenosyltransferase 1A in human hepatoma cells suppresses in vivo tumorigenicity in mice. *American Journal of Pathology* 176. 2456–2466.

Liao, Y.J., Liu, S.P., Lee, C.M., Yen, C.H., Chuang, P.C., Chen, C.Y., Tsai, T.F., et al. (2009) Characterization of a glycine N-methyltransferase gene knockout mouse model for hepatocellular carcinoma: implications of the gender disparity in liver cancer susceptibility. *International Journal of Cancer* 124, 816–826.

Lieber, C.S. (1977) Cytochrome P-4502E1: its physiological and pathological role. *Physiological Reviews* 77, 517–544.

Lu, S.C. and Mato, J.M. (2008) S-Adenosylmethionine in cell growth, apoptosis and liver cancer. *Journal of Gastroenterolology and Hepatology* 23, S73–S77.

Lu, S.C., Alvarez, L., Huang, Z.Z., Chen, L., An, W., Corrales, F.J., Avila, M.A., et al. (2001) Methionine adenosyltransferase 1A knockout mice are predisposed to liver injury and exhibit increased expression of genes involved in proliferation. *Proceedings of the National Academy of Sciences USA* 98, 5560–5565.

Lu, S.C., Ramani, K., Ou, X., Lin, M., Yu, V., Ko, K., Park, R., et al. (2009) S-Adenosylmethionine in the chemoprevention and treatment of hepatocellular carcinoma in a rat model. *Hepatology* 50, 462–471.

Luka, Z., Mudd, S.H. and Wagner, C. (2009) Glycine N-methyltransferase and regulation of S-adenosylmethionine levels. *Journal of Biological Chemistry* 284, 22507–22511.

Markham, G.D. and Pajares, M.A. (2009) Structure-function relationships in methionine adenosyltransferase. *Cellular and Molecular Life Sciences* 66, 636–648.

Martínez-Chantar, M.L., Corrales, F.J., Martínez-Cruz, L.A., García-Trevijano, E.R., Huang, Z.Z., Chen, L., Kanel, G., et al. (2002) Spontaneous oxidative stress and liver tumors in mice lacking methionine adenosyltransferase 1A. *FASEB Journal* 16, 1292–1294.

Martínez-Chantar, M.L., García-Trevijano, E.R., Latasa, M.U., Martín-Duce, A., Fortes, P., Caballería, J., Avila, M.A., et al. (2003) Methionine adenosytransferase II β subunit gene expression provides a proliferative advantage in human hepatoma. *Gastroenterology* 124, 940–948.

Martínez-Chantar, M.L., Vázquez-Chantada, M., Garnacho, M., Latasa, M.U., Varela-Rey, M., Dotor, J., Santamaría, M., et al. (2006) S-adenosylmethionine regulates cytoplasmic HuR via AMP-activated kinase. *Gastroenterology* 131, 223–232.

Martínez-Chantar, M.L., Vázquez-Chantada, M., Ariz, U., Martínez, N., Varela, M., Luka, Z., Capdevila, A., et al. (2008) Loss of the glycine N-methyltransferase gene leads to steatosis and hepatocellular carcinoma in mice. *Hepatology* 47, 1191–1199.

Martínez-Chantar, M.L., Lu, S.C., Mato, J.M., Luka, Z., Wagner, C., French, B.A. and French, S.W. (2010) The role of stem cells/progenitor cells in liver carcinogenesis in glycine N-methyltransferase deficient mice. *Experimental and Molecular Pathology* 88, 234–237.

Mato, J.M. and Lu, S.C. (2007) Role of S-adenosyl-L-methionine in liver health and injury. *Hepatology* 45, 1306–1312.

Mato, J.M., Cámara, J., Fernández de Paz, J., Caballería, L., Coll, S., Caballero, A., García-Buey, L., et al. (1999) S-adenosylmethionine in alcoholic liver cirrhosis: a randomized, placebo-controlled, double-blind, multicenter clinical trial. *Journal of Hepatology* 30, 1081–1089.

Mato, J.M., Corrales, F.J., Lu, S.C. and Avila, M.A. (2002) S-Adenosylmethionine: a control switch that regulates liver function. *FASEB Journal* 16, 15–26.

Mato, J.M., Martínez-Chantar, M.L. and Lu, S.C. (2008) Methionine metabolism and liver disease. *Annual Review of Nutrition* 28, 273–293.

Mikol, Y.B., Hoover, K.L., Creasia, D. and Poirier, L.A. (1983) Hepatocarcinogenesis in rats fed methyl-deficient, amino acid-defined diets. *Carcinogenesis* 4, 1619–1629.

Mudd, S.H., Cerone, R., Schiaffino, M.C., Fantasia, A.R., Minniti, G., Caruso, U., Lorini, R., et al. (2001) Glycine N-methyltransferase deficiency: a novel inborn error causing persistent isolated hypermethioninemia. *Journal of Inherited Metabolic Disease* 24, 448–464.

Parks, E.J. and Hellerstein, M.K. (2006) Thematic review series: Patient-oriented research. Recent advances in liver triacylglycerol and fatty acid metabolism using stable isotope labeling techniques. *Journal of Lipid Research* 47, 1651–1660.

Ramani, K., Yang, H., Xia, M., Ara, A.I., Mato, J.M. and Lu, S.C. (2008) Leptin's mitogenic effect in human liver cancer cells requires induction of both methionine adenosyltransferase 2A and 2beta. *Hepatology* 47, 521–531.

Reid, A.E. (2001) Nonalcoholic steatohepatitis. *Gastroenterology* 121, 710–723.

Robert, K., Nehmé, J., Bourdon, E., Pivert, G., Friguet, B., Delcayre, C., Delabar, J.M., et al. (2005) Cystathionine beta synthase deficiency promotes oxidative stress, fibrosis, and steatosis in mice liver. *Gastroenterology* 128, 1405–1415.

Rontree, C.B., Senadheera, S., Mato, J.M., Crooks, G.M. and Lu, S.C. (2008) Expansion of liver cancer cells during aging in methionine adenosyltransferase 1A-deficient mice. *Hepatology* 47, 1288–1297.

Santamaria, E., Avila, M.A., Latasa, M.U., Rubio, A., Martin-Duce, A., Lu, S.C., Mato, J.M., et al. (2003) Functional proteomics of nonalcoholic steatohepatitis: mitochondrial proteins as targets of S-adenosylmethionine. *Proceedings of the National Academy of Sciences USA* 100, 3065–3070.

Sontag, J.M., Nunbhakdi-Craig, V., Montgomery, L., Arning, E., Bottiglieri, T. and Sontang, E. (2008) Folate deficiency induces in vitro and mouse brain region-specific downregulation of leucine carboxyl methyltransferase-1 and protein phosphatase 2A Bα subunit expression that correlates with enhanced Tau phosphorylation. *Journal of Neurosciences* 28, 11477–11487.

Sreekumar, A., Poisson, L.M., Rajemdiran, T.M., Khan, A.P., Cao, Q., Yu, J., Laxman, B., et al. (2009) Metabolomic profiles delineate potential role for sarcosine in prostate cancer progression. *Nature* 457, 910–914.

Taub, R. (2004) Liver regeneration: from myth to mechanism. *Nature Reviews Molecular Cellular Biology* 5, 836–847.

Tomasi, M.L., Iglesias-Ara, A., Yang, H., Ramani, K., Feo, F., Pascale, M.R., Martínez-Chantar, M.L., et al. (2009) S-adenosylmethionine regulates apurinic/apyrimidinic endonuclease 1 stability: implication in hepatocarcinogenesis. *Gastroenterology* 136, 1025–1036.

Tomasi, M.L., Ramani, K., Lopitz-Otsoa, F., Rodríguez, M.S., Li, T.W., Ko, K., Yang, H., et al. (2010) S-adenosylmethionine regulates dual-specificity mitogen-activated protein kinase phosphatase expression in mouse and human hepatocytes. *Hepatology* 51, 2152–2161.

Vander Heiden, M.G., Cantley, L.C. and Thompson, C.B. (2009) Understanding the Warburg effect: the metabolic requirements of cell proliferation. *Science* 324, 1029–1033.

Varela-Rey, M., Fernández-Ramos, D., Martínez López, N., Embade, N., Gómez-Santos, L., Beraza, N., Vázquez-Chantada, M., et al. (2009a) Impaired liver regeneration in mice lacking glycine N-methyltransferase. *Hepatology* 50, 443–452.

Varela-Rey, M., Embade, N., Ariz, U., Lu, S.C., Mato, J.M. and Martínez-Chantar, M.L. (2009b) Nonalcoholic steatohepatits and animal models: understanding the human disease. *International Journal of Biochemistry & Cell Biology* 41, 969–976.

Varela-Rey, M., Martínez-López, N., Fernández, D., Embade, N., Calvisi, D.F., Woodhoo, A., Rodríguez, J., et al. (2010) Fatty liver and fibrosis in glycine N-methyltransferase knockout mice is prevented by nicotinamide. *Hepatology* 52, 105–114.

Vázquez-Chantada, M., Ariz, U., Varela-Rey, M., Embade, N., Martínez-López, N., Gómez-Santos, L., Lamas, S., et al. (2009) Evidence for LKB1/AMP-activated protein kinase/endothelial nitric oxide synthase cascade regulated by hepatocyte growth factor, S-adenosylmethionine, and nitric oxide in hepatocyte proliferation. *Hepatology* 49, 608–617.

Vázquez-Chantada, M., Fernández-Ramos, D., Embade, N., Martínez-López, N., Varela-Rey, M., Woodhoo, A., Luka, Z., et al. (2010) HuR/methyl-HuR and AUF1 regulate the MAT expressed during liver proliferation, differentiation and carcinogenesis. *Gastroenterology* 138, 1943–1953.

Viollet, B., Athea, Y., Mounier, R., Guigas, B., Zarrinpashne, E., Horman, S., Lantier, L., et al. (2009) AMPK: Lessons from transgenic and knockout animals. *Frontiers in Bioscience* 14, 19–44.

Yang, H., Ara, A., Magilnick, N., Xia, M., Ramani, K., Chen, H., Lee, T.D., et al. (2008) Expression pattern, regulation, and functions of methionine adenosyltransferase 2beta splicing variants in hepatoma cells. *Gastroenterology* 134, 281–291.

Yuang, J.M., Lu, S.C., Van Den Berg, D., Govindarajan, S., Zhang, Z.Q., Mato, J.M. and Yu, M.C. (2007) Genetic polymorphisms in the methylenetetrahydrofolate reductase and thymidylate synthase genes and risk of hepatocellular carcinoma. *Hepatology* 46, 749–758.

Zhao, Y., Su, B., Jacobs, R.L., Kennedy, B., Francis, G.A., Waddington, E., Brosnan, J.T., et al. (2009) Lack of phosphatidylethanolamine N-methyltransferase alters VLDL phospholipids and attenuates atherosclerosis in mice. *Atherosclerosis, Thrombosis, and Vascular Biology* 29, 1349–1355.

Zong, C., Young, G.W., Wang, Y., Lu, H., Deng, N., Drews, O. and Ping, P. (2008) Two-dimensional electrophoresis-based characterization of post-translational modifications of mammalian 20S proteasome complexes. *Proteomics* 8, 5025–5037.

Part II

Dynamics

11 Amino Acid Transport Across Each Side of the Blood–Brain Barrier

R.A. Hawkins,[1]* J.R. Viña,[2] D.R. Peterson,[1] R. O'Kane,[3] A. Mokashi[1] and I.A. Simpson[4]

[1]Department of Physiology & Biophysics, The Chicago Medical School, Rosalind Franklin University of Medicine and Science, North Chicago, USA; [2]Departamento de Bioquímica & Biología Molecular, Facultad de Medicina/Fundación de Investigación Hospital Clinico-INCLIVA, Universidad de Valencia, Valencia, España; [3]Natural and Applied Science Department, La Guardia Community College/CUNY, Long Island City, USA; [4]Department of Neural and Behavioral Sciences, Milton S. Hershey Medical Center, Pennsylvania State University College of Medicine, Hershey, USA

11.1 Abstract

Brain capillary endothelial cells form the blood–brain barrier (BBB). They are connected by extensive tight junctions, and are polarized into luminal (blood-facing) and abluminal (brain-facing) plasma membrane domains. The polar distribution of transport proteins mediates amino acid (AA) homeostasis in the brain. The existence of two facilitative transporters for neutral amino acids (NAA) on both membranes provides the brain access to essential AA. Four Na$^+$-dependent transporters of NAA exist in the abluminal membranes of the BBB. Together these systems have the capability to actively transfer every naturally occurring NAA from the extracellular fluid (ECF) to endothelial cells and thence to the circulation. The presence of Na$^+$-dependent carriers on the abluminal membrane provides a mechanism by which NAA concentrations in the ECF of brain are maintained at about 10% of those of the plasma. Also present on the abluminal membrane are at least three Na$^+$-dependent systems transporting acidic AA (EAAT) and a Na$^+$-dependent system transporting glutamine (N). Facilitative carriers for glutamine and glutamate are found only in the luminal membrane of the BBB. This organization promotes the net removal of acidic and nitrogen-rich AA from brain, and accounts for the low level of glutamate penetration into the central nervous system (CNS). The presence of a γ-glutamyl cycle at the luminal membrane and Na$^+$-dependent AA transporters at the abluminal membrane may serve to modulate movement of AA from blood to brain. The γ-glutamyl cycle is expected to generate pyroglutamate within the endothelial cells. Pyroglutamate stimulates secondary active AA transporters at the abluminal membrane, thereby reducing net influx of AA to the brain. It is now clear the BBB participates in the active regulation of the AA content of the brain.

---

* E-mail address: RAH@post.harvard.edu

11.2 Introduction

The brain is sheltered from the changing metabolite concentrations in the blood by a blood–brain barrier (BBB) that surrounds the entire central nervous system (CNS) including the spinal cord (Fig. 11.1). The BBB is necessary to provide an optimal chemical environment for cerebral function. Several layers exist between blood and brain: capillary endothelial cells; a basement membrane comprising type IV collagen, fibronectin, and laminin that completely covers the capillaries; pericytes that are embedded in the basement membrane; and astrocyte processes that surround the basement membrane. Each of these layers could, potentially, restrict the movement of solutes (Fig. 11.2).

Endothelial cells were demonstrated to be the site of the BBB when it was observed that horseradish peroxidase could not pass the endothelial layer from either direction (Reese and Karnovsky, 1967; Brightman and Reese, 1969; Brightman *et al.*, 1971). Pappenheimer (1970a) challenged this concept, arguing that the astrocytes were a more likely site of the barrier. Crone decided the issue by demonstrating that brain capillaries from amphibians, which have no surrounding layer of astrocytes, have high electrical impedance, $\approx 2000 \, \Omega \times cm^2$ indicative of a restriction to the movement of ions. The cerebral endothelium is now accepted as the site of the BBB in higher animals (Crone and Olesen, 1982).

Cerebral capillary endothelial cells differ from other mammalian capillary endothelial cells; they have few cytoplasmic vesicles, more mitochondria (Oldendorf and Brown, 1975), and a larger number of tight junctions between overlapping cells. The tight junctions inhibit paracellular movement, prevent membrane molecules from moving from one cell to another (van Meer *et al.*, 1986), and divide the membranes of the endothelial cells into two distinct sides: luminal (blood side), and abluminal (brain side) (van Meer and Simons, 1986). Different populations of both lipids and intrinsic proteins (e.g. transporters) exist on the luminal and abluminal side (Betz and Goldstein, 1978; Betz *et al.*, 1980; Tewes and Galla, 2001). Therefore, hydrophilic nutrients must pass two sheaths of membrane, the combined characteristics of which determine which particles traverse the barrier and how quickly. Pappenheimer and Setchell (1973) recognized the implication of molecules having to pass two membranes in series to gain entry to the CNS, and Oyler *et al.* (1992) demonstrated the effect of two membranes in series by computer simulation.

Various methods are used to study the transport of solutes across the BBB *in vivo* and *in vitro* including single-pass indicator diffusion (Crone, 1963, 1965); the brain uptake index (Oldendorf, 1970); *in situ* brain perfusion (Takasato *et al.*, 1984); isolated brain microvessels (Brendal and Meezan, 1974; Goldstein *et al.*, 1975); and cultured endothelial cells (DeBault and Cancilla, 1980; Vinters *et al.*, 1985; Dehouck *et al.*, 1992). These techniques give valuable information about transport, but they did not distinguish between the different functions of the luminal and abluminal membranes.

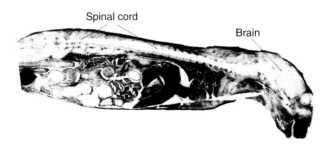

Fig. 11.1. The blood–brain barrier extends throughout the central nervous system. This saggital section through a mouse shows the distribution pattern of I^{131} labelled Renografin™, an hydrophilic dye that does not pass the blood–brain barrier, 15 min after injection. All tissues take up the dye except the entire central nervous system including the spinal cord (Nair and Roth, 1961). Photo courtesy of Professor V. Nair, Rosalind Franklin University of Medicine and Science. (A similar figure was previously published in IUBMB Life.)

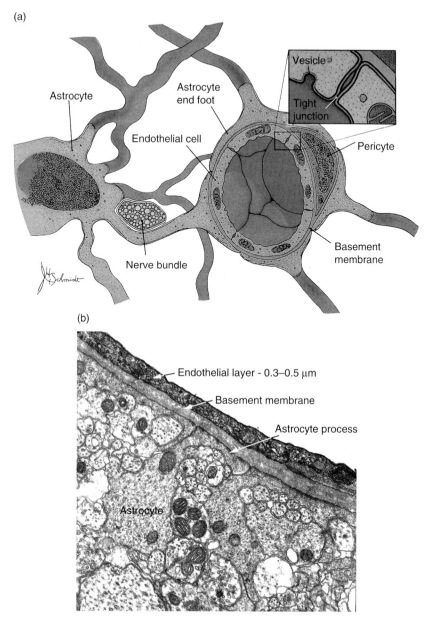

Fig. 11.2. (a) The BBB exists at the level of the endothelial cells of cerebral capillaries. The endothelial cells are joined together by an extensive network of tight junctions and surrounded by a basement membrane, within which pericytes reside. Astrocytic processes (commonly called end-feet) surround cerebral capillaries (previously published in IUBMB Life). (b) An electron micrograph of a cerebral capillary shows the basic elements. The electron micrograph was provided through the courtesy of Robert Page, MD; Professor, Neurosurgery and Anatomy, Pennsylvania State University College of Medicine. (A similar figure was previously published in the *Journal of Nutrition*.)

The studies *in vivo* led to the concept that the BBB, at least with regard to metabolites, was a passive system. The various facilitative transporters were considered to play a role in the regulation of brain metabolism through their ability to limit access (Pardridge, 1983). On the other hand it was known that active transport of ions exists. Bicarbonate and other

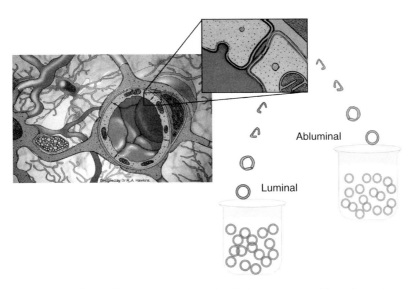

Fig. 11.3. Isolated luminal and abluminal membranes. Capillaries are separated from the bovine cerebral corticies, and the membranes detached. The membranes are divided into two fractions on the basis of differential centrifugation into luminal and abluminal fractions. The membranes form spheres that are suitable for the study of transport (Sánchez del Pino et al., 1992, 1995). It is possible, for instance, to load the vesicles with K^+ thereby forming transmembrane potentials. External Na^+ and substrate can be manipulated at will thereby testing for the presence of Na^+-dependent transport systems.

ions are actively secreted across the BBB (Pappenheimer, 1970b; Bradbury, 1979). (Na^+/K^+)-ATPase is present in the abluminal membrane (Vorbrodt, 1988). One of the most important functions of (Na^+/K^+)-ATPase is to maintain the high concentration gradient of Na^+ (external > internal) so Na^+-dependent transport can occur. Furthermore, cerebral endothelial cells have a high density of mitochondria compared with other endothelial cells and, therefore, the capacity for greater energy production (Oldendorf and Brown, 1975).

11.3 A New Approach to Studying the BBB

Betz et al. (1980) developed a procedure to separate the respective plasma membrane domains: they convincingly demonstrated a polarity between the two sides. Sánchez del Pino and associates recognized the potential of using these membranes to study transport under controlled conditions (Sánchez del Pino et al., 1992, 1995a,b). On isolation, luminal and abluminal membranes form sealed spherical vesicles that are predominantly right-side-out, and are suitable for the study of transport in vitro (Sánchez del Pino et al., 1992, 1995b) (Fig. 11.3). The isolated membranes maintain functional transport properties, and thus may be used to characterize the contribution of each membrane domain to BBB activity under controlled conditions in vitro. For instance the ionic composition inside and outside the vesicles permits the exploration of such conditions as the influence of the transmembrane potential and Na^+-dependence. This advance allowed the study of the BBB in a completely different manner and resulted in a change in the concept of the BBB and the synergy between its two membranes. The following sections illustrate that the BBB is an active participant in the regulation of the brain's amino acid (AA) content.

11.4 Facilitative Amino Acid Transporters of the BBB

Early studies of AA transport in vivo identified facilitative transporters on the luminal membrane that were saturable and stereoselective (Oldendorf, 1971a,b, 1973). Luminal carriers of AA have no dependence on Na$^+$ gradients (Battistin *et al.*, 1971; Oldendorf, 1971; Schain and Watanabe, 1972; Sershen and Lajtha, 1976; Christensen 1979; Smith and Stoll 1998). Three broad classes of facilitative carriers exist: large neutral amino acids (LNAA), cationic AA (CAA) and acidic AA (AAA) (Oldendorf and Szabo, 1976). Currently, four facilitative carriers have been identified: L1, y$^+$, x$_G$-, and n. L1 and y$^+$ are present in both membranes (Sánchez del Pino *et al.*, 1995a), while x$_G$- and n are restricted to the luminal membrane (Lee *et al.*, 1998).

11.4.1 Facilitative transport of large essential neutral amino acids: system L1

Early studies of transport *in vivo* revealed a distinct pattern of LNAA uptake by the brain: movement of essential NAA (neutral amino acids) from blood to brain was greater than non-essential NAA (Battistin *et al.*, 1971; Oldendorf, 1971b); the movements of the latter were minimal (Oldendorf and Szabo, 1976). Transport was facilitative, Na$^+$-independent and NAA were preferred (Oldendorf and Szabo 1976). Therefore, the carrier seems to belong to the L-system (leucine preferring) originally described by Oxender and Christensen (Oxender and Christensen, 1963) and it is probably the high affinity form currently referred to as L1 (Smith and Stoll, 1998; Boado *et al.*, 1999; Segawa *et al.*, 1999; Killian and Chikhale, 2001). Measurements in membranes indicate L1 is present in both membranes in a 2:1 ratio (luminal-to-abluminal) (Sánchez del Pino *et al.*, 1995). The substrates carried by L1 include leucine, valine, methionine, histidine, isoleucine, tyrosine, tryptophan, phenylalanine and threonine, most of which are essential. The affinity constants (K$_m$) are in the µM range and similar to the plasma concentrations (Smith and Stoll, 1998). Glutamine has also been described as a substrate of L1, but glutamine transport is not completely inhibited by BCH (2-aminobicyclo(2,2,1)-heptane-2-carboxylic acid), a specific inhibitor of the L1 system. Therefore it seems likely that glutamine is also transported by system N (Lee *et al.*, 1998).

L1 is undoubtedly the most important source by which essential NAA gain access to the brain. Fernstrom and Wurtman (1972) demonstrated the important role of the L1 system and the competition amongst LNAA by showing that brain tryptophan and serotonin contents were correlated with the ratio of tryptophan-to-LNAA existing in plasma. They concluded that competition between tryptophan and other LNAA for entry to the brain is an important factor in determining the content of serotonin in brain.

11.4.2 Facilitative transport of cationic amino acids: system y$^+$

Smith (1991) concluded that system y$^+$ is the primary CAA transporter of the BBB from experiments conducted *in vivo* that examined the BBB only from the luminal side. More recent study of plasma membranes isolated from bovine brain microvessels allowed characterization of the CAA transporters on both sides of the BBB to be studied in close detail (O'Kane *et al.*, 2006).

Two families of proteins: Cat, commonly referred to as the system y$^+$, and Bat, which comprise systems b$^{0,+}$ (Van Winkle *et al.*, 1985, 1988, 1990), B$^{0,+}$ (Van Winkle *et al.*, 1985), and y$^+$L (Deves *et al.*, 1998; Deves and Boyd, 1998; Palacin *et al.*, 1998) have been found to transport CAA in various tissues. Transporter system B$^{0,+}$ is the only Na$^+$-dependent carrier that carries CAA, as well as some NAA (although with less affinity) (Van Winkle *et al.*, 1985). There is no evidence for system B$^{0,+}$ in the BBB and no evidence of Na$^+$-dependence of CAA transport (O'Kane and Hawkins 2003; O'Kane *et al.*, 2006). In this regard the CAA are unique because all other naturally occurring AAA and NAA examined to date have Na$^+$-dependent transporters on the abluminal membrane that are capable of coupling the Na$^+$ gradient existing between the extracellular fluid (ECF) of brain and BBB endothelial cells to transport AA out of the ECF (Hawkins et al., 2006a). Facilitative transport seems to be the only mechanism in the BBB to allow the movement of CAA.

No evidence was found for the presence of Na$^+$-independent systems b$^{0,+}$, or of y$^+$L systems in the BBB (O'Kane et al., 2006). Therefore as posited by Smith (1991) only system y$^+$ is available to transport CAA. In addition to transporting CAA, y$^+$ exhibits weak interactions with NAA if Na$^+$ is present and hence it is referred to as y$^+$ (White, 1985; Mann et al., 2003). In the BBB y$^+$ may transport several essential NAA (phenylalanine, threonine, histidine, valine and methionine) as well as non-essential NAA (serine, glutamine, alanine, and glycine) but the affinity constants are about tenfold greater than those of system L1 (O'Kane et al., 2006). Thus while y$^+$ may contribute to the 'first-order' transport component observed in studies of AA transport (Pardridge, 1983), system L1 must be considered the principal provider of essential NAA while y$^+$ is primarily a purveyor of arginine.

The ability of system y$^+$ to transport several non-essential amino acids (serine, glutamine, alanine and glycine), with affinity values similar to their plasma concentrations, may explain the small, but finite, permeability of the BBB to small NAA (Oldendorf, 1971a).

Both membranes of the BBB contain y$^+$, but its activity is greater on the abluminal side and it is voltage sensitive (O'Kane et al., 2006). The affinity of y$^+$ is much greater for arginine compared with the other CAA and y$^+$ is probably important in the provision of arginine for nitric oxide (NO) synthesis, a diffusible gas, originally called endothelium-derived relaxing factor. NO regulates numerous physiological actions including smooth muscle contraction, blood flow and pressure (Palmer et al., 1987). NO also acts as a signal to regulate gene expression, apoptosis, cell cycle and differentiation (Hemish et al., 2003). The biosynthesis of NO requires L-arginine and O$_2$ for the NO synthase (NOS) catalysed reaction. Three isoforms of NOS have been identified: neuronal (nNOS), inducible (iNOS), and endothelial (eNOS) (Wu and Meininger, 2002). Real-time PCR and Western blotting techniques established the presence of all three known NOS in cerebral endothelial cells, suggesting that NO can be produced in brain endothelial cells (O'Kane et al., 2006).

Endothelial cells do not have the ability to synthesize arginine de novo (Wu and Meininger, 1993). They must therefore rely on an external source of arginine; it seems likely that the availability of arginine is the determining factor in NO production by endothelial cells (Wu and Meininger, 1993, 2002).

11.4.3 Facilitative transport of glutamine: system n

Lee et al. (1998) described facilitative transport of glutamine across the luminal membrane of the BBB that was not inhibited by BCH and did not demonstrate transstimulation. This transport system is similar to system n described in hepatic plasma membrane vesicles (Pacitti et al., 1993). The BBB system n is inhibited by asparagine and histidine (Hawkins et al., 2006a) as was found in hepatic vesicles by Pacitti et al. (1993). System n exists solely on the luminal membrane (Lee et al., 1998).

11.4.4 Facilitative transport of acidic amino acids: system x$_G^-$

Benrabh and Lefauconnier (1996) studied glutamate uptake in vivo and found no evidence of Na$^+$-dependent transport when glutamate was presented to the luminal membrane. They concluded the carrier was facilitative and probably the x$_G^-$ form because no evidence for the cystine–glutamate exchanger x$_C^-$ could be found: this was confirmed in isolated luminal membranes. Cystine did not compete with glutamate for uptake while aspartate did. Furthermore, cystine did not accelerate glutamate uptake in vesicles preloaded with 2 mmol L-cystine (Hawkins et al., 2006a).

Lee et al. (1998) measured facilitative glutamate transport in both luminal and abluminal membranes, and found facilitative glutamate transport only on the luminal border in a position to allow the release of glutamate from endothelial cells to the plasma.

A compilation of the substrates carried by the various facilitative systems is presented in Table 11.1 and their kinetic characteristics in Table 11.2. The organization of the transporters is depicted in Fig. 11.4.

Table 11.1. Amino acids transported by facilitative transport systems.

System	L1	y^+	n	x_G^-
Non-essential				
Glycine		*		
Alanine		*		
Serine		*		
Proline				
Asparagine	+		+	
Glutamine	+	*	+	
Aspartate				+
Glutamate				+
Arginine		+		
Ornithine		+		
Essential in brain				
Lysine		+		
Histidine	+	*	+	
Threonine	+	*		
Cysteine		*		
Methionine	+	*		
Valine	+	*		
Leucine	+			
Isoleucine	+			
Phenylalanine	+	*		
Tyrosine	+			
Tryptophan	+			

AA transported, or shown to inhibit transport, are indicated by a +. Facilitative transport (weak) of NAA by y^+ in the presence of Na^+ is indicated by *. Systems L1 and y^+ exist on both membranes while systems x_G^- and n are restricted to the luminal membrane (Lee *et al.*, 1998). AA in italics are essential in brain (Laterra *et al.*, 1999). The distribution of these transporters is depicted in Fig. 11.4.

11.5 Amino Acid Gradients between Brain and Plasma

The concentrations of all naturally occurring AA in the cerebrospinal fluid (CSF), presumably similar to the ECF, with the exception of glutamine, are about 10% or less than the plasma concentrations (Fig. 11.5) (Laterra *et al.*, 1999). This situation cannot be explained by the consumption of AA by the brain because the arteriovenous differences of most AA across the brain are imperceptible (Felig *et al.*, 1972; Drewes *et al.*, 1977; Sacks *et al.*, 1982) as are the arteriovenous differences of ammonia (NH_4^+), a by-product of AA catabolism (Cooper and Plum, 1987). These observations indicate that AA leave the brain against a concentration gradient. From this it may be concluded that active (e.g. Na^+-dependent) systems on the abluminal membrane have an important role in maintaining both homeostasis of brain AA content as well as the lower concentration in the extracellular fluid. Based on similar observations Bradbury wrote 'there is a strong indirect argument in favour of the hypothesis that most AA must be moved against a concentration gradient from interstitial fluid to blood' (Bradbury, 1979).

11.6 Na$^+$-dependent Transport Systems of the BBB

Several Na^+-dependent systems have been identified to date in the abluminal membrane of the BBB. They include: A (alanine preferring), which was first characterized and shown to actively transport small non-essential NAA (Betz and Goldstein, 1978; Sánchez del Pino *et al.*, 1992; O'Kane *et al.*, 2004); ASC (alanine,

Table 11.2. Kinetic characteristics of facilitative amino acid transporters on the blood–brain barrier.

Transporter (substrate)	Apparent K_m (mmol l^{-1})	Apparent V_{max} (pmol mg^{-1} min^{-1})	Clearance (µl mg^{-1} min^{-1})	Position
L1 (Phe)	0.012 ± 0.02	94 ± 9	8	Luminal & abluminal
y^+ (Lys)	0.8 ± 0.3	5800 ± 1600	7	Luminal & abluminal
n (Gln)	1 ± 0.5	1100 ± 230	1	Luminal
x_G^- (Glu)	0.9 ± 0.9	700 ± 300	1	Luminal

The radiolabelled substrate used for measurements are in parentheses. Clearance was calculated to the nearest integer as $V_{max} \div K_m$. Values were taken from Sánchez del Pino *et al.* (1992, 1995b).

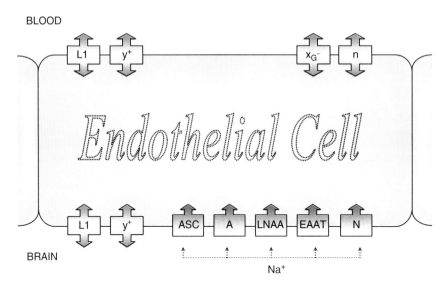

Fig. 11.4. Amino acid transporters of the BBB. The brain gains access to all essential AA through the facilitative systems L1 and y⁺ that exist on each membrane. Facilitative transporters x_G^- and n exist only on the luminal membrane and in a position to allow glutamate, aspartate and glutamine egress. Each facilitative transporter carries several substrates (see Table 11.1). The Na⁺-dependent transport systems provide mechanisms for the elimination of non-essential AA, toxic AA, as well as maintaining the optimal concentrations of all other AA. As with the facilitative systems there is considerable overlap of substrates (please see Table 11.3). All naturally occurring AA, except basic AA, are transported by at least one system and some by as many as three. A, Na⁺-dependent system A; N, Na⁺-dependent system N; EAAT, Na⁺-dependent glutamate transporter; x_G^-, facilitative glutamate transporter; n, facilitative glutamine transporter. (A similar figure was previously published in the *Journal of Nutrition*.)

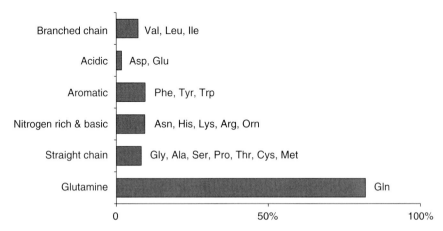

Fig. 11.5. Amino acid concentrations in plasma and brain. The plasma and CSF concentrations were grouped and the CSF-to-plasma ratio expressed as percentages of the plasma. CSF concentrations are assumed to approximate brain ECF (Davson and Welch, 1971; Laterra *et al.*, 1999). With the exception of glutamine, the concentrations of all AA in the ECF are much lower than the concentrations of AA in plasma. (A similar figure was previously published in the *Journal of Nutrition*.)

serine, and cysteine preferring) (Tayarani et al., 1987; Hargreaves and Pardridge, 1988; Tovar et al., 1988; O'Kane et al., 2004); N (e.g. glutamine, asparagine, and histidine preferring) (Lee et al., 1998; O'Kane et al., 2004); the excitatory acidic AA family (EAAT, e.g. aspartate and glutamate preferring) (Hutchison et al., 1985; O'Kane et al., 1999); and a recently described system that primarily transports essential LNAA (O'Kane and Hawkins, 2003). The latter system has not been named and is referred to as Na$^+$-LNAA.

Na$^+$-dependent transport of AA exists only in abluminal membranes. No Na$^+$ dependency has been detected in luminal membranes, which appear to have only facilitative carriers (Oldendorf, 1971a,b; Sershen and Lajtha, 1976; Christensen, 1979; Smith and Stoll, 1998). Therefore, the Na$^+$-dependent transporters are in a position to remove AA from the brain, utilizing the Na$^+$-gradient that exists between the ECF and the endothelial cells of brain capillaries comprising the BBB.

11.6.1 Na$^+$-dependent transport of large neutral amino acids: system Na$^+$-LNAA

Initial studies by Sánchez del Pino et al. (1995b) found Na$^+$-dependent phenylalanine transport that was inhibited by BCH. Studies by Van Winkle et al. (1985) had demonstrated that system B$^{0,+}$ is a Na$^+$-dependent carrier which recognizes NAA and is inhibited by BCH. Because of this characteristic and the observed inhibition, the authors thought carrier system B$^{0,+}$ was likely to be responsible for the transport activity. A characteristic of system B$^{0,+}$ is the ability to transport CAA (Van Winkle et al., 1985). However, the rate of lysine transport was not inhibited by the presence of BCH of up to 10 mmol l^{-1} concentrations, casting doubt on the presence of system B$^{0,+}$ (O'Kane and Hawkins, 2003). Further investigation led to the discovery of Na$^+$-LNAA as the carrier responsible for the BCH-inhibited, Na$^+$-dependent phenylalanine transport and other LNAA (O'Kane and Hawkins, 2003).

Na$^+$-LNAA was discovered as a distinct transporter in abluminal membrane microvessels, and its kinetic characteristics cannot be ascribed to any other currently known systems (O'Kane and Hawkins, 2003). Na$^+$-LNAA has a high affinity for leucine (K$_m$ = 21 µM ± 7 SE) and is inhibited by other NAA including glutamine, histidine, methionine, phenylalanine, serine, threonine, tryptophan and tyrosine. Transport is Na$^+$ dependent, voltage sensitive, and inhibited by BCH. The spectrum of AA carried by Na$^+$-LNAA is similar to the facilitative system L1 that allows the entry of essential LNAA down their concentration gradients (compare Tables 11.1 and 11.3). The presence of a Na$^+$-dependent carrier on the abluminal membrane, capable of removing LNAA (most of which are essential) from the brain, seems to provide a mechanism for the control of the LNAA content of brain.

11.6.2 Na$^+$-dependent transport of small non-essential neutral amino acids: system A

The activity of system A, named for its preference for transporting alanine (Oxender and Christensen, 1963) may be distinguished from other Na$^+$-dependent carriers by its acceptance of MeAIB (N-methylamino-isobutyric acid) as a unique substrate (Christensen et al., 1967). System A is voltage sensitive; three positive charges are translocated per MeAIB molecule (O'Kane et al., 2004). System A is inhibited by small non-essential AA such as proline, alanine, histidine, serine, asparagine and glutamine, as well as by the essential AA histidine. Some laboratories (Oxender and Christensen, 1963; Betz and Goldstein, 1978) reported a similar AA spectrum for system A but also included glycine. Glycine transport was not mediated by system A in isolated membrane vesicles but was a putative substrate of system ASC (O'Kane et al., 2004).

11.6.3 Na$^+$-dependent transport of some large and small neutral amino acids: system ASC

ASC activity was measured in abluminal membranes, after blocking system A with MeAIB, confirming the findings of others who have reported its presence (Tayarani et al., 1987; Hargreaves and Pardridge, 1988; Tovar et al., 1988). In addition to alanine, serine, cysteine and glycine, several essential AA were putative substrates including methionine, valine, leucine, isoleucine and threonine (O'Kane et al., 2004). ASC activity is independent of the transmembrane potential (O'Kane et al., 2004).

11.6.4 Na⁺-dependent transport of nitrogen-rich amino acids: system N

System N has a preference for NAA that are nitrogen-rich, such as glutamine, histidine and asparagine, hence its designation (Kilberg et al., 1980, 1993). BBB abluminal membranes also transport serine via this system. System N was not affected by the transmembrane potential (O'Kane et al., 2004). Li⁺ could substitute for Na⁺, suggesting that system N in the BBB is similar to system N in liver cells (Kilberg et al., 1980; O'Kane et al., 2004).

11.6.5 Na⁺-dependent transport of acidic amino acids: the EAAT family

Na⁺-dependent glutamate transporters exist on the abluminal membrane. They are voltage dependent, and collectively have an apparent K_m of 14 µM at a transmembrane potential of –61 mV (Lee et al., 1998; O'Kane et al., 1999). Analysis of mRNA demonstrated that three transporters were expressed (EAAT1, 2, and 3) in brain capillary endothelial cells. Western blot analysis confirmed the glutamate transporters to be present only on the abluminal membranes; none were detectable on luminal membranes (O'Kane et al., 1999). The activity of the three transporters was 1:3:6, EAAT1: EAAT2: EAAT3, respectively. Collectively the EAAT family is the most powerful of the Na⁺-dependent AA transporters; they show the greatest ability to clear AA at low concentrations (Table 11.4).

11.7 Organization of the Various Transport Systems

The brain gains access to all essential AA through the facilitative systems L1 and y⁺.

There is considerable substrate overlap within the facilitative systems as well as within the Na⁺-dependent systems (Tables 11.1 and 11.3).

Five Na⁺-dependent AA transport systems are present exclusively on the abluminal membrane of the BBB (Fig. 11.4), and the capacities of these transporters are similar or greater than those of the facilitative transporters. Because the electrochemical gradient for Na⁺ is oriented to flow from the extracellular fluid into the endothelial cells, these Na⁺-dependent transport systems are in a position to export AA from the brain extracellular fluid.

Thus, AA that pass both endothelial cell membranes and enter the basement membrane space could be actively, and selectively, pumped back across the abluminal membrane. This asymmetrical distribution of Na⁺-dependent carriers has the potential, therefore, to reduce the content of AA in brain.

Table 11.3. Amino acids transported by Na⁺-dependent systems of the abluminal membrane.

System	A	N	ASC	Na⁺-LNAA	EAAT
Non-essential					
Glycine			+	+	
Alanine	+		+	+	
Serine	+	+	+		
Proline	+				
Asparagine	+	+			
Glutamine	+	+			
Aspartate					+
Glutamate					+
Essential in brain					
Histidine	+	+		+	
Threonine			+	+	
Cysteine			+		
Methionine				+	
Valine				+	
Leucine				+	
Isoleucine				+	
Phenylalanine				+	
Tyrosine				+	
Tryptophan				+	

AA that are transported, or shown to inhibit transport, are indicated by a +. Values for systems A, N, and ASC are from O'Kane et al. (2004). Values for Na⁺-LNAA are from O'Kane and Hawkins (2003). Values for the EAAT1-3 family are from O'Kane et al. (1999). AA in italics are essential in brain (Laterra et al., 1999).

Table 11.4. Kinetic characteristics of Na⁺-dependent amino acid transporters in abluminal membranes.

Transporter (substrate)	Apparent K_m (mmol l^{-1})	Apparent V_{max} (pmol mg^{-1} min^{-1})	Clearance (µl mg^{-1} min^{-1})	Voltage sensitivity
A (MeAIB)	0.4 ± 0.16	500 ± 60	1*	Yes
N (Gln)	1.3 ± 0.4	4400 ± 700	3	No
ASC (Ala)	0.11 ± 0.06	660 ± 70	6	No
Na⁺-LNAA (Leu)	0.021 ± 0.007	114 ± 6	5*	Yes
EAAT (Glu)	0.014 ± 0.004	151 ± 20	11*	Yes

The radiolabelled AA used for measurements are in parentheses. Clearance was calculated as V_{max}/K_m. Kinetic values were from: Na⁺-LNAA, (O'Kane and Hawkins, 2003); EAAT1-3, (O'Kane et al., 1999); A, ASC and N (O'Kane et al., 2004). Values marked by an asterisk were measured at a transmembrane potential of –61 mV. MeAIB (20 mmol l^{-1}) was included in measurements of systems N and ASC to exclude transport by system A.

The Na⁺-dependent transport systems provide a mechanism for the elimination of non-essential AA and toxic AA, as well as maintaining the optimal concentrations of all other AA. As with the facilitative systems, there is considerable substrate overlap. All naturally occurring AA are transported by at least one system and some by as many as three (Table 11.3). The kinetic characteristics are summarized in Table 11.4. The following sections illustrate how both membranes of the BBB may play an active role in maintaining homeostatic concentrations.

11.8 Branched-chain Amino Acids and Brain Function

It has been suggested that the plasma concentrations of branched-chain AA (BCAA) may influence brain function and affect appetite (Fernstrom, 1985); physical and mental fatigue (Newsholme et al., 1992; Newsholme and Blomstrand, 1996; Yamamoto and Newsholme, 2000); mental performance (Castell et al., 1999); physical endurance (Blomstrand et al., 1991; Hassmen et al., 1994); sleep (Castell et al., 1999); and hormonal function, blood pressure and affective state (Fernstrom, 2005). Presumably, BCAA influence brain function by altering the availability of aromatic AA (Fernstrom and Wurtman, 1972). As mentioned, transport of LNAA is mediated by the facilitative system L1, which is shared by several LNAA; BCAA are especially effective in competing with aromatic AA for entry. Consequently, when plasma BCAA concentrations rise – which can occur in various normal and abnormal situations – they impair the entry of aromatic AA, notably tryptophan (Fernstrom, 2005). Serotonin synthesis in brain depends directly on the availability of tryptophan. Therefore, when plasma BCAA concentrations rise, the contents of brain tryptophan and serotonin fall (Fernstrom, 2005). While the focus of LNAA transport has been on the facilitative system L1, the recent discoveries that Na⁺-dependent carrier systems are present on the abluminal membrane of the BBB (O'Kane and Hawkins, 2003; O'Kane et al., 2004) adds new elements that must be considered. These Na⁺-dependent carriers are capable of propelling all NAA, including BCAA and aromatic AA, back towards the plasma. Thus, future directions should consider mechanisms that affect the retention of AA by the brain once they have entered.

11.9 Glutamate in Plasma and Brain

Glutamate, a non-essential amino acid, is the most abundant free AA in the brain (Meldrum, 2000). In CNS, glutamate functions as a neurotransmitter (Meldrum, 2000); as a link between the redox states of the pyridine nucleotides (NAD⁺ and NADP⁺) (Krebs and Veech, 1969); and as a fuel reserve (Miller et al., 1975). The oxidation of glutamate to oxaloacetate yields 12 ATP per molecule. Therefore, when the brain has insufficient glucose levels, or glycolytic flux is reduced, it mobilizes glutamate as a fuel (Miller et al., 1975).

11.9.1 Compartmentation of glutamate

In CNS glutamate exists as the free AA divided between two separate metabolic compartments located in astrocytes and neurons. These compartments were first recognized in the brain on the basis of radioisotope precursor–product relationships between glutamine and glutamate (Balazs et al., 1972a,b; Martinez-Hernandez et al., 1977; Cooper et al., 1979; Cooper and Plum, 1987). Compartmentation is almost absent at birth and develops in parallel with glial cells (Balazs et al., 1972b) since glutamine synthetase is found only in astrocytes (Martinez-Hernandez et al., 1977).

Neuronal glutamate is contained in at least two pools: in neuronal perikarya and dendrites, and in nerve terminals (vesicles) (Balazs et al., 1972a,b; Meldrum, 2000). Nerve impulses trigger release of glutamate from the pre-synaptic cell, which in turn binds to the glutamate receptors on the opposing post-synaptic cell. Neurotransmission is terminated by astrocytes and neurons that take up glutamate. Very little glutamate is believed to diffuse away from the synapse.

11.9.2 Excitotoxicity hypothesis of neuronal death

Early studies that used pharmacological doses of glutamate demonstrated damage to areas of the brain that were not protected by the BBB (Olney and Sharpe, 1969; Price et al., 1981). These studies led to the concept that neuronal death could be produced by overstimulation of excitatory AA receptors (Schwarcz et al., 1984; Kirino, 1989; Albin and Greenamyre, 1992). Subsequently, this hypothesis became a popular explanation of the pathogenesis of neuronal death in a variety of acute conditions. However, the source of glutamate arises from within the brain in most circumstances. For instance, during an ischaemic episode, release of glutamate from brain cells (Choi et al., 1987; Castillo et al., 1996) may result in an excessive concentration of glutamate in the ECF (Martin et al., 1994; Rothstein et al., 1996). The extreme excitation of neurons by glutamate may in turn result in the opening of receptor-coupled ionophores, of which calcium channels are of particular importance. A large influx of calcium associated with impaired intracellular calcium sequestration mechanisms (which activate catabolic enzymes) may ultimately result in neuronal death (Benveniste et al., 1984). However, plasma glutamate is stable and does not change much unless glutamate is raised by artificial means.

11.9.3 Glutamate in circulation

Plasma glutamate concentrations are in the range of 50–100 µM in humans and other species (Laterra et al., 1999). Even when relatively large quantities of monosodium glutamate are added to the food of mice, monkeys or humans, only small changes in the plasma concentration of glutamate were found (Stegink et al., 1982, 1983, 1985; Tsai and Huang, 2000).

11.10 Facilitative and Active Transport Systems for Glutamate in the BBB

Early studies of the BBB, using whole brain perfusions or animals in vivo, identified facilitative transporters in the BBB membrane that are saturable and stereoselective (Oldendorf, 1970, 1971b). Because the substrate was presented to the capillary lumen it may be deduced that these transporters are present at least in the luminal membrane. On the other hand, it has been shown in several studies that glutamate does not enter the brain in material quantities, except in the circumventricular organs (Drewes et al., 1977; Hawkins et al., 1995; Viña et al., 1997). Until recently this has been a puzzle. Why should there be a transport system for an AA that is synthesized within the brain in large quantities? Examining the luminal and abluminal membranes separately provided an explanation.

11.10.1 Facilitative transport of glutamate in the luminal membrane

Lee et al. (1998) measured facilitative glutamate transport separately in luminal and abluminal membranes, and found that facilitative glutamate transport exists only in the luminal border in a position to allow transport in both directions between plasma and endothelial cells. However, the function of a transporter for AAA that had a high affinity and a low capacity (Pardridge, 1983; Benrabh and Lefauconnier, 1996; Smith, 2000) was not clear: both glutamate and aspartate are nonessential amino acids that are synthesized and accumulated in high concentrations in brain.

11.10.2 Active transport systems expel glutamate from the ECF

Ordinarily, ECF glutamate is kept very low ($\approx$ 0.5–2 µM) (Meldrum, 2000). In fact the concentration of glutamate and aspartate in CSF is lower than any other AA group (Fig. 11.5). The large gradient between brain cells and ECF is maintained by a family of Na^+-dependent glutamate transporters known as EAAT. These transporters couple the steep Na^+ gradient that normally exists between the ECF and brain cells. Currently five members of the EAAT family have been identified (Eliasof et al., 1998; Meldrum, 2000). They reside in the plasma membranes of astrocytes (Rothstein et al., 1994, 1996; Swanson et al., 1997; Meldrum, 2000); neurons (Kanai and Hediger, 1992, 2004; Lehre et al., 1995; Velaz-Faircloth et al., 1996; Attwell, 2000; Meldrum, 2000); and the BBB (O'Kane et al., 1999). The Na^+-dependent transporters work at the limit of their ability to maintain the glutamate gradient between the brain cells and ECF, and of course, the steep Na^+ gradient as well (extracellular >> intracellular) that is maintained by Na^+/K^+-ATPase. If the oxygen supply is insufficient to maintain ATP levels, membrane Na^+/K^+-ATPase cease to function. Under these circumstances the Na^+ gradient is dissipated and glutamate is released from both astrocytes and neurons by reversal of the EAAT family of transporters. If ECF glutamate rises, nerve cells may be damaged.

Of the five known Na^+-dependent glutamate transporters (EAATs 1–5) (Shigeri et al., 2004), at least three are proven to exist in the abluminal membrane of the BBB (Hutchison et al., 1985; O'Kane et al., 1999), and the transcript of EAAT 4 has been found in the BBB (Enerson and Drewes, 2006). The EAATs are voltage dependent, and collectively have an apparent K_m of 14 µM (Lee et al., 1998; O'Kane et al., 1999). Western blot analysis confirmed the glutamate transporters to be present exclusively in the abluminal membranes (O'Kane et al., 1999). Collectively the EAAT family is the most powerful of the Na^+-dependent AA transporters found in the abluminal membrane to date (Table 11.4).

11.10.3 Current concept of glutamate transport across the BBB

The current concept is that when glutamate concentrations increase above optimal in the ECF, the abluminal membrane of the BBB pumps glutamate into the endothelial cells. The facilitative transport system in the luminal membrane allows glutamate egress to the circulation (Fig. 11.6).

The organization of the BBB explains why various investigators have found that glutamate entry to brain is almost undetectable (Drewes et al., 1977; Hawkins et al., 1995; Viña et al., 1997; Smith, 2000). Glutamate may enter the endothelial cells, but net movement of glutamate from endothelial cells to brain is nearly impossible. This is a consequence of the steep Na^+-gradient that powers the EAAT family of glutamate transporters at the border between the ECF and the abluminal membrane of the endothelial cells. Because of this organization the BBB is virtually impermeable to the net movement of glutamate from the circulation into the brain.

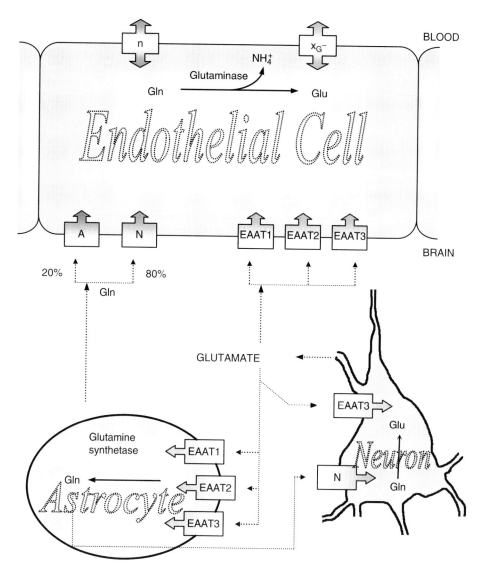

Fig. 11.6. Glutamate and glutamine transport between neurons, astrocytes, and endothelial cells. The presence of Na$^+$-dependent carriers capable of pumping glutamine and glutamate from brain into endothelial cells, glutaminase within endothelial cells to hydrolyze glutamine to glutamate and NH$_4^+$, and facilitative carriers for glutamine and glutamate at the luminal membrane provides a mechanism for removing nitrogen and nitrogen-rich AA from brain (Lee *et al.*, 1998). EAAT1, 2, and 3 are present in endothelial cells (O'Kane *et al.*, 1999), and astrocytes (Miralles *et al.*, 2001). A transcript of EAAT4 has also been found in endothelial cells (Enerson and Drewes 2006). EAAT3 is present in nerve cells (Rothstein *et al.*, 1994). A, Na$^+$-dependent system A; N, Na$^+$-dependent system N; EAAT, Na$^+$-dependent glutamate transporter; x$_G$-, facilitative glutamate transporter; n, facilitative glutamine transporter. (A similar figure was previously published in the *Journal of Nutrition*.)

11.11 Glutamine and Ammonia Balance

Glutamine is the second most abundant AA in brain, about 6.2 µmol g^{-1} (Hawkins and Mans, 1983). As mentioned, glutamine differs from other amino acids insofar as the CSF and plasma concentrations are similar (Fig. 11.4). Glutamine is synthesized in the mitochondria of astrocytes from α-ketoglutamate and NH_4^+ that constantly enters the brain from the circulation, as well as from recycled NH_4^+ that arises from glutamine metabolism by neurons (Fig. 11.6). Astrocytes are the sole source of glutamine because glutamine synthetase is only found in their mitochondria: no other brain cells have the capability to synthesize glutamine (Martinez-Hernandez et al., 1977; Norenberg and Martinez-Hernandez, 1979).

11.11.1 Facilitative transport of glutamine at the luminal membrane

Lee et al. (1998) described facilitative transport of glutamine across the luminal membrane of the BBB that was not inhibited by BCH and did not demonstrate trans-stimulation. This transport system is similar to system n described in hepatic plasma membrane vesicles (Pacitti et al., 1993). The BBB system n is inhibited by asparagine and histidine (Hawkins et al., 2006a) as was found in hepatic vesicles by Pacitti et al. (1993). System n exists solely on the luminal membrane (Lee et al., 1998). Glutamine is also transported weakly by system L1 (see below) in competition with many of the essential NAA.

11.11.2 Na$^+$-dependent transport of glutamine at the abluminal membrane

There are two Na$^+$-dependent systems that transport glutamine, systems A and N, both of which are located exclusively on the abluminal membrane. System N has a preference for NAA that are nitrogen-rich, such as glutamine, histidine and asparagine, hence its designation (Kilberg et al., 1980, 1993). BBB abluminal membranes also transport serine to some degree via this system. System A is named for its preference for transporting alanine (Oxender and Christensen, 1963). In addition to glutamine and alanine, system A also transports small non-essential amino acids such as proline, alanine, serine and asparagine, as well as the essential AA histidine. There are, therefore, two Na$^+$-dependent transport systems capable of moving glutamine from the ESF to the endothelial cells. Glutamine is free to diffuse to the plasma, facilitated primarily by system N and to a lesser degree by system L1. Thus it may be surmised that the Na$^+$-dependent systems of the abluminal membranes, together with the facilitative system n in the luminal membrane, remove glutamine from the brain (Fig. 11.5).

11.11.3 Ammonia balance

The organization of the BBB also provides an explanation for a long-standing puzzle regarding brain NH_4^+ metabolism. Various measurements have shown that 20–50% of the NH_4^+ circulating through the blood vessels in the brain passes the BBB and is incorporated quantitatively into the amide group of glutamine by astrocytes (Cooper et al., 1979; Cooper and Plum, 1987). It is intriguing, however, that it has not been possible to consistently measure arteriovenous differences of NH_4^+ (Cooper and Plum, 1987). If there were no mechanism for the removal of glutamine it would accumulate in the brain, thereby raising the osmolarity and causing swelling. For instance, taking cerebral blood flow to be 1 ml min^{-1} g^{-1} and plasma NH_4^+ to be 50–100 µmol l^{-1}, it may be calculated that glutamine accumulation could be 14–72 µmol g^{-1} each day. Clearly this would be an osmotic challenge for the brain. The situation is now clearer. Glutamine may be pumped from ECF into endothelial cells and is at least partially metabolized to NH_4^+ and glutamate. The remaining glutamine, as well as NH_4^+ and glutamate, are free to diffuse across the luminal membrane into the blood (Lee et al., 1998; O'Kane et al., 1999). This would provide an explanation of why the rate of NH_4^+ uptake and release are balanced.

This new knowledge also explains how the entry of glutamine (and glutamate) to the

CNS is restricted (Hawkins et al., 1995; Hawkins, 2009) even though carrier activities for both amino acids have been described (Oldendorf and Szabo, 1976; Smith et al., 1987). Glutamine and glutamate can traverse the luminal membrane on facilitative systems. However, movement into the brain, across the abluminal membrane, is small because of the lack of facilitative carriers in the abluminal membrane. Furthermore, the three Na^+-dependent carriers in the abluminal membrane that are driven by the steep Na^+ gradient that exists between brain ECF and the cell interior forcefully oppose glutamate entry and promote its removal from the brain.

The BBB seems to be arranged in such a manner as to not only restrict the entry of glutamine and glutamate into the brain, but also actively to export these amino acids and NH_4^+ to the circulation (Fig. 11.5). Therefore, the BBB participates in the regulation of brain nitrogen metabolism, and protects against the development of neurotoxicity by preventing the accumulation of glutamate as well as the accumulation of NH_4^+.

11.12 The γ-Glutamyl Cycle and the Role of Pyroglutamate on Na^+-dependent Carriers

The γ-glutamyl cycle proposed by Meister (Orlowski and Meister, 1970; Meister, 1973) accounts for the synthesis and degradation of reduced glutathione (GSH) and has been shown to influence AA transport in various tissues. The original suggestion that the cycle is involved directly in AA translocation into cells is controversial, having received both support and criticism. However, studies using lactating mammary glands and placenta of pregnant rats showed that pyroglutamate (also known as oxoproline), an intermediate of the γ-glutamyl cycle, serves to stimulate Na^+-dependent AA transport (Viña et al., 1985, 1989).

The first reaction of the cycle occurs extracellularly and is catalysed by γ-glutamyl transpeptidase (GGT) (Fig. 11.7) (Meister, 1973). The substrates for GGT are glutathione, which is exported across the luminal membrane of endothelial cells to the plasma side, and extracellular AA in the plasma. The γ-glutamyl-AA that results enters cells by a transport system that is not shared by free AA. Intracellularly, γ-glutamyl-AA are substrates of γ-glutamyl cyclotransferase, which converts the γ-glutamyl-AA into pyroglutamate and the corresponding free AA. Subsequently pyroglutamate is hydrolyzed to glutamate by oxoprolinase (Van Der Werf et al., 1974).

Using abluminal membrane vesicles from the BBB, it was shown that pyroglutamate stimulates the Na^+-dependent system A by 70% in a concentration-dependent manner (Lee et al., 1996). Thus, the affinity for MeAIB was increased by 50%, with no change in V_{max}. Pyroglutamate had no effect on luminal transport of L-phenylalanine (a representative substrate of the facilitative transport system L1); the effect of pyroglutamate was restricted to the Na^+-dependent AA transport systems of the abluminal membrane (Lee et al., 1996).

The effect of pyroglutamate on the other Na^+-dependent transporters of the BBB was studied recently (Hawkins et al., 2006b). It was found that preloading membrane vesicles with 2 mmol L-pyroglutamate stimulated all Na^+-dependent AA transport systems with the exception of system N, which transports glutamine. The latter is interesting because glutamine is the only AA present in similar concentrations in plasma and ECF, and is synthesized from NH_4^+ that enters brain continuously (Cooper and Plum, 1987). Also of interest was the finding that pyroglutamate stimulated y^+, a transporter that transports cationic AA, but also transports a range of NAA in the presence of Na^+ (White, 1985; Mann et al., 2003).

The presence of GGT in the BBB has been an enigma. GGT activity is high in tissues that actively transport AA, such as the brush border of the proximal convoluted tubules of the kidney (Curto et al., 1988), the lactating mammary gland (Curto et al., 1988), and the apical portion of the intestinal epithelium. The BBB differs from these tissues in that it is not associated with active AA uptake from plasma. While brain requires essential AA for its function and growth, their supply is not much greater than the demand, and it is difficult to detect arteriovenous differences of AA across

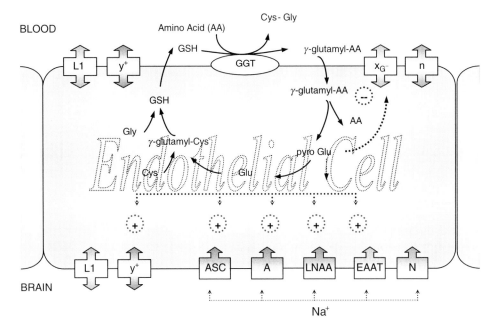

Fig. 11.7. The influence of pyroglutamate on AA transport across the blood–brain barrier. γ-Glutamyl-AAs are formed at the outer surface of luminal membranes of the endothelial cells by GGT that transfers the γ-glutamyl moiety of glutathione to most AA thereby forming a γ-glutamyl-AA. The γ-glutamyl-AA enters endothelial cells where the AA is released and pyroglutamate is formed. The Na^+-dependent transport systems A, ASC, and Na^+-LNAA, EAAT and y+, all located on the abluminal side, are activated by pyroglutamate. N was the only system not stimulated. L1 is present on both the luminal and abluminal membrane and is not affected by pyroglutamate (Lee et al., 1996). A, Na^+-dependent system A; N, Na^+-dependent system N; EAAT, Na^+-dependent glutamate transporter; x_G^-, facilitative glutamate transporter; n, facilitative glutamine transporter. (A similar figure was previously published in the Journal of Nutrition.)

the brain (Drewes et al., 1977; Sacks et al., 1982). It has, therefore, been puzzling why brain capillaries have such high GGT activity.

The data support the hypothesis that the γ-glutamyl cycle influences AA transport systems indirectly through pyroglutamate, produced intracellularly as an intermediary metabolite of the γ-glutamyl cycle. Pyroglutamate, in turn, acts to stimulate Na^+-dependent AA transport systems. The γ-glutamyl cycle and GGT may serve to monitor the availability of AA to the brain, and constitute the first step in a control mechanism that influences the accessibility and content of brain AA (Fig. 11.7). The question arises whether the pyroglutamate concentrations that exist in vivo are sufficient to stimulate Na^+-dependent transport. While data on the concentrations of pyroglutamate in cerebral microvessels seem to be unavailable, the concentrations in normal human plasma and various tissue extracts are between 20 and 50 μM (Van Der Werf et al., 1974; Van Der Werf and Meister, 1975), and as high as 6 mmol l^{-1} in plasma and CSF in pathological conditions (Meister and Anderson, 1983). Stimulation of the Na^+-dependent transport of system A was a linear function of the pyroglutamate concentration up to 2 mmol l^{-1}, a range that does not seem unreasonable.

The transpeptidation activity of GGT is a function of the plasma concentration and spectrum of AA (Allison and Meister, 1981), both of which may vary considerably depending on nutritional status. This provides a feedback mechanism in which the γ-glutamyl-AA produced by GGT enter cerebral capillary endothelial cells and are converted to pyroglutamate, which in turn activates four of the five Na^+-dependent systems at the abluminal membrane. Since these systems are oriented to remove AA from the brain in an energy-dependent fashion, their up-regulation could provide at least a part of a control mechanism to guard against elevations of AA in the brain when their availability is excessive. This is of particular interest with regard to smaller non-essential AA for which systems A and ASC have a relatively high affinity. Thus, this process may serve to modulate the entry of AA that serve as neurotransmitters, or their precursors.

transport systems capable of transporting NAA and acidic AA (Broer and Brookes, 2001; Miralles et al., 2001; Schousboe, 2003). These systems are actively involved in regulating AA concentrations in ECF and are especially important in the maintenance of low concentrations of neurotransmitter AA such as glutamate, aspartate and glycine. On the other hand, it now seems clear that BBB also participates in the active regulation of brain ECF composition, and the abluminal membrane is especially important in this role.

11.13 Concluding Comments

The present-day view of the BBB is that cerebral endothelial cells participate actively in regulating the composition of brain ECF and the AA content of the brain. The luminal and abluminal membranes work in a complementary fashion, with Na^+-dependent transport of AA occurring at the abluminal membrane and facilitative transport at the luminal, or in the case of LNAA, at both membranes (Hawkins et al., 2002).

While the BBB determines the availability and therefore the brain content of essential AA, astrocytes and neurons participate in maintaining the extracellular concentrations. Astrocytes and neurons have Na^+-dependent

11.14 Acknowledgements

Some sections of this article, and Figures 11.1, 11.2a, 11.5 and 11.6 are from an article published in IUBMB Life (Hawkins et al., 2002). Figures 11.2b, 11.4, 11.5, 11.6 and 11.7 were from an article published in the Journal of Nutrition (Hawkins et al., 2006a). The authors express their gratitude to Mary Regina DeJoseph for her skilled technical assistance. Financial support: portions of these works were supported by: National Institutes of Health Grants NS 31017 (R.A.H); NS 041405 (I.A.S); the Ministerio de Educación y Ciencia, Plan Nacional I+D+i(BFU2007-62036) (J.R.V); the International Glutamate Technical Committee (R.A.H).

References

Albin, R.L. and Greenamyre, J.T. (1992) Alternative excitotoxic hypotheses. *Neurology* 42, 733–738.
Allison, R.D. and Meister, A. (1981) Evidence that transpeptidation is a significant function of gamma-glutamyl transpeptidase. *Journal of Biological Chemistry* 256, 2988–2992.
Attwell, D. (2000) Brain uptake of glutamate, food for thought. *Journal of Nutrition* 130, 1023–1025.
Balazs, R., Machiyama, Y. and Patel, A.J. (1972a) Compartmentation and the metabolism of gamma-aminobutyrate. In: Balazs, R. and Cremer, J.E. (eds) *Metabolic Compartmentation in the Brain*. John Wiley & Sons, New York, pp. 57–70.
Balazs, R., Patel, A.J. and Richter, D. (1972b) Metabolic compartmentation in the brain: their properties and relation to morphological structures. In: Balazs, R. and Cremer, J.E. (eds) *Metabolic Compartmentation in the Brain*. John Wiley & Sons, New York, pp. 167–186.
Battistin, L., Grynbaum, A. and Lajtha, A. (1971) The uptake of various amino acids by the mouse brain in vivo. *Brain Research* 29, 85–99.
Benrabh, H. and Lefauconnier, J.M. (1996) Glutamate is transported across the rat blood-brain barrier by a sodium-independent system. *Neuroscience Letters* 210, 9–12.
Benveniste, H., Drejer, J. Schousboe, A. and Diemer, N.H. (1984) Elevations of the extracellular concentrations of glutamate and aspartate in rat hippocampus during transient cerebral ischemia monitored by intracerebral microdialysis. *Journal of Neurochemistry* 43, 1369–1374.

Betz, A.L. and Goldstein, G.W. (1978) Polarity of the blood-brain barrier: neutral amino acid transport into isolated brain capillaries. *Science* 202, 225–226.

Betz, A.L., Firth, J.A. and Goldstein, G.W. (1980) Polarity of the blood-brain barrier: distribution of enzymes between the luminal and antiluminal membranes of brain capillary endothelial cells. *Brain Research* 192, 17–28.

Blomstrand, E., Hassmen, P., Ekblom, B. and Newsholme, E.A. (1991) Administration of branched-chain amino acids during sustained exercise–effects on performance and on plasma concentration of some amino acids. *European Journal of Applied Physiology and Occupational Physiology* 63, 83–88.

Boado, R.J., Li, J.Y. Nagaya, M., Zhang, C. and Pardridge, W.M. (1999) Selective expression of the large neutral amino acid transporter at the blood-brain barrier. *Proceedings of the National Academy of Sciences USA* 96, 12079–12084.

Bradbury, M. (1979) *The Concept of a Blood-Brain Barrier*. John Wiley & Sons, New York, p. 162.

Brendal, K. and Meezan, E. (1974) Isolated brain microvessels: a purified, metabolically active preparation from bovine cerebral cortex. *Science* 185, 953–955.

Brightman, M.W. and Reese, T.W. (1969) Junctions between intimately apposed cell membranes in the vertebrate brain. *Journal of Cell Biology* 40, 648–677.

Brightman, M.W., Reese, T.S. and Feder, N. (1971) Assessment with the electronmicroscope of the permeability to peroxidase of cerebral endothelium and epithelium in mice and sharks. *Journal of Neuropathology and Experimental Neurology* 30, 137–138

Broer, S. and Brookes, N. (2001) Transfer of glutamine between astrocytes and neurons. *Journal of Neurochemistry* 77, 705–719.

Castell, L.M., Yamamoto, T., Phoenix, J. and Newsholme, E.A. (1999) The role of tryptophan in fatigue in different conditions of stress. *Advances in Experimental Medicine* 467, 697–704.

Castillo, J., Davalos, A., Naveiro, J., and Noya, M. (1996) Neuroexcitatory amino acids and their relation to infarct size and neurological deficit in ischemic stroke. *Stroke* 27, 1060–1065.

Choi, D.W., Maulucci-Gedde, M. and Kriegstein, A.R. (1987) Glutamate neurotoxicity in cortical cell culture. *Journal of Neuroscience* 7, 357–368.

Christensen, H.N. (1979) Developments in amino acid transport, illustrated for the blood-brain barrier. *Biochemical Pharmacology* 28, 1989–1992.

Christensen, H.N., Liang, M. and Archer, E.G. (1967) A distinct Na^+-requiring transport system for alanine, serine, cysteine, and similar amino acids. *Journal of Biological Chemistry* 242, 5237–5246.

Cooper, A.J. and Plum, F. (1987) Biochemistry and physiology of brain ammonia. *Physiological Reviews* 67, 440–519.

Cooper, A.J., McDonald, J.M, Gelbard, A.S. Gledhill, R.F. and Duffy, T.E. (1979) The metabolic fate of 13N-labeled ammonia in rat brain. *Journal of Biological Chemistry* 254, 4982–4992.

Crone, C. (1963) The permeability of capillaries in various organs as determined by use of the 'indicator diffusion' method. *Acta Physiologica Scandinavica* 58, 292–305.

Crone, C. (1965) Facilitated transfer of glucose from blood into brain tissue. *Journal of Physiology* 181, 103–113.

Crone, C. and Olesen, S.P. (1982) Electrical resistance of brain microvascular endothelium. *Brain Research* 241, 49–55.

Curto, K.A., Sweeney, W.E., Avner, E.D., Piesco, N.P., and Curthoys, N.P. (1988) Immunocytochemical localization of gamma-glutamyl transpeptidase during fetal development of mouse kidney. *Journal of Histology and Cytochemistry* 36, 159–166.

Davson, H. and Welch, K. (1971) The relations of blood, brain and cerebrospinal fluid. In: Siesjo, B.K. and Sorensen, S.C. (eds) *Ion Homeostasis of the Brain*. Munksgaard, Copenhagen, pp. 9–21.

DeBault, L.E. and Cancilla, P.A. (1980) γ-Glutamyl transpeptidase in isolated brain endothelial cells: induction by glial cells in vitro. *Science* 207, 653–655.

Dehouck, M.-P., Jolliet-Riant, P., Bree, F., Fruchart, J.-C., Cecchelli, R. and Tillement, J.-P. (1992) Drug transfer across the blood-brain barrier: correlation between in vitro and in vivo models. *Journal of Neurochemistry* 58, 1790–1797.

Deves, R. and Boyd, C.A. (1998) Transporters for cationic amino acids in animal cells: discovery, structure, and function. *Physiological Reviews* 78, 487–545.

Deves, R., Angelo, S. and Rojas, A.M. (1998) System y+L: the broad scope and cation modulated amino acid transporter. *Experimental Physiology* 83, 211–220.

Drewes, L.R., Conway, W.P. and Gilboe, D.D. (1977) Net amino acid transport between plasma and erythrocytes and perfused dog brain. *American Journal of Physiology* 233, E320–E325.

Eliasof, S., Arriza, J., Leighton, B., Amara, S. and Kavanaugh, M. (1998) Localization and function of five glutamate transporters cloned from the salamander retina. *Vision Research* 38, 1443–1454.

Enerson, B.E. and Drewes, L.R. (2006) The rat blood-brain barrier transcriptome. *Journal of Cerebral Blood Flow and Metabolism* 26, 959–973.

Felig, P., Wahren, J., and Ahlborg, G. (1972) Uptake of individual amino acids by the human brain (36994). *Proceedings of Experimental Biology and Medicine* 142, 230–231.

Fernstrom, J.D. (1985) Dietary effects on brain serotonin synthesis: relationship to appetite regulation. *American Journal of Clinical Nutrition* 42, 1072–1082.

Fernstrom, J.D. (2005) Branched-chain amino acids and brain function. *Journal of Nutrition* 135, 1539S–1546S.

Fernstrom, J.D. and Wurtman, R.J. (1972) Brain serotonin content: physiological regulation by plasma neutral amino acids. *Science* 178, 4l4–4l6.

Goldstein, G.W., Wolinsky, J.S., Csejtey, J. and Diamond, I. (1975) Isolation of metabolically active capillaries from rat brain. *Journal of Neurochemistry* 25, 715–717.

Hargreaves, K.M. and Pardridge, W.M. (1988) Neutral amino acid transport at the human blood-brain barrier. *Journal of Biological Chemistry* 263, 19392–19397.

Hassmen, P., Blomstrand, E., Ekblom, B. and Newsholme, E.A. (1994) Branched-chain amino acid supplementation during 30-km competitive run: mood and cognitive performance. *Nutrition* 10, 405–410.

Hawkins, R.A. (2009) The blood-brain barrier and glutamate. *American Journal of Clinical Nutrition* 90, 867S–874S.

Hawkins, R.A. and Mans, A.M. (1983) Intermediary metabolism of carbohydrates and other fuels. In: Lajtha, A. (ed.) *Handbook of Neurochemistry*. Plenum Press, New York, pp. 259–294.

Hawkins, R.A., DeJoseph, M.R. and Hawkins, P.A. (1995) Regional brain glutamate transport in rats at normal and raised concentrations of circulating glutamate. *Cell and Tissue Research* 281, 207–214.

Hawkins, R.A., Peterson, D.R. and Viña, J.R. (2002) The complementary membranes forming the blood-brain barrier. *IUBMB Life* 54, 101–107.

Hawkins, R.A., O'Kane, R.L., Simpson, I.A. and Viña, J.R. (2006a) Structure of the blood-brain barrier and its role in the transport of amino acids. *Journal of Nutrition* 136, 218S–226S.

Hawkins R.A., Simpson I.A., Mokashi A. and Viña J.R. (2006b) Pyroglutamate stimulates Na^+-dependent amino-acid transport across the blood-brain barrier. *FEBS Letters* 580, 4382–4386.

Hemish, J., Nakaya, N., Mittal, V. and Enikolopov, G. (2003) Nitric oxide activates diverse signaling pathways to regulate gene expression. *Journal of Biological Chemistry* 278, 42321–48329.

Hutchison, H.T., Eisenberg, H.M. and Haber, B. (1985) High-affinity transport of glutamate in rat brain microvessels. *Experimental Neurology* 87, 260–269.

Kanai, Y. and Hediger, M.A. (1992) Primary structure and functional characterization of a high-affinity glutamate transporter. *Nature* 360, 467–471.

Kanai, Y. and Hediger, M.A. (2004) The glutamate/neutral amino acid transporter family SLC1: molecular, physiological and pharmacological aspects. *Pflugers Archiv* 447, 469–479.

Kilberg, M.S., Handlogten, M.E. and Christensen, H.N. (1980) Characteristics of an amino acid transport system in rat liver for glutamine, asparagine, histidine, and closely related analogs. *Journal of Biological Chemistry* 255, 4011–4019.

Kilberg, M.S., Stevens, B.S. and Novak, D.A. (1993) Recent advances in mammalian amino acid transport. *Annual Review of Nutrition* 13, 137–165.

Killian, D.M. and Chikhale, P.J. (2001) Predominant functional activity of the large, neutral amino acid transporter (LAT1) isoform at the cerebrovasculature. *Neuroscience Letters* 306, 1–4.

Kirino, T. (1989) Neuronal degeneration and glutamate. *Rinsho Shinkeigaku* 29, 1522–1525.

Krebs, H.A. and Veech, R.L. (1969) Equilibrium relations between pyridine nucleotides and adenine nucleotides and their roles in the regulation of metabolic processes. *Advances in Enzyme Regulation* 7, 397–413.

Laterra, J., Keep, R., Betz, A.L. and Goldstein, G.W. (1999) Blood-brain-cerebrospinal fluid barriers. In: Siegel, G.J., Agrampff, B.W., Albers, R.W., Fisher, S.K. and Uhler M.D. (eds) *Basic Neurochemistry*. 6th edition, Lippincott-Raven, Philadelphia, Pennsylvania, USA, pp. 671–689.

Lee, W.J., Hawkins, R.A., Peterson, D.R. and Viña, J.R. (1996) Role of oxoproline in the regulation of neutral amino acid transport across the blood-brain barrier. *Journal of Biological Chemistry* 271, 19129–19133.

Lee, W.J., Hawkins, R.A., Viña, J.R. and Peterson, D.R. (1998) Glutamine transport by the blood-brain barrier: a possible mechanism for nitrogen removal. *American Journal of Physiology* 274, C1101–C1107.

Lehre, K.P., Levy, L.M., Ottersen, O.P., Storm-Mathisen, J. and Danbolt, N.C. (1995) Differential expression of two glial glutamate transporters in the rat brain: quantitative and immunocytochemical observations. *Journal of Neuroscience* 15, 1835–1853.

Mann, G.E., Yudilevich, D.L. and Sobrevia, L. (2003) Regulation of amino acid and glucose transporters in endothelial and smooth muscle cells. *Physiological Reviews* 83, 183–252.

Martin, R.L., Lloyd, H.G. and Cowan, A.I. (1994) The early events of oxygen and glucose deprivation: setting the scene for neuronal death? *Trends in Neurosciences* 17, 251–257.

Martinez-Hernandez, A., Bell, K.P. and Norenberg, M.D. (1977) Glutamine synthetase: glial localization in brain. *Science* 195, 1356–1358.

Meister, A. (1973) The enzymology of amino acid transport. *Science* 180, 33–39.

Meister, A. and Anderson, M.E. (1983) Glutathione. *Annual Review of Biochemistry* 52, 711–760.

Meldrum, B.S. (2000) Glutamate as a neurotransmitter in the brain: review of physiology and pathology. *Journal of Nutrition* 130, 1007S–1015S.

Miller, A.L., Hawkins, R.A. and Veech, R.L. (1975) Decreased rate of glucose utilization by rat brain in vivo after exposure to atmospheres containing high concentrations of CO_2. *Journal of Neurochemistry* 25, 553–558.

Miralles, V.J., Martinez-Lopez, I., Zaragoza, R., Borras, E., Garcia, C. Pallardo, F.V. and Viña, J.R. (2001) Na+ dependent glutamate transporters (EAAT1, EAAT2, and EAAT3) in primary astrocyte cultures: effect of oxidative stress. *Brain Research* 922, 21–29.

Nair, V. and Roth, L.J. (1961) Autoradiography of whole animals as an experimental tool in pharmacological research. In: Rothchild, S. (ed.) *Advances in Tracer Methodology*. Plenum Press, New York, pp. 309–313.

Newsholme, E.A. and Blomstrand, E. (1996) The plasma level of some amino acids and physical and mental fatigue. *Experientia* 52, 413–415.

Newsholme, E.A., Blomstrand, E. and Ekblom, B. (1992) Physical and mental fatigue: metabolic mechanisms and importance of plasma amino acids. *British Medical Bulletin* 48, 477–495.

Norenberg, M.D. and Martinez-Hernandez, A. (1979) Fine structural localization of glutamine synthetase in astrocytes of rat brain. *Brain Research* 161, 303–310.

O'Kane, R.L. and Hawkins, R.A. (2003) Na+-dependent transport of large neutral amino acids occurs at the abluminal membrane of the blood-brain barrier. *American Journal of Physiology* 287, E622–629.

O'Kane, R.L., Martinez-Lopez, I., DeJoseph, M.R., Viña, J.R. and Hawkins, R.A. (1999) Na(+)-dependent glutamate transporters (EAAT1, EAAT2, and EAAT3) of the blood-brain barrier. A mechanism for glutamate removal. *Journal of Biological Chemistry* 274, 31891–31895.

O'Kane, R.L., Viña, J.R., Simpson, I. and Hawkins, R.A. (2004) Na+-dependent neutral amino acid transporters (A, ASC and N) of the blood-brain barrier: mechanisms for neutral amino acid removal. *American Journal of Physiology* 287, E622–E629.

O'Kane R.L., Viña, J.R., Simpson, I.A., Zaragoza, R., Mokashi, A. and Hawkins, R.A. (2006) Cationic amino acid transport across the blood-brain barrier is mediated exclusively by system y+. *American Journal of Physiology* 291, E412–419

Oldendorf, W.H. (1970) Measurement of brain uptake of radiolabeled substances using a tritiated water internal standard. *Brain Research* 24, 372–376.

Oldendorf, W.H. (1971a) Brain uptake of radiolabeled amino acids, amines, and hexoses after arterial injection. *American Journal of Physiology* 221, 1629–1639.

Oldendorf, W.H. (1971b) Uptake of radiolabeled essential amino acids by brain following arterial injection. *Proceedings of the Society for Experimental Biology and Medicine* 136, 385–386.

Oldendorf, W.H. (1973) Stereospecificity of blood-brain barrier permeability to amino acids. *American Journal of Physiology* 224, 967–969.

Oldendorf, W.H. and Brown, W.J. (1975) Greater number of capillary endothelial cell mitochondria in brain than in muscle. *Proceedings of the Society for Experimental Biology and Medicine* 149, 736–738.

Oldendorf, W.H. and Szabo, J. (1976) Amino acid assignment to one of three blood-brain barrier amino acid carriers. *American Journal of Physiology* 230, 94–98.

Olney, J.W. and Sharpe, L.G. (1969) Brain lesions in an infant rhesus monkey treated with monosodium glutamate. *Science* 166, 386–388.

Orlowski, M. and Meister, A. (1970) The γ-glutamyl cycle: a possible transport system for amino acids. *Proceedings of the National Academy of Sciences* 67, 1248–1255.

Oxender, D.L. and Christensen, H.N. (1963) Distinct mediating systems for the transport of neutral amino acids by the Ehrlich cell. *Journal of Biological Sciences* 238, 3686–3699.

Oyler, G.A., Duckrow, R.B. and Hawkins, R.A. (1992) Computer simulation of the blood-brain barrier: a model including two membranes, blood flow, facilitated and non-facilitated diffusion. *Journal of Neuroscience Methods* 44, 179–196.

Pacitti, A.J., Inoue, Y. and Souba, W.W. (1993) Characterization of Na(+)-independent glutamine transport in rat liver. *American Journal of Physiology* 265, G90–98.

Palacin, M., Estevez, R. and Zorzano, A. (1998) Cystinuria calls for heteromultimeric amino acid transporters. *Current Opinion in Cell Biology* 10, 455–461.

Palmer, R.M., Ferrige, A.G. and Moncada, S. (1987) Nitric oxide release accounts for the biological activity of endothelium-derived relaxing factor. *Nature* 327, 524–526.

Pappenheimer, J.R. (1970a) On the location of the blood-brain barrier. *Proceedings of a Symposium on the Blood-Brain Barrier*. Truex Press, Oxford, pp. 66–84.

Pappenheimer, J.R. (1970b) Osmotic reflection coefficients in capillary membranes. In: Crone, C. and Lassen, N.A. (eds) *Capillary Permeability. The Transfer of Molecules and Ions between Capillary Blood and Tissue*. Munksgaard, Copenhagen, pp. 454–458.

Pappenheimer, J.R. and Setchell, B.P. (1973) Cerebral glucose transport and oxygen consumption in sheep and rabbits. *Journal of Physiology* 233, 529–551.

Pardridge, W.M. (1983) Brain metabolism: A perspective from the BBB. *Physiological Reviews* 63, 1481–1535.

Price, M.T., Olney, J.W., Lowry, O.H. and Buchsbaum, S. (1981) Uptake of exogenous glutamate and aspartate by circumventricular organs but not other regions of brain. *Journal of Neurochemistry* 36, 1774–1780.

Reese, T.S. and Karnovsky, M.J. (1967) Fine structural localization of a blood-brain barrier to exogenous peroxidase. *Journal of Cell Biology* 34, 207–217.

Rothstein, J.D., Martin, L., Levey, A.I., Dykes-Hoberg, M., Jin, L., Wu, D., Nash N., et al. (1994) Localization of neuronal and glial glutamate transporters. *Neuron* 13, 713–725.

Rothstein, J., Dykes-Hoberg, M., Pardo, C., Bristol, L., Jin, L., Kuncl, R. Kanai, Y., et al. (1996) Knockout of glutamate transporters reveals a major role for astroglial transport in excitotoxicity and clearance of glutamate. *Neuron* 16, 675–686.

Sacks, W., Sacks, S., Brebbia, D.R. and Fleischer, A. (1982) Cerebral uptake of amino acids in human subjects and rhesus monkeys in vivo. *Journal of Neuroscience Research* 7, 431–436.

Sánchez del Pino, M.M., Hawkins, R.A. and Peterson, D.R. (1992) Neutral amino acid transport by the blood-brain barrier: membrane vesicle studies. *Journal of Biological Chemistry* 267, 25951–25957.

Sánchez del Pino, M.M., Hawkins, R.A. and Peterson, D.R. (1995a) Biochemical discrimination between luminal and abluminal enzyme and transport activities of the blood-brain barrier. *Journal of Biological Chemistry* 270, 14907–14912.

Sánchez del Pino, M.M., Hawkins, R.A. and Peterson, D.R. (1995b) Neutral amino acid transport characterization of isolated luminal and abluminal membranes of the blood-brain barrier. *Journal of Biological Chemistry* 270, 14913–14918.

Schain, R.J. and Watanabe, K.S. (1972) Distinct patterns of entry of two non-metabolizable amino acids into brain and other organs of infant guinea pigs. *Journal of Neurochemistry* 19, 2279–2288.

Schousboe, A. (2003) Role of astrocytes in the maintenance and modulation of glutamatergic and GABAergic neurotransmission. *Neurochemical Research* 28, 347–352.

Schwarcz, R., Foster, A.C., French, E.D., Whetsell, W.O. Jr and Kohler, C. (1984) Excitotoxic models for neurodegenerative disorders. *Life Sciences* 35, 19–32.

Segawa, H., Fukasawa, Y., Miyamoto, K., Takeda, E., Endou, H. and Kanai, Y. (1999) Identification and functional characterization of a Na+-independent neutral amino acid transporter with broad substrate selectivity. *Journal of Biological Sciences* 274, 19745–19751.

Sershen, H. and Lajtha, A. (1976) Capillary transport of amino acids in the developing brain. *Experimental Neurology* 53, 465–474.

Shigeri, Y., Seal, R.P. and Shimamoto, K. (2004) Molecular pharmacology of glutamate transporters, EAATs and VGLUTs. *Brain Research Brain Research Reviews* 45, 250–265.

Smith, Q.R. (1991) The blood-brain barrier and the regulation of amino acid uptake and availability to brain. In: Vranic, M. (ed.) *Fuel Homeostasis and the Nervous System*. Plenum Press, New York, pp. 55–71.

Smith, Q.R. (2000) Transport of glutamate and other amino acids at the blood-brain barrier. *Journal of Nutrition* 130, 1016S–1022S.

Smith, Q.R., Momma, S., Aoyagi, M. and Rapoport, S.I. (1987) Kinetics of neutral amino acid transport across the blood-brain barrier. *Journal of Neurochemistry* 49, 1651–1658.

Smith, Q.R. and Stoll, J. (1998) Blood-brain barrier amino acid transport. In: Pardridge, W.M. (ed.) *Introduction to the Blood-Brain Barrier: Methodology, Biology, and Pathology.* Cambridge University Press, Cambridge, pp. 188–197.

Stegink, L.D., Filer, L.J., Jr and Baker, G.L. (1982) Plasma and erythrocyte amino acid levels in normal adult subjects fed a high protein meal with and without added monosodium glutamate. *Journal of Nutrition* 112, 1953–1960.

Stegink, L.D., Filer, L.J., Jr and Baker, G.L. (1983) Plasma amino acid concentrations in normal adults fed meals with added monosodium L-glutamate and aspartame. *Journal of Nutrition* 113, 1851–1860.

Stegink, L.D., Filer, L.J., Jr and Baker, G.L. (1985) Plasma glutamate concentrations in adult subjects ingesting monosodium L-glutamate in consomme. *American Journal of Clinical Nutrition* 42, 220–225.

Swanson, R., Liu, J., Miller, J., Rothstein, J., Farrell, K., Stein, B. and Longuemare, M. (1997) Neuronal regulation of glutamate transporter subtype expression in astrocytes. *Journal of Neuroscience* 17, 932–940.

Takasato, Y., Rapoport, S.I. and Smith, Q.R. (1984) An in situ brain perfusion technique to study cerebrovascular transport in the rat. *American Journal of Physiology* 247, H484–H493.

Tayarani, I., Lefauconnier, J.-M., Roux, F. and Bourrer, J.-M. (1987) Evidence for alanine, serine, and cystine system of transport in isolated brain capillaries. *Journal of Cerebral Blood Flow and Metabolism* 7, 585–591.

Tewes, B.J. and Galla, H.-J. (2001) Lipid polarity in brain capillary endothelial cells. *Endothelium* 8, 207–220.

Tovar, A.J., Tews, K., Torres, N. and Harper, A.E. (1988) Some characteristics of the threonine transport across the blood-brain barrier of the rat. *Journal of Neurochemistry* 51, 1285–1293.

Tsai, P.J. and Huang, P.C. (2000) Circadian variations in plasma and erythrocyte glutamate concentrations in adult men consuming a diet with and without added monosodium glutamate. *Journal of Nutrition* 130, 1002S–1004S.

Van Der Werf, P. and Meister, A. (1975) The metabolic formation and utilization of 5-oxo-L-proline (L-pyroglutamate, L-pyrrolidone carboxylate). *Advances in Enzymology* 43, 519–554.

Van Der Werf, P., Stephani, R.A. and Meister, A. (1974) Accumulation of 5-oxoproline in mouse tissues after inhibition of 5-oxoprolinase and administration of amino acids: evidence for function of the gamma-glutamyl cycle. *Proceedings of the National Academy of Sciences* 71, 1026–1029.

van Meer, G. and Simons, K. (1986) The function of tight junctions in maintaining differences in lipid composition between the apical and the basolateral cell surface domains of MDCK cells. *EMBO Journal* 5, 1455–1464.

van Meer, G., Gumbiner, B. and Simons, K. (1986) The tight junction does not allow lipid molecules to diffuse from one epithelial cell to the next. *Nature* 322, 639–641.

Van Winkle, L., Christensen, H. and Campione, A. (1985) Na^+-dependent transport of basic, zwitterionic, and bicyclic amino acids by a broad-scope system in mouse blastocysts. *Journal of Biological Chemistry* 260, 12118–12123.

Van Winkle, L.J., Campione, A.L. and Gorman, J.M. (1988) Na^+-independent transport of basic and zwitterionic amino acids in mouse blastocysts by a shared system and by processes which distinguish between these substrates. *Journal of Biological Chemistry* 263, 3150–3163.

Van Winkle, L., Campione, A. and Farrington, B. (1990) Development of system $B^{0,+}$ and a broad-scope Na-dependent transporter of zwitterionic amino acids in preimplantation mouse conceptuses. *Biochimica et Biophysica Acta* 1025, 225–233.

Velaz-Faircloth, M., McGraw, T.S., Malandro, M.S., Fremeau, R.T., Kilberg, M.S. and Anderson, K.J. (1996) Characterization and distribution of the neuronal glutamate transporter EAAC1 in rat brain. *American Journal of Physiology* 270, C67–C75.

Viña, J.R., Puertes, I.R., Montoro, J.B., Saez, G.T. and Viña, J. (1985) Gamma-glutamyl amino acids as signals for the hormonal regulation of amino acid uptake by the mammary gland of the lactating rat. *Biology of the Neonate* 48, 250–256.

Viña, J.R., Palacin, M., Puertes, I.R., Hernandez, R. and Viña, J. (1989) Role of the γ-glutamyl cycle in the regulation of amino acid translocation. *American Journal of Physiology* 257, E916–E922.

Viña, J.R., DeJoseph, M.R., Hawkins, P.A. and Hawkins, R.A. (1997) Penetration of glutamate into brain of 7-day-old rats. *Metabolic Brain Disease* 12, 219–227.

Vinters, H.V., Beck, D.W., Bready, J.V., Maxwell, K., Berliner, J.A., Hart, M.N. and Cancilla, P.A. (1985) Uptake of glucose analogues into cultured cerebral microvessel endothelium. *Journal of Neuropathology and Experimental Neurology* 44, 445–458.

Vorbrodt, A.W. (1988) Ultrastructural cytochemistry of blood-brain barrier endothelia. *Progress in Histochemistry and Cytochemistry* 18, 1–99.

White, M.F. (1985) The transport of cationic amino acids across the plasma membrane of mammalian cells. *Biochimica et Biophysica Acta* 822, 355–374.

Wu, G. and Meininger, C.J. (1993) Regulation of L-arginine synthesis from L-citrulline by L-glutamine in endothelial cells. *American Journal of Physiology* 265, H1965–1971.

Wu, G. and Meininger, C.J. (2002) Regulation of nitric oxide synthesis by dietary factors. *Annual Review of Nutrition* 22, 61–86.

Yamamoto, T. and Newsholme, E.A. (2000) Diminished central fatigue by inhibition of the L-system transporter for the uptake of tryptophan. *Brain Research Bulletin* 52, 35–38.

12 Inter-organ Fluxes of Amino Acids

M.C.G. van de Poll* and C.H.C. Dejong
Department of Surgery, Maastricht University Medical Centre, Maastricht, the Netherlands

12.1 Abstract

Plasma amino acid pools are regulated by production and disposal. Whereas essential amino acids are dependent on protein breakdown for their plasma flux, non-essential amino acids are produced *de novo* within the body. In many instances these production processes are encased in metabolic cycles, such as the urea cycle, that do not interact with the plasma pool. However when cells or organs lack the enzymes to complete a full cycle they must take up their substrate from the circulation and release the products of their metabolism back to it. In this way these organs regulate plasma pools of certain amino acids. In addition an intricate flux of amino acids between different organs exists by virtue of this phenomenon.

Glutamine is generated within the muscle and taken up by the kidney and the gut, where it is converted to ammonia. Intestinal-derived ammonia is taken up by the liver and detoxified to glutamine, and probably to a lesser extent to urea, which is generated from amino nitrogen and molecular ammonia generated within the liver itself. Since the liver extracts all ammonia generated by the intestines from the circulation, the kidneys are the only ammonia-producing organs that release ammonia to the systemic circulation.

Another product of intestinal glutamine metabolism is citrulline, which is released into the portal vein and largely passes the liver unchanged. Subsequently citrulline provides substrate for the kidneys that convert it to arginine. However, this process contributes only partly to systemic arginine flux. Moreover, many cells metabolize and generate arginine in an NO-cycle that is independent of plasma arginine.

Enteral administration of glutamine is accompanied by increased production of citrulline by the gut, and urea by the liver. Since hepatic arginase activity is compartmentalized within the urea cycle, hepatic extraction of enterally administered arginine is limited, and enteral arginine supplementation is feasible.

Since the intestinal conversion of glutamine to citrulline is crucial for total plasma citrulline flux, reduction of intestinal functional mass leads to low citrulline levels. Although the role of citrulline as a marker of enterocyte mass is becoming more and more established, the potential benefit of its supplementation in short-bowel patients is still unclear.

---

* E-mail address: mcg.vandepoll@ah.unimaas.nl

12.2 Introduction

Apart from being mere building blocks of protein, virtually all free amino acids fulfil specific functions, for example in neurotransmission, signal transduction, or cell proliferation (van de Poll *et al.*, 2005). Consequently, maintenance of the free amino acid pool within the body is of vital importance. The free amino acid pool is separated in extracellular (plasma) and intracellular compartments which are connected and equilibrated by several transporters situated on the cell membrane. These regulate amino acid uptake from the plasma into the cell or secretion from the cell into the plasma, thereby maintaining transmembrane gradients. All free amino acids are metabolized continuously, and therefore their different pools must be replenished at a similar rate to keep them at a constant level. The plasma concentration of an amino acid is a poor reflector of its flux. For example, increased plasma levels of glutamine are found during exogenous supplementation (higher influx) but also during liver failure (lower clearance); conversely, lower glutamine concentrations during experimental sepsis are initially accompanied by an increased flux of glutamine from the muscles to the liver (Bruins *et al.*, 2003).

The appearance of essential amino acids in the free amino acid pool depends completely on protein breakdown, whereas non-essential amino acids can be formed from other amino acids by specific enzymatic processes or by transamination. Such enzymatic processes may be encased in metabolic cycles within a single cell, such as the urea cycle which continuously turns over citrulline, arginine and ornithine within the hepatocyte. These cycles are highly compartmentalized and therefore do not contribute to the appearance rate of amino acids in the plasma (Cheung *et al.*, 1989). When there is no full enzymatic cycle present within a single cell, it must take up its substrate from the plasma. In line with this, non-essential amino acids that cannot be further metabolized are excreted.

These non-cyclic amino acid conversions are particularly important in the regulation of the extracellular free amino acid pool. Due to the tissue-specific distribution of most enzymes, non-essential amino acids are produced and released by specific organs. This leads to an intricate flux of amino acids between various organs resulting in the exchange of substrate through the bloodstream, thus forming inter-organ pathways. In some instances even cells within a single organ are distributed along the bloodstream in a way that allows them to exchange substrate efficiently. This is most strikingly exemplified by the differential distribution of glutaminase and glutamine synthetase within parenchymal cells lining the hepatic sinusoid. Appreciation of enzymatic distribution is crucial to the understanding of these intra- and inter-organ pathways of amino acid metabolism.

In this chapter some of the most important of these pathways will be outlined. In past years many data specifically concerning inter-organ nitrogen exchange in humans have emerged. Although similarities between different species are remarkable, so are some differences. In this chapter recent data that have elucidated and quantified inter-organ pathways of amino acid and nitrogen flux between the liver, intestines, kidney and skeletal muscle in health and disease will be reviewed.

12.3 Glutamine and Ammonia

12.3.1 Metabolism

Glutamine is the most abundant free amino acid in plasma and is central in amino acid metabolism as a nitrogen donor and transporter (Fig. 12.1). It is used as an energy source for enterocytes and immune cells, and amongst others plays a role in the regulation of cell size. In postabsorptive conditions it is released into the plasma at a rate of approximately 250 µmol kg^{-1} h^{-1} in healthy adults, which is amply sufficient to fulfil physiological demand (van de Poll *et al.*, 2007a). Therefore glutamine is a non-essential amino acid under normal physiological conditions. It is derived from protein breakdown and synthesized from glutamate and ammonia by the enzyme glutamine synthetase, particularly found in skeletal muscle and the liver. It is broken down again in a reverse reaction to glutamate and ammonia by the

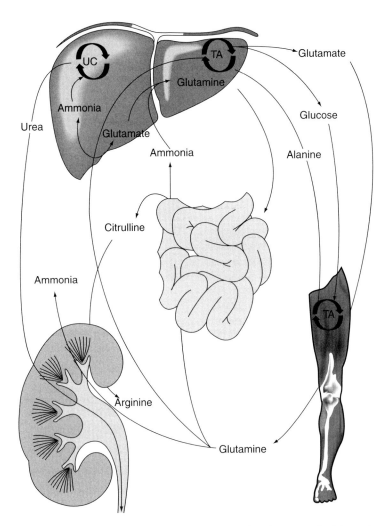

Fig. 12.1. Physiology of inter-organ amino acid exchange. Central is glutamine which is produced by skeletal muscle from glutamate. Glutamine is taken up by the gut, the kidneys, and the intestines. Ammonia is formed by glutaminase activity in these organs. Renal-derived ammonia is released into the systemic circulation, intestinal-derived ammonia is transported to the liver and eventually converted to glutamine again by perivenous glutamine synthetase. Hepatic glutaminase activity, which is confined to the periportal hepatocytes, serves to provide molecular ammonia to the urea cycle. The glutamate yielded in this process is used for glutamine synthesis by perivenous glutamine synthetase activity. Alternatively, the liver takes up glutamine as a nitrogen donor for the urea cycle and to serve gluconeogenesis after deamination. Ammonia released during gluconeogenesis is partly bound to glutamate and excreted to prevent loss of nitrogen via urea synthesis. Urea is released to the systemic circulation and excreted in the urine. Glucose is released into the systemic circulation and utilized ubiquitously. The carbon skeleton of glucose can be recycled to alanine within the muscle and subsequently serve hepatic gluconeogenesis again, thus creating an alanine-glucose cycle. Thirteen per cent of glutamine metabolized by the intestines is converted to citrulline. This is transported to the kidney where it is converted to arginine which is released into the systemic circulation. UC, urea cycle; TA, transamination.

enzyme glutaminase, which is predominantly present in the kidney, gut, and again in the liver.

Most endogenously synthesized plasma glutamine is derived from skeletal muscle glutamine synthetase activity. The ammonia needed for this process is mainly derived from amino acid breakdown within the muscle itself, since under normal circumstances skeletal muscle glutamate uptake by far exceeds ammonia uptake from the bloodstream (Olde Damink et al., 2002a). Although in the postabsorptive situation skeletal muscle is the most important glutamine producer, the liver is in fact the most active site of glutamine metabolism. However as mentioned above, the liver expresses both glutamine synthetase and glutaminase, and since their activity is approximately similar, net hepatic glutamine uptake or release is negligible (van de Poll et al., 2007a). Within the hepatic lobule glutaminase and glutamine synthetase are differentially expressed, with glutaminase being located in hepatocytes around the branches of the portal vein (upstream) and glutamine synthetase being located in hepatocytes that line the perivenous (downstream) part of the hepatic sinusoid. This distribution leads to an intercellular, but intrahepatic pathway of glutamine breakdown and synthesis that facilitates urea synthesis and ammonia clearance (Haussinger, 1986). This mechanism will be discussed in detail later in this chapter.

Net glutamine uptake is found within the intestines and the kidneys. In both organ systems, glutamine is deamidated by glutaminase to glutamate and ammonia immediately after uptake in the cell, and consequently both organ systems release ammonia to their venous effluent, the portal and renal veins, respectively (van de Poll et al., 2008b). Glutamate is further metabolized intracellularly and can either serve as a nitrogen donor for transamination processes or be metabolized further to form other non-essential amino acids.

Intestinal ammonia production is stoichiometrically related to intestinal net glutamine uptake, which both approximate 30 µmol kg^{-1} h^{-1} in the postabsorptive state. Intestinal ammonia production exceeds renal ammonia production threefold. However, ammonia – which is released from the intestines into the portal vein – must pass the liver before it can reach the systemic circulation. In the absence of portosystemic shunting, all ammonia that is released from the intestines is easily taken up by the liver which has two potential 'ammonia detoxification mechanisms'. The first and most important of these is the urea cycle which turns over at a rate of approximately 200 µmol kg^{-1} h^{-1} and that binds one molecule of ammonia per turn. The other is glutamine synthesis which occurs at a rate of approximately 75 µmol kg^{-1} h^{-1} (van de Poll et al., 2007a,c).

Considering the activity of hepatic glutamine synthetase and the activity of the urea cycle, it can be calculated that the liver can bind at least 275 µmol kg^{-1} h^{-1} of molecular ammonia in the postabsorptive state. From this it can easily be conceived that the 30 µmol kg^{-1} h^{-1} of ammonia that is generated by the intestines is only a minor substrate for hepatic nitrogen disposal. Urea synthesis is quantitatively the most important and also the only definitive way of disposing of nitrogen. Urea can readily be excreted in the urine by the kidney, whereas glutamine, like any other amino acid, does not get excreted from the body in significant amounts in subjects with a normal renal function. The urea cycle metabolizes one molecule of free ammonia per turn (Fig. 12.2). As indicated, regarding the low portal ammonia flux when compared to the total ammonia flux in the liver, the portal venous ammonia load is no driving force behind hepatic ammonia metabolism. Instead, the urea synthesis rate is closely regulated by the supply of amino nitrogen (Vilstrup, 1980) which is, next to molecular ammonia, the other source of nitrogen for urea synthesis (Fig. 12.2). In line with this, the primary function of the urea cycle appears to be the detoxification and disposal of amino nitrogen derived from degraded amino acids rather than to scavenge molecular ammonia derived from intestinal glutamine metabolism. Additionally, since net hepatic ammonia uptake is only a fraction of urea production, most of the molecular ammonia that is used in urea synthesis must be generated within the liver itself. This occurs within the

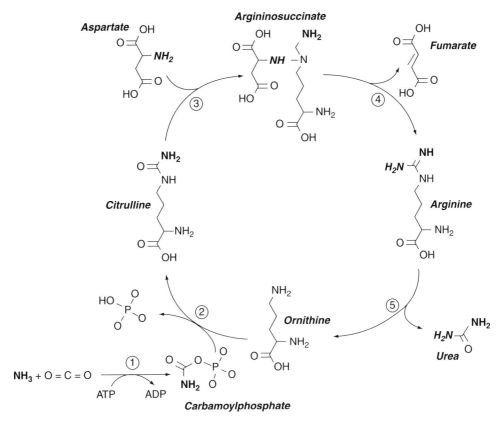

Fig. 12.2. Enzymes and substrates of the urea cycle. (1) Carbamoylphosphate synthetase. (2) Ornithine transcarbamylase. (3) Argininosuccinate synthetase. (4) Argininosuccinate lyase. (5) Arginase. The liver is the only organ that expresses all enzymes of the urea cycle. A full cycle requires the input of a single molecule of ammonia (marked bold throughout the cycle), and of an amino nitrogen group (marked with bold italics throughout the cycle) derived from amino acid transamination. The urea cycle does not require the input of carbon skeletons of amino acids from outside. Some organs express one or more urea cycle enzymes. These organs do require whole amino acids as a substrate. Examples of such organs are the intestines that express carbamoylphosphate synthetase and ornithine transcarbamylase which catalyse the conversion of ornithine to citrulline. Ornithine is a breakdown product of the metabolism of glutamine, which is taken up by the intestines from the blood stream or the gut lumen. Since argininosuccinate synthase activity in the intestines is low, citrulline is excreted from the cell to the plasma. The kidneys, unable to generate citrulline, do express argininosuccinate synthase and lyase and consequently generate arginine that is released in the blood due to limited arginase activity within the kidneys. Consequently, the intestines and the kidneys together express an almost complete urea cycle which facilitates the production of arginine from citrulline (and glutamine).

periportal hepatocytes, amongst other sites, by glutaminase activity (Fig. 12.3).

Hepatic ammonia production and disposal is a tightly regulated process, and in fact the hepatic venous ammonia concentration equals the arterial ammonia concentration, meaning that the net ammonia balance across the entire splanchnic region (intestines plus liver) equals zero. Since intestinal-derived ammonia does not gain access to the systemic circulation owing to its hepatic detoxification, glutaminase activity in the kidneys is the only process in the human body that substantially adds ammonia to the systemic circulation

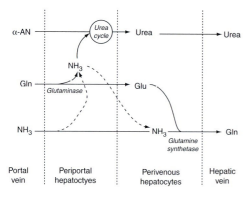

Fig. 12.3. Zonation of glutamine metabolism in the liver. In the periportal hepatocytes amino nitrogen (α-AN) is taken up and converted to urea, together with molecular ammonia, partly derived from periportal glutaminase activity. Portal venous ammonia is only a minor contributor to hepatic ureagenesis and may be the primary substrate for perivenous glutamine synthesis from glutamate that is produced by periportal glutaminase activity or transamination processes. The amount of glutamine being released in the hepatic vein is identical to the amount of glutamine taken up by the liver. The amount of ammonia taken up by the liver is equal to the amount of ammonia produced by the intestines.

(van de Poll et al., 2008b). This even holds true after an acute reduction of up to 70% of functional liver mass following surgical resection, illustrating the tremendous reserve capacity of the liver for ammonia detoxification. Interestingly, at the same timepoint an increase of plasma amino acid levels occurs, reflecting a reduction in hepatic nitrogen clearance capacity. This again underlines the fact that urea synthesis is driven by amino nitrogen rather than by molecular (intestinal-derived) ammonia (van de Poll et al., 2007c).

Finally, the liver produces and consumes glutamate during glutamine breakdown and synthesis, at a rate that is imperatively equal with glutamine turnover. Therefore the combined actions of glutaminase and glutamine synthetase would lead to a zero net balance of glutamate uptake and release across the liver. Despite this, the liver is a net releaser of glutamate to the circulation. The glutamate that is released into the hepatic vein is not derived from glutamine metabolism, but arises by transamination of gluconeogenic amino acids. By this mechanism, the amino nitrogen that is released from glutamine and particularly alanine during gluconeogenesis is preserved within the circulation. Glutamate will be converted to glutamine again in skeletal muscle. Another nitrogen-preserving process is the so-called alanine glucose cycle, which consists of an intricate exchange of carbon chains between the liver and skeletal muscle. Glucose which is transported from the liver yields two pyruvate molecules upon oxidation by the muscle. These pyruvate molecules get transaminated to alanine within the muscle. After being transported to the liver, alanine is deaminated again to yield pyruvate and glucose.

12.3.2 Pathophysiology

12.3.2.1 Critical illness and trauma

Critical illness and trauma result in an acute catabolic state. Under such conditions increased skeletal muscle breakdown leads to a higher plasma appearance of most amino acids. In addition, an increment of skeletal muscular endogenous glutamine production by increased glutamine synthase activity has been found in a pig model of early sepsis (Bruins et al., 2003). In the same experiment an increased *de novo* synthesis of alanine by skeletal muscle was found. The enhanced glutamine and alanine fluxes were accompanied by an increase of hepatic glucose production. Increased gluconeogenesis from amino acids is accompanied by the production of amino nitrogen. A simultaneous rise of the transamination rate of α-ketoglutarate to glutamate and a higher efflux of glutamate from the liver can be regarded as an attempt to prohibit nitrogen wasting and to preserve nitrogen balance. None the less, ureagenesis and hence nitrogen loss is higher during acute illness. The increased amino acid fluxes during catabolic states are seemingly contradictory, accompanied by a decline in plasma concentrations of most amino acids, particularly of glutamine. The lowered plasma concentrations may indicate that increased substrate demands are insufficiently compensated for by the increased supply from endogenous supplies. Consequently, low glutamine levels are seen by many as a sign of (impending) glutamine deficiency. Therefore glutamine is generally considered a conditionally (or semi-) essential amino acid, and indeed, in some selected patient categories such as surgical ICU patients and those suffering from severe burns, the positive effects of glutamine supplementation on clinical outcome parameters have been shown (Singer et al., 2009).

Interestingly, the catabolic response to trauma or illness and the increased flux of amino acids from peripheral to central organs is tightly orchestrated by a series of transcription factors and signalling molecules, and cannot be simply reversed by nutritional interventions (Tisdale, 2005). Moreover, attempts to reduce catabolism and improve the nitrogen balance in septic patients by growth hormone administration not only resulted in an attenuation of muscle wasting, but also in increased mortality (Takala et al., 1999).

12.3.2.2 Hyperammonaemia

In patients with liver disease, increased amounts of amino nitrogen and ammonia are found in the blood. This is associated with the development of hepatic encephalopathy. The increased amount of amino nitrogen can be ascribed to hepatocellular dysfunction and a decreased nitrogen clearance rate, since a higher load of amino nitrogen is needed to maintain urea synthesis (Vilstrup 1980). In contrast, the hyperammonaemia which is characteristic for liver disease, and which is commonly used as a clinical parameter for liver function, must in most cases not be ascribed to metabolic liver dysfunction but rather to increased portosystemic shunting consequent to portal hypertension. Owing to the large reserve capacity of the liver for ammonia detoxification, only in severe cases of (acute) liver failure does hepatocellular dysfunction directly influence hepatic ammonia clearance and systemic ammonia levels. The first important cause of hyperammonaemia in chronic liver disease is portosystemic shunting. Due to portosystemic shunting, portal venous blood and hence ammonia produced in the intestines can access the systemic circulation without passing through the liver, thus escaping hepatic ammonia detoxification mechanisms (Olde Damink et al., 2002b).

Apart from portosystemic shunting, renal ammonia production is an important source of hyperammonaemia. As outlined above, under normal conditions the kidney is the only source of ammonia in the systemic circulation, owing to its high glutaminase activity. The hyperaminoacidaemia which accompanies liver disease leads to an increase of renal ammonia production. It has been shown that in patients with chronic liver disease and a portosystemic shunt, renal ammonia production is as important as total splanchnic ammonia production (i.e. intestinal ammonia production minus hepatic ammonia uptake) for the total systemic ammonia flux (Olde Damink et al., 2002b). On the other hand, it has been shown in an experimental model of liver failure that urinary ammonia excretion can be increased while systemic ammonia release is reduced (Dejong et al., 1993). As such, the kidney appears to change from an ammonia-producing organ to one that causes a net removal of ammonia from the body, providing an alternative to urea synthesis and urinary urea excretion. An acute reduction of systemic ammonia release from the kidneys, observed in patients with chronic liver disease who received a transjugular intrahepatic portosystemic shunt, seems to confirm these experimental data (Olde Damink et al., 2006). As outlined above, skeletal muscle takes up only a limited amount of ammonia from the blood under normal conditions. In patients with hyperammonaemia due to chronic liver disease and portocaval shunting, however, skeletal muscle converts plasma ammonia to glutamine. In fact skeletal muscle consumes as much ammonia as the liver in such patients (Olde Damink et al., 2002b). However, since the body is not capable of excreting glutamine as a whole, this is only a temporary means of ammonia detoxification. Renal glutaminase activity and urinary ammonia excretion is mandatory to complete this alternative pathway of nitrogen disposal.

12.4 Glutamine, Citrulline and Arginine

12.4.1 Physiology

12.4.1.1 Glutamine and citrulline

After its deamidation to glutamate and ammonia in the gut, the carbon skeleton becomes metabolized further. Intestinal glutamine uptake is correlated with glutamine influx and therefore intestinal glutamine metabolism appears to be a substrate-driven process that can be stimulated by increasing glutamine plasma concentration. In the postabsorptive state, 13% of the glutamine taken up by the gut is eventually converted to ornithine and subsequently to citrulline. This comes down to a rate of approximately 4 µmol $kg^{-1}h^{-1}$. The enzymes that catalyse this process (carbamoylphosphate synthase and ornithine transcarbamylase) are identical to those that catalyse the conversion of ornithine to citrulline in the liver as part of the urea cycle. The human gut does express the arginine-synthesizing enzymes argininosuccinate synthase and argininosuccinate lyase, and therefore it does possess the intrinsic capacity to generate arginine from citrulline (and glutamine). However, after infancy the activities of these enzymes rapidly disappear and the adult human intestines produce only limited amounts of arginine (Kohler et al., 2008). Since the gut cannot further metabolize citrulline, most of the citrulline is released into the portal vein after its generation.

On a whole-body level, plasma citrulline flux depends for 60–90% on intestinal citrulline production (van de Poll et al., 2007b). Citrulline is also synthesized within the liver by the urea cycle, at a rate that exceeds its plasma flux by a factor of 50. However, given the cyclic and compartmentalized nature of this process, it does not lead to net citrulline release. In contrast to prior assumptions, recent findings indicate that the liver takes up citrulline from the portal circulation (van de Poll et al., 2007a,b) although the aim of hepatic citrulline metabolism outside the urea cycle remains unclear.

In addition to its focal intestinal production, citrulline is generated throughout the body during nitric oxide (NO) synthesis, which occurs by the conversion of arginine to citrulline in a reaction that is catalysed by one of three isoforms of the enzyme nitric oxide synthase (NOS) (Fig. 12.2). Nitric oxide is a pluripotent signalling molecule that is generated, amongst other sites, by the vascular endothelium and macrophages. It plays a role in the regulation of vascular tone, organ perfusion and in regulation and mediation of the inflammatory response. Insufficient NO production has been implicated in a wide array of clinical conditions including sepsis and ischaemia-reperfusion injury. Since arginine is the immediate precursor for NO synthesis, arginine supplementation is widely studied as a method to modulate NO synthesis.

Human studies with isotopically labelled tracers show that 1 µmol $kg^{-1}h^{-1}$ of citrulline generated during NO synthesis is released into the circulation (Castillo et al., 1996). This thus accounts for approximately 20% of total citrulline plasma flux. The total rate of the conversion of citrulline being produced during NO synthesis within the entire body, however, is difficult to determine since in many cells NOS is co-localized with argininosuccinate lyase and synthase. Because of this, citrulline can be resynthesized to arginine within the single cell where it is generated. As such an NO cycle is formed that does not depend on the exchange of citrulline and arginine across the cell membrane to maintain intracellular substrate supply (Mori, 2007). In fact it has been shown that activated macrophages are able to produce nitric oxide in an arginine-depleted medium, using glutamine as a nitrogen donor (Murphy and Newsholme, 1998). Due to the limited exchange between the citrulline plasma pool and the citrulline carbon skeletons that are confined to the NO cycle (Fig. 12.4), the total amount of citrulline that is generated during nitric oxide synthesis cannot accurately be assessed by classical intravenous tracer methods (Castillo et al., 1996).

Since plasma citrulline flux relies so heavily on intestinal glutamine metabolism, impairment of glutamine availability or reduction of intestinal function or mass are immediately reflected by changes in plasma

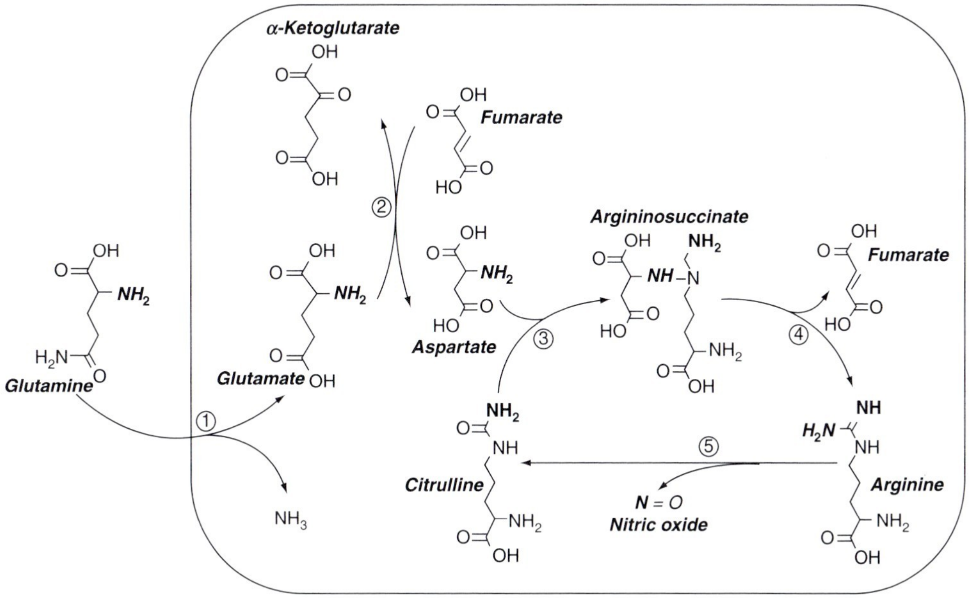

Fig. 12.4. Enzymes and substrates of the nitric oxide cycle. (1) Glutaminase. (2) Aminotransferase. (3) Argininosuccinate synthetase. (4) Argininosuccinate lyase. (5) Nitric oxide synthetase. Nitric oxide arises by the conversion of arginine to citrulline, catalysed by nitric oxide synthase. In many cells that express argininosuccinate synthase and argininosuccinate lyase, they are co-localized and also induced simultaneously, facilitating a rapid production of nitric oxide. Note that during this process only the input of a single amino nitrogen derived from amino acid transamination (bold italics) is required as input for the cycle, while the carbon skeleton and amino group (bold) of citrulline and arginine remains unaffected and is not transported across the cell membrane. Glutamine is probably the most important nitrogen donor for this cycle.

flux and concentration of citrulline. It has been found that experimental glutamine depletion leads to diminished citrulline levels in humans (Rouge *et al.*, 2007). In addition, diminished citrulline fluxes have been found in association with low glutamine levels in septic patients (Luiking *et al.*, 2009). Even more striking is the close correlation between citrulline and functional enterocyte mass that is firmly established in patients who had undergone extensive small bowel resection (Crenn *et al.*, 2000); patients with coeliac disease (Crenn *et al.*, 2003); and the treatment of oncological patients suffering from radiation-induced enteritis (Lutgens *et al.*, 2005). Although citrulline flux and levels decrease markedly in these patients, no evidence of the occurrence of clinically relevant citrulline depletion has been found to date.

12.4.1.2 Citrulline and arginine

Citrulline is taken up from the systemic circulation by the kidneys at a rate that approximately equals the intestinal release of citrulline. The kidneys convert citrulline to arginine by the consecutive actions of argininosuccinate synthase and argininosuccinate lyase, and release arginine to the circulation. This forms an inter-organ pathway between the intestines (which take up glutamine and release citrulline) and the kidneys (which take up citrulline and release arginine). Through this pathway glutamine becomes the ultimate precursor for endogenous arginine production. The enzymatic steps of the pathway are almost identical to those of the urea cycle, but owing to the distribution throughout different organs its intermediates enter the circulation and may thereby become available for other metabolic processes. Almost 70% of endogenously produced plasma arginine is derived from this inter-organ pathway (van de Poll et al., 2007a,b; Ligthart-Melis et al., 2008). The importance of intestinal citrulline production for renal arginine synthesis is illustrated by the fact that a reduction in intestinal citrulline production leads to diminished renal arginine synthesis (Luiking et al., 2009). On the other hand it must be pointed out that endogenous renal arginine synthesis (9 µmol kg^{-1} h^{-1}) accounts for only 10% of total plasma arginine flux (Castillo et al., 1993), which depends for the largest part on protein breakdown. Moreover, only 1% of plasma arginine flux serves NO synthesis. Considering this low number and the putatively high rate of intracellular NO cycling, the importance of renal arginine synthesis for NO synthesis remains to be elucidated.

12.4.2 Metabolism after enteral administration

12.4.2.1 Glutamine

Since enterocytes express such high glutaminase activity, enterally administered glutamine is rapidly metabolized during absorption. In fact, the proportion of glutamine that is metabolized by the intestines during absorption from the intestinal lumen (50%) is threefold higher than the proportion of glutamine that is metabolized by the intestines during a single pass, while being supplied through the bloodstream (Ligthart-Melis et al., 2007). Enteral glutamine supplementation therefore results in a lower rate of glutamine appearance in the plasma and in a lower systemic glutamine concentration than parenteral glutamine supplementation. On the other hand, enteral glutamine administration results in increased intestinal citrulline production and to increased plasma levels of citrulline and glutamate, compared to parenteral glutamine supplementation (Melis et al., 2005). In contrast, no differences in arginine production or plasma level have been found between subjects receiving either enteral or parenteral glutamine supplementation. This can be explained by the small proportion of intestinal glutamine metabolism (13%) that is involved in the glutamine–citrulline–arginine pathway and by the limited influence renal arginine synthesis exerts on total plasma arginine flux (10%).

Simultaneous with the increased amount of glutamine-derived amino acids that is released into the systemic circulation after enteral glutamine administration, an increased rate of glutamine oxidation and urea synthesis can be found. This indicates that a substantial part of the glutamine undergoes transamination and serves gluconeogenesis after enteral administration. In conclusion it must be assumed that enteral and parenteral administration of glutamine are two completely different entities, which also explains the diverse clinical effects that are exerted by both interventions.

12.4.2.2 Arginine

Like glutamine, arginine is considered by many to be an essential amino acid, although the indications for supplementation of arginine are much less defined than those of glutamine. Positive effects of arginine supplementation in experimental studies are most frequently ascribed to its role as the precursor for NO synthesis. Concerns have been raised regarding the systemic availability of enterally administered arginine. Although the intestines only show limited arginine metabolism and almost all enterally administered arginine becomes available in the portal vein, it is believed by many that systemic availability of enterally administered arginine is limited by hepatic arginase activity. However, as underlined earlier, hepatic arginase activity is part of the urea cycle which is highly compartmentalized. This means that there is little or no exchange between the arginine that is being formed and broken down within the urea cycle, and the arginine that reaches the liver through the portal vein. Indeed there is some hepatic arginine uptake, but the fractional extraction of arginine approximates a mere 10%, which is within the same range as the fractional extraction of citrulline and other amino acids. Therefore hepatic arginine uptake appears to be a physiological process that is not substrate driven.

Most arginine extracted by the liver is probably used for protein synthesis. In addition it is pragmatically shown that enteral arginine supplementation does effectively increase systemic arginine levels.

Hepatic arginase can only affect systemic arginine availability when it is released from injured hepatocytes into the circulation. However the specific activity and plasma half-life of arginase is very low, and in fact the only clinical situation where a relation between increased plasma arginase activity and diminished arginine levels was convincingly shown is the immediate reperfusion phase after liver transplantation. Increased plasma arginase levels due to other causes of hepatocellular injury or to red blood cell injury does not result in arginase activity of any clinical importance (van de Poll et al., 2008a).

12.4.2.3 Citrulline

The assumptions that arginine deficiency may occur in certain conditions and that arginine levels cannot effectively be raised by enteral arginine supplementation have led to the hypothesis that enteral citrulline supplementation, by stimulation of renal arginine synthesis, may be a more effective way of increasing systemic arginine levels than enteral arginine supplementation itself. Indeed, it has been shown that arginine plasma levels do increase after citrulline supplementation. However, at a citrulline dosage that exceeds endogenous citrulline flux five times, the plasma arginine concentration increased twofold while plasma citrulline concentration increased fivefold (Rouge et al., 2007). Moreover renal citrulline uptake and arginine production seem to be limited at high citrulline doses (Moinard et al., 2008). In contrast, in rats with short bowel syndrome, citrulline supplementation restored citrulline and arginine levels as well as nitrogen balance more effectively than did arginine supplementation (Osowska et al., 2004). These experimental data suggest that citrulline may become a conditionally essential amino acid under certain conditions, although it is far from clear that the effects of citrulline on nitrogen homeostasis are mediated by increased renal arginine synthesis.

12.5 Recommendations for Future Research

The physiological aspects of inter-organ flux of amino acids in humans seems to be firmly established. Data on the metabolism of glutamine and arginine after enteral administration and absorption from the lumen, however, are not that clear yet. Some very recent studies in a murine stable isotope model indicate that the carbon skeleton of enterally administered glutamine does not get converted to citrulline. The same experiments suggested that arginine, rather than glutamine, is the major dietary source for citrulline synthesis (Marini et al., 2010). Obviously these intriguing findings contrast sharply with existing views and warrant careful pursuit, since (if confirmed in other species and using intravenous tracers), they may ultimately lead to a rewriting of the textbooks.

Moreover, the physiological and clinical importance of renal arginine synthesis in the light of the much larger arginine flux from protein breakdown should be addressed. The question remains whether enhancement of renal arginine production (for example by glutamine or citrulline supplementation) is a fruitful way to increase arginine availability. In line with this question, and the relative inaccessibility of the intracellular NO cycle for plasma arginine, it remains to be seen if enhancement of plasma arginine levels is useful at all.

In past decades many studies have been performed that attempted to modify substrate metabolism by increasing substrate supply. The results of most of these studies have been disappointing. Given the fact that many processes (including NO synthesis in most cells) are enzyme rather than substrate driven, the rationale for substrate supplementation may be flawed. Pharmacological induction of enzymatic pathways (with or without additional supplementation of substrate) may prove to become an interesting alternative to increase metabolic conversions, especially when these metabolic conversions are captured in intracellular cycles that are not freely accessible for plasma amino acids.

12.6 Conclusions

Intercellular and inter-organ amino acid exchange occurs via an intricate network that serves to maintain plasma amino acid pools and nitrogen homeostasis. Glutamine produced by the muscles is taken up by the liver to provide substrate for ureagenesis, which is driven by amino nitrogen supply and not by intestinal ammonia production. Glutamate released from the liver preserves nitrogen, and again is the precursor for muscular glutamine synthesis. Sepsis leads to an increased flux of substrate from the muscle to the liver, partly due to increased muscle protein catabolism and partly to increased amino acid synthesis. Reversal of this catabolic response by anabolic steroids does not improve survival. During liver insufficiency, muscular ammonia uptake and urinary ammonia excretion increase, to detoxify the ammonia that escapes liver metabolism due to portosystemic shunting.

The intestines convert glutamine to citrulline, which subsequently gets converted to arginine by the kidney. This inter-organ pathway is particularly important for whole body citrulline plasma flux and for endogenous renal arginine synthesis. However, it comprises only 13% of intestinal glutamine metabolism and only 10% of whole-body arginine plasma flux, which is much more dependent on protein breakdown. The true synthesis rates of citrulline and arginine, however, remain elusive since the largest turnover of these amino acids occurs within intracellular cycles such as the urea cycle and the NO cycle.

Enteral supplementation of glutamine is followed by significant first-pass extraction, largely serving hepatic oxidation. It is accompanied by an increased production of citrulline, but not of arginine. The bioavailability of enterally supplied arginine is not limited by hepatic arginase activity, although the indications for arginine supplementation remain to be established. Citrulline supplementation leads to increased arginine levels at very high doses. It remains to be seen, however, if the putatively beneficial effects of citrulline supplementation in experimental settings are mediated via its conversion to arginine.

Future research should be aimed at elucidating the fate of enterally administered glutamine and at the modulation of metabolic pathways by enzyme induction, rather than by enhancing substrate supply.

References

Bruins, M.J., Deutz, N.E. and Soeters, P.B. (2003) Aspects of organ protein, amino acid and glucose metabolism in a porcine model of hypermetabolic sepsis. *Clinical Science* 104, 127–141.

Castillo, L., Chapman, T.E., Sanchez, M., Yu, Y.M., Burke, J.F., Ajami, A.M., Vogt, J., et al. (1993) Plasma arginine and citrulline kinetics in adults given adequate and arginine-free diets. *Proceedings of the National Academy of Science USA* 90, 7749–7753.

Castillo, L., Beaumier, L., Ajami, A.M. and Young, V.R. (1996) Whole body nitric oxide synthesis in healthy men determined from [15N] arginine-to-[15N]citrulline labeling. *Proceedings of the National Academy of Science USA* 93, 11460–11465.

Cheung, C.W., Cohen, N.S. and Raijman, L. (1989) Channeling of urea cycle intermediates in situ in permeabilized hepatocytes. *Journal of Biological Chemistry* 264, 4038–4044.

Crenn, P., Coudray-Lucas, C., Thuillier, F., Cynober, L. and Messing, B. (2000) Postabsorptive plasma citrulline concentration is a marker of absorptive enterocyte mass and intestinal failure in humans. *Gastroenterology* 119, 1496–1505.

Crenn, P., Vahedi, K., Lavergne-Slove, A., Cynober, L., Matuchansky, C. and Messing, B. (2003) Plasma citrulline: A marker of enterocyte mass in villous atrophy-associated small bowel disease. *Gastroenterology* 124, 1210–1219.

Dejong, C.H., Deutz, N.E. and Soeters, P.B. (1993) Renal ammonia and glutamine metabolism during liver insufficiency-induced hyperammonemia in the rat. *Journal of Clinical Investigation* 92, 2834–2840.

Haussinger, D. (1986) Regulation of hepatic ammonia metabolism: the intercellular glutamine cycle. *Advances in Enzyme Regulation* 25, 159–180.

Kohler, E.S., Sankaranarayanan, S., van Ginneken, C.J., van Dijk, P., Vermeulen, J.L., Ruijter, J.M., Lamers, W.H., *et al.* (2008) The human neonatal small intestine has the potential for arginine synthesis; developmental changes in the expression of arginine-synthesizing and -catabolizing enzymes. *BioMed Central; Developmental Biology* 8, p. 107.

Ligthart-Melis, G.C., van de Poll, M.C., Dejong, C.H., Boelens, P.G., Deutz, N.E. and van Leeuwen, P.A. (2007) The route of administration (enteral or parenteral) affects the conversion of isotopically labeled L-[2-15N]glutamine into citrulline and arginine in humans. *Journal of Parenteral and Enteral Nutrition* 31, 343–348; discussion 349–350.

Ligthart-Melis, G.C., van de Poll, M.C., Boelens, P.G., Dejong, C.H., Deutz, N.E. and van Leeuwen, P.A. (2008) Glutamine is an important precursor for de novo synthesis of arginine in humans. *American Journal of Clinical Nutrition* 87, 1282–1289.

Luiking, Y.C., Poeze, M., Ramsay, G. and Deutz, N.E. (2009) Reduced citrulline production in sepsis is related to diminished de novo arginine and nitric oxide production. *American Journal of Clinical Nutrition* 89, 142–152.

Lutgens, L.C., Blijlevens, N.M., Deutz, N.E., Donnelly, J.P., Lambin, P. and de Pauw, B.E. (2005) Monitoring myeloablative therapy-induced small bowel toxicity by serum citrulline concentration: a comparison with sugar permeability tests. *Cancer* 103, 191–199.

Marini, J.C., Cajo Didelija, I., Castillo, L. and Lee, B. (2010) Glutamine: precursor or nitrogen donor for citrulline synthesis? *American Journal of Physiology - Endocrinology and Metabolism* 299, E69–79.

Melis, G.C., Boelens, P.G., van der Sijp, J.R., Popovici, T., De Bandt, J.P., Cynober, L. and van Leeuwen, P.A. (2005) The feeding route (enteral or parenteral) affects the plasma response of the dipetide Ala-Gln and the amino acids glutamine, citrulline and arginine, with the administration of Ala-Gln in preoperative patients. *British Journal of Nutrition* 94, 19–26.

Moinard, C., Nicolis, I., Neveux, N., Darquy, S., Benazeth, S. and Cynober, L. (2008) Dose-ranging effects of citrulline administration on plasma amino acids and hormonal patterns in healthy subjects: the Citrudose pharmacokinetic study. *British Journal of Nutrition* 99, 855–862.

Mori, M. (2007) Regulation of nitric oxide synthesis and apoptosis by arginase and arginine recycling. *Journal of Nutrition* 137, 1616S–1620S.

Murphy, C. and Newsholme, P. (1998) Importance of glutamine metabolism in murine macrophages and human monocytes to L-arginine biosynthesis and rates of nitrite or urea production. *Clinical Science* 95, 397–407.

Olde Damink, S.W., Deutz, N.E., Dejong, C.H., Soeters, P.B. and Jalan, R. (2002a) Interorgan ammonia metabolism in liver failure. *Neurochemistry International* 41, 177–188.

Olde Damink, S.W., Jalan, R., Redhead, D.N., Hayes, P.C., Deutz, N.E. and Soeters, P.B. (2002b) Interorgan ammonia and amino acid metabolism in metabolically stable patients with cirrhosis and a TIPSS. *Hepatology* 36, 1163–1171.

Olde Damink, S.W. Dejong, C.H., Deutz, N.E., Redhead, D.N., Hayes, P.C., Soeters, P.B. and Jalan, R. (2006) Kidney plays a major role in ammonia homeostasis after portasystemic shunting in patients with cirrhosis. *American Journal of Physiology. Gastrointestinal and Liver Physiology* 291, G189–194.

Osowska, S., Moinard, C., Neveux, N., Loi, C. and Cynober, L. (2004) Citrulline increases arginine pools and restores nitrogen balance after massive intestinal resection. *Gut* 53, 1781–1786.

Rouge, C., Des Robert, C., Robins, A., Le Bacquer, O., Volteau, C., De La Cochetiere, M.F. and Darmaun, D. (2007) Manipulation of citrulline availability in humans. *American Journal of Physiology; Gastrointestinal and Liver Physiology* 293, G1061–1067.

Singer, P. Berger, M.M., Van den Berghe, G., Biolo, G., Calder, P., Forbes, A., Griffiths, R., *et al.* (2009) ESPEN guidelines on parenteral nutrition: intensive care. *Clinical Nutrition* 28, 387–400.

Takala, J., Ruokonen, E., Webster, N.R., Nielsen, M.S., Zandstra, D.F., Vundelinckx, G. and Hinds, C.J. (1999) Increased mortality associated with growth hormone treatment in critically ill adults. *New England Journal of Medicine* 341, 785–792.

Tisdale, M.J. (2005) The ubiquitin-proteasome pathway as a therapeutic target for muscle wasting. *Journal of Supportive Oncology* 3, 209–217.

van de Poll, M.C.G., Luiking, Y.C., Dejong, C.H.C. and Soeters, P.B. (2005) Amino acids; specific functions. In: Caballero, B., Allen, L. and Prentice, A. (eds) *Encyclopedia of Human Nutrition*. Academic Press, San Diego, California, pp. 92–100.

van de Poll, M.C., Ligthart-Melis, G.C., Boelens, P.G., Deutz, N.E., van Leeuwen, P.A. and Dejong, C.H. (2007a) Intestinal and hepatic metabolism of glutamine and citrulline in humans. *Journal of Physiology* 581, 819–827.

van de Poll, M.C., Siroen, M.P., van Leeuwen, P.A., Soeters, P.B., Melis, G.C., Boelens, P.G., Deutz, N.E., et al. (2007b) Interorgan amino acid exchange in humans: consequences for arginine and citrulline metabolism. *American Journal of Clinical Nutrition* 85, 167–172.

van de Poll, M.C., Wigmore, S.J., Redhead, D.N., Beets-Tan, R.G., Garden, O.J., Greve, J.W., Soeters, P.B., et al. (2007c) Effect of major liver resection on hepatic ureagenesis in humans. *American Journal of Physiology; Gastrointestinal and Liver Physiology* 293, G956–962.

van de Poll, M.C., Hanssen, S.J., Berbee, M., Deutz, N.E., Monbaliu, D., Buurman, W.A. and Dejong, C.H. (2008a) Elevated plasma arginase-1 does not affect plasma arginine in patients undergoing liver resection. *Clinical Science* 114, 231–241.

van de Poll, M.C., Ligthart-Melis, G.C., Olde Damink, S.W., van Leeuwen, P.A., Beets-Tan, R.G., Deutz, N.E., Wigmore, S.J., et al. (2008b) The gut does not contribute to systemic ammonia release in humans without portosystemic shunting. *American Journal of Physiology; Gastrointestinal and Liver Physiology* 295, G760–765.

Vilstrup, H. (1980) Synthesis of urea after stimulation with amino acids: relation to liver function. *Gut* 21, 990–995.

13 Cellular Adaptation to Amino Acid Availability: Mechanisms Involved in the Regulation of Gene Expression

J. Averous, S. Lambert-Langlais, C. Chaveroux, L. Parry, V. Carraro, A.-C. Maurin, C. Jousse, A. Bruhat and P. Fafournoux*

Unité de Nutrition Humaine, Institut National de la Recherche Agronomique de Theix, France

13.1 Abstract

In mammals, the impact of nutrients on gene expression has become an important area of research. Nevertheless, the current understanding of amino acid-dependent control of gene expression is limited. Amino acids have multiple and important roles, so their homeostasis has to be finely maintained. However, the blood amino acid content can be affected by certain nutritional conditions or various forms of pathology. It follows that mammals have to adjust several of their physiological functions involved in the adaptation to amino acid availability by regulating expression of numerous genes. The aim of this review is to examine the role of amino acids in regulating mammalian gene expression and physiological functions.

A limitation for several individual amino acids strongly increases the expression of target genes such as insulin-like growth factor-binding protein1 (IGFBP-1), C/EBP homologous protein (CHOP) and asparagine synthetase (ASNS) genes. The molecular mechanisms involved in the regulation of CHOP and ASNS gene transcription in response to amino acid starvation have been partly identified. In particular, a signalling pathway requiring the protein kinase general control non-derepressive 2 (GCN2) and the activating transcription factor 4 (ATF4) has been described as sensing the amino acid limitation. In the case of an amino acid-imbalanced food source, this pathway has been shown to decrease food intake by activating a neuronal circuit. Taken together, the results discussed in this review demonstrate that amino acids by themselves can act as 'signal' molecules, with important roles in the control of gene expression and physiological functions.

13.2 Introduction

Regulation of metabolism is achieved by coordinated actions between cells and tissues, and also by mechanisms operating at the cellular level. These mechanisms involve the conditional regulation of specific genes in the presence or absence of appropriate nutrients. In multicellular organisms, the control of gene expression involves complex interactions of hormonal, neuronal, and nutritional factors.

---

* E-mail address: pierre.fafournoux@clermont.inra.fr

Although not as widely appreciated, nutritional signals play an important role in controlling gene expression in mammals. It has been shown that major (carbohydrates, fatty acids, sterols) and minor (minerals, vitamins) dietary constituents participate in the regulation of gene expression (Towle, 1995; Foufelle *et al.*, 1998; Pégorier, 1998; Duplus *et al.*, 2000; Vaulont *et al.*, 2000; Grimaldi, 2001). In the last decade, significant progress has been achieved in the understanding of molecular mechanisms involved in the control of mammalian gene expression in response to amino acid availability (Jousse *et al.*, 2004; Kimball and Jefferson, 2004; Kilberg *et al.*, 2005). This review summarizes recent work on the effect of amino acid availability in the regulation of biological functions. On the basis of the physiological concepts of amino acids homeostasis, we will discuss specific examples of the role of amino acids in the regulation of physiological functions, particularly focusing on the mechanisms involved in the amino acid regulation of gene expression.

13.3 Regulation of Amino Acid Metabolism and Homeostasis in the Whole Animal

Mammals are composed of a series of organs and tissues with different functions and, consequently, different metabolic demands. As a consequence, the regulation of protein and amino acid metabolism in the whole animal is made up of the sum of the regulatory responses in all individual parts of the body, and is achieved through a series of reactions that are both integrated and cooperative. Enzymes regulating the reactions of amino acid metabolism are distributed differently in various tissues. Consequently, there is a continuous exchange of amino acids between tissues, and metabolic regulation responds to the flow of compounds arriving at each cell. For example, arginine is mainly synthesized by liver and kidney but can be degraded by nitric oxide synthase in most of the tissues. Arginine is also catabolized by arginase, which is primarily found in the liver (Cynober, 2007).

In healthy adult humans, nine amino acids (valine, isoleucine, leucine, lysine, methionine, phenylalanine, threonine, histidine and tryptophan) cannot be synthesized *de novo* and are designated as indispensable (or essential) amino acids and have to be supplied by the food (Munro, 1970; Young *et al.*, 1994). In addition, under a particular set of conditions certain non-indispensable amino acids may become indispensable. These amino acids are called 'conditionally indispensable'. For example, enough arginine is synthesized by the liver (urea cycle) and by the kidney (from citrulline) to meet the needs of an adult but not those of a growing child. Second, there are no large and specific stores of amino acids. Consequently, when necessary, an organism has to hydrolyse muscle protein to produce free amino acids. This loss of protein will be at the expense of essential elements. Therefore, complex mechanisms that take these amino acid characteristics into account are needed for maintaining the free amino acid pools.

13.3.1 Free amino acid pool

The size of the cellular pool of each amino acid is the result of a balance between input and removal (Fig. 13.1). The metabolic outlets for amino acids are protein synthesis and amino acid degradation, whereas the inputs are *de novo* synthesis (for non-indispensable amino acids), protein breakdown, and dietary supply. Changes in the rates of these systems lead to an adjustment in nitrogen balance. For example, the plasma concentration of amino acids has been reported to rise following the administration of a protein-containing meal to animals or humans. The concentration of leucine and some other amino acids approximately doubles in peripheral blood following a protein-rich meal (Aoki et al., 1976) and reaches much higher concentrations within the portal vein (Fafournoux *et al.*, 1990). It has been well demonstrated that the increased concentrations of circulating amino acids resulting from a protein-rich meal ingestion is involved in the regulation of protein turn-over (Yoshizawa *et al.*, 1995; Svanberg *et al.*, 1997).

Due to the properties of amino acids (indispensable AA cannot be synthesized and there is no AA storage), adjustment of the amino acid metabolism is even more critical

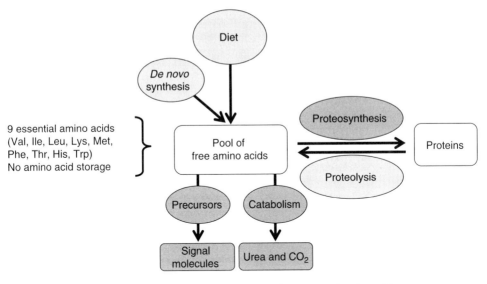

Fig. 13.1. Biochemical systems involved in the homeostasis of proteins and amino acids.

in case of protein malnutrition. A dramatic drop in the plasma concentrations of certain indispensable amino acids has been shown to occur following insufficient amino acid or protein intake.

13.3.2 Specific examples of the role of amino acids in the adaptation to protein deficiency

13.3.2.1 Protein undernutrition

Prolonged feeding on a low-protein diet causes a fall in the plasma level of most indispensable amino acids. For example, leucine and methionine concentrations can be reduced from about 100–150 µM and 18–30 µM to 20 µM and 5 µM, respectively, in plasma of children affected by kwashiorkor (Grimble and Whitehead, 1970; Baertl et al., 1974). It follows that individuals have to adjust several physiological functions in order to adapt to this amino acid deficiency. Protein undernutrition has its most devastating consequences during growth. One of the main consequences of feeding a low-protein diet is the dramatic inhibition of growth. Growth is controlled by a complex interaction of genetic, hormonal, and nutritional factors. A large part of this control is due to growth hormone (GH) and insulin-like growth factors (IGF). The biological activities of IGF are modulated by the IGF-binding proteins (IGFBP) that specifically bind IGF-I and IGF-II (Lee et al., 1993; Straus, 1994). Straus et al. (1993) demonstrated that a dramatic overexpression of IGFBP-1 was responsible for growth inhibition in response to prolonged feeding on a low-protein diet. Known regulators of IGFBP-1 expression are GH, insulin, or glucose. However, the high IGFBP-1 levels found in response to a protein-deficient diet cannot be explained by these factors. It has been demonstrated that a fall in the amino acid concentration was directly responsible for IGFBP-1 induction (Straus et al., 1993; Jousse et al., 1998). Therefore, amino acid limitation, as occurring during dietary protein deficiency, participates in the down-regulation of growth through the induction of IGFBP-1.

13.3.2.2 Imbalanced diet

The ability to synthesize protein is essential for survival, and protein synthesis is dependent on the simultaneous supply of the 20 precursor amino acids. Because mammals cannot synthesize all of the amino acids, the diet must provide the remainder. Thus, in the event of a deficiency in one of the indispensable amino acids, body proteins are broken down to provide the limiting amino acid (Munro, 1976). It follows that mammals need mechanisms that provide for selection of a balanced diet. Amino acid-imbalanced diets can be a frequent nutritional situation for wild omnivorous animals. For example, rodents are often confronted with poor food availability with a single plant protein source, which is most likely partially deficient for one indispensable amino acid.

After eating an amino acid-imbalanced diet, animals first recognize the amino acid deficiency and then respond by reducing their food intake (see Chapter 19). Recognition and anorexia resulting from an amino acid-imbalanced diet take place very rapidly (Harper et al., 1970; Rogers and Leung, 1977; Gietzen, 1993). The mechanisms that underlie the recognition of protein quality must act by the way of the free amino acids resulting from intestinal digestion of proteins. The decrease in the blood concentration of the limiting amino acid become apparent as early as few minutes after feeding an imbalanced diet, and depends on the extent of deficiency. The anorectic response is correlated with a decreased concentration of the limiting amino acid in the plasma. Several lines of evidence have suggested that the fall in the limiting amino acid concentration is detected in the brain. Gietzen (1993, 2000) reviews the evidence that a specific brain area, the anterior pyriform cortex (APC), can sense the variations of the amino acid concentrations. This recognition phase is associated with a localized decrease in the concentration of the limiting amino acid and changes in protein synthesis rate and gene expression. Subsequent to recognition of the deficiency the second step, development of anorexia, involves another part of the brain.

These two examples suggest that a variation in blood amino acid concentration can regulate several physiological functions including growth and appetite, and the expression of target genes (IGFBP-1). Recent progress has been made in understanding the mechanisms by which amino acid limitation controls the expression of several genes. The present review focuses on the regulatory role of low amino acid availability. The effects of an excess of amino acids are not considered here.

13.4 Molecular Mechanisms Involved in the Regulation of Gene Expression by Amino Acid Limitation

In mammalian cells, specific mRNAs that are induced following amino acid deprivation have been reported (Marten et al., 1994). Most of the molecular mechanisms involved in the amino acid regulation of gene expression have been obtained by studying the up-regulation of C/EBP homologous protein (CHOP), asparagine synthetase (ASNS), and the cationic amino acid transporter (Cat-1) genes.

Three distinct mechanisms of regulation of gene expression have been identified so far:

1. A post-transcriptional component involving stabilization of mRNA under starved conditions has been shown for CHOP and ASNS, but the molecular mechanisms involved in this process have not been fully identified (Gong et al., 1991; Bruhat et al., 1997; Aulak et al., 1999).
2. A translational control. It was shown that translation of the arginine/lysine transporter Cat-1 mRNA increases during AA starvation via the presence of internal ribosome entry site (IRES) located in the 5'UTR (Fernandez et al., 2001). It has also been shown that translation of the Cat-1 transcript can be regulated by miRNA (Bhattacharyya et al., 2006).
3. A transcriptional control. Most of the information we have concerning the regulation of gene transcription by AA availability has been obtained studying CHOP and asparagine synthetases genes. In this article we will focus on the transcriptional control of gene expression in response to amino acid deficiency.

13.4.1 Transcriptional activation of mammalian genes by amino acid starvation

It was established that the increase in CHOP or ASNS mRNA following amino acid starvation is due mainly to an increased transcription

(Hutson and Kilberg, 1994; Bruhat et al., 1997). By first identifying the genomic cis-elements and then the corresponding transcription factors responsible for regulation of these specific target genes, it is anticipated that one can progress backwards up the signal transduction pathway to understand the individual steps required.

13.4.1.1 Regulation of the human CHOP gene by amino acid starvation

CHOP encodes a ubiquitous transcription factor that heterodimerizes avidly with the other members of the C/EBP (Fawcett et al., 1996) and jun/fos (Ubeda et al., 1999) families. The CHOP gene is tightly regulated by a wide variety of stresses in mammalian cells (Luethy and Holbrook, 1992; Sylvester et al., 1994; Wang et al., 1996). Leucine limitation in human cell lines leads to induction of CHOP mRNA and protein in a dose-dependent manner (Bruhat et al., 1997).

We have identified a cis-positive element located between -313 and -295 that is essential for amino acid regulation of its transcription in the CHOP promoter (Bruhat et al., 2000) (Fig. 13.2). This short sequence can regulate a basal promoter in response to starvation of several individual amino acids and so can be called an amino acid regulatory element (AARE). The sequence of the CHOP AARE region shows some homology with the specific binding sites of the C/EBP and ATF/CREB transcription factor families. Using gel shift experiments and chromatin immunoprecipitation, we have shown that several transcription factors belonging to the ATF or C/EBP family and regulatory proteins have the ability to bind to the CHOP AARE (ATF2, ATF3, ATF4, and CCAAT/enhancer-binding proteinβ (C/EBPβ)). Among these factors, ATF2 and ATF4 are indispensable for the amino acid control of CHOP expression: in cell knockout for these two proteins, the amino acid regulation of CHOP expression is abolished (Bruhat et al., 2000; Averous et al., 2004).

13.4.1.2 Regulation of the asparagine synthetase gene by amino acid starvation

At the same time, the Kilberg laboratory identified a sequence in the ASNS promoter (between -70 to -62) responsible for its regulation in response to amino acid starvation. This sequence was referred to as the nutrient-sensing response element-1 (NSRE-1) (Barbosa-Tessmann et al., 1999, 2000). Further promoter analysis indicated that a second sequence, 11 nucleotides downstream from NSRE-1, was also required for activation of the ASNS promoter by both amino acid starvation and endoplasmic reticulum (ER) stress. This sequence was referred to as NSRE-2. The genomic unit encompassing NSRE-1 and NSRE-2 was named NSRU, for nutrient-sensing response unit. NSRU is also responsible for the induction of ASNS by glucose starvation or ER stress. The same group demonstrated that several transcription factors and regulatory proteins (including ATF3, ATF4, C/EBPβ, TBP, and TFII) bind ASNS-NSRE-1. Using a chromatin immunoprecipitation approach they analysed precisely the time course of interaction between these transcription factors and the ASNS promoter (Chen et al., 2004).

Comparison between CHOP and ASNS transcriptional control elements shows that ASNS NSRE-1 and CHOP AARE share a similar nucleotide sequence (Bruhat et al., 2002) (Fig. 13.2). The core sequences of CHOP AARE and ASNS NSRE-1 differ only by two nucleotides (Fig. 13.3). It is thus expected that a common set of transcription factors bind to both ASNS-NSRE-1 and CHOP-AARE.

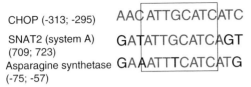

CHOP (-313; -295)   AAC ATTGCATC ATC
SNAT2 (system A)   GAT ATTGCATC AGT
(709; 723)
Asparagine synthetase GA AATTTCATC ATG
(-75; -57)

Fig. 13.2. Cis-acting elements required for induction of CHOP, SNAT2, and ASNS genes following amino acid starvation. Sequence comparison of the CHOP AARE with the ASNS NSRE-1 and the SNAT2 AARE. The positions of sequences from the transcription start site are shown in brackets. The minimum (core) sequence required for the response to amino acid starvation is within the box. Identical nucleotides to the CHOP sequence are underlined.

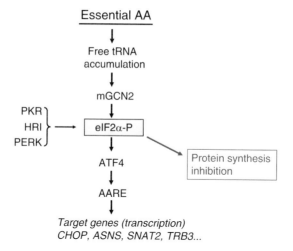

Fig. 13.3. The mammalian GCN2/ATF4 signalling pathway. The signal transduction pathway triggered in response to amino acid starvation is referred to as the amino acid response (AAR). The initial step in AAR is activation by uncharged tRNAs of GCN2 kinase which phosphorylates the α subunit of translation initiation factor eIF2 (eIF2α) on serine 51. This phosphorylation decreases protein synthesis by inhibiting the formation of the pre-initiation complex. However, eIF2α phosphorylation also triggers the translation of specific mRNAs including ATF4. Once induced, ATF4 induces transcription of specific target genes such as *CHOP, ASNS, TRB3* or *SNAT2*. In mammals, three other eIF2α kinases leading to ATF4 expression have been identified: PKR (double-stranded RNA dependent protein kinase) which is activated by double-stranded RNA during viral infection, HRI (haem-regulated translational inhibitor) which is activated by heme deficiency, and PERK (PKR-like endoplasmic reticulum kinase) which is activated by protein load in the endoplasmic reticulum.

13.4.1.3 Transcription factors binding the AARE

Several transcription factors have been described for their ability to bind the CHOP or the NSRE1- AARE. However, only ATF4 is indispensable for the amino acid regulation of ASNS expression, and both ATF2 and ATF4 are indispensable for the regulation of the CHOP-AARE.

13.4.1.3.1 ATF 4.
ATF4 belongs to the basic region/leucine zipper (bZIP) family of transcription factors that also includes members of the Jun/Fos (AP-1) family (Karpinski *et al.*, 1992; Ameri and Harris, 2008). Its key role in amino acid regulated transcription has been clearly established in the past few years (Chen *et al.*, 2004; Averous *et al.*, 2004; Kilberg *et al.*, 2005; Pan *et al.*, 2007). In the case of CHOP, it has been shown that:

1. the expression of ATF4 and its binding to CHOP AARE sequences are increased following amino acid starvation;
2. in cells devoid of ATF4 expression, the induction of CHOP upon amino acid starvation is completely lost; and
3. when over-expressed, ATF4 by itself is able to activate the CHOP AARE-dependent transcription.

13.4.1.3.2 ATF 2.
ATF2 belongs to the bZIP family of transcription factors and is an important member of activating protein 1 (AP-1) (Wagner, 2001). The transactivation capacity of the N terminal domain of this transcription factor can be enhanced through phosphorylation of two threonine residues, Thr-69 and Thr-71 (Gupta *et al.*, 1995; Livingstone *et al.*, 1995; Ouwens *et al.*, 2002). The role of ATF2 has been studied in the context of CHOP regulation by amino acid starvation (Bruhat *et al.*, 2000; Averous *et al.*, 2004; Bruhat *et al.*, 2007). It was shown that:

1. in cells devoid of ATF2 expression, the induction of CHOP transcription upon amino acid starvation is lost;

2. ATF2 binds to the CHOP AARE in both starved and unstarved conditions; and
3. ATF2 phosphorylation is necessary for the activation of the CHOP AARE-dependent transcription.

In a further study, it has been reported using a chromatin immunoprecipitation approach that *in vivo* binding of phospho-ATF2 to CHOP AARE is associated with acetylation of histones H4 and H2B in response to amino acid starvation (Bruhat et al., 2007). A time course analysis revealed that ATF2 phosphorylation precedes histone acetylation, ATF4 binding, and the increase in CHOP mRNA. Using cells devoid of ATF2 expression, it has also been demonstrated that ATF2 is essential for the acetylation of histones H4 and H2B within AARE sequences in response to amino acid starvation. Phosphorylation of this transcription factor may have a key role in stimulating an unidentified histone acetyl transferase (HAT) activity. Thus, ATF2 appears to be involved in promoting the modification of the chromatin structure to enhance CHOP transcription in response to amino acid starvation.

13.4.1.3.3 ROLE OF ATF4 AND ATF2 IN THE CONTROL OF THE AARE-DEPENDENT TRANSCRIPTION. Although the CHOP AARE and NSRE1 are very similar, some differences prompt us to think that CHOP and ASNS induction following amino acid starvation do not entirely occur through a unique and common mechanism:

1. no *cis*-DNA sequence equivalent of NSRE2 has been identified in the CHOP gene;
2. it has been shown (Bruhat et al., 2002) that ATF2 does not bind the ASNS NSRE; and
3. the amino acid specificity in relation to the degree of induction of these two genes is different (Jousse et al., 2000).

Hence, CHOP AARE and ASNS NSRE-1 are structurally related but functionally distinct.
Identification and studies of AARE sequences located in other genes allowed the identification of two sets of AARE-regulated genes (Bruhat et al., 2002; Chaveroux et al., 2009). Both are dependent on ATF4 but only one depends on ATF2 for its regulation. For example, regulation of *CHOP* and *ATF3* transcription by leucine starvation depends on the expression of both ATF4 and ATF2, whereas regulation of ASNS and SNAT2 is dependent on ATF4 but not on ATF2 (Averous et al., 2004; Chen et al., 2004; Palii et al., 2004, 2006; Bruhat et al., 2007). These last genes contain an AARE that is identical or very homologous to CHOP or ATF3 AARE in sequence, and binds ATF4 but not ATF2. Taken together, these results demonstrate that the flanking sequences of the AARE are important for precise control of AARE-dependent transcription. These differences in mechanism would permit flexibility among amino acid-regulated genes in terms of the rapidity, magnitude, and cell specificity of the transcriptional response for the same initial signal.

13.4.2 Signalling pathways regulated by amino acid limitation

In mammals, the signalling pathways that mediate regulation of gene expression in response to amino acid starvation are partially understood. A pathway leading to the up-regulation of ATF4 protein has been described at molecular level, and a second pathway leading to ATF2 phosphorylation has recently been identified.

13.4.2.1 The GCN2/ATF4 pathway (the AAR pathway)

In mammals, limiting the extracellular supply of an indispensable amino acid or blocking the synthesis of an otherwise non-indispensable one results in activation of a signal transduction pathway that is referred to as the amino acid response (AAR). Ron's group identified this signalling pathway for regulating gene expression in mammals (Harding et al., 2003). The AAR is homologous to the well-characterized yeast general control response to amino acid deprivation (Dever et al., 1992). Its components include the mammalian homologue of GCN2 kinase, the initiation factor of translation eIF2α, and ATF4 (Fig. 13.3). The initial step in AAR is activation by uncharged tRNA of mammalian GCN2 protein kinase, which phosphorylates eIF2α on serine 51 (Dever et al., 1992). This phosphorylation decreases the cap-dependent translation of most mRNAs. Like the GCN4 transcript, ATF4 mRNA contains uORFs in its 5'UTR that allow translation when cap-dependent translation is inhibited (see Lu *et al.*, 2004 and Vattem and Wek, 2004 for the molecular mechanisms). Therefore, under circumstances of amino acid starvation, transcription factor ATF4 is translationally up-regulated. Once induced, ATF4 directly or indirectly induces transcription of specific target genes.

13.4.2.2 Signalling pathway leading to ATF2 phosphorylation

Several data (described above) established that ATF2 is phosphorylated in response to amino acid starvation (Bruhat *et al.*, 2000; Averous *et al.*, 2004). Collectively, these data suggested the existence of a specific amino acid-regulated pathway leading to phosphorylation of ATF2. This pathway was partially identified recently (Chaveroux *et al.*, 2009). We first showed that the MAPK module MEKK1/MKK7/JNK2 is responsible for ATF2 phosphorylation in response to leucine starvation. Then we progressed backwards up the signal transduction pathway and showed that GTPase Rac1/Cdc42 and protein Gα12 control the MAPK module, ATF2 phosphorylation, and AARE-dependent transcription.

13.4.2.3 Other signalling pathways

In yeast, the mechanisms involved in amino acid detection have been well documented (Hinnebusch, 1988) and several signalling pathways identified. By homology to yeast we can imagine that pathways other than mGCN2 are involved in sensing amino acid availability in mammals. Notably, mTOR is well known to be involved in the regulation of translation by amino acid availability. However, several studies have shown that mTOR is not widely involved in regulation of gene expression (Peng *et al.*, 2002; Deval *et al.*, 2009). Recent studies suggest that other signalling mechanisms could be involved in regulation of gene expression in response to amino acid limitation. These conclusion were obtained either by measuring the response of gene expression to deprivation of different amino acids (Palii *et al.*, 2008) or by using transcription profiling from cells devoid of GCN2 expression (Deval *et al.*, 2009). In addition, it has been shown that amino acids can interfere directly or indirectly with signalling pathways and/or various transcription factors (distinct from the AAR). In particular, it was shown that glutamine, the most abundant amino acid, modulated activity of various transcription factors through mechanisms that remain to be identified (see Brasse-Lagnel *et al.*, 2009 for review). Hence we can conclude here that the response to amino acid starvation in mammals is a complex process that involves different regulatory processes.

13.5 Control of Physiological Function by the GCN2/ATF4 Pathway

Although several signalling mechanisms modulated by amino acid starvation have been described, the GCN2/ATF4 pathway is the most studied and is likely to be the most important (Deval *et al.*, 2009). In this chapter we focus on the role the GCN2/ATF4 pathway plays in the control of several physiological functions.

13.5.1 Amino acid deficiency sensing by GCN2 triggers food aversion

Food intake results from a complex behavioural pattern in which innate factors play an important role, particularly in the case of omnivores. A remarkable example of an innate mechanism governing food choice is presented by the fact that omnivorous animals will consume substantially less of an otherwise identical experimental meal lacking a single indispensable amino acid (see Chapter 19) (Leung *et al.*, 1968; Harper *et al.*, 1970). Although it seems likely that the signalling pathway leading to this response comprises the sensing of amino acid variations, the basis for this innate aversive response is poorly understood. Blood concentration of an indispensable amino acid decreases rapidly when it is missing in the diet. As a consequence, the protein kinase GCN2, which is ubiquitously expressed, could be activated in most tissues. Therefore GCN2 could be an important sensor of amino acid homeostasis inside cells and could activate downstream-rectifying responses mediated by phosphorylated eIF2α (Hinnebusch, 1994; Harding *et al.*, 2000; this review).

Recent results (Hao *et al.*, 2005; Maurin *et al.*, 2005) establish that the aversive response of wild-type mice to a diet deficient in one indispensable amino acid is likewise blunted in GCN2–/– mice (Fig. 13.4a), whereas serum amino acid levels are decreased to similar levels by the imbalanced diet in both genotypes (Fig. 13.4b). These results indicate an altered response to amino acid deficiency in mice lacking GCN2 activity. Using conditional GCN2 knockout mice, we further demonstrated that GCN2 ablation specifically in the brain also impairs the aversive response to an imbalanced diet. Thus, even if the consumption of an imbalanced meal also activates GCN2 and promotes eIF2α in peripheral tissues, particularly in the liver, our observation implicates brain GCN2 signalling in initiating the aversive response.

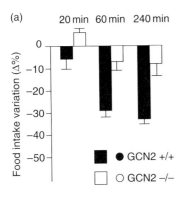
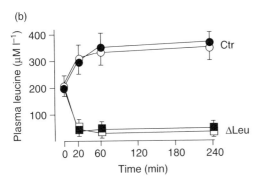

Fig. 13.4. Mice lacking the GCN2 kinase are impaired in their aversive response to amino acid-imbalanced food. (a) Relative consumption of balanced diet (Ctr) and diet lacking leucine (ΔLeu) for 20, 60 or 240 minutes after the beginning of the meal. Results from GCN2+/+ mice are shown as dark bars and mutant GCN2–/– mice as open bars. Results are expressed as the ratio of consumption (Δ% ±SEM) of the ΔLeu diet versus the consumption of the Ctr by the same animal. For example, 60 minutes after the beginning of the meal, wild-type mice consumed 30% less of the ΔLeu diet compared to the Ctr diet, whereas the GCN2–/– mice consumed both diets equally. (b) Plasma leucine levels (µM) of mice fed the indicated diet (circles: control diet; squares: leucine-devoid diet). Results from GCN2+/+ mice are shown as dark symbols and mutant GCN2–/– mice as open symbols.

13.5.2 Role of GCN2 in the regulation of neuronal plasticity

Several studies have shown a link between messenger RNA translation, learning, and memory (Kandel, 2001). Costa-Mattioli *et al.* (2005, 2007) provided evidence that GCN2 regulate synaptic plasticity, as well as learning and memory. The molecular basis for enhanced memory in GCN2–/– mice with reduced eIF2α phosphorylation is explained by the fact that GCN2-mediated eIF2α phosphorylation causes an increase in translation of ATF4 mRNA in the brain. ATF4 suppresses memory because it inhibits transcription factor c-AMP response element binding (CREB) protein-mediated gene expression. It is likely that the basal activity of GCN2 is required for its function. Modulation of GCN2 activity in the brain by various factors has not been addressed in these studies.

13.5.3 Role of GCN2 in the regulation of fatty-acid homeostasis during leucine deprivation

Guo and Cavener (2007) brought to light the role of GCN2 in the regulation of lipid metabolism in the liver during deprivation of an indispensable amino acid. These authors showed that expression of lipogenic genes in the liver were repressed and lipid stores in adipose tissue were mobilized upon leucine deprivation. In contrast, GCN2-deficient mice developed liver steatosis and exhibited reduced lipid mobilization. Liver steatosis in GCN2−/− mice was found to be caused by unrepressed expression of lipogenic genes, including Srebp-1c. The signalling pathway linking GCN2 activity to the regulation of Srebp-1c expression is not identified at present.

In the same way, two recent articles demonstrated that phosphorylation of eIF2α was a key regulator of several aspects of intermediary metabolism. Oyadomari et al. (2008) demonstrated that eIF2α phosphorylation signalling in the liver was regulating transcription factors involved in carbohydrate and lipid metabolism. The Kaufman group showed that translation attenuation through eIF2α phosphorylation prevented oxidative stress and optimized ER protein folding to support insulin production in pancreatic β cells (Back et al., 2009).

13.5.4 Role of GCN2 in the immune system

It was shown recently that the AAR pathway was involved in several aspects of regulation of the immune response (Mellor and Munn, 2004, 2008; Pierre, 2009). In particular, associated with the induction of indoleamine 2,3-dioxygenase (IDO initiates the degradation of tryptophan), AAR is involved in communication between cells. For example, after stimulation, IDO-expressing antigen presenting cells (APC) cells reduce extracellular tryptophan concentrations so that adjacent T-cells, which depend on tryptophan from the extracellular environment, are unable to activate and proliferate upon encountering antigens. Therefore IDO might play a role in preventing the initiation of autoimmune disease by enforcing T-cell tolerance by suppressing their proliferation (Moffett and Namboodiri, 2003). Hence, high local expression of IDO by IDO-expressing APC may represent an anti-inflammatory and immunosuppressive mechanism attempting to counterbalance tissue damage (Wolf et al., 2004). In addition, IDO/GCN2 activities are implicated in several other contexts, such as the inhibition of maternal T-cell immunity to fetal tissues during mammalian gestation (Munn et al., 1998) and T-cell tolerance to tumours (Friberg et al., 2002; Uyttenhove et al., 2003).

Taken together, these examples highlight the need for relying on physiological observations to molecular events described *in vitro* to improve our knowledge on physiological consequences of nutritional status.

13.6 Conclusions

The idea that amino acids can regulate gene expression is now well established. In concert with hormones, amino acids can by themselves play an important role in the control of physiological function; however, the underlying processes have only begun to be discovered. Defining the precise cascade of molecular events by which the cellular concentration of an individual amino acid regulates gene expression will be an important contribution to our understanding of metabolic control in mammalian cells.

The molecular basis of gene regulation by dietary protein intake is an important field of research for study of the regulation of physiological functions of individuals living under conditions of restricted, imbalanced, or excessive food intake. Beyond gaining a basic understanding of the amino acid control of biological mechanisms, the characterization of how these processes contribute to the pathology of various diseases represents an important field of investigation in molecular nutrition.

References

Ameri, K. and Harris, A.L. (2008) Activating transcription factor 4. *International Journal of Biochemistry & Cell Biology* 40, 14–21.

Aoki, T.T., Brennan, M.F., Muller, W.A., Soeldner, J.S., Alpert, J.S., Saltz, S.B., Kaufmann, R.L., et al. (1976) Amino acid levels across normal forearm muscle and splanchnic bed after a protein meal. *American Journal of Clinical Nutrition* 29, 340–350.

Aulak, K.S., Mishra, R., Zhou, L., Hyatt, S.L., de Jonge, W., Lamers, W., Snider, M., et al. (1999) Post-transcriptional regulation of the arginine transporter Cat-1 by amino acid availability. *Journal of Biological Chemistry* 274, 30424–30432.

Averous, J., Bruhat, A., Jousse, C., Carraro, V., Thiel, G. and Fafournoux, P. (2004) Induction of CHOP expression by amino acid limitation requires both ATF4 expression and ATF2 phosphorylation. *Journal of Biological Chemistry* 279, 5288–5297.

Back, S.H., Scheuner, D., Han, J., Song, B., Ribick, M., Wang, J., Gildersleeve, R.D., et al. (2009) Translation attenuation through eIF2alpha phosphorylation prevents oxidative stress and maintains the differentiated state in beta cells. *Cell Metabolism* 10, 13–26.

Baertl, J.M., Placko, R.P. and Graham, G.G. (1974) Serum proteins and plasma free amino acids in severe malnutrition. *American Journal of Clinical Nutrition* 27, 733–742.

Barbosa-Tessmann, I.P., Chen, C., Zhong, C., Schuster, S.M., Nick, H.S. and Kilberg, M.S. (1999) Activation of the unfolded protein response pathway induces human asparagine synthetase gene expression. *Journal of Biological Chemistry* 274, 31139–31144.

Barbosa-Tessmann, I.P., Chen, C., Zhong, C., Siu, F., Schuster, S.M., Nick, H.S., et al. (2000) Activation of the human asparagine synthetase gene by the amino acid response and the endoplasmic reticulum stress response pathways occurs by common genomic elements. *Journal of Biological Chemistry* 275, 26976–26985.

Bhattacharyya, S.N., Habermacher, R., Martine, U., Closs, E.I. and Filipowicz, W. (2006) Relief of microRNA-mediated translational repression in human cells subjected to stress. *Cell* 125, 1111–1124.

Brasse-Lagnel, C., Lavoinne, A. and Husson, A. (2009) Control of mammalian gene expression by amino acids, especially glutamine. *FEBS Journal* 276, 1826–1844.

Bruhat, A., Jousse, C., Wang, X.Z., Ron, D., Ferrara, M. and Fafournoux, P. (1997) Amino acid limitation induces expression of CHOP, a CCAAT/enhancer binding protein-related gene, at both transcriptional and post-transcriptional levels. *Journal of Biological Chemistry* 272, 17588–17593.

Bruhat, A., Jousse, C., Carraro, V., Reimold, A.M., Ferrara, M. and Fafournoux, P. (2000) Amino acids control mammalian gene transcription: activating transcription factor 2 is essential for the amino acid responsiveness of the CHOP promoter. *Molecular and Cellular Biology* 20, 7192–7204.

Bruhat, A., Averous, J., Carraro, V., Zhong, C., Reimold, A.M., Kilberg, M.S. and Fafournoux, P. (2002) Differences in the molecular mechanisms involved in the transcriptional activation of chop and asparagine synthetase in response to amino acid deprivation or activation of the unfolded protein response. *Journal of Biological Chemistry* 25, 25.

Bruhat, A., Cherasse, Y., Maurin, A.C., Breitwieser, W., Parry, L., Deval, C., Jones, N., et al. (2007) ATF2 is required for amino acid-regulated transcription by orchestrating specific histone acetylation. *Nucleic Acids Research* 35, 1312–1321.

Chaveroux, C., Jousse, C., Cherasse, Y., Maurin, A.C., Parry, L., Carraro V., Derijard, B., et al. (2009) Identification of a novel amino acid response pathway triggering ATF2 phosphorylation in mammals. *Molecular and Cellular Biology* 29, 6515–6526.

Chen, H., Pan, Y.X., Dudenhausen, E.E. and Kilberg, M.S. (2004) Amino acid deprivation induces the transcription rate of the human asparagine synthetase gene through a timed program of expression and promoter binding of nutrient-responsive basic region/leucine zipper transcription factors as well as localized histone acetylation. *Journal of Biological Chemistry* 279, 50829–50839.

Costa-Mattioli, M., Gobert, D., Harding, H., Herdy, B., Azzi, M., Bruno, M., Bidinosti, M., et al. (2005) Translational control of hippocampal synaptic plasticity and memory by the eIF2alpha kinase GCN2. *Nature* 436, 1166–1173.

Costa-Mattioli, M., Gobert, D., Stern, E., Gamache, K., Colina, R., Cuello, C., Sossin, W., et al. (2007) eIF2alpha phosphorylation bidirectionally regulates the switch from short- to long-term synaptic plasticity and memory. *Cell* 129, 195–206.

Cynober, L. (2007) Pharmacokinetics of arginine and related amino acids. *Journal of Nutrition* 137, 1646S–1649S.

Deval, C., Chaveroux, C., Maurin, A.C., Cherasse, Y., Parry, L., Carraro, V., Milenkovic, D., et al. (2009) Amino acid limitation regulates the expression of genes involved in several specific biological processes through GCN2-dependent and GCN2-independent pathways. *FEBS Journal* 276, 707–718.

Dever, T.E., Feng, L., Wek, R.C., Cigan, A.M., Donahue, T.F. and Hinnebusch, A.G. (1992) Phosphorylation of initiation factor 2 alpha by protein kinase GCN2 mediates gene-specific translational control of GCN4 in yeast. *Cell* 68, 585–596.

Duplus, E., Glorian, M. and Forest, C. (2000) Fatty acid regulation of gene transcription. *Journal of Biological Chemistry* 275, 30749–30752.

Fafournoux, P., Remesy, C. and Demigne, C. (1990) Fluxes and membrane transport of amino acids in rat liver under different protein diets. *American Journal of Physiology* 259, E614–625.

Fawcett, T.W., Eastman, H.B., Martindale, J.L. and Holbrook, N.J. (1996) Physical and functional association between GADD153 and CCAAT/enhancer-binding protein beta during cellular stress. *Journal of Biological Chemistry* 271, 14285–14289.

Fernandez, J., Yaman, I., Mishra, R., Merrick, W.C., Snider, M.D., Lamers, W.H. and Hatzoglou, M. (2001) Internal ribosome entry site-mediated translation of a mammalian mRNA is regulated by amino acid availability. *Journal of Biological Chemistry* 276, 12285–12291.

Foufelle, F., Girard, J. and Ferre, P. (1998) Glucose regulation of gene expression. *Current Opinion Clinical Nutrition and Metabolic Care* 1, 323–328.

Friberg, M., Jennings, R., Alsarraj, M., Dessureault, S., Cantor, A., Extermann, M., Mellor, A.L., *et al.* (2002) Indoleamine 2,3-dioxygenase contributes to tumor cell evasion of T cell-mediated rejection. *International Journal of Cancer* 101, 151–155.

Gietzen, D.W. (1993) Neural mechanisms in the responses to amino acid deficiency. *Journal of Nutrition* 123, 610–625.

Gietzen, D.W. (2000) Amino acid recognition in the central nervous system. In: Berthoud, H.-R. and Seeley, R.J. (eds) *Neural and Metabolic Control of Macronutrient Intake*. CRC Press, New York, pp. 339–357.

Gong, S.S., Guerrini, L. and Basilico, C. (1991) Regulation of asparagine synthetase gene expression by amino acid starvation. *Molecular and Cellular Biology* 11, 6059–6066.

Grimaldi, P.A. (2001) Fatty acid regulation of gene expression. *Current Opinion in Clinical Nutrition and Metabolic Care* 4, 433–437.

Grimble, R.F. and Whitehead, R.G. (1970) Fasting serum-aminoacid patterns in kwashiorkor and after administration of different levels of protein. *Lancet* 1, 918–920.

Gupta, S., Campbell, D., Derijard, B. and Davis, R.J. (1995) Transcription factor ATF2 regulation by the JNK signal transduction pathway. *Science* 267, 389–393.

Hao, S., Sharp, J.W., Ross-Inta, C.M., McDaniel, B.J., Anthony, T.G., Wek, R.C., Cavener, D.R., *et al.* (2005) Uncharged tRNA and sensing of amino acid deficiency in mammalian piriform cortex. *Science* 307, 1776–1778.

Harding, H.P., Novoa, I.I., Zhang, Y., Zeng, H., Wek, R., Schapira, M. and Ron, D. (2000) Regulated translation initiation controls stress-induced gene expression in mammalian cells. *Molecular Cell* 6, 1099–1108.

Harding, H.P., Zhang, Y., Zeng, H., Novoa, I., Lu, P.D., Calfon, M., Sadri, N., *et al.* (2003) An integrated stress response regulates amino acid metabolism and resistance to oxidative stress. *Molecular Cell* 11, 619–633.

Harper, A.E., Benevenga, N.J. and Wohlhueter, R.M. (1970) Effects of ingestion of disproportionate amounts of amino acids. *Physiological Review* 50, 428–558.

Hinnebusch, A.G. (1988) Mechanisms of gene regulation in the general control of amino acid biosynthesis in Saccharomyces cerevisiae. *Microbiological Review* 52, 248–273.

Hinnebusch, A.G. (1994) Translational control of GCN4: an in vivo barometer of initiation-factor activity. *Trends in Biochemical Sciences* 19, 409–414.

Jousse, C., Bruhat, A., Ferrara, M. and Fafournoux, P. (1998) Physiological concentration of amino acids regulates insulin-like- growth-factor-binding protein 1 expression. *Biochemical Journal* 334, 147–153.

Jousse, C., Bruhat, A., Ferrara, M. and Fafournoux, P. (2000) Evidence for multiple signaling pathways in the regulation of gene expression by amino acids in human cell lines. *Journal of Nutrition* 130, 1555–1560.

Jousse, C., Averous, J., Bruhat, A., Carraro, V., Mordier, S. and Fafournoux, P. (2004) Amino acids as regulators of gene expression: molecular mechanisms. *Biochemical and Biophysical Research Communications* 313, 447–452.

Kandel, E.R. (2001) The molecular biology of memory storage: a dialogue between genes and synapses. *Science* 294, 1030–1038.

Karpinski, B.A., Morle, G.D., Huggenvik, J., Uhler, M.D. and Leiden, J.M. (1992) Molecular cloning of human CREB-2: an ATF/CREB transcription factor that can negatively regulate transcription from the cAMP response element. *Proceedings of the National Academy of Sciences USA* 89, 4820–4824.

Kilberg, M.S., Pan, Y.X., Chen, H. and Leung-Pineda, V. (2005) Nutritional control of gene expression: how mammalian cells respond to amino acid limitation. *Annual Review of Nutrition* 25, 59–85.

Kimball, S.R. and Jefferson, L.S. (2004) Amino acids as regulators of gene expression. *Nutrition and Metabolism* 1, 3.

Lee, P.D., Conover, C.A. and Powell, D.R. (1993) Regulation and function of insulin-like growth factor-binding protein-1. *Proceedings of the Society for Experimental Biology and Medicine* 204, 4–29.

Leung, P.M., Rogers, Q.R. and Harper, A.E. (1968) Effect of amino acid imbalance on dietary choice in the rat. *Journal of Nutrition* 95, 483–492.

Livingstone, C., Patel, G. and Jones, N. (1995) ATF-2 contains a phosphorylation-dependent transcriptional activation domain. *EMBO Journal* 14, 1785–1797.

Lu, P.D., Harding, H.P. and Ron, D. (2004) Translation reinitiation at alternative open reading frames regulates gene expression in an integrated stress response. *Journal of Cell Biology* 167, 27–33.

Luethy, J.D. and Holbrook, N.J. (1992) Activation of the gadd153 promoter by genotoxic agents: a rapid and specific response to DNA damage. *Cancer Research* 52, 5–10.

Marten, N.W., Burke, E.J., Hayden, J.M. and Straus, D.S. (1994) Effect of amino acid limitation on the expression of 19 genes in rat hepatoma cells. *FASEB Journal* 8, 538–544.

Maurin, A.C., Jousse, C., Averous, J., Parry, L., Bruhat, A., Cherasse, Y., Zeng, H., *et al.* (2005) The GCN2 kinase biases feeding behavior to maintain amino acid homeostasis in omnivores. *Cell Metabolism* 1, 273–277.

Mellor, A.L. and Munn, D.H. (2004) IDO expression by dendritic cells: tolerance and tryptophan catabolism. *Nature Reviews Immunology* 4, 762–774.

Mellor, A.L. and Munn, D.H. (2008) Creating immune privilege: active local suppression that benefits friends, but protects foes. *Nature Reviews Immunology* 8, 74–80.

Moffett, J.R. and Namboodiri, M.A. (2003) Tryptophan and the immune response. *Immunology and Cell Biology* 81, 247–265.

Munn, D.H., Zhou, M., Attwood, J.T., Bondarev, I., Conway, S.J., Marshall, B., Brown, C. *et al.* (1998) Prevention of allogeneic fetal rejection by tryptophan catabolism. *Science* 281, 1191–1193.

Munro, H.N. (1970) *Mammalian Protein Metabolism.* Vol. 4, Academic Press, New York and London.

Munro, H.N. (1976) Second Boyd Orr Memorial Lecture. Regulation of body protein metabolism in relation to diet. *Proceedings of the Nutrition Society* 35, 297–308.

Ouwens, D.M., de Ruiter, N.D., van der Zon, G.C., Carter, A.P., Schouten, J., van der Burgt, C., Kooistra, K., *et al.* (2002) Growth factors can activate ATF2 via a two-step mechanism, phosphorylation of Thr71 through the Ras-MEK-ERK pathway and of Thr69 through RalGDS-Src-p38. *EMBO Journal* 21, 3782–3793.

Oyadomari, S., Harding, H.P., Zhang, Y., Oyadomari, M. and Ron, D. (2008) Dephosphorylation of translation initiation factor 2alpha enhances glucose tolerance and attenuates hepatosteatosis in mice. *Cell Metabolism* 7, 520–532.

Palii, S.S., Chen, H. and Kilberg, M.S. (2004) Transcriptional control of the human sodium-coupled neutral amino acid transporter system A gene by amino acid availability is mediated by an intronic element. *Journal of Biological Chemistry*, 279, 3463–3471.

Palii, S.S., Thiaville, M.M., Pan, Y.X., Zhong, C. and Kilberg, M.S. (2006) Characterization of the amino acid response element within the human sodium-coupled neutral amino acid transporter 2 (SNAT2) System A transporter gene. *Biochemistry Journal*, 395, 517–527.

Palii, S.S., Kays, C.E., Deval, C., Bruhat, A., Fafournoux, P. and Kilberg, M.S. (2009) Specificity of amino acid regulated gene expression: analysis of genes subjected to either complete or single amino acid deprivation. *Amino Acids* 37, 79–88.

Pan, Y.X., Chen, H., Thiaville, M.M. and Kilberg, M.S. (2007) Activation of the ATF3 gene through a co-ordinated amino acid-sensing response programme that controls transcriptional regulation of responsive genes following amino acid limitation. *Biochemical Journal* 401, 299–307.

Pégorier, J.P. (1998) Regulation of gene expression by fatty acids. *Current Opinion in Clinical Nutrition & Metabolic Care* 1, 329–334.

Peng, T., Golub, T.R. and Sabatini, D.M. (2002) The immunosuppressant rapamycin mimics a starvation-like signal distinct from amino acid and glucose deprivation. *Molecular and Cellular Biology* 22, 5575–5584.

Pierre, P. (2009) Immunity and the regulation of protein synthesis: surprising connections. *Current Opinion in Immunology* 21, 70–77.

Rogers, Q.R. and Leung, P.M.B. (1977) *The Control of Food Intake: When and How are Amino Acids Involved?* Vol. 213, Academic Press, New York.

Straus, D.S. (1994) Nutritional regulation of hormones and growth factors that control mammalian growth. *FASEB Journal* 8, 6–12.

Straus, D.S., Burke, E.J. and Marten, N.W. (1993) Induction of insulin-like growth factor binding protein-1 gene expression in liver of protein-restricted rats and in rat hepatoma cells limited for a single amino acid. *Endocrinology* 132, 1090–1100.

Svanberg, E., Jefferson, L.S., Lundholm, K. and Kimball, S.R. (1997) Postprandial stimulation of muscle protein synthesis is independent of changes in insulin. *American Journal of Physiology* 272, E841–847.

Sylvester, S.L., ap Rhys, C.M., Luethy-Martindale, J.D., and Holbrook, N.J. (1994) Induction of GADD153, a CCAAT/enhancer-binding protein (C/EBP)-related gene, during the acute phase response in rats. Evidence for the involvement of C/EBPs in regulating its expression. *Journal of Biological Chemistry* 269, 20119–20125. [Published erratum appears in *Journal of Biological Chemistry* 270, 14842.]

Towle, H.C. (1995) Metabolic regulation of gene transcription in mammals. *Journal of Biological Chemistry* 270, 23235–23238.

Ubeda, M., Vallejo, M. and Habener, J.F. (1999) CHOP enhancement of gene transcription by interactions with Jun/Fos AP-1 complex proteins. *Molecular and Cellular Biology* 19, 7589–7599.

Uyttenhove, C., Pilotte, L., Theate, I., Stroobant, V., Colau, D., Parmentier, N., Boon, T., *et al.* (2003) Evidence for a tumoral immune resistance mechanism based on tryptophan degradation by indoleamine 2,3-dioxygenase. *Nature Medicine* 9, 1269–1274.

Vattem, K.M. and Wek, R.C. (2004) Reinitiation involving upstream ORFs regulates ATF4 mRNA translation in mammalian cells. *Proceedings of the National Academy of Sciences USA* 101, 11269–11274.

Vaulont, S., Vasseur-Cognet, M. and Kahn, A. (2000) Glucose regulation of gene transcription. *Journal of Biological Chemistry* 275, 31555–31558.

Wagner, E.F. (2001) AP-1: Introductory remarks. *Oncogene* 20, 2334–2335.

Wang, X.Z., Lawson, B., Brewer, J.W., Zinszner, H., Sanjay, A., Mi, L.J., Boorstein, R., *et al.* (1996) Signals from the stressed endoplasmic reticulum induce C/EBP-homologous protein (CHOP/GADD153). *Molecular and Cellular Biology* 16, 4273–4280.

Wolf, A.M., Wolf, D., Rumpold, H., Moschen, A.R., Kaser, A., Obrist, P., Fuchs, D., *et al.* (2004) Overexpression of indoleamine 2,3-dioxygenase in human inflammatory bowel disease. *Clinical Immunology* 113, 47–55.

Yoshizawa, F., Endo, H., Ide, H., Yagasaki, K. and Funabiki, R. (1995) Translational regulation of protein synthesis in the liver and skeletal muscle of mice in response to refeeding. *Nutrional Biochemistry* 6, 130–136.

Young, V.R., El-Khoury, A.E., Melchor, S. and Castillo, L. (1994) The biochemistry and physiology of protein and amino acid metabolism, with reference to protein nutrition. In: Niels, C.R.R. (ed.) *Protein Metabolism During Infancy*. Vol. 33, Nestec Ltd: New York; Raven Press Ltd: Vevey, pp. 1–28.

Part III

Nutrition

14 Endogenous Amino Acids at the Terminal Ileum of the Adult Human

P.J. Moughan*

Riddet Institute, Massey University, Palmerston North, New Zealand

14.1 Abstract

During the digestion of food very considerable quantities of proteins of body origin (endogenous protein) are voided into the digestive tract of the adult human. Much of this material is recycled, with the protein being digested and the amino acids reabsorbed. Nevertheless large quantities of endogenous protein, peptides and amino acids remain unabsorbed at the end of the small intestine, and these along with endogenous protein originating from the colon, are largely catabolized by the colonic microflora, and represent a loss of amino acids from the body. In the adult human around 2 g d^{-1} of endogenous nitrogen (13 g protein) flow from the terminal ileum into the colon, and such a loss of amino acids is of importance metabolically.

This chapter reviews methods which may be applied in humans for collecting ileal digesta and measuring the endogenous protein component. Literature estimates of endogenous ileal nitrogen flow in humans are reviewed and factors influencing the endogenous flows discussed. The practical relevance of the estimates of endogenous N flow, both physiologically and nutritionally, is discussed in the context of gut and body metabolic rate, the daily amino acid requirement and the determination of estimates of ileal amino acid digestibility.

14.2 Introduction

During the digestion of food copious quantities of nitrogen-containing materials originating from the body are voided into the lumen of the digestive tract. These are referred to as the endogenous nitrogen and are significant metabolically.

Sources of endogenous nitrogen include digestive enzymes, bile salts, phospholipids, desquamated cells, mucoproteins, urea, proteins and amino acids originating from lysed cells, plasma proteins (especially serum albumen), and other nitrogenous compounds found in the gastrointestinal secretions. Although strictly 'non-dietary' as opposed to 'endogenous', microbial nitrogen is often included as part of the endogenous measure. The overall amounts of material entering the digestive tract from different sources are not known precisely, with estimates varying widely. Table 14.1 provides some approximate values based on the wider literature. In the adult human, it is considered that endogenous

---

* E-mail address: p.j.moughan@massey.ac.nz

Table 14.1. Approximate amounts of endogenous nitrogen from different sources entering the digestive tract of the adult human.

	Endogenous nitrogen (g d^{-1})[a]
Saliva	0.2
Gastric juice	1.5
Bile	1.5
Pancreatic secretions	2.5
Urea	5.0
Mucus	2.0
Epithelial enzymes/sloughed cells	5.5
Total	18.0

[a]Based on literature data for growing pig and adult human.

nitrogen flowing through the digestive tract to the terminal ileum amounts to some 11–16 g d^{-1} (FAO et al., 2007), values consistent with the estimates for the total tract given in Table 14.1.

During the digestive process, endogenous sources of nitrogen become mixed with proteins of dietary origin. Nasset (1965) suggested that a considerable amount of nitrogen in the duodenal digesta is of endogenous origin, and a study with humans (Nixon and Mawer, 1970) showed that after a protein meal as much as 53% of intraluminal protein in the small intestine was of endogenous origin. Johansson (1975) found endogenous protein to be about one third of the amount of that from the diet.

Much of the endogenous protein entering the gut lumen is digested and the amino acids reabsorbed, with the absorbed amino acids representing a significant supply of amino acids for metabolism. Up to 80% of endogenous nitrogen has been reported to be reabsorbed by the end of the small intestine (Krawielitzki et al., 1990; Souffrant et al., 1993). Based on such a rate of reabsorption and an endogenous nitrogen inflow (mouth to terminal ileum) of 13.5 g d^{-1} (mean of 11 and 16 gN d^{-1} (FAO et al., 2007)), this would equate to a loss of endogenous nitrogen from the small bowel of 2700 mg N d^{-1}. Such a value is higher than an estimate given by Chacko and Cummings (1988) of 1000 mg nitrogen d^{-1}, but is in line with more recent estimates obtained in subjects receiving protein-containing test diets (see below). A terminal ileal loss of 2700 mg N d^{-1} equates to a loss of endogenous protein of around 17 g d^{-1}, which is quantitatively significant.

The nitrogen-containing material remaining undigested at the end of the ileum, of both endogenous and dietary origin, passes into the colon where it is catabolized extensively by the resident microflora. Amino acids are not considered to be absorbed as such from the mammalian large bowel in quantitatively significant amounts (Wrong et al., 1981; McNeil, 1988), and thus amino acid absorption studies and studies of endogenous secretion and excretion have centred on the upper digestive tract (Moughan, 2003). The objectives of this contribution are to outline recent developments in the methodology for measuring endogenous ileal nitrogen loss in humans and the practical importance of such measures, and to give an overview of current estimates of endogenous ileal nitrogen and amino acid losses, and factors influencing endogenous nitrogen flow.

14.3 Endogenous Ileal Amino Acid Losses – How Should They be Determined?

14.3.1 The collection of ileal digesta

The determination of endogenous ileal amino acid losses from the terminal ileum into the colon necessitates the collection of samples of fresh ileal digesta. The total collection or sampling of digesta flowing at the terminal ileum (end of small intestine) is more easily undertaken with animal models (laboratory rat or growing pig) than with human subjects. With animal models digesta may be collected via surgically implanted cannulas, or directly from the deeply anaesthetized or euthanized animal, the latter being a common method with birds and smaller mammals. With humans, a number of workers have enlisted the cooperation of ileostomates, who have undergone an ileostomy operation usually due to ulcerative colitis. After colorectomy, the distal small bowel is attached to the abdominal wall as a fistula, and this allows a total collection of ileal digesta. A strength of this method is that no dietary markers are required to relate the sample of digesta collected to the food intake. A major drawback, however, is the largely unknown effects that the surgery or underlying disease states may have on endogenous protein loss. Colorectomy leads to physiological and metabolic adaptations (Christl and Scheppach, 1997), and it is well known that there is a very considerable microbial colonization of at least the lower small intestine in ileostomates (Gorbach et al., 1967). In this case, observations obtained using ileostomates as a model must be interpreted with some caution.

An alternative approach is naso-intestinal intubation (Schedl and Clifton, 1961; Modigliani et al., 1973) which allows the sampling of ileal digesta from conscious human volunteers with an intact digestive tract. The method consists of inserting a triple-lumen polyvinyl chloride (PVC) tube via the nose to the stomach, progressing down to the terminal ileum aided by peristalsis and by a terminal inflatable balloon containing mercury. Digesta are collected continuously by siphoning or by slight aspiration through the distal opening of the tube. The method relies on the use of a non-absorbable marker of the liquid phase, and may thus be subject to greater error than total collection methods. Further potential concerns with the method are whether the presence of a tube in the gut alters food transit rate and whether the method allows representative sampling of digesta. The second concern, at least, has been addressed experimentally (Deglaire, 2008), where it was concluded that the method allows accurate estimation of intestinal fluid flows and representative samples of digesta. The method, however, remains time-consuming, expensive and certainly not routine.

Given the difficulties with collecting ileal digesta samples from humans, it is not surprising that animal models have been evaluated for application in studying digestion in man. The growing pig, a meal-eating omnivore, has been shown to be a particularly useful model (Moughan et al., 1992, 1994; Rowan et al., 1994; Deglaire et al., 2009) and can be used routinely to provide samples of ileal digesta.

14.3.2 Quantification of the endogenous component

Having obtained a representative sample of ileal digesta, it is then necessary to distinguish endogenous sources of nitrogen from materials of undigested dietary origin. To this end a number of methods have been developed. Such methods have been the subject of comprehensive review (Moughan, et al., 1998). Those that would seem most applicable to humans are:

1. feeding the subject a protein-free diet;
2. the enzyme hydrolysed protein/ultrafiltration method; and
3. the isotope dilution method (^{15}N labelled diet).

All three methods have inherent strengths and weaknesses.

14.3.2.1 Protein-free diet

When a diet formulated to be devoid of protein is fed to a human subject for several days, all of the nitrogen and amino acids recovered in the terminal ileal digesta must, by definition, be of endogenous origin. Questions have been raised however about the physiological normality of the protein-depleted state and it is generally considered that the use of protein-free diets leads to lowered ileal endogenous nitrogen flows compared with protein-containing diets (Moughan et al., 2005). Also, the absence of protein in the diet can induce enhanced gut-endogenous losses of the amino acid proline.

14.3.2.2 Enzyme hydrolysed protein/ ultrafiltration method

The enzyme-hydrolysed protein method, sometimes referred to as the peptide alimentation method, was proposed by Moughan et al. (1990). It allows endogenous ileal nitrogen and amino acid flows to be determined in subjects fed a diet containing dietary peptides and free amino acids as the sole source of nitrogen. Usually, the subject or animal is fed an enzymatically hydrolysed casein (EHC)-based diet, containing a mixture of free amino acids and oligopeptides with no peptides being larger than 5000 Da, and thus simulating the products of gastric digestion. Digesta are collected from the terminal ileum and first centrifuged and then physically ultrafiltered, thus removing any material with a molecular weight lower than the filtration cut-off of 10,000 Da. This removes any undigested dietary peptides and free amino acids. The high molecular weight fraction (>10,000 Da) contains the endogenous material. An advantage of the peptide alimentation method over several other methods used to determine endogenous flows is that it allows the endogenous flows of total nitrogen and all amino acids to be determined directly.

With the peptide alimentation method, however, there may be some loss of small peptides and free amino acids of endogenous origin when the ultrafiltrate is discarded, leading to an underestimation of the total endogenous amino acid flow. Such underestimation is considered to be of a relatively small magnitude. The method has been criticized by some workers as leading potentially to inflated estimates of endogenous loss, as the hydrolysed casein may present a higher concentration of bioactive peptides to the gut lumen than would occur with the natural digestion of the parent casein. Further, the extent of hydrolysis of the casein hydrolysate may affect the outcome. A critical assumption with the enzymatically hydrolysed protein method is that the hydrolysed protein source, as fed, simulates the products of gastric digestion. Recent experimental findings with the laboratory rat and adult human (Deglaire *et al.*, 2008) suggest that the latter concerns are unfounded, with the administration of an extensively hydrolysed casein leading to similar endogenous ileal amino acid and nitrogen flows as found when intact casein was given. The enzymatically hydrolysed protein method allows the determination of endogenous nitrogen and amino acid flows associated with the ingestion of peptide-containing dry matter, under seemingly physiologically normal conditions. Dietary factors such as antinutritional factors (ANF) and fibre will lead to enhanced endogenous amino acid excretions above the basal level determined with this method. The effects of these factors cannot be readily determined using the enzymatically hydrolysed protein method, other than using purified diets and isolated ANF and fibre sources.

14.3.2.3 Isotope dilution

The use of stable isotopes allows determination of the endogenous nitrogen at the terminal ileum while the subject is fed a diet containing protein or peptides. Either the subject's body nitrogen pool or the food protein may be labelled, but in human studies it has been more common to label the food source. Use of the stable isotope of nitrogen (^{15}N) has been particularly popular. The technique has been used in animal studies and with humans (Mahé *et al.*, 1994) and over the years the spectrum of ^{15}N-labelled proteins has increased greatly.

When the food proteins are labelled, it is assumed that the labelled and unlabelled food amino acids are absorbed equally, and that endogenous nitrogen secreted into the gut during digestion does not become labelled to a significant extent during the course of the experiment. Leterme *et al.* (1996) have reported, however, that a proportion of the absorbed labelled dietary amino acids is rapidly synthesized into body protein and resecreted as gut-endogenous proteins. This will lead to an underestimation of the endogenous loss value. In more recent work with the growing pig and adult human (Deglaire, 2008), the extent of recycling of the dietary ^{15}N label has been determined. Some 10–20% of ileal endogenous protein was ^{15}N-labelled due to tracer recycling, contributing to a likely underestimation of endogenous ileal nitrogen flow of around 6–13%.

The ^{15}N isotope dilution method is a valuable method for determining gut-endogenous protein flows and in particular for allowing study of the relative *in situ* effects of dietary factors such as plant fibre and ANF that influence the recovery of endogenous protein in ileal digesta.

14.4 Determined Estimates of Endogenous Ileal Nitrogen and Amino Acid Losses in Humans

A number of studies using either the isotope dilution method (^{15}N-labelled diet), the enzyme hydrolysed protein ultrafiltration method, or

Table 14.2. Mean estimates[a] of endogenous ileal nitrogen flow in the adult human.

Endogenous loss	Methodology Digesta collection	Nitrogen flow (mg d^{-1})	Study reference
Protein-free	Ileostomate	836	Rowan et al. (1993)
Protein-free	Ileostomate	719	Fuller et al. (1994)
Protein-free	Ileostomate	845	Moughan et al. (2005)
Hydrolysed protein/ ultrafiltration	Ileostomate	1736	Moughan et al. (2005)
Isotope dilution (^{15}N milk protein)	Naso-ileal intubation	1638	Gaudichon et al. (2002)
Isotope dilution (^{15}N casein)	Naso-ileal intubation	2184	Deglaire (2008)
Isotope dilution (^{15}N hydrolysed casein)	Naso-ileal intubation	1851	Deglaire (2008)

Overall mean (protein-free) = 800 mg d^{-1}.
Overall mean (protein or peptides) = 1852 mg d^{-1}.
[a]Some data were initially reported in units of mg 8h^{-1}. The experimental meal was then assumed to represent one third of the daily food intake, and gut-endogenous flows were assumed to be constant over 24 h.

the protein-free diet approach have been conducted with human subjects. In some cases the cooperation of ileostomates has been sought, whereas in other studies the naso-ileal intubation method has been applied. Data from these studies, for estimates of endogenous nitrogen flow at the terminal ileum, are presented in Table 14.2. There is good agreement between the three protein-free values and the four protein/peptide values, respectively. It is clear that there is a significant effect of dietary protein or peptides, with the proteinaceous estimates being at least double those determined using a protein-free diet. Information on endogenous ileal amino acid flows in humans determined under proteinaceous feeding conditions is also available in the literature (e.g. Gaudichon et al., 2002; Moughan et al., 2005; Deglaire, 2008).

An informative study on the proteinaceous components of terminal ileal digesta collected from the growing pig has been published recently (Miner-Williams et al., 2009). A surprisingly large fraction of the total protein in the digesta appears to be bacterial protein (60.9%), with cellular protein contributing 6.7%, soluble free protein 18.2%, and mucin protein 14.1%.

14.5 Factors Influencing Endogenous Ileal Amino Acid Losses

The secretion of endogenous protein into the digestive tract and its subsequent digestion and reabsorption are influenced by a number of factors both related to the subject (e.g. body weight) but especially to the diet. Most studies investigating the influence of dietary factors on endogenous ileal nitrogen and amino acid flow conducted to date have used animals, and such studies have been the subject of review (Boisen and Moughan, 1996; Nyachoti et al., 1997). It seems that dietary dry matter intake, protein content, dietary fibre (amount and type), and the presence of ANF (e.g. lectins, tannins and enzyme inhibitors) can significantly influence the endogenous amino acid flow at the terminal ileum. This has particular implications for developing countries where foods such as cereals, starchy roots, legumes, and pulses make up a disproportionate contribution to the total daily protein supply. The latter types of food contain plant fibre, and may contain ANF, both of which may increase metabolic losses of amino acids from the body and lead either directly or indirectly to lowered digestibility and bioavailability of the dietary amino acids.

14.6 Practical Relevance of Measures of Endogenous Ileal Nitrogen

14.6.1 Metabolic cost

The gut is a highly active organ metabolically, and the synthesis and excretion of endogenous protein makes a significant contribution to overall gut and therefore body metabolism. Gut-endogenous amino acid losses contribute to maintenance amino acid and energy requirements, and also to the efficiency of utilization of dietary amino acids for body protein retention. A higher production of endogenous protein in the digestive tract caused by dietary factors (e.g. fibre, ANF), will be accompanied by a higher rate of gut protein turnover, an increased transport of nutrients and rate of blood flow through the intestinal tissue, and therefore increased energy expenditure. It is known that higher intakes of dietary protein are associated with higher flows of endogenous protein at the terminal ileum (Hodgkinson et al., 2000; Hodgkinson and Moughan, 2007), which in turn implies higher rates of gut metabolic activity and energy expenditure. This is one of several reasons why high protein diets may support body weight loss.

Zebrowska and Kowalczyk (2000) have calculated that for a 30 kg body weight pig, gut protein synthesis accounts for some 8% of the total maintenance energy requirement. Nyachoti et al. (1997) calculated that the energy cost of synthesizing endogenous gut proteins in a 13 kg body weight pig ranged from 6% to 13% of the maintenance energy requirement, dependent upon dietary composition. The gastrointestinal tract is estimated to account for around 25% of total body oxygen consumption in the 3.5 month old pig (Yen et al., 1989). There is no doubt, therefore, that gut-endogenous amino acid losses, which are highly variable and dependent upon a number of dietary factors, can have a significant bearing on the maintenance energy requirement. This often goes unrecognized.

It has also been reported that gut-secreted proteins may account for as much as 25% of total daily body protein synthesis (Simon et al., 1983) and that gut-endogenous amino acid losses are the single most important factor contributing to the maintenance amino acid requirement (de Lange et al., 1995).

14.6.2 Contribution to amino acid requirement

How important are the gut-endogenous amino acid losses as contributors to the daily amino acid requirement of the adult human?

In a paper presented at the 18th International Congress of Nutrition, Moughan (2005) attempted to calculate the contribution of the gut losses for the two dietary essential amino acids, lysine and threonine. Current best estimates for ileal endogenous lysine and threonine losses for the adult human consuming a normal protein-containing diet were taken to be 657 and 960 mg kg^{-1} food dry matter intake, respectively. These values were increased by around 10% to allow for hindgut-endogenous losses (estimates in the literature suggest that hindgut protein loss is 10% of that in the foregut) to give values of 723 and 1056 mg kg^{-1} food dry matter intake, respectively, for the endogenous losses over the total digestive tract. It was assumed that the amino acid compositions of the hindgut and foregut losses are similar. Data presented by Schulze (1994) were used to allow calculation of the effect of dietary fibre. It was assumed that a 1 g kg^{-1} increase in dietary neutral detergent fibre (NDF) would lead to a 0.22% increase in endogenous ileal protein excretion (Tamminga et al., 1995). The latter authors assuming calculated endogenous N losses of 0.04 and 15g per g diet fibre or tannin, respectively.

The calculated total gut-endogenous lysine and threonine flows are given in Table 14.3 and highlight how factors such as daily food dry matter intake and dietary composition (in this case plant fibre) can greatly influence gut amino acid losses and thus the daily amino acid requirement. The daily amino acid requirement is not a constant. The highest predicted gut lysine loss presented in Table 14.3 accounts for some 73% of the stated daily requirement value for lysine in the adult (FAO et al., 1985) and some 29% of the more recent MIT estimated requirement value (see Waterlow, 1996). The highest predicted threonine loss exceeds the corresponding requirement value (FAO et al., 1985) and, in line with the high concentration of threonine in digesta, is 86% of the MIT estimate. The gut-endogenous amino acid losses clearly make a significant contribution to the daily amino acid requirement.

A similar analysis has been conducted by Gaudichon et al. (2002) who concluded that amino acid losses at the terminal ileum of the adult human are substantial and depend on the type of protein ingested. Their estimates of endogenous amino acid loss made up a substantial proportion of current estimates of the daily amino acid requirement for adult humans.

14.6.3 True ileal amino acid digestibility

It is now widely accepted that for simple stomached animals including humans, the digestibility of dietary protein and amino acids should be determined based on the collection of ileal digesta (terminal ileum) rather than faeces (Moughan, 2003). Faecal amino acid digestibility values may be quite misleading, either overestimating (usually the case) or underestimating digestibility. When digestibility is determined at the end of the small intestine, however, it needs to be recognized that the digesta contain large quantities of endogenous amino acids and nitrogen, and ideally this should be corrected for when determining digestibility.

If total amino acids in ileal digesta are simply deducted from the dietary amino acids ingested, 'apparent' estimates of digestibility are obtained. Apparent estimates of digestibility are strongly influenced by the protein content of the test diet, and can thus be misleading. 'True' estimates of amino acid digestibility (i.e. corrected for the endogenous amino acid component), however, are independent of the dietary protein concentration and are a fundamental property of the food itself. True digestibility is a superior measure for determining the dietary amino acids that are absorbed from the gut.

It is particularly important when determining the protein digestibility–corrected amino acid score (PDCAAS) for human foods that standardized true digestibility coefficients be used, otherwise significant unintended biases may occur.

A range of true ileal protein digestibility values for humans is given in Table 14.4. Protein and amino acid digestibility can vary widely. Most ileal protein digestibility values in humans to date have been determined on

Table 14.3. Influence of food dry matter intake and high and low dietary fibre contents on the predicted endogenous lysine and threonine losses (mg kg^{-1} bodyweight d^{-1}) from the total digestive tract in adult 70 kg body weight humans.

	Low DMI[a] (350 g d^{-1})		High DMI (700 g d^{-1})	
	Low fibre (0% NDF)[b]	High fibre (10% NDF)	Low fibre (0% NDF)	High fibre (10% NDF)
Lysine	3.6	4.4	7.2	8.8
Threonine	5.3	6.4	10.6	12.9

[a]DMI, dry matter intake.
[b]NDF, neutral detergent fibre.

Table 14.4. Selected values for the true ileal digestibility of dietary nitrogen in humans.

	Protein source							
	Raw egg[a]	Rapeseed isolate[b]	Peas[c]	Lupins[c]	Soya-protein isolate[c]	Cooked egg[a]	Cow's milk[c]	Casein[d]
True ileal digestibility (%)	51.3	87.1	89.4	91.0	91.0	90.9	95.5	97.6

[a]Evenepoel et al. (1998).
[b]Bos et al. (2007).
[c]Gausserès et al. (1997); Bos et al. (1999); Mariotti et al. (1999, 2002).
[d]Deglaire et al. (2009).

Table 14.5. Gross lysine and true ileal digestible lysine contents (g kg^{-1}) of four types of breakfast cereal[a].

Cereal product	Lysine	
	Gross	Digestible[b]
Wheat-based (shredded)	1.74	0.8
Corn-based (flaked)	0.45	0.2
Rice-based (puffed)	1.22	0.6
Mixed-cereal (rolled)	3.65	1.9

[a]Adapted from Rutherfurd et al. (2006).
[b]Based on a digestibility value (laboratory rat) determined using reactive lysine values in diet, ileal digesta, and ileal endogenous protein.

relatively well digested foods. In developing countries, where less-refined cereals and grain legumes are used as major sources of protein, much lower values for true digestibility can be expected (Sarwar Gilani et al., 2005).

Many foods consumed by humans have been processed, including thermal processing, and during processing amino acids can undergo structural changes rendering them less digestible and also lowering their availability. Lysine, often the first-limiting amino acid, is particularly susceptible to damage. By way of example, the data given in Table 14.5 for cereal products show that lysine availability can be greatly affected by processing. These results imply a major extent of damage to lysine in what are staple foods commonly consumed by both adults and children. In some cases more than half of the lysine in the food, usually considered to be nutritionally available, is unavailable, largely due to the formation of Maillard and Maillard-like complexes. The latter data highlight the crucial need to have better information on the digestibility of amino acids in human foods. Such decreases in nutritional value have important consequences for the assessment of diets in the developing world where dietary protein and lysine intakes may be marginal.

14.7 Conclusions

The amounts of endogenous nitrogen entering the human digestive tract are substantial, and gut protein turnover makes a significant contribution to total body metabolism. In particular the energetic costs associated with the synthesis and secretion of the various proteins makes up a significant proportion of the maintenance energy requirement.

Whereas much of the material entering the gut is digested with the amino acids being absorbed, relatively large amounts of undigested endogenous amino acids are found at the terminal ileum along with undigested dietary amino acids. The loss of these endogenous amino acids into the colon, with subsequent catabolism by the colonic microbes, represents a loss of amino acids from the body which needs to be replaced. The endogenous amino acid flow at the terminal ileum, therefore, is an important measure in terms of the daily amino acid requirement.

Moreover, as the terminal ileal amino acid flow is highly variable, dependent upon a number of dietary influences, this implies that the daily amino acid requirement is also variable and strongly influenced by dietary habit.

It is also important to have accurate estimates of endogenous ileal amino acids to allow the correction of 'apparent' amino acid digestibility to 'true' digestibility. True amino acid digestibility varies among food sources, with vegetable proteins generally having a lower digestibility than animal proteins. Vegetable proteins, containing fibre and sometimes containing active ANF, also induce higher losses of endogenous amino acids at the terminal ileum. Amino acid digestibility, and particularly that of lysine, may be especially impaired in proteins that have been heat-treated during processing.

Traditionally protein digestibility in human foods has been based on a faecal digestibility assay. This approach, however, is known to be flawed, and true ileal amino acid digestibility represents a considerable step forward in dietary protein quality evaluation.

There is a general lack of information on ileal endogenous amino acid flow in humans and on the true ileal digestibility of amino acids in diverse foods. Particularly lacking is sound information on true ileal amino acid digestibility in proteinaceous foods commonly consumed in developing countries.

For the gut-endogenous amino acid losses, studies with humans are required to determine the relationship between ileal endogenous amino acid loss and food dry-matter intake, and to elucidate how these losses are affected by variables such as body weight, age, and physiological state. There is virtually no information available from studies in humans on the effects of plant fibre and various ANF on ileal amino acid flow. Also, the contribution that the hindgut tissue itself makes to endogenous amino acid losses in humans is unknown.

Over recent years, it has become evident that gut microbes can synthesize essential amino acids, which are absorbed and available for metabolism. It is unclear, however, as to what source of material the microbes utilize for such synthesis, and whether the microbial synthesis represents a meaningful net contribution to the host's amino acid supply. This is an area that requires further elucidation.

Finally, it is doubtful, at least in the foreseeable future, that true ileal amino acid digestibility measures will be made on a routine basis with human subjects. This necessitates adoption of an animal model for humans, and in this context the growing pig has a number of advantages. Predictive equations, relating amino acid digestibility for a wide range of foods in humans with that in the pig, would be particularly valuable. At the moment there is only a limited set of published observations of digestibility in the two species.

References

Boisen, S. and Moughan, P.J. (1996) Dietary influences on endogenous ileal protein and amino acid loss in the pig – A Review. *Acta Agriculturae Scandinavica* 46, 154–164.

Bos, C., Mahé, S., Gaudichon, C., Benamouzig, R., Gausserès, N., Luengo, C., Ferrière, F., *et al.* (1999) Assessment of net postprandial protein utilization of ^{15}N-labelled milk nitrogen in human subjects. *British Journal of Nutrition* 81, 221–226.

Bos, C., Airinei, G., Mariotti, F., Benamouzig, R., Bérot, S., Evrard, J., Fénart, E., *et al.* (2007) The poor digestibility of rapeseed protein is balanced by its very high metabolic utilization in humans. *Journal of Nutrition* 137, 594–600.

Chacko, A. and Cummings, J.H. (1988) Nitrogen losses from the human small bowel: obligatory losses and the effect of physical form of food. *Gut* 29, 809–815.

Christl, S.U. and Scheppach, W. (1997) Metabolic consequences of total colectomy. *Scandinavian Journal of Gastroenterology Supplement* 222, 20–24.

Deglaire, A. (2008) Gut endogenous protein flows and postprandial metabolic utilization of dietary amino acids in simple-stomached animals and humans. PhD Thesis, Massey University, Palmerston North, New Zealand.

Deglaire, A., Moughan P.J., Bos, C., Petzke, K., Rutherfurd, S.M. and Tomé, D. (2008) A casein hydrolysate does not enhance gut endogenous protein flows compared with intact casein when fed to growing rats. *Journal of Nutrition* 138, 556–561.

Deglaire, A., Bos, C., Tomé, D. and Moughan, P.J. (2009) Ileal digestibility of dietary protein in the growing pig and adult human. *British Journal of Nutrition* 102, 1752–1759.

de Lange, C.F.M., Mohn, S. and Nyachoti, C.M. (1995) Partitioning of protein and energy intake in grower-finisher pigs. In: Ivan, M. (ed.) *Animal Science Research and Development: Moving Towards a New Century.* Canadian Society of Animal Science, Ottawa, Canada, pp. 339–360.

Evenepoel, P., Geypens, B., Luypaerts, A., Hiele, M., Ghoos, Y. and Rutgeerts, P. (1998) Digestibility of cooked and raw egg protein in humans as assessed by stable isotope techniques. *Journal of Nutrition* 128, 1716–1722.

FAO, WHO, and UNU (1985) Energy and protein requirements. *Report of a Joint FAO/WHO/UNU Expert Consultation.* World Health Organization Technical Report Series 724, World Health Organization, Geneva, Switzerland.

FAO, WHO, and UNU (2007) Protein and amino acid requirements in human nutrition. *Report of a Joint FAO/WHO/UNU Expert Consultation.* WHO Technical Report Series 935, World Health Organization, Geneva, Switzerland.

Fuller, M.F., Milne, A., Harris, C.I., Reid, T.M. and Keenan, R. (1994) Amino acid losses in ileostomy fluid on a protein-free diet. *American Journal of Clinical Nutrition* 59, 70–73.

Gaudichon, C., Bos, C., Morens, C., Petzke, K.J., Mariotti, F., Everwand, J., Benamouzig, R., et al. (2002). Ileal losses of nitrogen and amino acids in humans and their importance to the assessment of amino acid requirements. *Gastroenterology* 123, 50–59.

Gausserès, N., Mahé, S., Benamouzig, R., Luengo, C., Ferrière, F., Rautureau, J. and Tomé, D (1997) [^{15}N]-labelled pea flour protein nitrogen exhibits good ileal digestibility and postprandial retention in humans. *Journal of Nutrition* 127, 1160–1165.

Gorbach, S.L., Nahas, L., Weinstein, L., Levitan, R. and Patterson, J.F. (1967) Studies of intestinal microflora. IV. The microflora of ileostomy effluent: A unique microbial ecology. *Gastroenterology* 53, 874–880.

Hodgkinson, S.M. and Moughan, P.J. (2007) An effect of dietary protein content on endogenous ileal lysine flow in the growing rat. *Journal of the Science of Food and Agriculture* 87, 233–238.

Hodgkinson, S.M., Moughan, P.J., Reynolds, G.W. and James, K.A.C. (2000) The effect of dietary peptide concentration on endogenous ileal amino acid loss in the growing pig. *British Journal of Nutrition* 83, 421–430.

Johansson, C. (1975) Studies of gastrointestinal interactions. VII Characteristics of the absorption pattern of sugar, fat and protein from composite meals in man. A quantitative study. *Scandinavian Journal of Gastroenterology* 10, 33–42.

Krawielitzki, K., Zebrowska, T., Schadereit, R., Kowalczyk, J., Hennig, U., Wunsche, J. and Herrmann, U. (1990) Determining of nitrogen absorption and nitrogen secretion in different sections of the pig's intestine by digesta exchange between ^{15}N-labelled and unlabelled animals. *Archiv fur Tierernahrung* 40, 25–37.

Leterme, P., Théwis, A., Francois, E., van Weerden, P., Wathelet, B. and Huisman, J. (1996) The use of ^{15}N-labelled dietary proteins for determining true ileal amino acid digestibilities is limited by their rapid recycling in the endogenous secretions of pigs. *Journal of Nutrition* 126, 2188–2198.

Mahé, S., Fauquant, J., Gaudichon, C., Roos, N., Maubois, J.L. and Tomé, D. (1994) 15N-labelling and preparation of milk, casein and whey proteins. *Lait* 74, 307–312.

Mariotti, F., Mahé, S., Benamouzig, R., Luengo, C., Daré, S., Gaudichon, C. and Tomé, D. (1999) Nutritional value of [^{15}N]-soy protein isolate assessed from ileal digestibility and postprandial protein utilisation in humans. *Journal of Nutrition* 129, 1992–1997.

Mariotti, F., Pueyo, M.E., Tomé, D. and Mahé, S. (2002) The bioavailability and postprandial utilization of sweet lupin (Lupinus albus) – flour protein is similar to that of purified soyabean protein in human subjects: a study using intrinsically ^{15}N-labelled proteins. *British Journal of Nutrition* 87, 315–323.

McNeil, N.I. (1988) Nutritional implications of human and mammalian large intestinal function. *World Review of Nutrition and Dietetics* 56, 1–42.

Miner-Williams, W., Moughan, P.J. and Fuller, M.F. (2009) Endogenous components of digesta protein from the terminal ileum of pigs for a casein-based diet. *Journal of Agricultural and Food Chemistry* 57, 2072–2078.

Modigliani, R., Rambaud, J.C. and Bernier, J.J. (1973) The method of intraluminal perfusion of the human small intestine. I. Principle and technique. *Digestion* 9, 176–192.

Moughan, P.J. (2003) Amino acid availability: Aspects of chemical analysis and bioassay methodology. *Nutrition Research Reviews* 16, 127–141.

Moughan, P.J. (2005) Physiological processes underlying the dietary amino acid requirements in humans. The role of the gut. In: Vorster, H.H., Blaauw, R., Dhansay, M.A., Kuzwayo, P.M.N., Moeng, L. and Wentzel-Viljoen, E. (eds) *Proceedings of the 18th International Congress of Nutrition*. Durban, South Africa, 10 pp.

Moughan, P.J., Darragh, A.J., Smith, W.C. and Butts, C.A. (1990) Perchloric and trichloroacetic acids as precipitants of protein in endogenous ileal digesta from the rat. *Journal of the Science of Food and Agriculture* 52, 13–21.

Moughan, P.J., Birtles, M.J., Cranwell, P.D., Smith, W.C. and Pedraza, M. (1992). The piglet as a model animal for studying aspects of digestion and absorption in milk-fed human infants. *World Review of Nutrition and Dietetics* 67, 40–113.

Moughan, P.J., Cranwell, P.D., Darragh, A.J. and Rowan, A.M. (1994) The domestic pig as a model animal for studying digestion in humans. In: Souffrant, W.B. and Hagemeister, H. (eds) *Proceedings of the 6th International Symposium on Digestive Physiology in Pigs*. EAAP, Bad Doberan, Germany, pp. 389–396.

Moughan, P.J., Souffrant, W.B. and Hodgkinson, S.M. (1998) Physiological approaches to determining gut endogenous amino acid flows in the mammal. *Archives of Animal Nutrition* 51, 237–252.

Moughan, P.J., Butts, C.A., Rowan, A.M. and Deglaire, A. (2005) Dietary peptides increase endogenous amino acid losses from the gut in adults. *American Journal of Clinical Nutrition* 81, 1359–1365.

Nasset, E.S. (1965) Role of the digestive system in protein metabolism. *Federation Proceedings* 24, 953–958.

Nixon, S.E. and Mawer G.E. (1970) The digestion and absorption of protein in man. 1. The site of absorption. *British Journal of Nutrition* 24, 227–240.

Nyachoti, C.M., de Lange, C.F.M., McBride, B.W. and Schulze, H. (1997) Significance of endogenous gut nitrogen losses in the nutrition of growing pigs: A review. *Canadian Journal of Animal Science* 77, 149–163.

Rowan, A.M., Moughan, P.J. and Wilson M.N. (1993) Endogenous amino acid flow at the terminal ileum of adult humans determined following the ingestion of a single protein-free meal. *Journal of the Science of Food and Agriculture* 61, 439–442.

Rowan, A.M., Moughan, P.J., Wilson, M.N., Maher, K. and Tasman-Jones, C. (1994) Comparison of the ileal and faecal digestibility of dietary amino acids in adult humans and evaluation of the pig as a model animal for digestion studies in man. *British Journal of Nutrition* 71, 29–42.

Rutherfurd, S.M., Torbatinejad, N.M., and Moughan, P.J. (2006) Available (ileal digestible reactive) lysine in selected cereal-based food products. *Journal of Agricultural and Food Chemistry* 54, 9453–9457.

Sawar Gilani, G., Cockell, K.A. and Sepehr, E. (2005) Effects of antinutritional factors on protein digestibility and amino acid availability in foods. *Journal of AOAC International* 88, 967–987.

Schedl, H.P. and Clifton, J.A. (1961) Kinetics of intestinal absorption in man: Normal subjects and patients with sprue. *Journal of Clinical Investigation* 40, 1079–1080

Schulze, H. (1994) Endogenous ileal nitrogen losses in pigs. PhD thesis, Wageningen University, the Netherlands, 147 pp.

Simon, O., Zebrowska, T., Bergner, H. and Munchmeyer, R. (1983) Investigation on the pancreatic and stomach secretion in pigs by means of continuous infusion of ^{14}C-amino acids. *Archives of Animal Nutrition* 33, 9–12.

Souffrant, W.B., Rérat, A., Laplace, J.P., Darcy-Vrillon, B., Kohler, R., Corring, T. and Gebhardt, G. (1993) Exogenous and endogenous contributions to nitrogen fluxes in the digestive tract of pigs fed a casein diet. III Recycling of endogenous nitrogen. *Reproduction Nutrition Development* 33, 373–382.

Tamminga, S., Schulze, H., Van Bruchem, J. and Huisman, J. (1995) The nutritional significance of endogenous N-losses along the gastro-intestinal tract of farm animals. *Archives of Animal Nutrition* 48, 9–22.

Waterlow, J.C. (1996) The requirements of adult man for indispensible amino acids. *European Journal of Clinical Nutrition* 50, 5151–5179.

Wrong, O.M, Edmonds, C.J. and Chadwick, V.S. (1981) *The Large Intestine: Its Role in Mammalian Nutrition and Homeostasis.* MTP Press Ltd, Lancaster, UK.

Yen, J.T., Neinaber, J.A., Hill, D.A. and Pond, W. (1989) Oxygen consumption by portal vein-drained organs and by whole animal in conscious growing swine. *Proceedings of the Society for Experimental Biology and Medicine* 190, 393–398.

Zebrowska, T. and Kowalczyk, J. (2000) Endogenous nitrogen losses in monogastrics and ruminants as affected by nutritional factors. *Asian-Australasian Journal of Animal Science* 13, 210–218.

15 Metabolic Availability of Amino Acids in Food Proteins: New Methodology

C.L. Levesque,[1]* R. Elango[2,3] and R.O. Ball[4,5]

[1]*Department of Animal and Poultry Science, Guelph, Canada;* [2]*Child & Family Research Institute, BC Children's Hospital, Vancouver, Canada;* [3]*Department of Pediatrics, Division of Gastroenterology, Hepatology and Nutrition, University of British Columbia, Vancouver, Canada;* [4]*Department of Agricultural, Food & Nutritional Sciences, University of Alberta, Edmonton, Canada;* [5]*Department of Nutritional Sciences, University of Toronto, Toronto, Canada*

15.1 Abstract

Protein quality is a term used to describe the capacity of food proteins to meet the amino acid requirement estimates for humans. It is a measure of the nutritional value of food protein sources which depends on the concentration and balance of amino acids and on the digestibility and availability of the food protein for metabolic processes. However, not all foods are equal in their capacity to supply protein and amino acids. The protein digestibility-corrected amino acid score (PDCAAS) was proposed as the method of choice for assessing protein quality in humans. Although it is an improvement over previous methods, the digestibility correction factor used to calculate PDCAAS is based on a rat fecal digestibility model and thus does not account for losses associated with incomplete digestion and absorption, gut endogenous amino acid losses, or absorbed amino acids which are unavailable due to the effect of heat processing and anti-nutritional factors on protein quality. Metabolic availability is a new method for protein quality evaluation utilizing the indicator amino acid oxidation technique. Oxidation of the indicator amino acid is inversely proportional to whole body protein synthesis, and responds rapidly to changes in the bioavailability of amino acids for metabolic processes, and therefore reflects the true metabolic availability (MA) of amino acids. MA is minimally invasive, determined directly in humans, and is based on minimal assumptions which have been validated in animals. It can be used to assess all protein sources, measures the bioavailability of individual amino acids and can be routinely applied in humans. Studies in animals and humans have demonstrated that MA provides an accurate estimate of the protein quality from various protein sources. Practical application of the MA method has the potential to significantly advance protein quality evaluation in humans.

15.2 Introduction

Practical application of amino acid requirement estimates for humans depends on the capacity of food proteins to meet the requirements

* E-mail address: crystal.levesque@uoguelph.ca

(Elango et al., 2009). The protein quality, or capacity of food proteins to meet the amino acid requirements, is a measure of their nutritional value, and this depends on the concentration and balance of amino acids (AA) and on their digestibility and availability for metabolic processes (i.e. growth or maintenance) (Humayun et al., 2007). The measurements of protein quality of food proteins demonstrate that protein sources are not equal in their ability to supply protein and AA (Schaafsma, 2005).

The quality of a protein is primarily determined by the relationship between the pattern of the AA composition of the protein source and the nitrogen and amino acid requirement of the subject (Schaafsma, 2005). Table 15.1 shows the differences in lysine, sulphur AA (methionine and cysteine) and threonine concentration in common foods. Cereals tend to be very low in lysine and threonine content, whereas legumes and animal foods are rich sources of lysine and threonine. Animal foods tend to have greater concentrations of essential AA compared to plant proteins. Peas have a similar lysine and threonine content as found in cereal grain, but are a very poor source of methionine and cystine. Therefore, a combination of protein sources is necessary to meet the daily nitrogen and amino acid requirements.

15.3 Methods to Estimate Protein Quality

Numerous methods have been used to estimate protein quality of food sources (Elango et al., 2009); however, the PDCAAS was proposed as the method of choice for assessing protein quality in humans (FAO, 1991). The PDCAAS is calculated as the proportion of limiting AA from a test protein expressed as a percentage of the content of the same AA in a reference pattern of essential AA, corrected for the digestibility of the test protein as measured in a rat fecal digestibility study (Schaafsma, 2005).

There are a number of limitations with PDCAAS: it utilizes fecal rather than ileal digestibility; it does not account for conditionally indispensable AA, for variations in digestibility between entire protein and individual AA, or for the effect of heat processing and antinutritional factors on digestibility (Elango et al., 2009). Due to these disadvantages of the PDCAAS method, new techniques need to be developed (Elango et al., 2009).

Stable isotope-based methods have the potential to more accurately estimate the nutritional value of food protein sources than PDCAAS. Within the last decade, three new technologies using stable isotope techniques have been developed: net postprandial protein utilization (NPPU) (Gaussères et al., 1997; Bos et al., 1999); postprandial protein utilization (PPU) (Millward et al., 2000, 2002); and MA (Moehn et al., 2005, 2007). Net postprandial protein utilization is calculated as the ileal digestibility of ^{15}N-labelled dietary protein corrected for ^{15}N-labelled AA deaminated in the body nitrogen pool, measured by plasma urea and urinary nitrogen (Gaussères et al., 1997). Although NPPU is a major advancement in protein quality evaluation,

Table 15.1. Concentration of selected amino acids in common food proteins (ISDA/ARS, 2006).

Food	Lysine		Methionine		Cystine		Threonine		Total protein
	g 100g^{-1a}	mg g^{-1b}	g 100g^{-1}	mg g^{-1}	g 100g^{-1}	mg g^{-1}	g 100g^{-1}	mg g^{-1}	g 100g^{-1}
Rice, white	0.258	36	0.168	24	0.146	21	0.255	36	7.1
Wheat flour	0.378	28	0.212	16	0.317	23	0.395	29	13.7
Peas	0.317	59	0.082	25	0.032	6	0.203	38	5.4
Chickpeas	1.291	67	0.253	13	0.259	13	0.716	37	19.3
Soybean, cooked	1.108	67	0.224	14	0.268	16	0.723	44	16.6
Egg, raw	0.914	72	0.380	30	0.272	22	0.556	44	12.6
Chicken, raw	1.818	85	0.592	28	0.274	13	0.904	42	21.4
Beef, raw	1.785	83	0.565	26	0.227	11	0.846	40	21.4

[a]Values are per 100g of food; [b]values are mg g^{-1} protein.

it is limited to foods which can be intrinsically labelled with ^{15}N, requires collection of ileal digesta via naso-intestinal intubation, and does not estimate digestibility of individual AA. These limitations suggest that routine or widespread application of this technique is unlikely. Postprandial protein utilization is expressed in terms of the efficiency of nitrogen utilization, i.e. nitrogen utilization/nitrogen intake (Millward et al., 2002). Nitrogen utilization is determined from leucine utilization (leucine intake minus cumulative leucine oxidation) assuming a leucine:nitrogen ratio of 625 mg g^{-1} nitrogen in body tissue protein. Leucine and nitrogen balances are estimated based on the oxidation of intravenously infused L-[1-^{13}C] leucine, using the cumulative difference between the postabsorptive and fed-state leucine oxidation rates. This method involves several assumptions which have not been validated. Since it is not possible to estimate the proportion of leucine oxidation in the 6 h postprandial period arising from exogenous (dietary) or endogenous sources, the PPU for nitrogen present in the test meal cannot be accurately determined (Kurpad and Young, 2003). Furthermore, the administration route of isotope labelled AA or proteins to estimate digestion and absorption of food proteins should be the same as that of the test protein (i.e. orally) (Ball et al., 1995).

Metabolic availability is determined by measuring the slope of the response (tracer oxidation) when a test protein is consumed, and calculating the ratio of the test response to the slope of the response of a reference protein or free amino acid (Elango et al., 2009). Metabolic availability utilizes the indicator amino acid oxidation (IAAO) technique in a slope ratio assay, which is considered the optimum method or comparison (Levesque et al., 2010). In addition, because the method measures the change in whole-body protein synthesis, it should account for all losses of AA during digestion, absorption, and metabolic utilization (Moehn et al., 2005). Therefore, this method has been called true metabolic bioavailability of AA in food protein. It is based on minimal assumptions which have been validated in animals, can be used to assess all protein sources, and measures bioavailability of individual AA. Metabolic availability is readily adaptable to routine use for evaluation of proteins in human nutrition because it is the least invasive of the new methods, and thus will be the focus of the remainder of this chapter.

15.4 Metabolic Availability of Amino Acids in Food Protein Sources

15.4.1 Concepts of indicator amino acid oxidation

The IAAO method is based on the principle that excess AA cannot be stored, so AA are either utilized for protein synthesis or must be oxidized. Therefore, the change in oxidation of the indicator AA is inversely proportional to the change in protein synthesis (Fig. 15.1) (Ball and Bayley, 1986). When one indispensible AA is deficient for protein synthesis, all other AA are therefore in excess and must be oxidized (Elango et al., 2008b). As the intake of the limiting AA increases, the oxidation of an indicator AA (another indispensible AA, typically [L-^{13}C]phenylalanine) decreases linearly until the requirement for the limiting AA is reached (Pencharz and Ball, 2003). Increases in intake of the test AA beyond the requirement do not increase protein synthesis further, and therefore there is no further change in oxidation of the indicator AA (Fig. 15.1); IAAO reaches a plateau. The inflection point between the linear decrease and plateau in oxidation represents the estimated average requirement (EAR) for the test amino acid and is determined with the use of bi-phase linear regression analysis (Elango et al., 2008a,b).

The IAAO technique has been extensively developed to determine AA requirements and was chosen as the gold standard by the World Health Organization for determination of AA requirements of humans (WHO, 2007; Pencharz and Ball, 2003). Initial development of the IAAO technique was in young pigs using ^{14}C phenylalanine to determine the requirement for histidine (Kim et al., 1983) and tryptophan (Ball and Bayley, 1984a) and was validated against the traditional method of nitrogen balance (Kim et al., 1983). Extensive work followed to adapt the IAAO technique to humans, including the use of stable rather

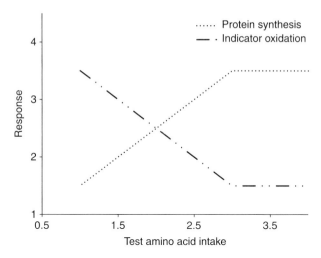

Fig. 15.1. Inverse relationship between protein synthesis and oxidation of an indicator amino acid with increasing intake of limiting amino acid. EAR, estimated average requirement. Adapted from Ball and Bayley (1986).

than radioactive isotope (Zello *et al.*, 1993); the route of isotope administration (intravenous versus oral delivery) (Bross *et al.*, 1998; Kriengsinyos *et al.*, 2002); the time of adaptation required for the level of test AA (Zello *et al.*, 1990, Elango *et al.*, 2009); and the time of adaptation necessary for the level of dietary protein (Thorpe *et al.*, 1999). Thus the current protocol involved a 2 d adaptation to a fixed daily protein intake followed by at least 8 h adaptation to the test AA intake on the day of study (Elango *et al.*, 2008a, 2009). The IAAO technique has been used in the pig model to assess the effect of enteral versus parenteral nutrition on AA requirements (e.g. Bertolo *et al.*, 1998), the development of advanced parenteral nutrition solutions (Brunton *et al.*, 2007), the effect of gut AA utilization on whole body AA requirements (Law *et al.*, 2007, Shoveller *et al.*, 2003), the availability of amino acid supplements (Shoveller *et al.*, 2010) and the inter-animal variability of AA requirements (Bertolo *et al.*, 2005; Moehn *et al.*, 2008).

Indicator AA oxidation relies on selection of an appropriate indicator AA. There are three key criteria when selecting an AA as indicator:

1. a dietary indispensable AA;
2. the labelled carbon is irreversibly lost as CO_2 during oxidation, preferably during the first steps of AA catabolism; and
3. the AA should undergo no other significant reactions apart from oxidation to CO_2 and incorporation into protein (Zello *et al.*, 1995).

Since accurate measurement of label in the free AA pool and the end products of degradation are essential to the oxidation technique, ubiquitously labelled carbon atoms would not be appropriate (Zello *et al.*, 1995). Although lysine (Ball and Bayley, 1984a), threonine (Soliman and King, 1969), [^{14}C-methyl]-methionine (Brookes *et al.*, 1972), and leucine (Kurpad *et al.*, 1998; Hsu *et al.*, 2006) have all been used as indicator AAs, in comparison to phenylalanine these have all been found to be less responsive or less accurate in determining the requirement of the test amino acid. Therefore, L-[1-^{13} or 1-^{14}C]-phenylalanine (Kim *et al.*, 1983; Ball and Bayley, 1984a,b), in the presence of excess tyrosine, has been used most often because it satisfies all three key criteria above. It also has a number of additional advantages: the free pool size is comparatively small, with a rapid turnover rate compared to other indispensable amino acids (Neale and Waterlow, 1974); and the size of the intracellular free phenylalanine pool is tightly regulated (Flaim *et al.*, 1982). Phenylalanine oxidation was more responsive to dietary changes than lysine or leucine (Neale and Waterlow, 1974; Hsu *et al.*, 2006). The advantage of the rapid turnover and small, tightly regulated size of the free phenylalanine pool is that it responds rapidly to changes in test AA intake. Ball and Bayley (1984b) showed in baby pigs that AA requirement could be determined with as little as 4 h of adaptation to the diet. In sows and growing pigs, phenylalanine oxidation responded within 1–2 d of a change in test AA intake, and remained constant for up to 10 d after a change in diet (Moehn et al., 2004). Therefore, 2 d of adaptation to a new dietary test AA level are deemed sufficient. Recently, Elango et al. (2009) showed in humans that the adaptation period to the test AA can be even shorter (~8 h), provided the subjects are adapted to a standard protein intake prior to receiving the test diet.

15.4.2 Application of indicator amino acid oxidation to determine metabolic availability of amino acids in food protein sources

The change in appearance of $^{13}CO_2$ or $^{14}CO_2$ in breath from oxidation of the indicator amino acid reflects the change in whole-body protein synthesis; therefore, the IAAO can be used to determine the MA of AA in foodstuffs. At a given AA intake below requirement, the change in indicator oxidation reflects the response of whole-body protein synthesis to graded levels (or intakes) of the limiting AA (Moehn et al., 2005). This slope indicates the change in IAAO per unit change in limiting AA. A shallower slope indicates that less AA per unit intake is available to support protein synthesis (Fig. 15.2). Therefore, the relative difference in the rate of change (slope) of IAAO between test and reference proteins will be proportional to the whole-body MA of the test AA for protein synthesis. Metabolic availability, therefore, takes into account all losses associated with incomplete digestion and absorption, gut endogenous AA losses, amino acid oxidation and absorbed AA which are unavailable due to anti-nutritional factors, damage caused during heat processing (Maillard reaction compounds), D-amino acids and cross-linked proteins such as lysinoalanine.

The MA method utilizes incremental increases in crystalline test AA to determine the reference slope. The true digestibility of crystalline (free) AA is essentially 100% (Baker, 1992). Thus, the slope of the indicator AA oxidation obtained with the crystalline form of the test AA represents the maximal unit increase in protein synthesis and is equivalent to 100% MA of the test AA. Oxidation of the indicator AA is regressed against the AA intake above that provided by the reference diet, supplied by crystalline test AA, and the protein source (Moehn et al., 2005). The ratio of the slope of the indicator

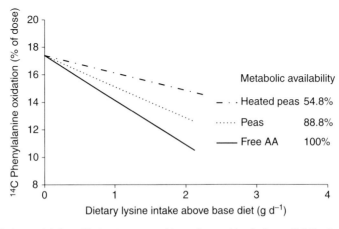

Fig. 15.2. Metabolic availability of lysine in peas and heated peas. Metabolic availability is calculated from the ratio of the slope from the test AA (i.e. peas or heated peas) to the slope of the free AA. Adapted from Moehn et al., 2005.

oxidation due to the test protein source compared to the indicator oxidation slope due to the free AA gives the MA of the food protein.

A number of key criteria must be met when determining MA:

1. the test AA must be first limiting to ensure that the intake of the test AA drives the change in indicator oxidation;
2. the change in indicator oxidation to incremental changes in test AA must be linear to allow calculation of availability; and
3. the observed response must not be influenced by other dietary nutrients in the test feed ingredient (Batterham, 1992; Littell et al., 1995). In addition, when applying the IAAO in a slope-ratio assay, an isotopic steady state must be achieved.

The determination of MA using the slope-ratio assay assumes a linear response to increasing test AA (Batterham, 1992). To ensure a linear response, the upper limit of test AA intake should be below the lower confidence interval of the requirement in every individual (Elango et al., 2009) or ~2 SD below the requirement (Moehn et al., 2005). Limiting the intake of the test amino acid to 2 SD below the animal's requirement ensures that each animal will respond to increasing intake in a linear fashion. If intake were to exceed the requirement, the slope would not be linear because oxidation of the indicator amino acid would be in the plateau phase. Figure 15.3 shows change in indicator oxidation with incremental changes in test AA intake above and below daily intake requirement. At AA intakes at least 2 SD below the daily intake requirement, there is a linear change in indicator oxidation.

One of the advantages of using the indicator amino acid oxidation technique to determine MA of AA in food proteins is the use of repeated measurements within each subject. Each study subjects receives each of a series of four reference diets supplying free test AA (crystalline form) at incremental increases to a maximum of 80% of the EAR of the test AA (Moehn et al., 2005). The reference diets supply all AA, except the test AA, in excess and identical in content to that supplied by the test proteins. Free AA is then replaced by protein-bound AA from the protein source being measured. Again, each subject receives the diet containing the protein-bound AA. The use of repeated measurements within the same subject reduces the effect of individual variability, and increases the sensitivity of the estimate accounting for between-subject variation which can be up to 30% in humans (Zello et al., 1993).

15.4.3 Validation of the metabolic availability method

The initial validation of MA methodology using the IAAO technique was conducted by Moehn et al. (2005) in growing pigs. The MA of lysine from peas and heat-treated peas in growing pigs (15–18 kg) was assessed by comparing the oxidation of the indicator AA to that when pigs were fed crystalline lysine. Replacing the free lysine with equal amounts of protein-bound lysine from peas and heated peas led to a lesser decrease in oxidation than addition of free lysine, as represented by a lower slope (Table 15.2; Fig. 15.2). This indicated an availability of lysine in peas (88.8%) and heated peas (54.8%) for protein synthesis. The MA of lysine in peas was similar to previously published estimates of the true ileal digestibility of lysine in peas (NRC, 1998). Ileal digestibility does not measure the reduction in bioavailability due to heat-damaged AA (Moughan and Rutherford, 2008); however, the MA of lysine in heated peas was comparable to the MA of lysine in similarly heated peas (48%), determined using slope ratio growth assay (van Barneveld et al., 1994). Similarly, Ball et al. (1995) reported impaired lysine availability in heated cottonseed meal, but found similar oxidation responses for lysine in soybean meal and for free lysine. However, in this experiment, the intake of lysine was in excess of the requirement and thus MA could not be calculated.

The MA method has been further validated with other protein sources in growing pigs (Moehn et al., 2007) and pregnant sows (Levesque, 2010) (Table 15.2). Using the method described by Moehn et al. (2005), the MA of

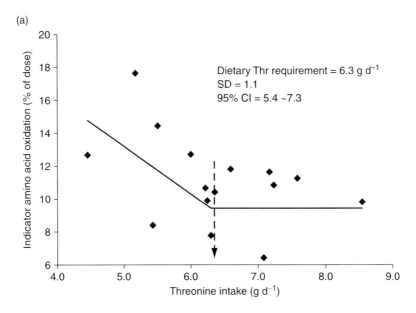

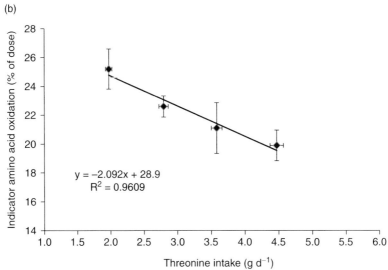

Fig. 15.3. The relationship between indicator amino acid oxidation and incremental increases in dietary threonine. (a) Decrease in indicator oxidation below requirement, plateau in indicator oxidation above daily intake requirement. (b) Linear decrease in indicator oxidation up to ~2 SD below requirement. Adapted from Levesque (2010).

threonine fed to pregnant sows was determined to be 88% in corn and 89.3% in barley. As with that observed for lysine (Moehn et al., 2005), addition of protein-bound threonine from corn or barley resulted in a slower rate of decrease in indicator oxidation than from crystalline threonine. The quality of a protein increases as the AA composition of the protein more closely matches the individual's requirement for different AA (Reeds and Beckett, 1996).

Table 15.2. Metabolic availability of amino acids in common protein sources fed to swine.

Amino acid intake	IAAO response (% of dose g^{-1} amino acid intake)	Metabolic availability (%)
Moehn et al., 2005[a]		
Crystalline lysine	−3.16 ± 0.39	100.0
Raw peas	−2.81 ± 0.44	88.8
Heated peas	−1.73 ± 0.41	54.8
Moehn et al., 2007[b]		
Crystalline lysine	−3.63 ± 0.43	100.0
Soybean meal	−3.18 ± 0.32	87.5
Canola meal	−2.59 ± 0.31	71.4
Cottonseed meal	−2.73 ± 0.38	75.1
Raw peas	−2.75 ± 0.29	75.8
Heated peas	−2.48 ± 0.30	68.3
Heated peas plus free lysine	−2.78 ± 0.27	76.5
Levesque, 2010[c]		
Crystalline threonine	−1.59 ± 0.53	100.0
Corn	−1.40 ± 0.62	88.0
Barley	−1.42 ± 0.81	89.2

[a]Values are mean ± SEM, $n = 4$ growing pigs.
[b]Values are mean ± SEM, $n = 8$ growing pigs.
[c]Values are mean ± SEM, $n = 6$ pregnant sows.

However, the relative requirements for different AA changes with developmental and physiological state, thus the quality of a protein source may not be constant if the physiological state of the animal changes (Reeds and Beckett, 1996). The MA of threonine in corn fed to growing pigs was 82.3%, similar to published estimates of the true ileal digestibility of threonine in corn (NRC, 1998), but lower than the MA of threonine from the same sample of corn when fed to adult sows (Levesque, 2010). Therefore, age appears to have an effect on the availability of AA from food sources in pigs.

The MA method has also been adapted for use in humans and was used to determine the MA of sulphur AA from casein and soy protein isolate (Humayun et al., 2007). Casein and soy protein isolates were tested at 60% of the total sulphur AA requirement. Oxidation of indicator AA when healthy young men were fed casein or soy protein isolate diets supplying 60% of the total sulphur AA requirement was compared to the IAAO response when the same subjects consumed diets supplemented with crystalline methionine. The study was repeated in the same subjects and the MA, unsupplemented and supplemented, respectively, for both casein (90.5 and 90.6%) and soy protein isolate (70.6 and 69.%) were obtained (Humayun et al., 2007). The methods commonly used in animals to determine AA availability are not ethical or applicable to humans and thus there are very few data in humans. The ability to routinely measure AA availability in humans in a non-invasive manner is important because AA availability is not currently used to adjust recommendations for amino acid intake in humans.

Using the IAAO in a slope-ratio assay allows determination of the availability of AA in vivo, and is capable, contrary to digestibility studies, of detecting reduced protein quality of heat-treated food sources. This method can also be used to measure the availability of amino acid supplements (Shoveller et al., 2006, 2010) and to detect differences in availability due to age.

15.5 Conclusions

Nutritional application of amino acid requirement estimates must be combined with an understanding of the capacity of food proteins to meet the amino acid requirements of humans. Although numerous methods for assessing protein quality have been developed, the MA method can be applied for rapid and routine use in humans. The MA method is minimally invasive, can be determined in the subject of interest (i.e. human) and accounts for all losses of AA during digestion, absorption, and metabolic utilization. It is based on minimal assumptions validated in animals, can be used to assess all protein sources, and measures the bioavailability of individual AA. Studies in animals and humans have demonstrated that the MA methodology provides an accurate estimate of the protein quality from various food protein sources.

References

Baker, D.H. (1992) Applications of chemically defined diets to the solution of nutrition problems. *Amino Acids* 2, 1–12.

Ball, R.O. and Bayley, H.S. (1984a) Tryptophan requirement of the 2.5-kg piglet determined by the oxidation of an indicator amino acid. *Journal of Nutrition* 114, 1741–1746.

Ball, R.O. and Bayley, H.S. (1984b) Time course of the total and radioactive carbon dioxide production by piglets receiving dietary [^{14}C]phenylalanine. *Canadian Journal of Physiology and Pharmacology* 63, 1170–1174.

Ball R.O. and Bayley, H.S. (1986) Influence of dietary protein concentration on the oxidation of phenylalanine by the young pig. *British Journal of Nutrition* 55, 651–658.

Ball, R.O., Batterham, E.S. and van Barneveld, R.J. (1995) Lysine oxidation by growing pigs receiving diets containing free and protein-bound lysine. *Journal of Animal Science* 73, 785–792.

Batterham, E.S. (1992) Availability and utilization of amino acids for growing pigs. *Nutrition Research Reviews*, 5, 1–18.

Bertolo, R.F.P., Chen, C.Z.L., Law, G., Pencharz, P.B. and Ball, R.O. (1998) Threonine requirement of neonatal piglets receiving total parenteral nutrition is considerably lower than that of piglets receiving an identical diet intragastrically. *Journal of Nutrition* 128, 1752–1759.

Bertolo, R.F., Moehn, S., Pencharz, P.B. and Ball, R.O. (2005) Estimate of the variability of the lysine requirement of growing pigs using the IAAO technique. *Journal of Animal Science* 83, 2535–2542.

Bos, C., Mahé, S., Gaudichon, C., Benamouzig, R., Gausserès, N., Luengo, C., Ferrière, F., *et al.* (1999) Assessment of net postprandial protein utilization of ^{15}N-labelled milk nitrogen in human subjects. *British Journal of Nutrition* 81, 221–226.

Brookes, I.M., Owens, F.N. and Garrigus, U.S. (1972) Influence on amino acid level in the diet upon amino acid oxidation by the rat. *Journal of Nutrition* 102, 27–36.

Bross, R., Ball, R.O. and Pencharz, P.B. (1998) Development of a minimally invasive protocol for the determination of phenylalanine and lysine kinetics in humans during the fed state. *Journal of Nutrition* 128, 1913–1919.

Brunton, J.A., Shoveller, A.K., Pencharz, P.B. and Ball, R.O. (2007) The indicator amino acid oxidation method identified limiting amino acids in two parenteral nutrition solutions in neonatal pigs. *Journal of Nutrition* 137, 1253–1259.

Elango, R., Ball, R.O. and Pencharz, P.B. (2008a) Individual amino acid requirement in humans: an update. *Current Opinions in Clinical Nutrition and Metabolic Care* 11, 34–39.

Elango, R., Ball, R.O. and Pencharz, P.B. (2008b) Indicator amino acid oxidation: concept and application. *Journal of Nutrition* 138, 243–246.

Elango, R., Ball, R.O. and Pencharz, P.B. (2009) Amino acid requirements in humans: with special emphasis on the metabolic availability of amino acids. *Amino Acids* 37, 19–27.

FAO (1991) Protein quality evaluation in human diets. *Report of a Joint FAO/WHO Expert Consultation*. FAO Food and Nutrition Paper 51, FAO, Rome.

Flaim, K.E., Peavy, D.E., Everson, W.V. and Jefferson, L.S. (1982) The role of amino acids in the regulation of protein synthesis in perfused rat liver. I. Reduction in rates of synthesis resulting from amino acid deprivation and recovery during flow-through perfusion. *Journal of Biological Chemistry* 257, 2932–2938

Gausserès, N., Mahé, S., Benamouzig, R., Luengo, C., Ferrière, F., Rautureau, J. and Tomè, D. (1997) [^{15}N]-labeled pea flour protein nitrogen exhibits good ileal digestibility and postprandial retention in humans. *Journal of Nutrition* 127, 1160–1165.

Hsu, J.W., Kriengsinyos, W., Wykes, L.J., Rafii, M., Goonewardene, L.A., Ball, R.O. and Pencharz, P.B. (2006) Leucine is not a good choice as an indicator for determining amino acid requirements in men. *Journal of Nutrition* 136, 958–964.

Humayan, M.A., Elango, R., Moehn, S., Ball, R.O. and Pencharz, P.B. (2007) Application of the indicator amino acid oxidation technique for the determination of metabolic availability of sulfur amino acids from casein versus soy protein isolate in adult men. *Journal of Nutrition* 137, 1874–1879.

ISDA/ARS (2006) Composition of foods: raw, processed, prepared. *USDA National Nutrient Database for Standard Reference*, US Department of Agriculture, Agricultural Research Service, Beltville, MA.

Kim, K.I., Elliott, J.I. and Bayley, H.S. (1983) Oxidation of an indicator amino acid by young pigs receiving diets with varying levels of lysine of threonine, and an assessment of amino acid requirements. *British Journal of Nutrition* 50, 383–390.

Kriengsinyos, W., Rafii, M., Wykes, L.J., Ball, R.O. and Pencharz, P.B. (2002) Long-term effects of histidine depletion on whole-body protein metabolism in healthy adults. *Journal of Nutrition* 132, 3340–3348.

Kurpad, A.V. and Young, V.R. (2003) What is apparent is not always real: lessons from lysine requirement studies in adult humans. *Journal of Nutrition* 133, 1227–1230.

Kurpad, A.V., El-Khoury, A.E., Beaumier, L., Srivatsa, A., Kuriyan, R., Ajami, A.M. and Young, V.R. (1998) An initial assessment, using [^{13}C]leucine kinetics, of the lysine requirement of healthy adult Indian subjects. *American Journal of Clinical Nutrition* 67, 58–66.

Law, G.K., Bertolo, R.F., Adjiri-Awere, A., Pencharz, P.B. and Ball, R.O. (2007) Adequate threonine is critical for mucin production and gut function in neonatal pigs. *American Journal of Physiology – Gastrointestinal and Liver Physiology* 292, 1293–1301.

Littell, R.C., Lewis, A.J. and Henry, P.R. (1995) Statistical evaluation of bioavailability assays. In: Ammerman, C.B., Baker, D.H., Lewis, A.J., (eds) *Bioavailability of Nutrients for Animals – Amino Acids, Minerals, Vitamins*. Academic Press Inc., San Diego, CA, pp. 5–34.

Levesque, C.L. (2010) Evaluation of the threonine requirement and the bioavailability of threonine in feedstuffs in pregnant sows. PhD thesis. University of Alberta, Edmonton, AB, Canada.

Levesque, C.L., Moehn, S., Pencharz, P.B. and Ball, R.O. (2010) Review of advances in metabolic availability of amino acids. *Livestock Science* doi:10.1016/j.livsci.2010.06.013.

Millward, D.J., Fereday, A., Gibson, N.R. and Pacy, P.J. (2000) Human adult amino acid requirement: [1-^{13}C] leucine balance evaluation of the efficiency of utilization and apparent requirement for wheat protein and lysine compared with those for milk protein in healthy adults. *American Journal of Clinical Nutrition* 72, 112–121.

Millward, D.J., Fereday, A., Bibson, N.R., Cox, M.C. and Pacy, P.J. (2002) Efficiency of utilization of wheat and milk protein in healthy adults and apparent lysine requirements determined by a single-meal [1-^{13}C]leucine balance protocol. *American Journal of Clinical Nutrition* 76, 1326–1334.

Moehn, S., Bertolo, R.F.P., Pencharz, P.B. and Ball, R.O. (2004) Indicator amino acid oxidation responds rapidly to changes inlysine or protein intake in growing and adult pigs. *Journal of Nutrition* 134, 836–841.

Moehn, S., Bertolo, R.F., Pencharz, P.B. and Ball, R.O. (2005) Development of the indicator amino acid oxidation technique to determine the availability of amino acids from dietary protein in pigs. *Journal of Nutrition* 135, 2866–2870.

Moehn, S., Bertolo, R.F.P., Martinazzo-Dallagnol, E., Pencharz, P.B. and Ball, R.O. (2007) Metabolic availability of lysine in feedstuffs determined using oral isotope delivery. *Livestock Science* 109, 24–26.

Moehn, S., Shoveller, A.K., Rademacher, M. and Ball, R.O. (2008) An estimate of the methionine requirement and its variability in growing pigs using the indicator amino acid oxidation technique. *Journal of Animal Science* 86, 364–369.

Moughan, P.J. and Rutherford, S.M. (2008) Available lysine in foods: a brief historical overview. *Journal of AOAC International* 91, 901–906.

Neale, R.J. and Waterlow, J.C. (1974) The metabolism of 14C-labelled essential amino acids given by intragastric or intravenous infusion to rats on normal and protein-free diets. *British Journal of Nutrition* 32, 11–25.

NRC (1998) *Nutrient Requirements of Swine*. 10th ed., National Academies Press, Washington, DC.

Pencharz, P.B. and Ball, R.O. (2003) Different approaches to define individual amino acid requirement. *Annual Review of Nutrition* 23, 101–116.

Reeds, P.J. and Beckett, P.R. (1996) Protein and amino acids. In: Ziegler, E.E. and Filer, L.J. (eds) *Present Knowledge in Nutrition*. 7th ed., ILSI Press, Washington, DC, pp. 67–86.

Schaafsma, G. (2005) The protein digestibility-corrected amino acid score (PDCAAS) – a concept for describing protein quality in foods and food ingredients: a critical review. *Journal of AOAC International* 88, 988–994.

Shoveller, A.K., Brunton, J.A., Pencharz, P.B. and Ball, R.O. (2003) The methionine requirement is lower in neonatal piglets fed parenterally than in those fed enterally. *Journal of Nutrition* 133, 1390–1397.

Shoveller, A.K., Brunton, J.A., Brand, O., Pencharz, P.B. and Ball, R.O. (2006) N-acetylcystein is a highly available precursor for cysteine in the neonatal piglet receiving parenteral nutrition. *Journal of Parenteral and Enteral Nutrition* 30, 23–42.

Shoveller, A.K., Moehn, S., Rademacher, M., Htoo, J.K. and Ball, R.O. (2010) Methionine-hydroxy analogue was found to be significantly less bioavailable compared to DL-methionine for protein deposition in growing pigs. *Animal* 4, 61–66.

Soliman, A.M. and King, K.W. (1969) Metabolic derangements in response of rats to ingestion of imbalanced amino acid mixtures. *Journal of Nutrition* 98, 255–270.

Thorpe, J.M., Roberts, S.A., Ball, R.O. and Pencharz, P.B. (1999) Effects of prior protein intake on phenylalanine kinetics. *Journal of Nutrition* 129, 343–348.

Van Barneveld, R.J., Batterham, E.S. and Norton, B.W. (1994) The effect of heat on amino acids for pigs 3. The availability of lysine for heat-treated filed peas (*Pisum sativum* cultivar Dindale) determined using the slope-ratio assay. *British Journal of Nutrition* 72, 257–275.

WHO (2007) Protein and amino acid requirements in human nutrition. *Report of a Joint WHO/FAO/UNU Expert Consultation*. WHO Technical Series Report 935, WHO, Geneva.

Zello, G.A., Pencharz, P.B. and Ball, R.O. (1990) Phenylalanine flux, oxidation and conversion to tyrosine in humans studies with L-[1-^{13}C] phenylalanine. *American Journal of Physiology* 259, E835–E843.

Zello, G.A., Pencharz, P.B. and Ball, R.O. (1993) Dietary lysine requirement of young adult males determined by oxidation of L-[1-^{13}C] phenylalanine. *American Journal of Physiology* 264, E677–E685.

Zello, G.A., Qykes, L.J., Ball, R.O. and Pencharz, P.B. (1995) Recent advances in methods of assessing dietary amino acid requirements for adult humans. *Journal of Nutrition* 125, 2907–2915.

16 Amino Acid Requirements: Quantitative Estimates

R.R. Pillai and A.V. Kurpad*

Division of Nutrition, St. John's Research Institute, St. John's National Academy of Health Sciences, Bangalore, India

16.1 Abstract

There are now several direct experimental methods that are available to measure indispensable amino acid (IAA) requirements. In all these, increasing intakes of amino acids are given until a change is observed in the response curve. The response could be nitrogen (N) balance or growth, although current methods measure amino acid oxidation or its surrogate by the use of stable isotope tracers. N balance or growth progressively increase until the requirement level of intake of the IAA is reached, after which it plateaus. Oxidation of the test IAA is measured as the primary route of loss of that amino acid, such that the IAA balance (intake–oxidation) can be measured. For oxidation, there is no change in response as graded levels of the IAA are fed below the requirement level. However, once the requirement level is reached there is a linear increase in oxidation. The IAA balance follows the same pattern as the N balance. However, both these methods have several requirements and assumptions, and are technically demanding. A third method has also been developed, related to measuring the oxidation of a selected amino acid whose kinetics are well described, in response to graded intakes of the test IAA. The selected amino acid (other than the test IAA) is called an indicator amino acid, and its oxidation (or balance) response is measured. The oxidation of the indicator, particularly in the fed state, is an index of protein synthesis, and will fall as increasing levels of the test IAA are fed until the requirement level is reached, after which there is no further change. The advantage of this method is that it is relatively non-invasive, and effectively is a breath test, since the oxidation of the tracer-labelled amino acid itself acts as a surrogate for whole-body amino acid oxidation. A modification of the indicator amino acid oxidation method relates to using the measured IAA balance as a surrogate for N balance, in 24-h indicator amino acid balance (IAAB) studies. Here, the balance response follows the same pattern as that of N balance and growth. The indicator amino acid oxidation (and balance) technique is now used primarily in both developed and developing countries, to derive estimates of amino acid requirements in humans. Values of IAA requirements based on the direct and indicator amino acid oxidation and balance (IAAO and IAAB) techniques are considerably higher than those derived from N balance studies, and these tracer-based estimates are now the basis of the recent WHO *et al.* (2007) recommendations for amino acid requirements.

---

* E-mail address: a.kurpad@sjri.res.in

16.2 Introduction

Determinations of human IAA requirements have been based on several strategies, and these offer insights into actual N balances, or surrogates of balance. The strategy of these determinations is to expose an individual or a group of individuals to different intakes of the experimental amino acid, ranging from below to above the putative requirement, and to look for quantifiable responses. An inspection of the intake-response curve should allow for the determination of a change in the response pattern, which could be interpreted within a plausible framework, to determine the requirement. Thus far, the methods that have been used include measurements of the N balance method, inspection of plasma amino acid responses to different intakes of amino acids, and a number of methods related to the use of stable isotopes to accurately quantify amino acid oxidation or flux. While the N balance method has been criticized and is difficult to perform, the amino acid response method is imprecise and no longer in general use, since better tracer techniques are now available. The more recent and precise stable isotopic techniques that have been used include direct measurements of amino acid oxidation (DAAO), and measurements of the oxidation of an indicator amino acid, which is presumed to indicate the status of other indispensable amino acids at different intakes (IAAO), as well as methods that measure the actual daily balance of indispensable amino acids. As with oxidation measurements, the measurements of balance could be associated with measurements related to the experimental amino acid (direct amino acid balance, DAAB) or measurements related to the balance of an indicator amino acid (indicator amino acid balance, IAAB). The latter measurements were usually made over a period of 1 d. In addition to all these methods, one can calculate the daily requirement of amino acids by a factorial method, based on the obligatory amino acid oxidative losses (OAAL, which can be predicted from the obligatory N loss from the body). Finally, more recently, short-term feeding and fasting studies of leucine oxidation and balance have also been applied to measurements of utilization of milk and wheat proteins in terms of the relative efficiency of postprandial protein utilization, from which the requirements for wheat protein and lysine have been derived. The different methods are described in more detail below.

16.3 Nitrogen Balance

Nitrogen balance is a deceptively simple concept, simply stated as the difference between the total nitrogen intake and total nitrogen excretion over a day. This technique has been used for many years in all aspects of protein and amino acid nutrition research, and remains the principal method used to estimate adult human protein requirements. However, there are several technical problems associated with measuring all the N intake and loss accurately (Manatt and Garcia, 1992). Measuring the N intake would appear to be easier, since it can be achieved by analysing duplicate portions of food and by careful attention to the collection of all food not consumed, such as spillage and residue on plates. If this error was present, it would lead to an overestimation of the N balance. On the other hand, exact N excretion is even more difficult to measure. While complete collections of urine and faeces are difficult but still possible, there are serious difficulties in determining the skin-based integumental and other minor or unmeasured routes of N loss such as hair, nails, and various bodily secretions. Attempts have been made to quantify these losses, and in a comprehensive and detailed study, Calloway and Margen (1971) concluded that dermal and miscellaneous losses amounted to about 0.5 g N daily (or about $7.1\,mg\,N\,kg^{-1}d^{-1}$) in sedentary, healthy young men. In older men these losses were found to be lower, at about $3\,mg\,N\,kg^{-1}d^{-1}$ (Zanni et al., 1979), and it is possible that the miscellaneous losses decline with advancing age. The precise magnitude of these miscellaneous losses cannot be stated with any confidence. The FAO et al. (1985) expert consultation proposed a value of $8\,mg\,N\,kg^{-1}d^{-1}$ for adults as a reasonable estimate of miscellaneous losses, but in the more recent WHO et al.

consultation (2007), a value of 5 mg N kg^{-1} d^{-1} was selected. The value assumed for the miscellaneous N loss could vary downward or upward (depending on environmental conditions or the nature of work the individual was engaged in).

Nevertheless, assuming different amounts of these miscellaneous N losses to add to the urinary and faecal N loss will affect the quantitative interpretation of N balance data in any individual study. For example, in a reanalysis of published N balance data in adult experiments designed to measure the amino acid requirement, Hegsted (1963) assumed an additional miscellaneous loss of 0.5 g N daily (amounting to about 8 mg N kg^{-1} d^{-1} in an individual weighing 60 kg). This meant that the N balances were made more negative by 0.5 g N daily. Based on this apparently small adjustment, the amino acid requirement values were significantly increased above those proposed in the original N balance experiments. The range of increase was in many cases quite dramatic; for example, the requirement for threonine and methionine increased by about 500%. If an even smaller value was used for the miscellaneous N loss, for example 0.3 g N daily or about 5 mg N kg^{-1} d^{-1}, Millward (1999) still found that there was an increase in the estimated amino acid requirement values, although the increases, as expected, were lower than when a daily miscellaneous loss of 0.5 g N d^{-1} was assumed. Nevertheless, these recalculations underline the importance of even small, unmeasured routes of N loss in N balance experiments. Adding N losses to the N balance estimate leads to different effects relating to the degree of slope of the N balances to the N intakes response, as the balances approach zero when the intake of the test amino acid is near adequate. If this is a relatively low slope, the effect of adjusting for a given value for miscellaneous N losses on the amino acid requirement estimate is even more dramatic. It is even likely that the response line is not linear and that the slope varies depending on the range of intakes being studied. For example, the gradient is higher at very low intakes, and declines appreciably as the balance point is approached (Young et al., 1973; Inoue et al., 1974). In essence, with a linear approach, it is likely that results from an experiment that included very low intakes are likely to lead to an underestimate of the requirement. It is therefore critical to study a range of intakes that encompass the putative requirement level. This is illustrated in a simulation (Rand et al., 1977; Rand and Young, 1999), in which different curve-fitting techniques were used on data acquired in an earlier study on the lysine requirement. Four different shaped curves: linear (A), logarithmic (B), square root (C), and exponential asymptotic (D) were fitted (Fig. 16.1). While all curves intersected at the same point, the intake value at which they reach the zero balance point was different. It is clear that curves B, C, and D had gradients that declined sharply as the zero balance point was approached, underlining the problem of selecting appropriate intakes to study. In addition, the median lysine requirements obtained by these three procedures were about 28–29 mg kg^{-1} d^{-1} when the miscellaneous N losses were assumed to be 8 mg kg^{-1} d^{-1}, and 20.4–22.7 mg kg^{-1} d^{-1} when miscellaneous losses of 5 mg N kg^{-1} d^{-1} were assumed. This illustrates the relatively high sensitivity of the nitrogen balance method to the assumed value of miscellaneous N losses.

The quantification of N losses may also be lower than expected because of unexplained losses. For example, it has often been found that there is a progressively better or more positive N balance with a continued increase in N intake, even above that known to be required to maintain body N equilibrium, including in adults who have ceased to grow and accrete protein (Hegsted, 1976; Kurpad and Vaz, 2000). A careful recovery study of N in piglets given alanine N infusions showed that even after accounting for expanded urea and α-amino nitrogen pools, the excretion of N was significantly lower than 100% (Davis et al., 2000). In addition, it has been thought that the IAA can be made available to the body by the gut microflora (Fuller and Garlick, 1994). It is known that there is some recycling of urea by intestinal bacteria (Jackson, 1993), and in humans, this is thought to occur to the extent of about 20% in subjects in whom the bacterial flora were reduced by antibiotics (Raj et al., 2008). There is also the question about the source of N needed for bacterial amino acid synthesis. If it

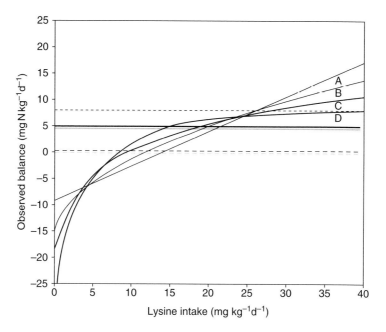

Fig. 16.1. Non-linear regression of N balance against lysine intake, using four different functions. The horizontal line at the balance of +5 mg N kg^{-1} d^{-1} represents the assumed additional miscellaneous N losses that were not measured. The dashed line at +8 mg N kg^{-1} d^{-1} represents another assumption of the miscellaneous N loss; the true value could lie between 5 and 8 mg N kg^{-1} d^{-1} depending on environmental conditions or nature of work. (From Rand and Young, 1999; actual data points removed for clarity.)

comes from the ingested dietary N in the form of amino acids in dietary protein, then the input of amino acids from microbial synthesis will not provide a net benefit to the host. The importance of the microbial source of amino acids is when nitrogenous end-products of no use to the host – such as urea or ammonia – are utilized by the microbes, or when the microbial IAA comes from surplus non-IAA N in the diet. In a recent study to assess the source of N used in microbial synthesis in the upper gut of normally nourished pigs fed their normal diets with additional pectin, it was found that preformed amino acids from dietary protein – as well as endogenous protein (from mucus glycoproteins and epithelial cell turnover) – contributed much more to microbial amino acids than *de novo* synthesis (Libao-Mercado *et al.*, 2009). Further, when human subjects are fed resistant starch along with adequate dietary N, it appears that there is no net extra IAA input into the body (Kurpad *et al.*, unpublished). Therefore, the nutritional significance of this finding, and in particular the extent to which this bacterial IAA can spare dietary IAA, is not yet clear. From a purely technical viewpoint, N balance approaches used in amino acid requirement experiments are beset by problems that may lead to an underestimate of those requirements (Young, 1987; Young *et al.*, 1989; Young and Marchini, 1990).

Experimental design also matters. The effect of dietary energy and energy balance on the N balance is well known, and the N balance experiments should typically be performed when subjects are in a near-zero energy balance. In the N balance-based estimates of amino acid requirements (Rose, 1957), one criticism was that the energy intakes in those studies were too high. This could account, at least in significant part, for an apparent underestimation of the minimum amino acid intakes actually needed to maintain body N equilibrium. Maintaining a perfect zero energy balance over many days is impractical and perhaps impossible. For example, Roberts *et al.* (1990) attempted to match precisely energy intake with estimated energy expenditure in one study, and found that they had overestimated the maintenance intake by about 3 kcal kg^{-1}d^{-1}. Although this overestimation might seem negligible, over short-term N balance experiments it would be sufficient to change N retention by about 6 mg N kg^{-1}d^{-1} (Young et al., 1992). In addition, adaptation to the new level of protein intake is important, as not only does metabolism take time to adapt to the new intake, but the body urea pool must also adjust to the change. Therefore, the length of the dietary adjustment period, and the degree to which the prior dietary intake differed from the experimental protocol intake, are also counted as important factors in the estimation of the N balance. This applies as a general principle to all studies in which a marker of equilibrium is sought on a particular amino acid intake, and will also be discussed under the other methods below. In N balance studies in experienced hands, where protein intake levels have been changed, a new and relatively steady state of N excretion is achieved, usually within about 4–6 d (Rand et al., 1976), and in general, this does not change by much with longer exposure to the changed protein intake (Rand et al., 1979, 1985). Other studies have been interpreted to indicate that a period of about 2 weeks or longer is necessary to achieve a new steady state N output with a change in total N intake (Quevedo et al., 1994). As detailed above, it is critical to ensure that confounders such as energy intake are adequately addressed in the design and interpretation of studies that seek to define N equilibrium at different N intakes.

In general, it would appear that the N balance approach is technically difficult and potentially confounded by many variables. For these various reasons the amino acid requirement values that were proposed by earlier N balance studies (Table 16.1) must be viewed with some caution, and more recent research with better techniques have indicated that the amino acid requirements are higher. Nevertheless, the N balance, when obtained via appropriately designed experiments, measured carefully, and the results analysed appropriately, can be a useful marker of the relative adequacy of dietary nitrogen or even of a specific, indispensable amino acid intake in comparison with an acceptable reference point.

Table 16.1. Estimates of adult indispensable amino acid requirements by the N balance method.

Amino acid	Requirement (mg kg^{-1} d^{-1})[a]
Isoleucine	10
Leucine	14
Lysine	12
Methionine	13
Phenylalanine + tyrosine	14
Threonine	7
Tryptophan	3.5
Valine	10

[a]Values from WHO et al. (2007).

16.4 Isotopic Tracer Methods

With advances in the measurement of stable isotope enrichment in biological matrices, and the expanded use of tracers enriched with these isotopes in human metabolic research, a second paradigm of measuring IAA requirements based on a stable isotope tracer technique to measure body amino acid balance was developed as the criterion of adequacy. A series of tracer studies was begun at MIT by Vernon Young and his colleagues in the early 1980s, to revisit the determination and estimation of the amino acid requirements in adults, using stable isotopic techniques to measure amino acid oxidation (Young and Bier, 1981; Young et al., 1984, 1987; Meguid et al., 1986a,b; Meredith et al., 1986). Amino acid oxidation studies are based on the principle that any amino acid, provided in excess of the needs of protein synthesis, is preferentially oxidized (Zello et al., 1995). This means that amino acid oxidation, measured in multiple amino acid intake experiments, will yield a pattern of a low or maintenance level of oxidation, which would increase as the intake of the test amino acid increased above the requirement level. The tracer used is an indispensable amino acid labelled at its carboxyl carbon (typically with ^{13}C for humans and ^{14}C for animals). This method relies on the assumption that the requirement of specific IAA in adults is the dietary intake of that amino acid which balances all routes of loss in which oxidation is primary.

Since that time, the paradigm has evolved into a number of different methods, all of which have used tracer-based studies of human amino acid requirements. These methods are both short and long term, and measure either the oxidation of the amino acid, or its daily balance. Studies that have used a tracer of the test dietary amino acid, with a measure of its rate of oxidation at various test intake levels are called the direct amino acid oxidation (DAAO) method, which can be extended to the measurement of the body ^{13}C-amino acid balance, or the direct amino acid balance (DAAB) method. These techniques have been used to assess the requirements for leucine, valine, lysine, and threonine (Young et al., 1989). Another key advance in the field is the use of an 'indicator' tracer to assess the status of whole-body amino acid oxidation (IAAO) or indicator amino acid balance (IAAB) at varying levels of a test dietary amino acid. An example of the IAAO approach is seen in the study by Zello et al. (1993) which included a determination of the rate of ^{13}C-phenylalanine oxidation at varying levels of lysine intake. Finally, and more recently, there have been studies designed to assess the retention of protein during the post-prandial phase of amino acid metabolism, using ^{13}C-leucine as a tracer (Millward, 2000; Millward et al, 2000). This is called the post-prandial protein utilization (PPU) approach. These tracer-based methods are described in sequence below.

16.4.1 Direct amino acid oxidation and balance

The potential advantage of the direct amino acid oxidation and balance (DAAO/DAAB) technique is that the rate of oxidation of the dietary amino acid of interest is directly estimated. This technique is based on the measurement of the irreversible oxidation of tracer-labelled test amino acids (Motil et al., 1981; Meguid et al., 1986a,b; Meredith et al., 1986; Zhao et al., 1986; Marchini et al., 1993; Hiramatsu et al., 1994), and involves correlating the measured oxidation rate with controlled diet studies at different levels of intake of the test amino acid. It is then possible to evaluate both the pattern of change in the oxidation rate of the test amino acid and the body balance (24 h intake–24 h predicted oxidation) of the test amino acid under study. The requirement level of the test amino acid is the minimum intake at which the estimate of daily balance was close to or equal to zero. Over a run-in period of up to a week in duration, the procedure involves giving subjects diets based on amino acid mixtures. These supply limiting to generous levels of the amino acid being tested, and the test amino acid balance at each level of test amino acid intake is measured. This balance could be measured by the intravenous infusion (or oral administration) of a stable isotope (^{13}C) labelled amino acid, such that the flux and the irreversible oxidation of the test amino acid could be measured. The measurement of this irreversible oxidation is based on the highly accurate quantification of the respiratory loss of oxidized tracer as carbon dioxide (by indirect calorimetry and isotope ratio mass spectrometry), as well as the measurement of the isotopic enrichment (by gas chromatography–mass spectrometry) of the precursor pool of the amino acid in the body.

This tracer approach was first applied in radio-tracer studies to determine the requirement for lysine in young rats (Brookes et al., 1972) and then later to estimate the requirement for leucine (Harper and Benjamin, 1984), threonine (Kang-Lee and Harper, 1978), and histidine (Kang-Lee and Harper, 1977) in growing rats, and lysine in young rats (Bergner et al., 1978) and pigs (Chavez and Bayley, 1976). These animal models revealed that oxidation of the amino acid remained low and relatively constant at sub-maintenance amino acid intakes and then began to increase as the intake approximated and then further exceeded the requirement for maximum growth. The amino acid oxidation rate continued to increase linearly with further increases in intake.

In humans, Young and co-workers used this approach in the 1980s, using stable isotope rather than radiolabelled tracers, for ethical and safety reasons. Until 1986, all of the published estimates of IAA requirements in adult humans had been obtained using either nitrogen balance or, for a few, using changes in plasma amino acid levels (Tontisirin et al., 1973; Young et al., 1971). In 1986, a series of DAAO studies were reported (Meguid et al., 1986a; Meredith et al., 1986; Zhao et al., 1986). Thereafter, a number of studies were performed with DAAO/DAAB methods (Table 16.2) to assess the selected IAA requirements in adults.

However, there are some limitations and disadvantages to this specific tracer approach (Table 16.3):

1. A precise determination of the rate of tracee oxidation is difficult to achieve, since for most amino acids, the isotopic enrichment of the pool directly supplying the substrate for oxidation is not actually known. For practical reasons, the isotopic enrichment of the venous plasma-free amino acid pool is routinely sampled and analysed for purposes of determining the oxidation rate. Except for leucine (El-Khoury et al., 1994a) and possibly methionine where the plasma enrichments of α-ketoisocaproate and homocysteine (MacCoss et al., 1999), respectively, can be used as an index of labelling in the intracellular pool of the parent amino acid, it is likely that the DAAO and DAAB approaches with other amino acids have underestimated oxidation and overestimated balance. However, it is likely that this is a systematic error, which would change the absolute value of the amino acid oxidation rate, but not the pattern of change in amino acid oxidation in response to altered intakes. Since the identification of the requirement level of the test amino acid is considered to be where the pattern of amino acid oxidation changes in response to altered amino acid intake, this may not necessarily be a major problem. However, for the accurate measurement of amino acid balance, it remains to be a problem.

2. Initial human studies of DAAO were of relatively short duration (about 3 h) and were conducted in subjects who were in the fed state (Meguid et al., 1986a,b; Meredith et al., 1986; Zhao et al., 1986). To estimate the DAAB, assumptions had to be made about the rates of amino acid oxidation during the remaining

Table 16.2. The estimation of IAA requirements with DAAO/DAAB method.

Amino acid	Method		Value obtained (range) mg kg^{-1} d^{-1}
	Short-term (3 h & 8 h)	24 h DAAB	
Leucine	Meguid et al. (1986a)	El-Khoury et al. (1994a)	39.6–40
	Cortiella et al. (1988)	El-Khoury et al. (1994b)	
	Krempf et al. (1993)	El-Khoury et al. (1995)	
	Young et al. (1991)	El-Khoury et al. (1996)	
		El-Khoury et al. (1997)	
		Kurpad et al. (2001c)	
		Kurpad et al. (2002)	
		Kurpad et al. (2003)	
Lysine	Meredith et al. (1986)	El-Khoury et al. (1998)	>20–30
Methionine + cysteine	Fukagawa et al. (1998)		6–13
	Raguso et al. (1997)		
	Raguso et al. (2000)		
	Storch et al. (1988)		
	Hiramatsu et al. (1994)		
Phenylalanine + tyrosine	Cortiella et al. (1992)	Sánchez et al. (1995)	>18.5–<39
		Sánchez et al. (1996)	
		Basile-Filho et al. (1997)	
		Basile-Filho et al. (1998)	
Threonine	Zhao et al. (1986)		10–20
Valine	Meguid et al. (1986b)		>16–20
	Pelletier et al. (1991)		

Table 16.3. DAAO/DAAB methods limitations and disadvantages.

- Prior adaptation is required
- Can only be used to determine the requirements of amino acids whose carboxyl group is directly released to the bicarbonate pool and so will appear in breath
- In short-term studies, measurements are made only after a few hours of feeding making it difficult to extrapolate findings to a normal day with no / any level of confidence; therefore whether fed state studies represent the daily (24 h) requirement is unclear
- The precursor pool from which oxidation takes place expands as the level of the test amino acid intake increases
- Infusion of nutritionally significant amounts of labelled amino acid is a potential problem
- 24-h studies are complex and difficult method to carry out, and limits the number of studies that can be conducted in any single subject

9 h of the fed period and then also during the 12-h post-absorptive period. These assumptions have been described (Meguid et al., 1986a) but a precise estimate of daily balance would require ideally use of a 24-h tracer protocol. A further reason is that the rate of amino acid oxidation during the fed period does not necessarily remain constant but can vary throughout the 12-h phase of the fed-fast cycle with the rhythm changing according to the adequacy of intake of the test amino acid (El-Khoury et al., 1994b; Sánchez et al., 1995). To measure the fasted state oxidation rate, a short, 8 h infusion protocol, in which no food is given for the first 3 h and small meals are given during the remaining 5 h, has been employed. This circumvents many of the problems associated with the fed-only procedure, as separate measurements are made for the fed and fasting states.

3. The stable isotopic label requires a higher amount of enrichment in the body amino acid or carbon dioxide pool for precise detection, because of the high background, or natural tracer enrichment that exists with these isotopes. This is in contrast to radioactive isotopes, in which this problem does not exist. Therefore, the stable isotope-labelled amino acid is given in larger or 'non-tracer' amounts, which effectively contribute to the test amino acid intake, with possible modification of the status of endogenous amino acid metabolism, particularly in the fasted state. Such effects may require relatively high tracer intakes, possibly equivalent to more than 10% of the plasma amino acid flux. In all recent ^{13}C tracer studies that have sought to measure balance, the tracer input has been included in the estimation of total test amino acid intake for purposes of estimating amino acid balance, but it is difficult to know whether the tracer, especially when given during a post-absorptive phase of amino acid metabolism, actually affects the rate of test amino acid oxidation. Later, more extensive DAAB studies with leucine (El-Khoury et al., 1994a) and lysine (El-Khoury et al., 2000) and additional metabolic studies on leucine and methionine (Raguso et al., 1999) suggest that the doses of labelled tracers usually given in these experiments do not significantly affect the oxidation rates of the trace. A more recent study has suggested that this error might not be important, as infusions of three different levels of leucine during the fasting phase were shown to have no significant effect on leucine oxidation (Kurpad et al., 2002a), suggesting that additional leucine would therefore be available for protein synthesis in the fasting state.

4. Although the short duration of study problem was solved through the deployment of 24-h protocols of measurement of amino acid balance (El-Khoury et al., 1994a,b, 1995, 2000; Kurpad et al., 2001c), such studies are complex and difficult to carry out, often limiting the number of repeat 24-h studies that can be conducted in any one single subject or the total number of 24-h studies that are feasible in any one investigation. It has been shown that the daily rate of protein oxidation, calculated from the leucine oxidation measured during this protocol, is closely similar to that derived from the measurement of nitrogen excretion in urine and faeces (El-Khoury et al., 1994a). The intake point at

which a zero balance is achieved is taken to be the requirement. Although this longer protocol answers questions about the shorter durations of the fasted-fed experiments, there is one controversy relating to the protocol, which involves the feeding of small meals for 12 h during the fed state in order to achieve a steady state of feeding. The question is whether this is representative of a 'normal' day, involving larger and fewer meals. This was tested in a study that compared the protocol described above with an otherwise similar protocol in which three discrete meals were given (El-Khoury et al., 1995). Despite receiving the same total dietary leucine intake with the two protocols, the daily leucine balances were quite different. Whereas the half-hourly small meal protocol gave an approximately zero balance, the discrete meal protocol gave a balance that was significantly positive. It is possible that the half-hourly small meals protocol is less conducive to protein retention and therefore might give rise to higher estimates of amino acid requirements. Nevertheless, in most 24-h studies, the small meal protocol has been used successfully, and was internally valid in that it demonstrated that an adequate intake of the test amino acid gave a zero leucine balance in adult men.

5. Although oxidation or conversion to other amino acids is by far the major route of disposal of IAA, some loss may occur via the urine, skin, and intestine. Intestinal losses have been estimated by collecting ileostomy fluid from subjects given a protein-free diet (Zello et al., 1993), suggesting that the intestine is potentially a major route of amino acid loss in these subjects. The unanswered question is how much of the ileal amino acids are subsequently reabsorbed in the colon. It is also possible that the amino acids synthesized in the intestine by intestinal microbes are made available to the body, as discussed above in the N-balance section. In this case, the increased intake would lead to higher oxidation. The apparent negative amino acid balance would give rise to an overestimate of the amount of dietary amino acid required to maintain balance. However, in both these cases, it is unlikely that these routes of amino acid loss or gain are very significant in normal nutrition.

6. There is some uncertainty over the measured rates of amino acid oxidation, because labelled CO_2 is sequestered in the body bicarbonate pool, leading to an incomplete recovery of the oxidized label in the breath. Then, the rate of labelled CO_2 output in the breath will be lower (by up to 30%), than the true cellular production rate. Typically, this incomplete recovery of label can be measured and corrected for by performing infusions of ^{13}C-labelled bicarbonate in prior experiments using the same fasting and fed protocol, preferably in the same subjects on the same diet. However, it is not certain how well intravenously infused bicarbonate mimics the endogenous production of bicarbonate in the cells where the metabolite of the labelled amino acid is oxidized, and this introduces a degree of imprecision in the method. The ^{13}C-enrichment of the natural CO_2 in the breath will also vary during the day, depending on the substrate being oxidized. This occurs because different dietary sources of carbon have different natural enrichments (for example, cane sugar and maize products have a much higher enrichment than potato or wheat products). Standardizing all diets with low enrichment ingredients minimizes this problem; in case a correction is required to improve precision, prior experiments can also be done with the same diet and subjects, in the same protocol, without any tracer, in which the natural variation in ^{13}C enrichment in breath CO_2 is characterized. The enrichments so obtained are then subtracted from those obtained during infusions of the labelled amino acid. This procedure is necessary to avoid serious systematic errors in the determination of oxidation rates, but as with the bicarbonate correction, it adds substantially to the overall variability of the method.

Despite these limitations, the 24-h tracer balance approach (DAAB) might be regarded currently as the most rigorous tracer-based paradigm for directly determining amino acid balance when its conditions are satisfied. Typically, this is for leucine only at present, and for this amino acid, is the method of choice for determining its requirement in adults.

16.4.2 Indicator amino acid oxidation and balance

The indicator amino acid oxidation (IAAO) method was applied initially in studies of amino acid requirements in young growing pigs and validated against traditional approaches based on criteria of growth, N balance, and body composition (Kim and Bayley, 1983; Kim et al., 1983a,b; Ball and Bayley, 1984). The requirement for a test IAA is determined from the pattern or rate of change in oxidation of another (indicator) amino acid (e.g. ^{13}C-phenylalanine). Therefore, unlike the carbon balance method, the test amino acid and the tracer are separate, and there is now no problem linked to the intake of nutritionally significant quantities of the tracer. It is also critical that the intake of the indicator amino acid is kept constant, since changes in amino acid concentrations in plasma or extracellular fluid can alter the rates of its transport into cells, such that the intracellular to extracellular or plasma enrichment ratio is changed (Mortimore et al., 1972). For amino acids such as phenylalanine and lysine, for which there are no surrogate measures of the intracellular enrichment – such as α-ketoisocaproate for leucine – the change in this ratio might confound the results. Thus, this method is not a direct measure of the maintenance requirement in the same way that the 24-h carbon balance method is, but is mainly a measure of the intake of the test amino acid as a proportion of its content in the amino acid mixture required for postprandial protein deposition.

Typically, when the intake of the test IAA is limiting, it is expected that there would be an increased oxidation pattern of all the other amino acids owing to inefficiency in protein synthesis. As the requirement level of the test IAA is approached, the excess oxidation of the indicator amino acid will decline, until it is at its lowest when the test IAA intake is at requirement. Thus, an inflection point occurs, at which the oxidation of the indicator amino acid reaches its nadir, and this is considered to be the requirement level of the test amino acid. Then, even if the intake of the test IAA goes above the requirement, the low rate of oxidation of the indicator amino acid will remain at its nadir. This of course assumes that the indicator amino acid, and indeed all other IAA, are being supplied at a constant requirement or above requirement level in the diet. The approach was first applied in adult humans in a study designed to determine the dietary requirement for lysine (Zello et al., 1993). It was extended to estimate the requirements of healthy adults for tryptophan (Lazaris-Brunner et al., 1998), threonine (Wilson et al., 2000), methionine with no cysteine (Di Buono et al., 2001a), minimum methionine with cysteine (Di Buono et al., 2001b; Ball et al., 2006), total branched-chain amino acids (Riazi et al., 2003), and total aromatic amino acids (phenylalanine, with no tyrosine) (Hsu et al., 2006; Pencharz et al., 2007), as well as a follow-up study on the lysine requirements of adults (Duncan et al., 1996), and a recent study on tyrosine-phenylalanine relationships (Roberts et al., 2001).

Two experimental approaches are followed in the IAAO method. The first is a short-term protocol, in which subjects are given an adequate, constant diet for a few days followed by ^{13}C-phenylalanine (or ^{13}C-lysine) tracer study at a test intake level of the amino acid whose requirement is being estimated, while the second is a longer term 24-h protocol (described below). The tracer protocol involves giving subjects small hourly meals for 7 h, beginning 3 h before the infusion of labelled indicator tracer. The enrichment of the breath $^{13}CO_2$ for the last 2 h of the 4-h tracer period is used to estimate the indicator amino acid oxidation rate. This is normalized for the amount of tracer given, and expressed as a proportion of the administered dose. Therefore, the actual oxidation of the tracee is not measured, since one is interested only in the oxidation of the tracer. Individual subjects are studied at multiple test amino acid intake levels, with as many as six or more levels in some of the investigations. If measurements of tracee oxidation are required, an invasive nature is added to the experiment, since enrichments of the precursor pool, normally estimated in the plasma, need blood samples. There have been attempts to use urinary enrichments to approximate the enrichment of the tracer amino acid in arterialized blood (Bross et al., 1998). Reasonably good correlations between plasma and urinary amino acid enrichments have been obtained with ^{13}C-leucine, ^{15}N-glycine, and ^{13}C-phenylalanine (De Benoist *et al.*, 1984; Wykes *et al.*, 1990; Zello *et al.*, 1994). Furthermore, Bross *et al.* (1998) developed an IAAO model which used oral dosing of tracer along with breath sampling alone in order to make the whole method completely non-invasive. Nevertheless, given the similar breakpoints obtained with the tracer or tracee oxidation response, it might seem reasonable to continue with the tracer oxidation method until further validations are performed for the tracee oxidation method.

There are a number of advantages to this short-term IAAO approach. In comparison to longer protocols which do not permit more than two or three studies at different test IAA intakes in a single subject, this method offers the possibility of carrying out a relatively large number of short-term tracer studies within the same subject, allowing for within-subject estimates to be made of the inflection point on the response curve. Given the assumptions of this method, problems arising from changes in pool sizes and kinetics that might affect the behaviour of a direct tracer and interpretation of the isotopic data obtained are largely avoided; there is no *a priori* reason to determine the actual rate of indicator amino acid oxidation, since the pattern of release of the ^{13}C label in expired air can provide the basis for requirement estimate derived from the inflection on the intake-oxidation response curve. A further advantage accrues from the fact that there is no need to measure the CO_2 recovery, in which some imprecision occurs.

Since the basis for the measurement of leucine kinetics is well validated, it might seem that only leucine is ideally suited as an indicator, as its carbon balance can be accurately measured. However, in the short-term IAAO method, actual balance of the indicator amino acid is not measured, allowing for the choice of other indicator amino acids, such as phenylalanine. This is also because of the low concentration of phenylalanine in blood and tissues, which allows its metabolism to be rapidly sensitive to changes in protein balance or other amino acid intake (Zello *et al.*, 1993).

It is important to understand that since $^{13}CO_2$ release occurs by tyrosine oxidation, which in turn is formed from phenylalanine, it is important to minimize the loss of ^{13}C into the protein-bound tyrosine pool by giving a high tyrosine diet prior to the study (Zello *et al.*, 1990, 1993). According to the concept on which this approach is based, this pattern of ^{13}C appearance as a result of oxidation of the tracer should, in theory, parallel that for the absolute oxidation rate of the indicator (tracee). In one study concerned with the lysine requirement of adult males (Duncan *et al.*, 1996) this was not found to be the case; while the absolute rate of phenylalanine oxidation showed a generally similar pattern to that of $^{13}CO_2$ release, the variation precluded use of this parameter to estimate the requirement for lysine. In other studies using leucine as an indicator for the phenylalanine requirement, however, the pattern of $^{13}CO_2$ release did mimic the pattern of leucine (indicator) oxidation.

The disadvantages of the short-term IAAO method are that it has been based essentially on a short-term fed-state model, even though it gives results similar to more complex models in many other studies. There is therefore uncertainty as to whether the same pattern of change or at least 'breakpoint' in IAAO response would apply similarly to a later (or even earlier) period within the 12 h fed phase as compared with the specific 2 h period used to elaborate the relationship between amino acid intake, oxidation, and requirements. From 24-h tracer studies (below) it is now clear that the rate of amino acid oxidation changes throughout a constant-fed period in a complex way depending upon the adequacy of amino acid intake (El-Khoury *et al.*, 1994b; Sánchez *et al.*, 1995). Second, Zello *et al.* (1995) state that the IAAO technique has the advantage of permitting oxidation measurements to be taken with no prior adaptation to the level of the test amino acid, in contrast to the DAAO and DAAB studies where adaptation periods of about 6–7 d have been included in the study design. This may not be a particular advantage of the IAAO technique, since the lack of a period of adaptation to a test amino acid intake level is potentially a serious design limitation.

El Khoury et al. (1994a,b) showed an adaptation of leucine oxidation in the fasting state over a twofold range after 6 d of leucine intakes at 89, 38, and 14 mg kg^{-1} d^{-1} at a constant nitrogen intake. These are similar to changes in fasting and fed nitrogen losses or leucine oxidation shown to occur in response to 2-week periods of widely varying protein intakes (Millward, 1999). Thus, adaptation should influence the overall need for amino acids, even when measurements are limited to the fed state. However, two separate studies of the lysine requirement at total protein intakes of 0.8 (Zello et al., 1993) or 1.0 g kg^{-1} d^{-} (Duncan et al., 1996) gave similar inflection points on the oxidation intake response curve. More recent studies on the pattern of $^{13}CO_2$ production after different periods of adaptation have shown that there really is no adaptive effect of prior feeding in the short-term protocol (Moehn et al., 2004). Furthermore, ^{13}C-phenylalanine oxidation, measured as F$^{13}CO_2$, was not significantly affected by 8 h, 3 d or 7 d of adaptation to a wide range of lysine intakes in healthy young men (Elango et al., 2009).

However, even if the potential drawback does exist, it must be recognized that at present several studies using this method give fairly similar answers about IAA requirements, in comparison to more rigorous and theoretically well-defined protocols of IAAO and IAAB (below). Millward (1998) has argued that, without a suitable adaptation period to a specific and lower test lysine intake, the IAAO approach would effectively give a higher value than the minimum physiological requirements for lysine. On the other hand, Young (1999) has argued the opposite, namely that the minimum requirement might, in theory, be underestimated when applying the IAAO approach under conditions where there is no adaptation to a lower intake than usual. Recent studies by Millward et al. (2000) on the post-prandial utilization of milk and wheat proteins would support this view; since their estimate of the nutritional quality of wheat protein was higher than the authors had predicted, presumably due to the 'buffering' effect of a significant and replete free tissue (perhaps muscle) lysine pool over the course of their short-term tracer study. Nevertheless, there is a need to establish whether or not, and for how long, an adaptation period should be included in studies involving the fed state and the IAAO technique. The strengths and limitations of the IAAO/IAAB methods have been summarized in Table 16.4.

In general, it is potentially useful to develop the short-term IAAO method for

Table 16.4. Strengths and limitations of IAAO/IAAB methods.

- Short-term IAAO measurements are made on only fed state method and is a short-term study with minimal complexity
- Short-term, minimally invasive IAAO can be applied on vulnerable groups such as malnourished children, pregnant or lactating women, and the elderly
- The requirement of any amino acid can be determined with a single indicator
- The pool from which oxidation takes place does not change in size as the level of the test amino acid is altered
- Prior adaptation to the level of the test amino acid is not needed in the short-term IAAO protocol, but this still needs to be rigorously evaluated
- A full range of intakes of the test amino acid can be used
- This method is not conditional on high levels of precision or accuracy in measurement of amino acid oxidation
- The demonstration of breakpoint is much less convincing since the net protein synthesis may be less than in a growing animal
- Choice of best indicator and oxidation is limited, at present phenylalanine (in the presence of an excess of tyrosine), lysine and leucine have been used; the only other possible choices are valine and isoleucine
- Fasted as well as in the fed state measurements can be performed in 24-h experiments
- 24-h studies require adaptation to the level of the test amino acid for 5–7 d; more invasive than the short-term IAAO method

further studies in low-resource, developing countries as well as in vulnerable groups such as children, pregnant or lactating women, and the elderly (Elango et al., 2008; Pillai et al., 2010). These estimates form the first direct experimental evidence of amino acid requirements in school-age children, where it was earlier estimated by a factorial method (Table 16.5). It has also been used in innovative ways to determine other metabolic indices. Recently, the IAAO method has adapted to determine protein requirements in adults, although this still needs to be validated (Humayun et al., 2007a). This method has also been applied recently to determine the metabolic availability of sulphur amino acid (SAA) from casein versus soy protein isolate using ^{13}C phenylalanine as an indicator amino acid (Humayun et al., 2007b).

To circumvent some of the limitations of the short-term IAAO technique, a 24-hour indicator amino acid oxidation balance (24-hour IAAO) and 24-hour IAAB approach was developed (Kurpad et al., 1998), the latter having an approach similar in concept to that of the IAAO technique but based on an indicator amino acid oxidation balance protocol conducted over an entire day, providing a true 24-h experimental observation. The 24-h IAAB could be regarded as a functional criterion of dietary amino acid adequacy in contrast to a measure of the short-term, fed state IAAO, which might be taken to be a biomarker of adequacy. This method has been applied in ^{13}C-leucine (indicator) tracer studies of the lysine requirement of adult Indian subjects (Kurpad et al., 1998; 2001a,b) and recently in studies of the threonine requirement in US adults (Borgonha et al., 2002) and Indian subjects (Kurpad et al., 2001b). The disadvantage of the 24-h IAAO and 24-h IAAB approaches relates to the complexity of the 24-h tracer study and possibly the rather stringent demands and restraints that it places on the experimental subject. Furthermore, the 24-h paradigm has been most often conducted using a 12-h fed-state period that involves giving small, frequent, isocaloric, isonitrogenous meals. Current meal patterns in most parts of the world tend toward a larger single, evening meal, and it is not known how this pattern of meal ingestion might impact on the minimum physiological requirement for amino acids. As stated above, leucine oxidation is lower when three discrete meals are used versus a multiple frequent meal schedule (El-Khoury, et al., 1995; Raguso et al., 1999). Hence, it raises the question of what might be the appropriate or best meal pattern for estimating amino acid requirements in adults when using the IAAO and IAAB techniques. Even with these caveats, it appears that the IAAO/IAAB method works best when the indicator (particularly in the case of leucine) is given at or just above the daily requirement level (Pencharz and Ball, 2003), since at higher intakes which approach the normal intake values, the IAAB balances response tends to be far more positive than can be explained (Kurpad et al., 2001b). Current data do not permit a sufficient resolution of this matter, but the best practice might be that the multiple, frequent meal paradigm is the most appropriate for the quantitative interpretation of current amino acid tracer data. Another issue of importance with respect to estimating the minimum physiological requirements of amino acids is the molecular form of the amino acid intake. The earlier amino acid requirement studies of Rose (1957) and of many of the other investigators (Irwin and Hegsted, 1971) used D- and L-amino acid mixtures as a principal source of amino acids. The more recent ^{13}C-tracer studies have generally used a mixture of L-amino acids. Studies of the comparative utilization of protein-bound versus free

Table 16.5. Estimation of IAA requirements by the IAAO in children.

Amino acid	Author's reference	Requirement (mg kg^{-1} d^{-1})
Lysine	Pillai et al. (2010)	33.5
	Elango et al. (2007)	35
Methionine (no cysteine, total SAA)	Turner et al. (2006)	12.9
Methionine (with cysteine)	Humayun et al. (2006)	5.8
Total BCAA (isoleucine + leucine + valine)	Mager et al. (2003)	147

leucine indicated better retention of the leucine when given in protein-bound form.

The amino acid requirement estimates generated from the ^{13}C-tracer 24-h DAAB, 24-h IAAB, and 24-h IAAO collectively provide the best primary estimates of the minimum physiological requirements for the indispensable amino acids. Table 16.6 gives the estimates for different amino acids that have been measured thus far. Nevertheless, the 24-h approach is open to the criticism in that it may not be an entirely physiological construct. In addition, the short-term IAAO method also gives estimates of IAA requirements that are consonant with the more rigorous 24-h methods. However, given the theoretical framework underpinning the 24-h IAAB technique (with its specific requirements), this method might be regarded as the reference method by which to validate other and possibly less complex tracer paradigms.

16.4.3 Post-prandial protein utilization

Short-term fast/fed tracer [1-^{13}C] leucine balance experiments have been used in another innovative way, to evaluate the utilization of wheat compared with milk protein, with a further calculation of the average requirement for lysine (Millward *et al.*, 2000). In theory, this approach could be adapted to estimate the requirements for other indispensable amino acids, especially if L-amino acid mixtures, or combinations of proteins and L-amino acids, were used in place of intact proteins. The tracer protocol lasts for 9 h with three consecutive 3-h phases: a post-absorptive phase, then a low protein meal phase, followed and terminated by a higher protein meal phase. The lysine requirement is derived from an estimate of the relative efficiency of wheat nitrogen retention compared with milk, assuming that lysine limits wheat utilization. This technique has the advantage of being based on an indicator tracer amino acid, in this case leucine. Thus, it has the potential for providing a reliable means of estimating the change in protein balance with protein intake in order to calculate the efficiency of post-prandial protein utilization (PPU) with one protein source and compare this with another.

There are areas where this protocol could be optimized for purposes of estimating the minimum daily requirement for an amino acid. Some of these are technical issues, which have been reviewed (Kurpad and Young, 2003a). For example Millward *et al.* (2000) found that at limiting intakes of an indispensable amino acid the estimate of PPU can differ with the passage of time within the meal-feeding phase. Also, it seems likely that the low-protein meal phase would influence the leucine balance that occurs during the succeeding high protein meal phase, so affecting the value of the PPU obtained.

Table 16.6. Estimation of different IAA requirements by the IAAO/IAAB method.

Amino acid	Method		Value obtained (range) mg kg^{-1} d^{-1}
	IAAO	IAAB	
Lysine	Zello *et al.* (1993)	Kurpad *et al.* (2001b)	29–45
	Duncan *et al.* (1996)	Kurpad *et al.* (2002a)	
	Kriengsinyos *et al.* (2002)	Kurpad *et al.* (2003a)	
	Kriengsinyos *et al.* (2004)	Kurpad *et al.* (2003c)	
Threonine	Wilson *et al.* (2000)	Borgonha *et al.* (2002)	15–19
		Kurpad *et al.* (2002b)	
Phenylalanine + tyrosine	Roberts *et al.* (2001)	Kurpad *et al.* (2006)	15–38
Tryptophan	Lazaris-Brunner *et al.* (1998)		4
Methionine	Di-Buono *et al.* (2001b)	Kurpad *et al.* (2003b)	13–16
		Kurpad *et al.* (2004)	
Valine		Kurpad *et al.* (2005)	17–20
BCAA	Riazi *et al.* (2003)		144

It might be critical to include changes in the size of the free leucine pool in estimating the change in protein-bound leucine balance; if not, the relative PPU may be overestimated, such that the apparent lysine requirement would be underestimated. Finally, when conducted in nutritionally replete individuals, the PPU of wheat protein would be expected to be higher than for individuals whose body, especially muscle, free lysine pool is lower as a consequence of an habitually lower intake of lysine. This underscores the fact that it is necessary to evaluate the question of an adaptation period, particularly with this method.

In summary, a number of different tracer techniques and protocols have been applied with the purpose of determining the requirement for specific indispensable amino acids in healthy adults. None are without important limitations. The 24-h IAAO and/or IAAB technique would appear to be the best current tracer-based approaches to date for estimation of adult amino acid requirements. Fundamentally, all of the methods used are surrogates for measuring protein synthesis, which is hard to measure directly. All the three different patterns of metabolic responses to graded intakes of an essential amino acid are summarized in Fig. 16.2.

16.5 Factorial Prediction of Amino Acid Requirements

One of the earlier paradigms for assessing IAA requirements was suggested by Young *et al.* (1989), based on estimates of the intakes of amino acids necessary to balance the minimum obligatory losses of amino acids (OAAL) as predicted from the composition of mixed body proteins (Table 16.7). In addition, when intakes of energy and other nutrients are adequate but the diet is essentially protein-free, the rate of body N loss, principally via urine and faeces, reaches a new, relatively steady-state level within about 1 week (Rand *et al.*, 1976). This new level is called the obligatory N loss (ONL) (FAO and WHO, 1973), and amounts to $54\,mg\,N\,kg^{-1}\,d^{-1}$ in healthy adults (FAO *et al.*, 1985). Moreover, various studies on obligatory nitrogen loss in different part of the world revealed that they are remarkably uniform (Bodwell *et al.*, 1979). Thus, it is assumed that the amounts of the different IAA contributing to these N losses occur in proportion to their concentrations in body mixed proteins, providing that those proteins contributing to the major proportion of the total N loss do not have amino acid patterns (concentrations) that differ markedly from the average of the body mixed proteins.

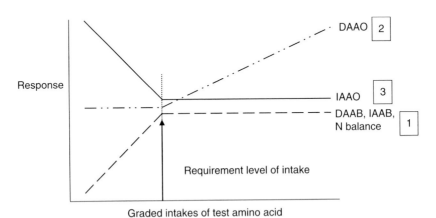

Fig. 16.2. The three different patterns of metabolic responses to graded intakes of an indispensable amino acid. Line 1 represents daily N balance, direct amino acid balance (DAAB) or indicator amino acid balance (IAAB). Line 2 represents the oxidation rate of the test amino acid (DAAO), in both short and 24-h measurements. Line 3 indicates the oxidation of an indicator amino acid (IAAO) in both short and 24-h measurements. The point of inflection of each line represents the requirement for the test amino acid. (Adapted from Pencharz and Ball, 2003.)

Table 16.7. Estimates of IAA requirements by the factorial prediction method.

Amino acid	Requirement (mg kg^{-1} d^{-1})[a]
Isoleucine	23
Leucine	40
Lysine	30
Methionine + cystine	13
Phenylalanine + tyrosine	39
Threonine	15
Tryptophan	6
Valine	20

[a]Values from Young et al. (1989).

The assumption that the amino acid requirement pattern for maintenance of protein nutritional status in adults is similar to that for mixed proteins in the whole body has been criticized (Millward et al., 1990; Fuller and Garlick, 1994; Waterlow, 1996). In addition, it was assumed that the efficiency of absorption of the IAA (at requirement level), in humans, was about 70%. This method is still used for those amino acids that have not yet been examined in tracer studies. The pattern of OAAL is assumed to be proportional to the relative concentrations of amino acids in whole-body mixed proteins. The question is whether the 70% value that has been assumed is valid for all the IAA. In general, however, there is a reasonable agreement between the body mixed protein–amino acid pattern and the estimations of the amino acid requirements in adults by tracer methods.

16.6 Estimates of the Amino Acid Requirement in Potentially Adapted States

From a homeostatic viewpoint, it might be anticipated that there would be a reduction in the body amino acid oxidation rate as a consequence of adaptation to the acute or chronic ingestion of decreased amounts of amino acid. That is indeed what is observed in the relatively acute conditions of the graded test intakes of amino acids described in the tracer section above, such that the oxidation of an amino acid reduces to a minimum when intakes of amino acid are below requirement. However, it might also be that under chronic conditions of under-nutrition, there is a constitutional decline in amino acid oxidation, as a conservation mechanism with lower than normal intakes. If this was the case, one might expect to observe an even greater reduction in oxidation at very low intakes, such that the degree of negativity of the amino acid balance at those low intakes is less than expected in the adapted individual. This was indeed the case in at least one set of comparisons of leucine balance at low intakes of leucine, between normal and chronically undernourished men (Kurpad et al., 2001c, 2003a). The chronically undernourished men were those with a low body mass index, and who came from a low socioeconomic stratum, living in slums in Bangalore, India. When comparing the response to graded intakes of leucine in these individuals, it becomes evident that the breakpoint for leucine requirement on the DAAB response line is about the same in both groups (Fig. 16.3). In this case, an adaptive response for conserving leucine only results in a shallower slope at leucine intakes that are very low and well below normal, since at subnormal intakes that are closer to the requirement level of 40 mg kg^{-1} d^{-1}, both groups have similar balances.

In effect, this does argue for an adaptive response, but one that is more evident or operative at very low intakes, in a manner that would improve survival, but probably not affect the actual requirement level. Given the issues with detecting a breakpoint in shallow response lines (discussed in the N balance section above, and Fig. 16.1), it might be that such a response could obtain a breakpoint in the response curve at a higher, rather than a lower intake. This emphasizes the need for measuring the amino acid oxidation or balance response at many intakes that cluster around the putative requirement, in order to define the breakpoint with more confidence. In any event, using the 24-h IAAB method in chronically undernourished men has yielded a higher breakpoint-based value for lysine intake, at about 45 mg kg^{-1} d^{-1}, in comparison with the normal value of 30 mg kg^{-1} d^{-1} (Kurpad et al., 2003b). In that case, however, it was found that intestinal parasites contributed to about half the increase in the

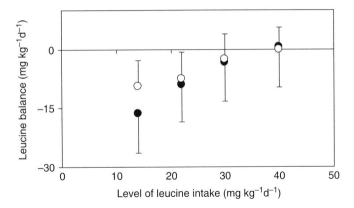

Fig. 16.3. Comparison of the 24-h leucine balance response to graded intakes of leucine in normal and chronically undernourished men. Filled circles, well-nourished subjects; open circles, undernourished subjects.

requirement, since de-worming the subjects reduced the requirement level (Kurpad *et al.*, 2003d), and it might be that under the physiologically 'perfect' experimental conditions during the 7 d adaptation period, there was some amount of tissue accretion, since the muscle mass in these subjects was also low. The same reasoning applies to children. In measurements of the lysine requirements in similar aged and otherwise healthy children in India (Pillai *et al.*, 2010) and Canada (Elango *et al.*, 2007), the daily requirements were the same, when measured by the relatively unadapted short-term IAAO method (Table 16.5), when ingesting their habitual levels of protein and energy intake. However, the Indian children were shorter and lighter than their Canadian counterparts, and this raises the question of how much the catch-up requirement of the children could be, under adapted and perfect conditions.

It is tempting to think that exposure to a chronically low and subnormal intake of protein and amino acids may result in adaptations that limit the oxidation of these amino acids, and therefore reduce the daily requirement. However, from the perspective of a requirement for optimal health in normal conditions, it is very likely that the requirement in such chronically undernourished individuals is the same, or even higher, than in normally nourished individuals, for the reasons stated above.

16.7 Conclusions

Depending on the method (N balance or tracer based), there appear to be greatly differing estimates of the IAA requirements. While the N balance method suffers from many technical difficulties and unresolved theoretical issues, the direct tracer-based methods potentially offer more accuracy and precision of measurement. The carbon balance method using ^{13}C-labelled amino acids is theoretically sound, but is subject to considerable uncertainty, with reasonably reliable estimates only available for amino acids that lose the label quantitatively and irreversibly when oxidized, and for which reliable estimates of precursor pool enrichment can be obtained. Another theoretically sound method is the adapted 24-h IAAB or carbon balance approach, in which most of the potential theoretical and practical problems for measuring the minimum physiological requirements have been addressed; in that sense, this is probably the closest one can get to a reference method. However, this method is difficult and cumbersome to use, particularly on vulnerable populations in whom IAA estimates are still based on factorial estimates. The short-term IAAO approach is easy to use and is effectively a breath test that can define the minimum requirements of an IAA, and has obtained estimates of IAA requirement that are close to those obtained by the 24-h adapted IAAB method (or the reference method). In that sense, it is probably the best method to deploy in resource poor environments, or in vulnerable populations. There is now a sufficient body of evidence based on the tracer methods that has led to a change in the estimates of human daily IAA requirements, and the currently accepted IAA requirements (WHO et al., 2007) are shown in Table 16.8. As always, additional studies on the quantitative aspects of the whole-body metabolism of indispensable and dispensable amino acids by these tracer approaches, particularly in subjects under different dietary conditions, are needed.

Table 16.8. Currently accepted IAA requirements (WHO et al., 2007).

Amino acid	Value (mg kg^{-1} d^{-1})
Leucine	39
Lysine	30
Threonine	15
Phenylalanine + tyrosine	25
Tryptophan	4
Methionine + cysteine	14
Valine	26
Isoleucine	20

References

Ball, R.O. and Bayley, H.S. (1984) Tryptophan requirement of the 2.5 kg piglet determined by the oxidation of an indicator amino acid. *Journal of Nutrition* 14, 1741–1746.

Ball, R.O., Courtney-Martin, G. and Pencharz, P.B. (2006) The in vivo sparing of methionine by cysteine in sulfur amino acid requirements in animal models and adult humans. *Journal of Nutrition* 136, 1682S–1693S.

Basile-Filho, A., El-Khoury, A.E., Beaumier, L., Wan, S.Y. and Young, V.R. (1997) Continuous twenty-four-hour L-[1-^{13}C]phenylalanine and L-[3,3-^{2}H$_2$]tyrosine oral tracer studies at an "intermediate" phenylalanine intake, to estimate requirements in adults. *American Journal of Clinical Nutrition* 65, 473–488.

Basile-Filho, A., Beaumier, L., El-Khoury, A.E., Yu, Y.M., Kenneway, M., Gleason, R.E. and Young, V.R. (1998) Twenty-four-hour L-[1-^{13}C]tyrosine and L-[3,3-^{2}H$_3$]phenylalanine oral tracer studies at generous, intermediate and low phenylalanine intakes to estimate aromatic amino acid requirements in adults. *American Journal of Clinical Nutrition* 67, 640–659.

Bergner, H., Simon, O. and Adam, K. (1978) Estimation of lysine requirements in growing rats from the rate of catabolism of ^{14}C and ^{15}N-labeled lysine. (Lysinbedarfs-bestimmung bei wachsenden Ratten anhand der Katabolisierungsrate von ^{14}C und ^{15}N-markiertem Lysin). *Archiv Tierenahrung* 28, 21–29.

Bodwell, C.E., Schuster, E.M., Kyle, E., Brooks, B., Womack, M., Steele, P. and Ahrens, R. (1979) Obligatory urinary and faecal nitrogen losses in young women, older men, and young men and the factorial estimation of adult human protein requirements. *American Journal of Clinical Nutrition* 32, 2450–59.

Borgonha, S., Regan, M.M., Oh, S.-H., Condon, M. and Young, V.R. (2002) Threonine requirements of healthy adults, evaluated by a 24h indicator amino acid balance technique. *American Journal of Clinical Nutrition* 75, 698–704.

Brookes, I.M., Owens, F.N. and Garrigus, U.S. (1972) Influence of amino acid level in the diet upon amino acid oxidation by the rat. *Journal of Nutrition* 102, 27–36.

Bross, R., Ball, R.O. and Pencharz, P.B. (1998) Development of a minimally invasive protocol for the determination of phenylalanine and lysine kinetics in humans during the fed state. *Journal of Nutrition* 128, 1913–9.

Calloway, D.H. and Margen, S. (1971) Variation in endogenous nitrogen excretion and dietary nitrogen utilization as determination of human protein requirements. *Journal of Nutrition* 101, 295–316.

Chavez, E.R. and Bayley, H.S. (1976) Amino acid metabolism in the piglet. 3. Influence of lysine level in the diet on energy metabolism and in vivo oxidation. *British Journal of Nutrition* 36, 369–380.

Cortiella, J., Matthews, D.E., Hoerr, R.A., Bier, D.M. and Young, V.R. (1988) Leucine kinetics at graded intakes in young men: quantitative fate of dietary leucine. *American Journal of Clinical Nutrition* 48, 998–1009.

Cortiella, J., Marchini, J.S., Branch, S., Chapman, T.E. and Young, V.R. (1992) Phenylalanine and tyrosine kinetics in relation to altered protein and phenylalanine and tyrosine intakes in healthy young men. *American Journal of Clinical Nutrition* 56, 517–525.

Davis, J.A., Greer, F.R. and Benevenga, N.J. (2000) Urea production is increased in neonatal piglets infused with alanine at 25, 50 and 75% of resting energy needs. *Journal of Nutrition* 130, 1971–1977.

De Benoist, B., Abdulrazzak, Y., Brooke, O.G., Halliday, D. and Millward, D.J. (1984) The measurement of whole body protein turnover in the preterm infant with intragastric infusion of L-[1-^{13}C]leucine and sampling of the urinary leucine pool. *Clinical Science* 66, 155–164.

Di Buono, M., Wykes, L.J., Ball, R.O. and Pencharz, P.B. (2001a) Dietary cysteine reduces the methionine requirement in men. *American Journal of Clinical Nutrition* 74, 761–766.

Di Buono, M., Wykes, L.J., Ball, R.O. and Pencharz, P.B. (2001b) Total sulfur amino acid requirement in young men as determined by indicator amino acid oxidation L-[1-^{13}C]phenylalanine. *American Journal of Clinical Nutrition* 74, 756–760.

Duncan, A.M., Ball, R.O. and Pencharz, P.B. (1996) Lysine requirement of adult males is not affected by decreasing dietary protein. *American Journal of Clinical Nutrition* 64, 718–725.

Elango, R., Humayun, M.A., Ball, R.O. and Pencharz, P.B. (2007) Lysine requirement of healthy school-age children determined by the indicator amino acid oxidation method. *American Journal of Clinical Nutrition* 86, 360–365.

Elango, R., Ball, R.O. and Pencharz, P.B. (2008) Individual amino acid requirements in humans: an update PB. *Current Opinion in Clinical Nutrition and Metabolic Care* 11, 34–39.

Elango, R., Humayun, M.A., Ball, R.O. and Pencharz, P.B. (2009) Indicator amino acid oxidation is not affected by period of adaptation to a wide range of lysine intake in healthy young men. *Journal of Nutrition* 139, 1–6.

El-Khoury, A.E., Fukagawa, N.K., Sánchez, M., Tsay, R.H., Gleason, R.E., Chapman, T.E. and Young, V.R. (1994a) Validation of the tracer-balance concept with reference to leucine: 24 El-Khoury hour intravenous tracer studies with L-(1-^{13}C)leucine and (^{15}N-^{15}N)urea. *American Journal of Clinical Nutrition* 59, 1000–1011.

El-Khoury, A.E., Fukagawa, N.K., Sánchez, M., Tsay, R.H., Gleason, R.E., Chapman, T.E. and Young, V.R. (1994b) The 24 hour pattern and rate of leucine oxidation, with particular reference to tracer estimates of leucine requirements in healthy adults. *American Journal of Clinical Nutrition* 59, 1012–1020.

El-Khoury, A.E., Sánchez, M., Fukagawa, N.K., Gleason, R.E., Tsay, R.H. and Young, V.R. (1995) The 24 hour kinetics of leucine oxidation in healthy adults receiving a generous leucine intake via three discrete meals. *American Journal of Clinical Nutrition* 62, 579–590.

El-Khoury, A.E., Ajami, A.M., Fukagawa, N.K., Chapman, T.E. and Young, V.R. (1996) Diurnal pattern of the interrelationships among leucine oxidation, urea production, and hydrolysis in humans. *American Journal of Physiology* 271, E563–E573.

El-Khoury, A.E., Forslund, A., Olsson, R., Branth, S., Sjodin, A., Anderson, A., Atkinson, A., *et al.* (1997) Moderate exercise at energy balance does not affect 24-h leucine oxidation or nitrogen retention in healthy men. *American Journal of Physiology* 273, E394–E407.

El-Khoury, A.E., Basile, A., Beaumier, L., Wang, S.Y., Al-Amiri, H.A., Selvaraj, A., Wong, S., *et al.* (1998) Twenty-four hour intravenous and oral tracer studies with L-[1-^{13}C]-2-aminoadipic acid and L-(1-^{13}C) lysine as tracers at generous nitrogen and lysine intakes in healthy adults. *American Journal of Clinical Nutrition* 68, 827–839.

El-Khoury, A.E., Pereira, P.C.M., Borgonha, S., Basile-Filho, A., Beaumier, L., Wang, S.Y., Metges, C.C., *et al.* (2000) Twenty-four-hour oral studies with L-[1-^{13}C]lysine at a low (15mg.kg^{-1}.d^{-1}) and intermediate (29mg.kg^{-1}.d^{-1})lysine intake in healthy adults. *American Journal of Clinical Nutrition* 72, 122–130.

FAO and WHO (1973) Energy and protein requirements. Report of a Joint FAO/WHO Ad Hoc Expert Committee, *Technical Report Series* 522. World Health Organization, Geneva.

FAO, WHO, and UNU (1985) Energy and protein requirements. Report of a Joint FAO/WHO/UNU Expert Consultation, *Technical Report Series* 724. World Health Organization, Geneva.

Fukagawa, N.K., Yu, Y.M. and Young, V.R. (1998) Methionine and cysteine kinetics at different intakes of methionine and cystine in elderly men and women. *American Journal of Clinical Nutrition* 68, 380–388.

Fuller, M.F. and Garlick, P. (1994) Human amino acid requirements: can the controversy be resolved? *Annual Review of Nutrition* 14, 217–241.

Harper, A.E. and Benjamin, E. (1984) Relationship between intake and rate of oxidation of leucine and α-ketoisocaproate in vivo in the rat. *Journal of Nutrition* 114, 431–440.

Hegsted, D.M. (1963) Variation in requirements of nutrients – amino acids. *Federation Proceedings* 22, 1424–1430.

Hegsted, D.M. (1976) Balance studies. *Journal of Nutrition* 106, 307–311.

Hiramatsu, T., Fukagawa, N.K., Marchini, J.S., Cortiella, J., Yu, Y.M., Chapman, T.E. and Young, V.R. (1994) Methionine and cysteine kinetics at different intakes of cystine in healthy adult men. *American Journal of Clinical Nutrition* 60, 525–533.

Hsu, J.W., Goonewardene, L.A., Rafii, M., Ball, R.O and Pencharz, P.B. (2006) Aromatic amino acid requirements in healthy men measured by indicator amino acid oxidation. *American Journal of Clinical Nutrition* 83, 82–88.

Humayun, M.A., Turner, J.M., Elango, R., Rafii, M., Langos, V., Ball, R.O. and Pencharz, P.B. (2006) Minimum methionine requirement and cysteine sparing of methionine in healthy school-age children. *American Journal of Clinical Nutrition* 84, 1080–1085.

Humayun, M.A., Elango, R., Ball, R.O. and Pencharz, P.B. (2007a) Re-evaluation of the protein requirement in young men with the indicator amino acid oxidation technique. *American Journal of Clinical Nutrition* 86, 995–1002.

Humayun, M.A., Elango, R., Moehn, S., Ball, R.O. and Pencharz, P.B. (2007b) Application of the indicator amino acid oxidation technique for the determination of metabolic availability of sulfur amino acid from casein versus soy protein isolate in adult men. *Journal of Nutrition* 137, 1874–1879.

Inoue, G., Fujita, Y., Kishi, K., Yamamoto, S. and Niiyama, Y. (1974) Nutritive values of egg protein and wheat gluten in young men. *Nutrition Reports International* 10, 202–207.

Irwin, M.I. and Hegsted, D.M. (1971) A conspectus of research on amino acid requirements of man. *Journal of Nutrition* 101, 539–566.

Jackson, A.A. (1993) Chronic malnutrition: protein metabolism. *Proceedings of the Nutrition Society* 8, 1617–1626.

Kang-Lee, Y.A.E and Harper, A.E. (1977) Effect of histidine intake and hepatic histidase activity on the metabolism of histidine in vivo. *Journal of Nutrition* 107, 1427–1443.

Kang-Lee, Y.A.E. and Harper, A.E. (1978) Threonine metabolism in vivo: Effect of threonine intake and prior induction of threonine dehydratase in rats. *Journal of Nutrition* 108, 163–175.

Kim, K.-I. and Bayley, H.S. (1983) Amino acid oxidation by young piglets receiving diets with varying levels of sulphur amino acids. *British Journal of Nutrition* 50, 383–390.

Kim, K.-I., McMillan, I. and Bayley, H.S. (1983a) Determination of amino acid requirements of young pigs using an indicator amino acid. *British Journal of Nutrition* 50, 369–382.

Kim, K.-I., Elliott, I.I. and Bayley, H.S. (1983b) Oxidation of an indicator amino acid by young pigs receiving diets with varying levels of lysine or threonine and assessment of amino acid requirements. *British Journal of Nutrition* 50, 391–399.

Krempf, M., Hoerr, R.A., Pelletier, V.A., Marks, L.M., Gleason, R. and Young, V.R. (1993) An isotopic study of the effect of dietary carbohydrate on the metabolic fate of dietary leucine and phenylalanine. *American Journal of Clinical Nutrition* 57, 161–169.

Kriengsinyos, W., Wykes, L.J., Ball, R.O. and Pencharz, P.B. (2002) Oral and intravenous tracer protocols of the indicator amino acid oxidation method provide the same estimate of the lysine requirement in healthy men. *Journal of Nutrition* 132, 2251–57.

Kriengsinyos, W., Wykes, L.J., Goonewardene, L.A., Ball, R.O. and Pencharz, P.B. (2004) Phase of menstrual cycle affects lysine requirement in healthy women. *American Journal of Physiology: Endocrinology and Metabolism* 287, E489–E496.

Kurpad, A.V. and Vaz, M. (2000) Protein and amino acid requirements in the elderly. *European Journal of Clinical Nutrition* 54, S131–S142.

Kurpad, A.V. and Young, V.R. (2003) What is apparent is not always real: lessons from lysine requirement studies in adult humans. *Journal of Nutrition* 133, 1227–1230.

Kurpad, A.V., El-Khoury, A.E., Beaumier, L., Srivatsa, A., Kuriyan, R., Raj, T., Borgonha, S., et al. (1998) An initial assessment, using 24 hour ^{13}C-leucine kinetics, of the lysine requirement of healthy adult Indian subject. *American Journal of Clinical Nutrition* 67, 58–66.

Kurpad, A.V., Raj, T., El-Khoury, A.E., Beaumier, L., Kuriyan, R., Srivatsa, A., Borgonha, S., et al. (2001a) Lysine requirements of healthy adult Indian subjects, measured by an indicator amino acid balance technique. *American Journal of Clinical Nutrition* 73, 900–908.

Kurpad, A.V., Regan, M.M., Raj, T., El-Khoury, A., Kuriyan, R., Vaz, M., Chandakudlu, D.V.G.V., et al. (2001b) The lysine requirement of healthy adult Indian subjects on longer term feeding and measured by the 24h indicator amino acid oxidation and balance technique. *American Journal of Clinical Nutrition* 73, 900–907.

Kurpad, A.V., Raj, T., El-Khoury, A., Kuriyan, R., Maruthy, K., Borgonha, S., Chandukudlu, D., et al. (2001c) The daily requirement for and splanchnic uptake of leucine in healthy adult healthy Indian subjects. *American Journal of Clinical Nutrition* 74, 747–755.

Kurpad, A.V., Regan, M.M., Raj, T., Maruthy, K., Gananou, J. and Young, V.R. (2002a) Intravenously infused 1-^{13}C leucine is retained in fasting healthy adult men. *Journal of Nutrition* 132, 1906–1908.

Kurpad, A.V., Regan, M.M., Raj, T., El-Khoury, A., Kuriyan, R., Vaz, M., Chandakudlu, D., *et al.* (2002b) Lysine requirements of healthy adult Indian subjects receiving long-term feeding measured with a 24-h indicator amino acid oxidation and balance technique. *American Journal of Clinical Nutrition* 76, 404–412.

Kurpad, A.V., Raj, T., Regan, M.M., Vasudevan., J., Caszo, B., Nazareth, D. and Young, V.R. (2002c) Threonine requirements of healthy Indian adults, measured by a 24-h indicator amino acid oxidation and balance technique. *American Journal of Clinical Nutrition* 76, 789–797.

Kurpad, A.V., Regan, M.M., Raj, T., Varalakshmi, S., Gnanou, J., Thankachan, P. and Young, V.R. (2003a) Leucine requirement and splanchnic uptake of leucine in chronically undernourished adult Indian subjects. *American Journal of Clinical Nutrition* 77, 861–867.

Kurpad, A.V., Regan, M.M., Raj, T., Vasudevan, J., Kuriyan, R., Gnanou, J. and Young, V.R. (2003b) Lysine requirements of chronically undernourished adult Indian men, measured by a 24-h indicator amino acid oxidation and balance technique. *American Journal of Clinical Nutrition* 77, 101–108.

Kurpad, A.V., Regan, M.M., Varalakshmi, S., Vasudevan, J., Gnanou, J., Raj, T. and Young, V.R. (2003c) Daily methionine requirements of healthy Indian men, measured by a 24-h indicator amino acid oxidation and balance technique. *American Journal of Clinical Nutrition* 77, 1198–205.

Kurpad, A.V., Regan, M.M., Nazareth, D., Nagaraj, S., Gnanou, J. and Young, V.R. (2003d) Intestinal parasites increase the dietary lysine requirement in chronically undernourished Indian men. *American Journal of Clinical Nutrition* 78, 1145–11451.

Kurpad, A.V., Regan, M.M., Varalakshmi, S., Gnanou, J. and Young, V.R. (2004) Daily requirement for total sulfur amino acids of chronically undernourished Indian men. *American Journal of Clinical Nutrition* 80, 95–100.

Kurpad, A.V., Regan, M.M., Raj, T., Gnanou, J., Rao, V. and Young, V.R. (2005) The daily valine requirement of healthy adult Indians determined by the 24-h indicator amino acid balance approach. *American Journal of Clinical Nutrition* 82, 373–379.

Kurpad, A.V., Regan, M.M., Raj, T., Rao, V., Gnanou, J. and Young, V.R. (2006) The daily phenylalanine requirement of healthy Indian adults. *American Journal of Clinical Nutrition* 83, 1331–1336.

Lazaris-Brunner, G., Rafii, M., Ball, R.O. and Pencharz, P.B. (1998) Tryptophan requirement in young adult women as determined by indicator amino acid oxidation with L-[^{13}C]phenylalanine. *American Journal of Clinical Nutrition* 68, 303–310.

Libao-Mercado, A.J.O., Zhu, C.L., Cant, J.P., Lapierre, H., Thibault, J., Sève, B., Fuller, M.F., *et al.* (2009) Dietary and endogenous amino acids are the main contributors to microbial protein in the upper gut of normally nourished pigs. *Journal of Nutrition* 139, 1088–1094.

MacCoss, M.J., Fukagawa, N.K. and Matthews, D.E. (1999) Measurement of homocysteine concentrations and stable isotope tracer enrichments in human plasma. *Analytical Chemistry* 71, 4527–4533.

Mager, D.R., Wykes, L.J., Ball, R.O. and Pencharz, P.B. (2003) Branched-chain acid requirements in school-aged children determined by indicator amino acid oxidation (IAAO). *Journal of Nutrition* 133, 3540–3545.

Manatt, M.W. and Garcia, P.A. (1992) Nitrogen balance: concepts and techniques. In: Nissen, S. (ed.) *Modern Methods in Protein Nutrition and Metabolism*. Academic Press, San Diego, CA, pp. 9–66.

Marchini, C.J., Cortiella, J., Hiramatsu, T., Chapman, T.E. and Young, V.R. (1993) Requirements for indispensable amino acids in adult humans: longer term amino acid kinetic study with support for the adequacy of the Massachusetts Institute of Technology amino acid requirement pattern. *American Journal of Clinical Nutrition* 58, 670–683.

Meguid, M.M., Matthews, D.E., Bier, D.M., Meredith, C.N., Soeldner, J.S. and Young, V.R. (1986a) Leucine kinetics at graded leucine intakes in young men. *American Journal of Clinical Nutrition* 43, 770–780.

Meguid, M.M., Matthews, D.E., Bier, D.M., Meredith, C.N. and Young, V.R. (1986b) Valine kinetics at graded valine intakes in young men. *American Journal of Clinical Nutrition* 43, 781–786.

Meredith, C.N., Wen, Z.-M., Bier, D.M., Matthews, D.E. and Young, V.R. (1986) Lysine kinetics at graded lysine intakes in young men. *American Journal of Clinical Nutrition* 43, 787–794.

Millward, D.J. (1998) Metabolic demands for amino acids and the human dietary requirement: Millward and Rivers (1988) revisited. *Journal of Nutrition* 128, 2563S–2576S.

Millward, D.J. (1999) The nutritional value of plant-based diets in relation to human amino acid and protein requirements. *Proceedings of the Nutrition Society* 58, 249–260.

Millward, D.J. (2000) Postprandial protein utilization: implications for clinical nutrition. In: Fürst, P. and Young, V.R. (eds) *Proteins, Peptides and Amino Acids in Enteral Nutrition*. Karger AG, Basel, pp. 135–155.

Millward, D.J., Price, G.M., Pacy, P.J.H. and Halliday, D. (1990) Maintenance protein requirements: the need for conceptual re-evaluation. *Proceedings of the Nutrition Society* 49, 473–487.

Millward, D.J., Fereday, A., Gibson, N.R. and Pacy, P.J. (2000) Human adult amino acid requirements: [1-^{13}C] leucine balance evaluation of the efficiency of utilization and apparent requirements for wheat protein and lysine compared with those for milk protein in healthy adults. *American Journal of Clinical Nutrition* 72, 112–121.

Moehn, S., Bertolo, R.F., Pencharz, P.B. and Ball, R.O. (2004) Indicator amino acid oxidation responds rapidly to changes in lysine or protein intake in growing and adult pigs. *Journal of Nutrition* 134, 836–41.

Mortimore, G.E., Woodside, K.H. and Henry, J.E. (1972) Compartmentation of free valine and its relation to protein turnover in perfused rat liver. *Journal of Biological Chemistry* 247, 2776–2784.

Motil, K.J., Bier, D.M., Matthews, D.E., Burke, J.F. and Young, V.R. (1981) Whole body leucine and lysine metabolism studied with [1-^{13}C]leucine and [1-^{15}N]lysine: response in healthy young men given excess energy intake. *Metabolism* 30, 783–791.

Pelletier, V., Marks, L., Wagner, D.A., Hoerr, R.A. and Young, V.R. (1991) Branched-chain amino acid interactions with reference to amino acid requirements in adult men: valine metabolism at different leucine intakes. *American Journal of Clinical Nutrition* 54, 395–401.

Pencharz, P.B. and Ball, R.O. (2003) Different approaches to define individual amino acid requirements. *Annual Review of Nutrition* 23, 101–116.

Pencharz, P.B., Hsu, J.W. and Ball, R.O. (2007) Aromatic amino acid requirements in healthy human subjects. *Journal of Nutrition* 137, 1576S–1578S.

Pillai, R.R., Elango, R., Muthayya, S., Ball, R.O., Kurpad, A.V. and Pencharz, P.B. (2010) Lysine requirement of healthy, school-aged Indian children determined by the indicator amino acid oxidation technique. *Journal of Nutrition* 140, 54–59.

Quevedo, M.R., Price, G.M., Halliday, D., Pacy, P.J. and Millward, D.J. (1994) Nitrogen homeostasis in man: diurnal changes in nitrogen excretion, leucine oxidation and whole body leucine kinetics during a reduction from a high to a moderate protein intake. *Clinical Science* 86, 185–193.

Raguso, C., Ajami, A.M., Gleason, R. and Young, V.R. (1997) Effect of cystine intake on methionine kinetics and oxidation, using oral tracers of methionine and cystine in healthy adults. *American Journal of Clinical Nutrition* 66, 283–292.

Raguso, C., El-Khoury, A.E. and Young, V.R. (1999) Leucine kinetics in reference to the effect of the feeding mode as three discrete meals. *Metabolism* 48, 1378–1386.

Raguso, C., Regan, M.M. and Young, V.R. (2000) Cysteine kinetics and oxidation at different intakes of methionine and cystine in young adults. *American Journal of Clinical Nutrition* 71, 491–499.

Raj, T., Dileep, U., Vaz, M., Fuller, M.F. and Kurpad, A.V. (2008) Intestinal microbial contribution to metabolic leucine input in adult men. *Journal of Nutrition* 138, 2217–2221.

Rand, W.M. and Young, V.R. (1999) Statistical analysis of N balance data with reference to the lysine requirement in adults. *Journal of Nutrition* 129, 1920–1926.

Rand, W.M., Young, V.R. and Scrimshaw, N.S. (1976) Change of urinary nitrogen excretion in response to low-protein diets in adults. *American Journal of Clinical Nutrition* 29, 639–644.

Rand, W.M., Scrimshaw, N.S. and Young, V.R. (1977) Determination of protein allowances in human adults from nitrogen balance data. *American Journal of Clinical Nutrition* 30, 1129–1134.

Rand, W.M., Scrimshaw, N.S. and Young, V.R. (1979) An analysis of temporal patterns in urinary nitrogen excretion of young adults receiving constant diets at two nitrogen intakes for 8 to 11 weeks. *American Journal of Clinical Nutrition* 32, 1408–1414.

Rand, W.M., Scrimshaw, N.S. and Young, V.R. (1985) A retrospective analysis of long term metabolic balance studies: Implications for understanding dietary nitrogen and energy utilization. *American Journal of Clinical Nutrition* 42, 1329–1350.

Riazi, R., Wykes, L.J., Ball, R.O. and Pencharz, P.B. (2003) The total branched-chain amino acid requirement in young healthy adult men determined by indicator amino acid oxidation by use of L-[1-^{13}C]phenylalanine. *Journal of Nutrition* 133, 1383–1389.

Roberts, S.B., Young, V.R., Fuss, P., Fiatarone, M.A., Richard, B., Rasmussen, H., Wagner, D.J., et al. (1990) Energy expenditure and subsequent nutrient intakes in overfed young men. *American Journal of Physiology* 259, R461–R469.

Roberts, S.B., Thorpe, J.M., Ball, R.O. and Pencharz, P.B. (2001) Tyrosine requirement of healthy men receiving a fixed phenylalanine intake determined by using indicator amino acid oxidation. *American Journal of Clinical Nutrition* 73, 276–282.

Rose, W.C. (1957) The amino acid requirements of adult man. *Nutrition Abstract and Review* 27, 631–647.

Sánchez, M., El-Khoury, A.E., Castillo, L., Chapman, T.E. and Young, V.R. (1995) Phenylalanine and tyrosine kinetics in young men throughout a continuous 24-h period, at a low phenylalanine intake. *American Journal of Clinical Nutrition* 61, 555–570.

Sánchez, M., El-Khoury, A.E., Castillo, L., Chapman, T.E., Basile, A., Beaumier, L. and Young, V.R. (1996) Twenty-four-hour intravenous and oral tracer studies with L-[1-^{13}C]phenylalanine and L-[3,3-^{2}H$_2$] tyrosine at a tyrosine-free generous phenylalanine intake in adults. *American Journal of Clinical Nutrition* 63, 532–545.

Storch, K.J., Wagner D.A., Burke J.F. and Young V.R. (1988) Quantitative study in vivo of methionine cycle in humans using [methyl-^{2}H$_3$]- and [1-^{13}C]methionine. *American Journal of Physiology* 255, E322–331.

Tontisirin, K., Young, V.R., Miller, M. and Scrimshaw, N.S. (1973) Plasma tryptophan response curve and tryptophan requirements of elderly people. *Journal of Nutrition* 103, 1220–1228.

Turner, J.M., Humayun, M.A., Elango, R., Rafii, M., Langos, V., Ball, R.O. and Pencharz, P.B. (2006) Total sulfur amino acid requirement of healthy school aged children as determined by indicator amino acid oxidation technique. *American Journal of Clinical Nutrition* 83, 619–623.

Waterlow, J.C. (1996) The requirements of adult man for indispensable amino acids. *European Journal of Clinical Nutrition* 50, S151–S179.

WHO, FAO, and UNU (2007) Protein and amino acid requirements in human nutrition. Report of a Joint WHO/FAO/UNU Expert Consultation. *World Health Organization Technical Report Series* 935, 1–265.

Wilson, D.C., Rafii, M., Ball, R.O., Pencharz, P.B. (2000) Threonine requirement of young men determined by indicator amino acid oxidation with use of L-[1-^{13}C]phenylalanine. *American Journal of Clinical Nutrition* 71, 757–764.

Wykes, L.J., Ball, R.O., Menendez, C.E. and Pencharz, P.B. (1990) Urine collection as an alternative to blood sampling: a noninvasive means of determining isotopic enrichment to study amino acid flux in neonates. *European Journal of Clinical Nutrition* 44, 605–608.

Young, V.R. (1987) McCollum Award Lecture. Kinetics of human amino acid metabolism: nutritional implications and some lessons. *American Journal of Clinical Nutrition* 46, 709–725.

Young, V.R. (1999) Amino acid flux and requirements: counterpoint; tentative estimates are feasible and necessary. In: *The Role of Protein and Amino Acids in Sustaining Enhancing Performance.* Committee on Military Nutrition Research, Food and Nutrition Board. Institute of Medicine, National Academies Press, Washington, DC, pp. 217–242.

Young, V.R. and Bier, D.M. (1981) Stable isotopes (^{13}C and ^{15}N) in the study of human protein and amino acid metabolism and requirements. In: Beers, R.F. and Bassett, E.G. (eds) *Nutritional Factors: Modulating Effects on Metabolic Processes.* Raven Press, New York, pp. 267.

Young, V.R. and Marchini, J.S. (1990) Mechanisms and nutritional significance of metabolic responses to altered adaptation in humans. *American Journal of Clinical Nutrition* 51, 270–289.

Young, V.R., Hussein, M.A., Murray, E. and Scrimshaw, N.S. (1971) Plasma tryptophan response curve and its relation to tryptophan requirement in young men. *Journal of Nutrition* 101, 45–60.

Young, V.R., Taylor, Y.S.M., Rand, W.M. and Scrimshaw, N.S. (1973) Protein requirements of man: efficiency of egg protein utilization at maintenance and sub maintenance levels in young men. *Journal of Nutrition* 103, 1164–1174.

Young, V.R., Wayler, A., Garza, C., Steinke, F.H., Murray, E., Rand, W.M. and Scrimshaw, N.S. (1984) A long-term metabolic balance study in young men to assess the nutritional quality of an isolated soy protein and beef proteins. *American Journal of Clinical Nutrition* 39, 8–15.

Young, V.R., Gucalp, C., Rand, W.M., Matthews, D.E. and Bier, D.M. (1987) Leucine kinetics during three weeks at submaintenance-to-maintenance intakes of leucine in men: adaptation and accommodation. *Human Nutrition: Clinical Nutrition* 41C, 1–18.

Young, V.R., Bier, D.M. and Pellett, P.L. (1989) A theoretical basis for increasing current estimates of the amino acid requirements in adult man, with experimental support. *American Journal of Clinical Nutrition* 50, 80–92.

Young, V.R., Wagner, D.A., Burini, R. and Storch, K.J. (1991) Methionine kinetics and balance at the 1985 FAO/WHO/UNU intake requirement in adult men studied with L-[^{2}H$_3$-methyl-1-^{13}C]methionine as tracer. *American Journal of Clinical Nutrition* 54, 377–385.

Young, V.R., Yu, Y.-M. and Fukagawa, N.K. (1992) Energy and protein turnover. In: Kinney, J.M. and Tucker, H.N. (eds) *Energy Metabolism: Tissue Determinants and Cellular Corollaries.* Raven Press, New York.

Zanni, E., Callow, D.H. and Zezulka, A.Y. (1979) Protein requirements of elderly men. *Journal of Nutrition* 109, 513–524.

Zello, G.A., Pencharz, P.B. and Ball, R.O. (1990) Phenylalanine flux, oxidation, and conversion to tyrosine in humans studies with L-[1-^{13}C]phenylalanine. *American Journal of Physiology* 259, E835–E843.

Zello, G.A., Pencharz, P.B. and Ball, R.O. (1993) Dietary lysine requirement of young adult males determined by oxidation of L-[1-^{13}C]phenylalanine. *American Journal of Physiology* 264, E677–E685.

Zello, G.A., Marai, L., Tung, A.S., Ball, R.O. and Pencharz, P.B. (1994) Plasma and urine enrichments following infusion of L-[1-^{13}C]phenylalanine and L-[ring-^{2}H$_5$]phenylalanine in humans: evidence for an isotope effect in renal tubular reabsorption. *Metabolism: Clinical and Experimental* 43, 487–491.

Zello G.A., Wykes, L.J., Ball, R.O. and Pencharz, P.B. (1995) Recent advances in method of assessing dietary amino acid requirements for adult humans. *Journal of Nutrition* 125, 2907–2915.

Zhao, X.-H., Wen, Z.-M., Meredith, C.N., Matthews, D.E., Bier, D.M. and Young, V.R. (1986) Threonine kinetics at graded threonine intakes in young men. *American Journal of Clinical Nutrition* 43, 795–802.

17 Amino Acid Supplements and Muscular Performance

T.A. Churchward-Venne, D.W.D. West and S.M. Phillips*

Exercise Metabolism Research Group, Department of Kinesiology, McMaster University, Hamilton, Canada

17.1 Abstract

Free form and protein source amino acid supplements are widely available, and are popular within the athletic community. Amino acids (AA) independently stimulate muscle protein synthesis (MPS) independently of hormones such as insulin, and suppress muscle protein breakdown (MPB) to a small degree. Concomitant with AA ingestion is an activation of cell-signalling pathways involved in the formation of translation-competent ribosomes, which occurs through the mammalian target of rapamycin (mTOR). As such, AA and protein (PRT) supplements represent a potentially effective strategy to increase skeletal muscle mass and strength, particularly when combined with anabolic modes of training such as resistance exercise (RE) training. The potential of these supplements is of great interest not only among athletes and their coaches, but also among researchers and clinicians as their application also represents a potentially effective strategy to counteract the loss of skeletal muscle mass that occurs with ageing (sarcopenia). Additionally, PRT and AA supplements have been reported to enhance endurance exercise (EE) performance, although this is a topic of considerable debate. In young subjects, PRT/AA supplements are capable of enhancing RE training-induced increases in skeletal muscle mass and strength; however, their role in facilitating similar adaptations in the elderly is less clear. Other factors such as timing (relative to exercise) of PRT/AA ingestion, PRT source or type and the AA composition may be particularly important in determining the efficacy of these supplements in the elderly. For example, the AA leucine is a key regulator of MPS that has been shown, in higher concentrations, to ameliorate the diminished anabolic sensitivity to AA that is characteristic of aged muscle. In addition, bovine milk and whey PRT, in particular, appear to be superior supplemental PRT sources capable of increasing MPS and enhancing RE-induced gains in lean mass. Overall PRT/AA supplements represent a convenient and effective means to stimulate MPS and enhance RE-induced gains in skeletal muscle mass; however, there is no evidence that they are more efficacious than consumption of a mixed meal containing high quality protein.

---

* E-mail address: phillis@mcmaster.ca

17.2 Introduction

There is great interest within the athletic community about the potential of nutritional interventions to enhance exercise training-induced increases in skeletal muscle mass and strength and/or improve endurance performance. In addition, both nutrition and exercise-based interventions to enhance muscle mass are of great interest clinically, as their application holds potential as an effective strategy to counteract the loss of muscle mass that occurs with ageing (sarcopenia) and other chronic diseases. Dietary supplements that purportedly increase skeletal muscle mass and strength, decrease fat mass, reduce fatigue or enhance athletic performance are widely available. Athletes in particular appear to be the greatest consumers of these supplements (Burke et al., 2006; Erdman et al., 2006; Huang et al., 2006), although individuals engaged in regular physical activity also report the use of such supplements (Morrison et al., 2004; Gaston and Correia, 2009), of which those containing PRT or AA appear to be the most popular (Gaston et al., 2009). But what is the scientific basis for the use of such supplements? The aim of this chapter is to examine the potential of AA/PRT supplements to support increases in skeletal muscle mass and strength, particularly in conjunction with RE, as well as to examine the potential for these supplements to augment EE performance and recovery. In addition, the potential of PRT/AA supplements in attenuating the loss in skeletal muscle mass that is characteristic of biological ageing will be examined. Important considerations such as timing of ingestion relative to exercise and the food source of dietary PRT supplements will be discussed, as these factors appear to modulate the anabolic response. This chapter will not specifically address the issue of protein requirements in resistance- and endurance-trained athletes and whether they are different from an average individual. Instead, we will simply highlight evidence supporting a role for PRT/AA supplements in augmenting adaptations to both RE and EE, and attempt to provide some insight into potential mechanisms.

17.3 Amino Acids and Protein Turnover

In addition to the well-recognized role of AA as substrate for protein synthesis, AA also stimulate the phosphorylation of various cell-signalling proteins and are capable of regulating protein synthesis (Fig. 17.1). Traditionally, AA have been classified as being either essential (indispensable) or non-essential (dispensable), based on requirements from the diet for attaining nitrogen balance. Thus, while non-essential AA may be synthesized *de novo*, essential AA (EAA) cannot be synthesized by the body and must be consumed through dietary intake. On average, the musculoskeletal system comprises 75% of the lean body mass of a healthy individual (Forbes, 1987), and so represents the largest reservoir for AA within the body. Although muscle is capable of oxidizing several AA, particularly the branched-chain amino acids (BCAA) (leucine, isoleucine, and valine) (Goldberg and Chang, 1978), AA contribute only ~2–5% of the energy contribution during prolonged dynamic exercise (Tarnopolsky, 2004; Rennie et al., 2006). Despite this relatively low energy contribution (as compared to carbohydrates and lipids), AA have a profound influence on skeletal muscle, particularly when combined with exercise. Body proteins are in a continuous state of turnover; that is, they are continuously being synthesized and degraded. The continual synthesis of new, and degradation of old proteins is an energetically expensive process that allows for damaged proteins to release their constituent AA into the local and systemic free pools where they may be used for the synthesis of new functional proteins, provide energy via gluconeogenesis, and/or direct oxidation.

The balance between MPS and MPB is the basis for determining the net protein balance (NPB) of a given tissue. When MPS > MPB, the result is a positive NPB and protein accretion. On the other hand, when MPB > MPS, NPB becomes negative and net tissue catabolism occurs. However, of the NPB equation, MPS is the variable that undergoes the greatest fold change in response to anabolic stimuli such as AA and RE (Chesley et al., 1992; Biolo et al., 1995; Biolo et al., 1997; Phillips et al., 1997; Phillips et al., 1999; Rasmussen and Phillips, 2003). Specifically, MPS undergoes changes

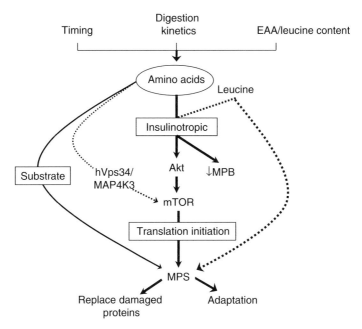

Fig. 17.1. Schematic showing the mechanism of action of exogenous amino acids in myofibre maintenance and adaptation. Dashed arrow pathways remain to be demonstrated convincingly in humans.

that are three- to fourfold greater than any change in MPB during the typical fasted- to fed-state transitions. This is not to say that MPB can be overlooked; however it plays a comparatively lesser role in determining muscle protein mass. As such, factors capable of augmenting both the magnitude and duration of MPS are likely to represent a relevant means to increase skeletal muscle mass.

17.4 Muscle Protein Synthesis

Protein synthesis involves the translation of ribonucleic acid (RNA) into a polypeptide before undergoing post-translational processing to produce the functional protein target. The translation of mRNA into a polypeptide involves the action of ribosomes and is conventionally described as consisting of three stages: initiation, elongation, and termination. Initiation brings the mRNA to the ribosome and involves a multitude of eukaryotic initiation factors that are involved in the assembly of the translation-ready ribosome. The elongation phase involves the addition of AA to the growing polypeptide chain and requires the presence of eukaryotic elongation factors. At the end of elongation, the newly synthesized polypeptide is released from the translational machinery when the termination codon is reached, thus completing the process of protein translation. Newly synthesized proteins can undergo post-translational modifications such as phosphorylation, carboxylation, or glycosylation that can modify the function of a given protein. Current research suggests that AA and exercise increase MPS primarily through increasing translation initiation, although alterations in the elongation stage of protein translation may also occur (Fujita *et al.*, 2007). The cell signalling pathways and the various proteins that respond to AA and exercise are discussed in further detail in the section 'Cell signalling response to amino acids and exercise' (below).

17.5 Enhancing Adaptations to Resistance Exercise with Amino Acid and Protein Supplements

High protein diets and the use of dietary protein supplements are largely grounded in the belief that such practices will increase skeletal muscle mass and strength and aid in recovery from exercise. A detailed review of protein requirements in strength and endurance trained athletes is beyond the scope of this chapter, however several reviews have been written on this topic elsewhere (Phillips, 2004; Phillips *et al.*, 2007). Briefly, strength athletes tend to habitually consume PRT in amounts that are far in excess of the current American and Canadian recommended dietary allowance (0.8 g kg^{-1} d^{-1}). Previously, it was thought that while exorbitant from a physiology standpoint, high PRT intakes were still contributing to a positive energy balance that was thought to be crucial to muscle anabolism. Furthermore, there is currently no tolerable upper limit for PRT, and since the conversion pathway of AA to lipid stores is biochemically more energetically expensive and inefficient compared to either excess carbohydrate or fat calories, energy from high PRO consumption may offer some advantage to athletes. Interestingly however, it has recently been observed that gains in lean mass can be achieved despite being in a negative energy balance (S.M. Phillips and A.R. Josse, unpublished observations). In addition, PRT consumed immediately after RE is able to augment adaptations to RE even when dietary PRT intake is as high as 1.4–1.5 g kg^{-1} d^{-1} (Hulmi *et al.*, 2009). Thus protein 'requirements' are likely to be dependent upon important outcomes such as lean mass accrual, fat mass loss, and strength, rather than attainment of nitrogen balance.

The remainder of this section will discuss the potential of PRT/AA supplements to enhance adaptations to RE training. It is important to state, however, that consumption of a mixed meal containing adequate amounts of high quality PRT is thought to be as efficacious as consumption of AA/PRT supplements in terms of facilitating adaptations to RE training (Rodriguez *et al.*, 2009). Indeed, provision of AA in close temporal proximity to a bout of RE increases MPS (Biolo *et al.*, 1997; Tipton *et al.*, 1999a, 2004; Bohe *et al.*, 2001, 2003; Katsanos *et al.*, 2006; Symons *et al.*, 2007; Wilkinson *et al.*, 2007; Tang *et al.*, 2009) and appears to enhance training-induced gains in skeletal muscle mass (Burke *et al.*, 2001; Candow *et al.*, 2006; Kerksick *et al.*, 2006; Cribb *et al.*, 2007; Hartman *et al.*, 2007; Willoughby *et al.*, 2007; Hulmi *et al.*, 2009; Josse *et al.*, 2010).

17.5.1 Acute studies

The provision of a complete mixture of AA, intravenously (Biolo *et al.*, 1997; Bohe *et al.*, 2001, 2003) or via oral ingestion (Tipton *et al.*, 1999a), has been shown to increase MPS. Likewise, ingestion of whole proteins is also capable of increasing MPS (Tipton *et al.*, 2004; Katsanos *et al.*, 2006; Symons *et al.*, 2007; Wilkinson *et al.*, 2007; Tang *et al.*, 2009). The shift from the fasted- (postabsorptive) to fed-state following AA provision results in a positive NPB and tissue protein accretion (Biolo *et al.*, 1997). The ability of AA to stimulate an increase in MPS forms the rationale for their use as a dietary supplement, particularly when combined with RE. For example, an acute bout of RE also stimulates an increase in MPS within as little as 2–4 h, but also increases the rate of MPB (Phillips *et al.*, 1997). This increase in MPS can be 40–150% above basal levels (Chesley *et al.*, 1992; Biolo *et al.*, 1995; Phillips *et al.*, 1997, 1999), and remain elevated for up to 48 h in the untrained state (Phillips *et al.*, 1997). However, when RE is performed in the fasted state, NPB remains negative because MPB is greater than MPS, despite MPS being stimulated to a greater extent (Biolo *et al.*, 1995; Phillips *et al.*, 1997). However, when PRT/AA are consumed following RE, NPB becomes positive due to large increases in MPS and a suppression of the normal exercise-induced rise in MPB (Biolo *et al.*, 1997). Biolo and colleagues reported that infusion of mixed AA after RE increased MPS >200% relative to basal rates, whereas AA infusion in the absence of prior exercise was associated with increases closer ~100% (Biolo *et al.*, 1997). Thus, the response to combined feeding and exercise is additive such that the increase in MPS is greater than that produced by either intervention alone (Biolo *et al.*, 1997). It is interesting, however, that the increase in MPS following AA provision can be attributed to the EAA, as non-essential AA appear to offer no further benefit (Tipton *et al.* 1999b; Borsheim *et al.*, 2002; Miller *et al.*, 2003). When performed chronically, RE and ingestion of quality PRT/ AA is thought to result in small net gains in muscle protein content that summate with each exercise/feeding session to produce gains in skeletal muscle mass (for review see Phillips, 2004).

17.5.2 Chronic studies

A valid question regarding the acute changes observed in MPS after RE and feeding is whether such findings, at least qualitatively, are predictive of long term changes in skeletal muscle mass following chronic training. While not definitively shown, there is evidence that the acute response of MPS to exercise and feeding is predictive of long-term changes in skeletal muscle mass following chronic exercise (Hartman *et al.*, 2007; Wilkinson *et al.*, 2007; West *et al.*, 2009, 2010). For instance, consumption of fluid milk after acute RE increases MPS to a greater extent than consumption of soy PRT (Wilkinson *et al.*, 2007). When examined chronically following 12 weeks of RE training, milk consumption was shown to translate into greater gains in fat and bone-free mass (i.e. muscle) than consumption of soy PRT (Hartman *et al.*, 2007) (Fig. 17.2).

In the absence of any planned dietary intervention, RE is able to increase skeletal muscle mass and strength in both young and old individuals (Frontera *et al.*, 1988; Fiatarone *et al.*, 1990; Kalapotharakos *et al.*, 2004; Kosek *et al.*, 2006). However, several studies have shown that PRT/AA supplements consumed in close temporal proximity RE increase skeletal muscle fibre cross-sectional area (CSA) following several weeks of training to a significantly greater degree than a carbohydrate- or energy-void placebo supplement (Anderson *et al.*, 2005; Bird *et al.*, 2006; Cribb *et al.*, 2007; Hartman *et al.* 2007). At the whole-body level, chronic consumption of PRT/AA supplements in the time period surrounding exercise also appears to increase lean tissue mass and muscle CSA following chronic RE training to a significantly greater extent than either carbohydrate or a non-energetic supplement (Burke *et al.*, 2001; Candow *et al.*, 2006; Kerksick *et al.*, 2006; Cribb *et al.*, 2007; Hartman *et al.*, 2007; Josse *et al.*, 2009; Willoughby *et al.*, 2007; Hulmi *et al.*, 2009). For example, Hartman and colleagues (2007) reported that consumption of fat-free fluid milk immediately and 1 h after

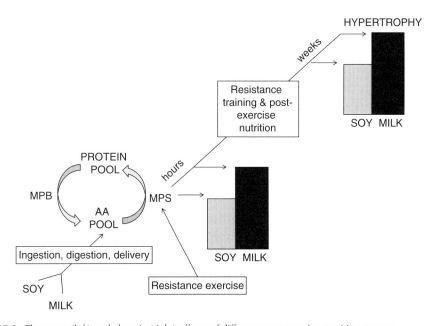

Fig. 17.2. The acute (left) and chronic (right) effects of different post-exercise nutrition sources.

RE resulted in significantly greater increases in type I and type II fibre CSA and lean body mass following 12 weeks of RE than consumption of isonitrogenous and isoenergetic soy beverages (Hartman et al., 2007). However, other studies have failed to report any benefit from supplemental PRT/AA on skeletal muscle fibre CSA or lean body mass following chronic RE (Godard et al., 2002; Candow et al., 2006a; Verdijk et al., 2009). Verdijk and colleagues (2009) reported no benefit in elderly men from 10 g of PRT both immediately before and after RE on lean body or limb mass or skeletal muscle fibre CSA, following 12 weeks of training. However, 10 g PRT post-workout is insufficient to maximize MPS (Moore et al., 2009a), particularly in the elderly who show a diminished sensitivity to the anabolic effects of AA (Cuthbertson et al., 2005) and pre-exercise protein is of questionable benefit (Tipton et al. 2007). Thus, the collective evidence suggests that when PRT/AA supplements are consumed in conjunction with chronic RE training, skeletal muscle mass (whole-body lean mass, and both limb muscle and fibre CSA) is increased to a greater degree than consumption of an energy-matched placebo/carbohydrate, at least in young subjects.

The roles that PRT/AA play in promoting gains in skeletal muscle mass with RE in the elderly are, however, less clear than in the young. Given that muscle in the elderly appears to be resistant to the anabolic effects of both RE (Kumar et al., 2009) and AA (Cuthbertson et al., 2005), factors such as timing of intake (Esmarck et al., 2001), PRT source (Dangin et al., 2003), leucine content (Katsanos et al., 2006), and PRT/AA dose (Katsanos et al., 2005) may be particularly important in the elderly population to maximize post-exercise MPS and promote training-induced gains in skeletal muscle mass.

17.5.3 Dose and distribution considerations to maximize MPS

Oral ingestion of ~20 g of complete high quality PRT appears sufficient to maximize the response of mixed MPS following acute RE in young men (Moore et al., 2009a). Consumption of twice as much PRT saw no further increase in MPS but increased leucine oxidation rate (Moore et al., 2009a). These findings are consistent with the dose-response relationship between EAA ingestion and the increase in myofibrillar protein synthesis reported during resting conditions (Cuthbertson et al., 2005). Cuthbertson and colleagues (2005) reported that 10 g of EAA were sufficient to maximize rates of myofibrillar protein synthesis in young and old men, an amount comparable to that found in 20 g of high quality PRT (~8.6 g). The amount of EAA required to maximize MPS after RE may actually be slightly less than requirements at rest. This is due to the elevation in MPB following RE that presumably allows for liberated AA to be re-utilized for the synthesis of new muscle proteins. In addition, meal distribution of PRT intake over the course of a day is also an important consideration from the perspective of maximizing gains in muscle protein content and minimizing AA oxidation and irreversible loss. However, current guidelines for dietary PRT do not address distribution of intake over the course of a day. Bohe and colleagues (2001) have shown that MPS becomes refractory despite continued elevations in aminoacidaemia. In addition, it is well known that increasing dietary PRT intake increases the activity of enzymes involved in AA catabolism (Das and Waterlow, 1974). Thus, 20 g PRT servings (or ~8–10 g EAA) spread out in even temporal intervals during the day may serve to maximize MPS and gains in RE-induced skeletal muscle protein gains in young subjects (Moore et al., 2009a). Intakes beyond this are unlikely to offer further benefit as far as maximizing the feeding-induced stimulation of MPS. However, given their reduced ability to elevate MPS in response to EAA (Cuthbertson et al., 2005), it appears that elderly muscle may require a higher dose of PRT to maximize MPS post-exercise.

17.6 Enhancing Endurance Exercise Performance and Recovery with Amino Acid and Protein Supplements

The oxidation of AA during EE contributes ~1–4% to the total energy provided, although sex and substrate availability from carbohydrate appear to influence the energy contribution from AA (Tarnopolsky, 2004; Rennie *et al.*, 2006). Despite the relatively minor contribution to energy provision from AA, several investigations have suggested that the addition of PRT to a carbohydrate beverage can improve EE performance (Ivy *et al.*, 2003; Saunders *et al.*, 2004; Saunders *et al.*, 2007). Other studies, however, have found no benefit to exercise performance from the addition of PRT to a carbohydrate beverage (van Essen and Gibala, 2006; Romano-Ely *et al.*, 2006; Osterberg *et al.*, 2008; Valentine *et al.*, 2008; Cermak *et al.*, 2009). However, as with RE, PRT consumption after EE has been shown to increase post-exercise MPS and NPB (Howarth *et al.*, 2009) and may thus represent an effective strategy to enhance the recovery process following EE (Fig. 17.3).

17.6.1 Amino acids and recovery from endurance exercise

Similar to RE, an acute bout of EE is associated with an increase in post-exercise MPS (Carraro *et al.*, 1990; Sheffield-Moore *et al.*, 2004). However unlike RE, EE training is not generally associated with increases in skeletal muscle mass. Wilkinson and colleagues (2008) examined the response of individual protein fractions (myofibrillar and mitochondrial) following 45 min of unilateral cycling exercise at 75% VO_2 max performed over several weeks. Regardless of the training status of the individuals, cycling exercise was associated with a pronounced increase in mitochondrial protein synthesis, yet no change in the synthesis of myofibrillar proteins (Wilkinson *et al.*, 2008). Thus the increase in mitochondrial (and to some extent sarcoplasmic) but not myofibrillar protein following EE is likely to play a vital role in facilitating the increases in aerobic capacity that are associated with this type of training.

Consumption of AA/PRT following EE may enhance the recovery process by increasing the synthesis of proteins involved in force production and energy metabolism (Rodriguez *et al.*, 2007), as well as by helping to restore muscle glycogen (van Loon *et al.*, 2000; Ivy *et al.*, 2002). When PRT is consumed immediately after EE, both skeletal muscle (Howarth *et al.*, 2009) and whole body (Levenhagen *et al.*, 2002)

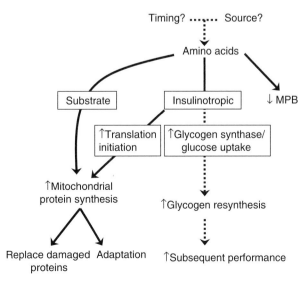

Fig. 17.3. Schematic showing the benefits of amino acids to endurance exercise. 'Insulinotropic' indicates activation of the insulin/IGF-1-derived pathway. 'Subsequent performance' refers to exercise or athletic event performed in close proximity (<24 h) to a previous bout. Dashed arrow pathways remain to be demonstrated convincingly in humans.

protein synthesis are increased. For example, Howarth and colleagues (2009) reported that co-ingestion of PRT with carbohydrate after cycling exercise increased mixed MPS and resulted in a more positive NPB than ingestion of a drink matched for carbohydrate or total energy content. Additionally, Koopman and colleagues (2004) reported that addition of PRT to a carbohydrate beverage improved whole-body NPB both during and after 6 h of ultra-endurance exercise, via increased protein synthesis and reduced protein breakdown. Thus, consumption of a source of AA with carbohydrate appears to increase MPS and improve whole-body NPB, but whether this practice enhances the adaptive response to chronic EE remains to be shown definitively. However, given that the mitochondrial protein fraction is sensitive to exogenous AA provision (Bohe et al., 2003), it may be inferred that PRT/AA immediately after EE is likely to represent an effective strategy to facilitate the adaptive response to EE by increasing the synthesis of mitochondrial proteins (Fig. 17.3).

In addition to promoting post-exercise protein synthesis, the addition of a source of AA to a carbohydrate beverage has been reported to modulate the synthesis of muscle glycogen (van Loon et al., 2000; Ivy et al., 2002). The increased rates of glycogen re-synthesis may be attributed to the insulinotropic effects of AA, which appears to enhance GLUT-4 translocation (the main insulin-sensitive glucose transporter) and stimulate glycogen synthase activity when carbohydrate is limiting (van Loon et al., 2000). Indeed, when carbohydrate content and rate of delivery are increased to 1.2 g $kg^{-1}h^{-1}$, glycogen synthesis was increased such that it was no different from the AA-containing solution (van Loon et al., 2000). A separate study from the same group (Jentjens et al., 2001) showed that when carbohydrate was increased and provided at a rate of 1.2 g $kg^{-1}h^{-1}$, addition of a source of AA (0.4 g $kg^{-1}h^{-1}$) did not increase rates of glycogen synthesis above that of carbohydrate. Thus, for those on a carbohydrate-restricted diet, provision of AA after exercise may represent an effective strategy to increase muscle glycogen while reducing the amount of carbohydrate intake.

17.6.2 Role of protein and amino acids in endurance exercise performance

Several studies have reported that PRT ingestion during exercise improves EE performance (Ivy et al., 2003; Saunders et al., 2004, 2007). Ivy and colleagues (2003) reported that adding PRT to a carbohydrate drink improved cycling endurance capacity (time to exhaustion) by ~30% compared to carbohydrate alone. However, other studies have failed to find any performance benefit from the addition of PRT to a carbohydrate beverage (van Essen and Gibala, 2006; Romano-Ely et al., 2006; Osterberg et al., 2008; Valentine et al., 2008; Cermak et al., 2009). For example, van Essen and Gibala (2006) found that addition of whey PRT to a carbohydrate solution did not improve cycling time trial performance relative to carbohydrate alone. Differences between these studies may relate to carbohydrate intake during exercise, and thus the rate of delivery. For instance, the studies demonstrating a benefit from added PRT (Ivy et al., 2003; Saunders et al., 2004, 2007) have typically provided carbohydrate at rates between 37 and 47 g carbohydrate h^{-1}. These rates are below peak exogenous oxidation rates for carbohydrate, which have been reported to be 60–72 g h^{-1} (Jentjens et al., 2004a,b,c). Thus, when carbohydrate is provided at a rate of 60 g carbohydrate h^{-1}, a rate considered optimal (Gibala, 2007), added PRT does not appear to improve cycling time-trial performance (van Essen and Gibala, 2006; Cermak et al., 2009) or alter markers of metabolic control such as muscle glycogen use, phosphocreatine hydrolysis, or tricarboxylic acid cycle intermediates (Cermak et al., 2009). In light of these recent data, use of AA or PRT with EE may best be directed to the post-exercise recovery period to enhance MPS, NPB, and glycogen re-synthesis.

17.7 Cell Signalling Responses to Amino Acids and Resistance Exercise

The molecular regulation of MPS in response to feeding and exercise is thought to involve multiple converging cell-signalling pathways.

Current understanding of the molecular regulation of MPS precludes the ability to predict quantitative changes in MPS based on acute cell-signalling responses to feeding and exercise. The cellular signalling response(s) to anabolic stimuli in the form of AA and/or RE remains to be fully elucidated, although this is currently an area of immense research interest. This section will provide an overview of current understanding of the ability of AA and RE to activate anabolic signalling pathways, with particular emphasis on mTOR and its downstream targets.

17.7.1 Cell signalling pathways involved in translation initiation and elongation

EAA stimulate MPS, an effect that is due to an increase in the concentration of extracellular EAA (Bohe *et al.*, 2003). The extracellular AA concentration (or changes in it) is somehow 'sensed', and a signal activates translation initiation. Insulin and EAA activate cell-signalling pathways that converge on mTOR, activate its downstream targets, and augment both translation initiation and elongation of protein synthesis (Fig. 17.1) (for review see Drummond *et al.*, 2009). That is, while insulin activates the phosphatidylinositol 3-kinase (PI3K) and protein kinase B (PKB/Akt) pathways, EAA can promote translation initiation in a manner that is independent of Akt (Wang *et al.*, 1998). Anthony and colleagues (2000) have shown that the mTOR inhibitor rapamycin is able to inhibit the leucine-induced stimulation of MPS and subsequent phosphorylation of p70S6k, supporting the notion that EAA such as leucine increase MPS through mTOR. Recently it has been proposed that hVps34, a class III PI3k, may play an important role in the AA-induced activation of mTOR and its downstream targets (Byfield *et al.*, 2005). Another study has shown a similar role for MAP4K3, a MAP kinase that may detect AA and signal mTOR independently of insulin (Findlay *et al.*, 2007). A role for either hVps34 or MAP4K3 in mediating the AA-induced activation of mTOR in human muscle remains to be shown.

17.7.2 Cell signalling response to amino acids

In human muscle, increases in MPS following ingestion of EAA and carbohydrate have been shown to be associated with activation of mTORC1 (complex 1) (Cuthbertson *et al.*, 2005; Fujita *et al.*, 2007). Fujita and colleagues (2007) have shown that a leucine-enriched mixture of EAA and carbohydrate increases MPS, concomitant with an increase in the phosphorylation of mTOR and its downstream targets p70S6k and 4E-BP1, and a decrease in eEF2. Leucine independently stimulates MPS in rats, and results in phosphorylation of factors associated with initiating mRNA translation primarily through the mTOR signalling pathway such as p70S6k and 4E-BP1 (Anthony *et al.*, 2002; Crozier *et al.*, 2005). Together, these findings suggest that provision of EAA and leucine are capable of increasing activation of components of the mTOR pathway including 4E-BP1 and p70S6k.

17.7.3 Cell signalling response to amino acids and exercise

It has been firmly established that RE stimulates MPS (Chesley *et al.*, 1992; Biolo *et al.*, 1995; Phillips *et al.*, 1997, 1999), and that this effect is synergistic with the provision of a source of AA (Biolo *et al.*, 1997; Dreyer *et al.*, 2008). Karlsson and colleagues (2004) demonstrated that p70S6k and S6 phosphorylation were increased post-exercise following the ingestion of EAA, as compared to exercise alone. In addition, PRT after acute RE results in greater phosphorylation of p70S6k than exercise performed without PRT (Koopman *et al.*, 2007). Leucine-enriched EAA and carbohydrate provided after acute RE have been shown to increase MPS and the phosphorylation status of Akt and components of the mTOR pathway including mTOR, p70S6k, and 4E-BP1, suggesting increased translation initiation (Dreyer *et al.*, 2008). Collectively, these findings support the notion that activation of the mTOR signalling pathway, and in particular phosphorylation of p70S6k, is associated with increases in MPS following RE.

17.8 Timing Considerations

Timing of nutrient intake involves the strategically planned consumption of either whole foods or dietary supplements, usually in the period surrounding an exercise stimulus in an attempt to enhance the adaptive response to exercise (Kerksick et al., 2008). Indeed, AA/PRT ingestion in close temporal proximity to a bout of RE appears to result in greater increases in lean body mass than nutrients provided at later times (Burk et al., 2009; Cribb and Hayes, 2006; Esmarck et al., 2001; Hartman et al., 2007). In this section we will discuss the relevance of timing of AA provision around an exercise stimulus and the potential of this strategy to augment adaptations to exercise.

17.8.1 Nutrient timing and acute exercise

An acute bout of RE stimulates an increase in MPS for up to 48 h (Phillips et al., 1997). Feeding any time within this 48-h window should simply add to this elevated rate of MPS to a greater extent than feeding during rested conditions in the absence of a previous bout of resistance exercise (Burd et al., 2009b). Indeed, Burd and co-workers (2009a) reported that acute RE results in enhanced anabolic sensitivity to AA provision that persists for 24 h post-exercise. However, early provision of AA after RE may confer greater benefit than delayed consumption, as MPS rates are elevated to a greater magnitude early after exercise (Phillips et al., 1997). In addition, cell-signalling proteins involved in increasing translation initiation after RE, such as mTOR and p70S6k are activated early and appear to undergo peak activation within 30–60 min after exercise (Camera et al., 2010). The exact duration of this 'anabolic window' is, however, not known. However, other reports suggest that this window may be at least 3 h long. For example, when 6 g of EAA and carbohydrate (35 g) were consumed at 1 or 3 h after RE, there was no difference in protein synthesis rates in young men (Rasmussen et al., 2000). In an early investigation, Tipton and colleagues (2001) reported greater increases in AA uptake across the leg when EAA were consumed before as opposed to after RE, and attributed the effect to a greater delivery of AA to the muscle as a result of exercise-induced hyperaemia. However, Fujita and colleagues (2009) reported no difference in the increase in post-exercise MPS relative to exercise without nutrients when EAA and carbohydrate were consumed before RE. Thus, the role of EAA ingestion prior to a bout of RE on post-exercise MPS appears to be less than the additive response that is observed with post-exercise feeding (see Drummond et al., 2009). The physiological relevance of providing a source of AA during acute exercise has also been investigated (Beelen et al., 2008). It appears that rates of MPS are reduced during the contractile activity associated with exercise (Dreyer et al., 2006). As both MPS and muscle contraction are energy-consuming processes, it has been suggested that the muscle contractile activity associated with physical exercise is of a higher metabolic priority than the synthesis of new proteins (Atherton and Rennie, 2009). However, co-ingestion of carbohydrate and PRT during exercise appears to increase MPS, although this increase was not associated with increased muscle protein accretion during subsequent overnight recovery (Beelen et al., 2008). Thus, AA/PRT consumption immediately after acute exercise appears to be more efficacious in promoting muscle protein accretion than consuming these nutrients immediately before or during exercise.

17.8.2 Nutrient timing and chronic exercise

In terms of long-term adaptations to chronic RE, Hartman and colleagues (2007) have shown that PRT consumption within 2 h following RE results in greater increases in muscle fibre hypertrophy and lean mass gains following 12 weeks of training, than consuming carbohydrate during this 2-h window (Hartman et al. 2007). Similarly, Cribb and Hayes (2006) examined changes in body composition and muscle strength following consumption of a supplement containing PRT, creatine and glucose immediately before and after RE relative to the same supplement consumed in the morning and evening. Following 10 weeks of training, the group consuming the supplement immediately before and after exercise experienced greater increases in lean body mass and strength, in conjunction with greater increases in type-II fibre CSA (Cribb and Hayes, 2006). Interestingly, Esmarck and colleagues (2001) reported that delaying PRT consumption after RE by only 2 h prevented training-induced gains in muscle mass and strength in older men, as compared to subjects who consumed a beverage containing PRT, fat, and carbohydrate immediately after workout. Overall, consuming a source of EAA immediately after RE (within 2 h) appears to result in greater gains in lean mass and strength than delayed consumption following several weeks of training; however, skeletal muscle appears to display enhanced sensitivity to the anabolic effects of AA for at least 24 h after exercise (Burd et al., 2009a).

17.9 Amino Acid Source

Sources of dietary PRT differentially affect the rate of whole-body (Boirie et al., 1997; Dangin et al., 2001) and skeletal MPS (Tang and Phillips 2009; Tang et al., 2009), as well as support RE-induced gains in lean mass (Cribb et al., 2006; Hartman et al., 2007). The mechanisms underpinning these differences are not entirely clear; however, important differences in the AA profile and/or differences in digestion/absorption kinetics may explain some of the observed differences. Bovine milk and whey PRT appear to support greater increases in MPS (Wilkinson et al., 2007; Tang et al., 2009) and training-induced lean mass accretion (Hartman et al., 2007; Cribb et al., 2006) than other sources of PRT or carbohydrate (see Phillips et al., 2009 for review).

17.9.1 Acute studies

Whey comprises ~20% of the proteins found in bovine milk (Ha and Zemel, 2003), with casein making up the other 80%. Whereas whey is acid soluble and digested quickly, casein coagulates in the stomach, a process delaying exit from the stomach and greatly slowing its absorption and subsequently the rate at which its constituent AA enter peripheral circulation. Thus whey is considered a 'fast' PRT that induces large but transient levels of hyperaminoacidaemia, whereas casein is a 'slow' PRT associated with a moderate but sustained rise in plasma AA (Boirie et al., 1997). Boirie and colleagues (1997) demonstrated that whey and casein differ in their ability to stimulate whole-body protein synthesis and attenuate whole body protein breakdown at rest. For example, ingestion of casein promoted a greater NPB than whey, due to a greater suppression of whole-body proteolysis (Boirie et al., 1997). Later work by Dangin and colleagues (2001) pointed to differences in the rate of PRT digestion (and subsequent hyperaminoacidaemia) between whey and casein as the key variable influencing the observed differences in whole-body protein kinetics. Interestingly, whole-body protein retention appears to be increased to a greater degree in the elderly following consumption of whey (Dangin et al., 2003). Thus, at the whole-body level, slowly digested proteins that induce a moderate but sustained rise in plasma AA appear to increase protein retention in young individuals. The elderly, however, respond differently, as whole body-protein retention is increased in response to a large but transient increase in plasma AA concentration (Dangin et al., 2003). Skeletal muscle accounts for ~25–30% of whole-body protein synthesis (Nair et al., 1988), with a turnover rate that is ~20-fold lower than both splanchnic (Nakshabendi et al., 1995, 1999) and plasma (Carraro et al., 1990a) proteins. Thus, it is not entirely clear if the whole-body protein data demonstrating differential effects of PRT source on whole-body synthesis and breakdown (Boirie et al., 1997) is indeed reflective of the anabolism of skeletal muscle proteins. To address this question, Tang and colleagues (2009) examined the effects of whey PRT hydrolysate, soy PRT isolate, and micellar casein on rates of mixed MPS at rest and after acute RE. Whey PRT stimulated mixed MPS to a greater degree at rest than casein, and to a greater degree than both soy and casein after exercise; however, soy was more effective than casein after RE (Tang et al., 2009). Interestingly, fat-free fluid milk increases MPS and net AA uptake across the leg to a greater degree than soy (Wilkinson et al., 2007). This finding is consistent with reports that milk and soy proteins are preferentially partitioned to different body pools for use following their ingestion (Fouillet et al., 2003). For example, soy appears to be preferentially directed towards the splanchnic tissues to support protein synthesis, while milk proteins are directed toward peripheral tissues (i.e. skeletal muscle) to support protein anabolism (Bos et al., 2003; Fouillet et al., 2003; Morens et al., 2003). Thus, differences between PRT sources may in part be explained by differences in digestion/absorption kinetics, and thus the rates at which AA enter circulation (Boirie et al., 1997; Dangin et al., 2001, 2003). However, whey PRT contains a greater amount of the BCAA leucine, a known regulator of the mTOR/p70S6k signalling cascade of translation initiation (Anthony et al., 2002). Thus, differences in leucine concentration may also affect the response of MPS following ingestion of different sources of high quality PRT. It is interesting to note that the anabolic effects of whey PRT are not simply due to its EAA content, as 15 g of whey PRT acutely increased muscle protein accrual in the elderly more than its constituent EAA content (6.72 g EAA) (Katsanos et al., 2008). The mechanism behind this finding is not clear, but may relate to the greater insulin response observed with whey as compared to EAA (Katsanos et al., 2008).

We conclude that in terms of increasing the anabolic effects of RE, consumption of whey or milk appears to be superior to consumption of micellar casein or soy (Fig. 17.2). Indeed, chronic RE training/feeding studies support this thesis (Cribb et al., 2006; Hartman et al., 2007).

17.9.2 Chronic studies

The acute responses that are observed following milk and whey in terms of their ability to promote greater muscle protein anabolism than soy and casein appear to be qualitatively predictive of the long-term hypertrophic response following chronic RE and feeding (Phillips et al., 2009). In young men, for instance, chronic consumption of fat-free fluid skim milk has been reported to result in greater lean mass accrual and greater fat mass loss than consuming soy, following 12 weeks of RE (Hartman et al., 2007). Additionally, Cribb and colleagues (2006) reported gains in muscle mass following 10 weeks of RE in recreational bodybuilders that were ~fivefold greater with whey PRT compared to casein. However, other studies have reported no effect of PRT source on gains in lean mass following a period of RE training. Supplemental whey and soy were reported to result in greater gains in lean mass than an isoenergetic placebo following 6 weeks of RE, but there was no effect of protein source (Candow et al., 2006). However, a comprehensive review of several RE studies concluded that consumption of both milk and whey are indeed associated with greater gains in lean muscle mass than consumption of soy or a carbohydrate/placebo, although soy appears to offer some benefit over carbohydrate (Phillips et al., 2009).

17.10 Role of Leucine and Amino Acid Supplements in the Sarcopenia of Ageing

Nutrition and exercise-based interventions to counteract the loss of muscle mass that occurs with ageing (sarcopenia) are of great interest clinically. Concurrent use of nutrition and RE-based interventions to promote MPS and muscle hypertrophy represent potentially effective therapeutic strategies to minimize, and potentially reverse, the loss of muscle mass and strength that occurs with ageing. Also important, however, is that a relatively large quantity of skeletal muscle may help to offset the morbidities associated with the sarcopenia of ageing such as type II diabetes, declines in aerobic capacity, and reductions in metabolic rate that can ultimately lead to fat-mass accumulation (Wolfe et al., 2006). Here we will discuss the potential role of leucine and AA/PRT supplements to help combat the loss of muscle mass that occurs in concert with biological ageing.

Current research supports a unique role for the AA leucine as a nutrient regulator of translation initiation of protein synthesis

(Anthony et al., 2002; Crozier et al., 2005). Leucine, isoleucine, and valine represent the BCAA that account for ~14% of the total AA found in skeletal muscle tissue (Riazi et al., 2003). In humans, infusion of a large dose of leucine is able to stimulate MPS (Smith et al., 1992). In rats, leucine alone stimulates MPS and phosphorylates factors associated with initiating mRNA translation, primarily through the mTOR signalling pathway such as p70S6k and 4E-BP1 (Anthony et al., 2002; Crozier et al., 2005). Plasma leucine concentration directs the peak activation of MPS in the post-prandial state. However, the length of time that MPS remains elevated following feeding is affected by other factors, which remain to be elucidated (Norton et al., 2009). Given the role of leucine as a primary regulator of MPS, an obvious avenue of research has been to investigate its potential as a nutritional intervention to attenuate age-related muscle wasting. Aged muscle has been shown to be resistant to the anabolic effects of AA (Cuthbertson et al., 2005) and the antiproteolytic effects of insulin (Wilkes et al., 2009). However, studies in both rats (Rieu et al., 2003) and humans (Katsanos et al., 2006; Rieu et al., 2006) have shown that a high concentration of leucine is able to restore rates of protein synthesis in aged muscle. For example, Katsanos and colleagues (2006) showed that the ingestion of 6.7 g of EAA (26% leucine) was unable to increase MPS above basal rates in the elderly, but effectively increased MPS in the young. However, when the leucine content was increased (41%), MPS was elevated above basal levels to the same extent as observed in young subjects. However, when larger doses of PRT are consumed, increased leucine does not appear to offer additional benefit (Tipton et al., 2009), suggesting that when leucine concentration is already high, additional leucine is not beneficial. In a long-term investigation, Verhoeven and colleagues (2009) reported that chronic (3 months) free-form leucine supplementation at 7.5 g d^{-1} (2.5 g at breakfast, lunch, and dinner) in the elderly did not increase lean muscle mass or strength as compared to an energy-matched placebo. In this context, it is interesting that other studies have reported increases in lean muscle mass in elderly subjects following chronic (3–16 months) mixed EAA supplementation (Borsheim et al., 2008; Solerte et al., 2008; Dillon et al., 2009). When leucine is provided in supplemental form, plasma levels of the other BCAA may become depleted (Dardevet et al., 2000); thus it has been suggested that a balanced mixture of BCAA may be more efficacious than free-form leucine supplementation (Balage and Dardevet, 2010). In addition, it may be that leucine supplementation is more effective when consumed in close proximity to acute RE. Moore and and co-workers (2009b) have shown that while PRT ingestion stimulates the synthesis of both the myofibrillar and sarcoplasmic protein fraction at rest, PRT consumption after RE is associated with an increase in the synthesis predominantly of the myofibrillar fraction of muscle protein. Thus, leucine supplementation is likely to be most efficacious when combined with RE, as it may potentiate the synthesis of myofibrillar proteins. In conclusion, both nutritional and exercise-based interventions represent potentially effective therapeutic strategies to enhance skeletal muscle mass in aged individuals. A combination of RE and AA/PRT feeding is likely to be more efficacious than either stimulus alone, but more research is needed to fully elucidate the conditions under which supplemental leucine may be most effective. However, aged muscle appears to be resistant to the anabolic effects of leucine at doses that stimulate MPS in the young (Katsanos et al., 2006), suggesting that the elderly may have a higher leucine 'threshold' to stimulate MPS. Thus, the elderly should focus on obtaining adequate protein at each meal to ensure an adequate leucine concentration to maximally stimulate MPS.

17.11 Conclusions and Future Directions

Exercise and AA, particularly in combination, have profound effects on muscle protein turnover and NPB. Athletes in particular report the use of AA/PRT supplements, although use of these supplements is also popular among physically active individuals in commercial exercise settings. Both feeding and RE are known to activate anabolic cell-signalling pathways, including the mTOR / p70S6k signalling cascade important in translation initiation. More research is required to fully elucidate these pathways and their respective proteins. Understanding how AA and RE are 'sensed' such that these anabolic signalling pathways are activated would greatly advance current understanding of the molecular basis of how muscle mass is regulated. It appears that in young subjects, PRT/AA supplements are more capable of enhancing RE-induced increases in skeletal muscle mass, and possibly strength, than are carbohydrate supplements. In particular, use of whey PRT and/or milk appears to result in greater gains in lean muscle mass than soy or carbohydrate when used in conjunction with RE. It is likely, however, that high-quality food-source animal proteins such as egg, chicken, or beef are also efficacious in this respect, although chronic studies incorporating these PRT sources are scarce (Campbell *et al.*, 1999; Haub *et al.*, 2002). The role of AA/PRT supplements in enhancing adaptations to RE in the elderly is a contentious issue and one that requires further investigation. Given that aged muscle is resistant to the anabolic effects of both RE and AA, factors such as PRT dose, leucine concentration, and timing of intake, may be of greater relevance to the elderly. Indeed, timed intake of a source of AA immediately post-exercise appears to result in greater muscle protein anabolism than intake at other times.

Although the addition of PRT to a carbohydrate beverage has been reported by some to increase EE performance, this is a very debatable issue. Indeed, there is currently no established mechanism to show how AA might be expected to acutely enhance EE performance. Future research needs to examine the role of PRT/AA supplements in enhancing EE-induced increases in oxidative capacity following a period of chronic training. In summary, AA/PRT supplements are efficacious in many respects. They clearly increase rates of MPS, and appear to enhance RE-induced gains in skeletal muscle mass in certain populations. Any benefits derived from these supplements, however, need to be weighed against the benefits of consuming PRT from a nutritionally balanced mixed meal. While these supplements may offer greater convenience under certain circumstances, they can be quite expensive. In addition, there is currently no evidence that these supplements are any more efficacious than high-quality food-source proteins such as milk, eggs, beef or chicken. Indeed, consumption of a complete meal is likely to provide other important macronutrients in addition to providing a complement of vitamins and minerals.

References

Andersen, L.L., Tufekovic, G., Zebis, M.K., Crameri, R.M., Verlaan, G., Kjaer, M., Suetta, C., *et al.* (2005) The effect of resistance training combined with timed ingestion of protein on muscle fiber size and muscle strength. *Metabolism* 54, 151–156.

Anthony, J.C., Yoshizawa, F., Anthony, T.G., Vary, T.C., Jefferson, L.S. and Kimball, S.R. (2000) Leucine stimulates translation initiation in skeletal muscle of postabsorptive rats via a rapamycin-sensitive pathway. *Journal of Nutrition* 130, 2413–2419.

Anthony, J.C., Lang, C.H., Crozier, S.J., Anthony, T.G., MacLean, D.A., Kimball, S.R. and Jefferson, L.S. (2002) Contribution of insulin to the translational control of protein synthesis in skeletal muscle by leucine. *American Journal of Physiology - Endocrinology and Metabolism* 282, E1092–E1101.

Atherton, P.J. and Rennie, M.J. (2009) It's no go for protein when it's all go. *Journal of Physiology* 587, 1373–1374.

Balage, M. and Dardevet, D. (2010) Long-term effects of leucine supplementation on body composition. *Current Opinion in Clinical Nutrition and Metabolic Care* 13, 265–270.

Beelen, M., Tieland, M., Gijsen, A.P., Vandereyt, H., Kies, A.K., Kuipers, H., Saris, W.H., *et al.* (2008) Coingestion of carbohydrate and protein hydrolysate stimulates muscle protein synthesis during exercise in young men, with no further increase during subsequent overnight recovery. *Journal of Nutrition* 138, 2198–2204.

Biolo, G., Maggi, S.P., Williams, B.D., Tipton, K.D. and Wolfe, R.R. (1995) Increased rates of muscle protein turnover and amino acid transport after resistance exercise in humans. *American Journal of Physiology* 268, E514–E520.

Biolo, G., Tipton, K.D., Klein, S. and Wolfe, R.R. (1997) An abundant supply of amino acids enhances the metabolic effect of exercise on muscle protein. *American Journal of Physiology* 273, E122–E129.

Bird, S.P., Tarpenning, K.M. and Marino, F.E. (2006) Independent and combined effects of liquid carbohydrate/essential amino acid ingestion on hormonal and muscular adaptations following resistance training in untrained men. *European Journal of Applied Physiology* 97, 225–238.

Bohe, J., Low, J.F., Wolfe, R.R. and Rennie M.J. (2001) Latency and duration of stimulation of human muscle protein synthesis during continuous infusion of amino acids. *Journal of Physiology* 532, 575–579.

Bohe. J., Low, A., Wolfe, R.R. and Rennie, M.J. (2003) Human muscle protein synthesis is modulated by extracellular, not intramuscular amino acid availability: a dose-response study. *Journal of Physiology* 552, 315–324.

Boirie, Y., Dangin, M., Gachon, P., Vasson, M.P., Maubois, J.L. and Beaufrere, B. (1997) Slow and fast dietary proteins differently modulate postprandial protein accretion. *Proceedings of the National Academy of Sciences of the USA* 94, 14930–14935.

Borsheim, E., Tipton, K.D., Wolf, S.E. and Wolfe, R.R. (2002) Essential amino acids and muscle protein recovery from resistance exercise. *American Journal of Physiology - Endocrinology and Metabolism* 283, E648–E657.

Borsheim, E., Bui, Q.U., Tissier, S., Kobayashi, H., Ferrando, A.A. and Wolfe, R.R. (2008) Effect of amino acid supplementation on muscle mass, strength and physical function in elderly. *Clinical Nutrition* 27, 189–195.

Bos, C., Metges, C.C., Gaudichon, C., Petzke, K.J., Pueyo, M.E., Morens, C., Everwand, J., et al. (2003) Postprandial kinetics of dietary amino acids are the main determinant of their metabolism after soy or milk protein ingestion in humans. *Journal of Nutrition* 133, 1308–1315.

Burd, N.A., Staples, A.W., West, D.W.D., Moore, D.R., Holwerda, A.M., Baker, S.K. and Phillips, S.M. (2009a) Latent increases in fasting and fed-state muscle protein turnover with resistance exercise irrespective of intensity. *Applied Physiology Nutrition and Metabolism* 34, 1122.

Burd, N.A., Tang, J.E., Moore, D.R. and Phillips, S.M. (2009b) Exercise training and protein metabolism: influences of contraction, protein intake, and sex-based differences. *Journal of Applied Physiology* 106, 1692–1701.

Burk, A., Timpmann, S., Medijainen, L., Vahi, M. and Oopik, V. (2009) Time-divided ingestion pattern of casein-based protein supplement stimulates an increase in fat-free body mass during resistance training in young untrained men. *Nutrition Research* 29, 405–413.

Burke, D.G., Chilibeck, P.D., Davidson, K.S., Candow, D.G., Farthing, J. and Smith-Palmer, T. (2001) The effect of whey protein supplementation with and without creatine monohydrate combined with resistance training on lean tissue mass and muscle strength. *International Journal of Sport Nutrition and Exercise Metabolism* 11, 349–364.

Burke, L., Cort, M., Cox, G., Crawford, R., Desbrow, B., Farthing, B.L., Minehan, M., et al. (2006) Supplements and sports foods. In: Burke, L. and Deakin, V. (eds) *Clinical Sports Nutrition*. 3rd ed., McGraw-Hill, Sydney, Australia, pp. 485–579.

Byfield, M.P., Murray, J.T. and Backer, J.M. (2005) hVps34 is a nutrient-regulated lipid kinase required for activation of p70 S6 kinase. *Journal of Biological Chemistry* 280, 33076–33082.

Camera, D.M., Edge, J., Short, M.J., Hawley, J.A. and Coffey, V.G. (2010) Early time-course of Akt phosphorylation following endurance and resistance exercise. *Medicine and Science in Sports and Exercise* 42, 1843–1852.

Campbell, W.W., Barton, M.L. Jr, Cyr-Campbell, D., Davey, S.L., Beard, J.L., Parise, G. and Evans, W.J. (1999) Effects of an omnivorous diet compared with a lactoovovegetarian diet on resistance-training-induced changes in body composition and skeletal muscle in older men. *American Journal of Clinical Nutrition* 70, 1032–1039.

Candow, D.G., Burke, N.C., Smith-Palmer, T. and Burke, D.G. (2006) Effect of whey and soy protein supplementation combined with resistance training in young adults. *International Journal of Sport Nutrition and Exercise Metabolism* 16, 233–244.

Candow, D.G., Chilibeck, P.D., Facci, M., Abeysekara, S. and Zello, G.A. (2006a) Protein supplementation before and after resistance training in older men. *European Journal of Applied Physiology* 97, 548–556.

Carraro, F., Stuart, C.A., Hartl, W.H., Rosenblatt, J. and Wolfe, R.R. (1990) Effect of exercise and recovery on muscle protein synthesis in human subjects. *American Journal of Physiology* 259, E470–E476.

Carraro, F., Hartl, W.H., Stuart, C.A., Layman, D.K., Jahoor, F. and Wolfe, R.R. (1990a) Whole body and plasma protein synthesis in exercise and recovery in human subjects. *American Journal of Physiology* 258, E821–E831.

Cermak, N.M., Solheim, A.S., Gardner, M.S., Tarnopolsky, M.A. and Gibala, M.J. (2009) Muscle metabolism during exercise with carbohydrate or protein-carbohydrate ingestion. *Medicine and Science in Sports and Exercise* 41, 2158–2161.

Chesley, A., MacDougall, J.D., Tarnopolsky, M.A., Atkinson, S.A. and Smith K. (1992) Changes in human muscle protein synthesis after resistance exercise. *Journal of Applied Physiology* 73, 1383–1388.

Cribb, P.J. and Hayes, A. (2006) Effects of supplement timing and resistance exercise on skeletal muscle hypertrophy. *Medicine and Science in Sports and Exercise* 38, 1918–1925.

Cribb, P.J., Williams, A.D., Carey, M.F. and Hayes, A. (2006) The effect of whey isolate and resistance training on strength, body composition, and plasma glutamine. *International Journal of Sport Nutrition and Exercise Metabolism* 16, 494–509.

Cribb, P.J., Williams, A.D., Stathis, C.G., Carey, M.F. and Hayes, A. (2007) Effects of whey isolate, creatine, and resistance training on muscle hypertrophy. *Medicine and Science in Sports and Exercise* 39, 298–307.

Crozier, S.J., Kimball, S.R., Emmert, S.W., Anthony, J.C. and Jefferson, L.S. (2005) Oral leucine administration stimulates protein synthesis in rat skeletal muscle. *Journal of Nutrition* 135, 376–382.

Cuthbertson, D., Smith, K., Babraj, J., Leese, G., Waddell, T., Atherton, P., Wackerhage, H., et al. (2005) Anabolic signaling deficits underlie amino acid resistance of wasting, ageing muscle. *FASEB Journal* 19, 422–424.

Dangin, M., Boirie, Y., Garcia-Rodenas, C., Gachon, P., Fauquant, J., Callier, P., Ballevre, O. et al. (2001) The digestion rate of protein is an independent regulating factor of postprandial protein retention. *American Journal of Physiology - Endocrinology and Metabolism* 280, E340–E348.

Dangin, M., Guillet, C., Garcia-Rodenas, C., Gachon, P., Bouteloup-Demange, C., Reiffers-Magnani, K., Fauquant, J., et al. (2003) The rate of protein digestion affects protein gain differently during ageing in humans. *Journal of Physiology* 549, 635–644.

Dardevet, D., Sornet, C., Balage, M. and Grizard, J. (2000) Stimulation of in vitro rat muscle protein synthesis by leucine decreases with age. *Journal of Nutrition* 130, 2630–2635.

Das, T.K. and Waterlow, J.C. (1974) The rate of adaptation of urea cycle enzymes, aminotransferases and glutamic dehydrogenase to changes in dietary protein intake. *British Journal of Nutrition* 32, 353–373.

Dillon, E.L., Sheffield-Moore, M., Paddon-Jones, D., Gilkison, C., Sanford, A.P., Casperson, S.L., Jiang, J., et al. (2009) Amino acid supplementation increases lean body mass, basal muscle protein synthesis, and insulin-like growth factor-1 expression in older women. *Journal of Clinical Endocrinology and Metabolism* 94, 1630–1637.

Dreyer, H.C., Fujita, S., Cadenas, J.G., Chinkes, D.L., Volpi, E. and Rasmussen, B.B. (2006) Resistance exercise increases AMPK activity and reduces 4E-BP1 phosphorylation and protein synthesis in human skeletal muscle. *Journal of Physiology* 576, 613–624.

Dreyer, H.C., Drummond, M.J., Pennings, B., Fujita, S., Glynn, E.L., Chinkes, D.L., Dhanani, S., et al. (2008) Leucine-enriched essential amino acid and carbohydrate ingestion following resistance exercise enhances mTOR signaling and protein synthesis in human muscle. *American Journal of Physiology - Endocrinology and Metabolism* 294, E392–E400.

Drummond, M.J., Dreyer, H.C., Fry, C.S., Glynn, E.L. and Rasmussen, B.B. (2009) Nutritional and contractile regulation of human skeletal muscle protein synthesis and mTORC1 signaling. *Journal of Applied Physiology* 106, 1374–1384.

Erdman, K.A., Fung, T.S. and Reimer, R.A. (2006) Influence of performance level on dietary supplementation in elite Canadian athletes. *Medicine and Science in Sports and Exercise* 38, 349–356.

Esmarck, B., Andersen, J.L., Olsen, S., Richter, E.A., Mizuno, M. and Kjaer, M. (2001) Timing of postexercise protein intake is important for muscle hypertrophy with resistance training in elderly humans. *Journal of Physiology* 535, 301–311.

Fiatarone, M.A., Marks, E.C., Ryan, N.D., Meredith, C.N., Lipsitz, L.A. and Evans, W.J. (1990) High-intensity strength training in nonagenarians. Effects on skeletal muscle. *Journal of the American Medical Association* 263, 3029–3034.

Findlay, G.M., Yan, L., Procter, J., Mieulet, V. and Lamb, R.F. (2007) A MAP4 kinase related to Ste20 is a nutrient-sensitive regulator of mTOR signalling. *Biochemical Journal* 403, 13–20.

Forbes, G.B. (1987) *Human Body Composition: Growth, Ageing, Nutrition and Activity*. 1st ed., Springer-Verlag, New York.

Fouillet, H., Mariotti, F., Gaudichon, C., Bos, C. and Tome, D. (2003) Peripheral and splanchnic metabolism of dietary nitrogen are differently affected by the protein source in humans as assessed by compartmental modeling. *Journal of Nutrition* 132, 125–133.

Frontera, W.R., Meredith, C.N., O'Reilly, K.P., Knuttgen, H.G. and Evans, W.J. (1988) Strength conditioning in older men: skeletal muscle hypertrophy and improved function. *Journal of Applied Physiology* 64, 1038–1044.

Fujita, S., Dreyer, H.C., Drummond, M.J., Glynn, E.L., Cadenas, J.G., Yoshizawa, F., Volpi, E. et al. (2007) Nutrient signaling in the regulation of human muscle protein synthesis. *Journal of Physiology* 582, 813–823.

Fujita, S., Dreyer, H.C., Drummond, M.J., Glynn, E.L., Volpi, E. and Rasmussen, B.B. (2009) Essential amino acid and carbohydrate ingestion before resistance exercise does not enhance postexercise muscle protein synthesis. *Journal of Applied Physiology* 106, 1730–1739.

Gibala, M.J. (2007) Protein metabolism and endurance exercise. *Sports Medicine* 37, 337–340.

Godard, M.P., Williamson, D.L. and Trappe, S.W. (2002) Oral amino-acid provision does not affect muscle strength or size gains in older men. *Medicine and Science in Sports and Exercise* 34, 1126–1131.

Goldberg, A.L. and Chang, T.W. (1978) Regulation and significance of amino acid metabolism in skeletal muscle. *Federation Proceedings* 37, 2301–2307.

Goston, J.L. and Correia, M.I. (2009) Intake of nutritional supplements among people exercising in gyms and influencing factors. *Nutrition* 26, 604–611.

Ha, E. and Zemel, M.B. (2003) Functional properties of whey, whey components, and essential amino acids: mechanisms underlying health benefits for active people (review). *Journal of Nutritional Biochemistry* 14, 251–258.

Hartman, J.W., Tang, J.E., Wilkinson, S.B., Tarnopolsky, M.A., Lawrence, R.L., Fullerton, A.V. and Phillips, S.M. (2007) Consumption of fat-free fluid milk after resistance exercise promotes greater lean mass accretion than does consumption of soy or carbohydrate in young, novice, male weightlifters. *American Journal of Clinical Nutrition* 86, 373–381.

Haub, M.D., Wells, A.M., Tarnopolsky, M.A. and Campbell, W.W. (2002) Effect of protein source on resistive-training-induced changes in body composition and muscle size in older men. *American Journal of Clinical Nutrition* 76, 511–517.

Howarth, K.R., Moreau, N.A., Phillips, S.M. and Gibala, M.J. (2009) Coingestion of protein with carbohydrate during recovery from endurance exercise stimulates skeletal muscle protein synthesis in humans. *Journal of Applied Physiology* 106, 1394–1402.

Huang, S.H., Johnson, K. and Pipe, A.L. (2006) The use of dietary supplements and medications by Canadian athletes at the Atlanta and Sydney Olympic Games. *Clinical Journal of Sport Medicine* 16, 27–33.

Hulmi, J.J., Kovanen, V., Selanne, H., Kraemer, W.J., Hakkinen, K. and Mero, A.A. (2009) Acute and long-term effects of resistance exercise with or without protein ingestion on muscle hypertrophy and gene expression. *Amino Acids* 37, 297–308.

Ivy, J.L., Goforth, H.W. Jr, Damon, B.M., McCauley, T.R., Parsons, E.C. and Price, T.B. (2002) Early postexercise muscle glycogen recovery is enhanced with a carbohydrate-protein supplement. *Journal of Applied Physiology* 93, 1337–1344.

Ivy, J.L., Res, P.T., Sprague, R.C. and Widzer, M.O. (2003) Effect of a carbohydrate protein supplement on endurance performance during exercise of varying intensity. *International Journal of Sport Nutrition and Exercise Metabolism* 13, 382–395.

Jentjens, R.L., van Loon, L.J., Mann, C.H., Wagenmakers, A.J. and Jeukendrup, A.E. (2001) Addition of protein and amino acids to carbohydrates does not enhance postexercise muscle glycogen synthesis. *Journal of Applied Physiology* 91, 839–846.

Jentjens, R.L., Achten, J. and Jeukendrup, A.E. (2004a) High oxidation rates from combined carbohydrates ingested during exercise. *Medicine and Science in Sports and Exercise* 36, 1551–1558.

Jentjens, R.L., Moseley, L., Waring, R.H., Harding, L.K. and Jeukendrup, A.E. (2004b) Oxidation of combined ingestion of glucose and fructose during exercise. *Journal of Applied Physiology* 96, 1277–1284.

Jentjens, R.L., Venables, M.C. and Jeukendrup, A.E. (2004c) Oxidation of exogenous glucose, sucrose, and maltose during prolonged cycling exercise. *Journal of Applied Physiology* 96, 1285–1291.

Josse, A.R., Tang, J.E., Tarnopolsky, M.A. and Phillips, S.M. (2010) Body composition and strength changes in women with milk and resistance exercise. *Medicine and Science in Sports and Exercise* 42, 1122–1130.

Kalapotharakos, V.I., Michalopoulou, M., Godolias, G., Tokmakidis, S.P., Malliou, P.V. and Gourgoulis, V. (2004) The effects of high- and moderate-resistance training on muscle function in the elderly. *Journal of Ageing and Physical Activity* 12, 131–143.

Karlsson, H.K., Nilsson, P.A., Nilsson, J., Chibalin, A.V., Zierath, J.R. and Blomstrand, E. (2004) Branched-chain amino acids increase p70S6k phosphorylation in human skeletal muscle after resistance exercise. *American Journal of Physiology Endocrinology and Metabolism* 287, E1–E7.

Katsanos, C.S., Kobayashi, H., Sheffield-Moore, M., Aarsland, A. and Wolfe, R.R. (2005) Ageing is associated with diminished accretion of muscle proteins after the ingestion of a small bolus of essential amino acids. *American Journal of Clinical Nutrition* 82, 1065–1073.

Katsanos, C.S., Kobayashi, H., Sheffield-Moore, M., Aarsland, A. and Wolfe, R.R. (2006) A high proportion of leucine is required for optimal stimulation of the rate of muscle protein synthesis by essential amino acids in the elderly. *American Journal of Physiology Endocrinology and Metabolism* 291, E381–E387.

Katsanos, C.S., Chinkes, D.L., Paddon-Jones, D., Zhang, X.J., Aarsland, A. and Wolfe, R.R. (2008) Whey protein ingestion in elderly persons results in greater muscle protein accrual than ingestion of its constituent essential amino acid content. *Nutrition Research* 28, 651–658.

Kerksick, C.M., Rasmussen, C.J., Lancaster, S.L., Magu, B., Smith, P., Melton, C., Greenwood, M., et al. (2006) The effects of protein and amino acid supplementation on performance and training adaptations during ten weeks of resistance training. *Journal of Strength and Conditioning Research* 20, 643–653.

Kerksick, C., Harvey, T., Stout, J., Campbell, B., Wilborn, C., Kreider, R., Kalman, D., et al. (2008) International Society of Sports Nutrition position stand: Nutrient timing. *Journal of the International Society of Sports Nutrition* 5, 17.

Koopman, R., Pannemans, D.L., Jeukendrup, A.E., Gijsen, A.P., Senden, J.M., Halliday, D., Saris, W.H., et al. (2004) Combined ingestion of protein and carbohydrate improves protein balance during ultra-endurance exercise. *American Journal of Physiology Endocrinology and Metabolism* 287, E712–E720.

Koopman, R., Pennings, B., Zorenc, A.H. and van Loon, L.J. (2007) Protein ingestion further augments S6K1 phosphorylation in skeletal muscle following resistance type exercise in males. *Journal of Nutrition* 137, 1880–1886.

Kosek, D.J., Kim, J.S., Petrella, J.K., Cross, J.M. and Bamman, M.M. (2006) Efficacy of 3 days/wk resistance training on myofiber hypertrophy and myogenic mechanisms in young vs. older adults. *Journal of Applied Physiology* 101, 531–544.

Kumar, V., Selby, A., Rankin, D., Patel, R., Atherton, P., Hildebrandt, W., Williams, J., et al. (2009) Age-related differences in dose response of muscle protein synthesis to resistance exercise in young and old men. *Journal of Physiology* 587, 211–217.

Levenhagen, D.K., Carr, C., Carlson, M.G., Maron, D.J., Borel, M.J. and Flakoll, P.J. (2002) Postexercise protein intake enhances whole-body and leg protein accretion in humans. *Medicine and Science in Sports and Exercise* 34, 828–837.

Miller, S.L., Tipton, K.D., Chinkes, D.L., Wolf, S.E. and Wolfe, R.R. (2003) Independent and combined effects of amino acids and glucose after resistance exercise. *Medicine and Science in Sports and Exercise* 35, 449–455.

Moore, D.R., Robinson, M.J., Fry, J.L., Tang, J.E., Glover, E.I., Wilkinson, S.B., Prior, T., et al. (2009a) Ingested protein dose response of muscle and albumin protein synthesis after resistance exercise in young men. *American Journal of Clinical Nutrition* 89, 161–168.

Moore, D.R., Tang, J.E., Burd, N.A., Rerecich, T., Tarnopolsky, M.A. and Phillips, S.M. (2009b) Differential stimulation of myofibrillar and sarcoplasmic protein synthesis with protein ingestion at rest and after resistance exercise. *Journal of Physiology* 587, 897–904.

Morens, C., Bos, C., Pueyo, M.E., Benamouzig, R., Gausseres, N., Luengo, C., Tome, D. et al. (2003) Increasing habitual protein intake accentuates differences in postprandial dietary nitrogen utilization between protein sources in humans. *Journal of Nutrition* 133, 2733–2740.

Morrison, L.J., Gizis, F. and Shorter, B. (2004) Prevalent use of dietary supplements among people who exercise at a commercial gym. *International Journal of Sport Nutrition and Exercise Metabolism* 14, 481–492.

Nair, K.S., Halliday, D. and Griggs, R.C. (1988) Leucine incorporation into mixed skeletal muscle protein in humans. *American Journal of Physiology Endocrinology and Metabolism* 254, E208–E213.

Nakshabendi, I.M., Obeidat, W., Russell, R.I., Downie, S., Smith, K. and Rennie, M.J. (1995) Gut mucosal protein synthesis measured using intravenous and intragastric delivery of stable tracer amino acids. *American Journal of Physiology Endocrinology and Metabolism* 269, E996–E999.

Nakshabendi, I.M., McKee, R., Downie, S., Russell, R.I. and Rennie, M.J. (1999) Rates of small intestinal mucosal protein synthesis in human jejunum and ileum. *American Journal of Physiology Endocrinology and Metabolism* 277, E1028–E1031.

Norton, L.E., Layman, D.K., Bunpo, P., Anthony, T.G., Brana, D.V. and Garlick, P.J. (2009) The leucine content of a complete meal directs peak activation but not duration of skeletal muscle protein synthesis and mammalian target of rapamycin signaling in rats. *Journal of Nutrition* 139, 1103–1109.

Osterberg, K.L., Zachwieja, J.J. and Smith, J.W. (2008) Carbohydrate and carbohydrate + protein for cycling time-trial performance. *Journal of Sports Sciences* 26, 227–233.

Phillips, S.M. (2004) Protein requirements and supplementation in strength sports. *Nutrition* 20, 689–695.

Phillips, S.M., Tipton, K.D., Aarsland, A., Wolf, S.E. and Wolfe R.R. (1997) Mixed muscle protein synthesis and breakdown after resistance exercise in humans. *American Journal of Physiology Endocrinology and Metabolism* 273, E99–E107.

Phillips, S.M., Tipton, K.D., Ferrando, A.A. and Wolfe, R.R. (1999) Resistance training reduces the acute exercise-induced increase in muscle protein turnover. *American Journal of Physiology Endocrinology and Metabolism* 276, E118–E124.

Phillips, S.M., Moore, D.R. and Tang, J.E. (2007) A critical examination of dietary protein requirements, benefits, and excesses in athletes. *International Journal of Sport Nutrition and Exercise Metabolism* 17, S58–S76.

Phillips, S.M., Tang, J.E. and Moore, D.R. (2009) The role of milk- and soy-based protein in support of muscle protein synthesis and muscle protein accretion in young and elderly persons. *Journal of the American College of Nutrition* 28, 343–354.

Rasmussen, B.B. and Phillips, S.M. (2003) Contractile and nutritional regulation of human muscle growth. *Exercise and Sport Sciences Reviews* 31, 127–131.

Rasmussen, B.B., Tipton, K.D., Miller, S.L., Wolf, S.E. and Wolfe, R.R. (2000) An oral essential amino acid-carbohydrate supplement enhances muscle protein anabolism after resistance exercise. *Journal of Applied Physiology* 88, 386–392.

Rennie, M.J., Edwards, R.H., Davies, C.T., Krywawych, S., Halliday, D., Waterlow, J.C. and Millward, D.J. (1980) Protein and amino acid turnover during and after exercise. *Biochemical Society Transactions* 8, 499–501.

Rennie, M.J., Bohe, J., Smith, K., Wackerhage, H. and Greenhaff, P. (2006) Branched-chain amino acids as fuels and anabolic signals in human muscle. *Journal of Nutrition* 136, S264–268.

Riazi, R., Wykes, L.J., Ball, R.O. and Pencharz, P.B. (2003) The total branched-chain amino acid requirement in young healthy adult men determined by indicator amino acid oxidation by use of L-[1-^{13}C]phenylalanine. *Journal of Nutrition* 133, 1383–1389.

Rieu, I., Sornet, C., Bayle, G., Prugnaud, J., Pouyet, C., Balage, M., Papet, I., *et al.* (2003) Leucine-supplemented meal feeding for ten days beneficially affects postprandial muscle protein synthesis in old rats. *Journal of Nutrition* 133, 1198–1205.

Rieu, I., Balage, M., Sornet, C., Giraudet, C., Pujos, E., Grizard, J., Mosoni, L. *et al.* (2006) Leucine supplementation improves muscle protein synthesis in elderly men independently of hyperaminoacidaemia. *Journal of Physiology* 575, 305–315.

Rodriguez, N.R., Vislocky, L.M. and Gaine, P.C. (2007) Dietary protein, endurance exercise, and human skeletal-muscle protein turnover. *Current Opinion in Clinical Nutrition and Metabolic Care* 10, 40–45.

Rodriguez, N.R., DiMarco, N.M. and Langley, S. (2009) American Dietetic Association; Dietetians of Canada; American College of Sports Medicine. Position of the American Dietetic Association, Dietitians of Canada, and the American College of Sports Medicine: Nutrition and athletic performance. *Journal of the American Dietetic Association* 109, 509–527.

Romano-Ely, B.C., Todd, M.K., Saunders, M.J. and St Laurent, T. (2006) Effect of an isocaloric carbohydrate-protein-antioxidant drink on cycling performance. *Medicine and Science in Sports and Exercise* 38, 1608–1616.

Saunders, M.J., Kane, M.D. and Todd, K.M. (2004) Effects of a carbohydrate-protein beverage on cycling endurance and muscle damage. *Medicine and Science in Sports and Exercise* 36, 1233–1238.

Saunders, M., Luden, M.D. and Herrick, J.E. (2007) Consumption of an oral carbohydrate-protein gel improves cycling endurance and prevents post-exercise muscle damage. *Journal of Strength and Conditioning Research* 21, 678–684.

Sheffield-Moore, M., Yeckel, C.W., Volpi, E., Wolf, S.E., Morio, B., Chinkes, D.L., Paddon-Jones, D. *et al.* (2004) Postexercise protein metabolism in older and younger men following moderate-intensity aerobic exercise. *American Journal of Physiology Endocrinology and Metabolism* 287, E513–E522.

Smith, K., Barua, J.M., Watt, P.W., Scrimgeour, C.M. and Rennie, M.J. (1992) Flooding with L-[1-13C] leucine stimulates human muscle protein incorporation of continuously infused L-[1-13C] valine. *American Journal of Physiology* 262, E372–E376.

Solerte, S.B., Gazzaruso, C., Bonacasa, R., Rondanelli, M., Zamboni, M., Basso, C., Locatelli, E., *et al.* (2008) Nutritional supplements with oral amino acid mixtures increases whole-body lean mass and insulin sensitivity in elderly subjects with sarcopenia. *American Journal of Cardiology* 101, 69E–7E.

Symons, T.B., Schutzler, S.E., Cocke, T.L., Chinkes, D.L., Wolfe, R.R. and Paddon-Jones, D. (2007) Ageing does not impair the anabolic response to a protein-rich meal. *American Journal of Clinical Nutrition* 86, 451–456.

Tang, J.E. and Phillips, S.M. (2009) Maximizing muscle protein anabolism: the role of protein quality. *Current Opinion in Clinical Nutrition and Metabolic Care* 12, 66–71.

Tang, J.E., Moore, D.R., Kujbida, G.W., Tarnopolsky, M.A. and Phillips, S.M. (2009) Ingestion of whey hydrolysate, casein, or soy protein isolate: effects on mixed muscle protein synthesis at rest and following resistance exercise in young men. *Journal of Applied Physiology* 107, 987–992.

Tarnopolsky, M. (2004) Protein requirements for endurance athletes. *Nutrition* 20, 662–668.

Tipton, K.D., Ferrando, A.A., Phillips, S.M., Doyle, D. Jr and Wolfe, R.R. (1999a) Postexercise net protein synthesis in human muscle from orally administered amino acids. *American Journal of Physiology* 276, E628–E634.

Tipton, K.D., Gurkin, B.E., Matin, S. and Wolfe, R.R. (1999b) Nonessential amino acids are not necessary to stimulate net muscle protein synthesis in healthy volunteers. *Journal of Nutritional Biochemistry* 10, 89–95.

Tipton, K.D., Rasmussen, B.B., Miller, S.L., Wolf, S.E., Owens-Stovall, S.K., Petrini, B.E. and Wolfe, R.R. (2001) Timing of amino acid-carbohydrate ingestion alters anabolic response of muscle to resistance exercise. *American Journal of Physiology Endocrinology and Metabolism* 281, E197–E206.

Tipton, K.D., Elliott, T.A., Cree, M.G., Wolf, S.E., Sanford, A.P. and Wolfe, R.R. (2004) Ingestion of casein and whey proteins result in muscle anabolism after resistance exercise. *Medicine and Science in Sports and Exercise* 36, 2073–2081.

Tipton, K.D., Elliot, T.A., Cree, M.G., Aarsland, A.A., Sanford, A.P. and Wolfe, R.R. (2007) Stimulation of net muscle protein synthesis by whey protein ingestion before and after exercise. *American Journal of Physiology Endocrinology and Metabolism* 292, E71–E76.

Tipton, K.D., Elliot, T.A., Ferrando, A.A., Aarsland, A.A. and Wolfe, R.R. (2009) Stimulation of muscle anabolism by resistance exercise and ingestion of leucine plus protein. *Applied Physiology Nutrition and Metabolism* 34, 151–161.

Valentine, R., Saunders, M.J., Todd, M.K. and St Laurent, T.G. (2008) Influence of carbohydrate-protein beverage on cycling endurance and indices of muscle disruption. *International Journal of Sport Nutrition and Exercise Metabolism* 18, 363–378.

van Essen, M. and Gibala, M.J. (2006) Failure of protein to improve a time trial performance when added to a sports drink. *Medicine and Science in Sports and Exercise* 38, 1476–1483.

van Loon, L.J., Saris, W.H., Kruijshoop, M. and Wagenmakers, A.J. (2000) Maximizing postexercise muscle glycogen synthesis: carbohydrate supplementation and the application of amino acid or protein hydrolysate mixtures. *American Journal of Clinical Nutrition* 72, 106–111.

Verdijk, L.B., Jonkers, R.A., Gleeson, B.G., Beelen, M., Meijer, K., Savelberg, H.H., Wodzig, W.K., *et al.* (2009) Protein supplementation before and after exercise does not further augment skeletal muscle hypertrophy after resistance training in elderly men. *American Journal of Clinical Nutrition* 89, 608–616.

Verhoeven, S., Vanschoonbeek, K., Verdijk, L.B., Koopman, R., Wodzig, W.K., Dendale, P. and van Loon, L.J. (2009) Long-term leucine supplementation does not increase muscle mass or strength in healthy elderly men. *American Journal of Clinical Nutrition* 89, 1468–1475.

Wang, X., Campbell, L.E., Miller, C.M. and Proud, C.G. (1998) Amino acid availability regulates p70 S6 kinase and multiple translation factors. *Biochemical Journal* 334, 261–267.

West, D.W., Kujbida, G.W., Moore, D., Atherton, P.J., Burd, N.A., Padzik, J.P., Delisio, M., *et al.* (2009) Resistance exercise-induced increases in putative anabolic hormones do not enhance muscle protein synthesis or intracellular signalling in young men. *Journal of Physiology* 587, 5239–5247.

West, D.W.D., Burd, N.A., Tang, J.E., Moore, D.R., Staples, A.W., Holwerda, A.M., Baker, S.K. *et al.* (2010) Elevations in ostensibly anabolic hormones with resistance exercise enhance neither training-induced muscle hypertrophy nor strength of the elbow flexors. *Journal of Applied Physiology* 108, 60–67.

Wilkes, E.A., Selby, A.L., Atherton, P.J., Patel, R., Rankin, D., Smith, K. and Rennie, M.J. (2009) Blunting of insulin inhibition of proteolysis in legs of older subjects may contribute to age-related sarcopenia. *American Journal of Clinical Nutrition* 10, 1343–1350.

Wilkinson, S.B., Tarnopolsky, M.A., MacDonald, M.J., Macdonald, J.R., Armstrong, D. and Phillips, S.M. (2007) Consumption of fluid skim milk promotes greater muscle protein accretion following resistance exercise than an isonitrogenous and isoenergetic soy protein beverage. *American Journal of Clinical Nutrition* 85, 1031–1040.

Wilkinson, S.B., Phillips, S.M., Atherton, P.J., Patel, R., Yarasheski, K.E., Tarnopolsky, M.A. and Rennie, M.J. (2008) Differential effects of resistance and endurance exercise in the fed state on signalling molecule phosphorylation and protein synthesis in human muscle. *Journal of Physiology* 586, 3701–3717.

Willoughby, D.S., Stout, J.R. and Wilborn, C.D. (2007) Effects of resistance training and protein plus amino acid supplementation on muscle anabolism, mass, and strength. *Amino Acids* 32, 467–477.

Wolfe, R.R. (2006) The underappreciated role of muscle in health and disease. *American Journal of Clinical Nutrition* 84, 475–482.

18 Amino Acids in Clinical and Nutritional Support: Glutamine in Duchenne Muscular Dystrophy

E. Mok and R. Hankard*
Pédiatrie Multidisciplinaire-Nutrition de l'Enfant, Centre Hospitalier Universitaire de Poitiers, Poitiers, France

18.1 Abstract

Nutritional support improves outcome in several clinical conditions. Glutamine (Gln), a non-essential amino acid, has distinct properties, apart from providing nitrogen for protein synthesis. This chapter aims to provide an in-depth review on the efficacy of oral Gln on protein metabolism and clinical outcomes in children with Duchenne muscular dystrophy (DMD), a severe muscle-wasting disease. Because muscle (the main source of endogenous Gln production) is severely reduced, DMD could be proposed as a 'model' for the role of muscle in whole-body Gln metabolism. Although short-term studies of supplemental Gln in DMD children suggest an acute 'protein-sparing' effect, resulting from a decrease in whole-body protein breakdown, the beneficial effects on protein metabolism have not been translated into prolonged benefits on clinical outcomes, such as muscle mass, muscle strength and muscle function. Better targeting of specific subgroups is necessary fully to evaluate the presence or absence of benefits of exogenous Gln in DMD children, particularly during acute 'stress', when demands of Gln might outweigh its endogenous synthesis.

18.2 Introduction

Glutamine (Gln) is the most abundant free amino acid in the muscle and plasma of humans (Bergstrom et al., 1974). Although Gln is a non-essential neutral amino acid, it is necessary for optimal growth of mammalian cells in tissue culture (Eagle et al., 1956) and has important physiological functions.

Apart from providing nitrogen (N) for protein synthesis, Gln is a precursor for nucleic acids, nucleotides (Newsholme et al., 1985), hexosamines (Neu, 2001), the nitric oxide precursor-arginine (Arg) (Ligthart-Melis et al., 2008) and the major antioxidant – glutathione (Neu, 2001; Duggan et al., 2002). Gln is also an important oxidative fuel for rapidly proliferating cells such as those of the gastrointestinal tract (Windmueller and Spaeth, 1980) and immune system (Newsholme et al., 1985), reticulocytes (Rapoport et al., 1971), fibroblasts (Darmaun et al., 1988) and so on. It plays a central role in N transport between tissues (Lacey and Wilmore, 1990), specifically from muscle to gut, kidney, and liver. In addition to its role as a gluconeogenic substrate (Nurjhan et al., 1995; Hankard et al., 1997; Mithieu, 2001),

---

* E-mail address: regis.hankard@free.fr

Gln is involved in the renal handling of ammonia, serving as a regulator of acid–base homeostasis (Welbourne et al., 1986) and might play a role in the regulation of protein synthesis (Hankard et al., 1996b). Present data also indicate that Gln functions as a signalling molecule (Curi et al., 2005), particularly under catabolic conditions.

Traditionally Gln is considered a non-essential amino acid, because it is synthesized from carbon (C) and N precursors in most tissue (skeletal muscle being the main producer and storage site) (Darmaun and Dechelotte, 1991, Neu et al., 1996). Gln synthetase catalyses the terminal step in Gln *de novo* synthesis and is a key enzyme in Gln metabolism (Labow et al., 1998, 1999) (Fig. 18.1). In mammals, Gln synthetase expression is regulated by transcriptional and post-transcriptional mechanisms, and increases Gln synthetase mRNA in response to stress (e.g. glucorticoids) and regulation of Gln synthetase protein turnover in response to its product (plasma Gln concentrations) (Labow et al., 2001).

Under normal conditions Gln is released into circulation for consumption by other tissues, whereas in serious diseases associated with acute catabolic stress the production of Gln may be insufficient to meet the increased requirements by other tissue (gut, immune system/inflammatory cells, liver, and kidneys). Demands are partly met by skeletal muscle proteolysis and the release of large amounts of Gln to maintain normal concentrations in the plasma, resulting in depletion of Gln stores. In those situations associated with acute 'stress' (Ziegler et al., 1992), Gln might become 'conditionally essential' (Lacey and Wilmore, 1990). Recent meta-analyses, however, failed to show any improvement in morbidity or mortality in children with gastrointestinal disease (Grover et al., 2007) or in premature babies (Tubman et al., 2008).

Whereas abundant literature has been published on Gln administration in critical care (e.g. premature infants of low birth weight), fewer data are available for other childhood diseases such as DMD. The purpose of this chapter is to provide an in-depth review on Gln administration in children with DMD, a serious muscle-wasting disease, and the most common muscular dystrophy of childhood. The effects of this muscle-wasting disease on Gln metabolism are discussed first, followed by a detailed discussion of the clinical studies that have examined the efficacy of oral Gln supplementation on protein metabolism, and clinical outcomes in DMD.

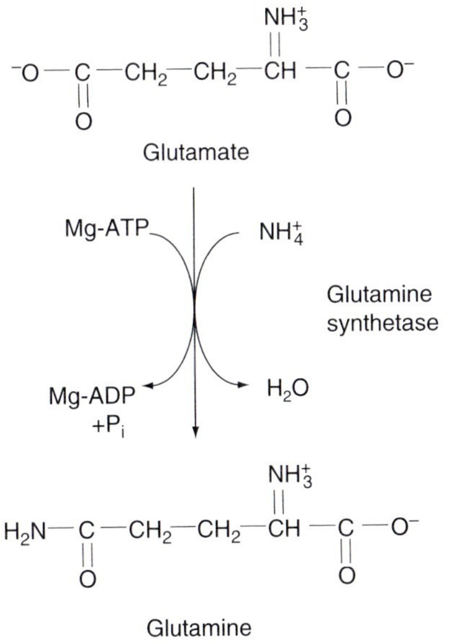

Fig. 18.1. Glutamine synthetase catalyses the terminal step in glutamine *de novo* synthesis and is a key enzyme in glutamine metabolism.

18.3 Duchenne Muscular Dystrophy: the Role of Muscle in Glutamine Metabolism

Duchenne muscular dystrophy is a serious X-linked disease caused by a defect in the gene encoding for the cytoskeletal protein dystrophin (Hoffman et al., 1988). The absence of dystrophin expression is associated with a progressive and severe loss of muscle mass and function. By the age of 10 years, muscle mass is reduced by 75% in DMD boys (Griffiths and Edwards, 1988, Hankard et al., 1996a, 1999).

Because of the dramatic muscle mass loss observed in this paediatric condition, we studied DMD as a 'model' to examine the role of muscle in both Gln and protein metabolism. Protein and Gln kinetics *in vivo* were assessed in DMD children and controls using stable non-radioactive isotope tracers (Hankard *et al.*, 1999). Whole-body protein kinetics can be determined from a primed continuous intravenous infusion of L-[1-^{13}C] labelled leucine (Leu) by measuring at isotopic steady state, plasma [1-^{13}C]Leu enrichment, expired $^{13}CO_2$ enrichment, and CO_2 production rate (Matthews *et al.*, 1980) (Fig. 18.2). After infusion [1-^{13}C]Leu is either oxidized and appears in the breath as $^{13}CO_2$ or is incorporated into tissue protein through protein synthesis. The isotope enrichment in expired air and plasma are determined by isotopic ratio mass spectrometry and gas chromatography mass spectrometry, and CO_2 production rate by indirect calorimetry. In the post-absorptive state, Leu appearance rate (Ra,Leu), an index of whole-body protein degradation, is determined from plasma [1-^{13}C]Leu enrichment. Similarly, Leu oxidation rate (OxLeu) is determined from $^{13}CO_2$ enrichment in expired air and CO_2 production rate. Estimates of whole-body protein synthesis are then calculated as Ra,Leu-OxLeu. For simultaneous determination of Leu and Gln kinetics, we infused L-[1-^{13}C] Leu with ^{15}N labelled Gln (i.e. L-[2-^{15}N]Gln) (Darmaun *et al.*, 1985, 1986). We observed that compared to control boys of the same age, the 75% muscle mass loss in DMD boys was associated with a 25% decrease in the rate of plasma Gln appearance in the postabsorptive state (resulting from a decrease in estimates of Gln *de novo* synthesis), and a more negative whole-body Leu balance (Hankard *et al.*, 1999), indicating that these children are in a state of hypercatabolism. Thus in DMD when muscle (the main Gln-producing organ) is severely reduced, Gln turnover is also reduced (Fig. 18.3).

Because skeletal muscle is the major source of endogenous Gln, Gln released into plasma from skeletal muscle must meet the Gln needs of other tissue. It is possible that in DMD, the lower Gln production might be the primary event (a direct consequence of the reduced muscle mass). With the progressive decline in muscle mass, the Gln needs of other tissue might outstrip the Gln synthetic capacity of skeletal muscle, particularly during increased 'stress' (Fig. 18.4). Similar observations were reported in DMD for another non-essential amino acid, alanine (Haymond *et al.*, 1978). Because the rate of Gln released from protein degradation was unaffected in DMD, decreased Gln turnover results from a decrease in Gln *de novo* synthesis. This supports the role of Gln synthetase in regulating Gln metabolism (Smith *et al.*, 1984). Likewise, decreased Gln *de novo* synthesis accounts for the decreased Gln appearance rate observed in healthy adults receiving exogenous Gln infusion (Hankard *et al.*, 1995), as well as in adults with short bowel syndrome (SBS) (Darmaun *et al.*, 1991). The latter condition might, however, represent an opposite 'model' to DMD, because the mass of the small intestine (a prominent Gln-consuming tissue) is severely reduced.

We studied SBS infants, and similar to DMD, we observed reduced Gln turnover (Gln appearance rate in the plasma) compared to control infants, whereas whole-body protein turnover (Leu appearance rate) was unaltered by intestinal resection (Hankard *et al.*, 1994). This suggests that for infants with SBS, Gln production is scaled down to meet a lower Gln demand by the gut (i.e. the lower Gln production rate is secondary to an initial decline in Gln needs for other tissue). Because Gln uptake by the gut can modulate muscle Gln production, the infant small intestine might also play a prominent role in Gln metabolism, but as a preferential user of Gln. This inter-organ adaptive process also supports the role of Gln

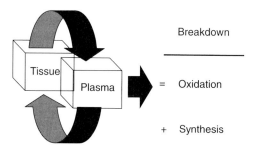

Fig. 18.2. Measurement of whole-body leucine metabolism (an index of whole-body protein metabolism) *in vivo*, determined from a primed continuous infusion of L-[1-^{13}C] leucine.

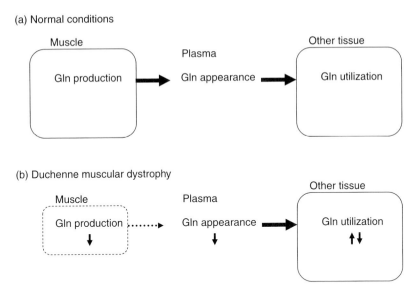

Fig. 18.3. Duchenne muscular dystrophy: a 'model' for the role of muscle in glutamine metabolism. (a) Under normal conditions, glutamine is released into circulation for consumption by other tissue (gut, immune system/inflammatory cells, liver, and kidneys). (b) In Duchenne muscular dystrophy, the severe reduction in muscle mass (the main source of endogenous glutamine production) is associated with a decrease in the rate of plasma glutamine appearance, resulting from a decrease in glutamine *de novo* synthesis. The lower glutamine production may be a direct consequence of reduced muscle mass.

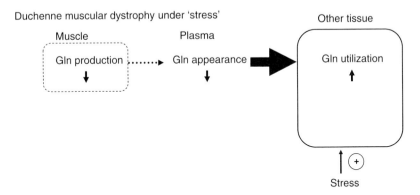

Fig. 18.4. Proposed model for the 'stressed' Duchenne muscular dystrophy patient. The progressive muscle mass depletion combined with increased 'stress' (e.g. prolonged use of corticosteroids) results in a persistent imbalance between glutamine utilization and glutamine production (i.e. during acute 'stress', demands of glutamine by other tissue outweigh glutamine *de novo* synthesis by muscle). This may ultimately result in a depletion of glutamine tissue stores, requiring exogenous support.

synthetase in regulating Gln metabolism, since plasma Gln concentration is known to exert feedback inhibition on Gln synthetase.

Because skeletal muscle is the body's main producer and exporter of Gln and muscle mass is drastically reduced in DMD, the need for Gln may be increased in persons who have this disease. Whereas the body has evolved normally effective mechanisms to maintain Gln homeostasis, it may fail to accomplish this homeostasis when muscle mass is severely depleted, limiting its ability to convert protein stores to free Gln (via Gln synthetase) (Labow et al., 2001). Furthermore in DMD, as in other protein-wasting conditions, the intramuscular Gln concentration is low (Rennie et al., 1989; Sharma et al., 2003). Sharma et al. (2003) suggested that this may be an underlying reason for muscle wasting in DMD. Thus in DMD, as in other acute 'stress' conditions, Gln might be considered a 'conditionally essential' amino acid.

18.4 Glutamine Supplementation in Children with Duchenne Muscular Dystrophy

While there is no cure for this fatal disease, current therapies aim at targeting downstream events in the pathologic progression of DMD muscle wasting. Nutritional support with amino acids (e.g. Gln, Arg, Leu) in conjunction with drug, cellular or gene therapy might have potential for slowing disease progression in these children (Archer et al., 2006; Payne et al., 2006). However, much of the data showing benefits are based on experimental evidence in the *mdx* mouse model (Granchelli et al., 2000; Barton et al., 2005; Chazalette et al., 2005; Voisin et al., 2005; Archer et al., 2006; Payne et al., 2006; Mok et al., 2008) and few randomized controlled trials have been conducted in DMD children (Mendell et al., 1984; Escolar et al., 2005; Mok et al., 2006, 2009).

18.4.1 Acute glutamine on protein metabolism

Studies on protein metabolism suggest that muscle wasting in DMD could result from a reduction in muscle protein synthesis, an increase in protein degradation, or from both (Rennie et al., 1982; Griggs and Rennie, 1983; Goldstein et al., 1989;). We conducted two separate studies using stable isotope methodology (Hankard et al., 1998; Mok et al., 2006), to test the effect of oral Gln on whole-body protein and Gln metabolism in DMD children during the postabsorptive state. In the initial study (Hankard et al., 1998), Leu and Gln kinetics were measured in six DMD boys aged 8–13 years on 2 consecutive days. Children received a 5-h oral administration of flavoured water (Kool-Aid) on the first study day, followed by Gln (0.6 g kg^{-1}) dissolved in the same flavoured water on study day 2. During Gln administration, Leu release from protein breakdown and Leu oxidation rate both decreased by 8% and 35% respectively ($P<0.01$), resulting in no change in non-oxidative Leu disposal (an index of protein synthesis). Whole-body Gln exchange in the plasma doubled ($P<0.01$), Gln from protein degradation and Gln *de novo* synthesis both decreasing during oral Gln administration. These preliminary data suggested that acute oral Gln might have an acute 'protein-sparing' effect in children with DMD, resulting from a decrease in whole-body protein degradation and Gln *de novo* synthesis. However, results should be viewed with caution, due to the small sample size. Additionally, the order of treatment allocation was not randomized and participants and assessors were not blinded to treatment. Moreover, the specificity of the effect of Gln on protein metabolism could not be tested, as measurements were not performed using an isonitrogenous control group as well.

We addressed these shortcomings more recently by conducting a double-blind randomized controlled trial (Mok et al., 2006) in 26 DMD boys (aged 7–15 y) to test whether the acute 'protein-sparing' effect of Gln persisted when oral Gln (0.5 g kg^{-1}d^{-1}) was given for 10 d, and whether the effect was specific to Gln, by comparing the Gln supplemented group to an isonitrogenous control (amino acid mixture). Whereas plasma Gln concentrations were not altered this time (since kinetic studies were performed 24 h after Gln or amino acid administration), the decrease in Leu release from protein breakdown persisted after 10 days of Gln supplementation (−9%, $P<0.05$), and endogenous Gln from protein degradation also decreased. Similar effects were observed after 10 days of amino acid supplementation; however, the magnitude of the decrease in whole-body proteolysis was less (−4%, $P<0.05$). There were no significant effects on other estimates of Leu or Gln turnover or on body composition (fat-free mass, % fat mass, muscle mass and weight) after 10 days of supplementation in either group. The lack of significant difference between Gln and isonitrogenous control could be explained by the variability in disease progression among the study population, since Gln treatment in DMD may have different effects depending on the stage of the disease process (Escolar et al., 2005). It is also possible that a higher dose or longer treatment duration may be necessary to demonstrate the specific effect of Gln, separate from its role of providing N. This highlights the need for dose and time-course data on Gln administration in DMD. Alternatively, the route of administration could partly explain the lack of significant difference, since the 'protein-sparing' effect of Gln may be less dramatic when it is given enterally (Darmaun et al., 1997; Parimi et al., 2004) as opposed to parenterally, as demonstrated in studies on protein metabolism in premature infants of low birth weight (des Robert et al., 2002; Kalhan et al., 2005).

18.4.2 Long-term glutamine on clinical outcomes

Based on experimental data showing that Gln improved performance in the *mdx* mouse model of DMD (Granchelli et al., 2000), Escolar et al. (2005) conducted a 6-month randomized double-blind placebo-controlled multi-centre study to test the efficacy and safety of oral Gln (0.6 g kg^{-1}d^{-1}) in 35 ambulant steroid naïve boys with DMD aged 4–10 years. While there were no significant differences in the primary outcome (manual muscle-testing score) or on quantitative measurements of muscle strength, subgroup analysis showed that in younger boys (<7 years) the Gln group had significantly less deterioration over 6 months in timed functional tests versus placebo. Although there was a trend toward less deterioration in quantitative and functional measures of muscle strength with Gln treatment over 6 months, the effect did not reach significance for the cohort as a whole. The inability to detect a significant difference in the primary outcome could be explained by the unexpected lack of strength deterioration in the placebo group (measured by manual muscle testing) over the 6-month trial. Thus the study may have been underpowered, since power calculations were based on previous natural history data of DMD (Brooke et al., 1983). The significant age-related results must be interpreted with caution as they were based on an unplanned subgroup analysis in a small group of patients. Larger trials incorporating *a priori* age stratification are required to test the disease-modifying effect of long-term Gln supplementation in DMD.

More recently, our group completed a multi-centre double-blind randomized crossover trial in 30 ambulatory DMD boys aged 2–10 years, to test whether 4 months' administration of oral Gln can slow the progressive loss in muscle mass and therefore provide functional benefit for these children (Mok et al., 2009). Subjects received 4 months' administration of Gln separated by a 1-month washout, followed by 4 months of placebo (malodextrin) or *vice versa*. The order of treatment allocation was randomized. Selection of the Gln dose (0.5 g kg^{-1}d^{-1}) was based on our previous studies in DMD boys (Hankard et al., 1998) and in healthy humans (Hankard et al., 1995, 1996b) that showed a twofold increase in plasma Gln concentrations during Gln administration. This same dose decreased whole-body protein degradation in DMD boys during Gln administration (Hankard et al., 1998), which persisted 24 h after supplementation ceased, while plasma Gln concentrations had returned to normal (Mok et al., 2006).

Overall, there was no apparent functional benefit as tested by comparing Gln versus placebo on change in walking speed at 4 months (primary outcome) or in secondary measures of muscle function (2-min walk test, work, power). We observed no differences in muscle mass (urinary creatinine), markers of protein breakdown (urinary 3-methylhistidine/creatinine) or serum creatine phosphokinase in the Gln group compared with placebo, except for a blunted increase in fat-free mass in the Gln group which led to a greater increase in fat mass percentage. Our findings that functional measures did not deteriorate during the 4-month placebo phase or over the course of the 9-month trial were not as expected. Based on natural history data

(Brooke et al., 1983), the trial was powered to detect a 10% difference in walking speed after 4 months of Gln compared to placebo. However, we did not consider the greater placebo effect reported in children (Rheims et al., 2008) which could have narrowed the expected effect size of Gln treatment.

Interestingly, subgroup analysis revealed a differential decline in functional measures in DMD boys taking corticosteroids (versus those not on corticosteroids) (Mok et al., 2009). For example, in the subgroup of boys taking corticosteroids (n=5), there was a 30% decrease in walking speed from baseline to 9 months ($P<0.05$), whereas those not on corticosteroids (n=25) showed no deterioration in function over time, similar to the cohort as a whole. There was also a significant effect of Gln treatment on functional measures in boys taking corticosteroids ($P<0.05$). Specifically, boys taking corticosteroids showed a significant decline in walking speed during the placebo phase (–40%, $P<0.05$), whereas walking speed remained stable when corticosteroid-treated boys received Gln treatment for 4 months. Although the findings must be interpreted with caution, because they derive from an unplanned analysis in a small subgroup of boys, they might suggest a rationale for Gln supplementation in conjunction with corticosteroid therapy (Hickson et al., 1995; Salehian et al., 2006), which needs to be investigated.

18.5 Conclusions and Future Research

DMD could be considered a 'model' for the role of muscle in Gln metabolism (Fig. 18.3). In DMD, the severe decrease in muscle mass (the main source of endogenous Gln production) is associated with a reduction in the rate of plasma Gln appearance (resulting from a decrease in Gln *de novo* synthesis).

Studies on protein metabolism in DMD children suggest a 'protein-sparing' effect of supplemental Gln, resulting from a decrease in whole-body proteolysis (Hankard et al., 1998; Mok et al., 2006). Although the acute benefits on protein metabolism (Hankard et al., 1998; Mok et al., 2006) and experimental data in *mdx* mice (Granchelli et al., 2000; Mok et al., 2008) indicate a role for Gln in the treatment of DMD, long-term supplemental Gln does not appear to improve muscle strength in DMD children (Escolar et al., 2005). However a disease-modifying effect of long-term Gln in younger DMD children cannot be ruled out. Our recent randomized crossover trial did not show added benefit on muscle mass or function, when oral Gln administered for 4 months was compared to placebo in ambulatory DMD boys (Mok et al., 2009). Hence, current data cannot support its routine use in this population as a whole. Better targeting of specific subgroups is necessary fully to evaluate the presence or absence of benefits, particularly in DMD children under 'stress'.

Over the long run, increased 'stress' (e.g. prolonged corticosteroid therapy) combined with progressive muscle mass depletion could result in a persistent imbalance between Gln utilization and Gln production, depleting Gln tissue stores (Fig. 18.4). A decrease in plasma Gln concentrations has also been observed in other diseases associated with acute 'stress' (e.g. neonates suffering from necrotizing enterocolitis (Becker et al., 2000)). In the 'stressed' DMD patient, Gln may be used in amounts exceeding the endogenous synthetic capacity of the remaining muscle, requiring exogenous support. Gln could therefore be considered a 'conditionally essential' amino acid in specific diseases such as DMD during acute 'stress'.

References

Archer, J.D., Vargas, C.C. and Anderson, J.E. (2006) Persistent and improved functional gain in mdx dystrophic mice after treatment with L-arginine and deflazacort. *FASEB Journal* 20, 738–740.

Barton, E.R., Morris, L., Kawana, M., Bish, L.T. and Toursel, T. (2005) Systemic administration of L-arginine benefits mdx skeletal muscle function. *Muscle Nerve* 32, 751–760.

Becker, R.M., Wu, G., Galanko, J.A., Chen, W., Maynor, A.R., Bose, C.L. and Rhoads, J.M. (2000) Reduced serum amino acid concentrations in infants with necrotizing enterocolitis. *Journal of Pediatrics* 137, 785–793.

Bergstrom, J., Furst, P., Noree, L.O. and Vinnars, E. (1974) Intracellular free amino acid concentration in human muscle tissue. *Journal of Applied Physiology* 36, 693–697.

Brooke, M.H., Fenichel, G.M., Griggs, R.C., Mendell, J.R., Moxley, R., Miller, J.P. and Province, M.A. (1983) Clinical investigation in Duchenne dystrophy: 2. Determination of the "power" of therapeutic trials based on the natural history. *Muscle Nerve* 6, 91–103.

Chazalette, D., Hnia, K., Rivier, F., Hugon, G. and Mornet, D. (2005) alpha7B integrin changes in mdx mouse muscles after L-arginine administration. *FEBS Letters* 579, 1079–1084.

Curi, R., Lagranha, C.J., Doi, S.Q., Sellitti, D.F., Procopio, J., Pithon-Curi, T.C., Corless, M. *et al.* (2005) Molecular mechanisms of glutamine action. *Journal of Cellular Physiology* 204, 392–401.

Darmaun, D. and Dechelotte, P. (1991) Role of leucine as a precursor of glutamine alpha-amino nitrogen in vivo in humans. *American Journal of Physiology* 260, E326–329.

Darmaun, D., Manary, M.J. and Matthews, D.E. (1985) A method for measuring both glutamine and glutamate levels and stable isotopic enrichments. *Analytical Biochemistry* 147, 92–102.

Darmaun, D., Matthews, D.E. and Bier, D.M. (1986) Glutamine and glutamate kinetics in humans. *American Journal of Physiology* 251, E117–126.

Darmaun, D., Matthews, D.E., Desjeux, J.F. and Bier, D.M. (1988) Glutamine and glutamate nitrogen exchangeable pools in cultured fibroblasts: a stable isotope study. *Journal of Cellular Physiology* 134, 143–148.

Darmaun, D., Messing, B., Just, B., Rongier, M. and Desjeux, J.-F. (1991) Glutamine metabolism after small intestinal resection in humans. *Metabolism* 40, 42–44.

Darmaun, D., Roig, J.C., Auestad, N., Sager, B.K. and Neu, J. (1997) Glutamine metabolism in very low birth weight infants. *Pediatric Research* 41, 391–396.

des Robert, C., Le Bacquer, O., Piloquet, H., Roze, J.C. and Darmaun, D. (2002) Acute effects of intravenous glutamine supplementation on protein metabolism in very low birth weight infants: a stable isotope study. *Pediatric Research* 51, 87–93.

Duggan, C., Gannon, J. and Walker, W.A. (2002) Protective nutrients and functional foods for the gastrointestinal tract. *American Journal of Clinical Nutrition* 75, 789–808.

Eagle, H., Oyama, V.I., Levy, M., Horton, C.L. and Fleischman, R. (1956) The growth response of mammalian cells in tissue culture to L-glutamine and L-glutamic acid. *Journal of Biological Chemistry* 218, 607–616.

Escolar, D.M., Buyse, G., Henricson, E., Leshner, R., Florence, J., Mayhew, J., Tesi-Rocha, C., *et al.* (2005) CINRG randomized controlled trial of creatine and glutamine in Duchenne muscular dystrophy. *Annals of Neurology* 58, 151–155.

Goldstein, M., Meyer, S. and Freund, H.R. (1989) Effects of overfeeding in children with muscle dystrophies. *Journal of Parenteral and Enteral Nutrition* 13, 603–607.

Granchelli, J.A., Pollina, C. and Hudecki, M.S. (2000) Pre-clinical screening of drugs using the mdx mouse. *Neuromuscular Disorders* 10, 235–239.

Griffiths, R.D. and Edwards, R.H. (1988) A new chart for weight control in Duchenne muscular dystrophy. *Archives of Disease in Childhood* 63, 1256–1258.

Griggs, R.C. and Rennie, M.J. (1983) Muscle wasting in muscular dystrophy: decreased protein synthesis or increased degradation? *Annals of Neurology* 13, 125–132.

Grover, Z., Tubman, R. and McGuire, W. (2007) Glutamine supplementation for young infants with severe gastrointestinal disease. Cochrane Database of Systematic Reviews, CD005947, DOI: 10.1002/14651858.CD005947.pub2.

Hankard, R., Goulet, O., Ricour, C., Rongier, M., Colomb, V. and Darmaun, D. (1994) Glutamine metabolism in children with short-bowel syndrome: a stable isotope study. *Pediatric Research* 36, 202–206.

Hankard, R., Darmaun, D., Sager, B.K., D'Amore, D., Parsons, W.R. and Haymond, M. (1995) Response of glutamine metabolism to exogenous glutamine in humans. *American Journal of Physiology* 269, E663–670.

Hankard, R., Gottrand, F., Turck, D., Carpentier, A., Romon, M. and Farriaux, J.P. (1996a) Resting energy expenditure and energy substrate utilization in children with Duchenne muscular dystrophy. *Pediatric Research* 40, 29–33.

Hankard, R., Haymond, M.W. and Darmaun, D. (1996b) Effect of glutamine on leucine metabolism in humans. *American Journal of Physiology* 271, E748–754.

Hankard, R., Haymond, M.W. and Darmaun, D. (1997) Role of glutamine as a glucose precursor in fasting humans. *Diabetes* 46, 1535–1541.

Hankard, R., Hammond, D., Haymond, M.W. and Darmaun, D. (1998) Oral glutamine slows down whole body protein breakdown in Duchenne muscular dystrophy. *Pediatric Research* 43, 222–226.

Hankard, R., Mauras, N., Hammond, D., Haymond, M. and Darmaun, D. (1999) Is glutamine a 'conditionally essential' amino acid in Duchenne muscular dystrophy? *Clinical Nutrition* 18, 365–369.

Haymond, M.W., Strobel, K.E. and DeVivo, D.C. (1978) Muscle wasting and carbohydrate homeostasis in Duchenne muscular dystrophy. *Neurology* 28, 1224–1231.

Hickson, R.C., Czerwinski, S.M. and Wegrzyn, L.E. (1995) Glutamine prevents downregulation of myosin heavy chain synthesis and muscle atrophy from glucocorticoids. *American Journal of Physiology* 268, E730–734.

Hoffman, E.P., Fischbeck, K.H., Brown, R.H., Johnson, M., Medori, R., Loike, J.D., Harris, J.B., et al. (1988) Characterization of dystrophin in muscle-biopsy specimens from patients with Duchenne's or Becker's muscular dystrophy. *New England Journal of Medicine* 318, 1363–1368.

Kalhan, S.C., Parimi, P.S., Gruca, L.L. and Hanson, R.W. (2005) Glutamine supplement with parenteral nutrition decreases whole body proteolysis in low birth weight infants. *Journal of Pediatrics* 146, 642–647.

Labow, B.I., Abcouwer, S.F., Lin, C.M. and Souba, W.W. (1998) Glutamine synthetase expression in rat lung is regulated by protein stability. *American Journal of Physiology* 275, L877–886.

Labow, B.I., Souba, W.W. and Abcouwer, S.F. (1999) Glutamine synthetase expression in muscle is regulated by transcriptional and posttranscriptional mechanisms. *American Journal of Physiology* 276, E1136–1145.

Labow, B.I., Souba, W.W. and Abcouwer, S.F. (2001) Mechanisms governing the expression of the enzymes of glutamine metabolism–glutaminase and glutamine synthetase. *Journal of Nutrition* 131, 2467S–2474S; discussion 2486S–2467S.

Lacey, J.M. and Wilmore, D.W. (1990) Is glutamine a conditionally essential amino acid? *Nutrition Reviews* 48, 297–309.

Ligthart-Melis, G.C., van de Poll, M.C., Boelens, P.G., Dejong, C.H., Deutz, N.E. and van Leeuwen, P.A. (2008) Glutamine is an important precursor for de novo synthesis of arginine in humans. *American Journal of Clinical Nutrition* 87, 1282–1289.

Matthews, D.E., Motil, K.J., Rohrbaugh, D.K., Burke, J.F., Young, V.R. and Bier, D.M. (1980) Measurement of leucine metabolism in man from a primed, continuous infusion of L-[1-3C]leucine. *American Journal of Physiology* 238, E473–479.

Mendell, J.R., Griggs, R.C., Moxley, R.T. 3rd, Fenichel, G.M., Brooke, M.H., Miller, J.P., Province, M.A. et al (1984) Clinical investigation in Duchenne muscular dystrophy: IV. Double-blind controlled trial of leucine. *Muscle Nerve* 7, 535–541.

Mithieux, G. (2001) New data and concepts on glutamine and glucose metabolism in the gut. *Current Opinion in Clinical Nutrition and Metabolic Care* 4, 267–271.

Mok, E., Eleouet-Da Violante, C., Daubrosse, C., Gottrand, F., Rigal, O., Fontan, J.E., Cuisset, J.M., et al. (2006) Oral glutamine and amino acid supplementation inhibit whole-body protein degradation in children with Duchenne muscular dystrophy. *American Journal of Clinical Nutrition* 83, 823–828.

Mok, E., Constantin, B., Favreau, F., Neveux, N., Magaud, C., Delwail, A. and Hankard, R. (2008) l-Glutamine administration reduces oxidized glutathione and MAP kinase signaling in dystrophic muscle of mdx mice. *Pediatric Research* 63, 268–273.

Mok, E., Letellier, G., Cuisset, J.M., Denjean, A., Gottrand, F., Alberti, C. and Hankard, R. (2009) Lack of functional benefit with glutamine versus placebo in Duchenne muscular dystrophy: a randomized crossover trial. *PLoS ONE* 4, e5448, doi:10.1371/journal.pone.0005448.

Neu, J. (2001) Glutamine in the fetus and critically ill low birth weight neonate: metabolism and mechanism of action. *Journal of Nutrition* 131, 2585S–2589S; discussion 2590S.

Neu, J., Shenoy, V. and Chakrabarti, R. (1996) Glutamine nutrition and metabolism: where do we go from here ? *FASEB Journal* 10, 829–837.

Newsholme, E.A., Crabtree, B. and Ardawi, M.S. (1985) Glutamine metabolism in lymphocytes: its biochemical, physiological and clinical importance. *Quarterly Journal of Experimental Physiology* 70, 473–489.

Nurjhan, N., Bucci, A., Perriello, G., Stumvoll, M., Dailey, G., Bier, D.M., Toft, I., et al. (1995) Glutamine: a major gluconeogenic precursor and vehicle for interorgan carbon transport in man. *Journal of Clinical Investigation* 95, 272–277.

Parimi, P.S., Devapatla, S., Gruca, L.L., Amini, S.B., Hanson, R.W. and Kalhan, S.C. (2004) Effect of enteral glutamine or glycine on whole-body nitrogen kinetics in very-low-birth-weight infants. *American Journal of Clinical Nutrition* 79, 402–409.

Payne, E.T., Yasuda, N., Bourgeois, J.M., Devries, M.C., Rodriguez, M.C., Yousuf, J. and Tarnopolsky, M.A. (2006) Nutritional therapy improves function and complements corticosteroid intervention in mdx mice. *Muscle Nerve* 33, 66–77.

Rapoport, S., Rost, J. and Schultze, M. (1971) Glutamine and glutamate as respiratory substrates of rabbit reticulocytes. *European Journal of Biochemistry* 23, 166–170.

Rennie, M.J., Edwards, R.H., Millward, D.J., Wolman, S.L., Halliday, D. and Matthews, D.E. (1982) Effects of Duchenne muscular dystrophy on muscle protein synthesis. *Nature* 296, 165–167.

Rennie, M.J., MacLennan, P.A., Hundal, H.S., Weryk, B., Smith, K., Taylor, P.M., Egan, C. *et al.* (1989) Skeletal muscle glutamine transport, intramuscular glutamine concentration, and muscle-protein turnover. *Metabolism* 38, 47–51.

Rheims, S., Cucherat, M., Arzimanoglou, A. and Ryvlin, P. (2008) Greater response to placebo in children than in adults: a systematic review and meta-analysis in drug-resistant partial epilepsy. *PLoS Medicine* 5, e166, DOI: 10.1371/journal.pmed.0050166.

Salehian, B., Mahabadi, V., Bilas, J., Taylor, W.E. and Ma, K. (2006) The effect of glutamine on prevention of glucocorticoid-induced skeletal muscle atrophy is associated with myostatin suppression. *Metabolism* 55, 1239–1247.

Sharma, U., Atri, S., Sharma, M.C., Sarkar, C. and Jagannathan, N.R. (2003) Skeletal muscle metabolism in Duchenne muscular dystrophy (DMD): an in-vitro proton NMR spectroscopy study. *Magnetic Resonance Imaging* 21, 145–153.

Smith, R.J., Larson, S., Stred, S.E. and Durschlag, R.P. (1984) Regulation of glutamine synthetase and glutaminase activities in cultured skeletal muscle cells. *Journal of Cellular Physiology* 120, 197–203.

Tubman, T.R., Thompson, S.W. and McGuire, W. (2008) Glutamine supplementation to prevent morbidity and mortality in preterm infants. *Cochrane Database of Systematic Reviews*, CD001457, DOI: 10.1002/14651858.CD001457.pub3.

Voisin, V., Sebrie, C., Matecki, S., Yu, H., Gillet, B., Ramonatxo, M., Israel, M., *et al.* (2005) L-arginine improves dystrophic phenotype in mdx mice. *Neurobiology of Disease* 20, 123–130.

Welbourne, T.C., Childress, D. and Givens, G. (1986) Renal regulation of interorgan glutamine flow in metabolic acidosis. *American Journal of Physiology* 251, R859–866.

Windmueller, H.G. and Spaeth, A.E. (1980) Respiratory fuels and nitrogen metabolism in vivo in small intestine of fed rats. Quantitative importance of glutamine, glutamate, and aspartate. *Journal of Biological Chemistry* 255, 107–112.

Ziegler, T.R., Young, L.S., Benfell, K., Scheltinga, M., Hortos, K., Bye, R., Morrow, F.D., *et al.* (1992) Clinical and metabolic efficacy of glutamine-supplemented parenteral nutrition after bone marrow transplantation. A randomized, double-blind, controlled study. *Annals of Internal Medicine* 116, 821–828.

19 Adverse Effects

J.P.F. D'Mello*
Formerly of SAC, University of Edinburgh King's Buildings Campus, Edinburgh, UK

19.1 Abstract

The adverse effects of amino acids in human nutrition and health have been reviewed in the context of the classical categories of imbalance, antagonism, and toxicity, first established in studies with animal models. This system has long existed as a conceptual framework primarily confined within the academic domain. However, there is now enhanced awareness that these categories may be relevant to a greater or lesser extent in human nutrition and health. A number of conclusions emerge in the light of this analysis, as detailed below.

It is suggested that two subdivisions, namely 'clinical amino acid imbalance' and 'excitotoxicity', are required within this classification to more accurately reflect observations in humans.

Clinical amino acid imbalance appears to be a regular feature of specific disease conditions. In patients with septic encephalopathy or with chronic liver disease, plasma ratios of branched-chain to aromatic amino acids are consistently reduced. Abnormal plasma amino acid patterns may also be seen in patients with cancer, cystinuria and Huntington's disease.

It is proposed that the category of antagonisms should include the effects of a wide range of plant non-protein amino acids. Canavanine, homoarginine and indospicine share structural similarity and compete with arginine for cellular transport and in the modulation of nitric oxide synthesis. Selenium analogues of the sulphur amino acids act by competing with methionine and cysteine at the levels of transport and protein synthesis. β-N-Oxalylamino-L-alanine and β-N-methylamino-L-alanine are potent glutamate receptor agonists implicated, respectively, in neurolathyrism and in amyotrophic lateral sclerosis and Parkinsonism-dementia (or Guam dementia). However, the aetiology of Guam dementia remains under review. On the other hand, it is widely acknowledged that hypoglycin A is associated with the seasonal incidence of a specific condition known as 'vomiting sickness'.

The category of toxicity is of particular significance in human health as it includes the adverse effects of glutamate, homocysteine, modified lysine residues and phenylalanine. The human health implications of these amino acids are reviewed later in this volume. Glutamate is the principal excitatory amino

---

* E-mail address: jpfdmello@hotmail.co.uk

acid implicated in neurodegenerative disorders. Thus, the status of excitotoxicity as the second significant subdivision in the classification of adverse effects of amino acids is amply justified.

Despite the adverse health implications cited above, there is increasing evidence that imbalance may be adapted for clinical purposes. In several studies, acute imbalance has been induced by the administration of drinks or mixtures rich in the indispensable amino acids but devoid of tryptophan or tyrosine and phenylalanine. This technique thus conforms with the classical method of precipitating amino acid imbalance. The resulting reductions in concentrations of the respective neurotransmitters provide a metabolic basis for psychiatric investigations. The potential of amino acid imbalance in cancer therapy has been briefly reviewed. The emerging consensus relates to the efficacy of branched-chain amino acid depletion in the inhibition of tumours in experimental models. However, the potential scope for specific non-protein amino acids in cancer therapy appears to be relatively more promising. Varying degrees of success have been reported with canavanine, sulphur amino acid analogues and mimosine. In experimental models, certain synthetic congeners of canavanine exhibit enhanced potential, but Se-methylselenocysteine is highly active, particularly in optimizing the therapeutic efficacy of anti-cancer drugs.

The wide interpretation of 'adverse effects' of amino acids adopted in this chapter thus allows a perspective for further consideration of clinical implications relating to cardiovascular, genetic and neurological disorders. Appropriate cross-referencing to subsequent chapters is provided for detailed review of these conditions.

19.2 Introduction

The distinctive and critical features of amino acids as multifunctional molecules have long been recognized and continue to be the subject of much research and innovative developments (see Chapters 1–13). As a corporate group, amino acids provide the building blocks for the biosynthesis of tissue proteins, but individual members play equally vital roles as signalling molecules and as precursors of specific neurotransmitters, hormones, purines, pyrimidines, creatine, haem and polyamines. Furthermore, arginine yields nitric oxide, while tryptophan is used to generate nicotinamide. Individual amino acids cannot be retained indefinitely as free molecules and must proceed along these synthetic pathways or follow catabolic routes involving deamination and synthesis of urea. The residual carbon skeletons are metabolized further in the processes of gluconeogenesis and/or ketogenesis. The metabolic fate of amino acids is often encapsulated in these terms in standard texts on biochemistry, and for most intents and purposes such a synopsis is eminently acceptable. Within such a benign scenario it is tacitly assumed that any surplus of amino acids is disposed of without harmful effects. However, this simplistic view is no longer tenable as increasingly more evidence accumulates to demonstrate the adverse effects of amino acids in several mammalian species, including humans.

The adverse effects of amino acids are well-established in studies with animals and the results extensively documented and reviewed (Harper, 1959; Harper et al., 1970; D'Mello, 2003). The literature relating to this field is in a reasonably advanced state. There are now compelling reasons to review the expanding evidence that these adverse effects may be replicated, to different degrees, in human subjects. The terminology developed with animal models is finding common usage in clinical sciences and it is opportune to examine the relevant data within the context of existing evidence.

19.3 Classification

In any scientific enquiry, classification of findings invariably facilitates a more orderly presentation and discussion of relevant data and this approach also applies to the question of adverse effects of amino acids. However, there are often notable exceptions to established schemes of rationalization which, equally, may deserve further exploration.

Using animal models, the diverse manifestations have been classified within three categories: imbalances, antagonisms and toxicity (Harper, 1959; Harper et al., 1970). As D'Mello (2003) observed, this system has long existed as a conceptual model primarily confined to the academic domain by virtue of its origin in contrived experiments with laboratory animals. However, there is now enhanced awareness that these categories of deleterious effects may be relevant to a greater or lesser extent in human nutrition and health. Accounts of adverse effects generally commence with the classification advanced by Harper (1959) and more fully expressed in the review of Harper (1964). The system emerged as a result of extensive research with a rat model (Table 19.1). His three-way framework has been retained in this chapter as many of the terms presented have become part of the terminology used in human nutrition and health.

It is immediately obvious that the classification was designed primarily to accommodate data obtained with the indispensable and dispensable amino acids (IAA and DAA, respectively). It is also apparent that in the development of this system, emphasis was placed on the adverse effects brought about solely by dietary manipulation of amino acids. Furthermore, no recognition was given to observations available at that time pertaining to those non-protein amino acids occurring in plants with the propensity to induce deleterious reactions in mammals (see D'Mello, 1991). Moreover, the system now requires updating to include particular amino acids that are considered to be risk factors in a number of human disorders, and efforts will be directed at integrating the associated effects into the classical three-way scheme presented in Table 19.1.

19.4 Amino Acid Imbalance

19.4.1 Concept

The term imbalance is relatively simple in concept, based on the premise that all amino acids must be available in balanced proportions at tissue level, with any deviation being accompanied by adverse effects. However, amino acid imbalance is often used out of context. There is, therefore, a need to begin with first principles to enable a more comprehensive discussion of the various issues that have appeared in the literature.

Amino acid imbalance is firmly embedded within the nutritional domain, where a precise definition has been applied for several decades. However, the term is also used in clinical investigations, where the terminology is less formal and has emerged independently of the nutritional work with animal models. It is intended to integrate observations from these parallel lines of investigation into a unifying framework. For the purposes of this review, it is intended to consider two forms of amino acid imbalance: dietary or nutritional and clinical.

19.4.2 Dietary or nutritional amino acid imbalance

Nutritional amino acid imbalance has been defined as a change in the dietary pattern of amino acids which results in the precipitation

Table 19.1. Classification of adverse effects of amino acids: a three-way model proposed by Harper (1964). (Based on nutritional studies with rats.)

Category	Dietary conditions
Imbalance	Addition of second-limiting amino acid; or addition of an incomplete amino acid mixture. Amelioration of gross effects by supplementation with first-limiting amino acid
Antagonism	Specific, conditionally reversible interactions induced by structurally-related indispensable amino acids, e.g. lysine and arginine; or by leucine, isoleucine and valine. Lysine antagonism reversed by arginine supplementation; leucine antagonism reversed by combinations of isoleucine and valine
Toxicity	Diverse effects of disproportionate levels of indispensable or dispensable amino acids, resulting in organ damage, e.g. renal or ocular lesions. Effects normally irreversible

of ill-effects that are completely reversed by supplementation with the first-limiting amino acid (Harper, 1964). The prerequisite for a limiting amino acid may be satisfied by the use of suitably deficient proteins such as casein, gelatin or zein, but more generally this condition is fulfilled by employing low-protein diets. The definition of imbalance was conceived and developed in studies with laboratory animals, but is now widely applied to the nutrition and well-being of human subjects even when the strict conditions of this phenomenon are not fulfilled. Thus, the precipitation of imbalance in animals has generally focused on IAA, whereas in the application to human health all amino acids are considered, irrespective of nutritional classification.

It is therefore, instructive to recall some of the fundamental tenets embodied within the original development of the concept of dietary amino acid imbalance. Two types of such imbalances are generally recognized (Table 19.2):

1. that induced by the addition of a relatively small quantity of IAA to a low-protein diet; and
2. that precipitated by an incomplete mixture of amino acids.

In the first type, there is normally a specific requirement that the agent inducing the imbalance should be the second-limiting amino acid (Winje *et al.*, 1954). A more reliable procedure involves the addition of an amino acid mixture devoid of one IAA to a low-protein diet limiting in that amino acid (Pant *et al.*, 1972). In both types, the effects of imbalances are rectified by supplementation with the first-limiting amino acid, which therefore acts as the antidote (Table 19.2). Other studies show that imbalances may also be created by the use of mixtures of DAA (Tews *et al.*, 1980). In such cases, the most reliable method involves the use of amino acids, individually or in mixtures, that compete with the dietary limiting amino acid for transport into the brain. Thus, the ratio of imbalancing amino acids to the limiting one is critical in this type of adverse effects. Therefore, the minimal requirements for unequivocal demonstration of an amino acid imbalance must involve the use of a suitable control, an imbalanced diet, and a corrected diet (Table 19.2).

Several studies with animal models indicate that amino acid imbalances may occur at the tissue level even though the diet may appear to be in ideal balance. These types of imbalances may, for example, occur with the use of crystalline amino acids in diets based on cereals. Such considerations may well apply in human nutrition if the intention is to provide a perfect balance at tissue level. It has long been recognized that free amino acids used as supplements are absorbed more rapidly than protein-bound amino acids, resulting in an imbalanced supply at the sites of protein synthesis (see D'Mello, 2003). For example, Leibholz *et al.* (1986) observed that the concentration of free lysine in plasma of pigs increased 1–2 h after feeding a diet containing pure lysine, declining thereafter, whereas the circulating concentrations of

Table 19.2. Effects of dietary amino acid imbalance on growth of rats fed low-protein diets. (Adapted from D'Mello, 2003.)

Protein source and amino acid supplements	First-limiting amino acid	Method of precipitating imbalance	Dietary regime	Growth response (proportion of control)	Reference
Egg albumen + Thr + Val	His	Addition of second-limiting amino acid (Lys)	Control Imbalanced Corrected	1.00 0.65 0.95	Winje *et al.* (1954)
Casein + Met	Trp	Addition of amino acid mixture devoid of Trp	Control Imbalanced Corrected	1.00 0.71 1.10	Pant *et al.* (1972)

other amino acids originating from the protein bound fraction of the diet peaked 2–6 h postprandial. In pigs fed once daily, this lack of synchrony in absorption would precipitate an imbalance at the cellular level. Under these circumstances growth and efficiency of dietary nitrogen utilization would be impaired, but the deleterious effects could be offset by more frequent feeding. This expectation was confirmed by Batterham (1974) who showed that the efficiency of utilization of free lysine supplements for growth of pigs fed once daily was only 0.43–0.67 of values recorded for pigs fed the same quantity of food in six equal portions at 3-hourly intervals. In contrast, no such benefit occurred on feeding the unsupplemented diet more frequently. Subsequent investigations by Partridge et al. (1985) extended the benefits of increased feeding frequency and lysine supplementation to improvements in nitrogen utilization.

19.4.2.1 Anorexia

Reports of amino acid imbalances conventionally focus on the growth-depressing effects in animal models (Harper, 1964; Tews et al. 1979). However, it has been consistently recorded that a predisposing factor is a rapid and marked reduction in food intake of affected animals. Thus, Harper and Rogers (1965) reported that rats fed an imbalanced diet reduced their food intake within 3–6 h, implying that appetite depression was the primary event responsible for the ensuing retardation of growth. A considerable body of evidence supports this hypothesis. If food intake in animals is increased by force-feeding, by insulin injections, by adjusting dietary protein to energy ratios, or by exposing animals to cold environmental temperatures, then commensurate improvements in growth also occur (D'Mello, 1994).

19.4.2.2 Dietary preferences

Alteration in dietary preference is another feature of nutritional amino acid imbalance, at least in the rat, with possible wider extrapolation to other mammals, including humans. When offered a choice, rats consume a balanced diet in preference to an imbalanced one, but more remarkably, select a protein-free diet incapable of supporting growth instead of an imbalanced diet which would allow growth, albeit at a low level (Sanahuja and Harper, 1962; Leung and Rogers, 1987).

19.4.2.3 Mechanisms

The biochemical mechanisms underlying the anorectic effects of amino acid-imbalanced diets have been described by Harper and Rogers (1965), following extensive studies with the rat. It was proposed that surplus amino acids arriving in the portal circulation following ingestion of the imbalanced diet stimulates synthesis or suppresses protein degradation in the liver, leading to enhanced retention of the limiting amino acid relative to that in control groups (Table 19.3). The supply of the limiting amino acid for utilization by peripheral tissues such as muscle is thereby reduced, but protein synthesis proceeds without interruption in these tissues. Ultimately, however, the free amino acid patterns of both muscle and blood plasma become so deranged as to invoke the intervention of the appetite-regulating system to reduce food intake. The growth-depressing effects are a direct consequence of reduced appetite and intake of nutrients. As D'Mello (2003) stated, this hypothesis is still accepted as a satisfactory explanation of the effects of amino acid imbalance in the rat. A central tenet within the hypothesis advanced by Harper and Rogers (1965) is the association between appetite depression and changes in tissue patterns of amino acids. In both blood plasma and muscle, concentrations of the limiting amino acid decline, while there is an accumulation of those amino acids added to create the imbalance. Since these events occur within a few hours of ingestion of imbalanced diets, it has been suggested that changes in the plasma amino acid pattern provide the metabolic signal that ultimately results in anorexia and abnormal feeding behaviour. In subsequent attempts to validate this hypothesis, the role of the first-limiting amino acid was placed in sharper focus. For example, preliminary work by Leung and Rogers (1969) indicated that the

Table 19.3. Nutritional amino acid imbalance: biochemical cascade leading to depressed appetite and growth in animal models. (Based on the hypothesis of Harper and Rogers, 1965.)

Site	Effects
Liver ↓	Surplus amino acids stimulate synthesis or suppress breakdown of proteins; efficient utilization of limiting amino acid
Muscle ↓	Protein synthesis continues normally; greater retention of limiting amino acid; deranged free amino acid pattern
Plasma ↓	Deranged free amino acid pattern
Brain ↓	Abnormal pattern in blood monitored by appetite-regulating regions; GCN2 signalling[a]
Whole-body responses	Depressed appetite ↓ Reduced nutrient intake ↓ Reduced growth

[a]See Chapter 13.

depression in appetite may be prevented by the infusion of a small quantity of the first-limiting amino acid via the carotid artery, whereas administration through the jugular vein was ineffective. These studies also provided the basis of the proposition that food intake and feeding behaviour may be linked with changes in brain uptake and metabolic disposition of critical amino acids. It was soon established that the concentration of the first-limiting amino acid declined more rapidly in cerebral tissues than in blood plasma (Peng *et al.*, 1972). This observation led to the proposal that the fall in brain concentrations of the limiting amino acid provides the signal that initiates the changes in food intake and dietary choice, although the definitive mechanism remains obscure (Leung and Rogers, 1987). However, the regions of the central nervous system sensitive to dietary amino acid imbalance have been delineated in the rat. These include the anterior prepyriform cortex, the medial amygdala, and certain sites of the hippocampus and septum. In particular, the sensitivity of the prepyriform cortex to amino acid imbalance has been extensively investigated by Gietzen *et al.* (1986) and Beverly *et al.* (1990a,b, 1991a). Thus the selection of a protein-free diet in preference to an imbalanced one is reversed when the limiting amino acid is directly injected into the prepyriform cortex. Beverly *et al.* (1991b) showed that injected dose levels are important, exerting separate effects on dietary selection and on intake of imbalanced diets. Gietzen *et al.* (1998) developed this concept further by demonstrating that different neural circuits mediate the initial recognition and secondary conditioned responses to amino acid imbalanced diets.

Amino acid imbalance may affect food intake and dietary selection by modulating the synthesis and metabolic disposition of neurotransmitters in the brain. In one study, feeding imbalanced diets reduced production of noradrenaline in the anterior prepyriform cortex of rats (Leung *et al.*, 1985). However, Harrison and D'Mello (1987) showed that an imbalance induced by the addition of a mixture devoid of tyrosine and phenylalanine to a diet deficient in these two amino acids reduced food intake of chicks, without affecting noradrenaline or dopamine levels in brain homogenates. This discrepancy may have more to do with neurotransmitter synthesis and metabolism at specific sites in the brain than with any genuine differences between species or type of imbalance used in the two studies.

19.4.2.4 Effects on nutrient utilization

The effect of amino acid imbalance on nutrient utilization continues to be the subject of some debate. An imbalance might be expected to impair overall efficiency of utilization of dietary protein. Studies with a rat model confirm this expectation, with N retention efficiency declining from 0.60 to 0.44 on addition of an imbalancing amino acid mixture to a control diet. However, further examination reveals that in rats pair-fed the control diet to match food intakes of the imbalanced group, efficiency of N retention decreased to 0.33, indicating that the effects of imbalance are mediated via reductions in appetite (Kumta et al., 1958). Despite these observations, the accepted consensus is that amino acid imbalances reduce the overall efficiency of protein utilization in other animals. Thus, Moughan (1991) attributed the low efficiency of protein utilization in pigs partly to dietary amino acid imbalance. In addition, Partridge et al. (1985) demonstrated that imbalances at the tissue level, induced by the differential absorption of amino acids from crystalline and protein-bound sources, can reduce overall efficiency of protein utilization in pigs fed once daily. Furthermore, Wang and Fuller (1989) maintained that manipulation of the composition of a mixture of amino acids to simulate the pattern in casein enhanced N retention in pigs by reducing imbalances. However, Langer and Fuller (1994) demonstrated that the addition of an imbalancing mixture containing leucine, isoleucine, and valine to a diet limiting in methionine enhanced N efficiency in growing pigs. This effect was attributed to increased metabolic availability of methionine due to inhibition of enzymes associated with methionine degradation (Langer et al., 2000). The concept of enhanced utilization of the limiting amino acid under such imbalances is not new. Thus Harper and Rogers (1965) reported that rats fed a threonine-imbalanced diet reduced oxidation of this amino acid. In subsequent studies, Yoshida et al. (1966) and Benevenga et al. (1968) demonstrated increased incorporation of the first-limiting amino acid into hepatic proteins of rats fed imbalanced diets. Thus both whole-animal and biochemical studies with rats have demonstrated enhanced utilization and retention of the limiting amino acid following feeding of amino acid imbalanced diets. Despite this evidence, other investigators continue to invoke such imbalances to explain reductions in utilization of limiting amino acids in high-protein (Abebe and Morris, 1990a,b) or imbalanced dietary regimes (Yuan et al., 2000). In the light of recent evidence, there may be some merit in reviewing the results of Abebe and Morris (1990a,b). A more plausible explanation for these observations may reside in recent reports indicating the formation of advanced glycation end-products (AGE) in high-protein dietary regimes (Uribarri and Tuttle, 2006). The synthesis of AGE via Maillard-type reactions, occurring under normal physiological conditions, would be accompanied by a depletion of metabolic pools of lysine and other amino acids, leading to the reported reductions in utilization of these amino acids. Furthermore, AGE might then induce nephrotoxicity and other physiological aberrations such as intestinal inflammation and endothelial dysfunction. Thus, reduced biochemical availability of critical amino acids and AGE-induced metabolic stress may well combine to produce the discrepant responses reported by Abebe and Morris, (1990a,b). The diverse effects of AGE are of sufficient biomedical significance to justify a full review in this volume (see Chapter 22).

19.5 Clinical Amino Acid Imbalance

Although the classification of adverse effects is firmly embedded in the nutritional literature, the term imbalance, in particular, is widely used in the context of human health. However, the concept of imbalance in human health has evolved along parallel lines with little or no overlap between studies on nutritional and clinical amino acid imbalance. There is no formal definition of the latter term, and a definitive review of this subject is therefore justified here. For the purposes of this chapter, clinical amino acid imbalance is used to represent abnormal patterns and ratios of amino acids in human subjects enduring a variety of disorders. Clinical amino acid imbalance is used here primarily to denote adverse ratios between two or more specific groups of amino acids in physiological fluids of patients. However, this term is also used to describe abnormal plasma variations in amino acid profiles of diseased patients, relative to those of control healthy individuals. In both sets of cases, it should be noted that the literature rarely contains any reports in which an explicit attempt has been made to identify the physiologically limiting amino acids associated with these abnormalities. Furthermore, there are only limited data as to whether restoration of normal ratios might improve outcomes in patients with manifestations of clinical amino acid imbalance. This contrasts with the complete efficacy of the limiting amino acid in the dietary form of imbalance (Table 19.2).

A summary of research on clinical amino acid imbalance in human subjects is shown in Table 19.4. The table is not designed to be comprehensive, but rather illustrative of the incidence of such imbalances in diverse syndromes and diseases ranging from septic encephalopathy to cancer.

19.5.1 Septic encephalopathy

Basler et al. (2002) reported that within 12 h of the onset of septic encephalopathy, plasma amino acids were altered, with a decrease in the ratio of branched-chain to aromatic amino acids, although no severe liver dysfunction was seen in any of the patients under observation. Nakamura et al. (2003) commented that metabolic alterations including amino acid imbalance are involved in the pathogenesis of septic encephalopathy and further showed that within 12 h of the development of the syndrome, plasma ratios of branched-chain to aromatic amino acids in septic patients with encephalopathy declined relative to ratios in septic patients without encephalopathy or those in healthy controls. It was concluded that such imbalances in patients with septic encephalopathy might serve as a marker for the severity of the septic syndrome.

Table 19.4. Research titles purporting to demonstrate the incidence of clinical amino acid imbalance in diverse human conditions.

Research titles	Reference
Amino acid imbalance early in septic encephalopathy	Basler et al. (2002)
Effects of polymyxin B-immobilized fibre haemoperfusion on amino acid imbalance in septic encephalopathy	Nakamura et al. (2003)
Amino acid imbalance and hepatic encephalopathy	Bernardini and Fischer (1982)
Albumin dialysis has a favourable effect on amino acid profile in hepatic encephalopathy	Kolvusalo et al. (2008)
Albumin dialysis improves hepatic encephalopathy and decreases circulating phenolic aromatic amino acids in patients with alcoholic hepatitis and severe liver failure	Pares et al. (2009)
Plasma amino acid imbalance in patients with liver disease	Cascino et al. (1978)
Evaluating responses to nutritional therapy using the branched-chain amino acid/tyrosine ratio in patients with chronic liver disease	Kawamura-Yasui et al. (1999)
Measurement of serum branched-chain amino acids to tyrosine ratio level is useful in prediction of a change of serum albumin level in chronic liver disease	Suzuki et al. (2007)
Plasma amino acid imbalance in patients with chronic renal failure on intermittent dialysis	Young and Parsons (1970)
Plasma amino acid imbalance in patients with lung and breast cancer	Cascino et al. (1995)
Amino acid imbalance in cystinuria	Asatoor et al. (1974)
Imbalance of the amino acid pattern in patients with AIDS: special treatment with adapted amino acid solution	Althoff et al. (1989)
Huntington's disease: imbalance of free amino acids in the cerebrospinal fluid of patients and offspring at risk	Oepen et al. (1982)
Sporadic ulcerative mutilating acropathy with imbalance of free amino acids in the cerebrospinal fluid	Monaco et al. (1975)

In view of the foregoing, it is instructive to consider the effects of one study designed to evaluate the effects of remedial procedures. Garcia-de-Lorenzo et al. (1997) examined the clinical and metabolic responses of parenteral administration of different amounts of branched-chain amino acids in septic patients. Overall, the results indicated that formulas rich in these amino acids induced a beneficial effect in septic patients.

19.5.2 Liver disorders

According to Kolvusalo et al. (2008), hepatic encephalopathy is generally regarded to be at least partly caused by an imbalance in plasma amino acid levels. The ratio between the branched-chain and aromatic amino acids correlates with the severity of hepatic encephalopathy. The lower the ratio, the greater is the manifestation of this disorder. Pares et al. (2009) confirmed this correlation and also showed the benefits of albumin dialysis in reducing circulating levels of aromatic amino acids in patients with alcoholic hepatitis and severe liver failure. These studies reflect earlier studies showing high plasma levels of aromatic and sulphur amino acids, and low levels of branched-chain amino acids, in cirrhotic patients (Cascino et al., 1978). Kawamura-Yasui et al. (1999) suggested that the branched-chain to tyrosine ratio may serve as a useful marker for monitoring the response to nutritional therapy in patients with chronic liver disease. A similar theme appeared in the investigation of Suzuki et al. (2007) who measured serum branched-chain amino acid to tyrosine ratios in patients with chronic liver disease. They concluded that the incidence of amino acid imbalance was significantly higher in subjects with liver cirrhosis, and that the ratio of these amino acids is useful for diagnostic purposes. The expression of the relationship between the branched-chain and aromatic amino acids is sometimes referred to as the Fischer ratio (Bernardini and Fischer, 1982; Kolvusalo et al., 2008). Thus, from the foregoing accounts, it may be concluded that an abnormal Fischer ratio is a primary manifestation of amino acid imbalance in patients with liver failure.

19.5.3 Cancer and other conditions

Plasma amino acid imbalance may occur during carcinogenesis. In patients with lung cancer, a significant reduction of glucogenic amino acids (threonine, serine and glycine) and a significant increase of free tryptophan and glutamate were found in plasma. In patients with breast cancer, plasma concentrations of ornithine, glutamate and tryptophan were significantly elevated (Cascino et al., 1995). Amino acid imbalance can be demonstrated in cystinuric patients. After consumption of a free amino acid mixture, plasma increments of lysine and arginine were reduced and those of many other amino acids were significantly higher than those found in control subjects (Asatoor et al., 1974). Cerebrospinal fluid has also been used to investigate amino acid imbalance. In Huntington's disease, significant reductions were recorded for asparagine, isoleucine, leucine, phenylalanine, histidine and arginine in patients with the condition, compared to non-choreic control subjects (Oepen et al., 1982). It was further suggested that amino acid imbalance is an early metabolic disturbance in Huntington's disease. On the other hand, the levels of most amino acids in cerebrospinal fluid were increased in a case of sporadic ulcerative mutilating acropathy (Monaco et al., 1975).

19.5.4 Appetite

In laboratory models, imposition of dietary amino acid imbalance is consistently accompanied by profound reductions in food intake, as described above. Dietary choice is also markedly affected. Loss of appetite is seen in patients with hepatic encephalopathy (Takeda et al., 1993) and with sepsis (Vary and Lynch, 2004). It is pertinent to enquire whether clinical amino acid imbalance is the cause or the effect of anorexia in these and other disorders reviewed above. Furthermore, it would be of considerable academic and practical interest to ascertain whether correction of clinical imbalance by parenteral administration of formulas rich in branched-chain amino acids would enhance appetite in septic patients

(Garcia-de-Lorenzo et al., 1997) or, indeed, in any of the hepatic disorders cited above.

19.6 Amino Acid Antagonisms

An amino acid antagonism has been defined as a deleterious nutritional interaction between structurally related amino acids. This category of adverse effects was devised to accommodate the unique and separate effects of lysine and leucine in the rat and in other animal models (D'Mello and Lewis 1970a,b,c). The effects are most pronounced when excesses of these antagonists are employed in diets that are deficient in their respective 'target' amino acids. The target for lysine is its structural analogue arginine, while valine and isoleucine are antagonized by leucine. Demonstrations of antagonisms have now been extended to a wide range of experimental models including avian species (D'Mello and Lewis, 1970a,b). In addition, it is now recognized that antagonisms may be precipitated by particular analogues occurring naturally in plants as non-protein amino acids. In most instances, the action of these analogues is targeted at the metabolism and utilization of specific structurally related IAA and DAA.

19.6.1 Branched-chain amino acid antagonisms

Demonstrations of the antagonisms involving the branched-chain amino acids (BCAA) in animal models have been sustained by the knowledge that food staples such as maize and sorghum grains contain disproportionate quantities of leucine. Other reports that leucine may be linked with the deficiency condition pellagra in humans has provided impetus for further research.

Following initial observations with leucine-induced antagonisms in the rat, much evidence has emerged to confirm the specificity and complexity of interactions among BCAA in other animal models, including avian species. In one study, D'Mello and Lewis (1970b) showed that excess dietary leucine permitted the growth response to the first-limiting amino acid, methionine, only in the presence of supplementary isoleucine. The specificity of the leucine–isoleucine antagonism was thus established for the first time. However, other results led D'Mello and Lewis (1970b) to conclude that the leucine–valine interaction was relatively more potent. That conclusion was based on growth and plasma amino acid levels. Circulating concentrations of valine were markedly more sensitive than isoleucine to excess leucine in the diet. Nevertheless, despite the primacy of the leucine–valine interaction, it is possible to devise dietary conditions to enhance the sensitivity of isoleucine in BCAA antagonisms (see D'Mello, 2003).

Based on studies principally with the rat, Harper et al. (1984) attributed the leucine-induced antagonism to increased oxidation of valine and isoleucine, having previously discounted any effects associated with competition for intestinal or renal transport. The catabolism of BCAA is initiated by a reversible aminotransferase reaction (Chapter 2). The branched-chain keto acids (BCKA) so formed then undergo irreversible oxidative decarboxylation to yield acyl-CoA compounds, which are degraded further in a series of reactions analogous to those involved in fatty acid oxidation. Harper et al. (1984) proposed that enhanced BCKA oxidation might account for the depletion of plasma pools of valine and isoleucine in animals fed excess leucine. Studies with preruminant lambs support this view, in that marked reductions in plasma concentrations of keto acids derived from valine and isoleucine were observed in response to excess leucine intake (Papet et al., 1988a). Furthermore, Papet et al. (1988b) showed enhanced activities of aminotransferases in the liver and jejunum in response to excess leucine, which also caused activation of BCKA dehydrogenase in the jejunum. BCAA-induced antagonisms may, additionally, deplete brain pools of other amino acids, particularly those that are the precursors of the neurotransmitters (Harrison and D'Mello, 1986). It is generally conceded that changes in brain metabolism of amino acids and their neurotransmitter derivatives may be associated with alterations in food intake and feeding behaviour (Leung and Rogers, 1987; Gietzen et al., 1998). Consistent with this concept has been the observation that a substantial element of the adverse effects of excess leucine resides in food intake depression (Calvert et al., 1982; Papet et al., 1988a), which subjugates effects arising from oxidative catabolism of isoleucine and valine.

19.6.1.1 Leucine and pellagra

Excess leucine intake from maize and sorghum grains has been implicated in pellagra, a condition associated with nicotinic acid deficiency. In a general review, Dickerson and Wiryanti (1978) imply that leucine excess may increase requirements for this vitamin, although there is no suggestion of a structural antagonism in the classical sense. It is of interest, however, that isoleucine is effective in improving electroencephalograms of pellagrins with mental disturbances (Krishnaswamy and Gopalan, 1971). It is relevant to enquire here whether valine might have further enhanced the efficacy of isoleucine, judging by the complexity of interactions among the BCAA in other species (D'Mello, 2003).

19.6.2 The lysine–arginine antagonism

The deleterious effects of lysine, particularly with respect to its target, arginine, is the classical example of an amino acid antagonism. The emergence of other analogues of arginine (see below) and continuing research on nitric oxide (NO) biosynthesis have re-focused interest in the lysine–arginine antagonism. Although this antagonism has been demonstrated in rats fed casein diets (Jones et al., 1966), its most potent form occurs in avian models (D'Mello and Lewis (1970a,c) since arginine is an indispensable amino acid for this species. The unique specificity of the lysine–arginine antagonism was examined in several experiments by D'Mello and Lewis (1970a), who designed basal diets that were first-limiting in methionine, tryptophan, histidine or threonine, with arginine marginally deficient. Addition of excess lysine to each of these diets precipitated a severe growth depression which, in every case, was reversed by arginine supplementation and not by the amino acid shown to be deficient in the basal diets. Plasma arginine was also specifically and consistently depressed on addition of excess lysine to these diets. However, a number of factors can affect the severity of this antagonism. For example, excess chloride augments the adverse effects, whereas alkaline salts of monovalent mineral cations reduce or eliminate the potency of this antagonism. As will be apparent later in this chapter, another analogue of arginine, namely canavanine, enhances the potency of the lysine–arginine antagonism.

By virtue of their uricotelism, avian species are unable to synthesize arginine and are, therefore, particularly sensitive to the lysine–arginine antagonism. The most significant factor in the avian manifestation of this antagonism is the enhanced activity of kidney arginase which results in increased catabolism of arginine. If arginase activity is suppressed by the use of a specific inhibitor, then the severity of the antagonism is also attenuated. A second factor is the depression in appetite, presumably caused by lysine-induced disruption of brain uptake and metabolism of other amino acids and their neurotransmitter derivatives. Secondary mechanisms include enhanced urinary excretion of arginine and inhibition of hepatic transamidinase activity, with consequent reduction of creatine biosynthesis (D'Mello, 2003). In addition, lysine may affect nitric oxide (NO) production from arginine.

It has been suggested that the arginine to lysine ratio might influence cholesterol concentrations in plasma and liver of humans. However, recent results with rats failed to support this contention (Spielmann et al., 2008).

19.6.2.1 Hyperlysinaemia

Although not a manifestation or a result of an antagonism, hyperlysinaemia is relevant here since there is potential for adverse effects (Woody, 1964). Despite some evidence to the contrary (Jones et al., 1966), there are reliable data to show that mammals are significantly less sensitive to the adverse effects of lysine than avian species (Edmonds and Baker, 1987; Tsubuku et al., 2004). This notion is corroborated by studies on patients with hyperlysinaemia. Dancis et al. (1983) examined patients with familial hyperlysinaemia caused by lysine-ketoglutarate reductase deficiency. No adverse physical or mental effects could be attributed to this condition. Similarly, Saudubray and Rabier (2007) reported that severe hyperlysinaemia in patients deficient in aminoadipic semialdehyde dehydrogenase was accompanied by minimal health consequences. However, biochemical studies are required to investigate any effects on transport of arginine and on NO production in these subjects. Luiking and Deutz (2007) maintain that lysine competes with arginine for transport into the cell, and it is logical to enquire whether arginine uptake and metabolism are affected in patients with hyperlysinaemia.

19.6.3 Antagonisms induced by non-protein amino acids

A wide array of amino acids, occurring naturally in unconjugated forms in plants (Table 19.5), may provoke adverse reactions in both animals and humans. These non-protein amino acids are ubiquitous in the plant, but the seed is normally the most concentrated source. Legumes contain higher concentrations and a more diverse range of non-protein amino acids than any other plant species (D'Mello, 1991). In many instances these compounds bear structural analogy with the physiologically important amino acids or their neurotransmitter derivatives. Consequently, manifestations of deleterious effects range from loss of appetite and reduced nutrient utilization to profound neurological disorders and even death (Table 19.6). Although the data are derived primarily from studies with rodent models, it is appropriate and instructive to consider the implications for human health as outlined in Table 19.7.

It will be apparent that the classification shown in Table 19.6 contains examples that are not consistent with the stringent definition of antagonisms. However, this scheme has been designed in order to integrate a wider range of the non-protein amino acids into a framework that would allow a comprehensive exposition of the diverse distribution, toxicology, and mechanisms of action of these amino acids. Furthermore, at least two of these amino acids may be regarded as potent glutamate receptor agonists and their activities are, therefore, of relevance here.

19.6.3.1 Analogues of arginine

19.6.3.1.1 CANAVANINE. Of the three analogues of arginine, canavanine is more ubiquitous (Table 19.5) and present in higher concentrations in leguminous seeds (D'Mello, 2003).

Table 19.5. Distribution of non-protein amino acids in plants. (Adapted from D'Mello, 1991.)

Category	Plant species	Non-protein amino acid
Legume	*Canavalia ensiformis*, *Medicago sativa* (lucerne; alfalfa), *Gliricidia sepium*, *Dioclea megacarpa*, *Robinia pseudoacacia*	Canavanine
	Lathyrus cicera	Homoarginine
	Indigofera spicata	Indospicine; canavanine
	Astragalus spp.	Se-Methylselenocysteine; selenocystathionine; selenomethionine
	Leucaena leucocephala (ipil ipil)	Mimosine
	Lathyrus sativus	β-N-Oxalylamino-L-alanine
	Vicia sativa	β-Cyanoalanine
	Lathyrus sylvestris	α,γ-Diaminobutyric acid
Brassica	*Brassica oleracea* (cabbage, Brussels sprouts)	S-Methylcysteine sulphoxide
	Brassica oleracea (broccoli)	Se-Methylselenocysteine
Other	*Cycas circinalis* (false sago palm)	β-N-Methylamino-L-alanine
	Blighia sapida (ackee)	Hypoglycin A

Table 19.6. Adverse effects of some non-protein amino acids in animals. (Adapted from D'Mello, 1991.)

Group	Non-protein amino acid	Adverse effects
Arginine analogues	Canavanine	Inhibition of growth and nitrogen retention; suppression of reduced glutathione levels
	Homoarginine	Inhibition of growth and nitrogen retention; hypersensitivity; modulation of NO production; death
	Indospicine	Teratogenic effects; liver damage; arginase inhibition
Analogues of sulphur amino acids	Selenocystine	Hepatotoxicity
	Selenomethionine	Pancreatic acinar cell necrosis; anorexia; dermatitis; hypothermia
	S-Methylcysteine sulphoxide	Haemolytic anaemia; organ damage; death (in ruminants)
Aromatic	Mimosine	Inhibition of hair growth; loss of facial hair; irregular or termination of oestrus cycling; teratogenic effects; reduced collagen synthesis; uterine perforations; deformities of cranium, thorax and pelvis in fetus
Neurotoxins	β-N-Oxalylamino-L-alanine	Tremors; convulsive seizures; death
	β-Cyanoalanine	Hyperactivity; tremors; convulsions; prostration; death
	α,γ-Diaminobutyric acid	Hyperirritability; tremors; convulsions; death
	β-N-Methylamino-L-alanine	Damage of motor neurons; excitotoxicity
Other	Hypoglycin A	Fetal malformations; inhibition of gluconeogenesis

Table 19.7. Plant non-protein amino acids implicated in human disorders or affecting metabolic processes. (See text for references.)

Amino acid	Adverse or metabolic effects
Canavanine	Reactivation of systemic lupus erythaematosus (presumption); inhibition of iNOS
Homoarginine	Inhibition of lysine and arginine transport
Indospicine	Inhibition of cNOS and iNOS
Selenomethionine	Cautious approach to use as a Se supplement to avoid cytotoxic effects
Mimosine	Hair loss; inhibition of DNA replication
β-N-Oxalylamino-L-alanine	Neurolathyrism: muscular rigidity, weakness and paralysis of leg muscles (epidemiological evidence); potent glutamate receptor agonist
β-N-Methylamino-L-alanine	Amyotrophic lateral sclerosis and Parkinsonism-dementia in Guam (inconclusive evidence); potent glutamate receptor agonist
Hypoglycin A	Vomiting, convulsions, coma, death; hepatic encephalopathy; hypoglycaemia

Canavanine is now recognized as an inhibitor of constitutive and inducible forms of NOS (Pass *et al.*, 1996). Canavanine contributes significantly to the toxicity of *Canavalia ensiformis* in avian species. Adverse effects may also arise after synthesis of canaline, a structural analogue of ornithine, by the action of arginase on canavanine. The mammalian metabolism of canavanine is analogous with that of arginine in the urea cycle (Fig. 19.1; D'Mello, 1991). Since this cycle is non-functional in avian species, they are unable to synthesize arginine and, consequently, readily succumb to the adverse effects of canavanine (Table 19.6). Arginine is an effective antidote and on the basis of this evidence,

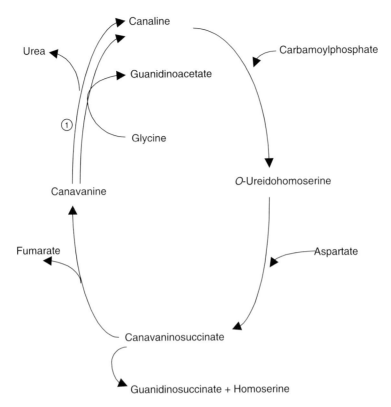

Fig. 19.1. The biochemical fate of canavanine in mammals. The analogy with arginine metabolism is unmistakable. Thus, the breakdown of canavanine is initiated by arginase, (1) Canaline, O-ureidohomoserine, and canavaninosuccinate are congeners of ornithine, citrulline, and argininosuccinate, respectively. (Adapted from D'Mello, 1991; for comparison with arginine metabolism, see pathways in Chapter 3.)

D'Mello (2003) proposed the existence of a canavanine–arginine antagonism analogous to that between lysine and arginine.

Canavanine also occurs in *Medicago sativa* (lucerne or alfalfa) seeds, regularly recommended as a herbal supplement. In monkeys, feeding lucerne sprouts induced haematological and serological abnormalities similar to those observed in human systemic lupus erythaematosus (SLE). Subsequent feeding of canavanine reactivated this condition in these monkeys (see Spencer and Berman, 2003). Notwithstanding the absence of direct definitive data, it is assumed here that canavanine might precipitate similar effects in humans consuming lucerne supplements (Table 19.7).

19.6.3.1.2 HOMOARGININE. The primary source of homoarginine is the seed of *Lathyrus cicera* (Table 19.5). In rodent models, homoarginine has been shown to induce hypersensitivity and mortality as well as a depression in brain concentrations of lysine (O'Kane *et al.*, 2006; Zinnanti *et al.*, 2007), ornithine, and arginine (Table 19.6; see also D'Mello, 1991). Kakoki *et al.* (2006) showed that homoarginine can influence NO production in endothelial cells by altering cellular arginine transport mechanisms. Homoarginine exacerbates the canavanine–arginine interaction in avian species (D'Mello, 2003), serving to illustrate the complexity of interactions among the analogues and antagonists of arginine. Since *L. cicera* (Table 19.5) is not a normal constituent of human diets, the toxicity of homoarginine is of minor relevance as regards health issues. Nevertheless, there is continuing research interest in the activities of the pure form of this amino acid as a substrate for modulation of NO production in infection and immunity (Degnan *et al.*, 1998), in human pregnancy (Valtonen *et al.*, 2008), and in the functional metabolism of the renal medulla (Kakoki *et al.*, 2004). Furthermore, Henningsson and Lundquist (1998) reported that homoarginine was less potent than arginine as an insulin secretagogue but equally effective for inducing glucagon release.

19.6.3.1.3 INDOSPICINE. It is widely acknowledged that indospicine is a powerful teratogen, inducing cleavage of the secondary palate and general somatic dwarfism in rats given a single oral dose of an extract of *Indigofera spicata* seeds (Tables 19.5 and 19.6). Furthermore, subcutaneous injections of indospicine precipitate fat deposition and cytological abnormalities in the liver of mice. The fat accretion can be prevented by simultaneous injections of arginine but not of canavanine (see D'Mello, 1991). In experimental models, indospicine has been shown to inhibit both constitutive and inducible forms of nitric oxide synthase (NOS) (Pass *et al.*, 1996) as well as arginase (Hey *et al.*, 1997). As *I. spicata* is not a normal component of human diets, it appears that interest in indospicine primarily resides in its ability to alter the partition of arginine metabolism between urea and NO production (Hey *et al.*, 1997).

19.6.3.2 Analogues of sulphur-containing amino acids

Arguably, the most striking structural analogues are those of methionine, cystine and cystathionine. When selenium replaces the sulphur atom of these amino acids in certain leguminous and brassica plants (Table 19.5), a number of congeners are formed. Those of primary interest here are selenomethionine, *Se*-methylselenocysteine, and selenocystine. Other analogues of the sulphur-containing amino acids include *S*-methylcysteine sulphoxide, also found in brassica plants (Table 19.5), and djenkolic acid, occurring in the djenkol bean (D'Mello, 1991).

19.6.3.2.1 SELENOAMINO ACIDS. The selenoamino acids are undoubtedly toxic to animals (Cukierski *et al.*, 1989). For example, selenomethionine is as harmful as selenite or selenate in acute tests (Schrauzer, 2000), precipitating pancreatic acinar cell necrosis in rats (Hietaranta *et al.*, 1990) and histopathological aberrations in liver and kidneys of juvenile white sturgeon (Tashjian *et al.*, 2006). Nakamuro *et al.* (2000) maintain that disturbances in the methylation reactions of the detoxification pathway (Fig. 19.2) may precede manifestations of hepatotoxicity. Selenomethionine is readily incorporated into tissue proteins of

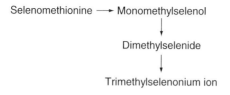

Fig. 19.2. Metabolism of selenomethionine, *S*-methylcysteine sulphoxide (in the plant) and hypoglycin A. (See text for further details and references.)

animals (Schrauzer, 2000), but the balance between synthetic and detoxification pathways is dependent upon methionine status. At sub-optimal intakes of methionine, selenomethionine is directed towards tissue protein incorporation. With adequate intakes of methionine, the Se analogue follows the pathway shown in Fig. 19.2. According to Schrauzer (2000), release of selenomethionine from body proteins by catabolic processes during illness should not result in toxicity, as a steady state is established which prevents the uncontrolled accumulation of Se.

19.6.3.2.2 S-METHYLCYSTEINE SULPHOXIDE. The deleterious effects of S-methylcysteine sulphoxide (SMCO) in ruminant animals fed mainly or solely on brassica forage are well recognized (see D'Mello, 1991). The condition haemolytic anaemia is precipitated by the synthesis of a reactive derivative during rumen fermentation by bacteria. In the plant, SMCO co-occurs with its metabolite, methyl methane thiosulphinate (Fig. 19.2). At doses of 0.5 and 1.0 mmol kg^{-1}, this metabolite was observed to induce severe toxicity in mice (Marks et al., 1993). There is no evidence that SMCO or methyl methane thiosulphinate exerts any adverse effects in humans consuming high levels of brassica vegetables.

19.6.3.3 Mimosine

Mimosine, present in *Leucaena leucocephala* (Table 19.5) is widely regarded as a structural analogue of tyrosine and its neurotransmitter derivatives, dopamine and norepinephrine. The biochemical or physiological evidence for such an assumption has yet to emerge. The extensive deleterious consequences of mimosine intake appear to be unrelated to any structural properties and include disruption of reproductive processes, teratogenic effects, and loss of hair. Similar reactions may be observed on feeding the seeds or foliage of *L. leucocephala* to laboratory animals (Table 19.6). The leaves, pods, and seeds of this legume are widely used in Central America, Indonesia, and Thailand to prepare a soup. Anecdotal evidence (Table 19.7) indicates that loss of hair is a frequent outcome among those individuals who regularly consume this broth. As will be elaborated later, current interest in mimosine has shifted to its role as an inhibitor of DNA replication and cell cycle progression (Dong and Zhang, 2003; Perry et al., 2005).

19.6.3.4 Neurotoxic amino acids

A number of neurotoxic amino acids occur in plants of economic importance (Table 19.5). β-N-Oxalylamino-L-alanine (BOAA) is a common constituent of *Lathyrus sativus*, while β-cyanoalanine and α,γ-diaminobutyric acid are components of *Vicia sativa* and *Lathyrus sylvestris*, respectively. The three amino acids are often referred to collectively as the neurolathyrogens. The structural homology of the lathyrogenic amino acids has been emphasized by D'Mello (1991). Another neurotoxic amino acid, β-N-methylamino-L-alanine (BMAA), occurs in the seed of *Cycas circinalis*.

19.6.3.4.1 β-N-OXALYLAMINO-L-ALANINE. There is overwhelming evidence that BOAA is one of the most potent neurotoxic amino acids found in plants. Neurological and biochemical lesions in animal models include tremors, convulsive seizures, and increased brain concentrations of ammonia and glutamine (Table 19.6; see also D'Mello, 1991). The precipitation of adverse effects is influenced by age and by physiological factors such as the induction of an acidotic state, but not by animal species. Other studies confirm that BOAA is a powerful glutamate receptor agonist (Andersson et al., 1997). Intake of BOAA via the grain of *L. sativus* has been positively associated with the incidence of neurolathyrism in humans living in India and in parts of China. This condition (Table 19.7) is characterized by muscular rigidity, weakness and paralysis of leg muscles. Neurolathyrism affects all ages and several members of the same family may be similarly affected (Spencer and Berman, 2003).

19.6.3.4.2 β-CYANOALANINE. The neurotoxicity of β-cyanoalanine is well established (Table 19.6) following systematic work with animal models (see D'Mello, 1991). Single doses of this amino acid are sufficient to provoke severe metabolic and neurological manifestations of toxicity.

Effects include cystathioninuria, hyperactivity, tremors, convulsions, rigidity, and death. Pyridoxal hydrochloride administration delays the onset of the neurological lesions and increases the dose required to induce adverse reactions. The role of β cyanoalanine in human neurolathyrism has been discounted as *V. sativa* generally only occurs as a contaminant of other legume grains.

19.6.3.4.3 α,γ-DIAMINOBUTYRIC ACID. Toxicological investigations with α,γ-diaminobutyric acid reveal increased susceptibility of mammals relative to avian species (D'Mello, 1991). Effects in the rat include upper extremity tremors, convulsions, and death. Biochemical changes may also occur, including increased ammonia concentrations in blood and brain, elevated glutamine levels in brain, and inhibition of ornithine carbamoyltransferase with reduced urea production. Human exposure to α,γ-diaminobutyric acid is limited as *L. sylvestris* is not a normal dietary component.

19.6.3.4.4 β-N-METHYLAMINO-L-ALANINE. Following extensive research, BMAA has been designated as a potent glutamate receptor agonist (Table 19.6; Andersson *et al.*, 1997) and, controversially, has been implicated in a specific neurodegenerative disorder in humans (Table 19.7). In a mouse model, BMAA induced neuronal cell death *in vivo* (Santucci *et al.*, 2009) while in dissociated rat brain cells, the amino acid caused an elevation in intracellular Ca levels (Brownson *et al.*, 2002). Using dissociated mixed spinal cord cultures, Rao *et al.* (2006) observed that pure BMAA selectively induced motor neuron loss via AMPA/kainate receptor activation, which was replicated with the use of cycad seed extracts. Spencer and Berman (2003) discounted any link between cycad-derived BMAA and the incidence of amyotrophic lateral sclerosis/Parkinsonism dementia complex (ALS/PDC) in Chamorro communities of Guam (Table 19.7). Instead, the co-occurring glycoside cycasin, in its aglycone form, was implicated in this condition. Others had previously concluded that processed cycad flour, as prepared by the Chamorros, contained extremely low levels of BMAA to account for the occurrence of ALS/PDC (Duncan *et al.*, 1990). However, contemporary views are that BMAA may well be the causative agent. Murch *et al.* (2004) found the amino acid in free form in 83% of ALS/PDC patients and in protein-bound form in 100% of these individuals. Both forms were also found in two Canadians who had died of progressive neurodegenerative disease. BMAA is now thought to be more ubiquitous, being a product of all cyanobacteria which are universally distributed in terrestrial, freshwater, and marine environments (see Santucci *et al.*, 2009). Thus, the amino acid can be biomagnified within the ecosystem and accumulate in the food chain. Furthermore, BMAA concentrations in the protein fraction of cycad seeds have hitherto been underestimated. In addition, evidence demonstrating similar efficacy of cycad seed extracts compared with the pure form of BMAA in precipitating motor neuron injury is consistent with the hypothesis that BMAA exerts a major role in the aetiology of ALS/PDC (Rao *et al.*, 2006). Nevertheless, it is still possible that BMAA and the aglycone of cycasin may act additively, synergistically or in a potentiating mode to precipitate ALS/PDC in Chamorro communities.

19.6.3.5 Hypoglycin A

The fruit of the ackee tree (*Blighia sapida*) is the source of hypoglycin A (Table 19.5) and its glutamyl derivative, hypoglycin B. In animal models, hypoglycin A induces fetal malformations and inhibits gluconeogenesis (Table 19.6). Research continues on the toxicology of hypoglycin A. For example, Blake *et al.* (2006) suggested that the form in which the amino acid is administered to rats could affect outcome in dose-response investigations, and concluded that for the purpose of risk assessment, hypoglycin A should be incorporated within the matrix of the fruit.

In the West Indies, consumption of the arils and seed of unripe fruits is associated with violent vomiting, convulsions, coma and mortality (Table 19.7; see also Spencer and Berman, 2003). Incidence of this 'vomiting sickness' tends to be familial, affecting undernourished children during periods of scarcity of mature fruits.

19.6.3.6 Mechanisms

There is overwhelming evidence to indicate that the adverse effects of non-protein amino acids are mediated via diverse mechanisms (Table 19.8). This polymorphism is observed individually and collectively for most of the non-protein amino acids present in plants. In addition, a number of structural analogues share common mechanisms. The following account represents an updated version of comprehensive reviews by D'Mello (1991), D'Mello (2003) and Spencer and Berman (2003).

19.6.3.6.1 ARGININE ANALOGUES. There are compelling arguments to support the hypothesis that the adverse effects of arginine

Table 19.8. Diverse mechanisms and reactions underlying the adverse effects of non-protein amino acids. Biochemical changes observed in animal models and/or humans. (See text for further details and references.)

Amino acid	Biochemical changes	Outcome/comments
Canavanine	Enhanced arginase activity	Increased arginine catabolism
	Reduced activity of ornithine decarboxylase following synthesis of canaline	Depressed polyamine synthesis
	Competition with lysine and arginine for transport	Reduced cellular levels of lysine and arginine
	Inhibition of transamidinase activity	Suppression of creatine synthesis
	Synthesis of aberrant proteins	Enhanced protein turnover[a]
	Inhibition of NO synthesis	Impaired immunocompetence[a]
	Depression of intracellular reduced glutathione	Effect unrelated to inhibition of NO synthesis
Homoarginine	Competition with lysine and arginine for transport	Reduced brain lysine levels; modulation of NO synthesis
Indospicine	Competitive inhibition of arginase	Hepatotoxicity
	Inhibition of amino acylation of arginine	Protein synthesis impaired
	Disruption of DNA synthesis (*in vitro* data)	Substantial reversal by increasing arginine supply
	NOS inhibitor	Diverse physiological effects
Selenoamino acids	Replacement of sulphur amino acids in protein synthesis	Reduced functional properties[a]
	Competition with sulphur amino acids for transport	Impaired intestinal absorption of sulphur amino acids
	Suppression of selenium methylation	Hepatotoxicity
S-Methylcysteine sulphoxide	Synthesis of reactive metabolites	Inactivation of key proteins; endocrine stimulation
Mimosine	Complex formation with pyridoxal phosphate	Cystathioninuria
	Inhibition of DNA replication	Reduced keratin synthesis[a]
β-N-Oxalylamino-L-alanine	Potent glutamate receptor agonist	Neurotoxicity
β-Cyanoalanine	Complex formation with pyridoxal phosphate	Cystathioninuria
α,γ-Diaminobutyric acid	Inhibition of ornithine carbamoyltransferase	Liver dysfunction; brain lesions
β-N-Methylamino-L-alanine	Potent glutamate receptor agonist	Neurotoxicity
Hypoglycin A	Synthesis of methylene cyclopropylacetyl-coenzyme A	Hypoglycaemia; organic acidaemia

[a]Speculative.

analogues are mediated via diverse and complex mechanisms (Table 19.8). The major route of canavanine metabolism in mammals follows the urea cycle, where the amino acid undergoes arginase-induced hydrolysis to canaline and urea (Fig. 19.1). Canavanine administration elicits striking increases in serum and urinary concentrations of ornithine. This pathway should, therefore, provide a mechanism for at least partial detoxification of canavanine. However, canaline forms a covalent complex with pyridoxal phosphate, thereby inhibiting the activities of enzymes dependent upon this cofactor. One such enzyme is ornithine decarboxylase, and its inhibition by canaline would account for the substantial accumulation of ornithine in body fluids. Ornithine decarboxylase is a key enzyme in the synthesis of specific polyamines required for regulation of cell growth and differentiation. Inhibition of polyamine synthesis by canaline thus provides an important focal point for the action of canavanine (Bence et al., 2002). Canavanine may also act by competing with lysine and arginine for transport across cell membranes. Other studies suggest that canavanine may, like lysine, act by inhibiting transamidinase activity, thus reducing creatine synthesis. It is widely recognized that canavanine can replace arginine during protein synthesis, resulting in the formation of aberrant macromolecules with modified functional properties. Thus in rats, canavanine is incorporated into liver enzymes and into brain components, yielding proteins of reduced activity. However, other studies with rats show negligible rates of canavanine incorporation into tissue proteins. D'Mello (1991) suggested that canavanyl proteins may be degraded as rapidly as they are formed. Any cycle of synthesis and degradation of these proteins might well result in increased protein turnover rates. Arguably, the most interesting biochemical feature to emerge is the inhibition of constitutive and inducible forms of NOS by canavanine (Pass et al., 1996; Rios-Santos et al., 2007). The consequences of this effect on essential physiological processes have yet to be elucidated, but will probably impact adversely on signalling, immunocompetence, and cardiovascular function. Finally, canavanine may act in glial cells by decreasing levels of reduced glutathione, an effect not related to inhibition of NOS (Riganti et al., 2003).

Current indications are that homoarginine competes with lysine for transport across the blood–brain barrier (O'Kane et al., 2006). In the work of Zinnanti et al. (2007), for example, brain lysine concentrations were reduced by 50%. In the perfused rat kidney, it has been shown that homoarginine can modulate NO production by altering cellular arginine transport via y^+ and y^+ L mechanisms (Kakoki et al., 2006).

Indospicine operates via at least four mechanisms. It acts as a competitive inhibitor of arginase (Hey et al., 1997), a property which accounts for the precipitation of hepatotoxicity in mammals owing to the critical role of this enzyme in the elimination of nitrogen in the urea cycle. Furthermore, indospicine strongly inhibits aminoacylation of arginine, whereas charging of leucine remains unaffected. Incorporation of arginine into proteins is thereby impaired. Other evidence suggests that DNA synthesis is inhibited by indospicine and that this effect may be substantially reversed by increasing arginine supply. Indospicine is another inhibitor of constitutive and inducible forms of NOS, a property it shares with canavanine (Pass et al., 1996). Thus indospicine has the capacity to alter the pathway of arginine utilization depending upon the cellular status of inducible NOS (Hey et al., 1997).

19.6.3.6.2 ANALOGUES OF THE SULPHUR-CONTAINING AMINO ACIDS. Three types of reactions have been associated with the selenoamino acids (Table 19.8):

1. replacement of sulphur amino acids in protein synthesis;
2. competition with sulphur amino acids for transport; and
3. suppression of selenium methylation.

Schrauzer (2000) suggested that substitution of methionine by its Se analogue does not significantly alter protein structure, but the functional properties may be affected if the replacement occurs near an active site. The release of Se stored in body proteins during illness is not considered to result in adverse effects, as no mechanism exists for the selective release of Se-methionine during degradative processes (Schrauzer, 2000). However, disturbances in the methylation pathway (Fig. 19.2) may lead to manifestation of selenosis (Nakamuro *et al.*, 2000).

In ruminant animals, toxicity of SMCO arises after its metabolism to a reactive metabolite (Table 19.8). In brassica vegetables, SMCO co-exists with its metabolite, methyl methane thiosulphinate (Fig. 19.2). At relatively high doses (0.5 and 1.0 mmol kg^{-1} bodyweight), this metabolite precipitated severe acute toxicity in mice (Marks *et al.*, 1993). SMCO itself is considered to be safe for humans; indeed, it may confer beneficial effects, as reported below.

19.6.3.6.3   MIMOSINE. The two features of mimosine commonly associated with its adverse effects are complex formation with pyridoxal phosphate, and inhibition of DNA replication (Table 19.8). Lin *et al.* (1996) noted that mimosine is an extremely effective inhibitor of DNA replication, and specifically indicated that it targets serine hydroxymethyltransferase, involved in the penultimate step of thymidylate biosynthesis. Perry *et al.* (2005) concluded that mimosine attenuates serine hydroxymethyltransferase transcription by chelating Zn, and considered the implications for inhibition of DNA replication. Other relevant studies include the effect of mimosine in cell cycle progression (Kulp and Vulliet, 1996; Dong and Zhang, 2003) and its role in the induction of apoptosis (Hallak *et al.*, 2008).

19.6.3.6.4   NEUROTOXIC AMINO ACIDS. Of the four neurotoxic amino acids listed in Table 19.8, two (BOAA and BMAA) act as potent glutamate receptor agonists (Andersson *et al.*, 1997). Brownson *et al.* (2002) suggest the involvement of a product of BMAA and CO_2 which mimics the structure of other excitatory amino acids, such as glutamate, in its mechanism of toxicity. Rao *et al.* (2006) demonstrated the capacity of BMAA to selectively damage motor neurons via AMPA/kainate receptor activation.

In the case of β-cyanoalanine, complex formation with pyridoxal phosphate appears to be the major mechanism of action. With α,γ-diaminobutyric acid, inhibition of ornithine carbamoyltransferase induces primary liver dysfunction accompanied by secondary brain lesions in mammals, while avian models are unaffected by this neurotoxin (D'Mello, 1991).

19.6.3.6.5   HYPOGLYCIN A. According to Spencer and Berman (2003), hypoglycin A metabolism (Fig. 19.2) results in inhibition of fatty acid transport, acyl-CoA dehydrogenases, and neoglucogenesis. Tanaka (2005) showed that glucose-6-phosphatase activity is also impaired. The resulting hypoglycaemia is a characteristic feature of hypoglycin A toxicity (Table 19.8).

19.6.3.6.6   UNDERLYING THEMES. A number of general rules may be formulated in the light of the evidence presented above. Urea cycle enzymes appear to be an important focal point for the action of at least three amino acids (Table 19.8). Canavanine enhances and indospicine inhibits arginase activity. In mammals, the effect of canavanine is observed after synthesis of canaline, which then precipitates the adverse effect, but the action of indospicine is more direct due to competitive inhibition of arginase, required for the proper functioning of the urea cycle. The inhibition of ornithine carbamoyltransferase by α,γ-diaminobutyric acid is also of significance in mammals due to disruption of the urea cycle.

Another common theme relates to the modulation of NO production by canavanine, homoarginine, and indospicine (Table 19.8), while competition during cellular amino acid transport is a feature of the individual actions of canavanine, homoarginine, and the selenoamino acids.

Despite their diverse nature, a number of non-protein amino acids, including canaline, mimosine, and β-cyanoalanine form complexes with pyridoxal phosphate and are thus associated with inhibition of certain aminotransferases and decarboxylases. The three amino acids also inhibit cystathionase, a feature which accounts for the cystathioninuria observed in rats administered with mimosine or with β-cyanoalanine (Table 19.8).

19.7 Amino Acid Toxicity

In the conventional classification of adverse effects, 'amino acid toxicity' has always represented a somewhat heterogeneous cluster, based on nutritional assessments of the most toxic individual amino acid. Disproportionate levels have been employed with the additional aim of discerning unique effects (see Benevenga and Steele, 1984 and D'Mello, 2003). Results have remained largely within the academic domain with methionine emerging as the most toxic IAA. A defining issue for this category, however, is that there is no simple antidote for reversing the ensuing adverse effects (Table 19.1). However, in human nutrition and health, the study of amino acid toxicity is, arguably, as important as that of imbalances or antagonisms. A number of examples are relevant in this context, including glutamate, homocysteine, modified lysine residues and phenylalanine. These topics are summarized below but considered more comprehensively in specified chapters of this volume.

19.7.1 Glutamate

Glutamate provides a prime example of investigations in amino acid toxicity that impact on human nutrition and health. Interest has arisen from its use as an additive and its role as an important excitatory neurotransmitter. The disquiet over the use of monosodium glutamate (MSG) in foods continues despite the conclusions of a consensus meeting indicating that the amino acid is 'harmless for the whole population' (Beyreuther et al., 2007). Indeed, it was suggested that glutamate salts may improve appetite in particular circumstances where such an effect is desirable, e.g. geriatric nutrition. However, others have questioned their use on the basis that hypothalamic regulation of appetite may be damaged (Hermanussen et al., 2006). Earlier evidence linking MSG to 'Chinese restaurant syndrome' has been adequately reviewed by Simon and Ishiwata (2003). Nevertheless, the 'umami' flavour of this additive continues to be the subject of research. McCabe and Rolls (2007) presented some elegant results based on functional brain imaging, and a comprehensive review appears in Chapter 20 of this volume.

Glutamate is also the principal excitatory neurotransmitter in the mammalian central nervous system. Lipton and Rosenberg (1994) stated that in several neurodegenerative disorders, injury to neurons may be caused, at least in part, by excessive activity of receptors for excitatory amino acids. The title of their paper, 'Excitatory amino acids as a final common pathway for neurologic disorders' provides a succinct analysis of emerging views concerning glutamate in particular (Pitt et al., 2000; Sarchielli et al., 2003). Thus, the concept of 'excitotoxicity' as a significant subset in the classification of adverse effects of amino acids is now firmly established. Further consideration of the pivotal role of excitatory amino acids in neurodegenerative disorders appears in Chapter 25.

19.7.2 Homocysteine

Homocysteine is considered to be an independent risk factor for cardiovascular disease, and recently Wagner and Koury (2007) questioned whether S-adenosylhomocysteine might be a better indicator for this disorder. Although there is no generally accepted mechanism for the pathophysiology involved, Wagner and Koury (2007) proceeded to consider various factors for the 'toxic action' of homocysteine. Hyperhomocysteinaemia has also been associated as an independent risk factor for cognitive impairment (Kim et al., 2007). A full review of factors affecting homocysteine status and health risks is presented in Chapter 21.

19.7.3 Modified lysine residues

As stated earlier in this chapter, amino acids may participate in the post-translational modification of proteins *in vivo* yielding AGE. Much information is available on the carboxymethyl and carboxyethyl residues of lysine in AGE and on the implications of these proteins in cardiovascular disease (Hartog *et al.*, 2007), acute lung injury (Calfee, 2008), renal dysfunction in diabetic patients (Lieuw-A-Fa *et al.*, 2004) and intestinal inflammation (Andrassy *et al.*, 2006). In addition, high dietary protein regimes may precipitate adverse reactions by increasing the AGE burden (Uribarri and Tuttle, 2006). These and related issues are of sufficient importance to merit detailed consideration (Chapter 22).

19.7.4 Phenylalanine

Inborn errors of amino acid metabolism may be regarded as manifestations of toxic reactions. Phenylketonuria (PKU) represents the classical and most significant example of such a genetic disorder, with detrimental effects arising from accumulation of phenylalanine and other catabolic intermediates in affected subjects. Issues such as the molecular basis of PKU, maternal influence, diet and compliance, and screening are under regular review. Clinical presentation and novel strategies relevant to this condition are discussed in Chapter 23.

19.8 Potential Applications

19.8.1 Neuropsychological investigations

The imposition of dietary amino acid imbalance is now increasingly and deliberately employed as a technique to investigate psychiatric disorders in humans. For example, Stadler *et al.* (2007) reported the results of a study on the effects of rapid tryptophan depletion on laboratory-provoked aggression in children with attention deficit/hyperactivity disorder (ADHD). Porter *et al.* (2007) used a similar technique to examine the effects of tryptophan depletion in patients recovered from depression, while Norra *et al.* (2008) investigated effects on acoustic startle response in females. In all cases, acute tryptophan depletion was induced by the administration of a drink or a mixture rich in IAA but devoid of tryptophan. This technique thus conforms with the classical method of precipitating amino acid imbalance as described earlier (Tables 19.1 and 19.2). Peripheral plasma tryptophan levels may fall by up to 80% within 5–7 hours (Porter *et al.*, 2007). Under these conditions, tissue and circulating levels of serotonin also decline and provide a metabolic basis for psychiatric investigations. Stadler *et al.* (2007) observed that there is an inverse relationship between serotonin and aggression in children with ADHD. Tryptophan depletion is reviewed in greater depth in Chapter 24. Acute tyrosine depletion has also been used in a similar context, with the aim of reducing metabolic pools of dopamine. In this instance, amino acid mixtures devoid of tyrosine and phenylalanine are provided in a drink. As before, this is another example of the imposition of an imbalance in the classical sense. In examining the effects of tyrosine depletion in normal healthy volunteers, McLean *et al.* (2004) considered the implications for unipolar depression, while Ellis *et al.* (2005) used a similar technique to investigate effects on working memory performance.

The procedure and effects are short term, but it is salutary to recall that in laboratory models, imposition of an imbalance is attended by unexpected and profound alterations in diet selection (see above). If similar effects occur in humans during amino acid depletion, then it is reasonable to enquire whether the responses observed in psychiatric investigations can be isolated from other underlying aspects of behaviour associated with imbalance.

19.8.2 Therapeutic aspects

Despite the negative attributes presented in this chapter, there is increasing evidence that imbalances and non-protein amino acids may be used for clinical benefit. The therapeutic potential of amino acid imbalance is presented in Table 19.9, which represents a selection of anti-cancer studies with animal or *in vitro* models and one clinical investigation with septic patients. An unmistakable feature is the use of BCAA deprivation in the quest

Table 19.9. Therapeutic potential of amino acid imbalance. (A selection of anti-cancer studies with animal or *in vitro* models and one clinical investigation with septic patients.)

Title of study	Reference
Clinical study of amino acid imbalance as an adjunct to cancer therapy	Goseki *et al.* (1982)
Anti-cancer therapy with valine-depleted amino acid imbalance solution	Nishihira *et al.* (1988)
Anti-cancer therapy with amino acid imbalance	Komatsu *et al.* (2001)
Effect of complex amino acid imbalance on growth of tumors in tumor-bearing rats	He *et al.* (2003)
Branched-chain amino acid imbalance selectively inhibits growth of gastric carcinoma cells *in vitro*	Sun *et al.* (2003)
Investigations of branched-chain amino acids and their metabolites in animal models of cancer	Baracos and Mackenzie (2006)
Parenteral administration of different amounts of branch-chain amino acids in septic patients: clinical and metabolic aspects	Garcia-de-Lorenzo *et al.* (1997)

for adjuncts to cancer therapy. It is clear that research has proceeded with the opposing objectives of restricting tumour growth but providing sufficient BCAA to replenish host tissue losses. Nishihira *et al.* (1988) reported that valine depletion elicited the most significant inhibition of hepatoma and mammary tumours in a rat model, and concluded that this treatment is a promising tool in cancer therapy. He *et al.* (2003) further showed that simultaneous omission of valine and methionine was more effective than either amino acid alone in reducing growth of tumours in rats. Sun *et al.* (2003) confirmed the efficacy of BCAA imbalance in selectively suppressing growth of gastric carcinoma cells *in vitro*. The role of amino acid imbalance in cancer therapy awaits further elucidation and evaluation in clinical trials.

Depressed BCAA to aromatic amino acid ratios appears to be a characteristic feature of septic encephalopathy and chronic liver disease (Table 19.4). It is logical to expect that BCAA supplementation might be beneficial in these conditions. The data of Garcia-de-Lorenzo *et al.* (1997) suggest that formulas rich in BCAA elicit ameliorative effects in septic patients.

The potential scope for specific non-protein amino acids in cancer therapy (Table 19.10) appears to be more promising than that for imbalance. Canavanine, *Se*-methylselenocysteine, *Se*-allylselenocysteine, selenomethionine, SMCO, mimosine and selected congeners have been tested in animal and *in vitro* models with varying degrees of efficacy. For example, NaPhuket *et al.* (1998) reported that several ester derivatives of canavanine were markedly more effective than the parent compound in suppressing the growth of cultured pancreatic carcinoma cells, whereas analogues based on modification of carbon chain length or of the terminal functional group were less successful. More substantive evidence is available for the selenoamino acids. Thus, Whanger (2002) concluded that *Se*-methylselenocysteine was most effective against mammary tumours, while Rustum *et al.* (2004) reported that this amino acid was highly effective in potentiating the efficiency of anti-cancer drugs and in protecting against drug-induced toxicity. Indeed, Azrak *et al.* (2007) suggested that the increased therapeutic efficacy of the anti-cancer drug, irinotecan, when in combination with methylselenocysteine, was dependent upon the dose of the amino acid. While there is good evidence of the therapeutic potential of methylselenocysteine (see also El-Bayoumy and Sinha, 2004; and Rayman, 2005), it should be recalled that in the studies of Ip *et al.* (1999), *Se*-allylselenocysteine was more effective than a number of other selenoamino acids for chemoprevention of mammary cancer in a rat methylnitrosourea model. Limited work points to the potential therapeutic use of selenomethionine (Kumar *et al.*, 2005), but Wu *et al.* (2009) recommended a cautious approach to minimize cytotoxic effects of the amino acid as a supplement. Marks *et al.*

Table 19.10. Therapeutic potential of non-protein amino acids. (Selected studies with animal and *in vitro* models and supporting reviews.)

Amino acid	Examples of investigations/conclusions	Reference
Canavanine	Synthesis and structure-activity studies of some antitumor congeners of L-canavanine	NaPhuket *et al.* (1998)
	Effects of NO donors and NO synthase substrates for possible use in myopia prevention	Beauregard *et al.* (2001)
	The anti-proliferative and immunotoxic effects of L-canavanine and L-canaline	Bence *et al.* (2002)
Se-Methylselenocysteine	Effective against mammary tumorigenesis	Whanger (2002)
	Highly effective in potentiating efficacy of anti-cancer drugs and protecting against drug-induced toxicity	Rustum *et al.* (2004) and Azrak *et al.* (2007)
	Appraisal of evidence relating to selenocysteine and methyl selenol	Rayman (2005)
Se-Allylselenocysteine	More effective than other selenoamino acids for chemoprevention of mammary cancer	Ip *et al.* (1999)
Selenomethionine	Prevents degeneration induced by overexpression of wild-type human α-synuclein during differentiation of neuroblastoma cells	Kumar *et al.* (2005)
	Efficacy of selenomethionine on genome stability and cytotoxicity	Wu *et al.* (2009)
S-Methylcysteine sulphoxide	Efficacy of S-methylcysteine sulphoxide and its metabolite, methyl methane thiosulphinate, on mouse genotoxicity	Marks *et al.* (1993)
Mimosine	Mimosine blocks cell cycle progression in asynchronous human breast cancer cells	Kulp and Vulliet (1996)
	Mimosine attenuates serine hydroxymethyltransferase transcription	Perry *et al.* (2005)
	Mimosine-induced apoptosis: molecular mechanism	Hallak *et al.* (2008)

(1993) examined the efficacy of SMCO and its metabolite, methyl methane thiosulphinate, on mouse genotoxicity, and concluded that these two organosulphur compounds may contribute to the anti-carcinogenic properties of brassica vegetables. However, epidemiological evidence only supports the case for prevention of gastric and lung cancers through consumption of these vegetables (Kim and Park, 2009). Finally, interest in mimosine as a potential anti-cancer agent is typified by three investigations cited in Table 19.10. It is well known that mimosine blocks cell cycle progression and the report of Kulp and Vulliet (1996) with asynchronous human breast cancer cells is consistent with this particular property. The work of Dong and Zhang (2003) provides data illustrating part of the mechanism for this effect. Mimosine attenuates serine hydroxymethyltransferase transcription by chelating Zn, and Perry *et al.* (2005) consider the implications for inhibition of DNA replication, a well-recognized effect of this non-protein amino acid (Lin *et al.*, 1996). The third investigation relates to mimosine-induced apoptosis. A molecular mechanism has been proposed involving oxidative stress and mitochondrial activation, with both factors exerting functional roles in the induction of cell death (Hallak *et al.*, 2008).

19.9 Conclusions

The traditional categories of imbalance, antagonism and toxicity established in nutritional studies with experimental models constitute a satisfactory basis for classifying the adverse effects of amino acids in human subjects. However, two subdivisions, namely 'clinical amino acid imbalance' and 'excitotoxicity', have been introduced to more accurately incorporate current interpretations of deleterious reactions observed in humans.

The concept of clinical amino acid imbalance has been advanced here to accommodate the incidence of adverse ratios of groups of amino acids in specific disease conditions. In patients with septic encephalopathy or with chronic liver disease, plasma ratios of branched-chain to aromatic amino acids are consistently reduced.

Antagonistic effects of a wide range of plant non-protein amino acids have also been reviewed. β-N-Oxalylamino-L-alanine occurs in the grain of *L. sativus*, while β-N-methylamino-L-alanine is a constituent of the seed of the false sago palm. Both amino acids are potent glutamate receptor agonists implicated, respectively, in neurolathyrism and in amyotrophic lateral sclerosis and Parkinsonism-dementia. However, the aetiology of ALS/PDC remains contentious and may be associated with other underlying factors. On the other hand, there is universal agreement that hypoglycin A is the dominant agent causing vomiting sickness with hypoglycaemia in individuals consuming the unripe fruit of the ackee tree.

The issue of toxicity is currently of much greater significance in human health than it has been in nutritional investigations with animal models. A number of examples have been highlighted here, including glutamate, homocysteine, lysine adducts, and phenylalanine. The human health implications of these amino acids are considered more comprehensively in specified chapters of this volume. Interest in glutamate, in particular, has arisen due to its dual role as a food additive and as the pre-eminent excitatory amino acid implicated in neurodegenerative disorders (Chapter 25). Thus, the introduction of excitotoxicity as the second significant subdivision in the classification of adverse effects of amino acids is fully justified.

Notwithstanding the overall theme of negativity in this chapter it is, nevertheless, important not to overlook a number of potential applications for clinical research. For example, the imposition of dietary amino acid imbalance is now deliberately employed as a technique to investigate behavioural and psychiatric disorders in humans. In several studies, acute imbalance has been induced by the administration of a mixture rich in IAA but devoid of tryptophan. This technique thus conforms with the classical method of precipitating amino acid imbalance. Under these conditions, tissue and circulating levels of serotonin decline and provide a metabolic basis for psychiatric investigations. The results are considered in greater depth in Chapter 24 of this volume. The potential of amino acid imbalance in cancer therapy has also been the subject of a limited number of investigations. A consistent feature is the efficacy of BCAA-depleted amino acid mixtures in the inhibition of tumours in laboratory models. However, the potential scope for specific non-protein amino acids in cancer therapy appears to be more promising than that for imbalance. Varying degrees of efficacy have been reported with canavanine, *Se*-methylselenocysteine, *Se*-allylselenocysteine, selenomethionine, SMCO, mimosine and selected congeners and metabolites in studies involving animal and *in vitro* models. Of these amino acids, *Se*-methylselenocysteine was most effective against mammary tumours, with the capacity of potentiating the efficacy of anti-cancer agents and protecting against drug-induced toxicity. Thus the interpretation of adverse effects of amino acids, as presented in this chapter, transcends the original conceptual model to accommodate significant food safety and clinical issues.

References

Abebe, S. and Morris, T.R. (1990a) Note on the effects of protein concentration on responses to dietary lysine by chicks. *British Poultry Science* 31, 255–260.

Abebe, S. and Morris, T.R. (1990b) Effects of protein concentration on responses to dietary tryptophan by chicks. *British Poultry Science* 31, 267–272.

Althoff, P.H., Schifferdecker, E., Forster, H., Michels, B., Helm, E. and Schoffling, K. (1989) Imbalance of the amino acid pattern in patients with AIDS – special treatment with adapted amino acid solution? *International Conference on AIDS* 5, 218.

Andersson, H., Lindqvist, E. and Olsen, L. (1997) Plant-derived amino acids increase hippocampus BDNF, NGF, *c-fos* and *hsp 70* mRNAs. *Neuroreport* 8, 1813–1817.

Andrassy, M., Igwe, J., Volz, C., Neurath, M.F., Schleicher, E. and Bierhaus, A. (2006) Post-translationally modified proteins as mediators of sustained intestinal inflammation. *American Journal of Pathology* 169, 1223–1237.

Asatoor, A.M., Freedman, P.S., Gabriel, J.R., Milne, M.D., Roberts, J.T. and Willoughby, C.P. (1974) Amino acid imbalance in cystinuria. *Journal of Clinical Pathology* 27, 500–504.

Azrak, R.G., Cao, S., Durrani, F.A. and Rustum, Y.M. (2007) Efficacy of increasing the therapeutic index of irinotecan, plasma and tissue selenium concentrations is methylselenocysteine dose dependent. *Biochemical Pharmacology* 73, 1280–1287.

Baracos, V.E. and Mackenzie, M.L. (2006) Investigations of branched-chain amino acids and their metabolites in animal models of cancer. *Journal of Nutrition* 136, 237S–242S.

Basler, T., Meier-Hellmann, A. and Bredle, D. (2002) Amino acid imbalance early in septic encephalopathy. *Intensive Care Medicine* 28, 293–298.

Batterham, E.S. (1974) The effect of frequency of feeding on the utilization of free lysine by growing pigs. *British Journal of Nutrition* 31, 237–242.

Beauregard, C., Liu, Q. and Chiou, G.C.Y. (2001) Effects of NO donors and NO synthase substrates on ciliary muscle contracted by carbachol and endothelin for possible use in myopia prevention. *Journal of Ocular Pharmacology and Therapeutics* 17, 1–9.

Bence, A.K., Worthen, D.R., Adams, V.R. and Crooks, P.A. (2002) The antiproliferative and immunotoxic effects of L-canavanine and L-canaline *in vitro*. *Anticancer Drugs* 13, 313–320.

Benevenga, N.J. and Steele, R.D. (1984) Adverse effects of excessive consumption of amino acids. *Annual Review of Nutrition* 4, 157–181.

Benevenga, N.J., Harper, A.E. and Rogers, Q.R. (1968) Effects of an amino acid imbalance on the metabolism of the most limiting amino acid in the rat. *Journal of Nutrition* 95, 434–444.

Bernardini, P. and Fischer, J.E. (1982) Amino acid imbalance and hepatic encephalopathy. *Annual Review of Nutrition* 2, 419–454.

Beverly, J.L., Gietzen, D.W. and Rogers, Q.R. (1990a) Effect of the dietary limiting amino acid in the prepyriform cortex on food intake. *American Journal of Physiology* 259, R709–R715.

Beverly, J.L., Gietzen, D.W. and Rogers, Q.R. (1990b) Effect of the dietary limiting amino acid in the prepyriform cortex on meal patterns. *American Journal of Physiology* 259, R716–R723.

Beverly, J.L., Hrupka, B.J., Gietzen, D.W. and Rogers, Q.R. (1991a) Distribution of the dietary limiting amino acid injected into the prepyriform cortex. *American Journal of Physiology* 260, R525–R532.

Beverly, J.L., Gietzen, D.W. and Rogers, Q.R. (1991b) Threonine concentration in the prepyriform cortex has separate effects on dietary selection and intake of a threonine-imbalanced diet by rats. *Journal of Nutrition* 121, 1287–1292.

Beyreuther, K., Fernstrom, J.D., Grimm, P., Steinhart, H. and Walker, R. (2007) Consensus meeting: monosodium glutamate - an update. *European Journal of Clinical Nutrition* 61, 304–313.

Blake, O.A., Bennink, M.R. and Jackson, J.C. (2006) Ackee (*Blighia sapida*) hypoglycin A toxicity: dose response assessment in laboratory rats. *Food and Chemical Toxicology* 44, 207–213.

Brownson, D.M., Mabry, T.J. and Leslie, S.W. (2002) The cycad neurotoxic amino acid, beta-N-methylamino-L-alanine (BMAA), elevates intracellular calcium levels in dissociated rat brain cells. *Journal of Ethnopharmacology* 82, 159–167.

Calfee, C.S. (2008) Plasma receptor for advanced glycation end products and clinical outcomes in acute lung injury. *Thorax* 63, 1080–1089.

Calvert, C.C., Klasing, K.C. and Austic, R.E. (1982) Involvement of food intake and amino acid catabolism in the branched chain amino acid antagonism in chicks. *Journal of Nutrition* 112, 627–635.

Cascino, A., Cangiano, C., Rossi-Fanelli, F. and Capocaccia, L. (1978) Plasma amino acid imbalance in patients with liver disease. *Digestive Diseases and Sciences* 23, 591–598.

Cascino, A., Muscaritola, M., Cangiano, C., Mequid, M.M. and Rossi-Fanelli, F. (1995) Plasma amino acid imbalance in patients with lung and breast cancer. *Anticancer Research* 15, 507–510.

Cukierski, M.J., Willhite, C.C., Lasley, B.L., Cox, D.N. and Henderickx, A.G. (1989) 30-Day oral toxicity study of L-selenomethionine in female long-tailed macaques (*Macaca fascicularis*). *Toxicological Sciences* 13, 26–39.

Dancis, J., Hutzler, J., Ampola, M.G., Shih, V.E., Kirby, L.T. and Woody, N.C. (1983) The prognosis of lysinemia: an interim report. *American Journal of Human Genetics* 35, 438–442.

Degnan, B.A., Palmer, J.M., Robson, T., Jones, C.E.D., Mellor, G.D., Diamond, A.G., Kehoe, M.A. *et al.* (1998) Inhibition of human peripheral blood mononuclear cell proliferation by *Streptococcus pyogenes* cell extract is associated with arginine deiminase activity. *Infection and Immunity* 66, 3050–3058.

Dickerson, J.W.T. and Wiryanti, J. (1978) Pellagra and mental disturbance. *Proceedings of the Nutrition Society* 37, 167–171.

D'Mello, J.P.F. (1991) Toxic amino acids. In: D'Mello, J.P.F., Duffus, C.M. and Duffus, J.H. (eds) *Toxic Substances in Crop Plants*. The Royal Society of Chemistry, Cambridge, pp. 21–48.

D'Mello, J.P.F. (1994) Amino acid imbalances, antagonisms and toxicities. In: D'Mello, J.P.F. (ed.) *Amino Acids in Farm Animal Nutrition*. CAB International, Wallingford, UK, pp. 63–97.

D'Mello, J.P.F. (2003) Adverse effects of amino acids. In: D'Mello, J.P.F. (ed.) *Amino Acids in Animal Nutrition*. CAB International, Wallingford, UK, pp. 125–142.

D'Mello, J.P.F. and Lewis, D. (1970a) Amino acid interactions in chick nutrition. 1. The interrelationship between lysine and arginine. *British Poultry Science* 11, 299–311.

D'Mello, J.P.F. and Lewis, D. (1970b) Amino acid interactions in chick nutrition. 2. The interrelationship between leucine, isoleucine and valine. *British Poultry Science* 11, 313–323.

D'Mello, J.P.F. and Lewis, D. (1970c) Amino acid interactions in chick nutrition. 3. Interdependence in amino acid requirements. *British Poultry Science* 11, 367–385.

Dong, Z. and Zhang, J.-T. (2003) E1F3p170, a mediator of the mimosine effect on protein synthesis and cell cycle progression. *Molecular Biology of the Cell* 14, 3942–3951.

Duncan, M.W., Steele, J.C., Kopin, I.J. and Markey, S.P. (1990) 2-Amino-3-(methylamino)-propanoic acid (BMAA) in cycad flour. An unlikely cause of amyotrophic lateral sclerosis and parkinsonism-dementia of Guam. *Neurology* 40, 767.

Edmonds, M.S. and Baker, D.H. (1987). Failure of excess lysine to antagonise arginine in young pigs. *Journal of Nutrition* 117, 1396–1401.

El-Bayoumy, K. and Sinha, R. (2004) Mechanisms of mammary cancer chemoprevention by organoselenium compounds. *Mutation Research* 551, 181–197.

Ellis, K.A., Mehta, M.A., Wesnes, K.A., Armstrong, S. and Nathan, P.J. (2005) Combined D_1/D_2 receptor stimulation under conditions of dopamine depletion impairs spatial working memory performance in humans. *Psychopharmacology* 181, 771–780.

Garcia-de-Lorenzo, A., Ortiz-Leyba, C., Planas, M., Nunez, R., Aragon, C. and Jimenez, F. (1997) Parenteral administration of different amounts of branched-chain amino acids in septic patients: clinical and metabolic aspects. *Critical Care Medicine* 25, 418–424.

Gietzen, D.W., Leung, P.M.B. and Rogers, Q.R. (1986) Noradrenaline and amino acids in prepyriform cortex of rats fed imbalanced amino acid diets. *Physiology of Behaviour* 36, 1071–1080.

Gietzen, D.W., Erecius, L.F. and Rogers, Q.R. (1998) Neurochemical changes after imbalanced diets suggest a brain circuit mediating anorectic responses to amino acid deficiency in rats. *Journal of Nutrition* 128, 771–781.

Goseki, N., Onodera, T., Mori, S. and Menjo, M. (1982) Clinical study of amino acid imbalance as an adjunct to cancer therapy. *Nippon Gan Chiryo Gakkai Shi* 17, 1908–1916.

Hallak, M., Vazana, L., Shpilberg, O., Levy, I., Mazar, J. and Nathan, I. (2008) A molecular mechanism for mimosine-induced apoptosis involving oxidative stress and mitochondrial activation. *Apoptosis* 13, 147–155.

Harper, A.E. (1959) Amino acid balance and imbalance. *Journal of Nutrition* 68, 405–418.

Harper, A.E. (1964) Amino acid toxicities and imbalances. In: Munro, H.N. and Allison, J.B. (eds) *Mammalian Protein Metabolism*. Vol. II, Academic Press, New York, pp. 87–134.

Harper, A.E. and Rogers, Q.R. (1965) Amino acid imbalance. *Proceedings of the Nutrition Society* 24, 173–190.

Harper, A.E., Benevenga, N.J. and Wohlheuter, R.M. (1970) Effects of ingestion of disproportionate amounts of amino acids. *Physiological Reviews* 50, 428–558.

Harper, A.E., Miller, R.H. and Block, K.P. (1984) Branched-chain amino acid metabolism. *Annual Review of Nutrition* 4, 409–454.

Harrison, L.M. and D'Mello, J.P.F. (1986) Large neutral amino acids in the diet and neurotransmitter concentrations in the chick. *Proceedings of the Nutrition Society* 45, 72A.

Harrison, L.M.and D'Mello, J.P.F. (1987) Zinc deficiency, amino acid imbalance and brain catecholamine concentrations in the chick. *Proceedings of the Nutrition Society* 46, 58A.

Hartog, J.W.L., Voors, A.A., Schalkwijk, C.G., Bakker, S.J.L., Smit, A.J. and van Veldhuisen, D.J. (2007) Clinical and prognostic value of advanced glycation end-products in chronic heart failure. *European Heart Journal* 28, 2879–2885.

He, Y.-C., Wang, Y.-H., Cao, J., Chen, J.-W., Pan, D.-Y. and Zhou, Y.-K. (2003) Effect of complex amino acid imbalance on growth of tumor in tumor-bearing rats. *World Journal of Gastroenterology* 9, 2772–2775.

Henningsson, R. and Lundquist, I. (1998) Arginine-induced insulin release is decreased and glucagon increased in parallel with islet NO production. *American Journal of Physiology – Endocrinology and Metabolism* 275, E500–E506.

Hermanussen, M., Garcia, A.P., Salazar, V. and Tresguerres, J.A.F. (2006) Obesity, voracity and short stature; the impact of glutamate on the regulation of appetite. *European Journal of Clinical Nutrition* 60, 25–31.

Hey, C., Boucher, J.-L., Goff, V.-L., Ketterer, G., Wessler, I. and Racke, K. (1997) Inhibition of arginase in rat and rabbit alveolar macrophages by N_ω-hydroxy-D,L-indospicine: effects on L-arginine utilization by NO synthase. *British Journal of Pharmacology* 121, 395–400.

Hietaranta, A.J., Nevalainen, T.J., Aho, H.J., Hamalainen, O.M. and Suortamo, S.H. (1990) Pancreatic acinar cell necrosis with intact storage of digestive enzymes in selenomethionine-treated rats. *Virchows Archives of Cell Pathology* 58, 397–403.

Ip, C., Zhu, Z., Thompson H.J., Lisk, D. and Ganther, H.E. (1999) Chemoprevention of mammary cancer with *Se*-allylselenocysteine and other selenoamino acids in the rat. *Anticancer Research* 19, 2875–2880.

Jones, J.D., Wolters, R. and Burnett, P.C. (1966) Lysine-arginine-electrolyte relationships in the rat. *Journal of Nutrition* 89, 171–188.

Kakoki, M., Kim, H.-S., Arendshorst, W.J. and Mattson, D.L. (2004) L-Arginine uptake affects nitric oxide production and blood flow in the renal medulla. *American Journal of Physiology - Regulators, Integrative and Comparative Physiology* 287, R1478–R1485.

Kakoki, M., Kim, H.-S., Edgell, C.J., Maeda, N., Smithies, O. and Mattson, D.L. (2006) Amino acids as modulators of endothelium-derived nitric oxide. *American Journal of Physiology - Renal Physiology* 291, F297–F304.

Kawamura-Yasui, N., Kaito, M., Nakagawa, N., Fujita, N., Watanabe, S. and Adachi, Y. (1999) Evaluating responses to nutritional therapy using the branched-chain amino acid/tyrosine ratio in patients with chronic liver disease. *Journal of Clinical Laboratory Analysis* 13, 31–34.

Kim, J., Park, M.H., Kim, E., Han, C., Jo, S.A. and Jo, I. (2007) Plasma homocysteine is associated with the risk of mild cognitive impairment in an elderly Korean population. *Journal of Nutrition* 137, 2093–2097.

Kim, M.K. and Park, J.H. (2009) Cruciferous vegetable intake and the risk of human cancer: epidemiological evidence. *Proceedings of the Nutrition Society* 68, 103–110.

Kolvusalo, A.M., Teikari, T., Hockerstedt, K. and Isoniemi, H. (2008) Albumin dialysis has a favourable effect on amino acid profile in hepatic encephalopathy. *Metabolism and Brain Disease* 23, 387–398.

Komatsu, H., Doi, H., Satomi, S. and Nishihira, T. (2001) Anti-cancer therapy with amino acid imbalance. *Japanese Journal of Clinical Medicine* 59, 895–898.

Krishnaswamy, K. and Gopalan, C. (1971) Effect of isoleucine on skin and electroencephalogram in pellagra. *Lancet* 2, 1167–1169.

Kulp, K.S. and Vulliet, P.R. (1996) Mimosine blocks cell cycle progression by chelating iron in asynchronous human breast cancer cells. *Toxicology and Applied Pharmacology* 139, 356–364.

Kumar, B., Nahreini, P., Hanson, A.J., Prasad, J.E. and Prasad, K.N. (2005) Selenomethionine prevents degeneration induced by overexpression of wild-type human α-synuclein during differentiation of neuroblastoma cells. *Journal of the American College of Nutrition* 24, 516–523.

Kumta, U.S., Harper, A.E. and Elvehjem, C.A. (1958) Amino acid imbalance and nitrogen retention in adult rats. *Journal of Biological Chemistry* 233, 1505–1508.

Langer, S. and Fuller, M.F. (1994) The effect of excessive amounts of branched-chain amino acids on amino acid utilization in growing pigs. *Proceedings of the Nutrition Society* 53, 108A.

Langer, S. Scislowski, P.W.D., Brown, D.S., Dewey, P. and Fuller, M.F. (2000) Interactions among the branched-chain amino acids and their effects on methionine utilization in growing pigs: effects on plasma amino- and keto-acid concentrations and branched-chain keto-acid dehydrogenase activity. *British Journal of Nutrition* 83, 49–58.

Leibholz, J., Love, R.J., Mollah, Y. and Carter, R.R. (1986) The absorption of dietary L-lysine and extruded L-lysine in pigs. *Animal Feed Science and Technology* 15, 141–148.

Leung, P.M.B. and Rogers, Q.R. (1969) Food intake: regulation by plasma amino acid pattern. *Life Sciences* 8, 1–9.

Leung, P.M.B. and Rogers, Q.R. (1987) The effect of amino acids and protein on dietary choice. In: Kawamura, Y. and Kate, M.R. (eds) *Umami: A Basic Taste*. Marcel Dekker, New York, pp. 565–610.

Leung, P.M.B., Gietzen, D.W. and Rogers, Q.R. (1985) Alterations in the amino acid profile of prepyriform cortex from rats fed amino acid-imbalanced diets. *Federation Proceedings* 44, 1523.

Lieuw-A-Fa, M.L.M., van Hinsberg, V.W.M., Teerlink, T., Twisk, J., Stehouwer, C.D.A. and Schalkwijk, C.G. (2004) Increased levels of N^ε-(carboxymethyl)lysine and N^ε-(carboxyethyl)lysine in type 1 diabetic patients with impaired renal function: correlation with markers of endothelial dysfunction. *Nephrology, Dialysis and Transplantation* 19, 631–636.

Lin, H-B., Falchetto, R., Mosca, P.J., Hunt, D.F. and Hamlin, J.L. (1996) Mimosine targets serine hydroxymethyltransferase. *Journal of Biological Chemistry* 271, 2548–2556.

Lipton, S.A. and Rosenberg, P.A. (1994) Excitatory amino acids as a final common pathway for neurologic disorders. *New England Journal of Medicine* 330, 613–622.

Luiking, Y.C. and Deutz, N.E.P. (2007) Biomarkers of arginine and lysine excess. *Journal of Nutrition* 137, 1662S–1668S.

Marks, H.S., Anderson, J.A. and Stoewsand, G.S. (1993) Effect of *S*-methyl cysteine sulphoxide and its metabolite methyl methane thiosulphinate, both occurring naturally in brassica vegetables, on mouse genotoxicity. *Food and Chemical Toxicology* 31, 491–495.

McCabe, C. and Rolls, E.T. (2007) Umami: a delicious flavour formed by convergence of taste and olfactory pathways in the human brain. *European Journal of Neuroscience* 25, 1855–1864.

McLean, A., Rubinsztein, J.S., Robbins, T.W. and Sahakian, B.J. (2004) The effects of tyrosine depletion in normal healthy volunteers: implications for unipolar depression. *Psychopharmacology* 171, 286–297.

Monaco, F., Riccio, A., Durelli, L., Giordana, M.T. and Palmucci, L. (1975) Sporadic ulcerative mutilating acropathy with imbalance of free amino acids in the cerebrospinal fluid. *Journal of Neurology, Neurosurgery and Psychiatry* 38, 740–744.

Moughan, P.J. (1991) Towards an improved utilization of dietary amino acids by the growing pig. In: Haresign, W. and Cole, D.J.A. (eds) *Recent Advances in Animal Nutrition*. Butterworths, London, pp. 45–64.

Murch, S.J., Cox, P.A., Banack, S.A., Steele, J.C. and Sacks, O.W. (2004) Occurrence of β-N-methylamino-L-alanine (BMAA) in ALS/PDC patients from Guam. *Acta Neurologica Scandinavica* 110, 267–269.

Nakamura, T., Kawagoe, Y., Matsuda, T., Ebihara, I. and Koide, H. (2003) Effects of polymyxin B-immobilized fiber haemoperfusion on amino acid imbalance in septic encephalopathy. *Blood Purification* 21, 282–286.

Nakamuro, K., Okuno, T. and Hasegawa, T. (2000) Metabolism of selenoamino acids and contribution of selenium methylation to their toxicity. *Journal of Health Science* 46, 418–421.

NaPhuket, S.R., Trifonov, L.S., Crooks, P.A., Rosenthal, G.A., Freeman, J.W. and Strodel, W.E. (1998) Synthesis and structure-activity studies of some antitumor congeners of L-canavanine. *Drug Development Research* 40, 325–332.

Nishihira, T., Takagi, T., Kawarabayashi, Y., Izumi, U., Ohkuma, S., Koike, N., Toyoda, T. et al. (1988) Anti-cancer therapy with valine-depleted amino acid imbalance solution. *Tohoku Journal of Experimental Medicine* 156, 259–270.

Norra, C, Becker, S., Herpertz, S.C. and Kunert, H.J. (2008) Effects of experimental acute tryptophan depletion on acoustic startle response in females. *European Archives of Psychology and Clinical Neuroscience* 258, 1–9.

Oepen, G., Cramer, H., Bernasconi, R. and Martin, P. (1982) Huntington's disease - imbalance of free amino acids in the cerebrospinal fluid of patients and offspring at risk. *European Archives of Psychiatry and Clinical Neuroscience* 231, 131–140.

O'Kane, R.L., Vina, J.R., Simpson, I., Zaragoza, R., Mokashi, A. and Hawkins, R.A. (2006) Cationic amino acid transport across the blood-brain barrier is mediated exclusively by system y$^+$. *American Journal of Physiology - Endocrinology and Metabolism* 291, E412–E419.

Pant, K.C., Rogers, Q.R. and Harper, A.E. (1972) Growth and food intake of rats fed tryptophan-imbalanced diets with or without niacin. *Journal of Nutrition* 102, 117–130.

Papet, I., Breuille, D., Glomot, F., and Arnal, M. (1988a) Nutritional and metabolic effects of dietary leucine excess in preruminant lambs. *Journal of Nutrition* 118, 450–455.

Papet, I., Lezebot, N., Arnal, M. and Harper, A.E. (1988b) Influence of dietary leucine content on the activities of branched-chain amino acid aminotransferase (EC 2.6.1.42) and branched-chain α-keto acid dehydrogenase (EC 1.2.4.4) complex in tissues of preruminant lambs. *British Journal of Nutrition* 59, 475–483.

Pares, A., Cisneros, L., Salmeron, J.M., Caballeria, J. and Mas, A. (2009) Albumin dialysis improves hepatic encephalopathy and decreases circulating phenolic aromatic amino acids in patients with alcoholic hepatitis and severe liver failure. *Critical Care* 13, R8.

Partridge, I.G., Low, A.G. and Keal, H.D. (1985) A note on the effect of feeding frequency on nitrogen use in growing boars given diets with varying levels of free lysine. *Animal Production* 40, 375–377.

Pass, M.A., Arab, H., Pollitt, S. and Hegarty, M.P. (1996) Effects of the naturally occurring arginine analogues indospicine and canavanine on NO mediated functions in aortic endothelium and peritoneal macrophages. *Natural Toxins* 4, 135–140.

Peng, Y., Tews, J.K. and Harper, A.E. (1972) Amino acid imbalance, protein intake and changes in rat brain and plasma amino acids. *American Journal of Physiology* 222, 314–321.

Perry, C., Sastry, R., Nasrallah, I.M. and Stover, P.J. (2005) Mimosine attenuates serine hydroxymethyltransferase transcription by chelating zinc. Implications for inhibition of DNA replication. *Journal of Biological Chemistry* 280, 396–400.

Pitt, D., Werner, P. and Raine, C.S. (2000) Glutamate excitotoxicity in a model of multiple sclerosis. *Nature Medicine* 6, 67–70.

Porter, R.J., Gallagher, P. and O'Brien J.T. (2007) Effects of rapid tryptophan depletion on salivary cortisol in older people recovered from depression. *Journal of Psychopharmacology* 21, 71–75.

Rao, S.D., Banack, S.A., Cox, P.A. and Weiss, J.H. (2006) BMAA selectively injures motor neurons via AMPA/kainate receptor activation. *Experimental Neurology* 201, 244–252.

Rayman, M.P. (2005) Selenium in cancer prevention: a review of the evidence and mechanism of action. *Proceedings of the Nutrition Society* 64, 527–542.

Riganti, C., Aldieri, E., Bergandi, L., Miraglia, E. and Ghigo, D. (2003) Nitroarginine methyl ester and canavanine lower intracellular reduced glutathione. *Free Radical Biology and Medicine* 35, 1210–1216.

Rios-Santos, F., Alves-Filho, J.C., Spiller, F., Freitas, A., Soares, M.B.P., dos Santos, R.R., Teixeira, M.M. *et al.* (2007) Down-regulation in severe sepsis is mediated by inducible nitric oxide synthase-derived nitric oxide. *American Journal of Respiratory and Critical Care Medicine* 175, 490–497.

Rustum, Y.M., Cao, S., Durrani, F.A. and Fakih, M. (2004) *Se*-(methyl)selenocysteine (MSC) potentiates the antitumor activity of irinotecan against human xenografts and protects against drug induced toxicity. *Journal of Clinical Oncology* 22, 2068.

Sanahuja, J.C. and Harper, A.E. (1962) Effect of amino acid imbalance on food intake and preference. *American Journal of Physiology* 202, 165–170.

Santucci, S., Zsurger, N. and Chabry, J. (2009) β-N-methylamino-L-alanine induced *in vivo* retinal cell death. *Journal of Neurochemistry* 109, 819–825.

Sarchielli, P., Greco, L., Floridi, A. and Gallai, V. (2003) Excitatory amino acids and multiple sclerosis: evidence from cerebrospinal fluid. *Archives of Neurology* 60, 1082–1088.

Saudubray, J.-M. and Rabier, D. (2007) Biomarkers identified in inborn errors for lysine, arginine, and ornithine. *Journal of Nutrition* 137, 1669S–1672S.

Schrauzer, G.N. (2000) Selenomethionine: a review of its nutritional significance, metabolism and toxicity. *Journal of Nutrition* 130, 1653–1656.

Simon, R.A. and Ishiwata, H. (2003) Adverse reactions to food additives. In: D'Mello, J.P.F. (ed.) *Food Safety. Contaminants and Toxins.* CAB International, Wallingford, UK, pp. 235–270.

Spencer, P.S. and Berman, F. (2003) Plant toxins and human health. In: D'Mello, J.P.F. (ed.) *Food Safety. Contaminants and Toxins.* CAB International, Wallingford, UK, pp. 1–23.

Spielmann, J., Noatsch, A., Brandsch, C., Stangl, G.I. and Eder, K. (2008) Effects of various dietary arginine and lysine concentrations on plasma and liver cholesterol concentrations in rats. *Annals of Nutrition and Metabolism* 53, 223–233.

Stadler, C., Zepf, F.D., Demisch, L., Schmitt, M., Landgraf, M. and Poustka, F. (2007) Influence of rapid tryptophan depletion on laboratory-provoked agression in children with ADHD. *Neuropsychobiology* 56, 104–110.

Sun, X., Zhang, N., Li, K., Lu, M., Zhi, X., Jiang, X. and Shou, N. (2003) Branched-chain amino acid imbalance selectively inhibits growth of gastric carcinoma cells *in vitro*. *Nutrition Research* 23, 1279–1290.

Suzuki, K., Koizumi, K., Ichimura, H., Oka, S., Takada, H. and Kuwayama, H. (2007) Measurement of serum branched-chain amino acids to tyrosine ratio level is useful in a prediction of a change of serum albumin level in chronic liver disease. *Hepatology Research* 38, 267–272.

Takeda, M., Tachibana, H., Okuda, B. and Sugita, M. (1993) Two cases of hepatic encephalopathy associated with a high-intensity area in the basal ganglia on T1-weighted MR images. *Nippon Ronen Igakkai Zasshi* 30, 709–713.

Tanaka, K. (2005) Inhibition of gluconeogenesis by hypoglycin: alternate interpretations. *Hepatology* 7, 1377–1379.

Tashjian, D.H., Teh, S.J., Sogomonyan, A. and Hung, S.S.O. (2006) Bioaccumulation and chronic toxicity of dietary L-selenomethionine in juvenile white sturgeon (*Acipenser transmontanus*). *Aquatic Toxicology* 79, 401–409.

Tews, J.K., Kim, Y.W.L. and Harper, A.E. (1979) Induction of threonine imbalance by dispensable amino acids: relation to competition for amino acid transport into brain. *Journal of Nutrition* 109, 304–315.

Tews, J.K., Kim, Y.W.L. and Harper, A.E. (1980) Induction of threonine imbalance by dispensable amino acids: relationships between tissue amino acids and diet in rats. *Journal of Nutrition* 110, 394–408.

Tsubuku, S., Mochizuki, M., Mawatari, K., Smriqa, M. and Kimura, T. (2004) Thirteen-week oral toxicity study of L-lysine hydrochloride in rats. *International Journal of Toxicology* 23, 113–118.

Uribarri, J. and Tuttle, K.R. (2006) Advanced glycation end products and nephrotoxicity of high-protein diets. *Clinical Journal of the American Society of Nephrology* 1, 1293–1299.

Valtonen, P., Laitinen, T., Heiskanen, N., Vanninen, E., and Heinonen, S. (2008) Serum L-homoarginine concentration is elevated during normal pregnancy and is related to flow-mediated vasodilation. *Circulation Journal* 72, 1879–1884.

Vary, T.C. and Lynch, C.J. (2004) Biochemical approaches for nutritional support of skeletal muscle protein metabolism during sepsis. *Nutrition Research Reviews* 17, 77–88.

Wagner, C. and Koury, M.J. (2007) S-Adenosylhomocysteine - a better indicator of vascular disease than homocysteine? *American Journal of Clinical Nutrition* 86, 1581–1585.

Wang, T.C. and Fuller, M.F. (1989) The optimum dietary amino acid pattern for growth in pigs. 1. Experiments by amino acid deletion. *British Journal of Nutrition* 62, 77–89.

Whanger, P.D. (2002) Selenocompounds in plants and animals and their biological significance. *Journal of the American College of Nutrition* 21, 223–232.

Winje, M.E., Harper, A.E., Benton, D.A., Boldt, R.E. and Elvehjem, C.A. (1954) Effect of dietary amino acid balance on fat deposition in the livers of rats fed low protein diets. *Journal of Nutrition* 54, 155–166.

Woody, N.C. (1964) Hyperlysinemia. *American Journal of Diseases of Children* 108, 543–553.

Wu, J., Lyons, G.H., Graham, R.D. and Fenech, M.F. (2009) The effect of selenium, as selenomethionine, on genome stability and cytotoxicity in human lymphocytes measured using the cytokinesis-block micronucleus cytome assay. *Mutagenesis* 24, 225–232.

Yoshida, A., Leung, P.M.B., Rogers, Q.R. and Harper, A.E. (1966) Effects of amino acid imbalance on the fate of the limiting amino acid. *Journal of Nutrition* 89, 80–90.

Young, C.A. and Parsons, F.M. (1970) Plasma amino acid imbalance in patients with chronic renal failure on intermittent dialysis. *Clinica Chimica Acta* 27, 491–496.

Yuan, J.H., Davis, A.J. and Austic, R.E. (2000) Temporal response of hepatic threonine dehydrogenase in chickens to the initial consumption of a threonine-imbalanced diet. *Journal of Nutrition* 30, 2746–2752.

Zinnanti, W.J., Housman, C., O'Callaghan, J.P., Simpson, I., Goodman, S.I., Jacobs, R.E. and Cheng, K.C. (2007) Mechanism of age-dependent susceptibility and novel treatment strategy in glutaric acidemia type I. *Journal of Clinical Investigation* 117, 3258–3270.

20 The Umami Taste of Glutamate

X. Li*

GPCR Biology, Senomyx, Inc., San Diego, California, USA

20.1 Abstract

Umami, the savoury taste of L-glutamate, is one of the five basic taste qualities detected by humans. The umami taste receptor is a heteromeric complex of two class-C G protein-coupled receptors, T1R1 and T1R3. Breakthrough discoveries have been made in the molecular biology of the mammalian taste system since identification of the first taste receptors a decade ago. This chapter provides an overview of the molecular biology and physiology of umami taste, including the identification and characteristic of the umami receptor, the signal transduction pathway and the recent attempts to understand the neuronal representation of umami taste in the brain. Particular focus is given to umami synergy, a unique feature of umami taste.

20.2 Introduction

Protein is considered one of the basic nutrients. Amino acids serve as building blocks for proteins and can also be used as an energy source. It is essential for animals to detect and consume protein-rich food. The appetite for protein-rich food is mediated primarily by the gustatory system in humans.

Humans can detect at least five basic taste qualities, including sweet, umami, bitter, salty, and sour. Umami taste is the specific taste quality dedicated to detection of selective L-amino acids. This taste quality was discovered by Kikunae Ikeda (Ikeda, 1909), who named it 'umami', a Japanese word meaning 'delicious'. The closest English words for umami are 'savoury' or 'meaty'. The primary umami tastant is L-glutamate, one of the most abundant free amino acids in protein-rich food. Other umami tastants include L-aspartate and purinic ribonucleotides, such as inosine-5′-monophosphate (IMP) (Kodama, 1913) and guanosine-5′-monophosphate (GMP) (Kuninaka, 1960).

The most unique feature of umami taste is the synergy (Kuninaka, 1960) among its natural ligands: the mixture of umami-tasting amino acid with purinic ribonucleotide gives a much stronger umami taste than the sum of the either class of umami tastants alone. In fact, sub-milimolar concentrations of IMP or GMP, which elicit no umami taste on their own, can greatly potentiate the

---

* E-mail address: xiaodong.li@senomyx.com

umami taste of glutamate or aspartate. IMP and GMP are thus considered umami taste 'enhancers', and probably the only known natural enhancers of any G protein-coupled receptors (GPCR).

In contrast to other four taste qualities, umami taste is a subtle sensation not so easy to describe. There has been a long debate over the validity of umami as the fifth basic taste quality. In fact, the concept was not generally accepted until the umami taste receptor was identified.

20.3 The Taste Sensory System

Taste is mediated by a group of specialized chemosensory cells known as the taste receptor cells (TRC). Clusters of 50–100 taste cells form a taste bud (Fig. 20.1), an onion-shaped assembly distributed on the surface of the tongue and soft palate. The majority of taste buds on the tongue sit on raised protrusions of the tongue surface called papillae. There are three types of taste papillae present in the human tongue:

1. Fungiform papillae: as the name suggests, these are slightly mushroom-shaped if viewed in longitudinal section. They are present mostly at the tip of the tongue, as well as at the sides, and are innervated by the chorda tympani nerve.

2. Circumvallate papillae: most people only have about 10–14 of these papillae. Located at the back of the oral part of the tongue, they are arranged in a circular row just in front of the sulcus terminalis of the tongue. They are associated with ducts of Von Ebner's glands and are innervated by the glossopharyngeal nerve.

3. Foliate papillae: these are ridges and grooves towards the posterior part of the tongue, and are found on lateral margins; they are innervated by the chorda tympani nerve (anterior papillae) and glossopharyngeal nerve (posterior papillae).

The cluster of elongated TRC project microvillae to the apical surface and form the 'taste pore' at the top of the taste bud. Taste receptor proteins are concentrated on the taste pore and exposed to the oral cavity. This is where the tastant molecules come into contact with the receptor proteins and taste detection is initiated. Taste stimuli activate the taste receptors, which trigger their specific signal transduction pathways and lead

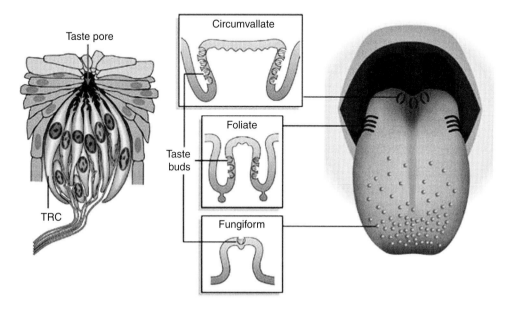

Fig. 20.1. Diagram of a human tongue, highlighting the structure of a single taste bud (left), the three different types of taste papillae (middle), and their corresponding topographic distribution (right). Reproduced with permission from Chandrashekar *et al.* (2006).

to activation of the TRC. The signal is relayed to the brain through either the chorda tympani or the glossopharyngeal nerves.

Cells in a taste bud can be categorized into three types based on their morphology (Fig. 20.2) (Murray, 1973; Finger, 2005):

1. Type I cells, sometimes called 'dark cells' extend lamellate processes around other types of taste cells and express glutamate–aspartate transporter (Lawton *et al.*, 2000). These features suggest a glial function for Type I cells, e.g. transmitter clearance and functional isolation of other taste cell types.
2. Type II taste cells have a characteristic large, round nucleus and express all of the elements of the taste transduction cascade for GPCR-mediated taste qualities (sweet, umami, and bitter) (Boughter *et al.*, 1997; Yang *et al.*, 2000b; Clapp *et al.*, 2001).
3. Type III cells are characterized by morphologically identifiable synaptic contacts with the gustatory nerve fibres and expression of the synaptic membrane protein SNAP25 (Yang *et al.*, 2000a), as well as the neural cell adhesion molecule (NCAM) (Nelson and Finger, 1993). The presence of a prominent synaptic contact implicates these cells in transmission of information to the nervous system.

The TRC can also be divided based on the taste quality they mediate. Each TRC expresses only a single type of taste receptor and can therefore only respond to the single specific taste quality, consequently being categorized as umami-, sweet-, bitter-, salty-, or sour-responding cells. There is no overlap among the five types of TRC (Chandrashekar *et al.*, 2006, 2010). This functional segregation of TRC is believed to be important for the brain to differentiate the taste qualities, as the cells are believed to be hard-wired to the brain (the labelled-line model) (Yarmolinsky *et al.*, 2009). The umami, sweet and bitter TRC belong to type II, while sour cells belong to type III.

20.4 The T1R Family of Taste Receptor

Multiple candidate receptors have been proposed for umami taste over the years. Only recently have molecular biology and mouse genetics studies demonstrated that the mammalian umami taste receptor is a heteromeric complex of T1R1/T1R3. There are three genes in the T1R family. T1R1 and T1R2 were identified in 1999 by sequencing a subtracted cDNA library derived from rat taste tissue (Hoon *et al.*, 1999), and T1R3 was identified in 2001 (Bachmanov *et al.*, 2001; Kitagawa *et al.*, 2001; Max *et al.*, 2001; Montmayeur *et al.*, 2001; Nelson *et al.*, 2001; Sainz *et al.*, 2001).

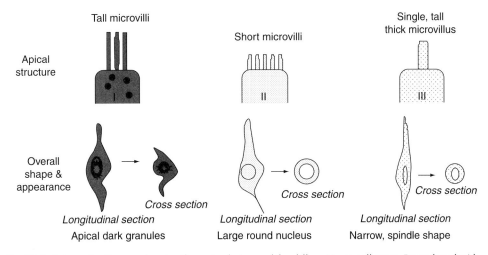

Fig. 20.2. Schematic diagram showing the major features of the different taste cell types. Reproduced with permission from Finger (2005).

In situ hybridization revealed selective expression of T1R in mouse taste tissue, with T1R1 more enriched in the fungiform taste buds and T1R2 in the circumvallate taste buds. T1R3 was also found to be selectively expressed in a subset of TRC. Although T1R1 and T1R2 are expressed in different cells, they are each coexpressed with T1R3 (Max *et al.*, 2001; Montmayeur *et al.*, 2001; Nelson *et al.*, 2001). Besides the T1R1/T1R3 and T1R2/T1R3 cells, a fraction of TRC expresses T1R3 only.

An important clue about the function of T1R came from the genetic locus of T1R3. Importantly, mouse T1R3 was mapped to a genomic interval containing *Sac* (Fuller, 1974), a locus that influences sweet-taste sensitivity in mice. Different inbred strains of mice are known to have different sweet-taste sensitivities. The difference was found to be dependent solely on the Sac locus. The dominant *Sac* allele (taster) is associated with higher taste sensitivity than the recessive allele (nontaster). To prove that the *Sac* locus does encode T1R3, transgenic mice were generated to introduce the T1R3 gene from a taster into a nontaster strain. As a result, the taste deficiency of nontaster mice was fully rescued, indicating that T1R3 was indeed the Sac gene (Nelson *et al.*, 2001).

The T1R belong to class-C GPCR (Fig. 20.3). Other renowned members of this class of GPCR include the metabotropic glutamate receptors (mGluR), γ-aminobutyric acid receptor B (GABA$_B$R), and calcium-sensing receptor (CaSR). The defining motif of this class of GPCR is the extracellular Venus flytrap (VFT) domain, which is their ligand-binding domain. The VFT domain is so named because of its structural resemblance to the leaves of the Venus flytrap plant, a carnivorous plant that catches animal prey. The crystal structures of mGluR VFT domains have been solved (Kunishima *et al.*, 2000; Tsuchiya *et al.*, 2002; Muto *et al.*, 2007). The domain is composed of two globular subdomains connected by a three-stranded flexible hinge. The bi-lobed architecture can form an 'open' or 'closed' conformation (Fig. 20.4). The closed conformation of the VFT domain is stabilized by glutamate, analogous to the closure of the Venus flytrap leaves with a trapped prey.

20.5 Functional Expression of T1R

Functional assays were developed for T1R in mammalian cell lines (Li *et al.*, 2002; Nelson *et al.*, 2001, 2002). According to their *in vivo* expression pattern, T1R2 and T1R1 were each

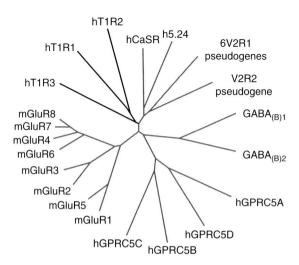

Fig. 20.3. Phylogenic tree of human class C G protein-coupled receptors.

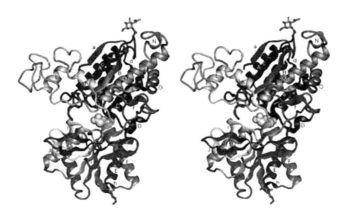

Fig. 20.4. Stereoview of mGluR1 VFT domain in a closed conformation. Reproduced with permission from Kunishima et al. (2000).

coexpressed with T1R3 in a HEK cell line that expresses Gα15, a promiscuous G protein. Binding of T1R agonists would activate Gα15, which leads to release of Ca^{2+} from intracellular stores. The elevated Ca^{2+} concentration can be monitored with a calcium-sensitive fluorescent dye. The cells were stimulated with different taste stimuli and the T1R receptor activities were monitored. The heteromeric human T1R2/T1R3 receptor selectively responded to all of the ~20 known sweeteners tested at physiologically relevant concentrations, and the responses were inhibited by lactisole (Li et al., 2002), a human sweet-taste inhibitor. Similarly, rat T1R2/T1R3 also responded to all of the dozen molecules that generate similar behavioural responses to sucrose (Li et al., 2002).

In contrast, human T1R1/T1R3 receptor selectively responded to L-glutamate (Li et al., 2002). The activities of human T1R1/T1R3 in the functional assay correlated well with umami taste (Fig. 20.5). The heteromeric receptor recognized glutamate with an EC_{50} closely matching the umami detection threshold. More importantly, the hallmark umami synergy is reconstituted in the assay: IMP or GMP can strongly potentiate the response of the receptor to glutamate or aspartate. The human receptor was highly selective for umami stimuli (Li et al., 2002), responding only to glutamate, aspartate, and L-AP4. Interestingly, mouse T1R1/T1R3 was found to be far more promiscuous (Nelson et al.,

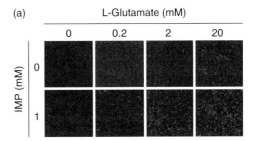

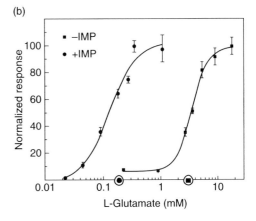

Fig. 20.5. Human T1R1/T1R3 activity correlated with umami taste. (a) Calcium imaging of T1R1/T1R3-expressing cells in response to glutamate with or without IMP. (b) T1R1/T1R3 dose response curves in the presence and absence of 0.2 mM IMP. The X axis circles represent average psychophysical detection threshold values for L-glutamate in the presence and absence of 0.2 mM IMP. Reproduced with permission from Li et al. (2002).

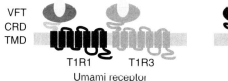
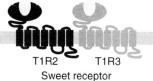

Fig. 20.6. Schematic drawing of umami and sweet receptors. T1R1 is used as an example to illustrate the overall domain structure of this class of GPCR. CRD, cys-rich domain; TMD, transmembrane domain; VFT, Venus flytrap domain.

2002), responding to virtually all L-amino acids in heterologous cells.

The same functional assays for human T1R1/T1R3 and T1R2/T1R3 were adopted for high-throughput screening of synthetic compound libraries. Multiple novel chemical classes of umami-tasting compounds, sweeteners, and sweet-taste enhancers have been identified through this effort (Zhang et al., 2008, 2010; Servant et al., 2010). These results validated the functional assay data. The human umami and sweet taste are mediated by related heteromeric receptors sharing one common subunit (Fig. 20.6).

20.6 T1R Knockout Mice

Behavioural and physiological studies using knockout mice demonstrated that T1R were required for rodent sweet and umami taste. Knockout mice were generated for each T1R gene (Zhao et al., 2003), and analysed using brief access taste tests and chorda tympani nerve recording. As expected, T1R1 null mice exhibited complete loss in preference for umami tastants; T1R2 null mice exhibited complete loss in preference for artificial sweeteners and greatly diminished preference for sugars; and T1R3 null mice lost preferences for both umami stimuli and artificial sweeteners completely, displaying greatly diminished responses to sugars. The CT nerve responses were consistent with the behavioural data.

Independently, a T1R3 knockout mouse model was generated and analysed using the two-bottle preference test (Damak et al., 2003). The results were somewhat different: the preference for monosodium glutamate (MSG) in T1R3-null mice was reduced but not abolished. The animals showed no preference for artificial sweeteners, and a diminished preference for sucrose, but essentially the same preferences for glucose and maltose as the wild-type mice.

The discrepancies between the behavioural results from these two reports could be due to the different taste test protocols. The brief access taste tests were carried out within 30 min and stimuli were presented in 5-s trials, while in two-bottle tests, the animals were exposed to the tastants for 48 h. It is now known that post-ingestive effects can greatly distort the outcome of two-bottle preference tests. Genetically engineered mice lacking the cellular machinery required for sweet-taste transduction can still develop a robust preference for sucrose solutions based solely on caloric content (de Araujo et al., 2006). The post-ingestive effect of MSG is also documented in the literature (Bachmanov et al., 2000; Zhao et al., 2003). Therefore, data from the brief access tests are more relevant to taste physiology.

20.7 The Molecular Mechanism of Umami Synergy

The unique feature of synergy in umami taste is scientifically intriguing. The molecular mechanism for the synergy has been revealed recently using a combination of chimeric receptors, mutagenesis and molecular modelling approaches (Zhang et al., 2008). The first step of this study was to discover the umami ligand binding sites on the receptor. Since the umami and sweet-taste receptors recognize different taste stimuli, the primary ligand binding sites should reside on the unique subunits T1R1 and T1R2, not the shared subunit T1R3. A chimeric receptor (Fig. 20.7) with the T1R1 N-terminal domain and the T1R2 transmembrane domain (T1R1-2) displayed essentially the same ligand specificity as the umami taste receptor, and the activity was enhanced by IMP. Conversely, chimera with T1R2 N-terminal domain and T1R1 transmembrane domain (T1R2-1) displayed the same ligand specificity as the sweet-taste receptor. These data indicate that the T1R1 N-terminal domain is critical for binding IMP as well as glutamate.

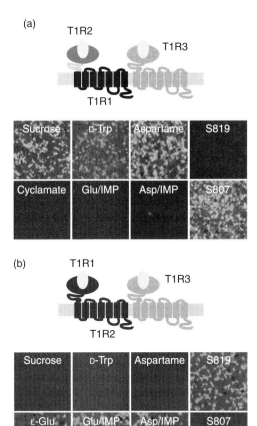

Fig. 20.7. Schematics of sweet–umami chimeric receptors and their ligand specificities. (a) T1R2-1/T1R3 chimeric receptor recognizes sweeteners. (b) T1R1-2/T1R3 chimeric receptor recognizes umami tastants. Reproduced with permission from Zhang et al. (2008).

Mutagenesis analysis further defined the binding site of glutamate and IMP to the VFT domain of T1R1. In the VFT domain of T1R1, 38 residues were mutated individually, and the mutants were tested for their response to glutamate and IMP. Among the 38 residues, four were found to be essential for glutamate recognition, and another set of four residues was found to be critical for IMP activity, suggesting that glutamate and IMP occupy different parts of the space within the VFT domain.

Molecular modelling of T1R1 VFT based on the crystal structure of metabotropic glutamate receptors revealed the relative positions of the eight critical residues. The four residues important for glutamate binding are located near the hinge region, while the four for IMP are located near the opening or 'lips' of the bi-lobed structure. It is known that the negatively charged phosphate group of IMP is important for its umami-enhancement activity. A cluster of positively charged residues was found near the lips of the T1R1 VFT. In fact, three of the four residues important for IMP activity are positively charged, and they could interact with the phosphate group of IMP through a salt bridge. A molecular model was constructed (Fig. 20.8), where both glutamate and IMP were positioned in the cleft of the T1R1 VFT domain. A mechanism for the synergy is proposed: glutamate binds close to the hinge region of the VFT domain, and induces the closure of the lobes and activates the receptor. IMP binds close to the opening of the VFT domain and coordinates the positively charged residues from both sides of the bi-lobed structure, thereby stabilizing the closed conformation and enhancing the activity of the receptor.

GPCR modulators can be categorized as orthosteric or allosteric, depending on their binding sites. The orthosteric modulators work on the same binding site as the natural ligand of the receptor, while the allosteric modulators work on different sites. In recent years, researchers have become more and more interested in allosteric modulators of GPCR as novel therapeutic agents. In many cases, allosteric modulators have advantages over orthosteric ones. For instance, the family of mGluR shares the same ligand and highly conserved ligand binding domain, making it very difficult to develop a selective orthosteric modulator for an individual receptor. Allosteric modulators, on the other hand, can target the less conserved portion of the receptors and achieve subtype selectivity. Many synthetic allosteric modulators for class-C GPCR have been developed over the years (Brauner-Osborne et al., 2007); however, all of them target the transmembrane domains. IMP is a naturally occurring allosteric modulator of the umami taste receptor, as it occupies a different part of the VFT binding pocket from glutamate. The cooperative binding of glutamate and IMP to the T1R1 VFT domain represents a novel mechanism, and could stimulate new ideas to allow the development of allosteric modulators of other class-C GPCR.

This mechanism of enhancement also applies to the sweet-taste receptor. Recently, synthetic enhancers have been identified for the human sweet-taste receptor through high-throughput screening (Servant et al., 2010). Similar to the umami enhancers, the sweet-taste enhancers elicit no sweet taste on their own, but can strongly potentiate the sweet taste of selective sweeteners in human taste test. A molecular mechanism of these molecules was proposed (Zhang et al., 2010) based on data from the same chimeric receptor, mutagenesis, and molecular modelling approaches, and turned out to be very similar to that of umami synergy. Using the sucralose enhancer SE-2 as an example (Fig. 20.9), sucralose binds deep inside the VFT domain of T1R2 and induces the closure of the two lobes by interacting with the hinge region, while the enhancer molecule binds near the lips of the Venus flytrap and stabilizes the closed conformation. SE-2 is not a charged molecule like IMP. Based on the model, it interacts with the T1R2 VFT domain mostly through hydrogen bonding and hydrophobic interactions.

Besides the VFT domain, other ligand interaction sites (Fig. 20.10) have also been identified on both umami and sweet-taste receptors in studies using similar chimeric

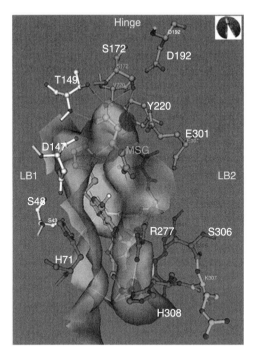

Fig. 20.8. A molecular model for the umami synergy. Glutamate and a potent analogue of IMP molecules are fitted inside the binding pocket of T1R1 VT domain. LB1 is the upper lobe of T1R1 VFT domain and LB2 the lower lobe. The cartoon of a clam shell in the upper right corner shows the overall orientation of the VFT domain.

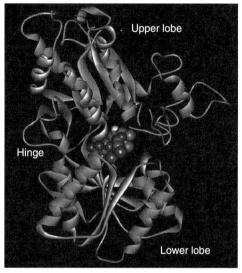

Fig. 20.9. A molecular model of the T1R2 VFT domain in closed conformation with bound sucralose and its enhancer molecule SE-2. Reproduced with permission from Zhang et al. (2010).

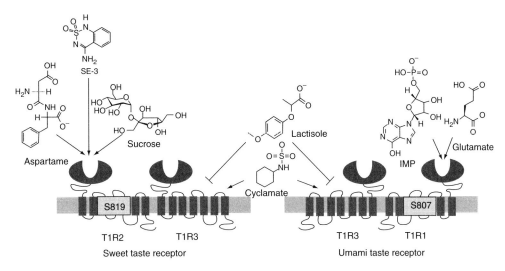

Fig. 20.10. Schematics of human sweet and umami receptor indicating the multiple ligand binding sites. S819 is a sweet compound identified in T1R2/T1R3 high throughput screening. S807 is an umami compound identified in T1R1/T1R3 high throughput screening.

receptor and mutagenesis analysis (Jiang et al., 2004, 2005a,b; Xu et al., 2004; Winnig et al., 2007; Zhang et al., 2008, 2010).

20.8 Umami Signal Transduction

A number of different signalling pathways have been proposed over the years for umami, sweet, and bitter taste (Gilbertson et al., 2000). It became clear only recently that the three groups of taste receptors share the same signal transduction cascade (Chandrashekar et al., 2006). Studies using mouse knockout models proved that gustducin (Wong et al., 1996), phospholipase Cβ2 (PLC-β2) (Zhang et al., 2003), inositol 1,4,5-trisphosphate receptor type 3 (IP3R3) (Hisatsune et al., 2007), and a transient receptor potential protein (TRPM5) (Zhang et al., 2003; Damak et al., 2006) are required for the pathway. Knockout of each component results in severe electrophysiological and behavioural defects in umami, sweet, and bitter taste.

The transduction cascade (Fig. 20.11) emerges after identification of the critical components: activation of umami receptor triggers conformation changes in the heterotrimeric G protein gustducin, leading to release of the Gβγ subunits (Huang et al., 1999; Zhang et al., 2003), which in turn activate PLC-β2. Two messenger molecules are generated by PLC-β2: inositol 1,4,5-trisphosphate (IP3) and diacylglycerol. IP3 binds to IP3R3 and leads to Ca^{2+} release from intracellular stores. The elevated Ca^{2+} level results in gating of the TRPM5 channel and depolarization of the taste-receptor cell. The depolarized TRC release neurotransmitter and the signal is transmitted to the chorda tympani or glossopharyngeal nerves.

Adenosine 5′-triphosphate (ATP) is believed to be the key neurotransmitter linking taste buds to the taste nerves (Finger et al., 2005). Stimulation of taste buds in vitro evokes release of ATP. The ionotropic purinergic receptors $P2X_2$ and $P2X_3$, which respond to ATP, are present on the taste nerve fibres (Bo et al., 1999; Finger et al., 2005). Knockout of the two receptors specifically eliminates the taste responses without affecting other responses to touch or temperature in the nerves (Finger et al., 2005; Eddy et al., 2009).

The umami, sweet and bitter TRC all belong to type II, which do not form morphologically identifiable synaptic contact with the taste nerves. It is not clear how neurotransmissions occur between type II cells and the nerves. One hypothesis is that type II cells use type III

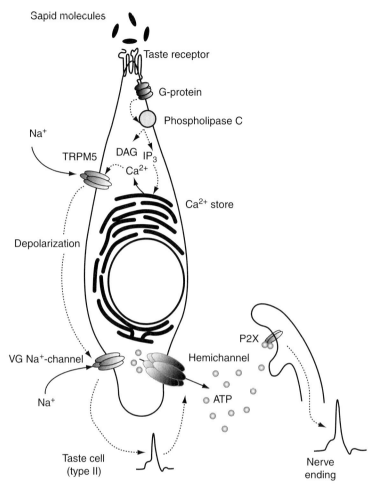

Fig. 20.11. Schematic model showing the sequence of intracellular events that are triggered by the binding of sapid molecules (tastants) to taste receptors and culminate in ATP release through hemichannels. Reproduced with permission from Romanov et al. (2007).

cells as intermediates for neurotransmission (Roper, 2006). However, data from transneuronal tracing experiments (Damak et al., 2008; Ohmoto et al., 2008) argue against the intermediate cell hypothesis. Transgenic mouse lines were engineered to express the transneuronal tracer wheat germ agglutinin (WGA), in sweet and umami TRC under the control of the mouse T1R3 gene promoter. WGA protein was transferred not laterally to other TRC, but directly to a subset of neurons in the geniculate and nodose/petrosal ganglia, and further conveyed to a subpopulation of neurons in the rostrocentral region of the nucleus of the solitary tract. Therefore, direct neurotransmissions exist between type II TRC and the taste nerves. Recently, it was proposed that ATP was released from type II taste cells via a non-exocytotic mechanism, most likely through the connexin or pannexin hemichannels (Fig. 20.11) (Huang et al., 2007; Romanov et al., 2007).

20.9 Functional Neuroimaging of Umami Taste

Umami tastants increase the palatability of a variety of foods. However, umami alone is not a pleasant taste. In fact, many find the taste of glutamate solution very unpleasant. It is clear that the pleasant taste perception associated with umami results from the integration of multiple sensory cues in the central nervous system. Recently, the mechanisms for the pleasantness associated with umami taste were investigated in humans using functional magnetic resonance imaging (fMRI) (McCabe and Rolls, 2007).

This study was based on findings from neuronal recordings in macaque monkeys. In primates, taste signals generated at the taste buds are transmitted to the primary taste cortex through relays at the nucleus of the solitary tract and taste thalamus (Rolls, 2009). A region of secondary taste cortex is found in the primate orbitofrontal cortex. More importantly, neurons in the orbitofrontal taste cortex appear to be related to food reward, as their activities are potentiated by hunger and inhibited by satiety (Rolls *et al.*, 1989; Critchley and Rolls, 1996).

Neurons that are best tuned to umami were identified in the primary taste cortex as well as the orbitofrontal cortex of macaques (Baylis and Rolls, 1991; Rolls *et al.*, 1996). These neurons responded to gustatory stimuli by glutamate or IMP. The neuronal representation of umami taste is separate from those of other taste qualities (sweet, sour, salty and bitter). Interestingly, the responses of some of these neurons decreased when the monkeys were fed to satiety with monosodium glutamate solution (Rolls *et al.*, 1996). Based on this inverse correlation between the sensory-specific neuronal activity and satiety, it was proposed that the pleasantness of umami is represented in the orbitofrontal cortex.

Human studies were carried out to address the fundamental questions of what makes umami pleasant and how the pleasantness correlates with the neuronal activities. fMRI revealed umami-responding neurons (de Araujo *et al.*, 2003) in the insular-opercular taste cortex, the putative human primary taste cortex, and the orbitofrontal cortex. The combination of glutamate and a consonant vegetable odour was found to result in a much more pleasurable response (McCabe and Rolls, 2007). More importantly, the combination of umami taste and the olfactory stimulus elicited synergistic effect on the activity of certain brain regions, i.e., the activity induced by the combination is significantly larger than the sum of either stimulus alone. This supralinear additivity was observed in the medial orbitofrontal cortex, and in a part of the ventral striatum which receives inputs from the orbitofrontal cortex. Activation of these brain regions correlated with the pleasantness (McCabe and Rolls, 2007). In contrast, the supralinear additivity was significantly less between salty taste and the vegetable odour.

There are likely to be many other ways to make umami taste pleasant. Sometimes it is just as simple as changing the label of the taste sample. The same sample was rated significantly more pleasant when labelled 'rich and delicious taste' than 'MSG' (Grabenhorst *et al.*, 2008), while the umami intensity rating was not significantly changed. Interestingly, this cognitive modulation also correlated with the neuronal activities in the medial orbitofrontal cortex: samples with the 'rich and delicious taste' label elicited much higher response in this brain region.

20.10 Conclusions

The last decade has witnessed many breakthrough discoveries in taste biology. Identification of the taste receptors led to revolutions in our understanding of the taste mechanism. Many important questions are being addressed by different research groups, including the mechanisms of signal transduction between TRC to the taste nerves, and the brain representation of the different taste qualities. As the labelled-line model becomes generally accepted, an interesting question arises: how is the specific wiring between the taste nerves and the TRC maintained, given the rapid turnover of TRC? Many other interesting questions still remain: is there any other more subtle taste quality besides the basic five, such as a fat taste? How do experience and cognition modulate people's taste sensations and food preferences?

The presence of taste receptors is not limited to taste buds. Specialized chemosensory cells expressing taste receptors and their downstream signalling elements have been found in many tissues, including the gastrointestinal tract (Wu et al., 2002; Kaske et al., 2007) and the respiratory tree (Finger et al., 2003; Kaske et al., 2007; Merigo et al., 2007; Lin et al., 2008; Sbarbati et al., 2009; Shah et al., 2009). Important functions of these chemosensory cells are being revealed (Kokrashvili et al., 2009; Tizzano et al., 2010).

References

Bachmanov, A.A., Tordoff, M.G. and Beauchamp, G.K. (2000) Intake of umami-tasting solutions by mice: a genetic analysis. *Journal of Nutrition* 130, 935S–941S.

Bachmanov, A.A., Li, X., Li, S., Neira, M., Beauchamp, G.K. and Azen, E.A. (2001) High-resolution genetic mapping of the sucrose octaacetate taste aversion (Soa) locus on mouse Chromosome 6. *Mammalian Genome* 12, 695–699.

Baylis, L.L. and Rolls, E.T. (1991) Responses of neurons in the primate taste cortex to glutamate. *Physiology & Behavior* 49, 973–979.

Bo, X., Alavi, A., Xiang, Z., Oglesby, I., Ford, A. and Burnstock, G. (1999) Localization of ATP-gated P2X2 and P2X3 receptor immunoreactive nerves in rat taste buds. *NeuroReport* 10, 1107–1111.

Boughter, J.D., Jr, Pumplin, D.W., Yu, C., Christy, R.C. and Smith, D.V. (1997) Differential expression of alpha-gustducin in taste bud populations of the rat and hamster. *Journal of Neuroscience* 17, 2852–2858.

Brauner-Osborne, H., Wellendorph, P. and Jensen, A.A. (2007) Structure, pharmacology and therapeutic prospects of family C G-protein coupled receptors. *Current Drug Targets* 8, 169–184.

Chandrashekar, J., Hoon, M.A., Ryba, N.J. and Zuker, C.S. (2006) The receptors and cells for mammalian taste. *Nature* 444, 288–294.

Chandrashekar, J., Kuhn, C., Oka, Y., Yarmolinsky, D.A., Hummler, E., Ryba, N.J. and Zuker, C.S. (2010) The cells and peripheral representation of sodium taste in mice. *Nature* 464, 297–301.

Clapp, T.R., Stone, L.M., Margolskee, R.F. and Kinnamon, S.C. (2001) Immunocytochemical evidence for co-expression of Type III IP3 receptor with signaling components of bitter taste transduction. *BMC Neuroscience* 2, 6.

Critchley, H.D. and Rolls, E.T. (1996) Olfactory neuronal responses in the primate orbitofrontal cortex: analysis in an olfactory discrimination task. *Journal of Neurophysiology* 75, 1659–1672.

Damak, S., Rong, M., Yasumatsu, K., Kokrashvili, Z., Varadarajan, V., Zou, S., Jiang, P., et al. (2003) Detection of sweet and umami taste in the absence of taste receptor T1r3. *Science* 301, 850–853.

Damak, S., Rong, M., Yasumatsu, K., Kokrashvili, Z., Perez, C.A., Shigemura, N., Yoshida, R., et al. (2006) Trpm5 null mice respond to bitter, sweet, and umami compounds. *Chemical Senses* 31, 253–264.

Damak, S., Mosinger, B. and Margolskee, R.F. (2008) Transsynaptic transport of wheat germ agglutinin expressed in a subset of type II taste cells of transgenic mice. *BMC Neuroscience* 9, 96.

de Araujo, I.E., Kringelbach, M.L., Rolls, E.T. and Hobden, P. (2003) Representation of umami taste in the human brain. *Journal of Neurophysiology* 90, 313–319.

de Araujo, I.E., Gutierrez, R., Oliveira-Maia, A.J., Pereira, A., Jr, Nicolelis, M.A. and Simon, S.A. (2006) Neural ensemble coding of satiety states. *Neuron* 51, 483–494.

Eddy, M.C., Eschle, B.K., Barrows, J., Hallock, R.M., Finger, T.E. and Delay, E.R. (2009) Double P2X2/P2X3 purinergic receptor knockout mice do not taste NaCl or the artificial sweetener SC45647. *Chemical Senses* 34, 789–797.

Finger, T.E. (2005) Cell types and lineages in taste buds. *Chemical Senses* 30, i54–55.

Finger, T.E., Bottger, B., Hansen, A., Anderson, K.T., Alimohammadi, H. and Silver, W.L. (2003) Solitary chemoreceptor cells in the nasal cavity serve as sentinels of respiration. *Proceedings of the National Academy of Sciences of the USA* 100, 8981–8986.

Finger, T.E., Danilova, V., Barrows, J., Bartel, D.L., Vigers, A.J., Stone, L., Hellekant, G., et al. (2005) ATP signaling is crucial for communication from taste buds to gustatory nerves. *Science* 310, 1495–1499.

Fuller, J.L. (1974) Single-locus control of saccharin preference in mice. *Journal of Heredity* 65, 33–36.

Gilbertson, T.A., Damak, S. and Margolskee, R.F. (2000) The molecular physiology of taste transduction. *Current Opinion in Neurobiology* 10, 519–527.

Grabenhorst, F., Rolls, E.T. and Bilderbeck, A. (2008) How cognition modulates affective responses to taste and flavor: top-down influences on the orbitofrontal and pregenual cingulate cortices. *Cerebral Cortex* 18, 1549–1559.

Hisatsune, C., Yasumatsu, K., Takahashi-Iwanaga, H., Ogawa, N., Kuroda, Y., Yoshida, R., Ninomiya, Y., et al. (2007) Abnormal taste perception in mice lacking the type 3 inositol 1,4,5-trisphosphate receptor. *Journal of Biological Chemistry* 282, 37225–37231.

Hoon, M.A., Adler, E., Lindemeier, J., Battey, J.F., Ryba, N.J. and Zuker, C.S. (1999) Putative mammalian taste receptors: a class of taste-specific GPCRs with distinct topographic selectivity. *Cell* 96, 541–551.

Huang, L., Shanker, Y.G., Dubauskaite, J., Zheng, J.Z., Yan, W., Rosenzweig, S., Spielman, A.I., et al. (1999) Ggamma13 colocalizes with gustducin in taste receptor cells and mediates IP3 responses to bitter denatonium. *Nature Neuroscience* 2, 1055–1062.

Huang, Y.J., Maruyama, Y., Dvoryanchikov, G., Pereira, E., Chaudhari, N. and Roper, S.D. (2007) The role of pannexin 1 hemichannels in ATP release and cell-cell communication in mouse taste buds. *Proceedings of the National Academy of Sciences of the USA* 104, 6436–6441.

Ikeda, K. (1909) On a new seasoning. *Journal of the Tokyo Chemical Society* 30, 820–836.

Jiang, P., Ji, Q., Liu, Z., Snyder, L.A., Benard, L.M., Margolskee, R.F. and Max, M. (2004) The cysteine-rich region of T1R3 determines responses to intensely sweet proteins. *Journal of Biological Chemistry* 279, 45068–45075.

Jiang, P., Cui, M., Zhao, B., Liu, Z., Snyder, L.A., Benard, L.M., Osman, R., et al. (2005a) Lactisole interacts with the transmembrane domains of human T1R3 to inhibit sweet taste. *Journal of Biological Chemistry* 280, 15238–15246.

Jiang, P., Cui, M., Zhao, B., Snyder, L.A., Benard, L.M., Osman, R., Max, M., et al. (2005b) Identification of the cyclamate interaction site within the transmembrane domain of the human sweet taste receptor subunit T1R3. *Journal of Biological Chemistry* 280, 34296–34305.

Kaske, S., Krasteva, G., Konig, P., Kummer, W., Hofmann, T., Gudermann, T. and Chubanov, V. (2007) TRPM5, a taste-signaling transient receptor potential ion-channel, is a ubiquitous signaling component in chemosensory cells. *BMC Neuroscience* 8, 49.

Kitagawa, M., Kusakabe, Y., Miura, H., Ninomiya, Y. and Hino, A. (2001) Molecular genetic identification of a candidate receptor gene for sweet taste. *Biochemical and Biophysical Research Communications* 283, 236–242.

Kodama, A. (1913) On a procedure for separating inosinic acid. *Journal of the Tokyo Chemical Society* 34, 751.

Kokrashvili, Z., Mosinger, B. and Margolskee, R.F. (2009) T1r3 and alpha-gustducin in gut regulate secretion of glucagon-like peptide-1. *Annals of the New York Academy of Sciences* 1170, 91–94.

Kuninaka, A. (1960) Studies on taste of ribonucleic acid derivatives. *Journal of the Agricultural Chemical Society of Japan* 34, 487–492.

Kunishima, N., Shimada, Y., Tsuji, Y., Sato, T., Yamamoto, M., Kumasaka, T., Nakanishi, S., et al. (2000) Structural basis of glutamate recognition by a dimeric metabotropic glutamate receptor. *Nature* 407, 971–977.

Lawton, D.M., Furness, D.N., Lindemann, B. and Hackney, C.M. (2000) Localization of the glutamate-aspartate transporter, GLAST, in rat taste buds. *European Journal of Neuroscience* 12, 3163–3171.

Li, X., Staszewski, L., Xu, H., Durick, K., Zoller, M. and Adler, E. (2002) Human receptors for sweet and umami taste. *Proceedings of the National Academy of Sciences of the USA* 99, 4692–4696.

Lin, W., Ogura, T., Margolskee, R.F., Finger, T.E. and Restrepo, D. (2008) TRPM5-expressing solitary chemosensory cells respond to odorous irritants. *Journal of Neurophysiology* 99, 1451–1460.

Max, M., Shanker, Y.G., Huang, L., Rong, M., Liu, Z., Campagne, F., Weinstein, H., et al. (2001) Tas1r3, encoding a new candidate taste receptor, is allelic to the sweet responsiveness locus Sac. *Nature Genetics* 28, 58–63.

McCabe, C. and Rolls, E.T. (2007) Umami: a delicious flavor formed by convergence of taste and olfactory pathways in the human brain. *European Journal of Neuroscience* 25, 1855–1864.

Merigo, F., Benati, D., Di Chio, M., Osculati, F. and Sbarbati, A. (2007) Secretory cells of the airway express molecules of the chemoreceptive cascade. *Cell and Tissue Research* 327, 231–247.

Montmayeur, J.P., Liberles, S.D., Matsunami, H. and Buck, L.B. (2001) A candidate taste receptor gene near a sweet taste locus. *Nature Neuroscience* 4, 492–498.

Murray, R.G. (1973) The ultrastructure of taste buds. In: Friedmann, I. (ed.) *The Ultrastructure of Sensory Organs*, North-Holland, Amsterdam, pp. 1–81.

Muto, T., Tsuchiya, D., Morikawa, K. and Jingami, H. (2007) Structures of the extracellular regions of the group II/III metabotropic glutamate receptors. *Proceedings of the National Academy of Sciences of the USA* 104, 3759–3764.

Nelson, G., Hoon, M.A., Chandrashekar, J., Zhang, Y., Ryba, N.J. and Zuker, C.S. (2001) Mammalian sweet taste receptors. *Cell* 106, 381–390.

Nelson, G., Chandrashekar, J., Hoon, M.A., Feng, L., Zhao, G., Ryba, N.J. and Zuker, C.S. (2002) An amino-acid taste receptor. *Nature* 416, 199–202.

Nelson, G.M. and Finger, T.E. (1993) Immunolocalization of different forms of neural cell adhesion molecule (NCAM) in rat taste buds. *Journal of Comparative Neurology* 336, 507–516.

Ohmoto, M., Matsumoto, I., Yasuoka, A., Yoshihara, Y. and Abe, K. (2008) Genetic tracing of the gustatory and trigeminal neural pathways originating from T1R3-expressing taste receptor cells and solitary chemoreceptor cells. *Molecular and Cellular Neuroscience* 38, 505–517.

Rolls, E.T. (2009) Functional neuroimaging of umami taste: what makes umami pleasant? *American Journal of Clinical Nutrition* 90, 804S–813S.

Rolls, E.T., Sienkiewicz, Z.J. and Yaxley, S. (1989) Hunger modulates the responses to gustatory stimuli of single neurons in the caudolateral orbitofrontal cortex of the macaque monkey. *European Journal of Neuroscience* 1, 53–60.

Rolls, E.T., Critchley, H.D., Wakeman, E.A. and Mason, R. (1996) Responses of neurons in the primate taste cortex to the glutamate ion and to inosine 5'-monophosphate. *Physiology & Behavior* 59, 991–1000.

Romanov, R.A., Rogachevskaja, O.A., Bystrova, M.F., Jiang, P., Margolskee, R.F. and Kolesnikov, S.S. (2007) Afferent neurotransmission mediated by hemichannels in mammalian taste cells. *EMBO Journal* 26, 657–667.

Roper, S.D. (2006) Cell communication in taste buds. *Cellular and Molecular Life Sciences* 63, 1494–1500.

Sainz, E., Korley, J.N., Battey, J.F. and Sullivan, S.L. (2001) Identification of a novel member of the T1R family of putative taste receptors. *Journal of Neurochemistry* 77, 896–903.

Sbarbati, A., Tizzano, M., Merigo, F., Benati, D., Nicolato, E., Boschi, F., Cecchini, M.P., et al. (2009) Acyl homoserine lactones induce early response in the airway. *Anatomical Record* (Hoboken) 292, 439–448.

Servant, G., Tachdjian, C., Tang, X.Q., Werner, S., Zhang, F., Li, X., Kamdar, P., et al. (2010) Positive allosteric modulators of the human sweet taste receptor enhance sweet taste. *Proceedings of the National Academy of Sciences of the USA* 107, 4746–4751.

Shah, A.S., Ben-Shahar, Y., Moninger, T.O., Kline, J.N. and Welsh, M.J. (2009) Motile cilia of human airway epithelia are chemosensory. *Science* 325, 1131–1134.

Tizzano, M., Gulbransen, B.D., Vandenbeuch, A., Clapp, T.R., Herman, J.P., Sibhatu, H.M., Churchill, M.E., et al. (2010) Nasal chemosensory cells use bitter taste signaling to detect irritants and bacterial signals. *Proceedings of the National Academy of Sciences of the USA* 107, 3210–3215.

Tsuchiya, D., Kunishima, N., Kamiya, N., Jingami, H. and Morikawa, K. (2002) Structural views of the ligand-binding cores of a metabotropic glutamate receptor complexed with an antagonist and both glutamate and Gd3+. *Proceedings of the National Academy of Sciences of the USA* 99, 2660–2665.

Winnig, M., Bufe, B., Kratochwil, N.A., Slack, J.P. and Meyerhof, W. (2007) The binding site for neohesperidin dihydrochalcone at the human sweet taste receptor. *BMC Structural Biology* 7, 66.

Wong, G.T., Gannon, K.S. and Margolskee, R.F. (1996) Transduction of bitter and sweet taste by gustducin. *Nature* 381, 796–800.

Wu, S.V., Rozengurt, N., Yang, M., Young, S.H., Sinnett-Smith, J. and Rozengurt, E. (2002) Expression of bitter taste receptors of the T2R family in the gastrointestinal tract and enteroendocrine STC-1 cells. *Proceedings of the National Academy of Sciences of the USA* 99, 2392–2397.

Xu, H., Staszewski, L., Tang, H., Adler, E., Zoller, M. and Li, X. (2004) Different functional roles of T1R subunits in the heteromeric taste receptors. *Proceedings of the National Academy of Sciences of the USA* 101, 14258–14263.

Yang, R., Crowley, H.H., Rock, M.E. and Kinnamon, J.C. (2000a) Taste cells with synapses in rat circumvallate papillae display SNAP-25-like immunoreactivity. *Journal of Comparative Neurology* 424, 205–215.

Yang, R., Tabata, S., Crowley, H.H., Margolskee, R.F. and Kinnamon, J.C. (2000b) Ultrastructural localization of gustducin immunoreactivity in microvilli of type II taste cells in the rat. *Journal of Comparative Neurology* 425, 139–151.

Yarmolinsky, D.A., Zuker, C.S., Ryba, N.J., Chandrashekar, J. and Hoon, M.A. (2009) Common sense about taste: from mammals to insects. *Cell* 139, 234–244.

Zhang, F., Klebansky, B., Fine, R.M., Xu, H., Pronin, A., Liu, H., Tachdjian, C. et al. (2008) Molecular mechanism for the umami taste synergism. *Proceedings of the National Academy of Sciences of the USA* 105, 20930–20934.

Zhang, F., Klebansky, B., Fine, R.M., Liu, H., Xu, H., Servant, G., Zoller, M., et al. (2010) Molecular mechanism of the sweet taste enhancers. *Proceedings of the National Academy of Sciences of the USA* 107, 4752–4757.

Zhang, Y., Hoon, M.A., Chandrashekar, J., Mueller, K.L., Cook, B., Wu, D., Zuker, C.S. et al. (2003) Coding of sweet, bitter, and umami tastes: different receptor cells sharing similar signaling pathways. *Cell* 112, 293–301.

Zhao, G.Q., Zhang, Y., Hoon, M.A., Chandrashekar, J., Erlenbach, I., Ryba, N.J. and Zuker, C.S. (2003) The receptors for mammalian sweet and umami taste. *Cell* 115, 255–266.

Part IV

Health

21 Homocysteine Status: Factors Affecting and Health Risks

L.M. Steffen[1]* and B. Steffen[2]

[1]*Division of Epidemiology and Community Health, University of Minnesota School of Public Health, Minneapolis, USA;* [2]*Department of Laboratory Medicine and Pathology, University of Minnesota, Minneapolis, USA*

21.1 Abstract

A significant finding in recent times is the classification of high homocysteine levels as a potential risk factor in a number of chronic vascular conditions, particularly cardiovascular disease – though neural tube defects and decreased cognitive performance have also been demonstrated. Several factors influence the level of homocysteine concentrations, including age, gender, smoking and diet. Interactions with folate and vitamin B_{12} may also be important in the risks imposed by high levels of homocysteine. Genetic factors also influence homocysteine metabolism, and therefore risk of vascular disease. Observational studies, both prospective and case-control, have shown a moderate risk between homocysteine and coronary heart disease, stroke and venous thromboembolism. The majority of randomized clinical trials testing the effectiveness of vitamin B on reducing homocysteine levels, and putatively decreasing the risk of vascular disease, are null. The epidemiological evidence is reviewed in this chapter.

21.2 Introduction and Objectives

Homocysteine is a sulphur-containing amino acid first identified for its role in methionine metabolism in the 1930s by DuVigneaud (1952) as well as others. But only recently have elevated homocysteine levels been associated with putative deleterious consequences, including cases of mental retardation, fatty liver, vascular lesions, thrombosis (McCully, 2005) and arterial stiffness (Nestel *et al.*, 2003).

In 1969, McCully identified the index case of methionine synthase deficiency associated with arteriosclerosis, which led to the theory of homocysteine-related arteriosclerosis. Since then, the influence of homocysteine on risk of cardiovascular disease, stroke, venous thromboembolism and cognitive function has been examined in observational studies and randomized clinical trials. Neural tube defects have also been associated with elevated homocysteine concentrations along with reduced levels of folate, vitamin B_6 and/ or vitamin B_{12}. The objective for this chapter is to review the epidemiology of homocysteine

* E-mail address: steffen@umn.edu

and its relation to chronic disease. Specifically, the topics reviewed include:

1. the metabolism of homocysteine;
2. the distribution of homocysteine in the US population;
3. the determinants of total serum homocysteine concentrations;
4. homocysteine as a risk factor for selected chronic diseases and conditions;
5. randomized clinical trials (RCT) testing the effectiveness of vitamin B supplementation to reduce the risk of chronic disease, including coronary heart disease, stroke and venous thromboembolism through the putative reduction in elevated homocysteine levels; and
6. a discussion of differences in study designs and methods that may influence results.

21.3 The Metabolism of Homocysteine

Homocysteine is a sulphur-containing amino acid formed during the metabolism of methionine (Chapter 10) and is either metabolized into cysteine through transsulphuration or into methionine through methylation, depending on methionine levels. When excess methionine is present, homocysteine is conjugated to cysteine by the enzymatic action of cystathionine β-synthase, requiring vitamin B_6 as a cofactor. When methionine levels are low, homocysteine is methylated by the enzyme methionine synthase that requires vitamin B_{12} as a cofactor, methyltetrahydrofolate as a co-substrate, adequate folate intake and the enzyme methylene tetrahydrofolate reductase (MTHFR) to form methionine (Selhub, 1999). Accumulation of homocysteine may occur through defects in either transsulphuration or remethylation (Herrmann, 2001).

21.4 Distribution of Homocysteine Concentrations in the US Population

Serum total homocysteine concentrations were measured in adolescents and adults (ages 12 to more than 80 years) attending the Third National and Health and Nutrition Examination Survey (NHANES III), phase 2. Generally, serum total homocysteine levels increased with age and were higher among males than females (Jacques et al., 1999a). Other investigators observed that higher oestrogen levels were associated with lower homocysteine levels, which may explain the male–female difference in levels (Morris et al., 2000). Mexican-American females across all ages had lower levels than non-Hispanic white or African-American females (7.4 μmol l^{-1} versus 7.9 μmol l^{-1} versus 8.2 μmol l^{-1}, respectively), whereas there were no race/ethnicity differences reported in men (ranging from 9.4 to 9.8 μmol l^{-1}) (Jacques et al., 1999a). Average serum homocysteine concentrations ranged from 6.1 μmol l^{-1} in those 12–15 years to 15.0 μmol l^{-1} in adults aged 80+ years. Plasma homocysteine ranged from 4.54 μmol l^{-1} in children less than 4 years to 6.89 for those aged 16–18 years (Ganji and Kafai, 2005). Clinically, normal values of homocysteine range from 5 μmol l^{-1} to less than 16 μmol l^{-1}, mild to moderately elevated levels range from 16 to 100 μmol l^{-1}, and severely elevated levels are above 100 μmol l^{-1} (Eikelboom et al., 1999).

21.5 The Determinants of Serum Total Homocysteine Concentrations

Serum homocysteine levels are influenced by genetics and environmental factors, including demographic characteristics, diet, smoking, chronic medical conditions and medication use.

21.5.1 Demographic characteristics

As previously discussed, total serum homocysteine concentrations have been shown to increase with age, in the male sex, and with menopause in women (Jacques et al., 1999a; Morris et al., 2000).

21.5.2 Diet

An important environmental factor influencing homocysteine levels is dietary intake of nutrients required for homocysteine metabolism, including folate (folic acid), vitamin B_6 (pyridoxine), and vitamin B_{12} (cyanocobalamin) (Malinow et al., 1999). Observational and clinical studies have demonstrated inverse associations of plasma or dietary folate and vitamins B_6 and B_{12} with total serum homocysteine concentrations (Homocysteine Lowering Trialists' Collaboration, 1998). Unsurprisingly, the majority of elderly adults and patients with elevated homocysteine levels are deficient in folate, vitamin B_6 and/or vitamin B_{12} (Selhub et al., 1993).

In a randomized, double-blind trial, 189 middle-aged and elderly, relatively healthy adults who did not consume dietary supplements were randomly assigned to a treatment group (daily consumption of one cup breakfast cereal fortified with 440 μg folic acid, 1.8 mg vitamin B_6, and 4.8 μg vitamin B_{12}) or a control group (no fortified cereal) for 12 weeks. Compared to the control group, the treatment group showed an increase in plasma levels of B vitamins – that is, plasma folate and vitamins B_6 and B_{12} – and a concomitant decrease in homocysteine levels overall, representing a 4.8% decrease in the prevalence of hyperhomocysteinaemia (Tucker et al., 2004).

Apart from folic acid, vitamin B deficiency has also been associated with elevated homocysteine concentrations. For example, vegetarian diets are low in vitamin B_{12}, and hyperhomocysteinaemia has frequently been observed in vegetarians (Mezzano, 2000). Supplementation with vitamin B_{12} corrects the hyperhomocysteinaemia. Whether this supplementation further improves the already reduced cardiovascular morbidity and mortality associated with a vegetarian diet has yet to be demonstrated. Expectedly, individuals consuming greater quantities of animal protein, i.e. red and processed meat and poultry, have higher levels of homocysteine (Gao et al., 2003).

In 1998, the US Food and Drug Administration mandated folate fortification of grain products in the United States to reduce the incidence of neural tube defects, a common birth defect in newborn infants. The effect of folate fortification on homocysteine levels was determined using pre- and post-fortification blood samples of adults enrolled in the Framingham Heart Study who did not consume vitamin supplements. The prevalence of mild hyperhomocysteinaemia was reduced by about 50% as a result of fortification (Jacques et al., 1999b). Similarly, in a study conducted among 2695 adolescents 5 years after the start of folate fortification, lower serum homocysteine levels were observed among adolescents consuming greater intakes of whole and refined grains and dairy products (Lutsey et al., 2006). These studies provide evidence that homocysteine levels are lowered by supplementation of folate, vitamin B_6 and B_{12}.

21.5.3 Smoking

In a population-based surveillance study of adults aged 40–67 years, current smokers had higher plasma homocysteine levels than non-smokers, with a dose response between the number of cigarettes smoked per day and level of homocysteine (Nygard et al., 1995). There was no difference in homocysteine levels between former smokers and non-smokers. Though the mechanism accounting for increased homocysteine levels in smokers remains unclear, a case control study of individuals less than 60 years old demonstrated that current smokers had lower levels of plasma folate, vitamin B_6 and vitamin B_{12} than non-smokers (O'Callaghan et al., 2002).

21.5.4 Medical conditions and medication use

Chronic disease may also alter homocysteine levels. Total serum homocysteine was found to be positively correlated with glomerular filtration rate, and higher levels have been observed in patients with kidney disease (van Guldener, 2006). Furthermore, elevated levels of homocysteine have been seen frequently in patients with coronary heart disease, stroke, venous thromboembolism, or other vascular disease (Makris, 2000), as well as in individuals with high blood pressure (Nygard et al., 1995), and retinal artery and vein occlusions (Wright et al., 2008).

Anticoagulated patients may be at risk of hyperhomocysteinaemia, since patients receiving oral anticoagulant therapy are normally asked to restrict vitamin K-rich foods, including green vegetables that are good sources of folate. Homocysteine levels significantly increased while folate levels decreased in individuals on anti-coagulation therapy with restricted vitamin K intake, thus raising the risk of thrombosis (Murua et al., 2001). Apart from anti-coagulation therapies, other medications including antiepileptic drugs, methotrexate, fibric acid derivatives, and metformin have been hypothesized to influence the absorption of vitamin B or interfere with the pathways involved in the metabolism of homocysteine, resulting in elevated homocysteine levels (Desouza et al., 2002).

21.5.5 Genetic factors

Some individuals are genetically predisposed to elevated homocysteine levels. A common genetic variant in methylenetetrahydrofolate reductase (MTHFR), an enzyme that regulates the conversion of homocysteine to methionine, is the 677C → T polymorphism, which has been shown to result in increased levels of homocysteine. Notably, the 677 C → T polymorphism is involved in two major functions of one-carbon metabolism, DNA synthesis and DNA methylation, which play key roles as cofactor substrates in one carbon metabolism. Additional genetic mutations may also influence the metabolism of homocysteine and folate, including defects in vitamin B_{12} metabolism or homozygous deficiency of folate, vitamin B_{12}, cystathionine β-synthase, or methionine synthase (Eikelboom et al., 1999). Current treatment for these mutations/conditions is ensuring adequate folate and vitamin B intakes.

21.6 Homocysteinaemia is a Risk Factor

21.6.1 Coronary heart disease, stroke and venous thromboembolism

It is well known that homocysteinuria, an inherited disorder of methionine metabolism, increases the risk for venous and arterial thrombosis. Individual observational studies have shown that moderately elevated homocysteine levels increase the risk of coronary heart disease (CHD), stroke, venous thromboembolism (VTE), and peripheral arterial disease, though reports are inconsistent. To increase the power and precision of these studies, meta-analyses of observational studies have been conducted to determine the predictive value of elevated homocysteine levels for incident CHD, stroke, and VTE. A recent meta-analysis of 18 nested case-control and 8 prospective observational studies showed a positive association between homocysteine and incident CHD (Humphrey et al., 2008). More specifically, the relative risk (RR) for incident CHD associated with each 5 µmol l^{-1} increase in homocysteine was 1.18 (95% C.I. 1.10–1.26). The RR was stronger for studies with follow-up less than 5 years (RR 1.39; 95% C.I. 1.20–1.62), while the RR for studies with follow-up time of 10 or more years was 1.13 (95% C.I. 1.00–1.28). Importantly, statistical models were adjusted for traditional risk factors for CHD, including age, gender, smoking, physical activity, blood pressure, and renal dysfunction. The major strength of this study was the inclusion of data from population-based prospective studies of incident CHD events. Other meta-analyses that included persons with known CVD reported similar findings (Boushey et al., 1995; Homocysteine Studies Collaboration, 2002; Wald et al., 2002). One such meta-analysis by Wald et al. (2002) included 72 observational studies that examined the prevalence of MTHFR genetic mutation in 16,849 cases and controls and 20 prospective studies (n = 3820) that examined homocysteine and risk of heart disease, stroke, and VTE. The odds for a 5 µmol l^{-1} increase in serum homocysteine for these vascular diseases ranged from 1.42 to 1.65 in the genetic studies and 1.32 to 1.59 in the prospective studies. An updated meta-analysis showed similar findings of prospective and genetic studies for VTE among first and recurrent events: a 20% increased risk for a first VTE event for those with the TT genotype compared to those with the CC genotype (den Heijer et al., 2005).

21.6.2 Cognitive function, dementia and Alzheimer's disease

Age is a major risk factor for the decline in cognitive function and incident dementia. According to estimations from the Aging, Demographics, and Memory Study in 2002, the prevalence of dementia and Alzheimer's disease (AD) was 13.9% and 9.7%, respectively, among US adults aged 70+ years (Plassman et al., 2007). Among adults aged 71–79 years, the prevalence of dementia was 5% and increased to 37.4% among those aged 90+ years. Apart from age, other risk factors for cognitive decline and dementia include cardiovascular risk factors such as obesity, hypertension, dyslipidaemia, diabetes, and hyperhomocysteinaemia (Lighart et al., 2010). Of these risk factors, hyperhomocysteinaemia was associated with AD and dementia as reported in several case-control and prospective studies (Van Dam and Van Gool, 2009). Thus, homocysteine may be an important modifiable risk factor that may delay the onset of cognitive decline and dementia, except in multimorbid elderly patients (Hengstermann et al., 2009).

The prevalence of hyperhomocysteinaemia among US adults aged 60+ years participating in NHANES III (1988–1994) was 43.2% in men and 46.5% in women (Jacques et al., 1999a). Janson et al. (2002) reported a higher prevalence of hyper–homocysteine, ranging from 66% to 75% in elderly men and women, respectively, who participated in a cross-sectional study. In a recent systematic review, higher homocysteine levels were reported in AD cases compared to controls, while the relative risk of hyperhomocysteinaemia with AD was 2.5 (95% C.I. 1.38–4.56, p <0.01) (Van Dam and Van Gool, 2009).

21.7 Clinical Efficacy of Folate and Vitamins B_6 and B_{12}

21.7.1 Homocysteine, folate, vitamin B_6, vitamin B_{12} and vascular disease

Dietary folate and vitamins B_6 and B_{12} are known to lower homocysteine concentrations. However, it is not clear whether homocysteine reduced by supplementation or dietary intake of the B vitamins influences the risk of a vascular event.

21.7.2 Coronary heart disease, stroke and venous thromboembolism

21.7.2.1 Observational studies

Briefly, the epidemiologic evidence has shown a moderate effect of dietary or supplemental vitamin B intakes on lowering the risk of CHD, stroke, and VTE (Rimm et al., 1998; Steffen et al., 2003, 2007).

21.7.2.2 Randomized clinical trials

Over the past 10 years, many large randomized clinical trials (RCT) have been conducted to evaluate the effectiveness of vitamin B supplementation in reducing homocysteine concentrations and putatively to lower the risk of recurrent CVD, including myocardial infarction (MI), stroke and CHD death (see Table 21.1). Generally, homocysteine-lowering treatment (folic acid, vitamin B_6 and vitamin B_{12} supplementation) versus placebo has not lowered the risk of vascular disease in study participants with pre-existing disease. A Cochrane review and meta-analysis reported the risk ratio and 95% confidence intervals for 8 RCT as 1.03 (0.94, 1.13) (Marti-Carvajal et al., 2009). Conversely, homocysteine-lowering treatment may lower the incidence of strokes. Lee et al. (2010) recently conducted a meta-analysis of 13 RCT that enrolled over 13,000 participants with or without a history of stroke. They reported an 11% lower risk of the incidence of stroke with vitamin B supplementation, while secondary prevention of stroke was not reduced with these supplements. Further, den Heijer et al. reported no effect of vitamin B supplements folic acid, vitamin B_6 and vitamin B_{12} in the secondary prevention of VTE (den Heijer et al., 2007).

21.7.3 Cognitive function, dementia and Alzheimer's disease

Haan et al. (2007) provide evidence from a prospective study that the association between hyperhomocysteinaemia and dementia over

Table 21.1. Summary of the major randomized clinical trials testing the effectiveness of vitamin B supplementation in reducing homocysteine concentrations to lower the risk of recurrent CVD.

Study	Population N = Number of centres	Health status	Age (y)	Data collection Intervention dose	Control treatment	Hcyst µmol l^{-1}	Duration (follow-up)	Outcome	Results Hcyst in treatment group; RR or HR (95% C.I.)
FOLARDA Liem et al., 2004	283 multicentre	Hx MI	59	N=140 Usual care 5 mg d^{-1} FA	N=143 Usual care	NR	1 year	Recurrent MI, revascularization CHD death	Hcyst no available No difference between groups (p=0.69)
GOES Liem et al., 2005	593 Single centre	Hx MI, unstable angina, revascular.	65	N=300 Usual care 0.5 mg d^{-1} FA	N=293 Usual care	12.0 µmol l^{-1}	42 months	Recurrent MI CVD death	Hcyst not available RR 0.85 (0.56, 1.31)
HOPE2 Investigators (2006)	5522 multicentre	Hx CVD	>55	N=2758 2.5 mg d^{-1} FA 50 mg d^{-1} B$_6$ 1 mg d^{-1} B$_{12}$	N=2764 Placebo	Baseline 12.2 µmol l^{-1}	5 years	Recurrent MI, stroke, Sudden death (CVD)	Hcyst ↓ 2.4 µmol l^{-1} CVD: RR 0.95 (0.8, 1.07); Stroke: 0.75 (0.59, 0.97)
NORVIT Bonaa et al., 2006	3749 multicentre	Hx MI	63	*n=937, Gp1 n=935, Gp2 n=934, Gp3	N=943 Placebo	NR	3.5 years	Recurrent MI, stroke, CVD death	Hcyst ↓ 3.5 µmol l^{-1} w/Gp1 and Gp2 RR1.22 (1.0, 1.50)
VISP Toole et al., 2004	3680 multicentre	Hx stroke	66	N=1827 2.5 mg d^{-1} FA 0.4 mg d^{-1} B$_{12}$ 25 mg d^{-1} B$_6$	N=1853 20 mcg d^{-1} FA 6 mcg d^{-1} B$_{12}$ 200 mcg c^{-1} B$_6$	25% of US stroke pop.	2 years	Recurrent stroke	Hcyst not available RR 1.0 (0.8, 1.3), p=0.80
WAFACS Albert et al., 2008	5442 women; multicentre	With or w/o CVD	≥42	N=2721 2.5 mg d^{-1} FA 1.0 mg d^{-1} B$_{12}$ 50 mg d^{-1} B$_6$	N=2721 Placebo	12.1–12.5 µmol l^{-1}	7.3 years	Incident/recurrent CVD	Hcyst ↓ 2 3 µmol l^{-1} CVD: RR 1.03 (0.9, 1.19)
WENBIT Ebbing et al., 2008	3096 multicentre	Hx CVD	≥18	**N=772 Gp1 N=772 Gp2 N=772 Gp3	N=780 Placebo	10.8 µmol l^{-1}	Median 38 months	Recurrent CVD	Hcyst ↓ 2.8 µmol l^{-1} Gp1,2: HR 1.09 (0.90,1.3) Gp 3: HR 0.90 (0.74,1.39)

Study	N	Inclusion	Age	Intervention	Control	Baseline Hcyst	Duration	Outcome	Result
SEARCH Collaborative Group (2000)	12064 multicentre	Hx MI	18–80	N=6033 2 mg d⁻¹ Fol, 1 mg d⁻¹ B₁₂	N=6031 Placebo	13.5 μmol l⁻¹	6.7 years	Recurrent MI or other vascular event	Hcyst ↓ 3.8 μmol l⁻¹ RR 1.04 (0.97, 1.12)
VITATOPS Trial Study Group (2010)	8164 multicentre	Hx stroke, TIA	62	N=4089 2 mg d⁻¹ Fol 500 mcg d⁻¹ B₁₂ 25 mg d⁻¹ B₆	N=4075 Placebo		3.4 years	Recurrent stroke, MI, or vascular death	Hcyst ↓ 1.1 μmol l⁻¹ in a subsample; RR 0.91 (0.82, 1.00), p=0.05
VITRO den Heijer et al., 2007	701 multicentre	Hx venous thrombosis	20–80	N=353 5 mg d⁻¹ Fol 0.4 mg B₁₂ 50 mg⁻¹ B₆	N=348 Placebo	6.5–15.6 μmol l⁻¹	2.5 years	Recurrent venous thrombosis	High Hcyst group: RR 0.84 (0.56, 1.26) Low Hcyst group: RR 0.58 (0.31, 1.07)
SU.FOL.OM3 Galan et al., 2003	3000 France	Hx CHD	45–80	FA B₁₂ B₆ Omega-3	Placebo		5 years	Recurrent CVD	In progress

B₆, vitamin B₆; B₁₂, vitamin B₁₂; CVD, cardiovascular disease; Fol, folic acid; Hcyst, homocysteine concentration; MI, myocardial infarction; HR, hazard ratio; Hx, history of; NR, not reported; RF, risk factors; RR, relative risk; TIA, transient ischaemic attack; 95% C.I., 95% confidence intervals.
*NORVIT: Gp1 = 0.8 mg d⁻¹ folic acid, 0.4 mg d⁻¹ B₁₂, 40 mg d⁻¹ B₆; Gp2 = 0.8 mg B₁₂ d⁻¹; Gp3 = 40 mg d⁻¹ B₆.
**WENBIT: Gp1 = 0.8 mg d⁻¹ folic acid, 0.4 mg d⁻¹ B₁₂, 40 mg d⁻¹ B₆; Gp2 = 0.8 mg d⁻¹ folic acid, 0.4 mg d⁻¹ B₁₂; Gp3 = 40 mg d⁻¹ B₆.

4.5 years of follow-up may be explained by lower levels of vitamin B_{12} but not low folate. However, in a randomized, double-blind, placebo-controlled trial, results showed that among 406 adults aged 50–70 years taking folic acid supplements for 3 years versus 413 adults assigned to the placebo group, homocysteine levels were lowered by 26% and cognitive function improved (Durga et al., 2007). Results from a meta-analysis of nine placebo-controlled randomized trials with a median duration of 6 months showed that folic acid with or without other B vitamins did not prevent cognitive decline in over 2835 participants (Wald et al., 2010). Similarly, two randomized controlled trials demonstrated that daily intake of high-dose B vitamin supplements for 6–18 months did not slow cognitive decline among elderly adults with mild to moderate AD (Sun et al., 2007; Aisen et al., 2008). Meanwhile, several randomized clinical trials are under way, testing whether folate, vitamin B_6, and vitamin B_{12} reduce levels of homocysteine and whether these will slow the progression of cognitive decline and dementia.

21.8 Neural Tube Defects

Neural tube defects (NTD) are severe congenital malformations that occur in early pregnancy. The development of NTD is multifactorial. Both genetic and environmental factors are involved in the metabolism of homocysteine in NTD, one potential pathway. Besides dietary intake, a number of environmental factors are associated with the development of NTD including socioeconomic status, geographic differences, and maternal characteristics, such as maternal medication use during pregnancy as well as status of maternal diabetes and obesity (Blom, 2009). One genetic risk factor associated with the development of NTD is ethnicity. After folate fortification of grain products in the United States in 1998, the prevalence of NTD was reduced by 50% to 70%, especially among non-Hispanic whites and Hispanics, but not among non-Hispanic blacks (Williams et al., 2005). Molloy et al. (2009) observed that low (i.e. deficient or inadequate intake) maternal vitamin B_{12} status was associated with increased risk for neural tube defects. Genetic factors may influence both homocysteine and folate metabolism. Despite the MTHFR 677T allele, adequate folate intake may reduce the risk of NTD, while inadequate intake of folate may have the opposite effect (Gueant et al., 2003). Further, the pathogenesis of NTD may be related to one-carbon metabolism that is influenced by intakes of folate and vitamin B_{12} and by several other genetic factors. Mechanisms that may play a role in the aetiology of NTD include folate receptor autoantibodies and methylation patterns. This literature has been reviewed by Blom (2009).

21.9 Methodological Issues

21.9.1 Differences among studies of homocysteine, B vitamins and vascular disease

Generally, the results from the majority of single RCT or meta-analyses that tested the effectiveness of vitamin B supplementation (including folate, vitamin B_6 and B_{12}) in reducing homocysteine levels did not influence the risk of recurrent CHD (Bazzano et al., 2006) and thus far, in most but not all trials, of cognitive dysfunction and dementia (Wald et al., 2010). For stroke, some benefit was demonstrated in some subgroups (Bazzano et al., 2006; Lee et al., 2010). In contrast, results from a meta-analysis of observational studies examining the relation between homocysteine levels and risk of vascular disease showed lower risk of CHD and stroke (Homocysteine Studies Collaboration, 2002).

Several factors that might explain these study results include differences in study design, study population, duration of follow-up, data collected (i.e., confounding factors), and study outcome. Cohort studies reported weaker relative risks of CVD outcomes than case-control studies, while the majority of RCT did not demonstrate an impact of supplements on the risk of a recurrent event. Another factor that influences the outcome of the study is the study population. Many of the reported studies on CHD included adults with a prior history of CHD or advanced vascular disease. For studies of dementia, the populations were those who had mild to moderate dementia or Alzheimer's disease, but did not include low-risk or intermediate-risk individuals. Even though homocysteine can be reduced with vitamin B supplementation in high risk patients, it may still not be possible to lower the risk of vascular disease in these individuals who are depleted of thioretinaco ozonide in cellular membranes (McCully, 1993). Sufficient sample size and power are needed to detect a significant difference between (treatment) groups. In some RCT, the sample size may have been inadequate or the observational studies inadequately powered considering the fortification of the US food supply with folic acid since 1998. Duration of follow-up is an important factor that affects the power of the study. Length of follow-up in published studies or RCT has varied from a few months to several years. Wang et al. (2007) found that greater benefit was shown with duration of vitamin B treatment greater than 36 months. Further, in the analysis of observational studies, the statistical models may not have been adjusted for the same confounding factors, such as the cardiovascular risk factors. Finally, in many of the studies, a variety of study outcomes was reported, instead of a single, defined outcome-of-interest. The primary endpoint for most of the trials testing the B vitamins to reduce risk was recurrent vascular disease, including CHD and stroke, while cognitive function and dementia were secondary endpoints for several of the studies. Similar methods are necessary for comparison of studies and to appropriately interpret the study results. Several meta-analyses have been conducted to synthesize the findings of the individual trials. One such study was a Cochrane review of the homocysteine-lowering interventions (Marti-Carvajal et al., 2009). Results from this meta-analysis provide no evidence to support homocysteine lowering to prevent CVD.

An important point to consider, however, is that folate may not be the most effective therapy or intervention to reduce risk of a recurrent event. As observed by Haan et al. (2007) in a prospective observational study, vitamin B_{12} appeared to provide the most benefit in reducing the risk of vascular events. Vitamin B_{12} status has also associated with lower risk of NTD in nested case-control studies (Molloy et al., 2009). Another potential therapy is the combination of omega-3 fatty acid and folic acid or vitamin B supplementation that may improve cognitive function or prevent dementia and Alzheimer's disease, as well as beneficially influencing CHD and stroke outcomes (Das, 2008). The SU.FOL.OM3 trial is evaluating the effect of supplementation of the B vitamins, folate, vitamin B_6 and vitamin B_{12}, with and without omega-3 fatty acids versus placebo on reducing the risk of recurrent ischaemic disease (Galan et al., 2003). However, more than one RCT is needed to test these hypotheses. Finally, the RCT have tested the effect of supplementation of the B vitamins on preventing recurrent disease, but not primary prevention. Epidemiologic evidence has shown, however, the cardiovascular benefits of a dietary pattern rich in fruit, vegetables, grain products and fish/seafood – foods that are rich in folate, vitamin B_6 and omega-3 fatty acids (Appel et al., 1997; Steffen et al., 2007).

21.10 Conclusions

Homocysteine is a risk factor for vascular disease and neural tube defects. Meta-analysis of the observational studies on homocysteine concentrations and risk of vascular events showed that a 5 µmol l^{-1} increase in homocysteine level conferred a 9–18% increase in risk for CHD, independent of CHD risk factors (Ganji and Kafai et al., 2006; Humphrey et al., 2008). Further, intakes of dietary folate or folic acid supplementation have been shown to lower homocysteine levels in adolescents and adults, both young and old. However, results have been null in the majority of RCT testing the effectiveness of folate, vitamin B_6 and vitamin B_{12} supplementation to reduce the risk of recurrent CHD, stroke, and VTE, as well as cognitive function or dementia. However, vitamin B supplementation may prevent the incidence of stroke events. Several RCT with large sample sizes are currently under way, and these may soon provide a definitive answer to these significant public health problems.

Although national folic acid fortification in the United States has been associated with over 50% lower prevalence of NTD, there are potentially other modifiable risk factors that may be targeted, including maternal status of obesity, diabetes and vitamin B_{12} status, to further reduce the risk of NTD. Large epidemiologic studies are warranted to further elucidate its multiple causes.

References

Aisen, P.S., Schneider, L.S., Sano, M., Dian-Arrastia, R., van Dyck, C.H. Weiner, M.F., Bottiglieri, T., et al. (2008) High-dose B vitamin supplementation and cognitive decline in Alzheimer disease: A randomized controlled trial. *Journal of the American Medical Association* 300, 1774–1783.

Albert, C.M., Cook, N.R., Gaziano, J.M., Danielson, E., Buring, J.E. and Manson, J.E. (2008) Effect of folic acid and B-vitamins on risk of cardiovascular events and total mortality among women at high risk for cardiovascular disease: A randomized trial. *Journal of the American Medical Association* 299, 2027–2036.

Appel, L.J., Moore, T.J. and Obarzanek, E. (1997) A clinical trial of the effects of dietary patterns on blood pressure. *New England Journal of Medicine* 336, 1117–1124.

Bazzano, L.A., Reynolds, K., Holder, K.N. and He, J. (2006) Effect of folic acid supplementation on risk of cardiovascular diseases: A meta-analysis of randomized controlled trials. *Journal of the American Medical Association* 296, 2720–2726.

Blom, H.J. (2009) Folic acid, methylation and neural tube closure in humans. *Birth Defects Research Part A: Clinical and Molecular Teratology* 85, 295–302.

Bonaa, K.H., Njolstad, I., Ueland, P.M., Schirmer, H., Tverdal, A., Steigen, T., Wang, H., Nordrehaug, J.E., Arnesen, E. and Rasmussen, K. (2006) Homocysteine lowering and cardiovascular events after acute myocardial infarction. *New England Journal of Medicine* 354, 1578–1588.

Boushey, C.J., Beresford, S.A., Omenn, G.S. and Motulsky, A.G. (1995) A quantitative assessment of plasma homocysteine as a risk factor for vascular disease: probable benefits of increasing folate acid intakes. *Journal of the American Medical Association* 274, 1049–1057.

Das, U.N. (2008) Folic acid and polyunsaturated fatty acids improve cognitive function and prevent depression, dementia, and Alzheimer's disease – But how and why? *Prostaglandins, Leukotrienes and Essential Fatty Acids* 78, 11–19.

den Heijer, M., Lewington, S. and Clarke, R. (2005) Homocysteine, MTHFR and risk of venous thromboembolism: a meta-analysis of published epidemiological studies. *Journal of Thrombosis and Haemostasis* 3, 292–299.

den Heijer, M., Willems, H.P.J., Blom, H.J., Gerrits, W.B.J., Cattaneo, M., Eichinger, S., Rosendaal, R.R. and Box, G.M.J. (2007) Homocysteine lowering by B vitamins and the secondary prevention of deep vein thrombosis and pulmonary embolism: a randomized, placebo-controlled, double-blind trial. *Blood* 109, 139–144.

Desouza, C., Keebler, M., McNamara, D.B. and Fonseca, V. (2002) Drugs affecting homocysteine metabolism: impact on cardiovascular risk. *Drugs* 62, 605–616.

Durga, J., Boxtel, M.P.J., Schouten, E.G., Kok, F.J., Jolles, J., Katan, M.B. and Verhoef, P. (2007) Effect of 3-year folic acid supplementation on cognitive function in older adults in the FACIT trial: a randomized, double blind, controlled trial. *Lancet* 369, 208–216.

Du Vigneaud V. (1952) *A Trail of Research in Sulfur Chemistry and Metabolism*. Cornell University Press, Ithaca, NY, pp. 25–56.

Ebbing, M., Bleie, Ø., Ueland, P.M., Nordrehaug, J.E., Nilsen, D.W., Vollset, S.E., Refsum, H., Redersen, E.K.R. and Nygard, O. (2008) Mortality and cardiovascular events in patients treated with homocysteine-lowering B vitamins after coronary angiography. *Journal of the American Medical Association* 300, 795–804.

Eikelboom, J.W., Lonn, E., Genest, J., Hankey, G. and Yusuf, S. (1999) Homocyst(e)ine and cardiovascular disease: A critical review of the epidemiologic evidence. *Annals of Internal Medicine* 131, 363–375.

Galan, P., de Bree, A., Mennen, L., Potier de Courcy, G., Preziozi, P., Bertrais, S., Castetbon, K., et al. (2003) Background and rationale of the SU.FOL.OM3 study: double-blind randomized placebo-controlled secondary prevention trial to test the impact of supplementation with folate, vitamin B6 and B12 and/or omega-3 fatty acids on the prevention of recurrent ischemic events in subjects with atherosclerosis in the coronary or cerebral arteries. *Journal of Nutrition, Health, and Aging* 7, 428–435.

Ganji, V. and Kafai, M.R. (2005) Population references for plasma total homocysteine concentrations for U.S. children and adolescents in the post-folic acid fortification era. *Journal of Nutrition* 135, 2253–2256.

Ganji, V. and Kafai, M.R. (2006) Population references for plasma total homocysteine concentrations in U.S. adults after the fortification of cereals with folic acid. *American Journal of Clinical Nutrition* 84, 989–994.

Gao, X., Yao, M., McCrory, M.A., Ma, G., Li, Y., Roberts, S.B. and Tucker, K.L. (2003) Dietary pattern is associated with homocysteine and B vitamin status in an urban Chinese population. *Journal of Nutrition* 133, 3636–3642.

Gueant, J.L., Gueant-Rodriguez, R.M., Anello, G., Bosco, R., Brunaud, L., Romano, C., Ferri, R., et al. (2003) Genetic determinants of folate and vitamin B12 metabolism: A common pathway in neural tube defect and down syndrome. *Clinical Chemistry and Laboratory Medicine* 41, 1473–1477.

Haan, M.N., Miller, J.W., Aiello, A.E., Whitner, R.A., Jagust, W.J., Mungas, D.M., Allen, L.H., et al. (2007) Homocysteine, B vitamins, and the incidence of dementia and cognitive impairment: results from the Sacramento Area Latino Study on Aging. *American Journal of Clinical Nutrition* 85, 511–517.

Hengstermann, S., Laemmler, G., Hanemann, A., Schweter, A., Steinhagen-Thiessen, E., Lun, A. and Schulz, R.-J. (2009) Total serum homocysteine levels do not identify cognitive dysfunction in multi-morbid elderly patients. *Journal of Nutrition, Health & Aging* 13, 121–126.

Herrmann W. (2001) The importance of hyperhomocysteinemia as a risk factor for diseases: an overview. *Clinical Chemistry in Laboratory Medicine* 39, 666–674.

Homocysteine Lowering Trialists' Collaboration (1998) Lowering blood homocysteine with folic acid based supplements: meta-analysis of randomised trials. *British Medical Journal* 316, 894–898.

Homocysteine Studies Collaboration (2002) Homocysteine and risk of ischemic heart disease and stroke: a meta-analysis. *Journal of the American Medical Association*, 288, 2015–2022.

HOPE (Heart Outcomes Prevention Evaluation) 2 investigators (2006) Homocysteine lowering with folic acid and B vitamins in vascular disease. *New England Journal of Medicine* 354, 1567–177.

Humphrey, L.L., Fu, R., Rogers, K., Freeman, M. and Helfand, M. (2008) Homocysteine level and coronary heart disease incidence: a systematic review and meta-analysis. *Mayo Clinic Proceedings* 83, 1203–1212.

Jacques, P.J., Rosenberg, I.H., Rogers, G., Selhub, J., Bowman, B.A., Gunter, E.W., Wright, J.D., et al. (1999a) Serum total homocysteine concentrations in adolescent and adult American: results from the third National Health and Nutrition Examination Survey. *American Journal of Clinical Nutrition* 69, 482–489.

Jacques, P.J., Selhub, J., Bostom, A.G., Wilson, P.W. and Rosenberg, I.H. (1999b) The effect of folic acid fortification on plasma folate and total homocysteine concentrations. *New England Journal of Medicine* 340, 1449–1454.

Janson, J.J., Galarza, C.R., Murua, A., Quintana, I., Przygoda, P.A., Waisman, G., Camera, L., et al. (2002) Prevalence of hyperhomocysteinemia in an elderly population. *American Journal of Hypertension* 15, 394–397.

Lee, M., Hong, K.-S., Chang, S.-C. and Saver, J.L. (2010) Efficacy of homocysteine-lowering therapy with folic acid in stroke prevention. *Stroke* 41, 1205–1212.

Liem, A., Reynierse-Buitenwerf, G.H., Zwinderman A.H., Jukema, J.W. and van Veldhuisen, D.J. (2003) Secondary prevention with folic acid: effects on clinical outcomes. *Journal of the American College of Cardiology* 41, 2105–2113.

Liem, A., Reynierse-Buitenwerf, G.H., Zwinderman, A.H., Jukema, J.W. and van Veldhuisen, D.J. (2005) Secondary prevention with folic acid: results of the GOES extension study. *Heart* 91, 1213–1214.

Lighart, S.A., van Charante, E.P.M., Van Gool, W.A. and Richard E. (2010) Treatment of cardiovascular risk factors to prevent cognitive decline and dementia: a systematic review. *Vascular Health and Risk Management*, 6, 775–785.

Lutsey, P.L. Steffen, L.M., Feldman, H.A., Hoelscher, D.H., Webber, L.S., Luepker, R.V., Lytle, L.A., et al. (2006) Serum homocysteine is related to food intake in adolescents: the Child and Adolescent Trial for Cardiovascular Health. *American Journal of Clinical Nutrition* 83, 1380–1386.

Makris, M. (2000) Hyperhomocysteinemia and thrombosis. *Clinical and Laboratory Haemotology* 22, 133–143.

Malinow, M.R., Bostom, A.G. and Krauss, R.M. (1999) Homocyst(e)ine, diet, and cardiovascular diseases: a statement for healthcare professionals from the Nutrition Committee, American Heart Association. *Circulation* 99, 178–182.

Marti-Carvajal, A.J., Sola, I., Lathyris, D. and Salanti G. (2009) Homocysteine lowering interventions for preventing cardiovascular events. *Cochrane Database of Systematic Reviews* Issue 4. Art. No.: CD006612. DOI: 10.1002/14651858.CD006612.pub2.

McCully, K.S. (1969) Vascular pathology of homocysteinemia: implications for the pathogenesis of arteriosclerosis. *American Journal of Pathology* 56, 111–128.

McCully, K.S. (1993) Chemical pathology of homocysteine. I. Atherogenesis. *Annals of Clinical Laboratory Science* 23, 477–493.

McCully, K.S. (2005) Hyperhomocysteinemia and arteriosclerosis: historical perspectives. *Clinical Chemistry and Laboratory Medicine* 43, 980–986.

Mezzano D., Kosiel, K., Martínez, C., Cuevas, A., Panes, O., Aranda, E., Strobel, P., *et al.* (2000) Cardiovascular risk factors in vegetarians: normalization of hyperhomocysteinemia with vitamin B12 and reduction of platelet aggregation with n-3 fatty acids. *Thrombosis Research* 100, 153–160.

Molloy, A.M., Kirke, P.N., Troendle, J.F., Burke, H., Sutton, M., Brody, L.C., Scott, J.M., *et al.* (2009) Maternal vitamin B12 status and risk of neural tube defects in a population with high neural tube defect prevalence and no folic acid fortification. *Pediatrics* 123, 917–923.

Morris, M.S., Jacques, P.F., Selhub, J. and Rosenberg, I.H. (2000) Total homocysteine and estrogen status indicators in the Third National Health and Examination Survey. *American Journal of Epidemiology* 152, 140–148.

Murua, A., Quintana, I., Galarza, C., Alfie, J. and Kordich, L. (2001) Unsuspected hyperhomocysteinemia in chronically anticoagulated patients. *Blood Coagulation and Fibrinolysis* 12, 79–80.

Nestel, P.J., Chronopoulos, A. and Cehun, M. (2003) Arterial stiffness is rapidly induced by raising plasma homocysteine concentration with methionine. *Atherosclerosis* 171, 83–86.

Nygard, O., Vollset, S.E., Refsum, H., Stensvold, I., Tverdal, A., Nordrehaug, J.E., Ueland, P.M., *et al.* (1995) Total plasma homocysteine and cardiovascular risk profile: The Hordaland Homocysteine Study. *Journal of the American Medical Association* 274, 1526–1533.

O'Callaghan, P., Meleady, R., Fitzgerald, T., Graham, I., *et al.* (2002) Smoking and plasma homocysteine. *European Heart Journal* 23, 1580–1586.

Plassman, B.L., Langa, K.M., Fisher, G.G., Heeringa, S.G., Weir, D.R., Ofstedal, M.B., Burke, J.R., *et al.* (2007) Prevalence of dementia in the United States: The Aging, Demographics, and Memory Study. *Neuroepidemiology* 29, 125–132.

Rimm, E.B., Willett, W.C., Hu, F.B., Sampson, L., Colditz, G.A., Manson, J.E., Hennekens, C., *et al.* (1998) Folate and vitamin B6 from diet and supplements in relation to risk of coronary heart disease among women. *Journal of the American Medical Association* 279, 359–364.

SEARCH (Study of the Effectiveness of Additional Reductions in Cholesterol and Homocysteine) Collaborative Group (2010) Effects of homocysteine-lowering with folic acid plus vitamin B12 vs. placebo on mortality and major morbidity in myocardial infarction survivors. *Journal of the American Medical Association* 303, 2486–2494.

Selhub, J. (1999) Homocysteine metabolism. *Annual Review of Nutrition* 19, 217–246.

Selhub, J., Jacques, P.F., Wilson, P.W., Rush, D. and Rosenberg, I.H. (1993) Vitamin status and intake as primary determinants of homocysteinemia in an elderly population. *Journal of the American Medical Association* 270, 2693–2698.

Steffen, L.M., Jacobs, D.R. Jr, Stevens, J., Shahar, E., Carithers, T. and Folsom, A.R. (2003) Associations of whole-grain, refined grain, and fruit and vegetable consumption with risk of all-cause mortality and incident coronary heart disease and ischemic stroke: The Atherosclerosis Risk in Communities (ARIC) Study. *American Journal of Clinical Nutrition* 78, 383–390.

Steffen, L.M., Folsom, A.R., Cushman, M., Jacobs, D.R. Jr, and Rosamond, W.D. (2007) Greater fish, fruit, and vegetable intakes are related to lower incidence of venous thromboembolism. The Longitudinal Investigation of Thromboembolism Etiology. *Circulation* 115, 188–195.

Sun, Y., Lu, C.-J., Chien, K.-L., Chen, S.-T. and Chen, R.-C. (2007) Efficacy of multivitamin supplementation containing vitamins B6 and B12 and folic acid as adjunctive treatment with a cholinesterase inhibitor in Alzheimer's Disease: A 26-week, randomized, double-blind, placebo-controlled study in Taiwanese patients. *Clinical Therapeutics* 29, 2204–2214.

Toole, J.F., Malinow, R., Chambless, L.E., Spence, J.D., Pettigrew, L.C., Howard, V.J., Sides, E.G., *et al.* (2004) Lowering homocysteine in patients with ischemic stroke to prevent recurrent stroke, myocardial infarction, and death: The Vitamin Intervention for Stroke Prevention (VISP) Randomized Controlled Trial. *Journal of the American Medical Association* 291, 565–575.

Tucker, K.L., Olson, B., Bakun, P., Dallal, G.E., Selhub, J. and Rosenberg, I.H. (2004) Breakfast cereal fortified with folic acid, vitamin B-6, and vitamin B-12 increased vitamin concentrations and reduces homocysteine concentrations: a randomized trial. *American Journal of Clinical Nutrition* 79, 805–811.

Van Dam, F. and Van Gool, W.A. (2009) Hyperhomocysteinemia and Alzheimer's disease: A systematic review. *Archives of Gerontology and Geriatrics* 48, 425–430.

van Guldener, C. (2006) Why is homocysteine elevated in renal failure and what can be expected from homocysteine-lowering? *Nephrology Dialysis Transplantation* 21, 1161–1166.

VITATOPS Trial Study Group (2010) B vitamins in patients with recent transcient ischaemic attack or stroke in the VITAmins TO Prevent Stroke (VITATOPS) trial: a randomized, double-blind, parallel, placebo-controlled trial. *Lancet Neurology* 9, 855–865.

Wald, D.S., Law, M. and Morris, J.K. (2002) Homocysteine and cardiovascular disease: evidence on causality from a meta-analysis. *British Medical Journal* 325, 1202–1206.

Wald, D.S., Kasturiratne, A. and Simmonds, M. (2010) Effect of folic acid, with or without other B vitamins, on cognitive decline: Meta-analysis of randomized trials. *American Journal of Medicine* 123, 522–527.

Wang, X., Qin, X., Demirtas, H., Li, J., Mao, G., Huo, Y., Sun, N., *et al.* (2007) Efficacy of folic acid supplementation in stroke population: a meta-analysis. *Lancet* 369, 1876–1882.

Williams, L.J., Rasmussen, S.A., Flores, A., Kirby, R.S. and Edmonds, L.D. (2005) Decline in the prevalence of spina bifida and anencephaly by race/ethnicity: 1995-2002. *Pediatrics* 116, 753–755.

Wright, A.D., Martin, N. and Dodson P.M. (2008) Homocysteine, folates, and the eye. *Eye* 22, 989–993.

22 Modified Amino Acid-Based Molecules: Accumulation and Health Implications

S. Bengmark*

Division of Surgery and Interventional Science, University College London, London, UK

22.1 Abstract

Industrial processing of food has not only improved the management and safety of foods, but also its taste. Unfortunately however, most of these processes – including plant breeding, gene manipulation, fractionation, separation, condensation, drying, freezing, heating, irradiation, roasting, microwaving, toasting, smoking, emulsification and homogenization – appear to be negative, as they reduce the nutritional quality of the food and also contribute significantly to increased vulnerability to development of diseases, especially those referred to as endemic and chronic.

This chapter deals especially with the negative consequences of heating and mainly with the impact of heat-produced glycated and lipoxidated molecules, often referred to as Maillard products. These products are more specifically referred to as advanced glycation end-products (AGE) and advanced lipoxidation end-products (ALE). The negative effects on health of other heat-produced compounds, such as heterocyclic aromatic amines, are outside the scope of this review.

Modern molecular biology has made it possible to explore the impact of these and other process-induced molecules on the body and its functions. The detection in 1992 of a specific receptor in the body for such products provided the opportunity for a better understanding of their effects in health and disease. This receptor for advanced glycation end products (RAGE) is recognized as a key member of the immunoglobulin superfamily of cell surface molecules. It functions as a master switch, induces sustained activation of NF-κB, suppresses a series of endogenous autoregulatory functions, and converts long-lasting pro-inflammatory signals into sustained cellular dysfunction and disease. Its activation is associated with much increased levels of dysfunctioning proteins in body fluids and tissues, and is strongly associated with a series of diseases from allergy and Alzheimer's disease to rheumatoid arthritis and urogenital disorders. It is important to observe that heat treatment and other forms of processing of foods will dramatically increase the content of these dysfunctional molecules, and thereby, with time, significantly contribute to the epidemic of chronic diseases seen around the world. An increased

---

* E-mail address: stig@bengmark.se

consumption of raw foods, fruits and vegetables; foods rich in polyphenols and other antioxidants; as well as live bacteria, probiotics and plant fibre seems appropriate in order to counteract these undesirable developments.

22.2 Introduction

Modern food is often extensively processed prior to distribution and sale. Drying, freezing, heating, irradiation, roasting, microwaving, toasting, emulsifying, homogenizing and the addition of numerous compounds are all aimed at enhancing the appeal of the food, its palatability and its shelf-life. The effects of each of these manipulations on human health are not fully explored, and even when documented, often not considered to the extent they should be, either by industry or the consumer.

Heating food to higher temperatures is generally regarded to improve both the taste and smell of the foods we eat. High temperature makes food proteins change structure: coagulate, aggregate and produce crusts. Modern food chemists, chefs and cooks use this information every day to produce delicious new foods.

The French biochemist Louis-Camille Maillard described the chemical process which occurs non-enzymatically in foods (Maillard, 1912), and which is much accelerated by heating. This process is now referred to as the Maillard reaction and its products collectively named Maillard products. Reducing sugars (fructose, glucose, glyceraldehyde, lactose, arabinose and maltose) will during the process bind to amino acids, nucleic acids, including DNA, RNA, peptides and proteins, to produce transitional compounds, most often referred to as Amadori products. In time these undergo complex changes: cyclization, dehydration, oxidation, condensation, cross-linking and polymerization, to form irreversible chemical products. In particular, reactive carbonyls such as glyoxal and methylglyoxal have been found to rapidly modify reactive side chains of proteins. Important amino acids such as lysine (essential amino acid) and histidine (essential for children) are often involved.

During the process significant amounts of pigments (melanoids) but also thousands of often good-tasting and good-smelling so-called volatile compounds will be released. These pigments often make the food or parts of the food look brown or black, which is why the process is sometimes referred to as 'browning'. Common browning products are bread crusts and roasted surfaces of fried meat and fish, all sorts of broths, irrespective of vegetable or animal origin, and all smoked food, as well as Asian sauces, balsamic products, Chinese soy, and cola products, all rich in brown/black Maillard products. But not all Maillard products are dark in colour; there are also white Maillard products, especially dairy products such as cheese and powdered milk. Maillard himself suggested that the Maillard process might be negative to health, as these products will accumulate in the body, as we now know, for many years and sometimes for the rest of life. The process might also reduce the availability in the body of important and essential amino acids.

22.3 Effects of Heating on Food Quality

Heat-induced alterations of foods are considered to commence at around 28°C – the highest processing temperature allowed for olive oil to be called virgin. Most enzymes in foods become deactivated after approximately 42°C. Some antioxidants are resistant to heat but a majority will disappear in the interval 30°–100°C, and almost all during microwaving. The heat-enhanced production of Maillard products – glycated and lipoxidated molecules – is said to start and accelerate from around 80°C. Similarly the heat-induced production of carcinogens such as heterocyclic amines is said to start from the interval 100°–130°C, after which the production accelerates dramatically.

Maillard products based on association of carbonyl groups in sugars and proteins are collectively referred to as AGE. Similar products, formed between reactive fatty acids and proteins, are referred to as ALE. Numerous such synthetic products are now identified, but two or three previously unknown compounds are each year added to the list. The most commonly studied AGE are pentosidine, N^ε-carboxymethyl-lysine (CML) and N^ε-(carboxyethyl)lysine (CEL).

It is important to note that the production of both AGE and ALE are not dependent on enzymes. The intensity in their production increases, not only with increase in temperature, but also with length of storage at elevated temperatures, and even at room temperature. The content of the AGE furosine increases dramatically with heat treatment such as pasteurization and especially with the production and storage of powdered milk (Baptista and Carvalho, 2004). Other industrial practices commonly used in food processing such as irradiation, ionization, microwaving and smoking also contribute significantly to increased production of AGE/ALE. Vegetable-based foods are no exception – industrial treatment of plant products, such as roasting, drying and 'curing' will lead to amounts of AGE/ALE that are as great as those found in animal products. One such example is roasted peanuts.

Fresh tobacco leaves, fresh coffee beans, and fresh peanuts are rich in powerful antioxidants, most of which will disappear during the industrial process ('curing', roasting) and be replaced by often large amounts of AGE/ALE. As the temperature increases above 130°C, carcinogens, especially heterocyclic amines, will also be produced, and their production increases dramatically as the temperature increases. AGE/ALE will not exclusively reach the body through the food we eat, or the smoke we inhale – they are also produced spontaneously in the body, especially in the presence of increased levels of sugars and fatty acids in body fluids and tissues, and in those suffering chronic diseases such as diabetes and chronic renal diseases.

22.4 AGE/ALE Accumulation in the Body

The accumulation of late/matured Maillard products – AGE/ALE – in the body is in principle irreversible; what is accumulated in the tissues persists for a very long time and most often forever. Hitherto, the finding of larger amounts of AGE/ALE in the tissues of elderly individuals has simply been regarded as a normal effect of ageing. However, it might not be so. Instead it might mainly be a result of the lifestyle chosen, smoking, and eating habits, and thus in theory preventable. Large to extreme increases in AGE/ALE are regularly observed in body fluids and tissues of patients with chronic diseases, particularly those with diabetes and chronic renal diseases, and in patients suffering complications of these diseases. It is commonly observed in diabetic patients, who suffer from reduced wound healing (Peppa et al., 2003), retinopathy, nephropathy (Zheng et al., 2002), and angiopathy (Vlassara et al., 2002; Lin et al., 2003). Accumulation of AGE/ALE in tissues is seen as intracellular or extracellular deposits referred to as tau proteins, amyloid β proteins (Smith et al., 1994) and in neurofibrillary tangles (Smith et al., 1994; Vitek et al., 1994). Such depositions in various body tissues were long regarded as degenerative but biologically inert structures. However, increasing evidence supports the conclusion that these structures are foci with very strong pro-inflammatory potential, which maintain the systemic chronic inflammation at a high level in the tissues, and thereby accelerate further production of AGE/ALE and exacerbation of disease.

22.5 Modern Molecular Biology: Essential for Understanding the Effects of AGE/ALE

Almost 100 years ago, Maillard suggested that accumulation in the body of AGE/ALE would significantly contribute to the progression of diseases, especially of chronic urinogenital diseases, and in particular uraemia. He created what he called an 'index of urinogenital imperfection', which he used to document the association between the degree of accumulation in the body of Maillard products and the severity of disease, especially chronic renal disease.

The time was, however, not opportune for such radical thinking, and the concept was largely ignored by scientists and clinicians of the time, remaining so for several decades to come. It was the introduction of modern molecular biology and particularly the identification of specific receptors in the body for these substances that would dramatically change the attitude and interest in these substances by both biologists and physicians. The turning point seems to be the identification in 1992 by the American Ann Marie Schmidt of a specific receptor for AGE/ALE named RAGE (Schmidt et al., 1992, 1993, 1994a,b). Since then increasing numbers of publications have appeared in the literature. From the year 2000, several international scientific organizations have become involved in the concept, arranging special symposia on RAGE and AGE/ALE, and publishing special issues relating to these topics. New societies have also been founded with the aim of specifically investigating the effects of food-derived AGE/ALE on health and well-being. The New York Academy of Science seems to have taken the lead and many scientific contributions on AGE/ALE are published each year in its *Annals*. Searches on PubMed relating to AGE and ALE reveal more than 5000 publications, of which more than 25% appeared in 2009. In addition almost 20,000 titles on PubMed are about glycated haemoglobin, HbA_{1c}.

Several methods are available for the measurement of content of AGE/ALE in body fluids and tissues: immunohistochemistry with polyclonal or monoclonal antibodies, high performance liquid chromatography (HPLC), and mass spectrography. A majority of these substances are auto-fluorescing even if not visible to the human eye, and so can be used for diagnostic purposes (Meerwaldt et al., 2005a,b). The fluorescence has its maximum at wavelengths between 350 and 440 nm (Meerwaldt, 2005b). Often-studied substances such as CML and CEL do not, unfortunately, show any fluorescing ability, nor do they have any colour. Despite this, measuring fluorescence is an excellent tool for clinical use, especially for screening of individuals with suspected high levels of AGE/ALE in the body, but also for screening of foods suspected to be rich in such dysfunctional proteins.

22.6 RAGE: a Master Switch and Key to Inflammation

RAGE is a prominent member of what has been called the immunoglobulin superfamily of cell-surface molecules. It is described as a 'master switch' with the ability to coordinate the inflammatory reaction in the body. RAGE induces a long-lasting activation of the pro-inflammatory transcription factor NF-κB and suppresses a series of endogenous auto-regulatory functions (Bierhaus et al., 2001, 2005a; Schmidt et al., 2001; Vlassara, 2005). Increased deposition of AGE/ALE in the tissues is suggested to be a key element in the development of the so-called metabolic syndrome (Koyama et al., 2005; Soldatos et al., 2005). Accumulation of AGE/ALE and subsequent activation of RAGE is reported to induce a significant down-regulation of leptin in adipose cells (Unno et al., 2004). RAGE activation induces effects on a great variety of tissues, but they are particularly pronounced in endothelial cells, where increased expression occurs of a long row of molecules such as VCAM-1, ICAM-1, E-selektin, eNOS and TGF-β. TNF-α, Il-6, PAI-1 and VEGF are seen (Bohlender et al., 2005). Strong RAGE-induced effects are often observed on immune cells, macrophages (Sunahori et al., 2006), and dendritic cells (de Leeuw et al., 2005; Ge et al., 2005), but also on smooth muscle, particularly in the walls of blood vessels, under the mucosa and in the skin (Aronson, 2003). These changes are associated with subsequent reduction in regenerative capacity and function of the cells, increased blood pressure, and development of chronic diseases and/or exacerbation of complications to chronic diseases (Monnier et al., 2005). However, the conditions vary from tissue to tissue, the most sensitive and vulnerable being those with low regenerative capacity and long-lived cells such as myelin- and collagen-rich structures, where the substances are likely to remain. Among these are brain, peripheral nerves, skeleton, muscles, tendons, joints, skin and eye, especially the lens.

Research in recent years has also demonstrated the existence of an endogenous soluble form of RAGE known as sRAGE, which has an important effect as a decoy for RAGE and has been shown to prevent accumulation of RAGE in body tissues (Bierhaus et al., 2005b). This suggests that chronic diseases are not only associated with increased levels of RAGE in the body, but also, and probably as important, with low levels of sRAGE.

22.7 Factors Underlying Enhanced Systemic Inflammation

The largest part of the immune system is, in contrast to what was earlier believed, to be found in the gastrointestinal (GI) system (Brandtzaeg *et al.*, 1989) as 70–80% of the Ig-producing cells are located within the GI tract. This explains why the food we eat has such a profound influence on our well-being and health. Although AGE/ALE seem to play a major role, it is also clear that numerous other food-related factors will influence the degree of systemic inflammation in the body, the sensitivity to develop disease and our daily well-being. Increasing evidence suggests that all these factors are additive and collectively contribute to development of a sustained, long-lasting, often discrete and unrecognized, exaggerated stage of inflammation in the body, commonly seen before and when a chronic disease is manifest. Such factors are:

- *Low vitamin D status*. There is a strong correlation between the level of vitamin D in the body, degree of inflammation and incidence of chronic diseases. Individuals living at higher latitudes such as Canada, Russia and Scandinavia, but also countries in the Southern hemisphere, such as Argentina, New Zealand and Uruguay are reported to have generally lower levels of vitamin D in serum, especially during the winter season. This phenomenon is associated with higher incidence of coronary–vascular diseases, acute coronary events (Zittermann *et al.*, 2005; McCarty, 2005) and other chronic diseases such as cancer (Mohr *et al.*, 2006, 2007, 2008).
- *Low levels in the body of antioxidants such as folic acid and glutathione, and increased levels of homocysteine*. Increase in serum levels of homocysteine is regularly associated with increased levels of systemic inflammation and chronic diseases (Mattson, 2003).
- *Impaired hormonal homeostasis*. Ageing as well as chronic diseases are commonly accompanied by hormonal disturbances of various kinds, sometimes to the extent that ageing has been referred to as a state of 'hormonal chaos' (Hertoghe, 2005). Hormonal disturbances are often accompanied by increased oxidative stress/increased release of free radicals, intracellular accumulation of 'waste products', inhibition of apoptosis, disturbed repair mechanisms, reduced gene polymorphism, premature shortening of telomeres and reduced immune defence. Reduced resistance to disease is often observed in premature ageing as well as in several chronic diseases (Hertoghe, 2005). In particular, 17β-estradiol, plentiful in dairy products, is known to induce a strong activation of RAGE mRNA in endothelial cells. This effect is abolished if an anti-oestrogen such as 4-OH tamoxiphen is supplied (Yamagishi *et al.*, 1998, Suzuma *et al.*, 1999). An impaired hormonal homeostasis is suggested to explain why chronic diseases are often aggravated during pregnancy, frequently seen as vascular and eye complications to diabetes (Suzuma *et al.*, 1999). Physical as well as mental stress also contributes to activation of RAGE, and increased release of noradrenaline is reported to reduce immune defence and increases sensibility to acquire infections by up to 4 logs (Cooper, 1946). Increased release of noradrenaline in the intestine will dramatically reduce the beneficial intestinal flora, and increase the virulence of potentially pathogenic micro-organisms (Kinney *et al.*, 2000; Alverdy *et al.*, 2003), changes, which most likely also contribute to increased RAGE activation. Permanently increased levels of noradrenaline are reported in chronic diseases such as Alzheimer's disease and also found to correlate well with severity of the disease (Peskind *et al.*, 1998). Parathyroid hormones constitute another example of hormones deeply involved in the inflammatory process. Significant elevations in IL-6 are observed in hyperparathyroidism as in other chronic conditions with increased systemic inflammation such as obesity (Flyvbjerg *et al.*, 2004).
- *Angiotensin/renin*. Oxidative stress and increased systemic inflammation is also strongly associated with increased release

of angiotensin, increased levels of free fatty acids in serum, and with reduction in beta-cell function in diabetes (Flyvbjerg et al., 2004; Allen et al., 2005; Tikellis et al., 2006). The observation that blockage of the angiotensin receptor will reduce production and accumulation of AGE both in vitro and in vivo is of great interest (Allen et al., 2005).

- *Larger intake of glutenoids.* Glutenoids are increasingly regarded as pro-inflammatory in the body (Tlaskalová-Hogenová et al., 2005), and suggested to occur even in the absence of intestinal changes (Brady and Hoggan, 2002; Sbarbati et al., 2003).
- *Low intake of plant antioxidants.*
- *High intake of carbohydrates.*
- *High intake of saturated and trans fatty acids.* A strong association is repeatedly documented between the average content of fat in food and morbidity and/or mortality in chronic diseases in a country, as demonstrated for breast cancer (Carroll, 1975), as well as other cancers and also chronic diseases such as coronary heart disease (Artaud-Wild et al., 1993; Moss and Freed, 1999) and diabetes (Dahl-Jorgensen et al., 1991). More than three quarters of the saturated fat consumed is of bovine origin, and thus it is not surprising that the incidence of various chronic diseases also correlates well with the amount of dairy products consumed (Ganmaa et al., 2002).

stronger pro-inflammatory effects such as high-fructose corn syrup (HFCS), seems to make the situation even worse. In the United States, the intake of HFCS in carbonated drinks and fast foods now exceeds that of sucrose (Gaby, 2005).

A recent study in mice is of particular interest. Over 4 months, RAGE knockout (KO) mice received either a standard diet (7% fat) or a Western 'fast-food'-like diet (21% fat) and were compared to wild-type mice, receiving the same diet. The Western-food-like diet was associated with significant cardiac hypertrophy, inflammation, mitochondrial-dependent superoxide production and accumulation of AGE in both strains, but significantly less in the RAGE-KO mice. Both strains demonstrated reduced levels of inflammation and oxidative stress, in association with reductions in AGE as well as RAGE on supply of an AGE inhibitor (alagebrium chloride, 1 mg kg^{-1} day^{-1} (Tikellis et al., 2008).

Much can be learnt from studies of Japan, which has during the last 50–60 years made similar, although not as extensive, changes in food habits as the West. The incidence of several chronic diseases has increased dramatically during this time. As an example, the incidence of prostate cancer has increased 25-fold during the last 50 years, much in parallel with an increase in the consumption of industrially produced agricultural foods: 7 times more eggs, 9 times as much meat, and 20 times as much dairy product (Ganmaa et al., 2002, 2003).

22.8 Dietary Choice

The incidence of most chronic diseases has increased dramatically during the last 150 years, much of it in parallel with the significantly altered intake of foods which has occurred since the year 1850: a doubling of intake of saturated fat, 50% reduction in intake of omega-3 fatty acids, and a more than doubling in intake of omega-6 fatty acids (Leaf and Weber, 1988). The intake of refined sugar has during the same time period increased from approximately 0.5 kg to about 50–60 kg per person per year. Furthermore, the transition in use of carbohydrates with

22.9 Dairy in Focus

Commonly, 10–20% and sometimes up to 70% of the amino acid lysine is reported to be modified during the common industrial treatment of milk (including sterilization, pasteurization and irradiation). Fructoselysine is the dominating modified molecule, but CML and pyrraline are also produced during the processing of milk. Sugar content, the level and time of elevated temperature, and storage time are the main factors behind the increased production of AGE/ALE in milk products.

Not only the industrial treatment of dairy products but also the feeds given to the cows have changed dramatically during the 20th century – from mainly forage-based to starch-rich and fast-absorbed carbohydrates such as corn, maize grains, barley, molasses and dextrose. Intensive feeding of cows with carbohydrates induces insulin resistance in animals as well as in humans. Should the animals be allowed to live long enough they would also show the same symptoms of Western diseases including manifest diabetes. It has been demonstrated that milk- and lactose-fed calves show signs of insulin resistance at a young age (Hostettler-Allen et al., 1994).

High levels of pro-inflammatory cytokines and various stress hormones are regularly observed in intensively fed animals. No information is available in the literature, however, to support the notion that elevated inflammatory molecules are transferred to humans by meat and dairy products from such animals. Today's dairy products come, much in contrast to the old days, up to about 80%, from pregnant cows, and consequently are rich in growth factors and various hormones, especially sex hormones (Malekinejad et al., 2006), some of which (like 17β-oestradiol) are potentially pro-inflammatory and carcinogenic. It is suggested that dairy-derived hormones and growth factors are important pathogenetic factors behind the development of hormone-dependent cancers, especially of the colon, prostate and breast (Outwater et al., 1997). These hormones follow the fat fraction and are thus more concentrated in condensed products such as butter, cheese, and powdered milk.

It has been demonstrated that vegans, in great contrast to meat-eaters and lacto-vegetarians, have lower levels of AGE/ALE. Lacto-vegetarians seem to have even higher levels of AGE/ALE than meat-eaters (Sebekova et al., 2001), which might be explained by a higher intake of dairy products, especially cheese, to compensate for not eating lean meat, but which might also be due to a higher intake of fructose. Significant health advantages are reported for vegans: lower levels of pro-inflammatory molecules, cytokines and acute phase proteins; lower systolic and diastolic blood pressure; lower total cholesterol; lower LDL-cholesterol; lower fasting blood sugar and triglycerides; and lower incidence of chronic diseases, especially diabetes and complications to diabetes (Barnard et al., 2009). It would be no surprise if the lowest levels of AGE/ALE are to be found in the group referred to as raw-eaters, especially if they avoid dairy-based foods, but unfortunately, this group has attracted few studies and none with regard to the content of AGE/ALE.

22.10 AGE/ALE and Disease

Increased accumulations of AGE/ALE in tissues have been reported in numerous chronic diseases, as detailed below. In addition, changes in the skin and oral cavity may serve as markers of health risks associated with AGE/ALE.

22.10.1 Allergy and autoimmune diseases

Thermal processing, curing, and roasting of foods are known to often increase allergenicity of pre-existing allergens and also to introduce new antigens. Sometimes, however, reduced allergenicity has been reported (Davis et al., 2001; Sancho et al., 2005). Common foods such as milk, peanuts and soy are reported to induce significant increases in AGE levels and to severely affect the IgE-binding capacity (Chung et al., 2001; Franck et al., 2002; Rautava and Isolauri, 2004). Significantly elevated urinary levels of the AGE pentosine are observed in allergic children in association with signs of exacerbation of atopic dermatitis (Tsukahara et al., 2003).

22.10.2 Alzheimer's disease and other neurodegenerative diseases

Alzheimer's disease (AD) is one of the most common chronic diseases, affecting approximately 5% of all individuals over 65 years of age and more than 35% of those over 80. Strong similarites exist between AD and type 2 diabetes (T2DM), to the extent that Alzheimer's has been called 'the diabetes of the brain', or type 3 diabetes. The incidence of AD is reported to to be increased two- to fivefold in TD2DM (Nicolls, 2004). An approximate threefold increase in content of AGE is observed in AD brains compared to age-matched controls (Moreira et al., 2005). A common feature of both diseases is accumulation of amyloid deposits, a process which progresses during the course of disease, and much relates to the stage of disease. Signs of amyloidosis, pertubation of neuronal properties and functions, amplification of glial inflammatory response, increased oxidative stress, increased vascular dysfunction, increased Aβ in the blood–brain barrier and induction of autoantibodies are regularly seen. Increased levels of AGE and signs of oxidative damage are almost regularly observed in the eyes, known to be early targets of AD (Moreira et al., 2005). Central to, if not the cause of AD, is the progressive oligomerization and deposition in the cells of amyloid β-peptides (Aβ), tau, prions and transthyretin, all glycated molecules with strong neurotoxic effects. Amyloid β-peptides accumulate extracellularly to form amyloid plaques, while tau protein deposits occur as neurofibrillary tangles within the cells. Increased levels of AGE/ALE are most often demonstrated with immunohistochemical methods in senile plaques, tau proteins, amyloid β proteins, and in neurofibrillary tangles (see below (Vitek et al., 1994; Moreira et al., 2005)). Accumulation of AGE/ALE in brain tissues has also been observed in Parkinson's disease (PD) (Castellani et al., 1996; Dalfo et al., 2005), and cytoplasmic proteinaceous inclusions composed of the protein α-synuclein (α-syn) and named Lewy bodies are regularly observed in PD. AGE/ALE are also implicated in the pathogenesis of other neurodegenerative diseases: amyotrophic lateral sclerosis (ALS) (Chou et al., 1998; Kikuchi et al., 2002; Kaufmann et al., 2004), Huntington's disease (Ma and Nicholson, 2004), stroke (Zimmerman et al., 1995), familial amyloidotic polyneuropathy (Gomes et al., 2005), and Creutsfeldt-Jakob disease (Sasaki et al., 2002). Early accumulation of AGE is also reported in Down's syndrome, and early antiglycation treatment is suggested to reduce cognitive impairments (Odetti et al., 1998; Thiel and Fowkes, 2005). It has also been suggested that bovine spongiform encephalopathy (BSE) a disease with its significant similarities to AD, might be associated with increased glycation and lipoxidation (Frey, 2002). Involvement of glycation products and activation of prion proteins are also suggested by other authors (Boratynski and Gorski, 2002; Choi et al., 2004). AGE, amyloid fibrils, and prions all seem to have the same target, RAGE, and all activate the NF-κB pathway. Interaction between RAGE and Aβ is most likely to be the most important implication in the development of AD, enhancing inflammation in blood vessel endothelium, inducing increased response of NF-κB, mediating transport of Aβ across the blood–brain barrier, suppressing cerebral blood flow, and inducing cell death (apoptosis). RAGE is known to mediate Aβ-induced migration of monocytes across the thin brain endothelium and into the brain tissues.

Increased cholesterol is suggested to contribute to the production of AD by increasing generation of beta-amyloid (Aβ), and animal studies suggest that cholesterol co-localizes with fibrillar Aβ in the amyloid plaques (Burns et al., 2003).

22.10.3 Atherosclerosis and other cardiovascular disorders

Oxidative stress, lipid peroxidation and protein glycation are repeatedly associated with extensive arteriosclerosis. Significant increases in both chemical AGE (carboxymethyllysine) and fluorescent AGE (spectrofluorometry) were observed in 42 patients with atherosclerosis when compared to 21 healthy controls ($p<0.001$) (Kalousova et al., 2005). Increased levels of malondialdehyde, lipid peroxides and pentosidine were seen in a study of 225 haemodialysis patients and these also correlated significantly with the degree of coronary artery calcifications (Taki et al., 2006). Significant lipid oxidation, deposition of AGE/ALE in the arterial walls and development of atherosclerosis, are reported in rabbits fed a diet containing 1% cholesterol. Deposition is further enhanced when 10% fructose is added to the diet (Tokita et al., 2005). Structural modifications of high density lipoproteins (HDL), lipoxidation, glycation, homocysteinylation, or enzymatic degradation will make HDL lose its anti-inflammatory and cyto-protective ability (Ferretti et al., 2006). This emphasizes its importance in the pathogenesis of arteriosclerosis, as in neurodegenerative diseases, diabetes and other autoimmune diseases (de Leeuw et al., 2005). Supplementing AGE-modified serum albumin to experimental animals will significantly increase secretion of pro-inflammatory cytokines, maturation of dendritic cells, and augment the capacity to stimulate T-cell proliferation (Ge et al., 2005). The AGE CML in plasma was followed for six years in 1270 people aged 65 and older. In this period, 227 (22.4%) died during the period, 105 of cardiovascular disease. This mortality was significantly associated with high CML levels (Semba et al., 2009).

22.10.4 Cancer

Individuals with high levels of oxidative stress, such as those with type 2 diabetes and significantly increased accumulation in the body of AGE/ALE, suffer a significantly increased risk of developing cancer (Abe and Yamagishi, 2008). The receptor RAGE and its multiple ligands are shown to be involved in the pathogenesis of multiple tumours: brain, breast, colon, colorectal, lung, prostate, oral squamous cell carcinoma and ovarian cancer, as well as lymphoma and melanoma (Takada et al., 2004; Genkinger et al., 2006; Logsdon et al., 2007). In vitro and animal studies, as well as preliminary clinical observations, support the view of a direct link between RAGE activation and proliferation, migration, invasion of tumour cells and survival (Logsdon et al., 2007; Abe and Yamagishi, 2008). RAGE expression is reported to be elevated in human cells with high metastatic ability and low in tumour cells with low metastatic ability (Takada et al., 2004). A tumour-suppressive function of RAGE has also been reported for some distinct cell types (Gebhardt et al., 2008). It is suggested that cytokines produced by cells of the innate immune system play an indispensable role in tumour-promoting inflammation, while protective anti-tumour effects derive largely from adaptive immune cells, particularly T cells (Dougan and Dranoff, 2008). An up-regulation of the gene S100P, known to be involved in the activation of RAGE, has been reported for several tumour tissues including lung, breast, pancreas, prostate, and colon (Rehbein et al., 2008). The RAGE ligand sRAGE, highly expressed in healthy lung tissues especially at the site of alveolar epithelium, is significantly down-regulated in lung carcinomas (Jing et al., 2010), but also in pancreatic cancer (Krechler et al., 2010). The relationship between RAGE expression in surgical specimens of primary tumours and prognosis of the patient was studied recently in 216 patients with oesophageal squamous cell carcinoma (Tateno et al., 2008). Those with positive RAGE expression in tumour cells exhibited a significantly better prognosis than those with negative RAGE expression (5-year survival, 52% versus 32%, respectively) (Tateno et al., 2008).

22.10.5 Cataract and other eye disorders

AGE/ALE accumulate with age in all ocular tissues including lacrimal glands, and trigger pathogenic events, especially in diabetics, in all parts of the eye (Stitt, 2005). The lens contains abundant proteins, which undergo translational modifications throughout the lifespan, contributing to ageing and cataract formation. Kynurenines are diffusible components of the lens that absorb UVA and UVB radiation, and are believed to protect the retina from light damage. However, it is also unstable under physiological conditions and undergoes deamination, its half-life being approximately 7 days. The deaminated products, known to affects lens proteins and modify specific amino acids, are believed to contribute to AGE formation, ageing of the lens, and to development of cataracts (Nagaraj et al., 2010). Age-related macular degeneration (AMD) is also strongly associated with increased oxidative stress, and with increased deposition of AGE/ALE. A recent study found signs of systemic AGE accumulation in patients with AMD, implicating a role for AGE/ALE in the pathophysiology of AMD (Mulder et al., 2010). The AGE CML and pentosidine are also shown to be significantly increased in AMD patients relative to healthy controls: CML (~54%), and pentosidine (~64%) ($p < 0.0001$) (Ni et al., 2009). RAGE and its ligands are also reported to be involved in retinal diseases (Barile and Schmidt, 2007) and in glaucoma (Tezel et al., 2007).

22.10.6 Diabetes

More than 6000 publications in PubMed deal with AGE/ALE and more than half of them particularly with their role in diabetes mellitus (DM). Several excellent reviews have been published recently (Meerwaldt et al., 2008; Orasanu and Plutzky, 2009; Yan et al., 2009). Over-consumption of fat and carbohydrates, not only of glucose, but also of other carbohydrates such as lactose and fructose, contribute in diabetics to a significantly increased accumulation of AGE/ALE in the tissues. The consumption of high-fructose corn syrup in the United States today exceeds that of sucrose. It is ten times more capable of producing AGE/ALE, and is suggested as a major contributor, not only to obesity and accumulation of fat in the liver, but specifically to development of type 2 diabetes as well as to severe complications of both type 1 and 2 diabetes (Gaby, 2005). Chronic hyperglycaemia is suggested to alter mitochondrial function through glycation of mitochondrial proteins. A direct relationship is demonstrated between excess intracellular formation of reactive species, intracellular formation of AGE from mitochondrial proteins, and decline in mitochondrial function (Rosca et al., 2005). Methylglyoxal (MGO), a highly reactive α-dicarbonil by-product of glycolysis, which readily reacts with arginine, lysine and sulfhydryl groups of both proteins and nucleic acids to form AGE, is significantly increased in diabetes (Ceriello, 2009). Diabetic complications such as retinopathy, nephropathy, and neuropathy are significantly associated with levels of AGE in the body. Increased levels of AGE in skin biopsies are found to be significantly associated with the outcome of micro-vascular complications (Genuth et al., 2005), and closely associated with incidence and severity of diabetic complications. Intensive control of glycaemia in insulin-dependent diabetes (IDDM) effectively delays the onset and slows down the progression of diabetic retinopathy, nephropathy, and neuropathy (DCCT, 1993). Five years of such treatment will significantly reduce various AGE/ALE in the body (30–32% lower furosine, 9% lower pentosidine, 9–13% lower CML), and increase the levels of soluble collagen (24% higher in acid-soluble collagen and 50% higher in pepsin-soluble collagen) (Monnier et al., 1999).

22.10.7 Endocrine disorders

Many, if not most, of the signs and symptoms of ageing, and age-associated diseases are strongly associated with multiple hormone deficiencies. Most consequences of ageing, such as excessive free radical formation, imbalance of the apoptosis systems, failure of repair systems, tissue accumulation of waste products, deficient immune system, poor gene polymorphisms and premature telomere shortening, are all associated, if not caused, by hormone deficiencies (Hertoghe, 2005). Up-regulation of putative pathological pathways, accumulation of advanced glycation end products, activation of the renin–angiotensin system, oxidative stress and increased expression of growth factors and cytokines are all intimately associated with ageing. However, little information is yet available about the content of AGE/ALE in endocrine organs and their influence on the body both in health or disease. With the exception of the ovaries, most of the endocrine organs – the pituitary gland, thyroids, parathyroids, adrenals and testes – are thus far almost totally unexplored. Increased serum AGE levels and increased activation of RAGE are reported in women with polycystic ovary syndrome (PCOS) (Diamanti-Kandarakis et al., 2005). A recent study reports that the content of AGE/ALE is twice as high in patients with PCOS as in healthy controls, and also strongly associated with signs of increased chronic inflammation; increases in homocysteine (Hcy), malonyldialdehyde (MDA), C-reactive protein (CRP) and with higher fasting insulin levels; and a higher homeostasis model assessment (HOMA) index (fasting glucose (mg dl^{-1}) x fasting insulin (mU ml^{-1}) x 0.055/22.5) (Kaya et al., 2009). Deposition of excess collagen in PCOS tissues that induce cystogenesis are suggested, at least in part, to be due to stimulation by AGE (Papachroni et al., 2009).

22.10.8 Gastrointestinal disorders

Various gastrointestinal cancers and their ability to grow and produce metastases are associated to increased levels of AGE/ALE in the body and to increased activity of RAGE. Little, however, is known about an eventual association between accumulation in the body of these molecules or activity of RAGE and common inflammatory and ulcerative conditions in the gut. The only exception seems to be a recent study, which reports that the urinary concentration of pentosidine is significantly elevated in active compared to inactive IBD, ulcerative colitis (0.12 versus 0.021 mg mg^{-1}), and Crohn's disease (0.071 versus 0.039 mg mg^{-1}) (Kato et al., 2008).

22.10.9 Liver disorders

Patients with liver cirrhosis demonstrate much increased AGE levels, which sometimes reach almost the same extent as in patients with end-stage renal disease (Sebekova et al., 2002). Serum levels of AGE (CML) are shown to be significantly affected by the stage of the disease in liver cirrhosis, and are closely associated with liver function capacity, as reported in a study of 110 patients with chronic liver disease (CLD) compared to 124 healthy controls (Yagmur et al., 2006). Furthermore, the level of AGE (CML) seemed to correlate well with levels of hyaluronic acid (HA) (r = 0.639, $P < 0.0001$). Glyoxal-derived adducts are suggested to be increased up to no less than 15 times in both portal and hepatic venous plasma of cirrhotic patients compared to healthy controls (Ahmed et al., 2005). A dramatic improvement is observed in patients after liver transplantation, although the AGE levels do not return to the levels seen in healthy controls (Sebekova et al., 2002). Animal studies suggest that blockage of RAGE is highly protective against hepatocellular necrosis and cell death, and to significantly increase the rate of survival (Zeng et al., 2004; Ekong et al., 2006). A significant increase in glutathione and pro-regenerative cytokines TNF-α and IL-6 are observed, in addition to decreased hepatic necrosis and increased survival (Ekong et al., 2006). Much remains to be done to define the role of AGE/ALE and RAGE in the progression of non-alcoholic fatty liver disease (NAFLD) to non-alcoholic steatohepatitis (NASH) and cirrhosis. However, recent observations of serum glyceraldehyde-derived AGE levels (U ml^{-1}) being significantly elevated in NASH patients (9.78) compared to those with simple steatosis (7, $P = 0.018$) and healthy controls (6.96, $P = 0.003$) are of significant interest (Hyogo et al., 2007). These authors also observed an inverse correlation to the level of adiponectin, an adipocytokine with insulin-sensitizing and anti-inflammatory properties. Immunohistochemistry of glyceraldehyde-derived AGE also showed increased staining in the livers of NASH patients.

22.10.10 Lung disorders

A variety of airway diseases such as asthma, acute respiratory distress syndrome (ARDS), chronic obstructive pulmonary disease (COPD), cystic fibrosis and idiopathic pulmonary fibrosis are all characterized by lack of homeostasis in the oxidant/antioxidant balance. Interaction of AGE/ALE and RAGE are well known to play a large, if not dominating, role in the depletion of antioxidants, particularly reduced glutathione (GSH) in lung epithelial lining and to play a key role in the pathogenesis of these disorders (Foell et al., 2003; Rahman et al., 2006a).

22.10.11 Rheumatoid arthritis and other skeletomuscular disorders

Among the highest levels of AGE in the body, and the strongest expression of RAGE, are found in inflamed tissues characterized for slow turnover, such as tendons, bone, cartilage, skin and amyloid plaques. These changes are associated with a slight change in colour towards yellow-brown and an increased fluorescence, all associated with increased expression of pro-inflammatory cytokines and matrix metalloproteinases (MMP), especially MMP-1 and MMP-9. These manifestations are regarded as being responsible for the observed increased tissue stiffness and brittleness in structures such as intervertebral discs, bones, tendons, cartilages, synovial membranes and skeletal muscles, and are regarded as major pathogenic factors behind diseases such as osteoarthritis (DeGroot, 2004; Steenvoorden, 2006), rupture of inter-vertebral discs (Hormel and Eyre 1991), rupture of Achilles tendons (Reddy, 2004), menisci and also in rheumatoid diseases (Hein et al., 2005; Sunahori, et al., 2006), such as rheumatoid arthritis (Matsumoto et al., 2007) and fibromyalgia (Hein and Franke, 2002; Rüster et al., 2005). A significant increase in glycation of myosin occurs with age (Ramamurthy et al., 2001), and is most likely to contribute to age-associated muscular disorders. High levels of AGE/ALE in the body are also reported in patients with osteoporosis; significantly elevated levels of pentosidine and CML in serum (Hein et al., 2003) and significantly increased pentosidine in cortical bone (Odetti et al., 2005) being observed. It has also been observed that the remodelling of senescent bone is impaired by AGE, with both stimulation of bone-resorbing cytokines and enhancement of bone resorption by osteoclasts being observed (Miyata et al., 1996). A recent American study reports a significantly reduced bone density in older women consuming > 3 cola drinks per week when compared to matched controls consuming similar amounts of other carbonated soft drinks (Tucker et al., 2006). This information is especially interesting when one considers that cola drinks, much in contrast to other soft drinks, are considered rich in AGE. A recent in vitro study reports profound effects by cola-derived AGE: activation of platelets, an up to 7.1-fold increase in CD62 expression, and an increase of up to 2.2-fold in CD63 at the platelet surface membrane, also accompanied by increases in RAGE expression (Gawlowski et al., 2009).

The common belief that bovine milk prevents osteoporosis is today much questioned. Instead, increasing documentation suggests that it has quite the opposite effect, and that negative interactions of RAGE and AGE/ALE play a larger role in the pathogenesis of osteoporosis than lack of minerals.

22.10.12 Skin and oral cavity issues

The skin is one of, if not the largest, organ in the body. The health condition of the skin has a similar ability to the gingiva in the mouth, to reflect the total health of the body. Skin autofluorescence seems to be a good measure of cumulative metabolic stress and accumulation of advanced glycation end products in the body (Meerwaldt et al., 2005a,b). Accumulation of AGE/ALE in the skin relates to the content of these proteins in the body, and so is an expression of the risk of developing chronic diseases, in particular coronary heart disease. A recent study found a significant correlation between coronary calcifications and AGE/ALE in the body measured as skin fluorescence, suggesting such measurements could serve both as a marker of risk but also as a measurement of therapeutic success when patients are treated (Conway et al., 2010). Skin autofluorescence is especially suggested to be a method for prediction of the risk for progression of diabetic complications such as angiopathy, nephropathy and retinopathy, and the severity of disease and mortality in haemodialysis patients (Meerwaldt et al., 2005b).

The skin has a high density of RAGE receptors. AGE/ALE are known to accumulate in dermal elastine and in collagens, and to interact with dermal fibroblasts, inhibiting their proliferation capacity. A tenfold reduction in proliferation rate is described to occur normally in humans from the second to seventh decade (Stamatas et al., 2006), and is suggested as explaining the reduced healing capacity of age-related wounds, and especially chronic wounds, such as those on the diabetic foot. RAGE and AGE/ALE-induced apoptosis and enhanced loss of fibroblasts and osteoblasts are also regarded as major pathogenic factors in periodontal pathology, especially in chronic periodontitis (Holla et al., 2001). A 50% increase is observed compared with controls in RAGE mRNA in gingiva of diabetic patients ($p<0.05$) (Katz et al., 2005).

22.10.13 Urogenital disorders

Nephropathy is today more common than ever before and continues to increase, much in parallel to the increase in diabetes. It is the single most important cause of end-stage renal failure in the western world (Ostergaard et al., 2005). Consequently it receives great interest from scientists. Today no less than 1000 papers in PubMed deal with RAGE and AGE/ALE in renal diseases. Diabetic nephropathy today affects 15–25% of patients with type 1 diabetes, and as much as 30–40% of patients with type 2 diabetes. The kidney appears as both culprit and target of AGE/ALE, and it is well documented that RAGE is significantly activated, and advanced AGE/ALE markedly elevated in renal failure patients. Patients with mild chronic uremic renal failure are reported to have plasma glycation-free adduct concentrations increased up to fivefold, patients with end-stage renal disease as much as 18-fold when on peritoneal dialysis, and up to 40-fold on haemodialysis (Agalou et al., 2005). A decrease in renal function and reduced clearance is observed much in parallel to increases in circulating AGE levels. AGE are involved in the structural changes observed in progressing nephropathies such as glomerulosclerosis, interstitial fibrosis and tubular atrophy (Bohlender et al., 2005). For detailed information, see recent excellent reviews (Vlassara et al., 2009; Daroux et al., 2010; Schepers et al., 2010). Kidney transplantation is reported to improve but does not fully correct the increased AGE/ALE levels in previously dialysed patients.

22.11 Foods Rich in AGE/ALE

It is a most interesting observation that increased accumulation of AGE/ALE in endothelial cells, and most likely also in some other tissues, can be significantly avoided or reduced by control of intake of foods known to contain these substances in large amounts. Thus far the information regarding content of AGE/ALE in foods is rather incomplete. Leading universities around the world are building institutions for studies of nutragenomics (how various food ingredients affect our health). However, from existing information it is clear that dysfunctioning proteins are especially rich in foods which have been subjected to industrial processing. The foods with the highest AGE content were animal-derived products exposed to high, dry heat such as broiling, frying and grilling. A detailed description of the database can be found in Goldberg et al. (2004). A brief summary is provided below.

- *Heated dairy products:* powdered milk (ice cream, baby and clinical nutrition formulas) cheese, especially when heated. High in pizza, tacos, nachos, salad dressings, fast food, sandwiches, sauces and brown cheeses.
- *Heated grain products:* bread (e.g. toasted bread, bread crusts, and crispbreads).
- *Heated meat, poultry, and fish:* especially bacon, sausages, fried and barbecued meat. The content of AGE/ALE increases as one goes from boiling to oven frying: boiling (1000 kU/serving) < roasting (4300 kU) < broiling (5250 kU) < deep frying (6700 kU) < oven frying (9000 kU/serving) (Goldberg et al., 2004).
- *Other heated foods:* egg yolk powder, lecithin powder, coffee (especially dark roasted), hard-cured teas, roasted and salted peanuts, dark and sugar-rich alcoholic beverages, broth, Chinese soy, balsamic vinegar, cola drinks, etc.

A recent study adds further and important information about dietary AGE (Uribarri et al., 2010). It should be observed that lean red meats and poultry contain high levels of dietary AGE. Even when cooked under dry heat, the explanation is that among the intracellular components of lean muscle there are highly reactive amino lipids, as well as reducing sugars such as fructose or glucose-6-phosphate. In the presence of heat, this combination rapidly accelerates new AGE formation (Uribarri et al., 2010). The highest AGE levels are observed in beef and cheeses followed by poultry, pork, fish, and eggs, while lamb ranked relatively low in AGE, at least when compared to other meats. Cheeses, butter, and different types of oils are AGE-rich, even in uncooked forms. High-fat spreads, including butter, cream cheese, margarine and mayonnaise, are also among the foods containing the highest AGE, followed by oils and nuts. It should especially be observed that olive oil, for example, contains large amounts of AGE when heated to 100°C for 5 min (Uribarri *et al.*, 2010). Carbohydrate-rich foods such as vegetables, fruits and whole grains contain relatively few AGE, even after cooking (Uribarri *et al.*, 2010).

22.12 Prevention and Treatment of AGE/ALE Accumulation

22.12.1 Changing food preparation habits

It is clear that significant benefits will be obtained by reducing the intake of cheese, meats, powdered milk, other processed foods such as heated oils, and also of bread; and instead increasing the consumption of vegetables and fruits, especially when raw. These recommendations are in line with the policy of various expert organizations with the aim to reduce chronic diseases such as cancer, heart diseases and hypertension (cancer: American Cancer Society, 2006; heart: Lichtenstein *et al.*, 2006; hypertension: US Department of Health and Human Services *et al.*, 2006). AGE formation in food is reduced when cooking on surfaces that provide no direct contact with metal; when foods are immersed in acid solutions such as tomato sauce and ketchup; and when there is contact with aminoguanidine, a known inhibitor of AGE formation (He *et al.*, personal communication, 2010). Eating foods raw or prepared at a low temperature (below 80°C), steam cooking or boiling, and minimal cooking are preferred over frying, grilling and microwaving, and also to roasting and salting. Recent information seems especially to warn against microwaving food, as this treatment dramatically accelerates the rate of AGE production (Visentin *et al.*, 2010). A trial designed to compare the potential metabolic effects of two different diets, one based on mild steam cooking and another based on high-temperature cooking was recently reported (Birlouez-Aragon *et al.*, 2010). A randomized crossover study assigned 62 volunteers (university students) to each of the two diets for four weeks. Consuming the steamed-cooked diet for 1 month induced significantly improved insulin sensitivity and also increased plasma levels of omega-3 fatty acids (217%, $p = 0.002$), vitamin C (213%, $p = 0.0001$), and vitamin E (28%, $p = 0.01$), in comparison to the high temperature diet. Furthermore, reduced concentrations of plasma cholesterol (5%, $p = 0.01$) and triglycerides (9%, $p = 0.01$) were also reported.

A challenge for the future in the Western world is to find techniques to produce bread at 100°C or below as the Chinese have done for centuries. Marinating for some hours at room temperature with ingredients such as antioxidant-rich herbs, garlic, tea, red wine, onions, olive oil and beer are also known to significantly reduce the development of AGE/ALE, and this was also recently demonstrated for heterocylic aromatic amines (Melo *et al.*, 2008). Reduction in total intake of proteins (Uribarri and Tuttle, 2006), and most likely a particular reduction in methionine and other sulphur-containing amino acids, are additional issues of relevance (McCarty *et al.*, 2009).

22.12.2 Energy restriction

Significant reduction in body content of AGE/ALE in comparison to controls (eating standard Western food) is observed in individuals, who for > 2 years practise what is called caloric restriction (CR). They eat only two thirds of what they would like to, and this is accompanied by significant health advantages compared to matched controls: lower blood pressure (102/61±7 versus 131/83 mm Hg), and lower levels of markers of inflammation such as CRP (0.3 versus 1.9 mg l^{-1}), TNF-α (0.8 versus 1.5 pg ml^{-1}), and TGF-β (29.4 versus 35.4 ng ml^{-1}) (Meyer *et al.*, 2006). Elevated RAGE and low sRAGE is reported in patients with active rheumatoid arthritis (RA), but patients with RA practising CR for about 2 months demonstrated not only lower levels of pentosidine (an often-measured AGE) in urine, but also lower disease activity (Iwashige *et al.*, 2004). Thirty-seven obese individuals (mean BMI of 28.3 ± 3.2) were treated with calorie restriction for 8 weeks. Reduction occurred in BMI (6.3%, $p < 0.001$), waist circumference (5.7%, $p < 0.002$), triglycerides (11.9 % ($p < 0.002$), and AGE (7.21%, $p < 0.001$) (Gugliucci et al., 2009). FEV1, an expression of respiratory capacity, almost doubled.

22.12.3   Antioxidants and vitamins

Provision of vitamins such as A, B (especially B_6 and B_{12}), C, D, E, and K, as well as glutathione and folic acid, is often emphasized. Many plant antioxidants, particularly those collectively defined as polyphenols, have documented oxidation-quenching properties up to ten times more powerful than conventional vitamins. They have also been shown to have great chemo-preventive properties, a marked ability to prevent accumulation in the body of AGE/ALE, and significant capacities to reduce inflammation in the body and to prevent reduction in organ function and premature ageing (Delmas et al., 2005; Osawa and Kato, 2005; Bengmark, 2006; Rahman et al., 2006b; Sun et al., 2010). Such plant antioxidants exist in nature in many thousands – most probably hundreds of thousands – of different compounds. More than 4000 flavonoids alone have been identified, and almost 1000 carotenoids. Here are the most studied: isothiocyanates in cruciferous vegetables; anthocyanins and hydroxycinnamic acids in cherries; epigallocatechin-3-gallate (EGCG) in green tea; chlorogenic acid and caffeic acid in fresh coffee beans and also in fresh tobacco leaves; capsaicin in hot chilli peppers; chalcones in apples; euginol in cloves; gallic acid in rhubarb; hisperitin and naringenin in citrus fruits; kaempferol in white cabbage; myricetin in berries; rutin and quercetin in apples and onions; resveratrol and other procyanidin dimers in red wine and virgin peanuts; various curcumenoids, the main yellow pigments in turmeric curry foods; and daidzein and genistein from the soy bean.

22.12.4   Supplementing histidine, taurine, carnitine or carnosine

Supplementing the diet with histidine, taurine, carnitine or carnosine has also been reported to assist in protecting the body from AGE/ALE (Nandhini et al., 2004, 2005). No vegetarian food contains taurine, with the exception of certain algae. This important amino acid is only obtained from eating animal-derived foods – meat, poultry and fish.

22.12.5   Pharmaceuticals

Several pharmaceuticals, especially those used for treatment of diabetes, are reported to reduce the content of AGE/ALE in the body, at least in short-lived tissues; that is, those with high turnover.

22.13   Pro- and Synbiotics

Probiotics and synbiotics have a dual role in reduction of dietary AGE/ALE as they both metabolize these substances (Erbersdobler et al., 1970; Finot and Magnenat, 1981; Faist and Erbersdobler, 2001; Faist et al., 2001; Wiame et al., 2002) and also release important vitamins and antioxidants with documented preventive effects against AGE and ALE. A rich intestinal flora is regarded as necessary for the release and absorption of various important antioxidants. However, the increased intake of refined food and deficient intake of fresh fruits and vegetables among Westerners has led to a significant reduction in both density and diversity of the flora. This reduction is especially pronounced for strong fibre-fermenting lactic acid bacteria (LAB) such as *Lactobacillus plantarum* and *L. paracasei*. Seventy-five per cent of omnivorous Americans and 25% of vegetarians in the United States lack *L. plantarum* (Finegold et al., 1983). A more recent Scandinavian study found *L. plantarum* in only 52% and *L. paracasei* in only 17% of healthy individuals (Ahrné et al., 1998). This information is particularly interesting, as *L. plantarum* and *L. paracasei* belong to the small group of intestinal bacteria with ability to break down semi-resistant fibres such as inulin (Müller and Lier, 1994), reduce inflammation, reduce infection, and eliminate pathogenic bacteria such as *Clostridium difficile* (Naaber et al., 2004). Some specific LAB might well have the ability to eliminate AGE/ALE from foods, in a way that is very similar to that demonstrated for gluten (di Cagno et al., 2005) and heterocyclic amines (Tavan et al., 2002). In vitro studies have shown that fructoselysine, the dominating AGE in heated milk, can be effectively eliminated when incubated with fresh intestinal flora (Erbersdobler et al., 1970).

22.14 Conclusions

There is growing consensus that the dietary intake or endogenous production of AGE/ALE is associated with a diverse range of disorders, although the underlying mechanisms remain largely obscure. This chapter has focused on the dietary sources of AGE/ALE and on the effects of heat treatment in the production of these dysfunctional adducts during the processing of foods. The accumulation of AGE has been documented in conditions such as Alzheimer's disease, cardiovascular disease, cancer, diabetes, lung disease, liver disease and other disorders, and this research evidence has also been reviewed in this chapter.

It is increasingly clear that the intestinal microflora and its more than 2 million metagenes play a key role in health and disease. Western lifestyle is clearly associated with a deranged microbionta, with reduced diversity and an increased quotient between gram-negative and gram-positive bacteria, which in association with reduced barrier function seems to contribute to the observed elevated systemic inflammation. Patients with metabolic derangements such as obesity and with chronic diseases are known to have increased blood levels of endotoxin, a product of gram-negative bacteria. Recent in vitro observations suggest that human AGE-modified albumin and lipopolysaccharide (LPS) exhibit a synergistic effect on proinflammatory cytokine/chemokine interleukin-6, interleukin-8, and monochemoattractant protein-1 production in human endothelial cells (Liu et al., 2009). A link exists between fat intake and accumulation of endotoxin in the blood (endotoxaemia), and recent studies demonstrate that intake of emulsified fat in particular (water-in-oil emulsions such as butter; free oil or dispersed fat inclusions in cheeses, cookies, ice cream and dressings), which is known to affect the kinetics of lipid absorption, increases both endotoxaemia and inflammation (Laugerette et al., 2010).

It is now well documented in the literature that a healthy lifestyle has profound effects on health and well-being. Control of what we eat is an important component within such a programme. Studies suggest reductions of as much as 83% in coronary heart disease (Stampfer et al., 2000), 91% in diabetes (Hu et al., 2001), and 71% in colon cancer (Platz et al., 2000) in patients adhering to a 'healthy lifestyle' (such as no use of tobacco, moderate use of alcohol, regular physical exercise, and controlled food intake). To these four factors must be added control of stress. Numerous studies demonstrate that both physical and mental stress increases the degree of inflammation in the body and activates RAGE (Kjaer, 2004; Bierhaus et al., 2006; Chida et al., 2006). Control of intake and endogenously produced AGE/ALE, will, together with restrictions on the intake of fat and carbohydrate-rich foods, significantly improve health and well-being. However, only a fraction of consumers are willing to consider this option. A study in the United States (Reeves and Rafferty, 2005), suggests that only about 3% adhere to the principles advocated above.

References

Abe, R. and Yamagishi, S. (2008) AGE-RAGE system and carcinogenesis. *Current Pharmaceutical Design* 14, 940–945.

Agalou, S., Ahmed, N. Babaei-Jadidi, R., et al. (2005) Profound mishandling of protein glycation degradation products in uremia and dialysis. *Journal of the American Society of Nephrology* 16, 1471–1485.

Ahmed, N., Lüthen, R., Häussinger, D., et al. (2005) Increased protein glycation in cirrhosis and therapeutic strategies to prevent it. *Annals of the New York Academy of Sciences* 1043, 718–724.

Ahrné, S., Nobaek, S., Jeppsson, B., et al. (1998) The normal Lactobacillus flora of healthy human rectal and oral mucosa. *Journal of Applied Microbiology* 85, 88–94.

Allen, T.J. and Jandeleit-Dahm, K.A. (2005) Preventing atherosclerosis with angiotensin-converting enzyme inhibitors: emphasis on diabetic atherosclerosis. *Current Drug Targets - Cardiovascular & Hematological Disorders* 5, 503–512.

Alverdy. J.C., Laughlin, R.S. and Wu, L. (2003) Influence of the critically ill state on host-pathogen interactions within the intestine: gut-derived sepsis redefined. *Critical Care Medicine* 31, 598–607.

American Cancer Society (2006) Choices for good health: American Cancer Society guidelines for nutrition and physical activity for cancer prevention. *CA – A Cancer Journal for Clinicians* 56, 310–312.

Aronsen, D. (2003) Cross-linking of glycated collagen in the pathogenesis of arterial and myocardial stiffening of aging and diabetes. *Journal of Hypertension* 21, 3–12.

Artaud-Wild, S.M., Connor, S.L., Sexton, G. and Connor, W.E. (1993) Differences in coronary mortality can be explained by differences in cholesterol and saturated fat intakes in 40 countries but not in France and Finland. A paradox. *Circulation* 88, 2771–2779.

Baptista, J.A.B. and Carvalho, R.C.B. (2004) Indirect determination of Amadori compounds in milk-based products by HPLC/ELSD/UV as an index of protein detorioration. *Food Research International* 37, 739–747.

Barile, G.R. and Schmidt, A.M. (2007) RAGE and its ligands in retinal disease. *Current Molecular Medicine* 7, 758–765.

Barnard, N.D., Cohen, J., Jenkins, D.J., et al. (2009) A low-fat vegan diet and a conventional diabetes diet in the treatment of type 2 diabetes: a randomized, controlled, 74-wk clinical trial. *American Journal of Clinical Nutrition* 89, 1588S–1596S.

Bengmark, S. (2006) Curcumin: an atoxic antioxidant and natural NF-κB, COX-2, LOX and iNOS inhibitor – a shield against acute and chronic diseases. *Journal of Parenteral and Enteral Nutrition* 30, 45–51.

Bierhaus, A., Schiekofer, S., Schwaninger, M., et al. (2001) Diabetes-associated sustained activation of the transcription factor nuclear factor –κB. *Diabetes* 50, 2792–2808.

Bierhaus, A., Humpert, P.M., Stern, D.M., et al. (2005a) Advanced glycation end product receptor-mediated cellular dysfunction. *Annals of the New York Academy of Sciences* 1043, 676–680.

Bierhaus, A., Humpert, P.M., Morcos, M., et al. (2005b) Understanding RAGE, the receptor for advanced glycation end products. *Journal of Molecular Medicine* 83, 876–886.

Bierhaus, A., Humpert, P.M. and Nawroth, P.P. (2006) Linking stress to inflammation. *Anesthesiology Clinics* 24, 325–340.

Birlouez-Aragon, I. and Tessier, F.J. (2003) Antioxidant vitamins and degenerative pathologies. A review of vitamin C. *Journal of Nutrition, Health & Aging* 7, 103–109.

Birlouez-Aragon, I., Saavedra, G., Tessier, F.J., Galinier, A., Ait-Ameur, L., Lacoste, F., Niamba, C.N., et al. (2010) A diet based on high-heat-treated foods promotes risk factors for diabetes mellitus and cardiovascular diseases. *American Journal of Clinical Nutrition* 91, 1220–1226.

Bohlender, J.M. Franke, S., Stein, G. and Wolf, G. (2005) Advanced glycation end products and the kidney. *American Journal of Physiology - Renal Physiology* 289, F645–659.

Boratynski, J. and Gorski. A. (2002) BSE: a consequence of cattle feeding with glycated molecules host-unknown? *Medical Hypotheses* 58, 276–278.

Brady, J. and Hoggan, R. (2002) *Dangerous grains*. Avery-Penguin Putnam, New York.

Brandtzaeg, P., Halstensen, T.S., Kett, K., et al. (1989) Immunobiology and immunopathology of human gut mucosa: Humoral immunity and intraepithelial lymphocytes. *Gastroenterology* 97, 1562–1584.

Burns, M., Gaynor, K. and Olm, V. (2003) Presenilin redistribution associated with aberrant cholesterol transport enhances beta-amyloid production in vivo. *Journal of Neuroscience* 23, 5645–5649.

Carroll, K.K. (1975) Experimental evidence of dietary factors and hormone-dependent cancers. *Cancer Research* 35, 3374–3383.

Castellani, R., Smith, M.A., Richey, P.J. and Perry, G. (1996) Glycoxidation and oxidative stress in Parkinson disease and diffuse Lewy body disease. *Brain Research* 737, 195–200.

Ceriello, A. (2009) Hypothesis: the "metabolic memory", the new challenge of diabetes. *Diabetes Research and Clinical Practice* 86, S2–S6.

Chida, Y., Sudo, N. and Kubo, C. (2006) Does stress exacerbate liver diseases? *Journal of Gastroenterology & Hepatology* 21, 202–208.

Choi, Y.G., Kim, J.I., Jeon, Y.C., et al. (2004) Nonenzymatic glycation at the N terminus of pathogenic prion protein in transmissible spongiform encephalopathies. *Journal of Biological Chemistry* 279, 30402–30409.

Chou, S.M., Wang, H.S., Taniguchi, A. and Bacula, R. (1998) Advanced glycation end products in neurafilament conglomeration of motorneurons in familial and sporadic amyotrophic lateral sclerosis. *Molecular Medicine* 4, 324–332.

Chung, S.Y. and Champagne, E.T. (2001) Association of end-product adducts with increased IgE binding of roasted peanuts. *Journal of Agricultural and Food Chemistry* 49, 3911–3916.

Conway, B., Edmundowicz, D., Matter, N., et al. (2010) Skin fluorescence correlates strongly with coronary artery calcification severity in type 1 diabetes. *Diabetes Technology & Therapeutics* 12, 339–345.

Cooper, E.V. (1946) Gas gangrene following injection of adrenaline. *Lancet* 247, 459–461.

Dahl-Jorgensen, K., Joner, G. and Hanssen, K.F. (1991) Relationship between cows' milk consumption and incidence of IDDM in childhood. *Diabetes Care* 14, 1081–1083.

Dalfo, E., Portero-Otin, M., Ayala, V., et al. (2005) Evidence of oxidative stress in the neocortex in incidental Lewy body disease. *Journal of Neuropathology & Experimental Neurology* 64, 816–830.

Daroux, M., Prévost, G., Maillard-Lefebvre, H., et al. (2010) Advanced glycation end-products: implications for diabetic and non-diabetic nephropathies. *Diabetes & Metabolism* 36, 1–10.

Davis, P.J., Smales, C.M. and James, D.C. (2001) How can thermal processing modify the antigenicity of proteins? *Allergy* 56, 56–60.

DCCT (Diabetes Control and Complications Trial) (1993) The effect of intensive treatment of diabetes on the development and progression of long-term complications in insulin-dependent diabetes mellitus. *New England Journal of Medicine* 329, 977–986.

DeGroot, J. (2004) The AGE of the matrix: chemistry, consequence and cure. *Current Opinion in Pharmacology* 4, 301–305.

De Leeuw, K., Kallenberg, C. and Bijl, M. (2005) Accelerated atherosclerosis in patients with systemic autoimmune diseases. *Annals of the New York Academy of Sciences* 1051, 362–371.

Delmas, D., Jannin, B. and Latruffe, N. (2005) Resveratrol: preventing properties against vascular alterations and ageing. *Molecular Nutrition & Food Research* 49, 377–395.

Diamanti-Kandarakis, E., Piperi, C., Kalofoutis, A. and Creatsas, G. (2005) Increased levels of serum advanced glycation end-products in women with polycystic ovary syndrome. *Clinical Endocrinology* 62, 37–43.

di Cagno, R., de Angelis, M., Alfonsi, G., et al. (2005) Pasta made from durum wheat semolina fermented with selected lactobacilli as a tool for a potential decrease of the gluten intolerance. *Journal of Agricultural and Food Chemistry* 53, 4393–4402.

Dougan, M. and Dranoff, G.(2008) Inciting inflammation: the RAGE about tumor promotion. *Journal of Experimental Medicine* 205, 267–270.

Ekong, U., Zeng, S., Dun, H., et al. (2006) Blockade of the receptor for advanced glycation end products attenuates acetaminophen-induced hepatotoxicity in mice. *Journal of Gastroenterology & Hepatology* 21, 682–688.

Erbersdobler, H., Gunsser, I. and Weber, G. (1970) Abbau von Fructoselysine durch die Darmflora. *Zentralblatt für Veterinärmedizin* A17, 573–575.

Faist, V. and Erbersdobler, H.F. (2001). Metabolic transit and in vivo effects of melanoidins and precursor compounds deriving from the Maillard reaction. *Annals of Nutrition and Metabolism* 45, 1–12.

Faist, V., Wenzel, E. and Erbersdobler, H.F. (2000) *In vitro* and *in vivo* studies on the metabolic transit of Nε-carboxymethyllysine. *Czech Journal of Food Sciences* 18, 116–119.

Ferretti, G., Bacchetti, T. and Negre-Salvayre, A. (2006) Structural modifications of HDL and functional consequences. *Atherosclerosis* 184, 1–7.

Finegold, S.M., Sutter, V.L. and Mathisen, G.E. (1983) Normal indigenous intestinal flora. In: Hentges, D.J. (ed.) *Human Intestinal Microflora in Health and Disease*. Academic Press, London, pp. 3–31.

Finot, P.A. and Magnenat, E. (1981) Metabolic transit of early and advanced Maillard products. *Progress in Food & Nutrition Science* 5, 193–207.

Flyvbjerg, A., Khatir, D.S., Jensen. L.J., et al. (2004) The involvement of growth hormone (GH), insulin-like growth factors (IGFs) and vascular endothelial growth factor (VEGF) in diabetic kidney disease. *Current Pharmaceutical Design* 10, 3385–3394.

Foell, D., Seeliger, S., Vogl, T., et al. (2003) Expression of S100A12 (EN-RAGE) in cystic fibrosis. *Thorax* 58, 613–617.

Franck, P., Moneret Vautrin, D.A., Dousset, B., et al. (2002) The allergenicity of soybean-based products is modified by food technologies. *International Archives of Allergy and Applied Immunology* 128, 212–219.

Frey, J. (2002) Bovine spongiform encephalopathy: are the cows mad or full of carbohydrate. *Clinical Chemistry and Laboratory Medicine* 40, 101–103.

Gaby, A.R. (2005) Adverse effects of dietary fructose. *Alternative Medicine Review* 10, 294–306.

Ganmaa, D., Li, X.M. and Wang, J. (2002) Incidence and mortality of testicular and prostatic cancers in relation to world dietary practices. *International Journal of Cancer* 98, 262–267.

Ganmaa, D., Li, X.M., Qin, L.Q., *et al.* (2003) The experience of Japan as a clue to the etiology of testicular and prostatic cancers. *Medical Hypotheses* 60, 724–730.

Gawlowski, T., Stratmann, B. and Ruetter, R. (2009) Advanced glycation end products strongly activate platelets. *European Journal of Nutrition* 48, 475–481.

Ge, J., Jia, Q., Liang, C., *et al.* (2005) Advanced glycosylation end products might promote atherosclerosis through inducing the immune maturation of dendritic cells. *Arteriosclerosis, Thrombosis, and Vascular Biology* 25, 2157–2163.

Gebhardt, C., Riehl, A., Durchdewald, M., Németh, J., Fürstenberger, G., Müller-Decker, K., Enk, A., *et al.* (2008) RAGE signaling sustains inflammation and promote tumor development. *Journal of Experimental Medicine* 205, 275–285.

Genkinger, J.M., Hunter, D.J., Spiegelman, D., *et al.* (2006) Dairy products and ovarian cancer: a pooled analysis of 12 cohort studies. *Cancer Epidemiology, Biomarkers & Prevention* 15, 364–372.

Genuth, S., Sun, W., Cleary, P., *et al.* (2005) Glycation and carboxymethyllysine levels in skin collagen predict the risk of future 10-year progression of diabetic retinopathy and nephropathy in the diabetes control and complications trial and epidemiology of diabetes interventions and complications participants with type 1 diabetes. *Diabetes* 54, 3103–3111.

Goldberg, T., Cai, W., Peppa, M., *et al.* (2004) Advanced glycoxidation end products in commonly consumed foods. *Journal of the American Dietetic Association* 104, 1287–1291.

Gomes, R., Sousa Silva, M., Quintas, A., *et al.* (2005) Argpyrimidine, a methylglyoxal-derived advanced glycation end-product in familial amyloidotic polyneuropathy. *Biochemical Journal* 385, 339–345.

Gugliucci, A., Kotani, K., Taing, J., *et al.* (2009), Short-term low calorie diet intervention reduces serum advanced glycation end products in healthy overweight or obese adults. *Annals of Nutrition and Metabolism* 54, 197–201.

Hein, G. and Franke, S. (2002) Are advanced glycation end-product-modified proteins of pathogenetic importance in fibromyalgia? *Rheumatology* 41, 1163–1167.

Hein, G., Wiegand, R., Lehmann, G., *et al.* (2003) Advanced glycation end-products pentosidine and N epsilon-carboxymethyllysine are elevated in serum of patients with osteoporosis. *Rheumatology* 42, 1242–1246.

Hein, G.E., Kohler, M., Oelzner, P., *et al.* (2005) The advanced glycation end product pentosidine correlates to IL-6 and other relevant inflammatory markers in rheumatoid arthritis. *Rheumatology International* 26, 137–141.

Hertoghe, T. (2005). The "multiple hormone deficiency" theory of aging: is human senescence caused mainly by multiple hormone deficiencies? *Annals of the New York Academy of Sciences* 1057, 448–465.

Holla, L.I., Kankova, K., Fassmann, A., *et al.* (2001) Distribution of the receptor for advanced glycation end products gene polymorphisms in patients with chronic periodontitis: a preliminary study. *Journal of Periodontology* 72, 1742–1746.

Hormel, S.E. and Eyre, D.R. (1991) Collagen in the ageing human intervertebral disc: an increase in covalently bound fluorophores and chromophores. *Biochimica et Biophysica Acta* 1078, 243–250.

Hostettler-Allen, R.L., Tappy, L. and Blum, J.W. (1994) Insulin resistance, hyperglycemia, and glucosuria in intensively milk-fed calves. *Journal of Animal Science* 72, 160–173.

Hu, F.B., Manson, J.E., Stampfer, M.J., *et al.* (2001) Diet, lifestyle and the risk of type 2 diabetes mellitus in women. *New England Journal of Medicine* 345, 790–797.

Hyogo, H., Yamagishi, S., Iwamoto, K., *et al.* (2007) Elevated levels of serum advanced glycation end products in patients with non-alcoholic steatohepatitis. *Journal of Gastroenterology & Hepatology* 22, 1112–1119.

Iwashige, K., Kouda, K., Kouda, M., *et al.* (2004) Calorie restricted diet and urinary pentosidine in patients with rheumatoid arthritis. *Journal of Physiological Anthropology and Applied Human Science* 23, 19–24.

Jing, R., Cui, M., Wang, J. and Wang, H. (2010) Receptor for advanced glycation end products (RAGE) soluble form (sRAGE): a new biomarker for lung cancer. *Neoplasma* 57, 55–61.

Kalousova, M., Zak, A. and Soukupova, J. (2005) Advanced glycation and oxidation products in patients with atherosclerosis. *Cas Lek Cesk* 144, 385–390 [in Czech].

Kato, S., Itoh, K., Ochiai. M., *et al.* (2008) Increased pentosidine, an advanced glycation end-product, in urine and tissue reflects disease activity in inflammatory bowel diseases. *Journal of Gastroenterology & Hepatology* 2, S140–S145.

Katz, J., Bhattacharyya, I., Farkhondeh-Kish, F., *et al.* (2005) Expression of the receptor of advanced glycation end products in gingival tissues of type 2 diabetes patients with chronic periodontal disease: a study utilizing immunohistochemistry and RT-PCR. *Journal of Clinical Periodontology* 32, 40–44.

Kaufmann, E., Boehm, B.O. and Sussmuth, S.D. (2004) The advanced glycation end-product N epsilon-(carboxymethyl)lysine level is elevated in cerebrospinal fluid of patients with amyotrophic lateral sclerosis. *Neuroscience Letters* 371, 226–229.

Kaya, C., Erkan, A.F., Cengiz, S.D., *et al.* (2009) Advanced oxidation protein products are increased in women with polycystic ovary syndrome: relationship with traditional and nontraditional cardiovascular risk factors in patients with polycystic ovary syndrome. *Fertility and Sterility* 92, 1372–1377.

Kikuchi, S., Shinpo, K., Ogata, A., *et al.* (2002) Detection of N-(carboxymethyl)lysine (CML) and non-CML advanced glycation end products in the anterior horn of amyotrophic lateral sclerosis spinal cord. *Amyotrophic Lateral Sclerosis and Other Motor Neuron Disorders* 3, 63–68.

Kinney, K.S., Austin, C.E., Morton, D.S. and Sonnenfeld, G. (2000) Norepinephrine as a growth stimulating factor in bacteria–mechanistic studies. *Life Science* 67, 3075–3085.

Kjaer, M. (2004) Role of extracellular matrix in adaptation of tendon and skeletal muscle to mechanical loading. *Physiological Reviews* 84, 649–698.

Koyama, H., Shoji, T., Yokoyama, H., *et al.* (2005) Plasma level of endogenous secretory RAGE is associated with components of the metabolic syndrome and atherosclerosis. *Arteriosclerosis, Thrombosis, and Vascular Biology* 25, 2587–2593.

Krechler, T., Jáchymová, M. and Mestek, O. (2010) Soluble receptor for advanced glycation end-products (RAGE) and polymorphisms of RAGE and glyoxalase I genes in patients with pancreas cancer. *Clinical Biochemistry* 43, 10–11.

Kurien, B.T., Hensley, K., Bachmann, M. and Scofield, R.H. (2006) Oxidatively modified autoantigens in autoimmune diseases. *Free Radical Biology & Medicine* 41, 549–556.

Lalla, E., Lamster, I.B., Stern, D.M. and Schmidt, A.M. (2001) Receptor for advanced glycation end products, inflammation, and accelerated periodontal disease in diabetes: mechanisms and insights into therapeutic modalities. *Annals of Periodontology* 6, 113–118.

Larsson, S.C., Bergkvist, L. and Wolk, A. (2004) Milk and lactose intakes and ovarian cancer risk in the Swedish Mammography Cohort. *American Journal of Clinical Nutrition* 80, 1353–1357.

Laugerette, F., Vors, C., Géloën, A., Chauvin, M.A., Soulage, C., Lambert-Porcheron, S., Peretti, N., *et al.* (2010) Emulsified lipids increase endotoxemia: possible role in early postprandial low-grade inflammation. *Journal of Nutritional Biochemistry* 22, 53–59.

Leaf, A. and Weber, P.C. (1988) Cardiovascular effects of n-3 fatty acids. *New England Journal of Medicine* 318, 549–557.

Lichtenstein, A.H., Brands, M., Franch, H.A., *et al.* (2006) Diet and lifestyle recommendations revision 2006. A scientific statement from the American Heart Association Nutrition Committee. *Circulation* 114, 82–96.

Lin, R.Y., Choudhury, W., Cai, W., *et al.* (2003) Dietary glycotoxins promote diabetic atherosclerosis in apolipoprotein E-deficient mice. *Atherosclerosis* 168, 213–220.

Liu, J., Zhao, S., Tang, J., *et al.* (2009) Advanced glycation end products and lipopolysaccharide synergistically stimulate proinflammatory cytokine/chemokine production in endothelial cells via activation of both mitogen-activated protein kinases and nuclear factor-kappaB. *FEBS Journal* 276, 4598–4606.

Logsdon, C.D., Fuentes, M.K., Huang, E.H. and Arumugam, T. (2007) RAGE and RAGE ligands in cancer. *Current Molecular Medicine* 7, 777–789.

Ma, L. and Nicholson, L.F. (2004) Expression of the receptor for advanced glycation end products in Huntington's disease caudate nucleus. *Brain Research* 1018, 10–17.

Maillard, L.C. (1912) Action des acids amine sur des sucres: formation des melanoides per voie methodique. *Comptes Rendus de l'Académie des Sciences* 154, 66–68.

Malekinejad, H., Scherpenisse, P. and Bergwerff, A.A. (2006) Naturally occurring estrogens in processed milk and in raw milk (from gestated cows). *Journal of Agricultural and Food Chemistry* 54, 9785–9791.

Matsumoto, T., Tsurumoto, T., Baba, H., *et al.* (2007) Measurement of advanced glycation end products in skin of patients with rheumatoid arthritis, osteoarthritis, and dialysis-related spondyloarthropathy using non-invasive methods. *Rheumatology International* 28, 157–160.

Mattson, M.P. (2003) Will caloric restriction and folate protect against AD and PD? *Neurology* 60, 690–695.

McCarty, M.F. (2005) Secondary hyperparathyroidism promotes the acute phase response – a rationale for supplementing vitamin D in prevention of vascular events in elderly. *Medical Hypotheses* 64, 1022–1026.

McCarty, M.F., Barroso-Aranda, J. and Contreras, F. (2009) The low-methionine content of vegan diets may make methionine restriction feasible as a life extension strategy. *Medical Hypotheses* 72, 125–128.

Meerwaldt, R., Links, T., Graaff, R., et al. (2005a) Simple noninvasive measurement of skin autofluorescence. *Annals of the Academy of Sciences* 1043, 290–298.

Meerwaldt, R., Hartog, J.W., Graaff, R., et al. (2005b) Skin autofluorescence, a measure of cumulative metabolic stress and advanced glycation end products, predicts mortality in hemodialysis patients. *Journal of the American Society of Nephrology* 16, 3687–3693.

Meerwaldt, R., Links, T., Zeebregts, C., et al. (2008) The clinical relevance of assessing advanced glycation endproducts accumulation in diabetes. *Cardiovascular Diabetology* 7, 29.

Melo, A., Viegas, O., Petisca, C., et al. (2008) Effect of beer/red wine marinades on the formation of heterocyclic aromatic amines in pan-fried beef. *Journal of Agricultural and Food Chemistry* 56, 10625–10632.

Meyer, T.E., Kovacs, S.J., Ehsani, A.A., et al. (2006) Long-term caloric restriction ameliorates the decline in diastolic function in humans. *Journal of the American College of Cardiology* 47, 398–402.

Miyata, T., Kawai, R., Taketomi, S. and Sprague, S.M. (1996) Possible involvement of advanced glycation end-products in bone resorption. *Nephrology Dialysis Transplantation* 11, 54–57.

Mohr, S.B., Gorham, E.D., Garland, C.F., et al. (2006) Are low ultraviolet B and high animal protein intake associated with risk of renal cancer? *International Journal of Cancer* 119, 2705–2709.

Mohr, S.B., Garland, C.F., Gorham, E.D., et al. (2007) Is ultraviolet B irradiance inversely associated with incidence rates of endometrial cancer: an ecological study of 107 countries. *Preventive Medicine* 45, 327–331.

Mohr, S.B., Garland, C.F., Gorham, E.D. and Garland, F.C. (2008) The association between ultraviolet B irradiance, vitamin D status and incidence rates of type 1 diabetes in 51 regions worldwide. *Diabetologia* 51, 1391–1398.

Monnier, V.M., Bautista, O., Kenny, D., et al. (1999) Skin collagen glycation, glycoxidation, and crosslinking are lower in subjects with long-term intensive versus conventional therapy of type 1 diabetes: relevance of glycated collagen products versus HbA1c as markers of diabetic complications. DCCT Skin Collagen Ancillary Study Group. Diabetes control and complications trial. *Diabetes* 48, 870–880.

Monnier, V.M., Sell, D.R. and Genuth, S. (2005) Glycation products as markers and predictors of the progression of diabetic complications. *Annals of the New York Academy of Sciences* 1043, 567–581.

Moreira, P.I., Smith, M.A., Zhu, X., et al. (2005) Oxidative stress and neurodegeneration. *Annals of the New York Academy of Sciences* 1043, 543–552.

Moss, M. and Freed, D.L. (1999) Survival trends, coronary event rates, and the MONICA project. Monitoring trends and determinants in cardiovascular disease. *Lancet* 354, 862–865.

Mulder, D.J., Bieze, M., Graaff, R., et al. (2010) Skin autofluorescence is elevated in neovascular age-related macular degeneration. *British Journal of Ophthalmology* 94, 622–625.

Müller, M. and Lier, D. (1994) Fermentation of fructans by epiphytic lactic acid bacteria. *Journal of Applied Bacteriology* 76, 406–411.

Naaber, P., Smidt, I., Stsepetova, J., et al. (2004) Inhibition of *Clostridium difficile* strains by intestinal *Lactobacillus* species. *Journal of Medical Microbiology* 53, 551–554.

Nagaraj, R.H., Padmanabha, S., Mailanko, M., et al. (2010) Modulation of advanced glycation endproduct synthesis by kynurenines in human lens proteins. *Biochimica et Biophysica Acta* 1804, 829–838.

Nandhini, A.T.A., Thirunavakkarasu, V. and Anuradha, C.V. (2004) Stimulation of glucose utilization and inhibition of protein glycation and AGE products by taurine. *Acta Physiologica Scandinavica* 181, 297–303.

Nandhini, A.T.A., Thirunavakkarasu, V. and Anuradha, C.V. (2005) Taurine prevents collagen abnormalities in high fructose-fed rats. *Indian Journal of Medical Research* 122, 171–177.

Ni, J., Yuan, X., Gu, J., et al. (2009) Plasma protein pentosidine and carboxymethyllysine, biomarkers for age-related macular degeneration. *Molecular & Cellular Proteomics* 8, 1921–1933.

Nicolls, M.R. (2004) The clinical and biological relationship between type II diabetes mellitus and Alzheimer's disease. *Current Alzheimer Research* 1, 47–54.

Odetti, P., Angelini, G., Dapino, D., et al. (1998) Early glycoxidation damage in brains from Down's syndrome. *Biochemical and Biophysical Research Communications* 243, 849–851.

Odetti, P., Rossi, S., Monacelli, F., et al. (2005) Advanced glycation end products and bone loss during aging. *Annals of the New York Academy of Sciences* 1043, 710–717.

Orasanu, G. and Plutzky, J. (2009) The pathologic continuum of diabetic vascular disease. *Journal of the American College of Cardiology* 53, S35–42.

Osawa, T. and Kato, Y. (2005) Protective role of antioxidative food factors in oxidative stress caused by hyperglycemia. *Annals of the New York Academy of Sciences* 1043, 440–451.

Ostergaard, J., Hansen, T.K., Thiel, S. and Flyvbjerg, A. (2005) Complement activation and diabetic vascular complications. *Clinica Chimica Acta* 361, 10–19.

Outwater, J.L., Nicholson, A. and Barnard, N. (1997) Dairy products and breast cancer: the IGF-I, estrogen, and bGH hypothesis. *Medical Hypotheses* 48, 453–461.

Papachroni, K.K., Piper, C., Levidou, G., Korkolopoulou, P., Pawelczyk, L., Diamanti-Kandarakis, E. and Papavassiliou, A.G. (2009) Lysyl oxidase interacts with AGEs signaling to modulate collagen synthesis in polycystic ovarian tissue. *Journal of Cellular and Molecular Medicine* 14, 2460–2469; doi: 10.1111/j.1582-4934.2009.00841.x.

Peppa, M., Brem, P., Ehrlich, J., et al. (2003) Adverse effects of glycotoxins on wound healing in genetically diabetic mice. *Diabetes* 52, 2805–2813.

Peskind, E.R., Elrod, R., Dobie, D.J., et al. (1998) Cerebrospinal fluid epinephrine in Alzheimer's disease and normal aging. *Neuropsychopharmacology* 19, 465–471.

Platz, E.A., Willett, W.C., Colditz, G.A., et al. (2000) Proportion of colon cancer risk that might be preventable in a cohort of middle-aged US men. *Cancer Causes Control* 11, 579–588.

Rahman, I., Biswas, S.K. and Kode, A. (2006a) Oxidant and antioxidant balance in the airways and airway diseases. *European Journal of Pharmacology* 533, 222–239.

Rahman, I., Biswas, S.K. and Kirkham, P.A. (2006b) Regulation of inflammation and redox signaling by dietary polyphenols. *Biochemical Pharmacology* 72, 1439–1452.

Ramamurthy, B., Hook, P., Jones, A.D. and Larsson, L. (2001) Changes in myosin structure and function in response to glycation. *FASEB Journal* 15, 2415–2422.

Rautava, S. and Isolauri, E. (2004) Cow's milk allergy in infants with atopic eczema is associated with aberrant production of interleukin-4 during oral cow's milk challenge. *Journal of Pediatric Gastroenterology and Nutrition* 39, 529–535.

Reddy, G.K. (2004) Cross-linking in collagen by nonenzymatic glycation increases the matrix stiffness in rabbit achilles tendon. *Experimental Diabesity Research* 5, 143–153.

Reeves, M.J. and Rafferty, A.P. (2005) Healthy lifestyle characteristics among adults in the United States 2000. *Archives of Internal Medicine* 165, 854–857.

Rehbein, G., Simm, A. and Hofmann, H.S. (2008) Molecular regulation of S100P in human lung adenocarcinomas. *International Journal of Molecular Sciences* 22, 69–77.

Rosca, M.G., Mustata, T.G., Kinter, M.T., et al. (2005) Glycation of mitochondrial proteins from diabetic rat kidney is associated with excess superoxide formation. *American Journal of Physiology - Renal Physiology* 289, F420–F430.

Rüster, M., Franke, S., Späth, M., et al. (2005) Detection of elevated N epsilon-carboxymethyllysine levels in muscular tissue and in serum of patients with fibromyalgia. *Scandinavian Journal of Rheumatology* 34, 460–463.

Sancho, A.I., Rigby, N.M., Zuidmeer, L., et al. (2005) The effect of thermal processing on the IgE reactivity of the non-specific lipid transfer protein from apple, Mal d 3. *Allergy* 60, 1262–1268.

Sasaki, N., Takeuschi, M., Choei, H., et al. (2002) Advanced glycation end products (AGE) and their receptor (RAGE) in the brain of patients with Creutzfeldt-Jacob disease with prion plaques. *Neuroscience Letters* 326, 117–120.

Sbarbati, A., Valleta, E., Bertini, M., et al. (2003) Gluten sensitivity and 'normal' histology: is the intestinal mucosa really normal? *Digestive and Liver Disease* 35, 768–773.

Schepers, E., Glorieux, G. and Vanholder, R. (2010) The gut: the forgotten organ in uremia? *Blood Purification* 29, 130–136.

Schmidt, A.M., Vianna, M., Gerlach, M., et al. (1992) Isolation and characterization of binding proteins for advanced glycosylation endproducts from lung tissue which are present on the endothelial cell surface. *Journal of Biological Chemistry* 267, 14987–14997.

Schmidt, A.M., Yan, S.D., Brett, J., et al. (1993) Regulation of mononuclear phagocyte migration by cell surface binding proteins for advanced glycosylation endproducts. *Journal of Clinical Investigation* 92, 2155–2168.

Schmidt, A.M., Mora, R., Cao, R., et al. (1994a) The endothelial cell binding site for advanced glycation end products consists of a complex: an integral membrane protein and a lactoferrin-like polypeptide. *Journal of Biological Chemistry* 269, 9882–9888.

Schmidt, A.M., Hasu, M., Popov, D., et al. (1994b) The receptor for Advanced Glycation End products (AGEs) has a central role in vessel wall interactions and gene activation in response to AGEs in the intravascular space. *Proceedings of the National Academy of Sciences USA* 91, 8807–8811.

Schmidt, A.M., Yan, S.D., Yan, S.F. and Stern, D.M. (2001) The multiligand receptor RAGE is a progression factor amplifying immune and inflammatory responses. *Journal of Clinical Investigation* 108, 949–955.

Sebekova, K., Krajcoviova-Kudlackova, M., Schinzel, R., et al. (2001) Plasma levels of advanced glycation end products in healthy, long-term vegetarians and subjects on a western mixed diet. *European Journal of Nutrition* 40, 275–281.

Sebekova, K., Kupcova, V., Schinzel, R. and Heidland, A. (2002) Markedly elevated levels of plasma advanced glycation end products in patients with liver cirrhosis – amelioration by liver transplantation. *Journal of Hepatology* 36, 66–71.

Semba R.D., Bandinelli, S., Sun, K., et al. (2009) Plasma carboxymethyl-lysine, an advanced glycation end product, and all-cause and cardiovascular disease mortality in older community-dwelling adults. *Journal of the American Geriatric Society* 57, 1874–1680.

Smith, M.A., Taneda, S., Rickey, P.L., et al. (1994) Advanced Maillard reaction end products are associated with Alzheimer pathology. *Proceedings of the National Academy of Sciences USA* 91, 5710–5714.

Soldatos, G., Cooper, M.E. and Jandeleit-Dahm, K.A. (2005) Advanced-glycation end products in insulin-resistant states. *Current Hypertension Reports* 7, 96–102.

Stamatas, G.N., Estanislao, R.B., Suero, M., et al. (2006) Facial skin fluorescence as a marker of the skin's response to chronic environmental insults and its dependence on age. *British Journal of Dermatology* 154, 125–132.

Stampfer, M.J., Hu, F.B., Manson, J.E., et al. (2000) Primary prevention of coronary heart disease in women through diet and lifestyle. *New England Journal of Medicine* 343, 16–22.

Steenvoorden, M.M., Huizinga, T.W., Verzijl, N., et al. (2006) Activation of receptor for advanced glycation end products in osteoarthritis leads to increased stimulation of chondrocytes and synoviocytes. *Arthritis & Rheumatism* 54, 253–263.

Stitt, A.L. (2005) The Maillard reaction in eye disease. *Annals of the New York Academy of Sciences* 1043, 582–597.

Sun A.Y., Wang, Q., Simonyi, A. and Sun, G.Y. (2010) Resveratrol as a therapeutic agent for neurodegenerative diseases. *Molecular Neurobiology* 41, 375–83.

Sunahori, K., Yamamura, M., Yamana, J., et al. (2006) Increased expression of receptor for advanced glycation end products by synovial tissue macrophages in rheumatoid arthritis. *Arthritis & Rheumatism* 54, 97–104.

Suzuma, K., Otani, A., Oh, H., et al. (1999) 17- Beta-estradiol increases VEGF receptor-2 and promotes DNA synthesis in retinal microvascular endothelial cells. *Investigative Ophthalmology & Visual Science* 40, 2122–2129.

Takada, M., Hirata, K., Ajiki, T., Suzuki, Y. and Kuroda, Y. (2004) Expression of receptor for advanced glycation end products (RAGE) and MMP-9 in human pancreatic cancer cells. *Hepatogastroenterology* 51, 928–930.

Taki, K., Takayama, F., Tsuruta, Y. and Niwa, T. (2006) Oxidative stress, advanced glycation end product, and coronary artery calcification in hemodialysis patients. *Kidney International* 70, 218–224.

Tateno, T., Ueno, S. and Hiwatashi, K. (2008) Expression of receptor for advanced glycation end products (RAGE) is related to prognosis in patients with esophageal squamous cell carcinoma. *Annals of Surgical Oncology* 16, 440–446.

Tavan, E., Cayuela, C., Antoine, J.M. and Cassand, P. (2002) Antimutagenic activities of various lactic acid bacteria against food mutagens: heterocyclic amines. *Journal of Dairy Research* 69, 335–341.

Tezel, G., Luo, C. and Yang, X. (2007) Accelerated aging in glaucoma: immunohistochemical assessment of advanced glycation end products in the human retina and optic nerve head. *Investigative Ophthalmology & Visual Science* 48, 1201–1211.

Thiel, R. and Fowkes, S.W. (2005) Can cognitive deterioration associated with Down syndrome be reduced? *Medical Hypotheses* 64, 524–532.

Tikellis, C., Cooper, M.E. and Thomas, M.C. (2006) Role of the renin-angiotensin system in the endocrine pancreas: implications for the development of diabetes. *The International Journal Of Biochemistry & Cell Biology* 38, 737–751

Tikellis, C., Thomas, M.C., Harcourt, B.E., Coughlan, M.T., Pete, J., Bialkowski, K., Tan, A., et al. (2008) Cardiac inflammation associated with a Western diet is mediated via activation of RAGE by AGEs. *American Journal of Physiology - Endocrinology and Metabolism* 295, E323–330.

Tlaskalová-Hogenová, H., Tucková, L., Stepánková, R., et al (2005) Involvement of innate immunity in the development of inflammatory and autoimmune diseases. *Annals of New York Academy of Science* 1051, 787–798.

Tokita, Y., Hirayama, Y., Sekikawa, A., et al. (2005) Fructose ingestion enhances atherosclerosis and deposition of advanced glycated end-products in cholesterol-fed rabbits. *Journal of Atherosclerosis and Thrombosis* 12, 260–267.

Tsukahara, H., Shibata, R., Ohta N., *et al.* (2003) High levels of urinary pentosidine, an advanced glycation end product, in children with acute exacerbation of atopic dermatitis: relationship with oxidative stress. *Metabolism* 52, 1601–1605.

Tucker, K.L., Morita, K., Qiao, N., *et al.* (2006) Colas, but not other carbonated beverages, are associated with low bone mineral density in older women: The Framingham Osteoporosis Study. *American Journal of Clinical Nutrition* 84, 936–942.

Unno, Y., Sakai, M., Sakamoto, Y., *et al.* (2004) Advanced glycation end products-modified proteins and oxidized LDL mediate down-regulation of leptin in mouse adipocytes via CD36. *Biochemical and Biophysical Research Communications* 325, 151–156.

Uribarri, J. and Tuttle, K.R. (2006) Advanced glycation end products and nephrotoxicity of high-protein diets. *Clinical Journal of the American Society of Nephrology* 1, 1293–1299.

Uribarri, J., Woodruff, S., Goodman, S., *et al.* (2010). Advanced glycation end products in foods and a practical guide to their reduction in the diet. *Journal of American Dietetic Association* 110, 911–916.

US Department of Health and Human Services, National Institutes of Health, and National Heart, Lung, and Blood Institute (2006) *Your Guide to Lowering Your Blood Pressure with Dietary Approach to Stop Hypertension (DASH)*. NIH Publication 06-4082, revision of 1st ed. (1988).

Visentin, S., Medana, C., Barge, A., *et al.* (2010) Microwave-assisted Maillard reactions for the preparation of advanced glycation end products (AGEs). *Organic & Biomolecular Chemistry* 21, 2473–2477.

Vitek, M.P., Bhattacharya, K., Gendening, J.M., *et al.* (1994) Advanced glycation end products contribute to amyloidosis in Alzheimer disease. *Proceedings of the National Academy of Sciences USA* 91, 4766–4770.

Vlassara, H. (2005) Advanced glycation in health and disease. Role of the modern environment. *Annals of the New York Academy of Sciences* 1043, 452–460.

Vlassara, H., Cai, J., Crandall, J., *et al.* (2002) Inflammatory mediators are induced by dietary glycotoxins, a major risk factor for diabetic angiopathy. *Proceedings of the National Academy of Sciences USA* 99, 15596–15601.

Vlassara, H., Torreggiani, M., Post, J.B., *et al.* (2009) Role of oxidants/inflammation in declining renal function in chronic kidney disease and normal aging. *Kidney International Supplement* 14, S3–11.

Wiame, E., Delpierre, G., Collard, F. and Van Schaftingen, E. (2002) Identification of a pathway for the utilization of the Amadori product fructoselysine in Escherichia coli. *Journal of Biological Chemistry* 277, 42523–42529.

Yagmur, E., Tacke., F., Weiss, C.P., *et al.* (2006) Elevation of Nepsilon-(carboxymethyl)lysine-modified advanced glycation end products in chronic liver disease is an indicator of liver cirrhosis. *Clinical Biochemistry* 39, 39–45.

Yamagishi, S., Fujimori, H., Yonekura, H., *et al.* (1998) Advanced glycation end products inhibit prostacyclin production and induce plasminogen activator inhibitor-1 in human microvascular endothelial cells. *Diabetologica* 41, 1435–1441.

Yan, S.F., Ramasamy, R. and Schmidt, A.M. (2009) Receptor for AGE (RAGE) and its ligands-cast into leading roles in diabetes and the inflammatory response. *Journal of Molecular Medicine* 87, 235–247.

Zeng, S., Feirt, N., Goldstein, M., *et al.* (2004) Blockade of receptor for advanced glycation end product (RAGE) attenuates ischemia and reperfusion injury to the liver in mice. *Hepatology* 39, 422–432.

Zheng, F., He, C., Cai, W., *et al.* (2002) Prevention of nephropathy in mice by a diet low in glycoxidation products. *Diabetes/Metabolism Research and Reviews* 18, 224–237.

Zimmerman, G.A., Meistrell, M., Bloom, O., *et al.* (1995) Neurotoxicity of advanced glycation endproducts during focal stroke and neuroprotective effects of aminoguanidine. *Proceedings of the National Academy of Sciences USA* 92, 3744–3748.

Zittermann, A., Schleithoff, S.S. and Koerfer, R. (2005) Putting cardiovascular disease and vitamin D insufficiency into perspective. *British Journal of Nutrition* 94, 483–492.

23 Phenylketonuria: Newborn Identification Through to Adulthood

R. Koch and K. Moseley*

Department of Pediatrics, Genetics Division, Keck School of Medicine, University of Southern California, Los Angeles, USA

23.1 Abstract

The discovery of phenylketonuria (PKU) in 1934 by Asbørn Følling has led to many advances involving identification, diagnosis, classification, and treatment not only for PKU, but for many other inborn errors of metabolism. It took 20 years after the discovery before the first amino acid mixture was introduced for treatment, and another ten years for newborn screening tests to become available in developed nations. The successful identification and treatment of PKU has reversed the profound mental retardation associated with this disorder, and those affected and treated can now lead essentially normal lives. It is remarkable to think that simple restriction of the amino acid phenylalanine (Phe) could have such an effect. However, the dietary treatment is not ideal and maternal PKU remains a problem. It is difficult for many women with PKU to achieve low blood Phe levels throughout the pregnancy. High levels are harmful to the baby and the diet is so restrictive it may be lacking in essential nutrients. However, the past ten years have seen a surge in research, new products, and new treatment modalities. There are many different forms of medical food products available that include flavoured powder, gels, bars, capsules, and tablets to make adherence easier. However, since much of the diet is synthetic there are reported nutrient deficiencies which affect growth and cognitive development. New treatment modalities are also available with the use of large neutral amino acids (LNAA) and glycomacropeptide. In 2007, Kuvan^R, a new drug for the treatment of PKU, was introduced. This is the synthetic form of tetrahydrobiopterin (BH$_4$) and acts on the phenylalanine hydroxylase which stimulates enzyme activity, lowering the blood Phe in those who respond. Gene therapy continues to be researched and enzyme substitution is currently in clinical trials. Looking back over 75 years since the discovery of this disorder, we have come a long way. With continuing research, new products and treatment modalities, new guidelines will need to be implemented and perhaps a new paradigm of treatment strategy will emerge.

23.2 Introduction

Asbørn Følling was a Norwegian physician who fortunately also had a biochemical background. His discovery of 'imbecillitas

---

* E-mail address: kmoseley@usc.edu

phenylpyruvica' laid the co-groundwork for the successful accomplishments involving identification, diagnosis, classification, treatment, and progress for the next 75 years, bringing the PKU story to an apparent conclusion (Følling, 1934). It is remarkable to realize the significant progress that has been made in conquering a newly identified metabolic disorder that in the past caused profound mental retardation, in comparison to our present situation when a newborn baby with PKU can be expected to develop normally, attend school, marry, have children, and live a normal life. Dr Følling's accomplishment provided the opportunity and stimulus to lay the ground-work for an entirely new approach to the diagnosis and care of children with various other metabolic disorders. Archibald Garrod (1902) is to be honoured for initiating an interest in metabolic disorders; however, it is unlikely that Dr Følling was aware of the work of Garrod. Følling's discovery of PKU has resulted in the salvaging of many affected persons, allowing them to live normal lives.

23.3 Background

Prior to Følling's identification of PKU and even 20 years afterward, affected persons in the United States were eventually institutionalized in large facilities because no treatment was available. In 1954 Dr Horst Bickel, at the Manchester Children's Hospital in the United Kingdom (Bickel, et al., 1953), developed the first Phe-restricted diet, which became the foundation for the treatment of PKU. It was found that young children with PKU improved clinically and psychologically when treated with this diet; however, older severely mentally retarded persons usually did not benefit substantially.

In 1960 Robert Guthrie (Guthrie and Susi, 1963) developed a newborn screening blood test to identify babies with PKU. He was motivated after his wife's niece was identified to have PKU through the use of a ferric chloride test of the child's urine. Unfortunately, this child was already mentally delayed by the time the diagnosis was made. Dr Guthrie subsequently obtained a grant from the United States Children's Bureau, a Federal agency, to establish the accuracy of this test for PKU. Surprisingly, the development of newborn screening for PKU created controversy among members of the medical profession. It was thought that the test was not very accurate. Some physicians believed treatment for PKU would not be beneficial, while others thought this was the beginning of socialized medicine.

Our experience in treating late-diagnosed children with PKU using the Phe-restricted diet demonstrated that their intelligence did not degenerate, but improved over time with treatment. In 1964, one of us (R.K.) applied for a Federal grant to document these preliminary findings (Azen et al., 1991). The Collaborative Study of Children Treated for PKU was a prospective study of infants. Two hundred and eleven newborns identified in 14 states were enrolled and monitored for 12 years. It was shown clearly that the subjects who were maintained on the Phe-restricted diet for ten years had superior intellectual function than those who maintained the diet for only five years. The data were published by Azen et al. (1991).

23.4 Current Problem: Maternal PKU Therapy

In 1980 Harvey Levy MD, the head of the Harvard PKU programme at Boston Children's Hospital, and R. Lenke (Lenke and Levy, 1980) were the first physicians to do a worldwide assessment of maternal PKU (MPKU) problems. Initially it was thought that women with PKU could have normal children, regardless of whether or not they were on a diet restricted in Phe. However the Levy report clearly showed that women with PKU who have blood Phe levels greater than 1200 μmol l^{-1} during pregnancy have a high possibility of giving birth to severely mentally retarded children. Levy reported that over 90% of the infants born to these women suffered from microcephaly and 12–14% had congenital heart disease. The rate of abnormality depended upon the blood Phe levels that were documented in the mothers. These data led physicians to advise women with PKU not to have their own children, but rather to adopt if they wanted a family.

At the Children's Hospital of Los Angeles, dietary treatment was never discontinued; accordingly, during pregnancy, women with PKU were kept on the diet and blood Phe levels of 120–360 μmol l^{-1} were recommended. Fortunately the rate of microcephaly in their infants was very low (2–3%) and congenital heart disease was 1%. As a result the National Institute of Child Health and Human Development decided to fund a long-term study on MPKU, which involved 430 pregnancies (Koch et al., 2003a). Unfortunately 90% of clinics were discontinuing dietary therapy between 1970 and 1980 because it was mistakenly thought that PKU patients could eat a normal diet because the brain growth was completed by the age of 6 years. (The reader is referred to *Pediatrics* 112 (6) December 2003 supplement for additional details.) Many of the mothers who were enrolled in the study had intelligence quotients between 70 and 90 and a significant number of them did not start the Phe-restricted diet until late in the first trimester. Four mothers did not actually join the study until they were in their third trimester. The overall results were disappointing. Twenty four percent of the offspring exhibited a head circumference of 32 cm or less and 7% of the women had babies with congenital heart disease. The study did demonstrate that women who planned their pregnancies and kept their blood Phe levels at 120–360 μmol l^{-1} had babies with normal head circumferences of 33–36 cm. The rate of congenital heart disease in this group was 1–2%.

23.5 The Role of Tetrahydrobiopterin (BH$_4$) Treatment for Patients with PKU

In 1999 Professor Shigeo Kure in Japan published the first paper on treatment of five children with PKU who received BH$_4$ therapy during infancy and demonstrated significant improvement in blood Phe levels (Kure et al. 1999). Historically, of course, BH$_4$ was discovered at the National Institute of Neurological Disorders in Bethesda, Maryland (Kaufman 1963). However nearly all of the earlier studies were performed on animals and it was not tried on humans until the discovery of BH$_4$ metabolic defects in 1974 (Kaufman et al., 1975). BH$_4$ was found to have no toxicity and to be well tolerated. There are six biochemical steps in the human body resulting in biopterin production. Fortunately defects in biopterin production are rare. In the first author's 55 years of caring for patients with PKU, the only patient we have seen with a biopterin defect died in early infancy. Thus it was not until Dr Kure published his initial results that BH$_4$ was used to treat patients with PKU. Why is BH$_4$ important in patients with PKU? BH$_4$ is a cofactor required by Phe hydroxylase (PAH) to convert Phe to tyrosine, which in turn is then converted into dopamine in human metabolism. It may be in some obscure way related to schizophrenia. In addition, BH$_4$ is a cofactor for nitric oxide synthase (NOS), an enzyme important in brain metabolism. NOS is involved in the transmission of signals between neurons. The reader is referred to Chapter 168 in Scriver et al. (2001) for further details regarding NOS metabolism.

At present we have only two years of experience with this new product, however it has created a great deal of excitement. Persons who have mild hyper Phe due to mild mutations of the PKU gene may actually go off diet restriction of Phe altogether. Persons with one mild mutation and one severe mutation may exhibit a significant reduction of the blood Phe levels – by as much as 30%. Persons with two severe mutations, such as R408W/R408W rarely show a reduction in blood Phe levels, but do feel better, have more energy, and display improvement in behaviour (first author's personal observation). So we do not yet know the extent of the usefulness of BH$_4$ in the treatment of PKU. The first author would predict that all patients with PKU will eventually be taking BH$_4$ in addition to dietary restriction of Phe. In addition, the role of BH$_4$ in maternal PKU may become very important.

23.6 Dietary Therapy

The dietary management of PKU is a success story. Diet therapy implemented shortly after birth prevents the devastating outcomes associated with untreated PKU which includes severe cognitive delays, neurological deterioration, eczema, seizures and epilepsy, and progressive motor disorder. The mainstay of the treatment has been the Phe-restricted diet. Careful management and adherence to the dietary recommendations are essential for a good outcome. To date there is considerable variation on the recommended plasma blood Phe concentrations to be maintained at various ages. But most countries, including the United States, recommend blood Phe levels <360 µmol l^{-1} under the age of six years (NIH, 2000; Schweitzer-Krantz and Burgard, 2000). Maintaining the blood Phe concentrations is based on tolerance, which is the amount of Phe 'tolerated' for blood Phe concentrations to remain in the recommended ranges. However, the Phe-restricted diet is not easy to maintain. The standard diet consists of an amino acid mixture that contains all the necessary nutrients for normal growth except for Phe. The diet restricts high protein foods such as meat, poultry, fish, pork legumes, nuts and dairy products. Fruits, vegetables and a limited amount of grains are used in combination with low protein foods to provide a regulated amount of Phe in order to keep blood Phe levels within the recommended range. For many individuals the taste of the amino acid mixture is unpalatable and the amount that must be consumed is unattainable. Because the majority of this diet is synthetic with very low amounts of natural food, the diet is suboptimal as impaired growth, bone density, and other nutritional deficiencies have been reported.

During the 1960s when the diet for PKU was being established, there were reports of poor growth which was attributed to 'Phenylalanine deficiency syndrome'. In fact, two infants were reported to have been fed the Phe-restricted diet in error during the first few weeks of life and suffered failure to thrive, eczema, listlessness, and developmental delay (Rouse, 1966). Hanley et al. (1970) also reported malnutrition in the first year of life due to over-restriction of Phe as possibly contributing to mental retardation. In addition, the insufficiency of Phe may have led to growth deficiencies, as reported in a study in Germany where height and head circumference were decreased significantly during the first two years of life despite adequate weight gain and protein intake (Schaefer et al., 1994). The National PKU Collaborative Study conducted from 1967 to 1983 showed that normal physical growth was achievable using a protocol with prescribed amounts of protein and energy (Holm et al., 1979). In North America the growth status in PKU individuals on the Phe-restricted diet has been essentially normal compared to growth data from the National Center for Health Statistics (NCHS) in height and head circumference. However, PKU males and females weighed more and the growth curves suggested that this weight difference was related to diet adherence. High blood Phe concentrations were associated with higher weights, especially in females (McBurnie et al., 1991). Additionally, high blood levels of leptin, a hormone associated with obesity, has been reported in individuals with PKU and high blood Phe concentrations (Schulpis et al., 2000). Nutrient intakes and physical growth were assessed in PKU individuals using three different amino acid mixtures (Acosta et al., 2003). Outcome of this report revealed no statistical difference in mean z scores for height and body mass index (BMI) between the three groups. However, there is a suggestion of a trend towards obesity in those with PKU.

Most clinics in the United States use the Ross Protocols (Acosta and Yannicelli, 2001) for initiating the protein prescription which can be as much as 110–130% over the recommended dietary intakes (RDI). Huemer et al. (2007) reported the results of growth and body composition in children with classic PKU, showing that there were no statistical differences in growth or body composition or in fat-free mass in PKU subjects and age/sex-matched controls. Phe-free amino acid mixtures exceeded the RDI by a mean 20–40%. There was also a significant correlation between fat-free mass and natural protein intake (Huemer et al., 2007). A significant correlation between natural protein intake and head circumference was also reported suggesting that improvement of protein quality may improve growth and body composition in PKU (Hoeksma *et al.*, 2005).

There are also a number of reports indicating subtle cognitive deficits in individuals with PKU who are well treated (Waisbren *et al.*, 1994; DeRoche and Welsh, 2008). A comprehensive review of executive abilities was performed in 2010 and reported a number of studies finding information-processing speed, fine motor control, perception, and visual-spatial abilities are compromised in those with PKU, with conflicting reports on assessing language, learning, and memory impairments (Janzen and Nguyen, 2010). There is no clear delineation on the specific mechanisms for these impairments. However, dopamine deficiency and white matter abnormalities are highly suggestive (Christ *et al.*, 2010). In contrast, the pathogenesis of cognitive dysfunction hypothesized by de Groot *et al.* (2010) is reduced cerebral neurotransmitter and protein synthesis, caused by impaired brain uptake of the non-Phe LNAA with elevated blood Phe concentrations. Looking at the dietary intake and nutrient deficiencies may provide some answers.

It is well known that docosahexaenoic acid (DHA) (22:6n-3) and arachidonic acid (ARA) (20:4n-6) are very important structural components of the central nervous system and are transferred across the placenta, accumulating in the brain and other organs during the development of the fetus (Martinez, 1992). Studies have shown that DHA is vital throughout pregnancy in the first few weeks of brain cell division and the last trimester, when the content of the cerebrum and cerebellum increase three- to fivefold. There is a significant rapid increase in brain DHA from birth to 2 years of age. DHA is also the most abundant omega-3 fatty acid in the retina of the eye, which has the highest DHA concentration of any other organ, and is important for visual acuity (Dobbing and Sands, 1973). DHA facilitates many functions in the body including the regulation of gene expression, regulation of synthesis of eicosanoids derived from ARA, maintenance of membrane fluidity, protection of neural cells from apoptotic death, and regulation of nerve growth factor and neuron size; it is also needed for dopaminergic and serotoninergic neurotransmission (Sinclair *et al.*, 2002). Deficiencies of this very important essential fatty acid have been reported in individuals with PKU.

As early as 1973 (Acosta *et al.*, 1973) long-chain polyunsaturated fatty acids (LCPUFA) have been found to be deficient in individuals with PKU, both treated and untreated (Galli *et al.*, 1991; Sanjurjo *et al.*, 1994; Giovannini *et al.*, 1995; Moseley *et al.*, 2002). Since then there have been many reports in the literature documenting deficiencies (specifically in DHA) and normalization after supplementation. A randomized controlled trial was conducted showing that supplementation of LCPUFA in infants with PKU prevented the decline in DHA (Agostoni *et al.*, 2006). It was also shown that supplementation of LCPUFA including DHA improved visual function in children with well-controlled blood Phe levels, as well as improvement in fine motor skill and coordination (Agostoni *et al.*, 2000; Beblo *et al.*, 2007; Koletzko *et al.*, 2009). The study of essential fatty acids, especially DHA, is an emerging field of study and may contribute to the neurocognitive deficits that are seen in treated PKU individuals. It will be interesting to see over time if the individuals who are now supplemented in early infancy have the same deficits.

Since the primary source of the Phe-restricted diet is a synthetic medical food product many nutrients may not be absorbed or bioavailable. Deficiencies of iron, zinc, selenium, and Vitamin B_{12} have also been found in individuals with PKU (Acosta, 1996, 2004; Lombeck *et al.*, 1996; Van Bakel *et al.*, 2000). Vitamin B_{12} deficiency was also reported in a young female who was not taking her medical food product on a consistent basis yet eating very low protein foods. She presented with spastic paraparesis, tremor disorientation, slurred speech and deteriorating mental function with megaloblastic anaemia (Hanley *et al.*, 1996). After routinely checking complete blood count, ferritin, MCV, B_{12} and RBC folate, another 12 individuals were found with suboptimal B_{12} levels. Supplementation reversed some of the symptoms in some individuals but not all. Deficiencies of Vitamin B_{12} were also found in patients on an unrestricted or relaxed diet

(Robinson *et al.*, 2000). Additionally, PKU patients on a strict low Phe diet had low levels of vitamin B_6, vitamin B_{12} and folate which resulted in high blood levels of homocysteine; this may contribute to coronary artery disease later in life (Schulpis *et al.*, 2002; Hvas *et al.*, 2006). All of these deficiencies may impair normal growth and cognitive development.

Another area of concern is the bone health of individuals with PKU on restricted diets. A recent study of 31 patients reported osteopaenia in 11 and osteoporosis in two of the subjects. Compromised bone density with no clear cause was found in 42% of the subjects (Modan-Moses *et al.*, 2007). Other studies also report decreased bone mineralization, increased excretion of bone resorption markers and high osteoclast activity with no clear cause in individuals with PKU (Hillman *et al.*, 1996; Przyrembel and Bremer, 2000; Millet *et al.*, 2005; Porta *et al.*, 2008). Therefore, it is critical to monitor other nutritional markers that warrant supplementation in addition to blood Phe levels for normal growth and development.

Within the last ten years research in the area of PKU has surged as well as the availability of new products and treatment modalities. Phe-free amino acid mixtures are available in flavoured and unflavoured powdered form, gels, capsules, tablets, amino acid bars, and juice box drinks. They are also available fat free, low calorie, low volume, and high protein and tailored to each individual's needs (see Table 23.1). A number of products are now also supplemented with omega-3 fatty acids and DHA. The low-protein foods available to be used in conjunction with the diet have increased greatly in variety. There are low-protein pizzas, pastas, burgers, hot dogs, tortillas, cheese, yogurt, egg substitutes, a large variety of breads (including bagels, rolls, and buns), as well as a variety of ready-to-eat foods. However, up until recently, these foods contained trans fatty acids and very few nutrients. Several new treatment modalities are now available with the large neutral amino acid therapy, glycomacropeptide and BH_4.

Table 23.1. Medical food manufacturers.

Manufacturer	Products	Website
Nutricia SHS International	Powder, capsules, tablets, ready-to-drink, amino acid bars, add-ins, LNAA, low-protein food products	www.nutricia-na.com www.myspecialdiet.com www.shs-nutrition.com
Abbott Nutrition	Powder	www.abbottnutrition.com
Mead Johnson	Powder	www.meadjohnson.com
Applied Nutrition	Powder, amino acid bars, amino acid blends, LNAA, low-protein food products	www.medicalfood.com
VitaFlo USA	Gel, powder, ready-to-drink (DHA added)	www.Vitafloweb.com
Solace	Tablets, powder, LNAA	www.solacenutrition.com
Cambrooke Foods	Ready-to-drink, glycomacropeptide products	www.cambrookefoods.com
Davisco Foods Intl. Inc.	Daviscofoods.com	www.daviscofoods.com
Arla Food Ingredients	Glycomacropeptide	www.arlafoodsingredients.com

Low-protein foods only
    Dietary Specialties
    Med Diet
    PKU Perspectives
    Taste Connections
    Ener-G-Foods
    Specialty Food Shop (Canada)
    Glutino (Canada)
    Promin-PKU (United Kingdom)
		www.dietspec.com
		www.med-diet.com
		www.pkuperspectives.com
		www.tasteconnections.com
		www.ener-g.com
		www.specialtyfoodshop.ca
		www.glutino.com
		www.promin-pku.com

23.6.1 Large neutral amino acids

The use of the large neutral amino acid (LNAA) therapy has increased within the last few years because adherence to the Phe-restricted diet has decreased in the adolescent and adult population (Walter et al., 2002). The LNAA are amino acids that share a common transporter into the brain and compete with one another. Since Phe is so high in the blood it overwhelms the carrier and other LNAA do not get on. By giving large doses of LNAA except Phe the concentrations of other amino acids is increased (Christensen, 1953; Pardridge and Olendorf, 1975; Andersen and Avins, 1976; Olendorf and Szabo, 1976; Pratt, 1980). Although the exact mechanism for the brain damage in PKU is not known, it is believed the cause is decreased brain protein synthesis due to the lack of other LNAA, which results in increased myelin turnover and abnormalities in amine neurotransmitter systems (Surtees and Blau, 2000). Many studies including magnetic resonance spectroscopy (MRS) that actually can measure Phe in the brain have shown that LNAA can block the entry of Phe into the brain thereby reducing brain Phe (Knudsen et al., 1995; Pietz et al., 1999). Our six-month study conducted on six individuals with PKU used LNAA with enhanced amounts of tyrosine and tryptophan, and was found to lower brain Phe and increase the blood levels of tyrosine, as well as reduce the Phe/Tyr ratio. However, there was no significant effect on blood Phe (Koch et al., 2003b). Another study conducted reported giving 0.5 g kg^{-1} in three divided doses to eight subjects and 1 g kg^{-1} to three patients for 1 week; blood Phe was reduced by 50% in both groups ((Matalon et al., 2006). He also conducted a double-blind placebo study in 20 patients for 1 week and reported an average 39% decline in blood Phe (Matalon et al., 2007). A double-blind placebo crossover study using LNAA and MRS was also performed showing no correlation between brain and blood Phe when the blood Phe was under 1200 µmol l^{-1}, but a positive effect on executive function (Schindeler et al., 2007).

The dietary aspects of the LNAA therapy are the opposite of the Phe-restricted diet. The amount of protein in the Phe-restricted diet is approximately 20% natural protein and 80% synthetic protein coming from the medical food product. In the LNAA therapy 20% comes from the medical food product and 80% comes from natural protein. We have used this therapy in our clinic for the past 7 years in adults and adolescents. However, it may be necessary to provide a protein source without Phe (medical food product) since many individuals may not eat enough natural protein to meet nutritional requirements. A list of manufacturers of the medical food products and low-protein foods is presented in Table 23.1.

23.6.2 Glycomacropeptide

Another new approach to dietary treatment is glycomacropeptide. This compound is a protein in cheese whey, contains 64 amino acids and the commercial product contains 2.5–5 mg Phe g^{-1} of protein (Table 23.1). Its branched-chain amino acids compare to average dietary protein and it contains high amounts of threonine and isoleucine. In studies using glycomacropeptide, PKU mice showed significant decreases in both blood and brain Phe concentrations. In one case report a 29-year-old male completed a 15-week trial comparing glycomacropeptide to his usual medical food product. The glycomacropeptide products were an orange sports beverage, a pudding and a snack bar and were well accepted. The amino acid profile showed significant increases in plasma concentrations of LNAA and a 10% reduction in blood Phe with glycomacropeptide compared to the usual medical food product (Kyungwha et al., 2007; Ney et al., 2008, 2009). Because glycomacropeptide is an abundant food ingredient, naturally low in Phe, it may provide improved protein synthesis for growth due to the higher quality of protein. Long-term studies are needed to evaluate those parameters.

23.6.3 Tetrahydrobiopterin

Kuvan® is the name of the new BH_4 drug approved by the FDA in the United States in 2007. The dose ranges from 5–20 mg kg^{-1} and is shown to be well tolerated and effective in those who respond. Individuals who respond experience a drop in blood Phe concentrations and an increase in tolerance as well. A response is considered a drop in blood Phe concentrations of at least 30% (Burton et al., 2007; Kuvan, 2007; Levy et al., 2007). The majority of individuals who respond have mild or moderate PKU and are able to increase their tolerance to allow more natural foods. A recent study reported that the use of BH_4 allowed the liberalization of the diet in individuals with mild and moderate PKU, and improved LCPUFA status (specifically DHA) (Vilaseca et al., 2010). The use of BH_4 in normalizing the diet may prevent many of the deficiencies now seen in the Phe-restricted diet. It may also be especially important in MPKU, as the diet is so restrictive and very difficult for many women to consume the medical food products. It is labelled as a 'Pregnancy Category C' by the FDA, indicated by animal reproduction studies showing adverse effects on the fetus at 600 mg kg^1 which is 30 times the recommended dose. There are limited studies in the literature. Recently we reported the use of BH_4 on two women who were also following the Phe-restricted diet and both had a normal outcome (Moseley et al., 2009). The authors have followed six women with PKU who were taking small doses of BH_4 (300–600 mg) along with the Phe-restricted diet, with normal outcomes.

23.7 Future Research

Gene therapy research in PKU has been ongoing for the last two decades and when a therapeutic agent that is not harmful is introduced it perhaps will be the cure. However, much more research is needed. Currently, PEGylated recombinant phenylalanine ammonia lyase (PEG-PAL) is in Phase 2 clinical trials. This is enzyme-substitution therapy. PAL acts as a surrogate for the deficient PAH and converts the excess Phe to non-toxic trans-cinnamic acid and insignificant levels of ammonia. This new treatment could improve current therapy (no diet restriction) and increase quality of life (Sarkissian et al., 2009).

23.8 Conclusions

There is no question that Dr Følling's discovery of PKU, Dr Bickel's development of the Phe-restricted diet and Dr Guthrie's discovery of the newborn screening test are significant events. The contributions of Dr Savio Woo for his discovery of the structure of the PAH gene; and those of Dr Charles Scriver for the development of the PKU gene map, cataloguing the various mutations of the gene, have provided significant possibilities in understanding and studying PKU.

The new discovery that BH_4 can improve treatment for many people with PKU has been a significant development. More studies need to be performed for use in pregnancy, as the use of BH_4 may improve the outcomes due to the action on nitric oxide which may improve neuronal development in the fetal brain. Additionally, for those who respond, it will allow the consumption of more natural protein while maintaining low Phe blood concentrations.

The dietary treatment of PKU has progressed and many products and treatment options are now available. Individuals with PKU who were diagnosed in early infancy and followed the recommendations can have a positive outcome. However, as stated earlier, many adults and adolescents are not following the recommendations and many are doing very well. This may be due to many factors such as strict diet adherence during formative years, continuance of medical food products into adolescence and adulthood but no phe-restriction, or just the many variations of PKU. Therefore, more studies are needed about ageing with PKU in order to develop sound recommendations. There are no clear guidelines as to how long the diet must be maintained and what the adult blood Phe concentrations should be. It has been 10 years since the National Institutes of Health (NIH) Consensus Conference for Phenylketonuria was conducted, and new information and treatments have emerged. Currently the NIH is putting together a task force and will be conducting another conference. Also, the Genetic Metabolic Dieticians International (GMDI) is collaborating with the Southeast Region Genetics Collaborative and the Health Resources and

Services Administration (HRSA) to develop nutrition guidelines. With the conglomeration of all reviews of the literature and our current knowledge of PKU in the development of these guidelines, perhaps a new paradigm of treatment strategy will be established.

References

Acosta, P.B. (1996) Nutrition studies in treated infants and children with Phenylketonuria: vitamins, minerals, trace elements. *European Journal of Pediatrics* 155, S136–S139.

Acosta, P.B. and Yannicelli, S. (2001) *The Ross Metabolic Formula System Nutrition Support Protocols*. 4th ed., Ross Products Division/Abbott Laboratories, Columbus, OH, p. 12.

Acosta, P.B., Alfin-Slater, R.B. and Koch, R. (1973) Serum lipids in children with Phenylketonuria (PKU). *Journal of the American Dietetic Association* 63, 631–635.

Acosta, P.B., Yannicelli, S., Singh, R., Mofidi, S., Steiner, R., DeVincentis, E., Jurecki, E., et al. (2003) Nutrient intakes and physical growth of children with phenylketonuria undergoing nutrition therapy. *Journal of the American Dietetic Association* 103, 1167–1173.

Acosta, P.B., Yannicelli, S., Singh, R.H., Elsas, L.J., Mofidi, S. and Steiner, R.D. (2004) Iron status of children with phenylketonuria undergoing nutrition therapy assessed by transferring receptors. *General Medicine* 2, 96–101.

Agostoni, C., Massetto, N., Biasucci, G., Rottoli, A., Bonvissuto, M., Bruzzese, M., Giovannini, M., et al. (2000) Effects of long-chain polyunsaturated fatty acid supplementation on fatty acid status and visual function in treated children with hyperphenylalaninemia. *Journal of Pediatrics* 137, 504–509.

Agostoni, C., Harvia, A., McCulloch, D.L., Demellweek, C., Cockburn, F., Giovannini, M., Murray, G., et al. (2006) A randomized trial of long-chain polyunsaturated fatty acid supplementation in infants with Phenylketonuria. *Development Medicine and Child Neurology* 48, 207–212.

Andersen, A.E. and Avins, L. (1976) Lowering brain Phenylalanine levels by giving other large neutral amino acids. *Archives of Neurology* 33, 684–686.

Azen, C.G., Koch, R., Friedman, E.G., Berlow, S., Coldwell, J., Krause, W., Matalon, R., et al. (1991) Intellectual development in 12 year old children treated for phenylketonuria. *American Journal of Diseases of Children* 145, 35–39.

Beblo, S., Reinhardt, H., Demmelmair, H., Muntau, A.C. and Koletzko, B. (2007) Effect of fish oil supplementation on fatty acid status, coordination and fine motor skills in children with phenylketonuria. *Journal of Pediatrics* 150, 479–84.

Bickel, H., Gerrard, J. and Hickmans, E.M. (1953) Influence of phenylalanine intake on phenylketonuria. *Lancet* 2, 812–813

Bredt, D. (2001) The nitric oxide synthases. In: Sinclair, A.J., Attar-Bashi, N.M. and Li, D. (eds) *The Metabolic Basis of Inherited Metabolic Disease*, 8th ed., McGraw-Hill, New York, pp. 4278–4287.

Burton, B.K., Grange, D.K., Milanowski, A., Vockley, G., Feillet, F., Crombez, E.A., Abadie, V., et al. (2007) The response of patients with phenylketonuria and elevated serum phenylalanine to treatment with oral sapropterin dihydrochloride (6R-tetrahydrobiopterin): a phase II, multicentre, open-label, screening study. *Journal of Inherited Metabolic Disease* 30, 700–707.

Christ, S.E., Huijbregts, S.C.J., Sonneville, L.M.J. and White, D.A. (2010) Executive function in early-treated phenylketonuria: Profile and underlying mechanisms. *Molecular Genetics and Metabolism* 99, S22–32.

Christensen, H.N. (1953) Metabolism of amino acids and proteins. *Annual Review of Biochemistry* 22, 235.

de Groot, J.M., Hoeksma, M., Blau, N., Reijngound, D.F. and van Spronsen, F.J. (2010) Pathogenesis of cognitive dysfunction in phenylketonuria: Review of hypotheses. *Molecular Genetics and Metabolism* 99, S86–S89.

DeRoche, K. and Welsh, M. (2008) Twenty-five years of research on neurocognitive outcomes in early-treated phenylketonuria: intelligence and executive function. *Developmental Neuropsychology* 33, 474–504.

Dobbing, J. and Sands, J. (1973) Quantative growth and development of the human brain. *Archives of Diseases in Children* 48, 757–767.

Følling, A. (1934) Über Ausscheidung von Phenylbrenztraubensäure in den Harn als Stoffwechselanomalie in Verbindung mit Imbezilliät. *Zeitschrift fur Physiologische Chemie* 227, 169–76.

Galli, C., Agostoni, C., Mosconi, C., Riva, E., Salari, P.C. and Giovannini, M. (1991) Reduced plasma C-20 and C-22 polyunsaturated fatty acids in children with Phenylketonuria during dietary intervention. *Journal of Pediatrics* 119, 562–567.

Garrod, A.E. (1902) The incidence of alkaptonuria: a study in chemical individuality. *Lancet* 2, 1616–1620.

Giovannini, M., Biasucci, G., Agostoni, C., Luotti, D. and Riva, E. (1995) Lipid status and fatty acid metabolism in Phenylketonuria. *Journal of Inherited Metabolic Disease* 18, 265–272.

Guthrie, R. and Susi, A. (1963) A simple phenylalanine method for detecting phenylketonuria in large populations of newborn infants. *Journal of Pediatrics* 32, 338–343.

Hanley, W.B., Feigenbaum, A.S., Clarke, J.T., Schoonhey, W.E. and Austin, V.J. (1996) Vitamin B_{12} deficiency in adolescents and young adults with Phenylketonuria. *European Journal of Pediatrics* 155, S145–S147.

Hanley, W.B., Linsao, L., Davidson, W. and Moes, C.A.F. (1970) Malnutrition with early treatment of Phenylketonuria. *Pediatric Research* 4, 318–327.

Huemer, M., Huemer, C., Möslinger, D., Huter, D. and Stockler-Ipsiroglu, S. (2007) Growth and body composition in children with classical phenylketonuria: Results in 34 patients and review of the literature. *Journal of Inherited Metabolic Disease* 30, 694–699.

Hillman, L., Schlotzhauer, C., Lee, D., Grasela, J., Witter, S., Allen, S. and Hillman, R. (1996) Decreased bone mineralization in children with Phenylketonuria under treatment. *European Journal of Pediatrics* 155, S148–S152.

Hoeksma, M., Van Rijn, M., Verkerk, P.H., Bosch, A.M., Mulder, M.F., de Klerk, J.P., de Koning, T.J., et al. (2005) The intake of total protein, natural protein and protein substitute and growth of height and head circumference in Dutch infants with phenylketonuria. *Journal of Inherited Metabolic Disease* 28, 845–854.

Holm, V., Kronmal, R.A., Williamson, M. and Roche, A.F. (1979). Physical growth in phenylketonuria: ii. growth of treated childrenin the PKU collaborative study from birth to 4 years of age. *Journal of Pediatrics* 63, 700–707.

Hvas, A.M., Nexo, E. and Nielsen, J.B. (2006). Vitamin B12 and vitamin B6 supplementation is needed among adults with Phenylketonuria (PKU). *Journal of Inherited Metabolic Disease* 29, 47–53.

Janzen, D. and Nguyen, M. (2010). Beyond executive function: Non-executive cognitive abilities in individuals with PKU. *Molecular Genetics and Metabolism* 99, S47–S51.

Kaufman, S. (1963) The structure of the phenylalanine-hydroxylation cofactor. *Proceedings of the National Academy of Sciences USA* 50, 1085–1093.

Kaufman, S., Holtzman, N.A., Milstien, S., Butler, L.J. and Krumholz, A. (1975) Phenylketonuria due to a deficiency of dihydropteridine reductase. *New England Journal of Medicine* 293, 785–90.

Knudsen, G.M., Hasselbalch, S., Toft, P.B.,Christensen, E., Paulson, O.B. and Lou, H. (1995) Blood-brain barrier transport of amino acids in healthy controls and in patients with Phenylketonuria. *Journal of Inherited Metabolic Disease* 18, 653–664.

Koch, R., de la Cruz, F. and Azen, C.G. (2003a). The maternal phenylketonuria collaborative study: new developments and the need for new strategies. *Pediatrics* 112, 1513–1587.

Koch, R., Moseley, K.D., Yano, S., Nelson, M. Jr and Moats, R.A. (2003b) Large neutral amino acid therapy and Phenylketonuria: a promising approach to treatment. *Molecular Genetics and Metabolism* 79, 110–113.

Koletzko, B., Beblo, S., Demmelmair, H., Müller-Felber, W. and Hanebutt, F.L. (2009) Does dietary DHA improve neural function in children? Observations in Phenylketonuria. *Prostaglandins Leukotrienes and Essential Fatty Acids* 81, 159–164.

Kure, S., Hou, D.C., Ohura, T., Iwamoto, H., Suzuki, S., Sugiyamo, N., Sakamoto, O., et al. (1999) Tetrahydrobiopterin-responsive phenylalanine hydroxylase deficiency. *Journal of Pediatrics* 135, 375–348.

Kuvan (2007) Kuvan Full Prescribing Information. BioMarin Pharmaceutical, www.kuvan.com/hcp/kuvan-full-prescribing-information.html, accessed May 2011.

Lenke, R.R. and Levy, H.L. (1980) Maternal phenylketonuria and hyperphenylalaninemia: an international survey of the outcome of untreated and treated pregnancies. *New England Journal of Medicine* 303, 1202–1208.

Levy, H.L., Milanowski, A., Chakrapani, A., Cleary, M., Lee, P., Trefz, F.K., Whitley, C.B., et al. (2007) Efficacy of sapropterin dihydrochloride (tetrahydrobiopterin, 6R-BH4) for reduction of phenylalanine concentration in patients with phenylketonuria: a phase III randomized placebo-controlled study. *Lancet* 370, 504–510.

Lim, K., van Calcar, S.C., Nelson, K.L., Gleason, S.T. and Ney, D.M. (2007) Acceptable low-Phenylalanine foods and beverages can be made with glycomacropeptide from cheese whey for individuals with PKU. *Molecular Genetics and Metabolism* 92, 176–178.

Lombeck, L., Jochum, E. and Terwolbeck, K. (1996) Selenium status in infants and children with Phenylketonuria and in maternal Phenylketonuria. *European Journal of Pediatrics* 155, S140–S144.

Martinez, M. (1992) Tissue levels of polyunstaturated fatty acids during early human development. *Journal of Pediatrics* 120, S129–138.

Matalon, R., Michals-Matalon, K., Bhatia, G., Grechanina, E., Novikov, P., McDonald, J.D., Grady, J., et al. (2006) Large neutral amino acids in the treatment of Phenylketonuria (PKU). *Journal of Inherited Metabolic Disease* 29, 732–738.

Matalon, R., Michals-Matalon, K., Bhatia, G., Burlina, A.B., Burlina, A.P., Braga, C., Fiori, L. et al. (2007) Double blind placebo control trial of large neutral amino acids in treatment of PKU: Effect on blood Phenylalanine. *Journal of Inherited Metabolic Disease* 30, 153–158.

McBurnie, M.A., Kronmal, R.A., Schuett, V.E., Koch, R.M. and Azeng, C.G. (1991) Physical growth of children treated for phenylketonuria. *Annuals of Human Biology* 18, 357–368.

Millet, P., Valaseca, M.A., Valls, C., Pérez-Dueńas, B., Artuch, R., Gŏmez, L., Lambuschini, N., et al. (2005) Is deoxypyridinolina a good resorption marker to detect osteopenia in Phenylketonuria? *Clinical Biochemistry* 38, 1127–1132.

Modan-Moses, D., Vered, I., Schwartz, G., Anikster, Y., Abraham, S., Segev, R. and Efrati, O. (2007) Peak bone mass in patients with phenylketonuria. *Journal of Inherited Metabolic Disease* 30, 202–208.

Moseley, K., Koch, R. and Moser, A.B. (2002) Lipid status and long-chain polyunsaturated fatty acid concentrations in adults and adolescents with Phenylketonuria on a Phenylalanine-restricted diet. *Journal of Inherited Metabolic Disease* 25, 56–64.

Moseley, K., Skrabal, J., Yano, S. and Koch, R. (2009) Sapropterin dihydrochloride (6R-BH4) and maternal phenylketonuria. *Infants Children and Adolescents Nutrition* 5, 262–266.

Ney, D.M., Hull, A.K., van Calcar, S.C., Liu, X. and Etzel, M.R. (2008) Dietary glycomacropeptide supports growth and reduces the concentrations of phenylalanine in plasma and brain in a murine model of phenylketonuria. *Journal of Nutrition* 138, 316–322.

Ney, D.M., Gleason, S.T., van Calcar, S.C., MacLeod, E.L., Nelson, K.L., Etzel, M.R., Rice, G.M., et al. (2009). Nutritional management of PKU with glycomacropeptide from cheese whey. *Journal of Inherited Metabolic Disease* 32, 32–39.

NIH (2000) Phenylketonuria (PKU): screening and management. *NIH Consensus Statement* 17, 1–33.

Olendorf, W.H. and Szabo, J. (1976) Amino acid assignment to one of three blood-brain barrier amino acid carriers. *American Journal of Physiology* 230, 94–98.

Pardridge, W.M. and Olendorf, W.H. (1975) Kinetic analysis of blood-brain barrier transport of amino acids. *International Journal of Biochemistry, Biophysics and Molecular Biology* 401, 128–136.

Pietz, J., Kries, R., Rupp, A., Mayatepek, E., Rating, D., Boesch, C. and Bremer, H.J. (1999) Large neutral amino acids block Phenylalanine transport into brain tissue in patients with Phenylketonuria. *Journal of Clinical Investigation* 103, 1169–1178.

Porta, F., Roato, I., Mussa, A., Repici, M., Gorassini, E., Spada, M. and Ferracini, R. (2008) Increased spontaneous osteoclastogenesis from peripheral blood mononuclear cells in Phenylketonuria. *Journal of Inherited Metabolic Disease* DOI 10.1007/s10545-008-0907-9.

Pratt, O.E. (1980) A new approach to the treatment of Phenylketonuria. *Journal of Mental Deficiency Research* 3, 539–543.

Przyrembel, H. and Bremer, H.J. (2000) Nutrition, physical growth, and bone density in treated Phenylketonuria. *European Journal of Pediatrics* 159, S129–S135.

Robinson, M., White, F.J., Cleary, M.A., Wraith, E., Lam, W.K. and Walter, J.H. (2000) Increased risk of vitamin B12 deficiency in paients with Phenylketonuria on a unrestricted or relaxed diet. *Journal of Pediatrics* 136, 545–547.

Rouse, B.M. (1966) Phenylalanine deficiency syndrome. *Journal of Pediatrics* 69, 246–249.

Sanjurjo, P., Perteagudo, L., Rodriguez Soriano, J., Vilaseca, A. and Campistol, J. (1994) Polyunsaturated fatty acid status in patients with Phenylketonuria. *Journal of Inherited Metabolic Disease* 17, 704–709.

Sarkissian, C.N., Gámez, A., Scriver, C.R. (2009) What we know that could influence future treatment of phenylketonuria. *Journal of Inherited Metabolic Disease* 32, 3–9.

Schaefer, F., Burgard, P., Batzler, U., Rupp, A., Schmidt, H., Gilli, G., Bickel, H. et al. (1994) Growth and skeletal maturation in children with phenylketonuria. *Acta Paediatrica* 83, 534–541.

Schindeler, S., Ghosh-Jerath, S., Thompson, S., Rocca, A., Joy, P., Kempt, A., Rae, C., et al. (2007) The effects of large neutral amino acid supplements in PKU: An MRS and neuropsychological study. *Molecular Genetics and Metabolism* 91, 48–54.

Schulpis, K.H., Papakonstantinou, E.D. and Tzamouranis, J. (2000) Plasma leptin concentrations in phenylketonuric patients. *Hormone Research* 53, 32–35.

Schulpis, K.H., Karikas, G.A. and Papakonstantinou, E. (2002) Homocysteine and other vascular risk factors in patients with Phenylketonuria on a diet. *Acta Paediatica* 91, 905–909.

Schweitzer-Krantz, S. and Burgard, P. (2000) Survey of national guidelines for the treatment of Phenylketonuria. *European Journal of Pediatrics* 159, S70–S73.

Sinclair, A.F., Attar-Bashi, N.M. and Li, D. (2002) What is the role of α-linolenic acid for mammals? *Lipids* 37, 1113–1123.

Surtees, R. and Blau, N. (2000) The neurochemistry of Phenylketonuria. *European Journal of Pediatrics*, 159, S109–113.

Van Bakel, M.M., Printzen, G., Wermuth, B. and Wiesmann, U.N. (2000) Antioxidant and thyroid hormone status in selenium-deficient phenylketonuric and hyperphenylalaninemic patients. *American Journal of Clinical Nutrition* 72, 976–981.

Vilaseca, M., Lambruschini, N., López-Gómez, L., Gutierea, A., Moreno, J., Tondo, M., Artuch, R. *et al.* (2010) Long-chain polyunsaturated fatty acid status in phenylketonuric patients treated with tetrahydrobiopterin. *Clinical Biochemistry* 43, 411–415.

Waisbren, S.E., Brown, M.J., de Sonneveille, L.M. and Levy, H.L. (1994) Review of neuropsychological functioning in treated phenylketonuria: an information processing approach. *Acta Paediatrica Supplement* 407, 98–103.

Walter, J.F., White, F.J., Hall, S.K., MacDonald, A., Rylance, G., Boneh, A., Francis, D.E., *et al.* (2002) How practical are the recommendations for dietary control in Phenylketonuria? *Lancet* 360, 55–57.

Woo, S.L., DiLella, A.G., Marvit, J. and Ledley, F.D. (1987) Molecular basis of phenylketonuria and recombinant DNA strategies for its therapy. *Enzyme* 38, 207–213.

24 Principles of Rapid Tryptophan Depletion and its Use in Research on Neuropsychiatric Disorders

F.D. Zepf[1,2]*

[1]*Department of Child and Adolescent Psychiatry, Psychosomatics and Psychotherapy, RWTH Aachen University, Aachen, Germany;*
[2]*JARA Translational Brain Medicine, Aachen + Jülich Germany*

24.1 Abstract

Serotonin (5-HT) is a neurotransmitter which plays an important role in many psychiatric disorders. Existing evidence on the central nervous effects of 5-HT relies to a great extent on pharmacological investigations. Many studies used the administration of selective serotonin reuptake inhibitors (SSRI), which allow the investigation of how an increase in central nervous 5-HT neurotransmission influences behavioural characteristics and neural functioning. However, in order to achieve a central nervous dysfunction in 5-HT neurotransmission in animals and humans, a different approach called rapid tryptophan depletion (RTD) can be used. The fundamental concept of RTD builds on the administration of a tryptophan-free diet within an amino acid drink lacking tryptophan, the physiological precursor amino acid of 5-HT. RTD allows a short-term depletion of 5-HT synthesis in the brain. Following this there is a close link between nutritional intake of essential large neutral amino acids (such as tryptophan) and serotonergic neurotransmission in humans. The depletion of central nervous 5-HT allows the study of behavioural and neural effects of this deficit by combining RTD with behavioural test procedures, genetic markers, and imaging techniques. The data obtained under depleted conditions in such studies can serve as a human model for a central nervous 5-HT deficit, which is thought to play a decisive role in a variety of neuropsychiatric disorders. The following chapter gives an overview on the basic principles of RTD and how it can be used in an experiment involving both healthy subjects and patient populations.

24.2 Introduction

The neurotransmitter serotonin (5-hydroxytryptamine (5-HT)) was shown to be involved in the underlying pathophysiology of a variety of neuropsychiatric disorders, including affective disorders (in particular depression), as well as behavioural constructs and symptoms such as impulsivity and aggression. A

---

* E-mail address: fzepf@ukaachen.de

considerable amount of evidence on central nervous 5-HT functioning comes from psychopharmacological investigations, in particular research involving the acute and/or ongoing systematic administration of selective serotonin reuptake inhibitors (SSRI). SSRI are frequently used in order to treat depressive symptoms in humans. However, neuropsychopharmacological research also used SSRI administration in order to study a variety of processes in the human brain (in particular cognitive and affective processes), with the aim of providing a link between behavioural constructs and symptoms observed in humans, and serotonergic neurotransmission (Tse and Bond, 2002; Harmer et al., 2003; Scoppetta et al., 2005). This approach is particularly relevant to mood disorders such as major depression, bipolar disorder and acute manic states (Zepf, 2009). The considerable literature available on SSRI administration and its effects on neural functioning in a variety of neuropsychiatric disorders mainly focuses on increasing central nervous 5-HT availability by inhibiting the reuptake of 5-HT into the pre-synaptic neuron (Loubinoux et al., 2002, 2005; New et al., 2004; Harmer et al., 2006; Lundberg et al., 2007; Marsteller et al., 2007; McClure et al., 2007; Wingen et al., 2008; Kim et al., 2009; Murphy et al., 2009; Simmons et al., 2009; McCabe et al., 2010; Windischberger et al., 2010). However, a considerable amount of research has studied a 'reversed' approach in terms of a reduction of central nervous 5-HT neurotransmission in humans (Young et al., 1988, 1996; Young and Teff, 1989; Pihl et al., 1995; Moore et al., 2000; Young and Leyton, 2002; Stadler et al., 2007; Zepf et al., 2008a,b; Zepf et al., 2009a,c,d; Zepf et al., 2010). One technique enabling such a lowering of central nervous 5-HT neurotransmission is the rapid tryptophan-depletion test (RTD), which allows a short-term reduction of 5-HT synthesis in the human brain. Other terms frequently used for this approach are 'acute tryptophan depletion' (ATD), 'tryptophan depletion' (TD) or simply 'serotonin depletion' (SD). In the following the term RTD is used as a synonym for all of the aforementioned items in order to describe fundamental principles of RTD in human neurobiological and neuropsychiatric research.

24.3 Basic Principles

The fundamental concept of RTD builds on the dietary administration of large neutral amino acids (so called LNAA). Of note, RTD can be used in both animals and humans. The LNAA administered compete with endogenous tryptophan (Trp), the physiological precursor amino acid of 5-HT, on the uptake over the blood–brain barrier into the central nervous system. The physiological uptake of amino acids into the brain uses the so-called L-1 transport system (Figure 24.1), which is saturated under physiological conditions. Tryptophan competes with other amino acids such as leucine, isoleucine, phenylalanine, tyrosine and valine on the unidirectional influx on L-1 into the central nervous system. Plasma concentrations of the LNAA which are administered influence the uptake of tryptophan over the blood–brain barrier (Wurtman et al., 1980). There are three different transport systems for managing the influx of amino acids into the central nervous system over the blood–brain barrier:

1. for neutral amino acids (L-1, ASC, A);
2. for cationic amino acids (y^+); and
3. for anionic amino acids (y^-) (Oldendorf and Szabo, 1976; Pardridge, 1983, 2002; Zepf et al., 2008c).

Tryptophan is transported sodium-independently into the central nervous system using L-1. L-1 can be found on the luminal and abluminal membrane of capillary endothelial cells. It is saturated under physiological conditions and can be found in all cell types in the human body. However, the L-1 located on capillary endothelial cells of the blood–brain barrier has a 100–1000 times increased affinity to the relevant amino acids which use it as a shuttle into the central nervous system, which makes it different from the L-1 in other cell types (Oldendorf and Szabo, 1976). The influx into the central nervous system at L-1 uses Michaelis–Menten kinetics with competitive substrate inhibition (Smith, 1967; Oldendorf and Szabo, 1976; Smith and Takasato, 1986; Smith et al., 1987; Smith and Stoll, 1998). The influx rate for all LNAA was calculated at about 50 nmol min^{-1} and per gram brain tissue (Smith and Takasato, 1986; for a summary see also Kewitz, 2002).

The diminished uptake of 5-HT into the central nervous system (which is achieved by competitive antagonism of the amino acids administered with endogenous tryptophan) leads in turn to a diminished substrate availability for the tryptophan hydroxylase 2 (TPH2), the rate-limiting enzyme in central nervous 5-HT synthesis (Fig. 24.1). This again results in reduced hydroxylation of tryptophan and a subsequent reduction in 5-hydroxytryptophan synthesis. The substrate availability in terms of cerebral tryptophan regulates brain 5-HT synthesis. Finally, the diminished availability of 5-hydroxytryptophan results in a reduced central nervous availability of 5-HT, as the 5-hydroxytryptophan decarboxylase also lacks sufficient substrate availability in analogy to the TPH2.

A further proportion of tryptophan uses passive diffusion in order to get into the central nervous system, which contributes at the level of about 10% to the overall influx of tryptophan under physiological conditions.

In humans the amino acid tryptophan is mostly protein-bound (about 95%), and a proportion of 5% relates to free tryptophan. This free proportion is essential for tryptophan availability in the central nervous system and regulates 5-HT synthesis in the brain (Tagliamonte et al., 1971, 1973; Gessa and Tagliamonte, 1974). The concept that 5-HT synthesis depends on tryptophan availability was proven in studies involving both animals and humans (Moreno et al., 2010; Tagliamonte et al., 1971, 1973, 1974; Biggio et al., 1974, 1975; Gessa et al., 1974, 1975; Moja et al., 1988; Young et al., 1988; Young and Teff, 1989; Delgado et al., 1990).

The following section will give a detailed description on the actual test protocol in order to provide a guide on how RTD studies can be conducted, in particular with respect to patient safety. The safety requirements mentioned should be met regardless of which RTD protocol is actually used, in accordance with Moja and colleagues (Moja et al., 1988), Moja-De (Zepf et al., 2008b), or with Young and co-workers (Young et al., 1989; Young and Teff, 1989).

24.4 RTD Protocol

Before RTD is used in both patients as well as in healthy populations, institutional board

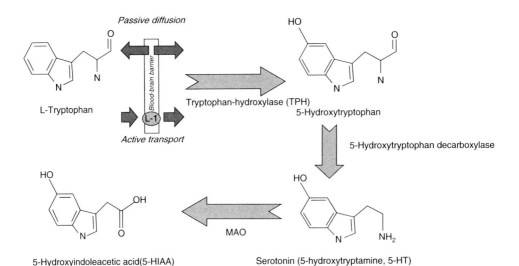

Fig. 24.1. Depicted are the two main influx mechanisms for the amino acid tryptophan over the blood–brain barrier into the human brain (passive diffusion and an active transport using the L-1 system; see main text for explanation).

review (IRB) should be obtained at the local ethics committee. Once IRB approval is available one should also think of having special insurance for the subjects enrolling in the study.

24.4.1 Before administration

Several safety requirements should be met before the amino acids are administered. Pregnancy tests in females as well as drug screenings (both immediately before amino acid administration) should be performed. Apart from the inclusion criteria for the particular study, the subjects should be screened (by interview) for several exclusion criteria, including developmental disorders, endocrine and metabolic disorders (diabetes, hypothyroidism, hyperthyroidism), schizophrenia, drug abuse and suicidal behaviour. There is currently no evidence that RTD endangers people using vehicles or large machines on the day of administration.

24.4.2 Administration of amino acids

The amino acids should be toxicologically tested before being mixed together in the required quantities with respect to the RTD procedure used. The creation of the amino acid mixtures for depletion and tryptophan-balanced placebo conditions should be done by a qualified person, in most cases a pharmacist. One should bear in mind that although the different composites of the amino acid drink can possibly be stored for almost a year before usage (if stored correctly, see below), once combined, the amino acid mixtures should be used within three months. It is advised that consultancy with a local pharmacist is sought before conducting RTD studies. Moreover, the amino acid mixtures should be stored in a refrigerator at approximately 5°C or below, in brown glass bottles with light-absorbing glass, until used. This is in order to prevent quality loss, because amino acids are rather sensitive to light. The fridge used for storage should be lockable in order to ensure that once the amino acids are stored no further components can be added or taken away. In addition, one should also ensure when using a tryptophan-balanced amino acid drink as a placebo condition that overall consistency, smell, and appearance should be as identical as possible. This can be achieved by mixing the amino acids of the RTD or placebo condition with other nutritional compounds (carbohydrates, salt) in order to achieve similar consistency and taste.

The amino acids should be administered in an aqueous suspension, and this is also the easiest way. An alternative could be capsules. However, because of the considerable amount of amino acids needed for sufficient depletion this would result in the intake of a relatively high number of capsules, which makes this an unsuitable method of administration, in particular when younger subjects are involved in the study. If the amino acids are administered in an aqueous suspension the amount of water should be kept to a minimum (approximately 200–300 ml) in order to keep the overall volume of the drink small. This makes it easier for the subjects to drink the amino acid mixture. They should also be advised to drink the mixture rather quickly, for once suspended in water, the amino acids very often tend to clump. A milk frother can be used in order to create smaller particles and thus help to minimize such unfavourable effects. Additional flavouring such as vanilla, peppermint, or raspberry, can be used if necessary in order to achieve a better taste. Other compounds such as oat flakes can be added in order to achieve similar consistency which may be required when aiming to compare RTD effects with 'real' placebo conditions (i.e. a sugar tablet) instead of using a tryptophan balanced amino acid load.

24.5 Effects on Mood

The RTD technique has been used in many studies involving animals and human subjects, including patients and healthy controls. With respect to the serotonin hypothesis of depression, one might be worried if significant mood changes occur if RTD is administered to healthy subjects. Overall, as reviewed by Moore and co-workers, the effects of RTD on mood ratings in healthy subjects are relatively small if measurable at all (Moore et al., 2000). As regards the use of RTD in children and adolescents, recent data showed no significant effects of RTD on mood in patients with attention deficit hyperactivity disorder (Zepf et al., 2009d). The picture changes when it comes to depressed patients; it is notable that it was shown that RTD leads to a depressive relapse in patients with major depressive disorder (Leyton et al., 2000).

24.6 Side Effects and Metabolic Complications

Side effects previously observed after the intake of conventional RTD protocols included nausea and vomiting in particular. Most of these events occurred in close temporal association with the intake of the RTD amino acids. The bad taste of some of the amino acids administered within the different RTD protocols was also a reason for drop-outs in some studies. Here the sulphuric side chain in methionine needs to be mentioned as a particular reason for the problems in taste just mentioned. Of note, recent developments have been promising as there is now a new RTD protocol available which has significantly fewer of the side effects outlined above. Known as Moja-De (a modification of the frequently used RTD protocol developed by Moja and colleagues), the protocol takes into account the body weight of the subjects. It evolved after the detection of a positive correlation between body weight and plasma concentrations of tryptophan in healthy adults (males and females) as well as in male children and adolescents (Demisch et al., 2002, 2004; Stadler et al., 2007; Zepf et al., 2008b). When administering the amino acids of the Moja-De protocol, they resemble approximately a single (or at the most, double) daily requirement of amino acids (Zepf et al., 2009b).

With respect to coenzyme metabolism one must note that RTD, when administered over a longer period of time (1 week or longer), may also have serious metabolic consequences. Niacin and NAD^+ are both tryptophan derived. Following this, a prolonged lack of tryptophan can have an effect on coenzyme metabolism and oxidative stress, in particular as NAD^+ is involved in a variety of redox reactions. A possible solution for such states evolving under RTD could be the supplementation of NAD^+. However, this should only be considered with caution, in particular because even small dosages can result in flush symptoms. In line with this, supplementation of NAD^+ requires extensive monitoring techniques as regards the assessment of the 5-HT metabolite 5-hydroxy-indole-acetic acid (5-HIAA) in the urine, as well as the serum concentrations of chromogranin-A. In patients with renal problems additional monitoring may also be required, since chromogranin-A can be falsely increased in such states. As a consequence, the assessment of additional renal parameters is highly recommended. An option for studies with single administration of RTD and/or a balanced amino acid drink for controlling purposes might be the administration of B_3 within a commercially available multivitamin tablet or drink (Zepf, 2008; Zepf et al., 2008a,b; Zepf et al., 2009a,b,c).

24.7 Positron Emission Tomography Studies

Several studies used positron emission tomography (PET) in order to study the central nervous effects of RTD in animals and humans. One study found a diminished activity in the ventral anterior cingulate, the caudate nucleus, and in the orbitofrontal cortex after RTD (Smith et al., 1999). Moreover, further studies found a diminished central nervous 5-HT synthesis after administration of RTD in animals and humans in various parts of the brain (Nishizawa et al., 1997, 1998; Shoaf et al., 1998; Diksic et al., 2000). One of these studies found that in males, mean 5-HT synthesis rate was about 52% higher compared to females (Nishizawa et al., 1997). Other measurements (H_2O^{15}-PET) showed a co-variation of activity in the habenula and dorsal raphe nuclei following RTD (Morris et al., 1999). A PET study using ^{18}F-Septoperone in healthy women showed a decreased 5-HT_2-receptor binding in the left insula, the left superior temporal, and superior frontal gyrus, as well as in the left fusiform gyrus (Yatham et al., 2001). However, the interpretation of such PET data obtained after administration of RTD is limited, because they are mainly related to the pre-synaptic serotonergic pool, and the results cannot provide information on overall serotonergic activity and synaptic 5-HT-release (Agren and Reibring, 1994).

24.8 Conclusions

It can be summarized that RTD is a physiological neurodietary interventional strategy in order to lower central nervous 5-HT synthesis, which allows one to gain insight on various processes in the human brain related to serotonergic neurotransmission. If the precautions mentioned are respected, RTD can be considered a safe procedure to lower central nervous neurotransmission in both healthy humans and many patient populations. Acutely ill patients (such as depressive patients, and those with schizophrenia) should not be included in these studies. The advantages of RTD are that it allows one to study a subject under a real central nervous 5-HT deficit, and that RTD can be combined with other measurements such as behavioural test batteries, genetic investigations and imaging techniques. Management of potential metabolic complications after prolonged depletion should be conducted by experienced clinicians. Future research using RTD will help to increase the understanding of neuropsychiatric disorders, building on significant changes in central nervous neurotransmission in humans.

References

Agren, H. and Reibring, L. (1994) PET studies of presynaptic monoamine metabolism in depressed patients and healthy volunteers. *Pharmacopsychiatry* 27, 2–6.

Biggio, G., Fadda, F., Fanni, P., Tagliamonte, A. and Gessa, G.L. (1974) Rapid depletion of serum tryptophan, brain tryptophan, serotonin and 5-hydroxyindoleacetic acid by a tryptophan-free diet. *Life Sciences* 14, 1321–1329.

Biggio, G., Corsini, G.U., Fadda, F., Ligouri, G. and Gessa, G.L. (1975) Role of tryptophan in the physiological regulation of brain serotonin synthesis. *Rivista di scienza e Tecnologia degli Alimenti e di Nutrizione Umana* 5, 219–222.

Delgado, P.L., Charney, D.S., Price, L.H., Aghajanian, G.K., Landis, H. and Heninger, G.R. (1990) Serotonin function and the mechanism of antidepressant action. Reversal of antidepressant-induced remission by rapid depletion of plasma tryptophan. *Archives of General Psychiatry* 47, 411–418.

Demisch, L.A.K., Schmeck, K., Sadigorsky, S., Barta, K., Dierks, T. and Poustka, F. (2002) Methodology of rapid tryptophan depletion (RTD): impact of gender and body weight. *European Archives of Psychiatry and Clinical Neuroscience* 252:I/25 (V105).

Demisch, L., Zepf, F., Schmitt, M., Demisch, D., Landgraf, M., Stadler, C. and Poustka, F. (2004) Experimentell induzierte Reduktion der zentralnervösen Serotonin Synthese durch den "Rapid Tryptophan Depletion-Test" (RTD) nach Moja et al.: Methodik, Entwicklung sowie Anwendung bei Kindern und Jugendlichen. *12th Annual Meeting on Biological Child and Adolescent Psychiatry*, Göttingen, Germany, 2–3 December 2004.

Diksic, M., Tohyama, Y. and Takada, A. (2000) Brain net unidirectional uptake of alpha-[14c]methyl-L-tryptophan (alpha-MTrp) and its correlation with regional serotonin synthesis, tryptophan incorporation into proteins, and permeability surface area products of tryptophan and alpha-MTrp. *Neurochemical Research* 25, 1537–1546.

Gessa, G.L. and Tagliamonte, A. (1974) Possible role of free serum tryptophan in the control of brain tryptophan level and serotonin synthesis. *Advances in Biochemical Psychopharmacology* 11, 119–131.

Gessa, G.L., Biggio, G., Fadda, F., Corsini, G.U. and Tagliamonte, A. (1974) Effect of the oral administration of tryptophan-free amino acid mixtures on serum tryptophan, brain tryptophan and serotonin metabolism. *Journal of Neurochemistry* 22, 869–870.

Gessa, G.L., Biggio, G., Fadda, F., Corsini, G.U. and Tagliamonte, A. (1975) Tryptophan-free diet: a new means for rapidly decreasing brain tryptophan content and serotonin synthesis. *Acta Vitaminologica et Enzymologica* 29, 72–78.

Harmer, C.J., Bhagwagar, Z., Perrett, D.I., Vollm, B.A., Cowen, P.J. and Goodwin, G.M. (2003) Acute SSRI administration affects the processing of social cues in healthy volunteers. *Neuropsychopharmacology* 28, 148–152.

Harmer, C.J., Mackay, C.E., Reid, C.B., Cowen, P.J. and Goodwin, G.M. (2006) Antidepressant drug treatment modifies the neural processing of nonconscious threat cues. *Biological Psychiatry* 59, 816–820.

Kewitz, A. (2002) Biochemische untersuchungen zur optimierung des "rapid tryptophan depletion-test" (RTD): eine physiologische method zur akuten verminderung der zentralnervösen serotoninsynthese in der psychobiologischen forschung. Johann Wolfgang Goethe-Universität, Frankfurt am Main, Germany.

Kim, W., Jin, B.R., Yang, W.S., Lee, K.U., Juh, R.H., Ahn, K.J., Chung, Y.A., et al. (2009) Treatment with selective serotonin reuptake inhibitors and mirtapazine results in differential brain activation by visual erotic stimuli in patients with major depressive disorder. *Psychiatry Investigation* 6, 85–95.

Leyton, M., Ghadirian, A.M., Young, S.N., Palmour, R.M., Blier, P., Helmers, K.F. and Benkelfat, C. (2000) Depressive relapse following acute tryptophan depletion in patients with major depressive disorder. *Journal of Psychopharmacology* 14, 284–287.

Loubinoux, I., Pariente, J., Boulanouar, K., Carel, C., Manelfe, C., Rascol, O., Celsis, P., et al. (2002) A single dose of the serotonin neurotransmission agonist paroxetine enhances motor output: double-blind, placebo-controlled, fMRI study in healthy subjects. *Neuroimage* 15, 26–36.

Loubinoux, I., Tombari, D., Pariente, J., Gerdelat-Mas, A., Franceries, X., Cassol, E., Rascol, O., et al. (2005) Modulation of behavior and cortical motor activity in healthy subjects by a chronic administration of a serotonin enhancer. *Neuroimage* 27, 299–313.

Lundberg, J., Christophersen, J.S., Petersen, K.B., Loft, H., Halldin, C. and Farde, L. (2007) PET measurement of serotonin transporter occupancy: a comparison of escitalopram and citalopram. *International Journal of Neuropsychopharmacology* 10, 777–785.

Marsteller, D.A., Barbarich-Marsteller, N.C., Patel, V.D. and Dewey, S.L. (2007) Brain metabolic changes following 4-week citalopram infusion: increased 18FDG uptake and gamma-amino butyric acid levels. *Synapse* 61, 877–881.

McCabe, C., Mishor, Z., Cowen, P.J. and Harmer, C.J. (2010) Diminished neural processing of aversive and rewarding stimuli during selective serotonin reuptake inhibitor treatment. *Biological Psychiatry* 67, 439–445.

McClure, E.B., Adler, A., Monk, C.S., Cameron, J., Smith, S., Nelson, E.E., Leibenluft, E., et al. (2007) fMRI predictors of treatment outcome in pediatric anxiety disorders. *Psychopharmacology* 191, 97–105.

Moja, E.A., Stoff, D.M., Gessa, G.L., Castoldi, D., Assereto, R. and Tofanetti, O. (1988) Decrease in plasma tryptophan after tryptophan-free amino acid mixtures in man. *Life Sciences* 42, 1551–1556.

Moore, P., Landolt, H.P., Seifritz, E., Clark, C., Bhatti, T., Kelsoe, J., Rapaport, M., et al. (2000) Clinical and physiological consequences of rapid tryptophan depletion. *Neuropsychopharmacology* 23, 601–622.

Moreno, F.A., Parkinson, D., Palmer, C., Castro, W.L., Misiaszek, J., El Khoury, A., Mathe, A.A., et al. (2010) CSF neurochemicals during tryptophan depletion in individuals with remitted depression and healthy controls. *European Neuropsychopharmacology* 20, 18–24.

Morris, J.S., Smith, K.A., Cowen, P.J., Friston, K.J. and Dolan, R.J. (1999) Covariation of activity in habenula and dorsal raphe nuclei following tryptophan depletion. *Neuroimage* 10, 163–172.

Murphy, S.E., Norbury, R., O'Sullivan, U., Cowen, P.J. and Harmer, C.J. (2009) Effect of a single dose of citalopram on amygdala response to emotional faces. *British Journal of Psychiatry* 194, 535–540.

New, A.S., Buchsbaum, M.S., Hazlett, E.A., Goodman, M., Koenigsberg, H.W., Lo, J., Iskander, L., et al. (2004) Fluoxetine increases relative metabolic rate in prefrontal cortex in impulsive aggression. *Psychopharmacology* 176, 451–458.

Nishizawa, S., Benkelfat, C., Young, S.N., Leyton, M., Mzengeza, S., de Montigny, C., Blier, P., et al. (1997) Differences between males and females in rates of serotonin synthesis in human brain. *Proceedings of the National Academy of Sciences of the USA* 94, 5308–5313.

Nishizawa, S., Leyton, M., Okazawa, H., Benkelfat, C., Mzengeza, S. and Diksic, M. (1998) Validation of a less-invasive method for measurement of serotonin synthesis rate with alpha-[11C]methyl-tryptophan. *Journal of Cerebral Blood Flow and Metabolism* 18, 1121–1129.

Oldendorf, W.H. and Szabo, J. (1976) Amino acid assignment to one of three blood-brain barrier amino acid carriers. *American Journal of Physiology* 230, 94–98.

Pardridge, W.M. (1983) Brain metabolism: a perspective from the blood-brain barrier. *Physiological Reviews* 63, 1481–1535.

Pihl, R.O., Young, S.N., Harden, P., Plotnick, S., Chamberlain, B. and Ervin, F.R. (1995) Acute effect of altered tryptophan levels and alcohol on aggression in normal human males. *Psychopharmacology* 119, 353–360.

Scoppetta, M., Di Gennaro, G. and Scoppetta, C. (2005) Selective serotonine reuptake inhibitors prevents emotional lability in healthy subjects. *European Review for Medical and Pharmacological Sciences* 9, 343–348.

Shoaf, S.E., Carson, R., Hommer, D., Williams, W., Higley, J.D., Schmall, B., Herscovitch, P., et al. (1998) Brain serotonin synthesis rates in rhesus monkeys determined by [11C]alpha-methyl-L-tryptophan and positron emission tomography compared to CSF 5-hydroxyindole-3-acetic acid concentrations. *Neuropsychopharmacology* 19, 345–353.

Simmons, A.N., Arce, E., Lovero, K.L., Stein, M.B. and Paulus, M.P. (2009) Subchronic SSRI administration reduces insula response during affective anticipation in healthy volunteers. *International Journal of Neuropsychopharmacology* 12, 1009–1020.

Smith, K.A., Morris, J.S., Friston, K.J., Cowen, P.J. and Dolan, R.J. (1999) Brain mechanisms associated with depressive relapse and associated cognitive impairment following acute tryptophan depletion. *British Journal of Psychiatry* 174, 525–529.

Smith, Q.R. and Takasato, Y. (1986) Kinetics of amino acid transport at the blood-brain barrier studied using an in situ brain perfusion technique. *Annals of the New York Academy of Sciences* 481, 186–201.

Smith, Q.R. and Stoll, J. (1998) Blood-brain barrier amino acid transport. In: Pardridge, W.M. (ed.) *Introduction to the Blood-Brain Barrier*, Cambridge University Press, Cambridge, pp. 188–197.

Smith, Q.R., Momma, S., Aoyagi, M. and Rapoport, S.I. (1987) Kinetics of neutral amino acid transport across the blood-brain barrier. *Journal of Neurochemistry* 49, 1651–1658.

Smith, S.E. (1967) Kinetics of neutral amino acid transport in rat brain in vitro. *Journal of Neurochemistry* 14, 291–300.

Stadler, C., Zepf, F.D., Demisch, L., Schmitt, M., Landgraf, M. and Poustka, F. (2007) Influence of rapid tryptophan depletion on laboratory-provoked aggression in children with ADHD. *Neuropsychobiology* 56, 104–110.

Tagliamonte, A., Tagliamonte, P., Perez-Cruet, J. and Gessa, G.L. (1971) Increase of brain tryptophan caused by drugs which stimulate serotonin synthesis. *Nature New Biology* 229, 125–126.

Tagliamonte, A., Biggio, G., Vargiu, L. and Gessa, G.L. (1973) Free tryptophan in serum controls brain tryptophan level and serotonin synthesis. *Life Sciences II* 12, 277–287.

Tagliamonte, A., Gessa, R., Biggio, G., Vargiu, L. and Gessa, G.L. (1974) Daily changes of free serum tryptophan in humans. *Life Sciences* 14, 349–354.

Tse, W.S. and Bond, A.J. (2002) Serotonergic intervention affects both social dominance and affiliative behaviour. *Psychopharmacology* 161, 324–330.

Windischberger, C., Lanzenberger, R., Holik, A., Spindelegger, C., Stein, P., Moser, U., Gerstl, F., et al. (2010) Area-specific modulation of neural activation comparing escitalopram and citalopram revealed by pharmaco-fMRI: a randomized cross-over study. *Neuroimage* 49, 1161–1170.

Wingen, M., Kuypers, K.P., van de Ven, V., Formisano, E. and Ramaekers, J.G. (2008) Sustained attention and serotonin: a pharmaco-fMRI study. *Human Psychopharmacology: Clinical and Experimental* 23, 221–230.

Wurtman, R.J., Hefti, F. and Melamed, E. (1980) Precursor control of neurotransmitter synthesis. *Pharmacological Reviews* 32, 315–335.

Yatham, L.N., Liddle, P.F., Shiah, I.S., Lam, R.W., Adam, M.J., Zis, A.P. and Ruth, T.J. (2001) Effects of rapid tryptophan depletion on brain 5-HT(2) receptors: a PET study. *British Journal of Psychiatry* 178, 448–453.

Young, S.N. and Teff, K.L. (1989) Tryptophan availability, 5HT synthesis and 5HT function. *Progress in Neuro-Psychopharmacology and Biological Psychiatry* 13, 373–379.

Young, S.N. and Leyton, M. (2002) The role of serotonin in human mood and social interaction. Insight from altered tryptophan levels. *Pharmacology Biochemistry and Behavior* 71, 857–865.

Young, S.N., Pihl, R.O. and Ervin, F.R. (1988) The effect of altered tryptophan levels on mood and behavior in normal human males. *Clinical Neuropharmacology* 11, S207–215.

Young, S.N., Ervin, F.R., Pihl, R.O. and Finn, P. (1989) Biochemical aspects of tryptophan depletion in primates. *Psychopharmacology* 98, 508–511.

Young, S.N., Pihl, R.O., Benkelfat, C., Palmour, R., Ellenbogen, M. and Lemarquand, D. (1996) The effect of low brain serotonin on mood and aggression in humans. Influence of baseline mood and genetic factors. *Advances in Experimental Medicine and Biology* 398, 45–50.

Zepf, F.D. (2008) Untersuchung zentralnervöser serotonerger Funktionen mit Hilfe des "Rapid Tryptophan Depletion-Test" (RTD) bei männlichen Kindern und Jugendlichen mit Aufmerksamkeits-Defizit/

Hyperaktivitäts-Syndrom (ADHS) - Einfluss einer akut verminderten Serotoninsynthese uaf laborexperimentelle Impulsivität und Aggression. Tectum Verlag, Marburg, Germany.

Zepf, F.D. (2009) Attention deficit-hyperactivity disorder and early-onset bipolar disorder: two facets of one entity? *Dialogues in Clinical Neuroscience* 11, 63–72.

Zepf, F.D., Wockel, L., Poustka, F. and Holtmann, M. (2008a) Diminished 5-HT functioning in CBCL pediatric bipolar disorder-profiled ADHD patients versus normal ADHD: susceptibility to rapid tryptophan depletion influences reaction time performance. *Human Psychopharmacology: Clinical and Experimental* 23, 291–299.

Zepf, F.D., Stadler, C., Demisch, L., Schmitt, M., Landgraf, M. and Poustka, F. (2008b) Serotonergic functioning and trait-impulsivity in attention-deficit/hyperactivity-disordered boys (ADHD): influence of rapid tryptophan depletion. *Human Psychopharmacology: Clinical and Experimental* 23, 43–51.

Zepf, F.D., Holtmann, M., Stadler, C., Demisch, L., Schmitt, M., Wockel, L. and Poustka, F. (2008c) Diminished serotonergic functioning in hostile children with ADHD: tryptophan depletion increases behavioural inhibition. *Pharmacopsychiatry* 41, 60–65.

Zepf, F.D., Wockel, L., Poustka, F. and Holtmann, M. (2009a) Dietary tryptophan depletion according to body weight - a new treatment option in acute mania? *Medical Hypotheses* 72, 47–48.

Zepf, F.D., Wockel, L., Herpertz-Dahlmann, B., Poustka, F. and Freitag, C.M. (2009b) Tryptophan depletion in bipolar mania: reduction of metabolic imbalance by administration according to body weight? *Bipolar Disorders* 11, 557–558.

Zepf, F.D., Holtmann, M., Stadler, C., Wockel, L. and Poustka, F. (2009c) Reduced serotonergic functioning changes heart rate in ADHD. *Journal of Neural Transmission* 116, 105–108.

Zepf, F.D., Holtmann, M., Stadler, C., Magnus, S., Wockel, L. and Poustka, F. (2009d) Diminished central nervous 5-HT neurotransmission and mood self-ratings in children and adolescents with ADHD: no clear effect of rapid tryptophan depletion. *Human Psychopharmacology: Clinical and Experimental* 24, 87–94.

Zepf, F.D., Gaber, T.J., Baurmann, D., Bubenzer, S., Konrad, K., Herpertz-Dahlmann, B., Stadler, C., et al. (2010) Serotonergic neurotransmission and lapses of attention in children and adolescents with ADHD: Availability of tryptophan influences attentional performance. *The International Journal of Neuropsychopharmacology* 13, 933–941.

25 Excitatory Amino Acids in Neurological and Neurodegenerative Disorders

G. Flores,[1] J.V. Negrete-Díaz,[1,2] M. Carrión,[2] Y. Andrade-Talavera,[2] S.A. Bello,[2] T.S. Sihra,[3] and A. Rodríguez-Moreno[2]*

[1]*Laboratorio de Neuropsiquiatría, Instituto de Fisiología, Universidad Autónoma de Puebla, Puebla, México;* [2]*Laboratorio de Neurociencia Celular y Plasticidad, Universidad Pablo de Olavide, Sevilla, España;* [3]*Department of Neuroscience, Physiology and Pharmacology, University College London, London, UK*

25.1 Abstract

Excitatory amino acids (glutamate and aspartate) form the mainstay of synaptic transmission in the central nervous system. By the same token, dysfunctional, excitotoxic activity of excitatory amino acids can lead to and/ or become instrumental in the progression of a number of neurological and neurodegenerative conditions. Dementia due to Alzheimer's disease (AD) is characterized by extracellular plaques containing amyloid (Aβ peptide) which, together with its disruption of dendritic morphology, affects glutamate (AMPA and NMDA) receptor function to alter glutamatergic transmission. The progressive neurodegeneration of nigrostriatal neurons in Parkinson's disease (PD) may in part arise as a result of overactivity of glutamatergic inputs from the cortex and subthalamic nuclei, presenting the utility of respective antagonism and agonism of stimulatory and inhibitory metabotropic glutamate receptors (mGluR) in PD therapeutics. Huntington's disease (HD) manifests as atrophy of the corpus striatum and cortex, with neurons containing the mutant *huntingtin* protein perhaps being more susceptible to excitotoxicity from corticostriatal inputs, as reflected by the NMDA receptor loss and interactions of huntingtin with facilitatory Group I mGluR. In schizophrenia, abnormalities in brain (dendritic) development and synaptic plasticity may precipitate the dysfunction of mesolimbic and mesocortical dopaminergic pathways. Here again, aberrations in glutamatergic transmission in the form of NMDA receptor hypofunction may underpin the pathophysiology, with inhibitory mGluR2/3 agonism presenting potential as a therapeutic recourse. Depression is classically attributed to defects in monoaminergic neurotransmission, but long-term changes in dendritic architecture in limbic areas arising from chronic stress may be subject to some influence of glucocorticoids on the glutamatergic input to hypothalamic neurons, and thus affect the hypothalamic/pituitary/adrenal axis and glucocorticoid secretion itself. Epilepsy is the perhaps the most clear example of excitatory transmission gone awry, with the manifest increases in cortical network activity during seizures. Increased glutamatergic activity is instrumental in the pathology, particularly

---

* E-mail address: arodmor@upo.es

given evidence of the convulsant associations of the kainate type glutamate receptors (KAR). Glutamatergic hyperactivity ultimately leads to excessive Ca^{2+} influx which can initiate the sequelae of events leading to neuronal damage and death. Thus the Ca^{2+}-permeable NMDA plays a villain's role in excitotoxic culling of motor neurons seen in amytrophic lateral sclerosis (ALS) and indeed the necrotic death of neurons following stroke and cerebral ischaemia. However, it is now increasingly evident that AMPA receptors and KAR, with subunit compositions that permit Ca^{2+}-permeability, may contribute significantly to neurodegenerative chaos when overactivated. Addressing the excitotoxic aspects of excitatory amino acids therefore represents a major challenge in any potential therapeutic intervention with a number of neuropathologies.

25.2 Introduction

In a number of neurological conditions, damage to neurons may be induced, at least in part, by excessive activation of receptors for the excitatory amino acids including glutamate and aspartate (Table 25.1). In other studies, it has been concluded that glutamate excitotoxicity may also damage the myelin-producing cells of the central nervous system. Aberrations in the glutamate system of neurotransmission may be the underlying thread in many neurological conditions. Here, we review the published evidence on neuropathologies where excitotoxicity might play a role in the instigation, perpetuation or final consequences of the disorder.

25.3 Alzheimer's Disease and Glutamate Receptors

Alzheimer's disease (AD) is an age-related disorder characterized by the dysfunction and death of neurons in brain regions such as the hippocampus and frontal cortex, critical structures in learning and memory processes. This neurological disease is the most common cause of dementia among the elderly and has a heterogeneous aetiology, involving genetic and environmental factors. AD is characterized by two major neuropathological hallmarks: extracellular plaques composed of the 40–42 residues Aβ peptide and neurofibrillary tangles, consisting of abnormal phosphorylated Tau protein (for review see Bayer and Wirths, 2010). Several studies have shown that neuronal death is limited in normal ageing, whereas in AD there is considerable neuronal loss (for review see Dickstein *et al.*, 2007). In addition, there is increasing evidence that Aβ peptide accumulates inside neurons, this being one of the mechanisms of neuronal degeneration (Gouras *et al.*, 2000), with Aβ peptide being able to induce the loss or alteration of neuronal dendritic spines (Knobloch and Mansuy, 2008).

At the neuronal level, the cholinergic system is one of the most affected in AD. Pyramidal cells in cortical and hippocampal areas are severely degenerated as well as those of the nucleus basalis of Maynert (Samuel *et al.*, 1994). The latter structure provides ~80% of the cholinergic neurons in the central nervous system (Samuel *et al.*, 1994). Several studies have demonstrated that in AD and other dementias,

Table 25.1. Neuropathologies associated with excitatory amino acids: receptors and effects.

Disease or neural state	Main receptors involved	Effects
Alzheimer's disease	NMDAR, AMPAR	No LTP, Inhibition
Parkinson's disease	NMDAR, mGluR	Loss of glutamatergic synapses
Huntington's disease	NMDAR, GABAR	Loss of NMDA and GABAergic transmission
Schizophrenia	NMDAR, AMPAR, mGluR	Hypofunction of receptors
Depression	NMDAR	Loss of glutamatergic transmission
Epilepsy	KAR, AMPAR, NMDAR	GABAergic inhibition
Amyotrophic lateral sclerosis	NMDAR, AMPAR	Motor neuron
Stroke	NMDAR	Excitoxicity

there are morphological changes in dendritic spine density, mainly observed in the prefrontal cortex (PFC) and the hippocampus (Uylings and de Brabander, 2002; Knobloch and Mansuy, 2008). The dendrites of AD brains show an increased curvature of processes, a decrease in dendritic length and spine density, and abruptly terminated dendritic endings (Dickstein et al., 2007, 2010). In addition, it has also been found that AD brains are characterized by reduced cell proliferation in the CA1 area of the hippocampus (Ferrer and Gullotta, 1990; Einstein et al., 1994; Scheff et al., 2007) and PFC (Shim and Lubec, 2002). Recently, alterations have been reported in the neuronal morphology of an AD mouse model (Aoki et al., 2007; Spires-Jones et al., 2007; Knafo et al., 2009). Taken together, AD brains are distinguished by the presence of dysmorphic dendrites in the pyramidal neurons of the hippocampus and PFC (for review see Dickstein et al., 2007).

It is known that Aβ protein binds to AMPA and NMDA receptors (AMPAR and NMDAR, respectively) to cause their internalization, leading to inhibition of long-term potentiation (LTP), which is an enhancement of synaptic strength that is correlated with memory (Snyder et al., 2005). In addition, a recent report has suggested that Aβ disruption of mitochondrial trafficking could contribute to AMPAR removal and trafficking defects, leading to synaptic inhibition (Rui et al., 2010). Moreover it has been suggested that it is possible to prevent Aβ-mediated synaptic plasticity disruption by using GluN2B subunit-containing NMDAR antagonists (Hu et al., 2009). Interestingly, Reelin, a signalling protein that is produced by interneurons in the brain, has an effect on synaptic function that is opposite to the Aβ protein, causing increased glutamatergic neurotransmission. Thus it is purported that Reelin signalling in glutamatergic synapses may restore normal synaptic plasticity, which is impaired by concentrations of oligomeric Aβ protein that lie well within the range present in the brains of AD patients (Durakoglugil et al., 2009). Finally, the treatment for AD has focused on symptomatic relief; however recent advances in molecular therapeutics have suggested specific new treatments, such as stem cell therapy, immunotherapy and neurotrophic factors with neuroprotection action that may alter the natural progression of this devastating illness.

25.4 Parkinson's Disease and Glutamate Receptors

Parkinson's disease is a progressive neurodegenerative disorder that is characterized by the degeneration of dopamine (DA) neurons of the substantia nigra pars compacta (SNc) (for review see Parent and Parent, 2010). The resultant degeneration of the nigrostriatal pathway is a main cause of the symptoms of PD, i.e. tremor, rigidity and bradykinesia (Deutch, 1993; Marsden, 1994). The main cells of the striatum, the medium spiny neurons, receive excitatory inputs from the cortex – especially from the PFC – and thalamus (for review see Vertes, 2004; Pennartz et al., 2009). The striatum comprises the caudate-putamen (CPu) and nucleus accumbens (NAcc). Both of these structures are interconnected by cell bridges (Heimer et al., 1991) and are densely innervated by dopaminergic projections (Anden et al., 1966; Beckstead et al., 1979; Voorn et al., 1986). The NAcc receives DA fibres mainly from mesolimbic neurons of the ventral tegmental area (Deutch et al., 1988), whereas the DA neurons of the SNc send projections to the medium spiny neurons of the CPu (Anden et al., 1964). Therefore, denervation of dopaminergic terminals to the medium spiny neurons of the CPu is the main event in PD (Deutch, 1993; Marsden, 1994). Taking into account the dopamine theory of PD, L-DOPA and dopaminergic agonists are generally used in PD therapy. However, in recent years, the role of glutamate in the pathophysiology of PD has been studied. Recent data from Solis et al. (2007) suggest that 6-OHDA-lesioned rats, an animal model of PD, may develop altered dendritic morphology in the CPu, NAcc and PFC, which may have participated in the emergence of the behavioural changes observed in these animals. The glutamatergic inputs from the cortex make an asymmetric synaptic contact with the heads of dendritic spines, and critically regulate the functions of the medium spiny neurons, the principal output neurons of the CPu (Ingham et al., 1989). DA afferents make synapses at the spine neck or dendritic shafts of the medium spiny neurons of the CPu, to regulate the excitatory drive of these neurons (for review see Arbuthnott et al., 2000). Thus it has been shown that alterations in dopaminergic inputs to the medium spiny neurons of the CPu may result in a reorganization of glutamatergic inputs into the CPu, and consequent changes in the functional properties of these neurons (Voulalas et al., 2005). An inappropriate functional interaction between SNc dopaminergic and cortical glutamatergic inputs on the medium spiny neurons of the CPu by the nigrostriatal dopaminergic disconnection may result in the selective loss of the glutamatergic synapse on the striatopallidal medium spiny neurons, as a recent report suggests (Day et al., 2006). In addition, the two CPu efferent systems, striatonigral (direct) and striato-pallido-subthalamo-nigral (indirect) pathways, oppositely regulate activity of the main output of the basal ganglia, the GABAergic nigrothalamic pathway. Interestingly, in the striato-pallido-subthalamo-nigral pathway, the subthalamic nucleus (STN) plays a critical role in the activity of the nigrothalamic projection. It is known that the glutamatergic neurons of the STN show an overactivity in the PD (for review see Blandini, 2001; Caudle and Zhang, 2009).

The pathophysiology of PD emphasizes that abnormalities of glutamatergic neurotransmission, especially the corticostriatal and STN hyperactivity, may be critical in local circuits that regulate the function of basal ganglia. Glutamatergic receptors are widely expressed in the basal ganglia, thus glutamatergic agents may modulate the activity of the medium spiny neurons of the CPu and STN neurons. Systemic or intrastriatal administration of group I (mGluR) antagonists (mGluR5 – MPEP, MTEP; mGluR1 – AIDA) were found to inhibit Parkinsonian-like symptoms (catalepsy, muscle rigidity) in animal models of PD. Similarly, ACPT-1, a group III mGluR agonist, administered into the striatum, globus pallidus or substantia nigra, inhibited the catalepsy (for review see Ossowska et al., 2007). In addition, Picconi et al. (2002) have reported that selective agonists of group II mGluR (i.e., mGluR2 and 3) potently decrease excitatory transmission at corticostriatal synapses via a presynaptic mechanism, and that the magnitude of this effect is enhanced after DA denervation. Therefore beneficial effects of group I mGluR antagonists, or group II and III mGluR agonists, observed in animal models of PD, could drive towards the reduction of both corticostriatal transmission and STN overactivity (for review see Bonsi, 2007). Moreover, systemic administration of NMDA receptor antagonists has been found to inhibit Parkinsonism symptoms in animal models of PD (Ossowska et al., 1994), emphasizing that targeting ionotropic glutamate receptor signalling may also be of therapeutic benefit in PD.

25.5 Huntington's Disease

Huntington's disease (HD) is an inherited autosomal-dominant genetic disorder, characterized by cognitive dysfunction and abnormal body movements (chorea or choreoathetosis), as well as by cognitive and emotional disturbances (depression, irritability, apathy and impulse control problems, for instance). Symptoms usually begin when patients are between 35 and 50 years old, although the onset may occur at any time. Death usually takes place 15–20 years after symptoms first appear. HD is also characterized by progressive neurodegeneration of the striatum but also involves other regions, basically the cerebral cortex. HD is considered to be an important disease for study, embodying many of the major themes in modern neuroscience, including molecular genetics, selective neuronal vulnerability, excitotoxicity, mitochondrial dysfunction, apoptosis, and transcriptional dysregulation.

Huntington's disease is caused by a mutation of a gene located on chromosome 4, which encodes a protein called huntingtin, in whose amino-terminal portion there is a repeated CAG triplet sequence, corresponding to a variable length string of polyglutamine, which in the normal population is between 12 and 36 residues in length. In patients with Huntington's disease there are an increased number of CAG triplets and therefore an increase in polyglutamine. This increase is variable and unstable, and the severity of the disease and age of onset correlate with and reverse, respectively, with the number of triplets. The number of triplets remains relatively stable, with variations smaller than ± 1 triplet in the mother–child transmission and in two thirds of parent–child transmission. In one third of the latter, however, there is an increase in the number of triplets that can be a few or several dozen. This explains why, while the children of a patient with Huntington's disease often have clinical features very similar to those of their mothers, in the case of father–child transmission an increase in the severity of the disease is possible.

Certain lines of evidence (from mouse studies) indicate that the major pathogenic mechanisms of HD involve a toxic gain of function by the mutant protein; the abnormal length of the polyglutamine repeat gives huntingtin a toxic property not found in the wild-type protein:

1. Like all the other polyglutamine repeat disorders, huntingtin has a dominant mode of inheritance, which is typically the result of gain-of-function mutations.
2. The age of onset for homozygotes for the HD mutation generally is not markedly less than the age of onset for cases with only one copy of comparable repeat length, although this is not necessarily the case in the other glutamine repeat diseases.
3. No cases of HD or related polyglutamine disorders have been identified with deletions or point mutations in any of the causative genes. In contrast, the fragile X phenotype can be caused by a triplet repeat expansion leading to impaired transcription, a deletion, or a point mutation; all three types of mutations result in loss of normal protein function. Finally, mice with targeted deletions of the HD gene resulting in expression that is a small fraction of normal, demonstrate developmental abnormalities rather than a progressive neurologic disorder.

The size of the CAG trinucleotide expansion is not the only thing that makes possible a prognostic on HD. Other elements of genetic origin are the polymorphisms of the glutamate receptors. It is possible, but so far unknown, that other genetic or environmental factors, as well as biological or pharmacological factors, may play a modulating role in the speed of the disease progression.

Various hypotheses have been advanced to explain the pathogenic mechanisms of mutant huntingtin-induced neuronal dysfunction and cell death, but none of these has gained universal support at present. A number of recent reports have concluded that oxidative stress also plays a key role in HD pathogenesis. Although there is no specific treatment available to block disease progression, treatments are available to help in controlling the chorea symptoms.

The nature of the motor symptoms changes over time, but generally speaking the *movement disorder* of HD can be said to consist of two components: *involuntary* movements and abnormal *voluntary* movements. These include some abnormal eye movements, such as slow, hypometric saccades and catchy pursuit; uncoordinated, arrhythmic, and slow fine motor movements; dysphagia and dysarthria; dysdiadochokinesis; rigidity; and gait disturbances. The most common clinical manifestation of HD is chorea. Chorea is defined as quick, vermicular movement, which may be superimposed on a purposeful act.

In contrast to AD, patients with HD seem to have trouble with retrieval rather than storage of memories. They are more apt than patients with AD to recognize words from a previously memorized list or to respond to other cues to help them recall information. All of these cognitive losses accumulate progressively. In patients with late-stage HD deficits in memory, visuospatial abilities, and judgment are observed to develop. Although attention impairment, problem solving, and verbal fluency are also described, along with memory deterioration over time, aside from dysfunction of the vocal apparatus, expressive and receptive language abilities may remain relatively stable or show only minimal disruption over the first few years of the disease. Anomia and aphasia, for example, are rare in early stages; the disease generally spares language functions, including comprehension, vocabulary, and general knowledge. As the disease progresses, language abilities begin to decline and combine with more severe exacerbation of early impairments to produce a general intellectual state that further causes mental retardation. Another behavioural alteration of HD is altered sexuality; the possible cause may be a delicate imbalance of hormones in the brain.

The most prominent atrophy in HD is found in the caudate nucleus and putamen, which together comprise the corpus striatum within the basal ganglia. Striatal atrophy leads to hydrocephalus *ex vacuo* and marked dilatation of the lateral ventricles. In addition, there is overall atrophy of the brain. Within the striatum, there is selective neuronal vulnerability, both in the anatomic pattern of regions affected and in the particular neurons lost. Loss of neurons in the caudate and putamen shows a gradient, with early and most severe loss in the dorsal and medial regions, and progressive loss of neurons in ventral and lateral regions, as the disease progresses. There is severe loss of medium spiny projection neurons, especially those synthesizing enkephalin and γ-aminobutyric acid, but relative preservation of large and medium aspiny interneurons. Neuronal loss is accompanied by reactive astrocytosis (gliosis). Other areas of the basal ganglia also become atrophic, especially the globus pallidus and subthalamic nucleus, although less than the striatum. Large cortical neurons appear to be most severely affected, and there is laminar specificity, with greatest loss in layer VI and significant loss in layers III and V. The neurons lost in the greatest numbers appear to project to the thalamus, whereas most neurons that project to the caudate and putamen lie in more superficial regions of layer V. In addition, the extent of cortical degeneration does not closely correlate to the severity of striatal degeneration. This set of observations indicates that the loss of neurons in the cortex does not arise simply from retrograde changes beginning in the striatum. Whereas the atrophy and neuronal cell loss of HD have been extensively studied, less attention has focused on the morphology of the surviving neurons. Contrary to expectations, application of the Golgi metal impregnation method to study neuronal morphology in the caudate and cortex from HD cases revealed evidence, in the surviving neurons, of 'regenerative' or 'plastic' changes. Relative to neurons in these regions from normal brains, surviving neurons in HD cases had more dendrites, more long recurved dendrites, greater density, and larger size of dendritic spines, and greater somatic area. A complete understanding of the pathogenesis of HD will need to encompass an explanation of these regenerative changes as well as neuronal death and brain atrophy (Kowall *et al.*, 1987; Sotrel *et al.*, 1993; Kim *et al.*, 1999; Ross and Margolis, 2002).

25.5.1 Animal models

There are several animal models available for HD, with a variety of advantages and limitations; these models mimic a number of HD symptoms to greater or lesser extent. There are various cascades contributing to HD pathogenesis and progression as well as drug targets, such as dopaminergic, γ-aminobutyric acid (GABA)ergic, glutamatergic, purinergic (adenosine), peptidergic and cannabinoid receptors, and adjuvant therapeutic drug targets such as oxidative stress and mitochondrial dysfunction that can be addressed in future experimental studies.

One approach is the use of the transgenic animal model. The first animal model for HD was generated in mice using exon 1 of huntingtin with a very long expanded repeat. These animals developed progressive neurologic deficits strikingly similar to those of HD, including incoordination, abnormal involuntary movements, seizures and weight loss. However, unlike patients with HD, neuronal cell loss is not prominent. These mice also developed intranuclear inclusions containing the truncated huntingtin transgene product, but not the endogenous huntingtin protein. The intranuclear inclusions are clearly distinct from the nucleolus, and no membrane separates them from the rest of the nucleus. The intranuclear inclusions are present at the time, and perhaps before, the animals have neurologic signs or brain or body weight loss (Schilling *et al.*, 1999).

Another HD mouse model has a truncated N-terminal fragment of huntingtin driven by the prion protein promoter, resulting in mice with features such as hypoactivity, incoordination and weight loss, and, on neuropathologic examination, show both intranuclear inclusions and neuritic aggregates. A transgene consisting of a full-length huntingtin cDNA driven by the CMV promoter resulted in a line of mice with a rather different phenotype, characterized by early weight gain and hyperactivity, but followed later by hypoactivity. These mice have both intranuclear inclusions and some loss of neurons (Reddy et al., 1998).

Perhaps the most promising mouse model of HD involves the use of yeast artificial chromosome (YAC) constructs, so the transgene consists of the entire human HD gene, including the human HD promoter and all introns, with an expanded repeat. These mice develop neurologic signs, electrophysiologic abnormalities, and a shortened lifespan. A single founder with a long repeat had striking evidence of selective striatal neurodegeneration and nuclear localization of N-terminal epitopes of huntingtin in striatal neurons. If additional lines can be generated, this model may be the closest to the human disease of any model yet generated. Another model of potential utility was generated by inserting an expansion of polyglutamine into the mouse huntingtin gene, thus avoiding the confounding factor of the presence of the human transgene. So far, these mice have not developed neurologic signs, and no neuronal loss has been detected (Hodgson et al., 1999). There is evidence of translocation of huntingtin into the nucleus in striatal neurons. Thus, these mice may model early aspects of HD pathogenesis and could provide a useful model for studying the initial features of the disease. The construction of an inducible mouse model of HD has yielded insight into HD pathogenesis. A transgene containing exon 1 of huntingtin with an expanded glutamine repeat under the control of the tet-off system was inserted so that the timing of transgene expression could be externally controlled by the presence or absence of an antibiotic in the animals' food (Yamamoto et al., 2000). With the transgene on, mice developed neurologic signs and neuropathologic changes including nuclear inclusions. Remarkably, when the expression of huntingtin was turned off, these abnormalities partially reversed. This surprising result suggests that the brain may have more restorative and plastic ability than previously appreciated, and that if the pathologic changes of HD could be halted, substantial repair would perhaps be possible. Apart from mice, some other models have been used, such as invertebrates, which offer the potential of using powerful genetic techniques to search for genetic factors that enhance or suppress an experimentally induced phenotype.

In reviewing HD, we can also consider alterations of neurotransmitter levels, especially glutamate, GABA and DA receptors. Altered expression of neurotransmitter receptors precedes clinical symptoms in transgenic mice and contributes to subsequent pathology. Inhibition of caspase activation prevents down-regulation of receptors, suggesting that caspases are mediators not only for cell death, but also for cell dysfunction. A faulty gene and excess glutamate may lead to damaging free radicals, which can harm the DNA of the nerve cell. Glutamate also may lead to detrimental Ca^{2+} influx, which can churn out its own supply of DNA-damaging free radicals. The free radicals also may injure neurofilaments, proteins that serve as the skeleton of the cell. In addition, the immune system may be involved in damaging neurons.

Referring to the role of glutamate, for instance, an 'excitotoxicity hypothesis' can be applied to HD. This hypothesis stipulates that increased glutamate release from cortical afferents and reduced uptake of glutamate by glia lead to excessive activation of glutamate receptors, or hypersensitivity of postsynaptic glutamate receptors on striatal projection neurons. This causes an alteration in intracellular Ca^{2+} homeostasis and mitochondrial dysfunction, resulting in neuronal dysfunction and death of striatal medium spiny neurons. Support for the excitotoxic hypothesis comes in part from radioligand binding studies in *post-mortem* HD brain tissue, which show a disproportionate loss of NMDAR from the striatum of patients in early symptomatic stages, and, in a few cases, pre-symptomatic stages of the disease. These studies suggest that striatal neurons with high NMDAR expression are the most vulnerable and are lost early during disease progression. Since NMDA receptors are intimately associated with excitotoxicity, they were one of the first glutamate receptors studied in mouse models of HD.

Early evidence suggests a decreased level of GABA and its synthesizing enzyme glutamic acid decarboxylase (GAD) in *post-mortem* HD brains. Whereas larger aspiny interneurons are unaffected in the early stages of HD, spiny neurons are severely diminished. The loss of striatal GABA receptors probably represents the loss of striatal neurons. However, the increase in GABA receptors in the GP external (GPe), an area that normally receives synaptic input from striatal projections, probably represents a measure of denervation supersensitivity. Disruptions in GABA systems are not limited to the striatum.

Glutamate release can be regulated by GABA receptors (GABAR) located on corticostriatal terminals. Activation of these receptors exerts a significant inhibitory effect. Although glutamate receptors are thought to contribute to excitotoxic neuronal loss in HD, it is still unclear whether group I mGluR activation could delay or accelerate HD, as different studies have reported contradictory data (DiFiglia, 1990; Beal *et al.*, 1991; Nicoletti *et al.*, 1996; Bruno *et al.*, 2001; Zeron *et al.*, 2002; Tang *et al.*, 2003; Schiefer *et al.*, 2004). Recently, it has been determined that group I mGluR interact with mutant huntingtin and that mGluR5 signalling was selectively uncoupled as a consequence of this interaction (Anborgh *et al.*, 2005). The neuronal cell loss that takes place in the striatum and cortex of HD patients is considered to be the primary cause of HD symptoms and eventual death of HD patients (Vonsattel *et al.*, 1985; Vonsattel and DiFiglia, 1998). It is still not clear why mutant huntingtin protein leads to selective neuronal cell death, and why there is a delayed loss of neurons late in life. mGluR1/5 can signal to activate different pathways that can be either protective or exacerbate neuronal cell death (Nicoletti *et al.*, 1996; Bruno *et al.*, 2001; Tang *et al.*, 2003; Baskys *et al.*, 2005). Thus, it is possible that alterations of receptor-mediated signalling pathways could contribute to protection or exacerbation of cell death cascades in the symptomatic and/or presymptomatic phases of HD. Some studies indicate that dysregulation of Ca^{2+} signalling is a common feature of HD mouse models, that mGluR5 signalling pathways are altered in HD, and that the adaptation in cell signalling favours the activation of pathways that promote striatal neuronal survival. What is postulated is that mGluR1/5 can signal to activate different pathways that can be either protective or exacerbate neuronal cell death.

25.6 Schizophrenia and Glutamate Receptors

Schizophrenia is a complex disorder of thought, perception, and social interactions affecting 1% of the world's population. The main diagnostics observed in schizophrenic patients comprise positive symptoms (e.g. thought disorder, delusions, hallucinations), negative symptoms (e.g. anhedonia, apathy, social withdrawal), and cognitive deficiencies, including attention deficit, impaired memory, and deficit in executive function. Various theories have been advanced to explain schizophrenia, and among these the dopamine theory postulates an overactive mesolimbic dopaminergic system in mediating some of the behavioural manifestations of the disorder. However, in recent years neuroimaging and neuropathological studies have provided strong evidence for structural and molecular changes in the PFC, hippocampal formation, and amygdala of schizophrenic brains, which are suggestive of abnormalities in brain development and plasticity. In addition, alterations in the cell pattern and orientation in the hippocampus of schizophrenic patients have been observed (Jacob and Beckman 1986). The volume of the amygdalo-hippocampal formation is decreased in schizophrenic patients in post-mortem brains (Bogerts *et al.*, 1985; Brown *et al.*, 1986; Jakob and Beckmann, 1986; Jeste and Lohr, 1989; Arnold *et al.*, 1991) and by *in vivo* analysis using magnetic resonance imaging (MRI) (De Lisi *et al.*, 1988; Suddath *et al.*, 1989, 1990; Rossi *et al.*, 1990).

Consistent with the hypothesis of altered cortical synaptic plasticity in schizophrenia, several reports have shown decreased dendritic arbour and spine density of prefrontal cortical pyramidal neurons in *post-mortem* schizophrenic brains (Garey *et al.*, 1998; Glantz and Lewis, 2000; Broadbelt *et al.*, 2002; Lewis *et al.*, 2003). Animal studies clearly indicate roles for hippocampal, amygdala and/or PFC inputs in modulating the activity of the medium spiny neurons of the NAcc (for review see Marcotte *et al.*, 2001; Lipska, 2004). For example, recent studies with neonatal lesions of the hippocampus or amygdala lesions in rats have revealed a reduction in the dendrites' parameters such as spines density and dendritic length in the pyramidal neurons of the PFC and medium spiny neurons of the NAcc (Flores *et al.*, 2005, Alquicer *et al.*, 2008, Solis *et al.*, 2009). Neuronal dendrites are instrumental in the formation and maintenance of neural networks, the regulation of synaptic plasticity and the integration of electrical inputs (for review, see Dickstein *et al.*, 2007). In addition, dendritic spines are small protrusions which are distinguished along the body of the dendrites of certain neurons and represent a site of excitatory synapses. The heads of dendritic spines comprise proteins involved in excitatory synaptic transmission, such as NMDAR, AMPAR, mGluR and associated signalling proteins (for review, see Kitanishi *et al.*, 2009). Therefore, pathophysiological theories of schizophrenia emphasize that abnormalities of glutamatergic neurotransmission, especially a hypofunction of NMDAR signalling, may be critical in local circuits that regulate the function of a given brain region, or control projections from one region to another (e.g. hippocampal–cortical projection) (for review, see Marek *et al.*, 2010). Interestingly, AMPAR expression is abnormally decreased in the schizophrenic hippocampus, and similar changes have been reported for KAR expression in the hippocampus as well as NMDAR in some cortical regions (for review, see Meador-Woodruff and Healy, 2000). A few studies have investigated the level expression of metabotropic glutamate receptor 2 (mGluR2) in *post-mortem* human brain of schizophrenic subjects, but the results have been conflicting thus far. While Ghose *et al.* (2008) reported an increase in mGluR2 expression in the PFC using *in situ* hybridization, Gonzalez-Maeso *et al.* (2008) showed lower levels of expression of mGluR2 using PCR. The expression of mGluR3 is unaffected in schizophrenia. However, agonists decreased both positive and negative symptoms of schizophrenia, raising hopes that glutamatergic mechanisms may provide therapeutic potential in this disease (for review, see Marek *et al.*, 2010).

25.7 Depression and Glutamate Receptors

Depression is a common, recurrent and chronic disorder that is a leading cause of functional impairment and disability. This disorder affects one in eight persons in the world and is projected to become the second leading cause of disability worldwide by the year 2020 (for review, see Gaynes *et al.*, 2009). Depression is not merely attributed to the functional defect of monoaminergic neurotransmission (e.g. serotonin, norepinephrine, and dopamine), but is also due to the structural impairment of neuroplasticity. Interestingly, chronic stress decreases dendritic arbor and dendritic spine density in the prefrontal cortex, hippocampus, and nucleus accumbens (Silva-Gómez *et al.*, 2003; Alquicer *et al.*, 2008), and neurotrophin levels (for review, see Calabrese *et al.*, 2009), precipitating or exacerbating depression. Conversely, antidepressant drugs increase expression of various neurotrophins (e.g. brain-derived neurotrophic factor). Therefore, effective treatments of depression should not be limited to their effects on the control of neurotransmitter release, but should seek to normalize defective mechanisms that sustain the impairment of neuronal plasticity (for review see Calabrese *et al.*, 2009).

The mechanism by which chronic stress induces long-term changes in dendritic architecture of neurons in the limbic regions such as PFC, hippocampus and NAcc is not clear. However, several reports suggest that increases in glucocorticoid levels, especially cortisol, and loss of glutamatergic synaptic transmission during chronic stress, may participate in this process (for review see Prager and Johnson, 2009). Interestingly, glucocorticoids exert an opposing rapid regulation of glutamate and GABA synaptic inputs to hypothalamic neurons via the activation of postsynaptic membrane-associated receptors (Di et al., 2009). In addition the hypothalamic–pituitary–adrenal axis is the key regulator of glucocorticoid levels. Dysregulation of this axis is thought to play a central role in the pathophysiology of depressive disorders (for review see Durand et al., 2008). Glutamate and its receptors (GluR) are found in all the hypothalamic areas critically involved in neuroendocrine functions. Similarly, the pituitary gland also expresses these excitatory amino acid receptors. In addition, several reports support the critical role of the GluR as regulators of hypothalamus-pituitary function (for review, see Durand et al., 2008). Therefore, accumulating evidence suggests that glutamatergic neurotransmission plays a critical role in the neurobiology of depression, and represents a key therapeutic target for this disease.

Clinical studies have demonstrated that the non-competitive NMDA receptor antagonist, ketamine, has rapid antidepressant effects in patients with depressive disorder, suggesting the role of glutamate in the pathophysiology of this disease (for review, see Hashimoto, 2010). Studies using animal models of depression have demonstrated that the agents which act at glutamate receptors such as NMDAR, AMPAR and mGluR might have antidepressant-like activities (for review see Hashimoto, 2010). Conversely, chronic treatment with antidepressants may modify the expression of the GluR in limbic regions (for review, see Machado-Vieira et al., 2009). For example, chronic desipramine treatment decreased AMPAR subunit GluR3 expression in PFC and hippocampus (Barbon et al., 2006), whereas chronic imipramine reduced the inhibitory properties of group II mGluR (Palucha et al., 2007). Neuropathological studies indicate that there is increased AMPA binding coupled with a decreased GluR1 subunit expression in the striatum of patients with mood disorder (Meador-Woodruff et al., 2001). In the PFC of patients with mood disorder, a reduction of GluR2 levels has also been reported (Scarr et al., 2003). Finally, several studies have reported intracellular protein changes associated with the postsynaptic density of the NMDA receptor complex (for review, see Machado-Vieira et al., 2009). For example, reduced expression of NR1 and NR2A subunits has been observed in hippocampus, striatum, and thalamus of patients with mood disorder (Clinton et al., 2004; Kristiansen and Meador-Woodruff, 2005; McCullumsmith et al., 2007).

25.8 Epilepsy and Glutamate Neurotransmission

Epilepsy affects 1–3% of people worldwide. Currently, there is little agreement as to the definition of the terms *seizure* and *epilepsy*. Nevertheless, the International League Against Epilepsy (ILAE) and the International Bureau for Epilepsy (IBE) have proposed definitions for these terms. *Epilepsy* is a disorder of the brain characterized by an enduring predisposition to the generation of epileptic seizures and by the neurobiologic, cognitive, psychological, and social consequences of this condition; an *epileptic seizure* is a transient occurrence of signs and/or symptoms due to abnormal excessive or synchronous neuronal activity in the brain. Such definitions are important for communication among professionals in many different fields (Fisher et al., 2005). Recently, the ILAE Commission on Classification and Terminology has revised concepts, terminology and approaches for classifying seizures and forms of epilepsy (Berg et al., 2010), but these will not be addressed here for reasons of space.

25.8.1 Excitatory amino acids in epilepsy

Little is known about the effects of seizures on brain amino acid metabolism. Altered release of amino acid and monoamine transmitters, caused by increased network activity during the initial stages of a seizure, can have a profound effect on the further course of that seizure. Increased release of glutamate can exacerbate or prolong pre-existing seizure activity, and may result in excitotoxicity. Increased γ-aminobutyric acid (GABA) release, on the other hand, may be a compensatory inhibitory mechanism in the epileptic focus and surrounding tissue, which limits the progression and spread of seizure activity. These studies have often focused on the hippocampus because of its involvement in the pathophysiology of temporal lobe seizures, the most common type of seizure in adults. Increases in hippocampal extracellular glutamate and GABA have consistently been observed during spontaneous seizures, as well as during different types of chemically and electrically induced seizures in rats (Meurs et al., 2008).

Alterations in the metabolism of several amino acids, especially glutamate, aspartate, and GABA, have been reported in the genetically epilepsy-prone rat. Lehmann (1989) studied basal and high potassium-stimulated release of endogenous amino acids measured using brain dialysis in the hippocampus of urethane-anesthetized seizure-resistant (SR) and seizure-susceptible (SS) rats. The basal extracellular concentrations of amino acids did not differ between SR and SS rats; however, aspartate release was higher in SS rats during stimulation with 100 mM K^+. In addition, aspartate was significantly elevated in the hippocampus, cortex and cerebellum of SS animals, concurrently with a depression in GABA concentrations in the hippocampus and cortex. Lasley (1991) compared seizure-naive and seizure-experienced genetically epilepsy-prone rats in order to distinguish transmitter amino acid changes related to seizure severity from those associated with seizure experience. GABA concentrations were lower in both moderate and severe seizures, compared to non-epileptic controls in each brain region examined. The low concentrations of GABA are consistent with a role for this amino acid in determination of seizure susceptibility. Aspartate content was elevated in brain areas in severe epilepsy compared to non-epileptic controls. Changes resulting from seizure experience consisted of increases in aspartate, glutamate, and glycine. Furthermore, the seizure-induced changes in aspartate and glutamate support the concept that these excitatory amino acids mediate changes in seizure predisposition.

Li et al. (2000), in a pentylenetetrazole (PTZ) model of epilepsy, studied the extracellular concentration of glutamate in the frontal cortex of freely-moving PTZ 'kindled' rats, using an *in vivo* microdialysis. A significant and sustained increase in glutamate levels was observed in the kindled rats. In contrast, a slight and delayed increase was observed in the non-kindled rats when the same grade seizure was induced by PTZ. Kindling is an experimental model of complex partial seizures followed by secondary generalization, which is characterized by the progressive development of electrographic after-discharge in response to repetitive and sub-threshold electrical stimulation of various brain structures, especially those from the limbic system including the cerebral cortex, hippocampus, and amygdala, where glutamate is the major excitatory neurotransmitter. The sub-threshold repetitive stimulation of these structures produces an enhancement of the cortical activity accompanied by the development of tonic–clonic seizures. The generalized seizures that are induced with this paradigm (Fig. 25.1) underlie a susceptibility state of the nervous system, which is permanently altered (Magdaleno-Madrigal et al., 2010).

Glutamate is the major fast excitatory amino acid transmitter in the central nervous system, and excessive glutamatergic neurotransmission has been considered an underlying factor in epilepsy. Glutamate exerts its action through receptors that function as ion channels such as NMDA receptors, AMPA receptors and KAR, and also through signalling cascades initiated by metabotropic receptors. KAR mediate most aspects of seizures pharmacologically induced by the neurotoxin and convulsant kainate, and thus are targets for antiepileptic drug action.

25.8.2 Kainate receptors in epilepsy

KAR are a family of glutamate receptors that participate in normal synaptic transmission. The actions of the defining agonist kainate (KA) at these receptors are mediated postsynaptically, to regulate excitatory synaptic transmission, and presynaptically, to modulate neurotransmitter release. In the latter context, KAR have been implicated in the modulation of both glutamate and GABA release in the hippocampus. The physiological properties of KAR and their roles in

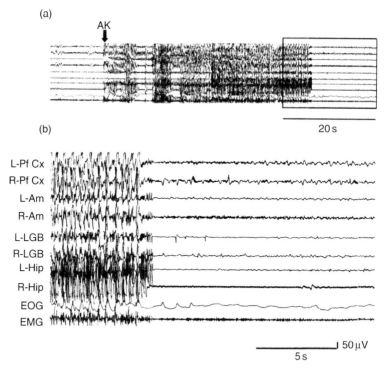

Fig. 25.1. Representative polygraph recording showing a generalized convulsive seizure (stage VI of kindling) in the cat. (a) Arrow indicates amygdaloid stimulation (AK). Part of the frame in the top panel is expanded below. (b) L-Pf Cx, left prefrontal cortices; R-Pf Cx, right prefrontal cortices; L-Am, left amygdalae; R-Am, right amygdalae; L-LGB, left lateral geniculate bodies; R-LGB, right lateral geniculate bodies; L-Hip, left hippocampi; R-Hip, right hippocampi; EOG, electrooculography; EMG, electromyography (modified with authorization of Magdaleno-Madrigal et al. (2010)).

synaptic transmission have been discerned only recently, and have been carried out mainly in the hippocampus (see Huettner, 2003, and Lerma, 2003 for reviews).

KA is a potent convulsive agent that, when administered *in vivo* leads to the generation of seizures. It has also been established that certain brain areas such as the CA3 and the CA1 regions of the hippocampus are particularly susceptible to the depolarizing actions of KA. When the granule cells therein are destroyed, there is a parallel reduction in the number of KA-binding sites and a decrease in the susceptibility to epileptogenic activity induced by the convulsant (see Lerma, 2003 for review).

Rodríguez-Moreno and Sihra (2004) described an increase in glutamate release at mossy fibre-CA3 (MF-CA3) synapses in the rat hippocampus induced by low KA concentrations. This regulation was mediated by the activation of an adenylyl cyclase (AC) (cAMP)/PKA cascade, but independently of G protein involvement. On the other hand, Negrete-Díaz et al. (2006) showed that the activation of presynaptic KAR at MF terminals by higher KA concentrations results in a long-lasting inhibition of glutamate release. This action of KAR seems to be mediated by the activation of a PTX-sensitive G protein, suggesting the coupling of KAR to a second messenger cascade involving the regulation of PKA activity. These observations therefore extend the metabotropic actions of KAR in the brain to include the AC (cAMP)/PKA signalling cascade. In addition,

Rodríguez-Moreno et al. (1997, 2000), using microcultured neurons and hippocampal slices, suggested that KAR on presynaptic GABAergic terminals reduce transmitter release by a G protein-mediated activation of phospholipase C and PKC. *In vivo* experiments using brain dialysis demonstrated that KA reversibly abolished recurrent inhibition and induced an epileptic-like electroencephalogram (EEG) activity. These results indicate that KAR activation down-regulates GABAergic inhibition by modulating the reliability of GABA synapses. The decrease in the efficacy of normal inhibition induced by KAR therefore promotes excitation and development of seizures.

Diverse studies on the effects of KAR activation on evoked excitatory postsynaptic currents (eEPSC) in the hippocampus have reported both decreases and increases of eEPSC amplitudes. Figure 25.2 shows the bidirectionality of the effects of a KA *in vitro* experiment using evoked field excitatory postsynaptic potential (fEPSP) recordings of hippocampal mossy fibres.

Finally, an important body of evidence at the molecular level has demonstrated the importance of KAR in epileptic pathology. For example, it has been discovered that allelic variants of the human KAR in certain subunits confer an increased susceptibility to the development of juvenile absence seizures, and that the level of KAR mRNA seems to be altered in the hippocampus of patients suffering from temporal lobe epilepsy (see Lerma, 2003 for review).

Overall, the role of glutamate in the pathogenesis of epilepsy is complex and

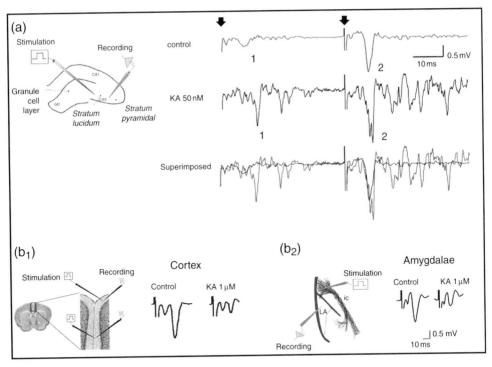

Fig. 25.2. KAR activation has a biphasic effect on glutamate release in hippocampal brain slices of the mouse. (a), Kainate receptors activation with low concentrations of KA (50 nM) enhanced the fEPSP amplitude and the excitability of mossy fibres in the hippocampus. Representative traces show single recordings of MF-CA3 synapses. A typical characteristic of the MF-CA3 synapse is its ability to display rapid and pronounced frequency facilitation with paired stimuli (1, 2), protocol at 40 ms interval (arrows). (b_1), KAR activation with higher concentrations of KA (1 μM) produces a decrease in fEPSP amplitude in the mouse prefrontal cortex and (b_2) lateral amygdalae (LA).

involves glutamate transporters, ionotropic, and metabotropic glutamate receptor activation; regulation of PKA and PKC; and may even be underpinned by inherited and acquired channelopathies (Bernard et al., 2004; Zhang et al., 2004; Negrete-Díaz et al., 2006; Fuortes et al., 2008; Karr and Rotecki, 2008). Crucially, the evidence suggests that KAR are excellent candidates as targets for future drug development in the treatment of epilepsy.

25.9 Amyotrophic Lateral Sclerosis and Excitatory Amino Acids

Amyotrophic lateral sclerosis (ALS) is a progressive neurodegenerative disease of middle and late life. The onset of ALS is age-related, with the highest rate of onset being between ages 55 and 75 years (Logroscino et al., 2008). A recent systematic review of ALS has found a relatively uniform incidence across the white populations of Europe and North America, and a lower incidence among African, Asian and Hispanic ethnicities. The degree to which these differences are due to lower ascertainment and/or lower life expectancy of the latter remains unclear. However, reduced mortality rates have been consistently observed in Hispanic and Asian groups compared with similar studies in white populations (Cronin et al., 2007). Existing evidence supports the concept of ALS as a complex genetic disease caused by multiple susceptibility genes interacting with a variety of environmental risks. European populations share common ancestral origins and, depending on the degree of relatedness, are likely to share a variety of rare 'at-risk' genes, combinations of which may increase susceptibility to the disease. Moreover, the population frequency of some rare at-risk genes may be higher in more homogenous populations, as has been demonstrated in Irish and Scottish ALS studies. Conversely, admixed populations, containing a much wider variety and different combinations of at-risk alleles, are therefore likely to experience a lower overall risk of developing the disease (Zaldívar et al., 2009). Although scant attention has been paid to variations in the frequency and natural history of neurodegenerative diseases outside ancestral European populations, there is evolving evidence that the prevalence of PD, for example, may be reduced in admixed populations, and that those of non-European or admixed origin with AD may differ from ancestral Europeans with respect to age at onset, phenotype, and survival (Prince et al., 2007; Miller et al., 2008).

ALS is characterized by a loss of motor neurons in the motor cortex, brainstem, and spinal cord. This results in progressive muscle weakness, and wasting and death – usually from respiratory failure – within 2–5 years. It has been recognized that motor neurons might be particularly susceptible to degeneration induced by toxicity because of their size, a somatic diameter of 50–60 μm with long axonal processes, and the high energy requirements of such a large cell. Approximately 10% of ALS cases are familial (FALS), and within this group, about 20% show mutations in the copper–zinc superoxide dismutase 1 (*SOD1*) gene (Rosen et al., 1993). The clinical features and pathology of the sporadic and familial forms of ALS are very similar, suggesting common mechanisms of neurodegeneration. Phenotypes of rodent models with mutations in SOD1 closely resemble those of the human disease (Cleveland and Rothstein, 2001; Bruijn et al., 2004). Hence, a number of studies have been carried out by modelling toxicity in ALS using mutant SOD1 (mSOD1) to elucidate the mechanism underlying selective motor neuronal death.

Current evidence suggests that there may be a complex interplay between several pathogenetic mechanisms underlying motor neuron degeneration. Although there are a number of possible aetiologies for ALS, including environmental agents such as toxic metals and viral infection, autoimmunity, oxidative stress and alteration in neurotrophic factors (Salasar et al., 1995; Arsac et al., 1996; Cookson and Shaw, 1999), there are several lines of circumstantial evidence implicating a disturbance of glutamatergic neurotransmission and excitotoxic mechanisms in the pathogenesis of ALS

(Heath and Shaw, 2002). In fact, mitigation of the effects of glutamate excitotoxicity in motor neurons is one of the most intensely investigated areas for the treatment of ALS, as excessive motor neuronal excitation by glutamate through ionotropic glutamate receptors has been demonstrated.

25.9.1 Glutamate receptors and excitotoxicity in ALS

Recent studies have shed light on the involvement of NMDAR in ALS motor neuronal excitotoxicity. A specific, non-competitive NMDA receptor blocker, memantin, was demonstrated to delay disease progression and prolong lifespan in the mSOD1 mouse model, through both subcutaneous and oral administrations. These data suggested that NMDAR-mediated excitability is involved in ALS pathogenesis, at least in part (Sasabe and Aiso, 2010). The reason for the discrepancy between effectiveness of NMDAR antagonists, and the relatively low expression of NMDAR in ALS remains uncertain, but an essential requirement for a co-agonist for the activity of these receptors should be considered.

Because glutamate-induced Ca^{2+} influx into neurons occurs mainly through NMDAR, they were initially considered to be uniquely responsible for the associated excitotoxicity. More recently, however, several lines of evidence demonstrate that some specific forms of AMPAR, lacking GluR2 subunits, also contribute to the Ca^{2+} influx and excitotoxicity (Choi, 1988; Hollmann et al., 1991; Burnashev, 1992). In fact, excitotoxic motor neuron death is mediated by extensive Ca^{2+} entry into the cell through Ca^{2+}-permeable AMPAR. The Ca^{2+} permeability of AMPAR is determined by the presence or absence of the GluR2 subunit in the receptor complex. However, there are contrasting studies in which lowering or overexpression of GluR2 subunits, respectively, aggravated or slowed down the motor neuron loss in a model of mutant SOD1-induced motor neuron degeneration in mice (Foran and Davide, 2010). The question arises as to whether genetically-determined differences in GluR2 expression could make humans more susceptible to diseases in which excitotoxicity is pathogenically involved.

GluR2 mRNA is regulated by editing, splicing, and the mRNA transported to dendrites where it can be locally translated. Non-NMDA receptors activate and desensitize rapidly and are primarily responsible for fast excitatory synaptic transmission. Thus, modulation of AMPAR properties can profoundly alter motor neuronal excitability. Most AMPAR are permeable to Na^+ and K^+, but impermeable to Ca^{2+}. Ca^{2+} impermeability is conferred by the presence of GluR2 subunits, because the subunit can undergo RNA editing to encode a positively charged arginine (R) at position 586 (Q/R site), while unedited subunits contain a glutamine (Q) residue at this position. In the context of ALS, this becomes particularly interesting as mutations in TDP-43 and FUS/TLS, which are RNA binding molecules, were recently discovered as genetic causes of the disease (Arai et al., 2006; Neumann et al., 2006; Lemmens et al., 2009).

Notwithstanding GluR2 mRNA editing as a developmentally regulated switch in AMPAR properties, the motor neuronal AMPA (and KA) receptor population is unusually Ca^{2+}-permeable and, therefore, vulnerable to excessive glutamate stimulation (Foran and Davide, 2010) because the expression of the GluR2 subunit is low or absent in motor neurons in any case. Thus, the assembly and incorporation of AMPAR complexes lacking the GluR2 into the synapse may be tightly regulated processes that could be disturbed in ALS and predispose patients to develop the disease. In addition, growth factors, secreted by cells surrounding motor neurons thought to play a dominant role in ALS pathogenesis, could also influence the expression level of the GluR2 subunit. For example, the vascular endothelial growth factor, secreted by astrocytes, is capable of inducing GluR2 expression levels. Consequently, such growth factors and other astrocytic mediators may modulate GluR2 expression in motor neurons and therefore determine their likely susceptibility to excitotoxicity.

25.9.2 Glutamate metabolism and transport in ALS

There is an underlying defect in glutamate metabolism in ALS. Studies of the fasting levels of glutamate in the plasma or serum have shown an increased level in ALS patients (Plaitakis et al., 1988) and oral loading with glutamate results in significantly greater elevations in plasma glutamate and aspartate in comparison with controls (Gredal and Moller, 1995; Plaitakis et al., 1988). Not all studies have confirmed these reports. A similar dichotomy exists in the studies of levels of glutamate in the cerebrospinal fluid (CSF) of ALS patients in comparison with controls. The level of glutamate in CSF has been reported to be raised in at least a subgroup of ALS patients, although not all laboratories have replicated this finding (Heath and Shaw, 2002).

There is evidence that some component in ALS plasma and CSF is toxic to neurons in culture. This toxicity appears to be mediated by non-NMDA glutamate receptors, suggesting that the toxic product is a non-NMDA receptor agonist. This concept is based on the evidence that the glutamate-release inhibitor, riluzole, is neuroprotective (Couratier et al., 1994). On the other hand, some studies have shown a decrease in glutamate levels in various regions of *post-mortem* CNS tissue in ALS patients in comparison with controls (Perry et al., 1987; Tsai et al., 1990). This suggests that there are some underlying disturbances in glutamate metabolism and transport in ALS. The failure to properly regulate glutamate may result in raised extracellular levels of glutamate and reduced levels within CNS tissue, but the abnormalities seen in levels of tissue or extracellular glutamate are not caused by derangement in the activity of the major synthesizing enzyme glutamate dehydrogenase. There is, however, evidence for altered expression and function of glial glutamate transporters in ALS, particularly the excitatory amino acid transporter 2 (EAAT2) (Heath and Shaw, 2002). Abnormal splice variants of EAAT2 have been detected in the human CNS. At present, it appears that alterations in the expression and function of EAAT2 do accompany the ALS disease state.

Overexpression of EAAT2 in a rodent SOD1 model delays the onset of motor neuron dysfunction (Guo et al., 2003), and treatment of mSOD1 mice with a beta-lactam antibiotic, which potently stimulates EAAT2 expression, increased their lifespan significantly with the delayed onset of neurodegeneration (Rothstein et al., 2005), supporting the idea that the loss of EAAT2 contributes to ALS pathogenesis. Overall, however, it remains unclear whether these changes represent a primary defect or part of an ascendant cycle of motor neuron injury, or if they occur as a secondary result of motor neuron loss and an attempted compensatory response to a failing motor system.

25.10 Stroke

25.10.1 Background

Stroke and cerebral ischaemia are the leading causes of death and permanent disability (Asplund et al., 1995), with no effective treatment currently known. Transient global cerebral ischaemia occurs during cardiac arrest, cardiopulmonary bypass surgery, and other situations that deprive the brain of oxygen and glucose for short periods. In both humans and animals, ischaemia damages neurons in vulnerable regions of the brain, including the hippocampus, striatum, cerebral cortex and cerebellum (Radenovic et al., 2008). Cerebral infarct is defined as a necrotic area that develops in sites where an acute ischaemic event has taken place, and can be divided into two forms: ischaemic or haemorrhagic. Haemorrhagic infarct is a consequence of the post-ischaemic reperfusion and can be a product of the re-opening of the artery, a partial occlusion of the artery, or because the blood is flowing from adjacent arteries. Acute ischaemia is associated with areas of complete infarct with tissue necrosis, oedema, and inflammation (Arango-Davila et al., 2004).

In general, cerebral ischaemia occurs when the amount of oxygen and other nutrients supplied by blood flow is insufficient to meet the metabolic demands of brain tissue. In ischaemic stroke, the blood supply to the brain is disrupted by cerebrovascular disease. For decades, extensive research and clinical approaches to combat stroke have focused on the vascular aspects of cerebral ischaemia. Therapeutic advances, including carotid endarterectomy, thrombolytic therapy, anticoagulation for cardiogenic stroke, antiplatelet agents and the treatment of risk factors such as hypertension and hyperlipaemia, have had significant effects on the morbidity and mortality of stroke. The final event in cerebral ischaemia is the death of neurons that can be of two forms: the first, which is closely related with energetic deprivation, is necrotic death; and the second, corresponding with the cellular programmed cell death, is apoptosis, which requires an adequate energetic supply in the neuron. In either case the result is an irreversible loss of neurologic function (Arango-Davila et al., 2004).

The advent of animal and tissue culture models of ischaemia has led to many new insights into the mechanisms by which ischaemic neurons die. If ischaemia is complete and prolonged, neuronal death is inevitable. However, it has become increasingly clear that many secondary biochemical changes that exacerbate injury occur in response to the initial insult. In models of cerebral ischaemia in rodents, as much as 50% or more of ischaemic brain may be spared from infarction by preventing these secondary biochemical events. Understanding of the mechanisms by which neuronal cell death takes place has resulted in a number of therapeutic strategies that aim to prevent secondary biochemical changes and thus decrease the damage that results from cerebral ischaemia. These basic mechanisms may also have relevance to other neurodegenerative diseases associated with excessive neuronal death.

25.10.2 Glutamate and glutamate receptors in cerebral ischaemia

It is well known that under physiologic conditions, glutamate participates in many neurologic functions, including memory, movement, sensation, cognition and synaptic plasticity (Lipton and Kater, 1989; Gasic and Hollmann, 1992; Martin and Wang, 2010). However, glutamate can also have a pathologic effect. Glutamate-mediated toxicity was first demonstrated by Olney and co-workers (Olney et al., 1971) by peripheral administration of an agonist that selectively killed neurons in the arcuate nucleus of the hypothalamus. These neurons contain high concentrations of glutamate receptors. Choi and co-workers demonstrated that micromolar extracellular concentrations of glutamate produce rapid increases in intraneuronal cytosolic Ca^{2+} concentrations. In accord, other studies have indicated that hippocampal neurons exposed to *in vitro* ischaemia exhibit increased Ca^{2+} accumulation following the activation of AMPA receptors. This accumulation is prevented by Joro spider toxin, a selective blocker of Ca^{2+} permeable AMPA receptors, and is associated with a higher vulnerability to AMPA-mediated excitotoxicity (Ying et al., 1997).

Blocking the translation of a gene that encodes a subunit of the NMDA receptor with intraventricular injection of antisense oligonucleotides also decreases infarction volume after middle cerebral artery occlusion in the rat (Wahlestedt et al., 1993). These data and many other studies support the hypothesis that excitotoxicity contributes to ischaemic injury *in vivo*. Extracellular glutamate may activate other receptors besides the NMDA channel. NMDAR facilitates an influx of both Na^+ and Ca^{2+}, whereas the non-NMDA receptors (AMPA and kainate receptors) primarily facilitate an influx of Na^+. However, some of the KAR and AMPA receptors are comprised of subunits that allow Ca^{2+} permeability. This may be relevant to ischaemic injury, because after cerebral ischaemia, the GluR2 subunit in neurons, responsible for non-NMDA receptors maintaining low Ca^{2+} permeability, is relatively depleted (Pellegrini-Giampietro et al., 1992). Accordingly, these non-NMDA receptors may become Ca^{2+} permeable after ischaemia. Type I metabotropic glutamate receptors may also increase intracellular Ca^{2+} by mobilizing Ca^{2+} from stores in the endoplasmic reticulum. Studies with antagonists of mGluR show that, depending on their subunit specificity, some, but not all, drugs of this class are neuroprotective in models of focal ischaemia (Lam et al., 1998; Bond et al., 1999). Thus, in vivo, excitotoxicity may be ameliorated by additional strategies besides inhibition of NMDAR.

Treatment with antagonists that compete with glutamate for the receptor (competitive NMDA antagonists) or antagonists that bind to the ion channel itself (non-competitive antagonists) can block Ca^{2+} entry into neurons and prevent cell death induced by glutamate (Hartley and Choi, 1989; Choi, 1990). Glycine is a co-agonist that is required in addition to glutamate to open the NMDA-Ca^{2+} channel (Thomson, 1989). Antagonists that bind to the glycine site on the NMDAR also block excitotoxicity in vitro (Smith and Meldrum, 1992). Compelling evidence is also available to indicate that excitotoxicity mediated by the NMDAR contributes to injury from cerebral ischaemia in vivo. A rapid and large increase in the concentration of extracellular amino acids can be monitored by microdialysis after cerebral ischaemia (Benveniste et al., 1984). Although NMDA antagonists are not effective in global ischaemia models in which temperature is carefully controlled (Buchan et al., 1991), a large number of studies have found that they decrease infarction volume in both permanent and temporary middle cerebral artery occlusion models in rodents (McCulloch, 1992).

Recent studies (Hardingham et al., 2002; Liu et al., 2007) suggest that a preferential activation of synaptically localized NMDAR, which predominantly contain NR2A, have a pro-survival role via activation of a neuronal survival signalling complex that is coupled to these receptors. In contrast, activation of extra-synaptic NMDA receptors, which predominantly contain NR2B (Tovar and Westbrook, 2002; Liu et al., 2007), may have a cell death-inducing role through stimulation of a neuronal death signalling complex. After stroke insult, the NMDAR complex interacts with death-associated protein kinase 1 (DAPK1), a member of a serine/threonine kinase family well known for its role in cell death (Bialik and Kimchi, 2006). DAPK1 directly interacts with the NMDA receptor via an interaction in the carboxyl tail region of the NR2B subunit. Future research is therefore important to determine how DAPK1 binding to NR2B induces cell death. Some data suggest that the binding is upstream of c-Jun N-terminal protein kinase (JNK) activation, an important step previously implicated in induction of neuronal death, but whether this is a consequence of DAPK1-dependent potentiation of NR2B-containing NMDA receptors, or direct activation of the neuronal death signalling cascade, is unclear (Martin and Wang, 2010). It is worth noting that specific antagonists of NR2B-containing NMDA receptors have shown little promise as a post-stroke therapeutic, suggesting that changes in channel conductance may not be critical in neuronal death at a later stage of stroke (Liu et al., 2007).

Intraneuronal Ca^{2+} increases not only depend on the activation of glutamate receptors, but also on the activation of voltage-gated Ca^{2+} channels (Choi, 1990). Drugs that prevent prolonged opening of P- and Q-type Ca^{2+} channel antagonists are also neuroprotective in animal models of stroke (Goldin et al., 1995). Hyperexcitation leads to the peri-infarct depolarization with the subsequent increase in the energetic failure, especially when the membrane is undergoing repolarization (Choi, 1992; Schiene et al., 1996; Back, 1998). Subsequently, increases in intraneuronal Ca^{2+} concentrations, peri-infarct depolarization and acidosis, contribute to the beginning of the processes that continue with inflammation and the activation of apoptotic mechanisms (Banasiak et al., 2000; White et al., 2000), amplifying the area of lesion and the death of adjacent healthy neurons. Mitochondria can buffer the large Ca^{2+} loads, but they do so at the expense of triggering injurious reactive oxygen species production. However, the final and definitive pathway to neuronal death has not yet been elucidated.

In addition to the direct downstream effects of enzymes that are activated by elevation of intracellular Ca^{2+}, a number of complex interactions and positive feedback loops augment the contribution of glutamate to ischaemic brain injury. For example, free arachidonic acid can potentiate NMDA-evoked currents in neurons and inhibit reuptake of glutamate by astrocytes (Miller *et al.*, 1992; Volterra *et al.*, 1992). In addition, platelet-activating factor, a phospholipase A2 metabolite, can stimulate the release of glutamate. Acidotic conditions favour the release of free iron, which can then participate in the metabolism of peroxide into the hydroxyl radical via the Fenton reaction. The pH sensitivity of the NMDA receptor has received increasing interest, since pH changes are extensively documented during ischaemia (Silver and Erecinska, 1992). The acidification associated with this latter pathological condition should serve to inhibit NMDA receptors, which may provide a negative feedback that minimizes their contribution to neurotoxicity. In addition, glutamate can interfere with the function of the cystine transporter. Inhibition of the cystine transporter results in decreased intracellular concentrations of glutathione and diminished intracellular endogenous antioxidant stores (Murphy *et al.*, 1989), which contribute to the excitotoxic damage.

Our knowledge of the mechanisms by which ischaemic neurons die has increased considerably. It is now clear that the toxic effects of glutamate exacerbate injury resulting from ischaemia. Antagonizing excitotoxicity via a variety of approaches can ameliorate injury in animal models of ischaemia. However, these treatments appear to be too toxic and are effective for too short an interval after the onset of ischaemia to be of practical use in treatments in humans. When ischaemia is transient or less severe, programmed cell death is activated. These events occur hours or days after the onset of ischaemia and thus may be more practical targets for treatment. Since there are multiple mechanisms involved in the ischaemic process, it is reasonable to assume that the combination of several drugs can have synergistic effects by blocking different steps in excitotoxicity. These combinations may include new and existing drugs able to limit neuronal depolarisation and abnormal Ca^{2+} and Na^+ loading of the neuron during energy deprivation. Further work is needed to determine the most effective and practical therapeutic strategies to prevent neuronal death after ischaemia.

25.11 Conclusions

Glutamatergic synaptic transmission is fundamental to the normal functioning of the central nervous system. Alterations to this normal functioning can precipitate diseases of the nervous system. Excitotoxity resultant from the overactivity of the glutamatergic system is seen to contribute to the aetiology of a number of neuropathologies discussed here. The propensity for excitotoxicity arises in the first instance from the pathological increase in extracellular glutamate concentrations produced by excessive release or inadequate uptake of the amino acid. A reduction in the energetic status of the neuron may contribute to this, in that lowered ATP levels (following ischaemia, for instance) can result in the cytosolic efflux of glutamate by reversal of glutamate transporters, as well as evoke exocytotic release due the failure of the compromised neuron to keep presynaptic cytosolic $[Ca^{2+}]$ low. The excitotoxic sequelae that follow increased extracellular glutamate are underpinned to a large degree by the cytosolic $[Ca^{2+}]$ issue, in that glutamate receptor-induced insults typically involve the pathophysiological activation of Ca^{2+}-permeable ionotropic glutamate receptors. This may be compounded by glutamate activation of type I mGluR, which instigate intracellular Ca^{2+} store mobilization. Altogether, the excessive cytosolic $[Ca^{2+}]$ initiates Ca^{2+}-dependent pathways that set neurodegeneration in motion. Regaining control of a glutamatergic system gone awry is therefore a clear and key objective in therapeutic interventions to either forestall or delay neurodegenerative processes underpinning neurological disorders. Pharmacologically, this could take the form of antagonists for the ionotropic glutamate receptors in principle; however, given the prevalence of these receptors and the generally pleiotropic effects of drugs targeted at them, better prospects may be forthcoming with the therapeutic development of agonists for the inhibitory metabotropic glutamate receptors, both pre- and post-synaptically. The challenge comes in determining when such interventions would be most efficacious given the complexity of the neuropathologies confronting us.

References

Alquicer, G., Morales-Medina, J.C., Quirion, R. and Flores, G. (2008) Postweaning social isolation enhances morphological changes in the Neonatal ventral hippocampal lesion rats. *Journal of Chemical Neuroanatomy* 35, 179–187.

Anborgh, P.H., Godin, C., Pampillo, M., Dhami, G.K., Dale, L.B., Cregan, S.P., Truant, R. and Ferguson, S.S.G. (2005) Inhibition of metabotropic glutamate receptor signaling by the huntingtin-binding protein optineurin. *Journal of Biological Chemistry* 280, 34840–34848.

Anden, N.E., Carlsson, A., Dahlstroem, A., Fuxe, K., Hillarp, N.A. and Larsson K. (1964) Demonstration and mapping out of nigro-neostriatal dopamine neurons. *Life Sciences* 3, 523–530.

Anden, N.E., Fuxe, K., Hamberger, B. and Hokfelt, T. (1966) A quantitative study on the nigro-neostriatal dopamine neuron system in the rat. *Acta Physiologica Scandinavica* 67, 306–312.

Aoki, C., Mahadomrongkul, V., Fujisawa, S., Habersat, R. and Shirao, T. (2007) Chemical and morphological alterations of spines within the hippocampus and entorhinal cortex precede the onset of Alzheimer's disease pathology in double knock-in mice. *Journal of Comparative Neurology* 505, 352–362.

Arai, T., Hasegawa, M., Akiyama, H., Ikeda, K., Nonaka, T., Mori, H., Mann, D., *et al.* (2006) TDP-43 is a component of ubiquitin-positive tau-negative inclusions in frontotemporal lobar degeneration and amyotrophic lateral sclerosis. *Biochemical and Biophysical Research Communications* 351, 602–611.

Arango-Davila, C., Escobar-Betancourt, M., Cardona-Gómez, G.P. and Pimienta-Jiménez, H. (2004) Pathophysiology of focal cerebral ischemia: Fundamental aspects and its projection on clinical practice. *Revista de Neurología* 39, 156–165.

Arbuthnott, G.W., Ingham, C.A. and Wickens, J.R. (2000) Dopamine and synaptic plasticity in the neostriatum. *Journal of Anatomy* 196, 587–596.

Arnold, S.E., Hyman, B.T., Van Hoesen, G.W. and Damasio, A.R. (1991) Some cytoarchitectural abnormalities of the entorhinal cortex in schizophrenia. *Archives of General Psychiatry* 48, 625–632.

Arsac, C., Raymond, C., Martin-Moutot, N., Dargent, B., Couraud, F., Pouget, J. and Seagar, M. (1996) Immunoassays fail to detect antibodies against neuronal calcium channels in amyotrophic lateral sclerosis serum. *Annals of Neurology* 40, 695–700.

Asplund, K., Bonita, R., Kuulasmaa, K., Rajakangas, A.M., Schaedlich, H., Suzuki, K., *et al.*, (1995) Multinational comparisons of stroke epidemiology. Evaluation of case ascertainment in the WHO MONICA Stroke Study. World Health Organization Monitoring Trends and Determinants in Cardiovascular Disease. *Stroke* 26, 355–360.

Back, T. (1998) Pathophysiology of the ischemic penumbra – revision of a concept. *Cellular and Molecular Neurobiology* 18, 621–638.

Banasiak, K., Xia, Y. and Haddad, G. (2000) Mechanisms underlying hypoxiainduced neuronal apoptosis. *Progress in Neurobiology* 62, 215–249.

Barbon, A., Popoli, M., La Via, L., Moraschi, S., Vallini, I., Tardito, D., *et al.* (2006) Regulation of editing and expression of glutamate alpha-amino-propionic-acid (AMPA)/kainate receptors by antidepressant drugs. *Biological Psychiatry* 59, 713–720.

Baskys, A., Bayazitov, I., Fang, L., Blaabjerg, M., Poulsen, F.R. and Zimmer, J. (2005) Group I metabotropic glutamate receptors reduce excitotoxic injury and may facilitate neurogenesis. *Neuropharmacology* 49, 146–156.

Bayer, T.A. and Wirths, O. (2010) Intracellular accumulation of amyloid-Beta – a predictor for synaptic dysfunction and neuron loss in Alzheimer's disease. *Frontiers in Aging Neuroscience* 2010, 2–8.

Beal, M.F., Ferrante, R.J., Swartz, K.J. and Kowall, N.W. (1991) Chronic quinolic acid lesions in rats closely resemble Huntington's disease. *Journal of Neuroscience* 11, 1649–1659.

Beckstead, R.M., Domesick, V.B. and Nauta, W.J. (1979) Efferent connections of the substantia nigra and ventral tegmental area in the rat. *Brain Research* 175, 191–217.

Benveniste, H., Drejer, J., Schousboe, A., *et al.* (1984) Elevation of the extracellular concentrations of glutamate and aspartate in rat hippocampus during transient cerebral ischemia monitored by intracerebral microdialysis. *Journal of Neurochemistry* 43, 1369–1374.

Berg, A.T., Berkovic, S.F., Brodie, M.J., Buchhalter, J., Cross, J.H., *et al.* (2010). Revised terminology and concepts for organization of seizures and epilepsies: Report of the ILAE Commission on Classification and Terminology, 2005–2009. *Epilepsia* 51, 676–685.

Bernard, C., Anderson, A., Becker, A., Poolos, N.P., *et al.* (2004) Acquired dendritic channelopathy in temporal lobe epilepsy. *Science* 305, 532–535.

Bialik, S. and Kimchi, A. (2006) The death-associated protein kinases: structure, function, and beyond. *Annual Review of Biochemistry 75*, 189–210.

Blandini, F. (2001) The role of the subthalamic nucleus in the pathophysiology of Parkinson's disease. *Functional Neurology* 16, 99–106.

Bogerts, B., Neertz, E. and Schonfeldt-Bausch, R. (1985) Basal ganglia and limbic system pathology in schizophrenia. A morphometric study of brain volume and shrinkage. *Archives of General Psychiatry* 42, 784–791.

Bond, A., Ragumoorthy, N., Monn, J.A., et al. (1999) Ly379268, a potent and selective group II metabotropic glutamate receptor agonist, is neuroprotective in gerbil global, but not focal, cerebral ischaemia. *Neuroscience Letters* 273, 191–194.

Bonsi, P., Cuomo, D., Picconi, B., Sciamanna, G., Tscherter, A., Tolu, M., Bernardi, G., et al. (2007) Striatal metabotropic glutamate receptors as a target for pharmacotherapy in Parkinson's disease. *Amino Acids* 32, 189–195.

Broadbelt, K., Byne, W. and Jones L.B. (2002) Evidence for a decrease in basilar dendrites of pyramidal cells in schizophrenic medial prefrontal cortex. *Schizophrenia Research* 58, 75–81.

Brown, R., Colter, N., Corsellis, J.A., Crow, T.J., Frith, C.D., Jagoe, R., Johnstone, E.C., et al. (1986) Postmortem evidence of structural brain changes in schizophrenia. Differences in brain weight, temporal horn area, and parahippocampal gyrus compared with affective disorder. *Archives of General Psychiatry* 43, 36–42.

Bruijn, L.I., Miller, T.M. and Cleveland, D.W. (2004) Unraveling the mechanisms involved in motor neuron degeneration in ALS. *Annual Review of Neuroscience* 27, 723–749.

Bruno, V., Battaglia, G., Copani, A., Cespédes, V.M., Galindo, M.F., Ceña, V., Sánchez-Prieto, J., et al. (2001) An activity-dependent switch from facilitation to inhibition in the control of excitotoxicity by group I metabotropic glutamate receptors. *European Journal of Neuroscience* 13, 1469–1478.

Buchan, A., Li, H. and Pulsinelli, W.A. (1991) The N-methyl-D-aspartate antagonist, mk-801, fails to protect against neuronal damage caused by transient, severe forebrain ischemia in adult rats. *Journal of Neuroscience* 11, 1049–1056.

Burnashev, N., Khodorova, A., Jonas, P., Helm, P.J., Wisden, W., Monyer, H., Seeburg, P.H., et al. (1992) Calcium-permeable AMPA-kainate receptors in fusiform cerebellar glial cells. *Science* 256, 1566–1570.

Calabrese, F., Molteni, R., Racagni, G. and Riva, M.A. (2009) Neuronal plasticity: a link between stress and mood disorders. *Psychoneuroendocrinology* 34, S208–216.

Caudle, W.M. and Zhang, J. (2009) Glutamate, excitotoxicity, and programmed cell death in Parkinson disease. *Experimental Neurology* 220, 230–233.

Choi, D.W. (1988) Glutamate neurotoxicity and diseases of the nervous system. *Neuron* 1, 623–634.

Choi, D.W. (1990) Cerebral hypoxia: some new approaches and unanswered questions. *Journal of Neuroscience* 10, 2493–501.

Choi, D.W. (1992) Excitotoxic cell death. *Journal of Neurobiology* 23, 1261–1276.

Cleveland, D.W. and Rothstein, J.D. (2001) From Charcot to Lou Gehrig: deciphering selective motor neuron death in ALS. *Nature Reviews Neuroscience* 2, 806–819.

Clinton, S.M. and Meador-Woodruff, J.H. (2004) Abnormalities of the NMDA receptor and associated intracellular molecules in the thalamus in schizophrenia and bipolar disorder. *Neuropsychopharmacology* 29, 1353–1362.

Couratier, P., Sindou, P., Esclaire, F., Louvel, E. and Hugon, J. (1994) Neuroprotective effects of riluzole in ALS CSF toxicity. *Neuroreport* 5, 1012–1014.

Cronin, S., Hardiman, O. and Traynor, B.J. (2007) Ethnic variation in the incidence of ALS: a systematic review. *Neurology* 68, 1002–1007.

Day, M., Wang. Z., Ding, J., An X., Ingham, C.A., Shering, A.F., Wokosin, D., et al. (2006) Selective elimination of glutamatergic synapses on striatopallidal neurons in Parkinson disease models. *Nature Neuroscience* 9, 251–259.

Deutch, A.Y. (1993) Prefrontal cortical dopamine systems and the elaboration of functional corticostriatal circuits: Implications for schizophrenia and Parkinson's disease. *Journal of Neural Transmission* 91, 197–221.

Deutch, A.Y., Goldstein, M., Baldino, F. Jr and Roth, R.H. (1988) The telencephalic projections of the A8 dopamine cell group. *Annals of the New York Academy of Sciences* 537, 27–50.

Di, S., Maxson, M.M., Franco, A. and Tasker, J.G. (2009) Glucocorticoids regulate glutamate and GABA synapse-specific retrograde transmission via divergent nongenomic signaling pathways. *Journal of Neuroscience* 29, 393–401.

Dickstein, D.L., Kabaso, D., Rocher, A.B., Luebke, J.I., Wearne, S.L. and Hof, P.R. (2007) Changes in the structural complexity of the aged brain. *Aging Cell* 6, 275–284.

Dickstein, D.L., Brautigam, H., Stockton, S.D. Jr, Schmeidler, J. and Hof, P.R. (2010) Changes in dendritic complexity and spine morphology in transgenic mice expressing human wild-type tau. *Brain Structure and Function* 214, 161–179.

DiFiglia, M. (1990) Excitotoxic injury of the neostriatum: a model for Huntington's disease. *Trends in Neurosciences* 13, 286–289.

Durakoglugil, M.S., Chen, Y., White, C.L., Kavalali, E.T. and Herz J. (2009) Reelin signaling antagonizes beta-amyloid at the synapse. *Proceedings of the National Academy of Sciences USA* 106, 15938–15943.

Durand, D., Pampillo, M., Caruso, C. and Lasaga, M. (2008) Role of metabotropic glutamate receptors in the control of neuroendocrine function. *Neuropharmacology* 55, 577–583.

Einstein, G., Buranosky, R. and Crain, B.J. (1994) Dendritic pathology of granule cells in Alzheimer's disease is unrelated to neuritic plaques. *Journal of Neuroscience* 14, 5077–5088.

Ferrer, I. and Gullotta, F. (1990) Down's syndrome and Alzheimer's disease: dendritic spine counts in the hippocampus. *Acta Neuropathologica* 79, 680–685.

Fisher, R.S., Emde Boas, W., Blume, W., Elger, C., Genton, P., et al. (2005) Epileptic seizures and epilepsy: definitions proposed by the International League Against Epilepsy (ILAE) and the International Bureau for Epilepsy (IBE). *Epilepsia* 46, 470–472.

Flores, G., Alquicer, G., Silva-Gómez, A.B., Rivera, G., Quirino, R. and Srivastava, L.K. (2005) Alterations in dendritic morphology of prefrontal cortical and nucleus accumbens neurons in adult rats after neonatal excitotoxic lesions of the ventral hippocampus. *Neuroscience* 133, 463–470.

Foran, E. and Davide, T. (2010) Glutamate transporters and the excitotoxic path to motor neuron degeneration in amyotrophic lateral sclerosis. *Antioxidants and Redox Signaling* 11, 1587–1602.

Fuortes, M.G., Faria, L.C. and Merlin, L.R. (2008) Impact of protein kinase C activation on epileptiform activity in the hippocampal slice. *Epilepsy Research* 82, 38–45.

García de Yébenes, J., Hernández, J. and Cantarero, S. (2002) Progresos en la enfermedad de Huntington. In: Segovia, J.M and Mora, F. (eds) *Enfermedades Neurodegenerativas*. Farmaindustria, Madrid, pp. 85–101.

Garey, L.J., Ong, W.Y., Patel, T.S., Kanani, M., Davis, A., Mortimer, A.M., Barnes, T.R., et al. (1998) Reduced dendritic spine density on cerebral cortical pyramidal neurons in schizophrenia. *Journal of Neurology, Neurosurgery & Psychiatry* 65, 446–453.

Gasic, G.P. and Hollmann, M. (1992) Molecular neurobiology of glutamate receptors. *Annual Review of Physiology* 54, 507–536.

Gaynes, B.N., Warden, D., Trivedi, M.H., Wisniewski, S.R., Fava, M. and Rush, A.J. (2009) What did STAR*D teach us? Results from a large-scale, practical, clinical trial for patients with depression. *Psychiatric Services* 60, 1439–1445.

Ghose, S., Crook, J.M., Bartus, C.L., Sherman, T.G., Herman, M.M., Hyde, T.M., Kleinman, J.E., et al. (2008) Metabotropic glutamate receptor 2 and 3 gene expression in the human prefrontal cortex and mesencephalon in schizophrenia. *International Journal of Neuroscience* 118, 1609–1627.

Glantz, A. and Lewis, D.A. (2000) Decreased dendritic spine density on prefrontal cortical pyramidal neurons in schizophrenia. *Archives of General Psychiatry* 57, 65–73.

Goldin, S.M., Subbarao, K., Margolin, L.D., et al. (1995) Neuroprotective use-dependent blockers of Na^+ and $Ca2^+$ channels controlling presynaptic release of glutamate. *Annals of the New York Academy of Sciences* 765, 210–229.

González-Maeso, J., Ang, R.L., Yuen, T., Chan, P., Weisstaub, N.V., López-Giménez, J.F., Zhou, M., et al. (2008) Identification of a serotonin/glutamate receptor complex implicated in psychosis. *Nature* 452, 93–97.

Gouras, G.K., Tsai, J., Naslund, J., Vincent, B., Edgar, M., Checler, F., Greenfield, J.P., et al. (2000) Intraneuronal Abeta 42 accumulation in human brain. *American Journal of Pathology* 156, 15–20.

Gredal, O. and Moller, S.E. (1995) Effect of branch chain amino acids on glutamate metabolism in amyotropic lateral sclerosis. *Journal of the Neurological Sciences* 129, 40–43.

Guo, H., Lai, L.E.M., Butchbach, R., Stockinger, M.P., Shan, X., Bishop, G.A. and Lin, C.L.G. (2003) Increased expression of the glial glutamate transporter EAAT2 modulates excitotoxicity and delays the onset but not the outcome of ALS in mice. *Human Molecular Genetics* 12, 2519–2532.

Hardingham, G.E., Fukunaga, Y. and Bading, H. (2002) Extrasynaptic NMDARs oppose synaptic NMDARs by triggering CREB shut-off and cell death pathways. *Nature Neuroscience* 5, 405–414.

Hartley, D.M. and Choi, D.W. (1989) Delayed rescue of N-methyl-D-aspartate receptor-mediated neuronal injury in cortical culture. *Journal of Pharmacology and Experimental Therapeutics* 250, 752–758.

Hashimoto, K. (2010) The role of glutamate on the action of antidepressants. *Progress in Neuropsychopharmacology & Biological Psychiatry* doi: 10.1016/j.pnpbp.2010.06.013.

Heath, P.R. and Shaw, P.J. (2002) Update on the glutamatergic neurotransmitter system and the role of excitotoxicity in amyotrophic lateral sclerosis. *Muscle and Nerve* 26, 438–458.

Heimer, L., Zahm, D.S., Churchill, L., Kalivas, P.W. and Wohltmann, C. (1991) Specificity in the projection patterns of accumbal core and shell in the rat. *Neuroscience* 41, 89–125.

Hodgson, J.G., Agopyan, N., Gutekunst, C.A., et al. (1999) A YAC mouse model for Huntington's disease with full-length mutant huntingtin, cytoplasmic toxicity, and selective striatal neurodegeneration. *Neuron* 23, 181–192.

Hollmann, M., Hartley, M. and Heinemann, S. (1991) Ca^{2+} permeability of KA-AMPA–gated glutamate receptor channels depends on subunit composition. *Science*, 252, 851–853.

Hu, N.W., Klyubin, I., Anwyl, R. and Rowan, M.J. (2009) GluN2B subunit-containing NMDA receptor antagonists prevent Abeta-mediated synaptic plasticity disruption in vivo. *Proceedings of the National Academy of Sciences* 106, 20504–20509.

Huettner, J.E. (2003) Kainate receptors and synaptic transmission. *Progress in Neurobiology* 70, 387–407.

Ingham, C.A., Hood, S.H. and Arbuthnott, G.W. (1989) Spine density on neostriatal neurones changes with 6-hydroxydopamine lesions and with age. *Brain Research* 503, 334–338.

Jacob, H. and Beckmann, H. (1986) Prenatal developmental disturbances in the limbic allocortex in schizophrenics. *Journal of Neural Transmission* 65, 303–326.

Jeste, D.V. and Lohr, J.B. (1989) Hippocampal pathologic findings in schizophrenia. A morphometric study. *Archives of General Psychiatry* 46, 1019–1024.

Karr, L. and Rotecki, P.A. (2008) Activity-dependent induction and maintenance of epileptiform activity produced by group I metabotropic glutamate receptors in the rat hippocampal slice. *Epilepsy Research* 81, 14–23.

Kim, M., Lee, H.S., LaForet, G., et al. (1999) Mutant huntingtin expression in clonal striatal cells: dissociation of inclusion formation and neuronal survival by caspase inhibition. *Journal of Neuroscience* 19, 964–973.

Kitanishi, T., Ikegaya, Y., Matsuki, N. and Yamada, M.K. (2009) Experience-dependent, rapid structural changes in hippocampal pyramidal cell spines. *Cerebral Cortex* 19, 2572–2578.

Knafo, S., Venero, C., Merino-Serrais, P., Fernaud-Espinosa, I., Gonzalez-Soriano, J., Ferrer, I., Santpere, G., et al. (2009) Morphological alterations to neurons of the amygdala and impaired fear conditioning in a transgenic mouse model of Alzheimer's disease. *Journal of Pathology* 219, 41–51.

Knobloch, M. and Mansuy, I.M. (2008) Dendritic spine loss and synaptic alterations in Alzheimer's disease. *Molecular Neurobiology* 37, 73–82.

Kowall, N.W., Ferrante, R.J. and Martin, J.B. (1987) Patterns of cell loss in Huntington's disease. *Trends in Neurosciences* 10, 24–29.

Kristiansen, L.V. and Meador-Woodruff, J.H. (2005) Abnormal striatal expression of transcripts encoding NMDA interacting PSD proteins in schizophrenia, bipolar disorder and major depression. *Schizophrenia Research* 78, 87–93.

Kumar, P., Harikesh, K. and Kumar, A. (2010) Huntington's disease: pathogenesis to animal models. *Pharmacological Reports* 62, 1–14.

Lam, A.G., Soriano, M.A., Monn, J.A., et al. (1998) Effects of the selective metabotropic glutamate agonist Ly354740 in a rat model of permanent ischaemia. *Neuroscience Letters* 254, 121–123.

Lasley, S.M. (1991) Roles of the neurotransmitter amino acids in seizure severity and experience in the genetically epilepsy-prone rat. *Brain Research* 560, 63–70.

Lehmann, A. (1989) Abnormalities in the levels of extracellular and tissue amino acids in the brain of the seizure-susceptible rat. *Epilepsy Research* 3, 130–137.

Lemmens, R., Race, V., Hersmus, N., Matthijs, G., Van Den Bosch, L., Van Damme, P., Dubois, B., et al. (2009) TDP-43 M311V mutation in familial amyotrophic lateral sclerosis. *Journal of Neurology, Neurosurgery & Psychiatry* 80, 354–355.

Lerma, J. (2003) Roles and rules of kainate in synaptic transmission. *Nature Reviews Neuroscience* 4, 481–495.

Lewis, D.A., Glantz, L.A., Pierri, J.N. and Sweet, R.A. (2003) Altered cortical glutamate neurotransmission in schizophrenia: evidence from morphological studies of pyramidal neurons. *Annals of the New York Academy of Sciences* 1003, 102–112.

Li, Z., Yamamoto, Y., Morimoto, T., Ono, J., Okada, S. and Yamatodani, A. (2000) The effect of pentylenetetrazole-kindling on the extracellular glutamate and taurine levels in the frontal cortex of rats. *Neuroscience Letters* 282, 117–119.

Lipska, B.K. (2004) Using animal models to test a neurodevelopmental hypothesis of schizophrenia. *Journal of Psychiatry & Neuroscience* 29, 282–286.

Lipton, S.A. and Kater, S.B. (1989) Neurotransmitter regulation of neuronal outgrowth, plasticity and survival. *Trends in Neurosciences* 12, 265–270.

Liu, Y., Wong, T.P., Aarts, M., Rooyakkers, A., Liu, L., Lai, T.W., Wu, D.C., et al. (2007) NMDA receptor subunits have differential roles in mediating excitotoxic neuronal death both *in vitro* and *in vivo*. *Journal of Neuroscience* 27, 2846–2857.

Logroscino, G., Traynor, B.J., Hardiman, O., Chio, A., Couratier, P., Mitchell, J.D., Swingler, R.J. and Beghi, E. (2008) Descriptive epidemiology of amyotrophic lateral sclerosis: new evidence and unsolved issues. *Journal of Neurology, Neurosurgery & Psychiatry* 79, 6–11.

Machado-Vieira, R., Salvadore, G., Ibrahim, L.A., Diaz-Granados, N. and Zarate, C.A. Jr (2009) Targeting glutamatergic signaling for the development of novel therapeutics for mood disorders. *Current Pharmaceutical Design* 15, 1595–1611.

Magdaleno-Madrigal, V.M., Martínez-Vargas, D., Valdés-Cruz, A., Almazán-Alvarado, S. and Fernández-Mas, R. (2010) Preemptive effect of nucleus of the solitary tract stimulation on amygdaloid kindling in freely moving cats. *Epilepsia* 51, 438–444.

Marcotte, E.R., Pearson, D.M. and Srivastava, L.K. (2001) Animal models of schizophrenia: a critical review. *Journal of Psychiatry & Neuroscience* 26, 395–410.

Marek, G.J., Behl, B., Bespalov, A.Y., Gross, G., Lee, Y. and Schoemaker, H. (2010) Glutamatergic (N-methyl-D-aspartate receptor) hypofrontality in schizophrenia: too little juice or a miswired brain? *Molecular Pharmacology* 77, 317–326.

Marsden, C.D. (1994) Parkinson's disease. *Journal of Neurology, Neurosurgery & Psychiatry* 57, 672–681.

Martin, G.S.H. and Wang, Y.T. (2010) Blocking the deadly effects of the NMDA receptor in stroke. *Cell* 140, 174–176.

McCulloch, J. (1992) Excitatory amino acid antagonists and their potential for the treatment of ischaemic brain damage in man. *British Journal of Clinical Pharmacology* 34, 106–114.

McCullumsmith, R.E., Kristiansen, L.V., Beneyto, M., Scarr, E., Dean, B. and Meador-Woodruff, J.H. (2007) Decreased NR1, NR2A, and SAP102 transcript expression in the hippocampus in bipolar disorder. *Brain Research* 1127, 108–118.

Meador-Woodruff, J.H. and Healy, D.J. (2000) Glutamate receptor expression in schizophrenic brain. *Brain Research Reviews* 31, 288–294.

Meador-Woodruff, J.H., Hogg, A.J. Jr and Smith, R.E. (2001) Striatal ionotropic glutamate receptor expression in schizophrenia, bipolar disorder, and major depressive disorder. *Brain Research Bulletin* 55, 631–640.

Meurs, A., Clinckers, R., Ebinger, G., Michotte, Y. and Smolders, I. (2008) Seizure activity and changes in hippocampal extracellular glutamate, GABA, dopamine and serotonin. *Epilepsy Research* 78, 50–59.

Miller, B., Sarantis, M., Traynelis, S.F., et al. (1992) Potentiation of NMDA receptor currents by arachidonic acid. *Nature* 355, 722–725.

Miller, L., Mehta, K.M., Yaffe, K., et al. (2008) Race/ethnic differences in AD survival in US Alzheimer's Disease Centers. *Neurology* 70, 1163–1170.

Murphy, T.H., Miyamoto, M., Sastre, A., et al. (1989) Glutamate toxicity in a neuronal cell line involves inhibition of cystine transport leading to oxidative stress. *Neuron* 2, 1547–1558.

Negrete-Díaz, J.V., Sihra, T.S., Delgado-García, J.M. and Rodríguez-Moreno, A. (2006) Kainate receptor-mediated inhibition of glutamate release involves protein kinase A in the mouse hippocampus. *Journal of Neurophysiology* 96, 1829–1837.

Neumann, M., Sampathu, D.M., Kwong, L.K., Truax, A.C., Micsenyi, M.C., Chou, T.T., Bruce, J., et al. (2006) Ubiquitinated TDP-43 in frontotemporal lobar degeneration and amyotrophic lateral sclerosis. *Science* 314, 130–133.

Nicoletti, F., Bruno, V., Copani, A., Casabona, G. and Knöpfel, T. (1996) Metabotropic glutamate receptors: a new target for the therapy of neurodegenerative disorders? *Trends in Neurosciences* 19, 267–271.

Olney, J.W., Ho, O.L. and Rhee, V. (1971) Cytotoxic effects of acidic and sulphur-containing amino acids on the infant mouse central nervous system. *Experimental Brain Research* 14, 61–76.

Ossowska, K., Lorenc-Koci, E. and Wolfarth, S. (1994) Antiparkinsonian action of MK-801 on the reserpine-induced rigidity: a mechanomyographic analysis. *Journal of Neural Transmission* 7, 143–152.

Ossowska, K., Konieczny, J., Wardas, J., Pietraszek, M., Kuter, K., Wolfarth, S. and Pilc, A. (2007) An influence of ligands of metabotropic glutamate receptor subtypes on parkinsonian-like symptoms and the striatopallidal pathway in rats. *Amino Acids* 32, 179–188.

Palucha, A., Branski, P., Klak, K. and Sowa, M. (2007) Chronic imipramine treatment reduces inhibitory properties of group II mGlu receptors without affecting their density or affinity. *Pharmacological Reports* 59, 525–530.

Parent, M. and Parent, A. (2010) Substantia nigra and Parkinson's disease: a brief history of their long and intimate relationship. *Canadian Journal of Neurological Sciences* 37, 313–319.

Pellegrini-Giampietro, D.E., Zukin, R.S., Bennett, M.V., *et al.* (1992) Switch in glutamate receptor subunit gene expression in CA1 subfield of hippocampus following global ischemia in rats. *Proceedings of the National Academy of Sciences USA* 89, 10499–10503.

Pennartz, C.M., Berke, J.D., Graybiel, A.M., Ito, R., Lansink, C.S., Van der Meer, M., Redish, A.D., *et al.* (2009) Corticostriatal interactions during learning, memory processing, and decision making. *Journal of Neuroscience* 29, 12831–12838.

Perry, T.L., Hansen, S. and Jones, K. (1987) Brain glutamate deficiency in amyotrophic lateral sclerosis. *Neurology* 37, 1845–1848.

Picconi, B., Pisani, A., Centonze, D., Battaglia, G., Storto, M., Nicoletti, F., Bernardi, G., *et al.* (2002) Striatal metabotropic glutamate receptor function following experimental parkinsonism and chronic levodopa treatment. *Brain* 125, 2635–2645.

Plaitakis, A., Constantakakis, E. and Smith, J. (1988) The neuroexcitotoxic amino acids glutamate and aspartate are altered in the spinal cord and brain in amyotrophic lateral sclerosis. *Annals of Neurology* 24, 446–449.

Prager, E.M. and Johnson, L.R. (2009) Stress at the synapse: signal transduction mechanisms of adrenal steroids at neuronal membranes. *Science Signalling* 2, 5.

Prince, M., Ferri, C.P., Acosta, D., *et al.* (2007) The protocols for the 10/66 dementia research group population-based research programme. *BMC Public Health* 7, 165.

Radenovic, L., Selacovic, V. and Andjus, P.R. (2008) Neuroprotection by MK-801 following cerebral ischemia in Mongolian gerbils. *Archives of Biological Sciences* 60, 341–346.

Reddy, P.H., Williams, M., Charles, V., *et al.* (1998) Behavioral abnormalities and selective neuronal loss in HD transgenic mice expressing mutated full-length HD cDNA. *Nature Genetics* 20, 198–202.

Rodríguez-Moreno, A. and Sihra, T.S. (2004) Presynaptic kainate receptor facilitation of glutamate release involves protein kinase A in the rat hippocampus. *Journal of Physiology* 557, 733–745.

Rodríguez-Moreno, A., Herreras, O. and Lerma, J. (1997) Kainate receptors presynaptically downregulate GABAergic inhibition in the rat hippocampus. *Neuron* 19, 893–901.

Rodríguez-Moreno, A., López-García, J.C. and Lerma, J. (2000) Two populations of kainate receptors with separated signalling mechanisms in hippocampal interneurons. *Proceedings of the National Academy of Sciences USA* 97, 1293–1298.

Rosen, D.R., Siddique, T., Patterson, D., Figlewicz, D.A., Sapp, P., Hentati, A., Donaldson, J., *et al.* (1993) Mutations in Cu/Zn superoxide dismutase gene are associated with familial amyotrophic lateral sclerosis. *Nature* 362, 59–62.

Ross, C.A. and Margolis, R.L. (2002) Huntington Disease. In: Davis, K.L., Charney, D., Coyle, J.T. and Nemeroff, C. (eds) *Neuropsychopharmacology: The Fifth Generation of Progress*. Lippincott Williams & Wilkins, New York, pp.1817–1830.

Rossi, A., Stratta, P., D'Albenzio, L., Tartaro, A., Schiazza, G., Di Michele, V., Bolino, F., *et al.* (1990) Reduced temporal lobe areas in schizophrenia: preliminary evidences from a controlled multiplanar magnetic resonance imaging study. *Biological Psychiatry* 27, 61–68.

Rothstein, J.D., Patel, S., Regan, M.R., Haenggeli, C., Huang, Y.H., Bergles, D.E., Jin, L., *et al.* (2005) Beta-lactam antibiotics offer neuroprotection by increasing glutamate transporter expression. *Nature* 433, 73–77.

Rui, Y., Gu, J., Yu, K., Hartzell, H.C. and Zheng J.Q. (2010) Inhibition of AMPA receptor trafficking at hippocampal synapses by beta-amyloid oligomers: the mitochondrial contribution. *Molecular Brain* doi: 10.1186/1756-6606-3-10.

Salasar, E.F. and Roos, R.P. (1995) Amyotrophic lateral sclerosis and viruses. *Clinical Neuroscience* 3, 360–367.

Samuel, W., Terry, R.D., DeTeresa, R., Butters, N. and Masliah, E. (1994) Clinical correlates of cortical and nucleus basalis pathology in Alzheimer dementia. *Archives of Neurology* 51, 772–778.

Sasabe, J. and Aiso, S. (2010) Aberrant control of motoneuronal excitability in amyotrophic lateral sclerosis: excitatory glutamate/D-serine vs. inhibitory glycine/γ-aminobutanoic acid (GABA). *Chemistry & Biodiversity* 7, 1479–1490.

Scarr, E., Pavey, G., Sundram, S., MacKinnon, A. and Dean, B. (2003) Decreased hippocampal NMDA, but not kainate or AMPA receptors in bipolar disorder. *Bipolar Disorders* 5, 257–264.

Scheff, S.W., Price, D.A., Schmitt, F.A., DeKosky, S.T. and Mufson, E.J. (2007) Synaptic alterations in CA1 in mild Alzheimer disease and mild cognitive impairment. *Neurology* 68, 1501–1508.

Schiefer, J., Sprünken, A., Puls, C., Lüesse, H.G., Milkereit, A., Milkereit, E., Johann, V., et al. (2004) The metabotropic glutamate receptor 5 antagonist MPEP and the mGluR2 agonist LY379268 modify disease progression in a transgenic mouse model of Huntington's disease. *Brain Research* 1019, 246–254.

Schiene, K., Bruehl, C., Zilles, K., Qü, M., Hagemann, G., Kraemer, M., et al. (1996) Neuronal hyperexcitability and reduction of GABAA-receptor expression in the surround of cerebral photothrombosis. *Journal of Cerebral Blood Flow & Metabolism* 16, 906–914.

Schilling, G., Becher, M.W., Sharp, A.H., et al. (1999) Intranuclear inclusions and neuritic aggregates in transgenic mice expressing a mutant N-terminal fragment of huntingtin. *Human Molecular Genetics* 8, 397–407.

Shim, K.S. and Lubec, G. (2002) Drebrin, a dendritic spine protein, is manifold decreased in brains of patients with Alzheimer's disease and Down syndrome. *Neuroscience Letters* 324, 209–212.

Silva-Gómez, A.B., Rojas, D., Juarez, I. and Flores, G. (2003) Decreased dendritic spine density on prefrontal cortical and hippocampal pyramidal neurons in postweaning social isolation rats. *Brain Research* 983, 128–136.

Silver, I.A. and Erecinska, M. (1992) Ion homeostasis in rat brain in vivo: intra- and extracellular $[Ca^{2+}]$ and $[Na^+]$ in the hippocampus during cortical neurons: implication for neuroprotective strategies. *Experimental Neurology* 147, 115–122.

Smith, S.E., Meldrum, B.S. (1992) The glycine-site NMDA receptor antagonist, r-cis-beta-methyl-3-amino-1-hydroxypyrrolid-2-one, l-687,414 is anticonvulsant in baboons. *European Journal of Pharmacology* 211, 109–111.

Snyder, E.M., Nong, Y., Almeida, C.G., Paul, S., Moran, T., Choi, E.Y., Nairn, A.C., et al. (2005) Regulation of NMDA receptor trafficking by amyloid-beta. *Nature Neuroscience* 8, 1051–1058.

Solis, O., Limón, D.I., Flores-Hernández, J. and Flores, G. (2007) Alterations in dendritic morphology of the prefrontal cortical and striatum neurons in the unilateral 6-OHDA-rat model of Parkinson's disease. *Synapse* 61, 450–458.

Solis, O., Vazquez-Roque, R.A., Camacho-Abrego, I., De la Cruz, F., Zamudio, S. and Flores, G. (2009) Decreased dendritic spine density of neurons of the prefrontal cortex and nucleus accumbens and enhanced amphetamine sensitivity in postpubertal rats after a neonatal amygdala lesion. *Synapse* 63, 1143–1159.

Sotrel, A., Williams, R.S., Kaufmann, W.E. and Myers, R.H. (1993) Evidence for neuronal degeneration and dendritic plasticity in cortical pyramidal neurons of Huntington's disease: a quantitative Golgi study. *Neurology* 43, 2088–2096.

Spires-Jones, T.L., Meyer-Luehmann, M., Osetek, J.D., Jones, P.B., Stern, E.A., Bacskai, B.J. and Hyman, B.T. (2007) Impaired spine stability underlies plaque-related spine loss in an Alzheimer's disease mouse model. *American Journal of Pathology* 171, 1304–1311.

Suddath, R.L., Casanova, M.F., Goldberg, T.E., Daniel, D.G., Kelsoe, J.R. Jr and Weinberger, D.R. (1989) Temporal lobe pathology in schizophrenia: a quantitative magnetic resonance imaging study. *American Journal of Psychiatry* 146, 464–472.

Suddath, R.L., Christison, G.W., Torrey, E.F., Casanova, M.F. and Weinberger, D.R. (1990) Anatomical abnormalities in the brains of monozygotic twins discordant for schizophrenia. *New England Journal of Medicine* 122, 789–794.

Tang, T.S., Tu, H., Chan, E.Y., Maximov, A., Wang, Z., Wellington, C.L., Hayden, M.R., et al. (2003) Huntington and huntingtin-associated protein 1 influence neuronal calcium signaling mediated by inositol-(1,4,5) triphosphate receptor type 1. *Neuron* 39, 227–239.

Thomson, A.M. (1989) Glycine modulation of the NMDA receptor/channel complex. *Trends in Neurosciences* 12, 349–353.

Tovar, K.R. and Westbrook, G.L. (2002) Mobile NMDA receptors at hippocampal synapses. *Neuron* 34, 255–264.

Tsai, G., Stauch-Slusher, B., Sim, L., Hedreen, J.C., Rothstein, J.D., Kuncl, R. and Coyle, J.T. (1990) Reductions in acidic amino acids and N-acetyl-aspartyl-glutamate (NAAG) in amyotrophic lateral sclerosis CNS. *Brain Research* 556, 151–156.

Uylings, H.B. and De Brabander, J.M. (2002) Neuronal changes in normal human aging and Alzheimer's disease. *Brain and Cognition* 49, 268–276.

Vertes, R.P. (2004) Differential projections of the infralimbic and prelimbic cortex in the rat. *Synapse* 51, 32–58.

Volterra, A., Trotti, D., Cassutti, P., *et al.* (1992) High sensitivity of glutamate uptake to extracellular free arachidonic acid levels in rat cortical synaptosomes and astrocytes. *Journal of Neurochemistry* 59, 600–606.

Vonsattel, J.P. and DiFiglia, M. (1998) Huntington disease. *Journal of Neuropathology & Experimental Neurology* 57, 369–384.

Vonsattel, J.P., Myers, R.H., Stevens, T.J., Ferrante, R.J., Bird, E.D. and Richardson, E.P. Jr (1985) Neuropathological classification of Huntington's disease. *Journal of Neuropathology & Experimental Neurology* 44, 559–577.

Voorn, P., Jorritsma-Byham, B., Van Dijk, C. and Buijs, R.M. (1986) The dopaminergic innervation of the ventral striatum in the rat: A light and electron-microscopical study with antibodies against dopamine. *Journal of Comparative Neurology* 251, 84–99.

Voulalas, P.J., Holtzclaw, L., Wolstenholme, J., Russell, J.T. and Hyman, S.E. (2005) Metabotropic glutamate receptors and dopamine receptors cooperate to enhance extracellular signal-regulated kinase phosphorylation in striatal neurons. *Journal of Neuroscience* 25, 3763–3773.

Wahlestedt, C., Golanov, E., Yamamoto, S., *et al.* (1993) Antisense oligodeoxynucleotides to NMDA-R1 receptor channel protect cortical neurons from excitotoxicity and reduce focal ischaemic infarctions. *Nature* 363, 260–263.

White, B., Sullivan, J., DeGracia, D., Oneil, B., Neumar, R., Grossman, L., *et al.* (2000) Brain ischemia and reperfusion: molecular mechanisms of neuronal injury. *Journal of the Neurological Sciences* 179, 1–33.

Yamamoto, A., Lucas, J.J. and Hen, R. (2000) Reversal of neuropathology and motor dysfunction in a conditional model of Huntington's disease. *Cell* 101, 57–66.

Ying, H.S., Weishaupt, J.H., Grabb, M., Canzoniero, L.M., Sensi, S.L., Sheline, C.T., Monyer, H., *et al.* (1997) Sublethal oxygen-glucose deprivation alters hippocampal neuronal AMPA receptor expression and vulnerability to kainate-induced death. *Journal of Neuroscience* 17, 9536–9544.

Zaldivar, T., Gutierrez, J., Lara, G., Carbonara, M., Logroscino, G. and Hardiman, O. (2009) Reduced frequency of ALS in an ethnically mixed population: A population-based mortality study. *Neurology* 72, 1640–1645.

Zeron, M.M., Hansson, O., Chen, N., Wellington, C.L., Leavitt, B.R., Brundin, P., Hayden, M.R. and Raymond, L.A. (2002) Increased sensitivity to N-methyl-Daspartate receptor-mediated excitotoxicity in a mouse model of Huntington's disease. *Neuron* 33, 849–860.

Zhang, G., Raol, Y.S., Hsu, F.C. and Brooks-Kayal, A.R. (2004) Long-term alterations in glutamate receptor and transporter expression following early-life seizures are associated with increased seizure susceptibility. *Journal of Neurochemistry* 88, 91–101.

26 Efficacy of L-DOPA Therapy in Parkinson's Disease

G. Sahin and D. Kirik*
Brain Repair And Imaging in Neural Systems (BRAINS), Section of Neuroscience, Department of Experimental Medical Science, Lund University, Lund, Sweden

26.1 Abstract

L-3,4-dihydroxyphenylalanine (L-DOPA) is a classical example of an amino acid that is an immediate precursor to dopamine and has been developed as an effective therapeutic agent for a neurodegenerative disease. Dopamine deficiency is known to be a core pathogenic event in Parkinson's disease (PD). It is the main neurotransmitter responsible for modulation of motor behaviour. Peripherally given, L-DOPA is transported into the brain and upon decarboxylation converted into dopamine. L-DOPA pharmacotherapy is used as a symptomatic treatment of PD as it restores dopamine neurotransmission. Since L-DOPA can also be decarboxylated in the periphery, and peripherally formed dopamine is not able to cross the blood–brain barrier, inhibition of the peripheral decarboxylation increases bioavailability of L-DOPA in the brain. An initial satisfactory clinical response to L-DOPA is invariably hampered later in the course of the disease, mainly due to progression of the neurodegenerative changes in the brain. In addition, side effects such as motor fluctuations and abnormal involuntary movements become a significant problem for patients with advanced disease. Moreover, it is thought that pulsatile administration of L-DOPA is one of the most important underlying trigger factors for induction and maintenance of these motor complications. This mode of stimulation is thought to lead to abnormal changes in basal ganglia neurons at the molecular level. These plastic changes can be reduced or avoided if dopaminergic replacement is done in a more continuous and physiologic manner. Currently, continuous dopaminergic stimulation can be achieved by using long-lasting drug formulations or continuous L-DOPA infusion pumps. In addition to these peripheral administration approaches, recently, viral-mediated intrastriatal 3,4-dihyroxyphenylalanine (DOPA) delivery strategies have been developed as an alternative treatment in Parkinson's disease.

26.2 Introduction

PD is a neurodegenerative disorder, first described in a monograph by James Parkinson (1817). Clinical features at onset typically include asymmetric bradykinesia (slowness

---

* E-mail address: Deniz.Kirik@med.lu.se

in movements), rigidity (stiffness in muscles), and tremor (shaking) at rest. The mean age of onset is 57 years and the disease affects 1–2% of the population over the age of 60 years, although it can also begin at a much younger age (Koller et al., 1987). The motor symptoms emerge when a significant proportion of dopamine-producing neurons in the substantia nigra have been lost and striatal dopamine has been reduced by 60–80% (Hornykiewicz, 1998; Lang, 2007). Other neuronal populations are also known to be lost in addition to the dopamine system, resulting in deficits in noradrenergic, serotonergic, and cholinergic neurotransmission. These are thought to underlie the non-motor symptoms including cognitive decline, sleep abnormalities, and depression, as well as gastrointestinal and genitourinary disturbances.

Dopamine deficiency in PD cannot be replaced by direct peripheral administration because dopamine has a very short half-life in the blood and does not cross the blood–brain barrier. Instead, dopaminergic drugs are used for replacement therapy. The uses of dopaminergic drugs improve motor function, significantly reduce both the morbidity and mortality of the affected individuals, and improve quality of life (Rajput, 2001).

26.3 L-DOPA

L-3,4-dihyroxyphenylalanine (L-DOPA), the naturally occurring isomer of aromatic amino acid 3,4-dihydrophenylalanine (DOPA), is a classical example of neurotransmitter replacement therapy in the brain. As a precursor of dopamine, L-DOPA is the mainstay of treatment in PD. Unlike dopamine, L-DOPA is transported into the brain by the large neutral amino acid transport system (Nutt and Fellman, 1984).

D,L-DOPA racemate was first synthesized in the laboratory in 1911. Two years later the L-isomer was isolated from legumes (seedlings of Vicia faba) by Guggenheim. Even though early pharmacological investigations suggested that L-DOPA was biologically inactive, in 1927 Hirai and Gondo found that it was an active compound causing hyperglycaemia and hypotension in rabbits. In 1938, Holtz and Credner demonstrated in mammalian tissue extracts that L-DOPA was decarboxylated by aromatic amino acid decarboxylase (AADC) (reviewed in Hornykiewicz, 2002).

Dopamine was identified in the brains of rats and other animals in 1957 (Montagu, 1957; Weil-Malherbe and Bone, 1957). In the same period the antipsychotic action of reserpine was discovered and Dr Arvid Carlsson (who was one of three to be awarded the Nobel Prize in Physiology or Medicine in 2000) started to study this potent drug that was able to deplete neurotransmitters. In 1957, Carlsson administered DOPA to reserpine-treated rabbits and mice in order to understand its action, and discovered that this amino acid had a central stimulant action and was able to reverse the akinetic and sedative actions of reserpine (Carlsson et al., 1957). Following this, Carlsson showed that dopamine was a normal brain constituent, and mapped its regional distribution (mainly in basal ganglia) (reviewed in Iversen and Iversen, 2007).

Based on Carlsson's discovery of dopamine, striatal dopamine deficiency in PD was described by Ehringer and Hornykiewicz in 1960, and, one year later, Birkmayer and Hornykiewicz showed that intravenous injection of single dose L-DOPA resulted in marked resolution of akinesia in 2–3 hours for up to 24 hours in PD patients (reprinted in English in Ehringer and Hornykiewicz, 1998; Birkmayer and Hornykiewicz, 2001). Later, Cotzias showed that oral administration of D, L-DOPA at a dose of 3–16 g day^{-1} was also effective, but four patients developed agranulocytopaenia (Cotzias et al., 1964, 1967). Subsequently he found that the use of the L-form was less toxic than the racemic D, L-DOPA mixture (Cotzias, 1968). These clinical studies established the efficacy of L-DOPA therapy in PD, and the US Food and Drug Administration approved L-DOPA as a treatment for PD in 1970.

It was only in 1975 when post-mortem analysis of brain tissue from L-DOPA-treated PD patients were found to have elevated levels of dopamine compared to untreated patients, that the effectiveness of L-DOPA was found to result from its metabolism to dopamine in the brain (Lloyd et al., 1975).

26.4 Dopamine Biosynthesis in Physiological Conditions

Tyrosine is an essential amino acid that is abundant in dietary proteins. Blood-borne tyrosine is taken up into the brain by the neutral amino acid transport system and subsequently from brain extracellular fluid into dopaminergic neurons (Elsworth and Roth, 1997). In the appropriate neuronal compartment, tyrosine is converted to DOPA by the tyrosine hydroxylase (TH) enzyme (Fig. 26.1). This reaction is the rate-limiting step in the synthesis of dopamine. The rate of tyrosine hydroxylation is not influenced by tyrosine availability *in vivo* under normal conditions in most dopaminergic neurons; however when the enzyme is activated by phosphorylation, or in dopamine neuronal systems that have a relatively high basal firing rate, tyrosine levels can affect the rate of conversion to DOPA. The activity of the TH enzyme is dependent on the presence of tetrahydrobiopterin, which acts as an essential cofactor and is formed from guanosine triphosphate (GTP) in a three-step enzymatic reaction. GTP cyclohydrolase 1 (GCH1) is the first and rate-limiting enzyme in tetrahydrobiopterin biosynthesis. During hydroxylation tetrahydrobiopterin is reduced to dihydrobiopterin by the activity of the dihydropteridin reductase enzyme.

Cytosolic DOPA is rapidly converted into dopamine by the pyridoxine-dependent aromatic AADC enzyme. Thus, under normal circumstances, the levels of DOPA in the brain are very low, typically below the detection limits of high-performance liquid chromatography (HPLC) assays. Needless to say, all endogenously formed DOPA in tissue is the L-isomer, whereas the D-isomer of the molecule does not act as a substrate for synthesis of dopamine. Importantly, however, not only dopamine neurons but also serotonin neurons, glia, and endothelial cells possess AADC activity and are known to contribute to the formation of dopamine, especially upon exogenous administration of L-DOPA (Melamed *et al.*, 1981; Mura *et al.*, 1995; Arai *et al.*, 1996).

Once dopamine is synthesized, it is transported from the cytoplasm to specialized storage vesicles by the help of vesicular monoamine transporter-2 (VMAT2). In the vesicular compartment dopamine is concentrated to approximately 0.1 M, much higher than its levels in the cytosol (Kelly, 1993; Peter *et al.*, 1995). Activation of the dopaminergic neuron by excitatory input causes influx of calcium ions that in turn give rise to fusion of vesicles with the synaptic membrane. The release of dopamine into the synaptic cleft stimulates its specific receptors located at both pre-synaptic and post-synaptic sites. This action is limited in duration by reuptake to the pre-synaptic terminal via the dopamine transporter. In addition, there is some evidence that glia and non-dopaminergic neurons may, to a limited extent, take up and metabolize extracellular dopamine (Hitri *et al.*, 1994).

Monoamine oxidase (MAO) and catechol-*O*-methyltransferase (COMT) are the main enzymes responsible for the metabolism of dopamine (Fig. 26.1). 3,4-dihydroxyphenylacetic acid (DOPAC) is formed either intraneuronally (dopamine and serotonin neurons) or extraneuronally (glial cells) by the MAO enzyme. Homovanillic acid (HVA) is the major end product of dopamine metabolism in the brain and is formed exclusively in the non-neuronal compartments via the COMT enzyme (Kopin, 1985).

26.5 Basic Principles of L-DOPA Pharmacotherapy in Parkinson's Disease

Although L-DOPA has the capability to cross the blood–brain barrier, only 1% of an orally administered dose of L-DOPA enters into the brain, because of the rapid conversion into dopamine in the periphery. After the discovery of the role of peripheral AADC in the metabolism of L-DOPA (Bartholini *et al.*, 1967), the addition of peripheral AADC inhibitors that do not cross the blood–brain barrier (carbidopa or benserazide) was found to significantly enhance the therapeutic efficacy, reduce the total dose required by approximately tenfold, and in turn lower the peripheral side effect profile (Cedarbaum, 1987; Pletscher and DaPrada, 1993). The therapeutic efficacy and side effects of these two AADC inhibitors when administered with L-DOPA have been thoroughly studied and

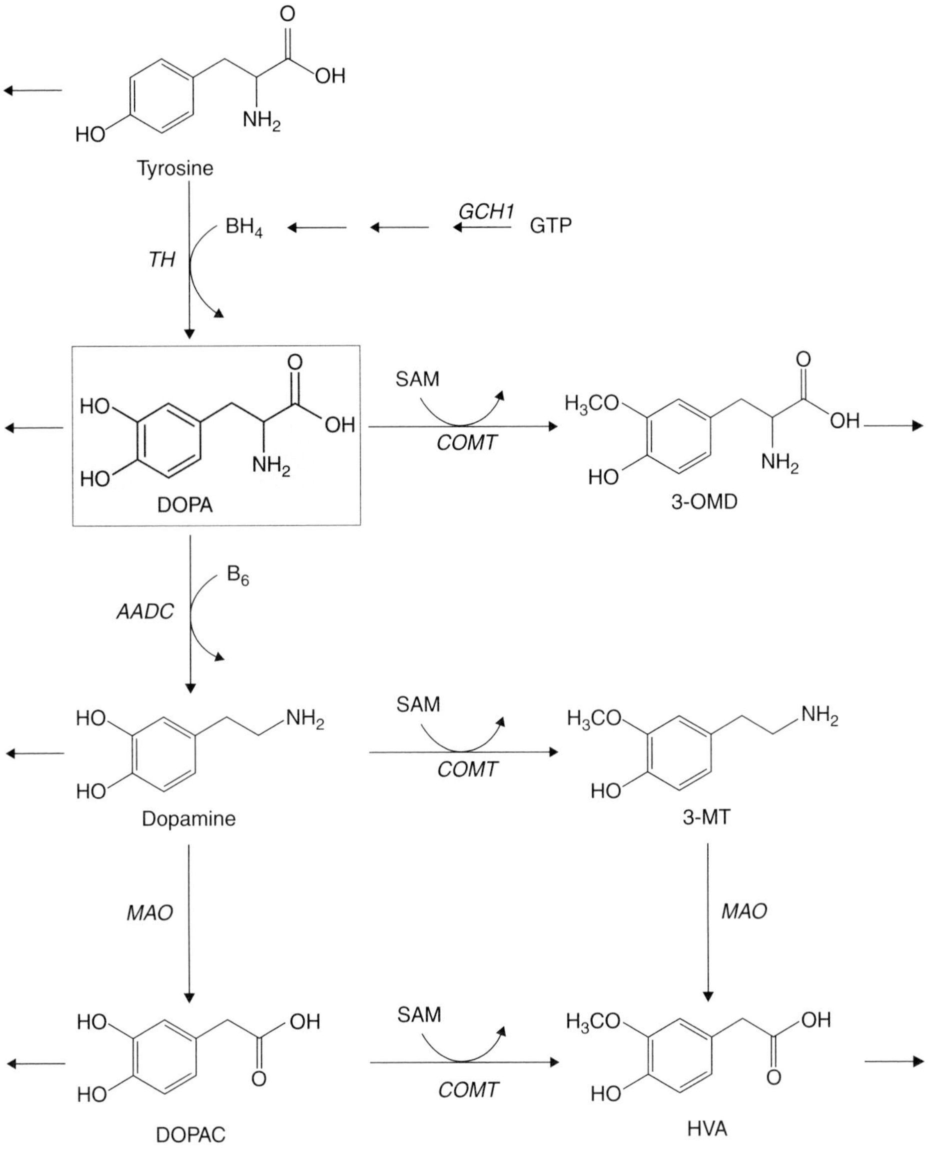

Fig. 26.1. Biosynthesis and metabolism of DOPA. Tyrosine, an essential amino acid obtained from dietary proteins, is converted to 3,4-dihyroxyphenylalanine (DOPA) by the tyrosine hydroxylase (TH) enzyme. Activity of the TH enzyme is dependent on the presence of tetrahydrobiopterin (BH_4), which acts as a cofactor and is synthesized from guanosine triphosphate (GTP) in a three-step enzymatic reaction. GTP cyclohydrolase 1 (GCH1) is the first and the rate-limiting enzyme in BH_4 biosynthesis. DOPA is either immediately converted into dopamine by the pyridoxine- (B_6) dependent aromatic amino acid decarboxylase (AADC) enzyme, or methylated to form 3-O-methyl-DOPA (3-OMD). The enzyme known as catechol-O-methyltransferase (COMT) catalyzes this methylation and S-adenosylmethionine (SAM) serves as the donor compound for the methyl group. Dopamine is metabolized to form either 3,4-dihydroxyphenylacetic acid (DOPAC) by the monoamine oxidase (MAO) or 3-methoxytyramine (3-MT) by the COMT enzymes. The end product of this metabolic pathway is homovanillic acid (HVA). The arrows on the left and right sides of the figure represent other synthesis and/or metabolism pathways, e.g. tyramine from tyrosine, melanin from DOPA, or norepinephrine from dopamine.

were found not to be significantly different (Greenacre et al., 1976).

In the presence of an AADC inhibitor, L-DOPA is substantially inactivated in the periphery by COMT enzyme to form 3-O-methyl-DOPA (3-OMD) (Fig. 26.1). Under these circumstances about 5–10% of the administered L-DOPA reaches the brain (Kaakkola, 2000). The 3-OMD metabolite is a large neutral amino acid with a long half-life (15 h). It crosses the blood–brain barrier but does not bind to the dopamine receptor and has no antiparkinsonian activity. The efficacy of L-DOPA can therefore be also enhanced by co-administration of a COMT inhibitor, which reduces O-methylation in the gut, increases L-DOPA absorption, and prolongs its half-life (Nutt et al., 1994). The first available COMT inhibitor in the market was tolcapone, but its usage was limited due to hepatic toxicity. Today entacapone is the most widely used COMT inhibitor and, when combined with L-DOPA, increases 'on' time and reduces 'off' time (Heikkinen et al., 2001).

26.6 Clinical Pharmacokinetics and Pharmacodynamics of L-DOPA Therapy

In clinical practice, L-DOPA is only available in a fixed-combination formulation with an AADC inhibitor. Between 80% and 90% of L-DOPA is absorbed in the proximal part of the small intestine by an active saturable carrier system for large neutral amino acids (Wade et al., 1973). The stomach has limited capacity for absorption but may be an important site of decarboxylation of L-DOPA, therefore the rate of gastric emptying is the principal determinant in the bioavailability of L-DOPA. L-DOPA alters the pattern of gastric emptying in healthy volunteers, explaining its erratic absorption from the gastrointestinal tract (Robertson et al., 1990). Gastric emptying may be delayed by food (especially fat), resulting in a threefold increase in the t_{max} of L-DOPA (Baruzzi et al., 1987). It should therefore be administered at least 30 min before meals.

Oral protein loads have shown to reverse the therapeutic effect of L-DOPA without reducing the plasma concentrations (Pincus and Barry, 1987). This is thought to be due to the competition between large neutral amino acids and L-DOPA for a common transport across the blood–brain barrier (Alexander et al., 1994). Dietary manipulations, including rescheduling of protein intake or protein restriction (e.g. 0.8 g of protein kg^{-1}), can be a simple and effective adjunct to the treatment, especially in the advanced PD patients (Karstaedt and Pincus, 1992).

In the early course of PD, L-DOPA therapy gives a sustained effect, which has been termed a long-duration response (LDR) (Zappia et al., 2000). This is a consequence of the ability of the nigrostriatal dopamine system to convert L-DOPA to dopamine, store it in the pre-synaptic vesicles, and release it in response to physiological stimuli. However, after a variable time period from months to years, this smooth clinical response is replaced with short-duration response (SDR), which provides an improvement in motor disability that lasts only a few hours after the administration of a single dose of L-DOPA. It is assumed that both type of responses are present when the treatment is initiated, but SDR may be unnoticed due to the masking effect of LDR (Nutt et al., 1992).

As the LDR is progressively lost and the clinical picture becomes dominated by the SDR, PD patients experience fluctuations in the clinical response to L-DOPA therapy. Motor fluctuations include delayed onset of L-DOPA's therapeutic effect or loss of efficacy between doses, termed 'wearing off'. L-DOPA benefit wearing off is characterized by the re-emergence of both the motor and various non-motor symptoms such as mood changes, anxiety, dysesthesias and diaphoresis (reviewed in Stocchi et al., 2010). L-DOPA-induced abnormal movements (dyskinesias) are the other motor complication of long-term L-DOPA therapy that has a significant impact on the quality of life of the patients.

26.7 L-DOPA-induced Dyskinesias

Dyskinesias are a central side effect of dopaminergic therapy and represent a major clinical problem in the management of patients with PD. Cotzias first observed 'the reversible induction of athetoid movements, which had been observed only in patients with PD and only when the therapeutic effect was significant' (Cotzias et al., 1967). Later observations clearly identified dyskinesias as a side effect of L-DOPA treatment (Barbeau, 1971). Based on published series, it has been estimated that PD patients treated for less than 5 years have an 11% risk of developing dyskinesias, those treated for 6–9 years have a risk of 32%, whereas patients treated for more than 10 years have a risk of 89% (Fabbrini et al., 2007).

The underlying mechanisms of L-DOPA-induced dyskinesias are still not fully understood. It is generally recognized that L-DOPA does not induce dyskinesias in PD patients (or in experimental animals) that have not been treated with dopaminergic medications previously. The process by which the brain becomes sensitized, such that each administration of dopaminergic therapy modifies the response to subsequent dopaminergic treatments, is called priming. Following priming, the development of dyskinesias largely depends on two additional factors, the pulsatile administration of L-DOPA, and the degree of dopaminergic denervation in the striatum (reviewed in Del Sorbo and Albanese, 2008). Current views suggest that both pre-synaptic (i.e., production, storage, controlled release and reuptake of dopamine by nigrostriatal dopaminergic neurons) and post-synaptic (i.e. status of receptors and second messenger signalling pathways in striatal neurons) components are critical in induction and maintenance of dyskinesias (reviewed in Cenci and Lundblad, 2006).

As the pre-synaptic dopaminergic neurodegeneration progresses in the parkinsonian brain (both in patients and in experimental models), other cell types start to take part in handling exogenously administered L-DOPA and its conversion to dopamine. In particular, serotonin neurons have recently been identified as playing a critical role. Serotonergic cells contain AADC enzyme and VMAT-2 transporter, and therefore possess not only the capability to convert L-DOPA to dopamine, but also to store it in synaptic vesicles as a false neurotransmitter (Arai et al., 1996). However, because they do not express the dopamine D2 auto-receptors and dopamine transporter, which are essential for the normal auto-regulatory feedback control of dopamine release from the pre-synaptic terminal, their activity is thought to lead to uncontrolled swings in extracellular dopamine concentrations. Importantly, it has been recently shown that dopamine released from serotonin terminals was responsible for the appearance of L-DOPA-induced dyskinesias in parkinsonian rats (Carta et al., 2007). Furthermore, either a lesion of the serotonin system by specific toxins, or pharmacological silencing of these neurons by selective serotonin 5-HT1A and 5-HT1B agonists, dramatically reduced or even completely abolished L-DOPA-induced dyskinesias in 6-hydroxydopamine (6-OHDA) lesioned rats and MPTP-treated monkeys (Munoz et al., 2008). These studies point to the deterministic role of the pre-synaptic dopamine-releasing compartment on the occurrence of dyskinesias.

Moreover, by using a novel system allowing the functional depletion of striatal dopamine while maintaining the structural integrity of the pre-synaptic compartment, we have shown that post-synaptic plastic changes caused by dopamine receptor stimulation occur as a consequence of the lack of dopamine, and do not require structural damage to the pre-synaptic dopaminergic terminals (Ulusoy et al., 2010). Importantly, although dyskinesias may be elicited as a function of the intrinsic cellular changes of the post-synaptic compartment, the striatal neurons respond normally to regulate dopamine release from an adequate pre-synaptic compartment.

26.8 Gene Therapy-mediated Continuous DOPA Delivery in the Parkinsonian Brain

In the light of these observations, it is plausible to think that the dyskinetic side effects of L-DOPA could be overcome by continuous delivery of L-DOPA. Actually, the proof-of-principle has already been obtained in the clinics. Intragastric, duodenal or intravenous infusions of L-DOPA have been shown to effectively decrease L-DOPA-induced dyskinesias

(Kurth et al., 1993; Nilsson et al., 1998; Stocchi et al., 2005; Olanow et al., 2006). These approaches support the basis for the concept of viral vector delivery of genes that encode enzymes critical for the synthesis of DOPA locally in the brain, as a tool for obtaining a source of continuous and physiological dopamine delivery locally in the brain.

Continuous DOPA delivery using viral vector-mediated gene transfer relies on the presence of a residual pool of endogenous AADC enzyme for synthesis of dopamine in the brain. The dopamine and serotonin terminals are two major sources of AADC in the striatum, while at least one additional minor non-neuronal pool is thought to be present as well. In the parkinsonian brain, the remaining dopamine axons and the serotonergic terminals are the two most likely places where conversion to (and release of) dopamine takes place. As the disease progresses, it is anticipated that fewer and fewer dopamine terminals will remain. Nevertheless, the serotonergic denervation of the striatum is significantly less than the dopaminergic one in PD patients and thus may remain as a reliable long-term source in a majority of the patients (Kish et al., 2008).

It is now established that not only TH, but also tetrahydrobiopterin (or the GCH1 gene), has to be provided for optimal DOPA synthesis ectopically in striatal neurons after gene transfer. By utilizing a new generation of recombinant-adeno-associated virus (rAAV2) vectors, the combined TH-GCH1 strategy provides therapeutic levels of DOPA synthesis in parkinsonian rats. At these levels of continuous DOPA synthesis, the animals not only recover in drug-induced rotation tests, but also show improvements on spontaneous motor tests (Kirik et al., 2002; Bjorklund et al., 2010). In line with these findings, it was recently shown that rAAV5-mediated DOPA delivery could reverse previously manifested L-DOPA-induced dyskinesias in rats (Carlsson et al., 2005). In this study, rats with an intrastriatal 6-OHDA lesion with moderate-to-severe behavioural impairments received daily pulsatile L-DOPA treatment until they became stably dyskinetic. After striatal injection of rAAV5-TH and rAAV5-GCH1, the severity of the abnormal dyskinetic movements gradually decreased to about 15% of the initial scores at 12 weeks post injection. The behavioural improvements, as well as the reversal of dyskinesias, would suggest that dopamine synthesized after this gene therapy approach should reach the post-synaptic receptors on striatal neurons in a physiological manner, and that the therapeutic effects are correlated with normalization of the dopamine neurotransmission. Indeed, dopamine D2 receptor ligand imaging using [^{11}C]Raclopride in AAV-treated rats showed normalization of dopamine D2 receptor binding and affinity, confirming this interpretation (Leriche et al., 2009). The ratio between TH and GCH1 availability is also important for optimization of continuous in vivo DOPA synthesis, and it was recently shown that optimal TH enzyme functionality requires GCH1/TH ratios of between 1/3 and 1/7 (Bjorklund et al., 2009).

Taken together, these data show that viral vector-mediated, continuous DOPA delivery is an attractive strategy for enzyme replacement in PD patients, and should be investigated further with the ultimate goal being clinically tested for efficacy.

26.9 Summary and Concluding Remarks

L-DOPA is a classic example of brain neurotransmitter replacement therapy. In the early stages, it gives a 'honeymoon' life to patients with PD. However, long-term motor complications constitute a major limiting factor in the treatment of advanced disease. Although patients experience these disabling side effects, they need continuous dopaminergic replacement therapy to have symptomatic relief. Use of L-DOPA in PD has been developed and improved by never-ending intensive research in the field, and optimization efforts are still ongoing. As the underlying mechanisms of long-term complications of L-DOPA are understood, new solutions are being developed and investigated for an optimized use in PD. Some of these include extending its half-life and improving efficacy by concomitant use with peripheral AADC and COMT inhibitors, attempts to develop oral long-lasting once-daily pills, transdermal formulations, and continuous infusion systems. Especially the latter approach is expected to have a big impact in quality of life for advanced PD patients. In this context, viral vector-mediated direct gene transfer techniques have been shown to provide continuous and stable dopamine synthesis in the experimental models of PD, and are currently being explored as a novel treatment modality in early clinical trials.

References

Alexander, G.M., Schwartzman, R.J., Grothusen, J.R. and Gordon, S.W. (1994) Effect of plasma levels of large neutral amino acids and degree of parkinsonism on the blood-to-brain transport of levodopa in naive and MPTP parkinsonian monkeys. *Neurology* 44, 1491–1499.

Arai, R., Karasawa, N. and Nagatsu, I. (1996) Aromatic L-amino acid decarboxylase is present in serotonergic fibers of the striatum of the rat. A double-labeling immunofluorescence study. *Brain Research* 706, 177–179.

Barbeau, A. (1971) Long-term side-effects of levodopa. *Lancet* 1 7695, 395.

Bartholini, G., Burkard, W.P. and Pletscher, A. (1967) Increase of cerebral catecholamines caused by 3,4-dihydroxyphenylalanine after inhibition of peripheral decarboxylase. *Nature* 215, 852–853.

Baruzzi, A., Contin, M., Riva, R., Procaccianti, G., Albani, F., Tonello, C., Zoni, E., *et al.* (1987) Influence of meal ingestion time on pharmacokinetics of orally administered levodopa in parkinsonian patients. *Clinical Neuropharmacology* 10, 527–537.

Birkmayer, W. and Hornykiewicz, O. (2001) The effect of l-3,4-dihydroxyphenylalanine (=DOPA) on akinesia in parkinsonism. 1961. *Wiener Klinische Wochenschrift* 113, 851–854.

Bjorklund, T., Hall, H., Breysse, N., Soneson, C., Carlsson, T., Mandel, R.J., Carta, M. and Kirik, D. (2009) Optimization of continuous in vivo DOPA production and studies on ectopic DA synthesis using rAAV5 vectors in Parkinsonian rats. *Journal of Neurochemistry* 111, 355–367.

Bjorklund, T., Carlsson, T., Cederfjall, E.A., Carta, M. and Kirik, D. (2010) Optimized adeno-associated viral vector-mediated striatal DOPA delivery restores sensorimotor function and prevents dyskinesias in a model of advanced Parkinson's disease. *Brain* 133, 496–511.

Carlsson, A., Lindqvist, M. and Magnusson, T. (1957) 3,4-Dihydroxyphenylalanine and 5-hydroxytryptophan as reserpine antagonists. *Nature* 180, 1200.

Carlsson, T., Winkler, C., Burger, C., Muzyczka, N., Mandel, R.J., Cenci, A., Bjorklund, A. and Kirik, D. (2005) Reversal of dyskinesias in an animal model of Parkinson's disease by continuous L-DOPA delivery using rAAV vectors. *Brain* 128, 559–569.

Carta, M., Carlsson, T., Kirik, D. and Bjorklund, A. (2007) Dopamine released from 5-HT terminals is the cause of L-DOPA-induced dyskinesia in parkinsonian rats. *Brain* 130, 1819–1833.

Cedarbaum, J.M. (1987) Clinical pharmacokinetics of anti-parkinsonian drugs. *Clinical Pharmacokinetics*, 13, 141–178.

Cenci, M.A. and Lundblad, M. (2006) Post- versus presynaptic plasticity in L-DOPA-induced dyskinesia. *Journal of Neurochemistry* 99, 381–392.

Cotzias, G.C. (1968) L-Dopa for Parkinsonism. *New England Journal of Medicine* 278, 630.

Cotzias, G.C., Papavasiliou, P.S., Vanwoert, M.H. and Sakamoto, A. (1964) Melanogenesis and extrapyramidal diseases. *Federation Proceedings*, 23, 713–718.

Cotzias, G.C., Van Woert, M.H. and Schiffer, L.M. (1967) Aromatic amino acids and modification of parkinsonism. *New England Journal of Medicine* 276, 374–379.

Del Sorbo, F. and Albanese, A. (2008) Levodopa-induced dyskinesias and their management. *Journal of Neurology* 255 Suppl 4, 32–41.

Ehringer, H. and Hornykiewicz, O. (1998) Distribution of noradrenaline and dopamine (3-hydroxytyramine) in the human brain and their behavior in diseases of the extrapyramidal system. *Parkinsonism & Related Disorders* 4, 53–57.

Elsworth, J.D. and Roth, R.H. (1997) Dopamine synthesis, uptake, metabolism, and receptors: relevance to gene therapy of Parkinson's disease. *Experimental Neurology* 144, 4–9.

Fabbrini, G., Brotchie, J.M., Grandas, F., Nomoto, M. and Goetz, C.G. (2007) Levodopa-induced dyskinesias. *Movement Disorders* 22, 1379–89; quiz 1523.

Greenacre, J.K., Coxon, A., Petrie, A. and Reid, J.L. (1976) Comparison of levodopa with carbidopa or benserazide in parkinsonism. *Lancet* 308, 381–384.

Heikkinen, H., Nutt, J.G., Lewitt, P.A., Koller, W.C. and Gordin, A. (2001) The effects of different repeated doses of entacapone on the pharmacokinetics of L-Dopa and on the clinical response to L-Dopa in Parkinson's disease. *Clinical Neuropharmacology* 24, 150–157.

Hitri, A., Hurd, Y.L., Wyatt, R.J. and Deutsch, S.I. (1994) Molecular, functional and biochemical characteristics of the dopamine transporter: regional differences and clinical relevance. *Clinical Neuropharmacology* 17, 1–22.

Hornykiewicz, O. (1998) Biochemical aspects of Parkinson's disease. *Neurology* 51, S2–9.

Hornykiewicz, O. (2002) L-DOPA: from a biologically inactive amino acid to a successful therapeutic agent. *Amino Acids* 23, 65–70.

Iversen, S.D. and Iversen, L.L. (2007) Dopamine: 50 years in perspective. *Trends in Neurosciences* 30, 188–193.

Kaakkola, S. (2000) Clinical pharmacology, therapeutic use and potential of COMT inhibitors in Parkinson's disease. *Drugs* 59, 1233–1250.

Karstaedt, P.J. and Pincus, J.H. (1992) Protein redistribution diet remains effective in patients with fluctuating parkinsonism. *Archives of Neurology* 49, 149–151.

Kelly, R.B. (1993) Storage and release of neurotransmitters. *Cell* 72 Suppl, 43–53.

Kirik, D., Georgievska, B., Burger, C., Winkler, C., Muzyczka, N., Mandel, R.J. and Bjorklund, A. (2002) Reversal of motor impairments in parkinsonian rats by continuous intrastriatal delivery of L-dopa using rAAV-mediated gene transfer. *Proceedings of National Academy of Sciences USA* 99, 1708–1713.

Kish, S.J., Tong, J., Hornykiewicz, O., Rajput, A., Chang, L.J., Guttman, M. and Furukawa, Y. (2008) Preferential loss of serotonin markers in caudate versus putamen in Parkinson's disease. *Brain* 131, 120–131.

Koller, W., O'Hara, R., Weiner, W., Lang, A., Nutt, J., Agid, Y., Bonnet, A.M., *et al.* (1987) Relationship of aging to Parkinson's disease. *Advances in Neurology* 45, 317–321.

Kopin, I.J. (1985) Catecholamine metabolism: basic aspects and clinical significance. *Pharmacological Reviews*, 37, 333–364.

Kurth, M.C., Tetrud, J.W., Tanner, C.M., Irwin, I., Stebbins, G.T., Goetz, C.G. and Langston, J.W. (1993) Double-blind, placebo-controlled, crossover study of duodenal infusion of levodopa/carbidopa in Parkinson's disease patients with 'on-off' fluctuations. *Neurology* 43, 1698–1703.

Lang, A.E. (2007) The progression of Parkinson disease: a hypothesis. *Neurology* 68, 948–952.

Leriche, L., Bjorklund, T., Breysse, N., Besret, L., Gregoire, M.C., Carlsson, T., Dolle, F., *et al.* (2009) Positron emission tomography imaging demonstrates correlation between behavioral recovery and correction of dopamine neurotransmission after gene therapy. *Journal of Neuroscience* 29, 1544–1553.

Lloyd, K.G., Davidson, L. and Hornykiewicz, O. (1975) The neurochemistry of Parkinson's disease: effect of L-dopa therapy. *Journal of Pharmacology and Experimental Therapeutics* 195, 453–464.

Melamed, E., Hefti, F., Pettibone, D.J., Liebman, J. and Wurtman, R.J. (1981) Aromatic L-amino acid decarboxylase in rat corpus striatum: implications for action of L-dopa in parkinsonism. *Neurology* 31, 651–655.

Montagu, K.A. (1957) Catechol compounds in rat tissues and in brains of different animals. *Nature* 180, 244–245.

Munoz, A., Li, Q., Gardoni, F., Marcello, E., Qin, C., Carlsson, T., Kirik, D., *et al.* (2008) Combined 5-HT1A and 5-HT1B receptor agonists for the treatment of L-DOPA-induced dyskinesia. *Brain* 131, 3380–3394.

Mura, A., Jackson, D., Manley, M.S., Young, S.J. and Groves, P.M. (1995) Aromatic L-amino acid decarboxylase immunoreactive cells in the rat striatum: a possible site for the conversion of exogenous L-DOPA to dopamine. *Brain Research* 704, 51–60.

Nilsson, D., Hansson, L.E., Johansson, K., Nystrom, C., Palzow, L. and Aquilonius, S.M. (1998) Long-term intraduodenal infusion of a water based levodopa-carbidopa dispersion in very advanced Parkinson's disease. *Acta Neurologica Scandinavica* 97, 175–183.

Nutt, J.G. and Fellman, J.H. (1984) Pharmacokinetics of levodopa. *Clinical Neuropharmacology* 7, 35-49.

Nutt, J.G., Woodward, W.R., Carter, J.H. and Gancher, S.T. (1992) Effect of long-term therapy on the pharmacodynamics of levodopa. Relation to on-off phenomenon. *Archives of Neurology* 49, 1123–1130.

Nutt, J.G., Woodward, W.R., Beckner, R.M., Stone, C.K., Berggren, K., Carter, J.H., Gancher, S.T., *et al.* (1994) Effect of peripheral catechol-O-methyltransferase inhibition on the pharmacokinetics and pharmacodynamics of levodopa in parkinsonian patients. *Neurology* 44, 913–919.

Olanow, C.W., Obeso, J.A. and Stocchi, F. (2006) Continuous dopamine-receptor treatment of Parkinson's disease: scientific rationale and clinical implications. *Lancet Neurology* 5, 677–687.

Parkinson, J. (1817) *An Essay on the Shaking Palsy*. Sherwood, Neely, and Jones, London (republished in *Journal of Neuropsychiatry and Clinical Neurosciences* 14, 223–236, 2002).

Peter, D., Liu, Y., Brecha, N. and Edwards, R.H. (1995) The transport of neurotransmitters into synaptic vesicles. *Progress in Brain Research* 105, 273–281.

Pincus, J.H. and Barry, K.M. (1987) Plasma levels of amino acids correlate with motor fluctuations in parkinsonism. *Archives of Neurology* 44, 1006–1009.

Pletscher, A. and DaPrada, M. (1993) Pharmacotherapy of Parkinson's disease: research from 1960 to 1991. *Acta Neurologica Scandinavica Supplementum* 146, 26–31.

Rajput, A.H. (2001) Levodopa prolongs life expectancy and is non-toxic to substantia nigra. *Parkinsonism & Related Disorders* 8, 95–100.

Robertson, D.R., Renwick, A.G., Wood, N.D., Cross, N., Macklin, B.S., Fleming, J.S., Waller, D.G., et al. (1990) The influence of levodopa on gastric emptying in man. *British Journal of Clinical Pharmacology* 29, 47–53.

Stocchi, F., Vacca, L., Ruggieri, S. and Olanow, C.W. (2005) Intermittent vs continuous levodopa administration in patients with advanced Parkinson disease: a clinical and pharmacokinetic study. *Archives of Neurology* 62, 905–910.

Stocchi, F., Jenner, P. and Obeso, J.A. (2010) When do levodopa motor fluctuations first appear in Parkinson's disease? *European Neurology* 63, 257–266.

Ulusoy, A., Sahin, G. and Kirik, D. (2010) Presynaptic dopaminergic compartment determines the susceptibility to L-DOPA-induced dyskinesia in rats. *Proceedings of National Academy of Sciences USA* 107, 13159–13164.

Wade, D.N., Mearrick, P.T. and Morris, J.L. (1973) Active transport of L-dopa in the intestine. *Nature* 242, 463–465.

Weil-Malherbe, H. and Bone, A.D. (1957) Intracellular distribution of catecholamines in the brain. *Nature* 180, 1050–1051.

Zappia, M., Oliveri, R.L., Bosco, D., Nicoletti, G., Branca, D., Caracciolo, M., Napoli, I.D., et al. (2000) The long-duration response to L-dopa in the treatment of early PD. *Neurology* 54, 1910–1915.

27 Amino Acid Profiles for Diagnostic Applications

T. Kimura,[1]* M. Takahashi,[2] A. Imaizumi,[2] Y. Noguchi[2] and T. Ando[3]

[1]R+D Planning Department; [2]Research Institute for Innovation; [3]AminoIndex Department, Ajinomoto Co., Inc., Tokyo, Japan

27.1 Abstract

We describe how amino acid profiles could be used for clinical diagnosis through the generation of an AminoIndex, a function composed of multiple amino acid concentrations. Early studies on the correlation of amino acids indicated that the relationships between certain amino acids changed with their physiological state. Initial animal studies suggested that a fractional function composed of multiple amino acids could be used to separate different disease and physiological states. We describe the various problems regarding analytical speed, sample handling, and algorithm that had to be overcome in order to apply the methodology to clinical diagnoses. Finally, the analysis of clinical data by the AminoIndex method is presented for liver fibrosis in type C hepatitis, metabolic syndrome, colon cancer and breast cancer. The results so far suggest that the AminoIndex has a potential to be used in a number of clinical diagnostic applications.

27.2 Introduction

Since the recognition of inborn errors in metabolisms over 100 years ago, it has been known that extreme cases of metabolic imbalance can lead to profound consequences (Garrod, 1909). Since then, the understanding of amino acid metabolism and the ability to quantify free amino acids have progressed. The measurement of amino acid concentrations in biological fluids and tissues has provided us with important biochemical and nutritional information that enables the diagnosis of diseases, especially metabolic deficiencies (Armstrong and Stave, 1973a,b,c; Deyl, 1986).

Recently, there has been much progress in genomics, transcriptomics, proteonomics, and metabolomics. Although there are comprehensive technologies for genomics, transcriptomics, and proteomics where universal methods are available to measure the relevant parameters, this is not yet the case in metabolomics.

One of the aims of metabolomics is to determine all, or as many as possible, of the relevant metabolites and to elucidate their relationships in a comprehensive manner. We have taken the view that useful information may be gained by the analysis of a metabolomic subset, such as the set of amino acids, and this type of approach has been called focused or targeted metabolomics (Kimura et al., 2008). Focused metabolomics has also been used in the analysis of the lipid metabolomic subset (German et al., 2007; Piomelli

---

* E-mail address: takeshi_kimura@ajinomoto.com

et al., 2007). The amino acid metabolomic subset seemed to be especially relevant in studying one of our interests – the effects of excessive intakes of amino acids, and how to determine safe upper intake levels. The amino acid metabolomic subset was also a convenient model for a study on how to analyse metabolomic data.

It was clear from earlier studies that plasma amino acid levels did not simply reflect the net intake of dietary amino acids (Moundras *et al.*, 1993; Forslund *et al.*, 2000), and that the final plasma level for each amino acid is determined by a multitude of factors including catabolic rates and transport rates into and out of various organs. We realized that one key concept was that when considering the relationships among metabolites, it was important to note that the various metabolites constituted networks within cells, tissues, or the whole organism. Much information regarding the network of relationships among the various metabolites would be lost by the traditional approach of averaging results from different individuals within a treatment group. This was especially so when considering the potential for genetic variability and variations in gene expression levels among individuals within a treatment group (Noguchi *et al.*, 2003).

27.3 Correlation-based Analysis of Amino Acids

Initial studies focused on data obtained from experiments where the protein contents of diets for rats were varied from deficiency to gross excess. Rats were fed for 2 weeks on diets where only the protein and carbohydrate contents were varied, with protein ranging from 5% to 70% of the diet. Two different types of protein, casein and purified egg protein, were used in parallel experiments. Blood samples were collected several hours after the end of the feeding period to minimize the effect of the postprandial rise in plasma amino acid levels. When analysing the data, it was found that when plasma amino acid concentrations from each rat were plotted against each other, most of the relationships were linear, or consisted of a combination of linear segments (Noguchi *et al.*, 2006). From these observations, if was found that the analysis of correlations between plasma amino acid levels in individual animals was a promising direction in the analysis of amino acid profiles. We have suggested that the use of correlation analysis could be useful in analysing metabolomic and other '-omics' data, as correlation is without units and can accommodate pseudo-quantitative data, such as the peak heights of unidentified metabolites (Noguchi *et al.*, 2003; Sakai *et al.*, 2004). The analysis of correlation has been further extended to studying the network of relationships between plasma amino acid concentrations, and the expression levels of genes related to amino acid metabolism of different organs (Noguchi *et al.*, 2008). As this type of analysis is totally data driven, we feel that correlation-based analysis will be extremely useful for the future development of the '-omics' technologies as the data become more quantitative. However, correlation-based analysis requires many data points in order to obtain a pattern of relationships, and is not suited for use in determining the particular physiological state of an individual organism. In theory, multiple blood samples could be used to generate a correlation-based picture of the metabolic network of an individual, but this would seem impractical.

27.4 Development of Amino Acid Diagnostics

27.4.1 Background

Amino acids, supplied as food intake or synthesized endogenously, play essential physiological roles both as basic metabolites and as regulators in many metabolic pathways (Felig, 1975; Brosnan, 2003; Cynober, 2004). These include protein synthesis, protein degradation, urea cycle, glucogenesis, NO production, as precursors for neurotransmitters in the central nervous system, and others. Since blood circulates as a medium linking all organ systems, the profiles of plasma amino acid concentration (aminogram) could be influenced by the metabolic variation of a particular organ system induced in a specific disease. Altered profiles of amino acid concentrations have been observed in various diseases including liver disease, cancer, diabetes, renal failure, and so on (Felig et al., 1970; Watanabe et al., 1984; Hong et al., 1998; Holm et al., 1999). However, the difference in any single plasma amino acid concentration between a normal state and a particular disease state, except for inborn errors of metabolism, may not be sufficient for gaining statistical significance due to factors including individual variability and heterogeneous backgrounds. Historically, as a first and simplest example of an amino acid-based diagnostic index, Fischer's ratio – the ratio between the branched-chain amino acids (BCAA) and aromatic amino acids (AAA), (Leu + Val + Ile) / (Tyr + Phe) – has been used for the diagnosis of hepatic encephalopathy and monitoring its drug treatment efficacy (Fischer et al., 1975, 1976). Although Fischer's ratio has been used in practice for clinical diagnosis, the extensive search for an optimal diagnostic index from a dataset of amino acid concentrations has not been exploited.

27.4.2 Initial studies

Initially, an attempt was made using available data to separate animals at a low protein state from those at a high protein state. It was found that a single amino acid could not act as a parameter to separate the two groups, especially if data for the two different types of protein were used. However when simple fractional functions similar in form to Fischer's ratio, and composed of the plasma amino acid concentrations, were screened by trial and error, it was found that a fractional function, (Thr + Lys + Leu) / Ser, could separate low-protein animals from high-protein animals. However, it could not be determined if this was the best function, as all possible combinations of amino acids had not been tested, so the expression was generalized and a computer programme was created to test all combinations of amino acids. When this program was applied to separate animals at a low-protein state from those at a high-protein state, the function, Ile / Glu + (Thr + His + Tau) / Ser, was found to be the best index for separation.

The first algorithm used to generate a diagnostic index was as follows (Noguchi et al., 2006):

1. Amino acids are classified into two groups on the basis of their positive or negative correlation with the target parameter, whether continuous, ordinal, or dichotomous, that represents the disease stage or physiological condition.

2. Amino acids from the positive correlation group are assigned to the numerator, and amino acids from the negative correlation group are assigned to the denominator, and all possible combinations for the fractional function in the form (A + B + C…) / (N + O + P…) + (D + E + F…) / (Q + R + T…)…, where letters A–M represent amino acids with a positive correlation to the target parameter, while letters N–X represent amino acids with negative correlation to the target parameter, are generated. The correlation with the target parameter is calculated for each combination. The fractional functions are selected for further processing by evaluation methods, such as the sum of squares due to error based on simple linear regression for continuous target parameters, or variance ratio for categorical target parameters.

3. The optimal fractional function is finally selected after cross-validation of a large set of candidate functions by using random sampling to attain robustness with respect to sample variability and noise (Hjourth, 1989; Lee et al., 2004). The resulting function is called an AminoIndex.

In order to validate the diagnostic potential of the AminoIndex, the program was applied in dichotomous mode to obtain functions that can discriminate diabetic model rats from normal rats. Goto-Kakizaki rats and streptozotocin-treated rats (Pain and Garlick, 1974) were used as the diabetic models, and it was found that the function (Tau + Cit + Lys) / (Asp + Ile) + (Thr + Tyr + His) / Glu could successfully discriminate between the diabetic and normal rats with a sensitivity of 98.6% and a specificity of 97.6%. Long-term insulin treatment of the streptozotocin-induced diabetic rats resulted in a statistically significant shift of the amino index toward normal values.

For continuous target variables, the program can generate an amino index with the best linear fit to the target variables. In order test this mode, dimethylnitrosamine-treated liver dysfunction model rats were used (Vendemiale et al., 2001). Liver hydroxyproline concentration, reported to be a marker for liver fibrosis (Rojkind and Kershenobich, 1976), was chosen as the target parameter. The linear regression to the hydroxyproline concentrations resulted in the amino index (Tau + Cit + Met + Arg) / (Ser + Leu) + (Phe + Orn) / (Glu + Trp) with a coefficient of determination (r^2) of 0.85. This compared favourably to Fischer's ratio which had a r^2 of 0.49 (Noguchi et al., 2006). The efficacy of this type of function may reflect the linear nature of the relationships of the amino acid concentrations found in the previously described correlation-based analysis. We have found it surprising that fitting to this type of simple fractional function, without coefficients, gives high correlations to biological parameters, and suspect that this type of function may be approximating some aspects of the true steady-state kinetics functions governing the behaviour of the amino acids. Given enough computing power it may be possible to derive the real function in a totally data-driven manner.

However, one drawback to the initial approach is that simple combinations of n variables give rise to 2^n-1 fractional functions; hence, calculation of all possible combinations of the amino acids to derive the optimal fractional function is time consuming. We have found that calculations with 30 amino acids would take all night on a personal computer, and although an increase in computing speed is effective in reducing the computing time for a given number of variables, it did not allow a great increase in the number of variables that could be handled, as the computing time increased exponentially with variable number.

In order to speed up analysis, various statistical methods have been incorporated in the analysis, and currently AminoIndex can be generated by a data-mining approach, through multi-variate statistical methods such as logistic regression, linear regression, linear discriminant analysis, support vector machine and Bayesian network (Hastie et al., 2001; Armitage et al., 2002), in addition to the fractional function approach (Fig. 27.1). Optimal variable selection and cross-validation methods are

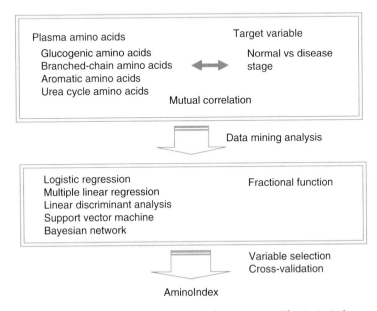

Fig. 27.1. Flowchart from plasma amino acids to AminoIndex generation. The AminoIndex generation proceeds from a dataset including amino acid profiles and target variables, through multi-variate statistical analysis, to the selection of AminoIndex with an optimal discriminating power.

used before finalization of the AminoIndex to ensure that the index is stable and robust.

27.4.3 Measurement of amino acids

Key historical developments in the analysis of amino acids was the use of paper chromatography (Martin and Synge, 1941), followed by the development of the amino acid analyser utilizing post-column ninhydrin reactions for detection (Spackman et al., 1958). Amino acid analysers currently available are being replaced with smaller and faster computerized operations and data processing, and advances in ion-exchanging resins has made it possible to analyse 41 plasma amino acids in 100 min. However, even though the analysis has been speeded up, at most only ten samples can be analysed in a day by one analyser. Because of such poor efficiency, it would not be suitable for handling large number of samples as required for routine diagnosis. In recent years, a wide variety of methods using pre-column derivatization of amino acids to replace the post-column ninhydrin reactions have increased the speed and sensitivity of amino acid analysis. We have developed new reagents for pre-column derivatization of amino acids so that separation can take place on reversed phase high-performance liquid chromatography (HPLC) for detection by mass spectrometry (Shimbo et al., 2009). This method can shorten the analysis time to about 7 min, which is less than one tenth of the post-column ninhydrin method.

27.5 Clinical Applications

27.5.1 Factors influencing stability of data

Early studies with clinical samples indicated that when collecting from different sites, the standardization of sample handling was essential. Otherwise, differences in amino acid concentrations reflecting differences in sample handling between different sites would give rise to AminoIndices that differentiated the clinical sites rather than the physiological conditions of the subjects.

Factors which influence the stability of the data needed to be examined.

There is generally an increase in plasma amino acid levels after a meal containing amino acids (Ozalp et al., 1972; Ljungqvist et al., 1978; Hegarty, 1982). It was therefore important to choose a time to collect blood when there was the least influence of the preceding meal. We have found that blood collected in the morning without breakfast, between 7 a.m. and 10 a.m., was consistent for an individual on separate days. The red blood cells and plasma have very different amino acid profiles so it is also important that there is no haemolysis of the blood sample. The blood contains enzymes that catabolize amino acids, and the time and temperature after blood collection was found to influence certain plasma amino acid concentrations. In order to avoid artefacts, it was found that cooling the samples on ice water immediately after blood collection and separating the plasma from the blood cells within 4 hours of blood collection gave stable results. It was also found that ethylendiamine tetraacetic acid disodium salt (EDTA 2Na) was superior to heparin as an anti-coagulant as it partly inhibited enzymes catabolizing amino acids. The plasma should be stored at −70°C rather than at −20°C, as certain amino acid concentrations decrease with time at −20°C. We have found that samples stored at −70°C can be thawed and restored up to three times without significant effects on plasma amino acid concentrations. Samples can be transported under dry ice for work with multiple sites.

27.5.2 Application of AminoIndex to liver fibrosis

The initial fractional function AminoIndex algorithm was first applied to the study of liver fibrosis to evaluate its usefulness in clinical diagnosis (Zhang et al., 2006). This study aimed to develop a non-invasive and effective method for the diagnosis of liver fibrosis using the plasma amino acid profiles. The background shows that among patients with chronic hepatitis C infection, the progression of liver fibrosis leads to cirrhosis and increases the risk of hepatocellular carcinoma (Poynard *et al.*, 2003). The grade of fibrosis influences the efficacy of current therapy, and therefore the accurate detection of the stage of fibrosis is needed for determining whether treatment is necessary, and what treatment is appropriate (Fried, 2002; Aspinall and Pockros, 2004; Shiffman, 2004). Although fibrosis grading by biopsy has been considered as a gold standard, there is a high demand for alternative effective and non-invasive methods (Imbert-Bismut *et al.*, 2001). In this study the liver specimens were analysed histologically, and graded with the METAVIR scoring system (Bedossa, 1994), where F0 means no fibrosis, F1 means portal fibrosis without septa, F2 means fibrosis with rare septa, F3 means portal fibrosis with numerous septa, and F4 means cirrhosis. The distribution of the 23 plasma amino acids of all 53 patients exhibiting the range of fibrosis stages is shown in Fig. 27.2 (from Zhang *et al.*, 2006). In the Kruskal–Wallis test for each amino acid, significant changes in the concentration of Phe, Val, Ile, Tyr, Gln, Leu, Met ($p < 0.01$) and

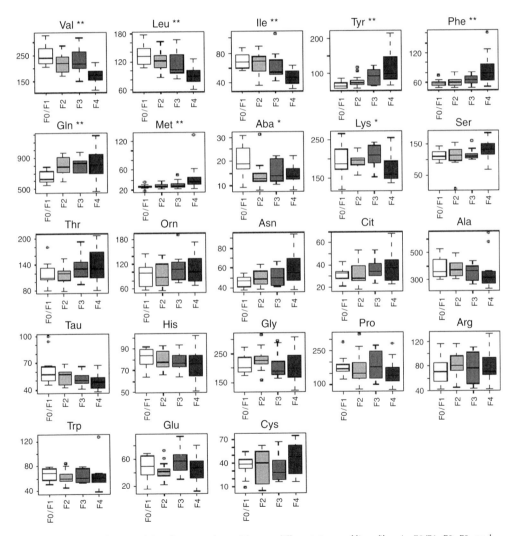

Fig. 27.2. The distribution of the plasma amino acids over different stages of liver fibrosis: F0/F1, F2, F3, and F4. The unit is µmol l^{-1}. The asterisks indicate the significance values by the Kruskal–Wallis test (** $p<0.01$, * $p<0.05$). Aba designates α-aminobutyric acid.

α ABA ($p < 0.05$) were observed between the different fibrosis stages. The dataset was analysed to give the AminoIndex, (Phe) / (Val) + (Thr + Met + Orn) / (Pro + Gly), that was optimized to be a surrogate marker to the liver stages obtained through biopsies. For the assessment of the surrogate AminoIndex, the area under the curve (AUC) of receiver operator characteristic (ROC) curve was used for evaluation. The AminoIndex showed high performance for discriminating advanced fibrosis (fibrosis stages F3 and F4) from the earlier stages F0–2, and also for discriminating cirrhosis (F4) from all other stages, with AUCs of 0.92 (95% CI 0.84–1.00) and 0.99 (0.96–1.00), respectively. Fischer's ratio has been reported for its good performance in assessing chronic hepatitis (Kano et al., 1991), and the comparison between it and AminoIndex is shown in Fig. 27.3 (modified from Zhang et al., 2006). The AminoIndex was generated to have a positive correlation with the degree of fibrosis, showing an inverse pattern to Fischer's ratio, and exhibited the larger values of ROC AUC than Fischer's ratio. The AminoIndex is a combination of two molar ratios, (Phe) / (Val) + (Thr + Met + Orn) / (Pro + Gly), and and the analysis in detail revealed that the former ratio mainly contributed to the F4 discrimination whereas the latter ratio mainly contributed to discrimination of advanced fibrosis (F3, F4). This is partially supported by the fact that the ratio Phe /Val correlated well with the inverse of Fischer's ratio ($r = 0.95$). Because BCAA had a tendency of mutual correlation, as did Tyr and Phe, it was confirmed that the substitution of Val with Leu or Ile or the substitution of Phe with Tyr showed similar discriminative power. These results suggested that the fibrosis AminoIndex based on plasma amino acid concentrations could be applied to evaluate liver fibrosis as an effective, less invasive method, than liver biopsy.

27.5.3 Application of AminoIndex to metabolic syndrome

Metabolic syndrome is a pathophysiological state consisting of hypertension, diabetes, and dyslipidaemia in combination, and is also a major risk factor for cardiovascular disease (Grundy et al., 2004; Després and Lemieux, 2006). With the high prevalence of metabolic syndrome in developed countries, where overeating and inactivity are common, metabolic syndrome is becoming a serious issue from the viewpoint of social medical care. The AminoIndex was also applied to the

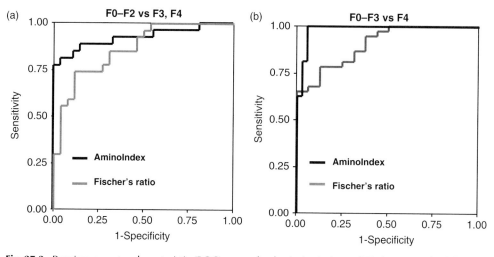

Fig. 27.3. Receiver operator characteristic (ROC) curves for the AminoIndex and Fischer's ratio for different fibrosis thresholds. The black and grey lines represent the ROC curves for the AminoIndex and Fischer's ratio, respectively. (a) F0–F2 versus F3 and F4; (b) F0–F3 versus F4.

study of metabolic syndrome (Takahashi et al., 2006) based on the observation that the plasma amino acids showed significant change associated with the metabolic syndrome subcomponents including obesity, dyslipidaemia, hypertension, and hyperglycaemia. From the viewpoint of metabolic networks, many amino acids play crucial roles as metabolic hubs, with highly linked metabolic nodes in all the metabolic pathways connecting glucose, lipid, and amino acids (Wagner and Fell, 2001). The elucidation of the metabolic state in metabolic syndrome is expected to lead to a deeper understanding of the physiological mechanism behind its aetiology.

In the study the criteria for extracting the metabolic syndrome group was based on the Examination Committee of Criteria for Metabolic Syndrome (2005), with the subcriteria:

1. waist circumference ≥ 85 for males and ≥ 90 cm for females;
2. systolic blood pressure ≥ 130 mmHg or diastolic blood pressure ≥ 85 mmHg;
3. triglycerides ≥ 150 mg dl^{-1} or HDL cholesterol < 40 mg dl^{-1}; and
4. fasting plasma glucose ≥ 110 mg dl^{-1}.

Metabolic syndrome is diagnosed if criterion 1 and at least two of criteria 2–4 are satisfied.

Plasma amino acids of 32 volunteers satisfying the metabolic syndrome criteria and 173 non-metabolic syndrome volunteers were analysed. When differences in individual amino acids were examined by t-test, significant increases in Ala, Glu, Tyr, Val and Trp, and significant decreases in Gly and Ser were seen in subjects with metabolic syndrome compared to non-metabolic syndrome subjects. Aminogram changes in glucogenic amino acids and branched-chain amino acids were similar to those in obesity and diabetes (Felig et al., 1969, 1970), and may reflect the metabolic modulation by insulin resistance, in which both the metabolic shift to protein catabolism and the up-regulation of gluconeogenesis in the liver would be induced (Chevalier et al., 2006). The optimal search of AminoIndex in the logistic regression analysis was performed for discriminating metabolic syndrome and gave the index, $-1.043 - 0.028$Gly $+ 0.011$Ala $+ 0.023$Thr $- 0.029$Ser $+ 0.020$Glu, with which the value of ROC AUC was 0.82 (95% CI 0.75–0.89), and the sensitivity and specificity were 0.81 and 0.75, respectively (Fig. 27.4). These results suggested that the AminoIndex for metabolic syndrome could reflect the nutritional and metabolic state as induced by the physiological changes including insulin resistance.

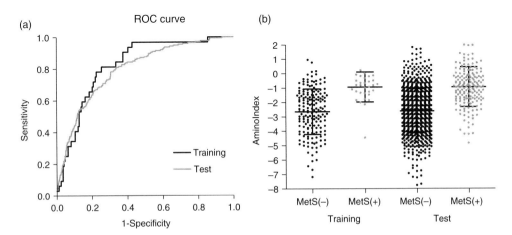

Fig. 27.4. Profiles of the AminoIndex for metabolic syndrome (MetS) discrimination. (a) Receiver operator characteristic (ROC) curves for training data (black) and test data (grey); (b) Distribution plots for MetS(−) and MetS(+) groups in training data (left) and test data (right). Bars are mean ± SD.

27.5.4 Application of AminoIndex to colorectal and breast cancer

It is well known that the metabolism of cancer cells is notably altered and that their plasma amino acid profiles are changed. There has been accumulating evidence of important effects on Arg levels in association with activities of the immune system in cancer patients. Several reports on cancer have mentioned increased production of arginase I, which catalyses the conversion of Arg to Orn and urea, and increased production of nitric oxide synthase, which catalyses the conversion of Arg to Cit and nitric oxide (NO) (Rodriguez et al., 2004; Yamaguchi et al., 2005). Plasma level of Arg would be affected by the change of arginase I activity (Vissers et al., 2005). It is also demonstrated that the central metabolism of cancer cells is changed drastically in studies measuring intracellular metabolites using capillary electrophoresis–mass spectrometry (CE–MS) (Hirayama et al., 2009). Therefore identification of metabolic changes using amino acid profiles was seen as a promising approach for detecting the presence of cancer. On the other hand, cachexia and malnutrition, typical symptoms observed in most patients with advanced cancer, also cause changes in plasma amino acid profiles. However, changes in the plasma levels of several amino acids are observed in cancer patients with little or no weight loss (Vissers et al., 2005). Therefore the changes in plasma amino acid profiles might be due not only to malnutrition, but to cancer-specific alterations of amino acid metabolism that occur even in early-stage cancer patients without cachexia and malnutrition.

Colorectal cancer is a major cause of morbidity and mortality worldwide, and is one of the most common causes of cancer deaths in Japan (Saito, 1996), while breast cancer is the most common cancer among Japanese women (Ohnuki et al., 2006). If diagnosed at an early stage, these kinds of cancer can be eliminated by surgical or endoscopic excision, without recurrence or metastases, in most patients.

AminoIndex was applied for early detection of colon and breast cancer patients (Okamoto et al., 2009). Plasma amino acid profiles were compared between cancer patients (who had colorectal cancer or breast cancer without any apparent symptoms) and control subjects for each type of cancer. The plasma concentrations of several amino acids in the colorectal cancer patients were significantly different from those observed in the controls. The concentrations of Thr, Cit, Val, Met, Ile, Leu, Tyr and Phe were reduced in the colorectal patients, while that of Glu was increased. The alteration of the plasma amino acid profile in breast cancer differed from that in colorectal cancer, with fewer changes observed. The levels of Met, Ile, Phe, and Arg decreased in the breast cancer patients, while those of Thr, Ser, Glu, α-ABA and Orn increased.

Multiple logistic regression analyses with selected variables were made using each data set. For colorectal cancer, discriminant-1 consisted of the six amino acids Val, Glu, Thr, α-ABA, Gln and Pro. For breast cancer, discriminant-2 consisted of the six amino acids Thr, Ala, α-ABA, Ile, Orn and Arg. When using training data sets, 0.860 of ROC AUC for colorectal cancer and 0.906 for breast cancer were obtained, respectively (Fig. 27.5, solid lines). To confirm the performance of the indices obtained, ROC curves from the split test data were also calculated. These reproduced the similar diagnostic performance, with AUC of 0.910 for colorectal cancer, and 0.865 for breast cancer, respectively (Fig. 27.5, broken lines). In the case of colorectal cancer, about 60% of the patients were categorized as early stage. In the case of breast cancer, most of the patients were also categorized as early stage. In both cases, the AminoIndex score in the early stages was not significantly different from those in the late stages. These results indicate that the AminoIndex is equally predictive for early and later stage patients, and may be useful for the early detection of colorectal and breast cancer.

27.6 Future Perspectives

Although the published applications of AminoIndex are still limited, the foundations for its use for diagnostic purposes are in progress as described above. Animal studies indicate that the AminoIndex concept is valid and can be used to separate physiological

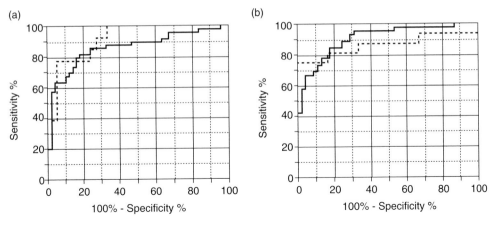

Fig. 27.5. ROC curves of discriminant-1 for colorectal cancer (a) and discriminant-2 for breast cancer (b) of training data (solid line) and test data (dotted line).

states, while studies with clinical data indicate that even with individual variability, the AminoIndex can be used to separate certain disease and physiological states. The practical aspects of the use of the AminoIndex as a diagnostic tool are also being addressed, with the development of improved analytical methods for amino acid quantification allowing higher throughput, and the standardization of sample handling conditions to minimize inter-site differences in data.

There is further scope for development in the analysis, such as the inclusion of parameters other than amino acids in the calculations.

We believe that there is potential benefit of the AminoIndex as a preliminary diagnostic screen for multiple diseases. By further accumulating data on multiple diseases and physiological conditions, it is hoped that multiple indices, each associated exclusively with a specific disease, can be generated without overlaps or crosstalk between the indices. It is also hoped that this type of analysis may be of great use in tailor-made medicine and nutrition, as it may be possible to discriminate populations for which certain pharmaceutical or nutritional interventions would be useful.

References

Armitage, P., Berry, G. and Matthews, J.N.S. (2002) *Statistical Methods in Medical Research*. 4th ed., Blackwell Science Ltd, Malden, MA.

Armstrong M.D. and Stave, U. (1973a) A study of plasma free amino acid levels. II. Normal values for children and adults. *Metabolism* 22, 561–569.

Armstrong M.D. and Stave, U. (1973b) A study of plasma free amino acid levels. IV. Characteristic individual levels of the amino acids. *Metabolism* 22, 821–825.

Armstrong, M.D. and Stave, U. (1973c) A study of plasma free amino acid levels. V. Correlations among the amino acids and between amino acids and some other blood constituents. *Metabolism* 22, 827–833.

Aspinall, R.J. and Pockros, P.J. (2004) The management of side-effects during therapy for hepatitis C. *Alimentary Pharmacology and Therapeutics* 20, 917–929.

Bedossa, P. (1994) Intraobserver and interobserver variations in liver biopsy interpretation in patients with chronic hepatitis C. The French METAVIR Cooperative Study Group. *Hepatology* 20, 15–20.

Brosnan, J.T. (2003) Interorgan amino acid transport and its regulation. *Journal of Nutrition* 133, 2068S–2072S.

Chevalier, S., Burgess, S.C., Malloy, C.R., Gougenon, R., Mailiss, E.B. and Morais, J.A. (2006) The greater contribution of gluconeogenesis to glucose production in obesity is related to increased whole-body protein catabolism. *Diabetes* 55, 675–681.

Cynober, L.A. (ed.) (2004) *Metabolic and therapeutic aspects of amino acids in clinical nutrition*, CRC Press, Boca Raton, FL.

Després, J.P. and Lemieux, I. (2006) Abdominal obesity and metabolic syndrome. *Nature*, 444, 881–887.

Deyl, Z., Hyanek, J. and Horakova, M. (1986) Profiling of amino acids in body fluids and tissues by means of liquid chromatography. *Journal of Chromatography* 379, 177–250.

Examination Committee of Criteria for Metabolic Syndrome (2005) Definition and criteria of metabolic syndrome. *Journal of the Japanese Society of Internal Medicine* 94, 794–809.

Felig, P. (1975) Amino acid metabolism in man. *Annual Reviews of Biochemistry* 44, 933–955.

Felig, P., Marliss, E. and Cahill, G.F. Jr, (1969) Plasma amino acid levels and insulin secretion in obesity. *New England Journal of Medicine* 281, 811–816.

Felig, P., Mariss, E., Ohman, J.L. and Cahill, C.F. Jr, (1970) Plasma amino acid levels in diabetic ketoacidosis. *Diabetes*, 19, 727–728.

Fischer, J.E., Funovics, J.M., Aguirre, A., James, J.H., Keane, J.M., Wesdorp, R.I., Yoshimura, N., et al. (1975) The role of plasma amino acids in hepatic encephalopathy. *Surgery*, 78, 276–290.

Fischer, J.E., Rosen, H.M., Ebeid, A.M., James, J.H., Keane, J.M. and Soeters, P.B. (1976) The effect of normalization of plasma amino acids on hepatic encephalopathy in man. *Surgery* 80, 77–91.

Forslund, A.H., Hambraeus, L., van Beurden, H., Holmback, U., El-Khoury, A.E., Hjorth, G., Olsson, R., et al. (2000) Inverse relationship between protein intake and plasma free amino acids in healthy men at physical exercise. *American Journal of Physiology Endocrinology and Metabolism* 278, E857–E867.

Fried, M.W. (2002) Side effects of therapy of hepatitis C and their management. *Hepatology* 36, S237–S244.

Garrod, A.E. (1909) *Inborn Errors of Metabolism*, Oxford University Press, London.

German, J.B., Gillies, L.A., Smilowitz, J.T., Zivkovic, A.M. and Watkins, S.M. (2007) Lipidomics and lipid profiling in metabolomics. *Current Opinion in Lipidology* 18, 66–71.

Grundy, S.M., Brewer, H.B. Jr, Cleeman, J.I., Smith, S.C. Jr and Lenfant, C. (2004) Definition of metabolic syndrome: report of the National Heart, Lung, and Blood Institute/American Heart Association conference on scientific issues related to definition. *Arteriosclerosis, Thrombosis and Vascular Biology* 21, e13–e18.

Hastie, T., Tibshirani, R. and Friedeman, J. (2001) *The Elements of Statistical Learning: Data Mining, Inference, and Prediction*. Springer-Verlag, New York.

Hegarty, J.E., Fairclough, P.D., Moriarty, K.J., Clark, M.L., Kelly, M.J. and Dawson, A.M. (1982) Comparison of plasma and intraluminal amino acid profiles in man after meals containing a protein hydrolysate and equivalent amino acid mixture. *Gut* 23, 670–674.

Hirayama, A., Kami, K., Sugimoto, M., Sugawara, M., Toki, N., Onozuka, H., Kinoshita, T., et al. (2009) Quantitative metabolome profiling of colon and stomach cancer microenvironment by capillary electrophoresis time-of-flight mass spectrometry. *Cancer Research* 69, 4918–4925.

Hjourth, U. (1989) On model selection in the computer age. *Journal of Statistical Planning Inference* 23, 101–115.

Holm, E., Sedlaczek, O. and Grips, E. (1999) Amino acid metabolism in liver disease. *Current Opinion in Clinical Nutrition and Metabolic Care* 2, 47–53.

Hong, S.Y., Yang, D.H. and Chang, S.K. (1998) The relationship between plasma homocysteine and amino acid concentrations in patients with end-stage renal disease. *Journal of Renal Nutrition* 8, 34–39.

Imbert-Bismut, F., Ratziu, V., Pieroni, L., Charlotte, F., Benharmou, Y. and Poynard, T. (2001) Biochemical markers of liver fibrosis in patients with hepatitis C virus infection: a prospective study. *Lancet* 357, 1069–1075.

Kano, T., Nagaki, M., Takahashi, T., Ohnishi, H., Saitoh, K., Kimura, K. and Muto, Y. (1991) Plasma free amino acid pattern in chronic hepatitis as a sensitive and prognostic index. *Gastroenterology Japan* 26, 344–349.

Kimura, T., Noguchi, Y., Shikata, N. and Takahashi, M. (2008) Plasma amino acid analysis for diagnosis and amino acid-based metabolic networks. *Current Opinion in Clinical Nutrition and Metabolic Care* 11, 1–5.

Lee, K., Hwang, D., Yokoyama, T., Stephanopoulos, G., Stephanopoulos, G.N. and Yarmush, M.L. (2004) Identification of optimal classification functions for biological sample and state discrimination from metabolic profiling data. *Bioinformatics* 20, 959–969.

Ljungqvist, B.G., Svanberg, U.S. and Young, V.R. (1978) Plasma amino acid response to single test meals in humans. II. Healthy young adults given synthetic amino acid mixtures. *Research in Experimental Medicine* 174, 13–28.

Martin, A.J.P. and Synge, R.L.M. (1941) A new form of chromatography employing two liquid phases. *Biochemical Journal* 35, 1358–1368.

Moundras, C., Remesy, C. and Demigne, C. (1993) Dietary protein paradox: decrease of amino acid availability induced by high-protein diets. *American Journal of Physiology* 264, G1057–G1065.

Noguchi, Y., Sakai, R. and Kimura, T. (2003) Metabolomics and its potential for assessment of adequacy and safety of amino acid intake. *Journal of Nutrition* 133, 2097S–2100S.

Noguchi, Y., Zhang, Q.W., Sugimoto, T., Furuhata, Y., Sakai, R., Mori, M., Takahashi, M., et al. (2006) Network analysis of plasma and tissue amino acids and the generation of an amino index for potential diagnostic use. *American Journal of Clinical Nutrition* 83, 513S–519S.

Noguchi, Y., Shikata, N., Furuhata, Y., Kimura, T. and Takahashi, M. (2008) Characterization of dietary protein dependent amino acid metabolism by linking free amino acids with transcriptional profiles through analysis of correlation *Physiological Genomics* 34, 315–26.

Ohnuki, K., Kurihara, S., Shoji, N., Nishio, Y., Tsuji, I. and Ohuchi, N. (2006) Cost-effectiveness analysis of screening modalities for breast cancer in Japan with special reference to women aged 40-49 years. *Cancer Science* 97, 1242–1247.

Okamoto, N., Miyagi, Y., Chiba, A., Akaike, M., Shiozawa, M., Imaizumi, A., Yamamoto, H., et al. (2009) Diagnostic modeling with differences in plasma amino acid profiles between non-cachectic colorectal/breast cancer patients and healthy individuals. *International Journal of Medicine and Medical Sciences* 1, 1–8.

Ozalp, I., Young, V.R., Nagchaudhuri, J., Tontisirin, K. and Scrimshaw, N.S. (1972) Plasma amino acid response in young men given diets devoid of single essential amino acids. *Journal of Nutrition* 102, 1147–1158.

Pain, V.M. and Garlick, P.J. (1974) Effect of streptozotocin diabetes and insulin treatment on the rate of protein synthesis in tissues of the rat in vivo. *Journal of Biological Chemistry* 249, 4510–4514.

Piomelli, D., Astarita, G. and Rapaka, R. (2007) A neuroscientist's guide to lipidomics. *Nature Reviews Neuroscience* 8, 743–754.

Poynard, T., Yuen, M.F., Ratziu, V. and Lai, C.L. (2003) Viral hepatitis C. *Lancet* 362, 2095–2100.

Rodriguez, P.C., Quiceno, D.G., Zabaleta, J., Ortiz, B., Zea, A.H., Piazuelo, M.B., Delgado, A., et al. (2004) Arginase I production in the tumor microenvironment by mature myeloid cells inhibits T-cell receptor expression and antigen-specific T-cell responses. *Cancer Research* 64, 5839–5849.

Rojkind, M. and Kershenobich, D. (1976) Hepatic fibrosis. *Progress in Liver Diseases*, 5, 294–310.

Saito, H. (1996) Screening for colorectal cancer by immunochemical fecal occult blood testing. *Japanese Journal of Cancer Research* 87, 1011–1024.

Sakai, R., Miura, M., Amao, M., Kodama, R., Toue, S., Noguchi, Y. and Kimura, T. (2004) Potential approaches to the assessment of amino acid adequacy in rats: a progress report. *Journal of Nutrition* 134, 1651S–1655S.

Shiffman, M.L. (2004) Management of patients with chronic hepatitis C virus infection and previous nonresponse. *Reviews in Gastroenterological Disorders* 4, S22–S30.

Shimbo, K., Oonuki, T., Yahashi, A., Hirayama, K. and Miyano, H. (2009) Precolumn derivatization reagents for high-speed analysis of amines and amino acids in biological fluid using liquid chromatography/electrospray ionization tandem mass spectrometry. *Rapid Communications in Mass Spectrometry* 23, 1483–1492.

Spackman, D.H., Stein, W.H. and Moore, S. (1958) Automatic recording apparatus for use in the chromatography of amino acids. *Analytical Chemistry* 30, 1190–1206.

Takahashi, M., Ando, T., Ishizaka, Y., Tani, M. and Yamakado, M. (2006) Usefulness of measurement of plasma amino acid at Ningen Dock (1): Diagnosis of metabolic syndrome. *Ningen Dock : Official Journal of the Japanese Society of Ningen Dock* 21, 589 (in Japanese).

Vendemiale, G., Grattagliano, I., Caruso M.L., Serviddio, G., Valentini, A.M., Pirelli, M. and Altomare E. (2001) Increased oxidative stress in dimethylnitrosamine-induced liver fibrosis in the rat: effect of N-acetylcysteine and interferon-alpha. *Toxicology and Applied Pharmacology* 175, 130–139.

Vissers, Y.L., Dejong, C.H., Luiking, Y.C., Fearon, K.C., Von Meyenfeldt, M.F. and Deutz, N.E. (2005) Plasma arginine concentrations are reduced in cancer patients: evidence for arginine deficiency? *American Journal of Clinical Nutrition* 81, 1142–1146.

Wagner, A. and Fell D.A. (2001) The small world inside large metabolic networks. *Proceedings of the Royal Society, London Series B-Biological Sciences* 268, 1803–1810.

Watanabe, A., Higashi, T., Sakata, T. and Nagashima, H. (1984) Serum amino acid levels in patients with hepatocellular carcinoma. *Cancer*, 54, 1875–82.

Yamaguchi, K., Saito, H., Oro, S., Tatebe, S., Ikeguchi, M. and Tsujitani, S. (2005) Expression of inducible nitric oxide synthase is significantly correlated with expression of vascular endothelial growth factor and dendritic cell infiltration in patients with advanced gastric carcinoma. *Oncology* 68, 471–478.

Zhang, Q., Takahashi, M., Noguchi, Y., Sugimoto, T., Kimura, T., Okumura, A., Ishikawa, T., *et al.* (2006) Plasma amino acid profiles applied for diagnosis of advanced liver fibrosis in patients with chronic hepatitis C infection. *Hepatology Research* 34, 170–177.

Part V

Conclusions

28 Emergence of a New Momentum

J.P.F. D'Mello*
Formerly of SAC, University of Edinburgh King's Buildings Campus, Edinburgh, UK

28.1 Abstract

It is appropriate and instructive to review the evidence presented in the preceding chapters of *Amino Acids in Human Nutrition and Health*. The purpose here is to integrate the individual sets of conclusions in a manner that emphasizes not only the underlying complexities of interdependence in amino acid metabolism and utilization, but also the relationship to diverse disorders and the potential for development of novel therapeutics. Enzyme expression and activity have been selected as the principal exponents of the impact of amino acid metabolism on nutrition and health.

An important function of the enzymes considered in this volume is the biosynthesis of the nutritionally dispensable amino acids. As a consequence of the action of these and other enzymes, glutamate, aspartate, arginine, glutamine, glycine, serine, tyrosine and cysteine need not be supplied in the diet. Nevertheless, glutamine supplementation may be beneficial in particular clinical conditions. Thus, the distinction between nutritional dispensability and clinical efficacy justifies further definition not only in relation to glutamine, but also to arginine. In other disorders, nutritional support comprising administration of branched-chain amino acids has been associated with consistent and positive responses. The position of glycine, specifically as an immunonutrient, has also been suggested. As further research is conducted on fundamental issues such as dynamics and metabolic regulation, nutritional support should emerge as a more consistent form of clinical intervention. This effort may well be enhanced by current studies designed to quantify requirements and endogenous losses of amino acids, and to assess nutritional adequacy of food proteins.

Notwithstanding the foregoing developments, a defining feature of recent research is the recognition of the critical role of several enzymes in eliciting normal, synchronized, aminoacidergic, monoaminergic and nitrergic neurotransmission in the central and peripheral nervous systems. For example, glutamatergic function is modulated by the interdependent activities of several enzymes reviewed in this volume, while nitrergic neurotransmission is determined by the competitive action of two key enzymes. The role of amino acid transporters is also of profound importance in these processes. Disruption of the major neurotransmission systems has been implicated in the pathophysiology of a diverse range of disorders. Thus, aberrations of the glutamatergic

---

* E-mail address: jpfdmello@hotmail.co.uk

system may contribute to conditions such as Alzheimer's disease, Parkinson's disease, multiple sclerosis, schizophrenia and some forms of epilepsy. Abnormalities of monoaminergic neurotransmission have been linked with cognitive impairment, psychiatric disorders and even obesity. Disruption of the nitrergic system has been implicated in multiple sclerosis and endothelial disorders. However, current research suggests that key enzymes and receptors associated with neurotransmission may emerge as potential targets for the development of novel therapeutics.

Progress in the nutritional and health sciences has been significantly enhanced by the development and application of innovative techniques, with the added benefit that even well-established syndromes, such as inborn errors of metabolism, are currently subject to reassessment. Another theme of contemporary work is the development of clinical methodologies for monitoring and risk assessment. Currently there is interest in employing homocysteine and post-translationally modified amino acid residues as indicators of cardiovascular disease and ornithine decarboxylase as a risk factor in carcinogenesis. Elevated plasma concentrations of aminotransferases may serve as markers for a variety of conditions including non-alcoholic fatty liver disease, insulin resistance, hazardous alcoholic consumption and atherosclerosis in rheumatoid arthritis.

There is thus unequivocal evidence of the emergence of a new momentum which should drive forward a comprehensive and dynamic agenda aimed at a more profound understanding of the functional metabolism and utilization of amino acids. Progress with this programme should enable the elucidation of the biochemical basis of a variety of amino acid-related disorders and the development of novel therapeutic and risk assessment strategies.

28.2 Rationale

The unprecedented scale of recent biochemical advances has provided the impetus for publication of this first edition of *Amino Acids in Human Nutrition and Health*. Even the most perfunctory inspection of the research literature will indicate a quantum shift in conceptual developments and published outcomes in virtually every discipline underpinning this title. New benchmarks have now been established across the breadth of the subject to provide new momentum for further research and clinical applications. Although occasional reviews have appeared before, it was deemed appropriate to formally acknowledge recent advances within a comprehensive volume. The recruitment of authors with exceptional merit constituted an integral part of this strategy.

The timing is opportune, as the programme embodying the concept of mammalian protein metabolism completes its full course. With a new ethos now emerging, focus has moved from nutritional questions associated with the indispensable amino acids to health and well being implications of the dispensable amino acids. However, even traditional issues, such as protein-energy malnutrition, are being investigated in the light of kinetics of specific amino acids, with reduced emphasis on whole-body protein dynamics. Against such a background, it was considered appropriate to secure reviews that would reflect a modernizing and progressive agenda in amino acid research.

28.3 Objectives and Approach

The purpose of this chapter is to review the principal findings of individual chapters in this volume and to consider the conclusions within a general interpretation of contemporary issues in human nutrition and health. Such an approach entails cross-referencing not only to chapters within this volume, but also to other relevant publications, with annotation as appropriate.

This chapter is divided into several broad categories, reflecting recent developments in enzyme characterization, molecular interactions, nutritional support, and diverse disorders associated with amino acid metabolism. Future initiatives relating to novel therapeutics are also of relevance and the chapter will end with a summary of salient points and comments on the outlook for further developments in a rapidly expanding field.

28.4 Key Enzymes and Pathways

The evidence presented in Chapters 1–10 demonstrates how profoundly classical perceptions of the characteristics and roles of enzymes in amino acid utilization have evolved over recent decades. The view that enzymes merely provide substrates for protein synthesis or mediate the disposal of excess dietary amino acids is no longer tenable. In this section, recent advances in the expression, characterization, and regulation of key enzymes are considered within the context of physiological, nutritional and clinical issues.

Amino acids of nutritional or endogenous origin are extensively metabolized in human tissues. Catabolic activity is significantly greater and more diverse than anabolic processes, owing to the inability of mammals to synthesize the carbon skeletons (or keto acids) of the nutritionally indispensable amino acids.

The major sites of amino acid metabolism are the gut, liver, muscle and brain. However, inter-organ flux of amino acids is important in determining the profile that reaches the ultimate sites of utilization and, in addition, membrane transport may influence availability of particular substrates. Amino acids cannot be retained indefinitely as free molecules and must follow anabolic routes to peptides, proteins, hormones and other bioactive compounds, or catabolic pathways to urea. In the breakdown of amino acids, the carbon skeletons are utilized in the synthesis of glucose and/or ketones. Thus, certain amino acids may serve as a source of energy.

A summary of the mammalian metabolism of amino acids, as depicted by a series of key enzyme-mediated reactions, is shown in Table 28.1. It will be apparent that diverse types of enzymes are involved in the metabolism of amino acids, including dehydrogenases, transferases, decarboxylases, synthetases and

Table 28.1. A selection of key enzymes and reactions associated with the mammalian metabolism of amino acids. The table provides a summary of enzymes and reactions that underpin several of the chapters in this volume.

Enzymes	Reactions
Glutamate dehydrogenase	Synthesis/breakdown of glutamate
Specific aminotransferases	Synthesis of a variety of amino acids, including aspartate and alanine
Glutamate decarboxylase	Synthesis of GABA
Glutamine synthetase	Synthesis of glutamine
Glutaminase	Breakdown of glutamine with synthesis of glutamate
Ornithine decarboxylase	Initiation of polyamine synthesis
Ornithine transcarbamylase	Synthesis of citrulline
Argininosuccinate synthetase	Synthesis of argininosuccinate
Argininosuccinate lyase	Arginine synthesis
Arginase	Breakdown of arginine to urea and ornithine
Nitric oxide synthase	Synthesis of nitric oxide
Histidine decarboxylase	Histamine synthesis
Serine racemase	Conversion of L- to D-serine
Phenylalanine hydroxylase	Synthesis of tyrosine
Tyrosine hydroxylase	Synthesis of DOPA
Aromatic decarboxylase	Dopamine synthesis
Tryptophan hydroxylase	Synthesis of 5-hydroxytryptophan
5-Hydroxytryptophan decarboxylase	Synthesis of 5-hydroxytryptamine (serotonin)
Tryptophan 2,3-dioxygenase	Kynurenine synthesis
Methionine adenosyltransferase	Formation of S-adenosylmethionine
S-Adenosylhomocysteine hydrolase	Homocysteine synthesis
Methionine synthase	Remethylation of homocysteine to yield methionine
Cystathionine β-synthase	Cystathionine synthesis
Cystathionine γ-lyase	Formation of cysteine

hydroxylases. A number of enzymes exist in isoforms, associated with distinctive functional properties and cellular localization. This section provides an appropriate opportunity to summarize the isozymes of importance in the biochemistry of amino acids (Table 28.2). However, it is also important to recognize the neuronal role of a number of these enzymes (Table 28.3). The clinical significance of enzymes associated with amino acid metabolism is a recurring theme in this volume. However, relevant evidence will be considered in the section pertaining to disorders.

28.4.1 Glutamate dehydrogenase

Glutamate dehydrogenase (GDH) is a pivotal enzyme in amino acid metabolism due to its involvement in both the synthesis and

Table 28.2. Isoforms of key enzymes catalysing the metabolism of amino acids. Sources of information are provided in the text of this chapter and elsewhere in this volume.

Enzyme	Isoform
Glutamate dehydrogenase (GDH)	GDH 1 (housekeeping)
	GDH 2 (nerve-specific)
Branched-chain aminotransferase (BCAT)	$BCAT_m$ (mitochondrial)
	$BCAT_c$ (cytosolic, neuronal)
Alanine aminotransferase (ALT)	ALT 1 (cytosolic)
	ALT 2 (mitochondrial)
Aspartate aminotransferase (AST)	AST_c (cytosolic)
	AST_m (mitochondrial)
Glutamic acid decarboxylase (GAD)	GAD 65 (65 kDa isoform)
	GAD 67 (67 kDa isoform)
Glutaminase (GA)	KGA (kidney isoform)
	GAC (colon, heart, pancreas, placenta)
	LGA (liver isoform)
	GAB (brain, breast cancer cells, pancreas)
Arginase	Arginase I (cytosolic)
	Arginase II (mitochondrial)
Nitric oxide synthase (NOS)	iNOS (inducible)
	cNOS (constitutive)
	eNOS (endothelial)
	nNOS (neuronal)
Tryptophan hydroxylase (TPH)	TPH 1 (in peripheral tissues and pineal body)
	TPH 2 (neuronal form)
Methionine adenosyltransferase (MAT)	MAT I and MAT III (hepatic isoforms)
	MAT II (extra-hepatic isoform)

Table 28.3. The neuronal role of enzymes involved in the metabolism of amino acids. A summary based on studies reviewed in this volume.

Enzyme	Neurobiochemical function
Glutamate dehydrogenase	Supply of neuronal glutamate
Glutamate decarboxylase	Synthesis of GABA
Glutamine synthetase	Participant in the glutamate–glutamine cycle in the CNS
Glutaminase	Participant in the glutamate–glutamine cycle in the CNS
Nitric oxide synthase	Astrocyte-derived NO implicated in multiple sclerosis
Histidine decarboxylase	Provision of neuronal histamine
Serine racemase	Yields D-serine, a modulator of glutamatergic neurotransmission
Tyrosine hydroxylase	Initiates pathway to dopamine biosynthesis
Tryptophan hydroxylase	Initiates pathway to serotonin biosynthesis

breakdown of glutamate in a reversible reaction (Chapter 1). Thus glutamate is broken down to and re-synthesized from α-ketoglutarate and ammonia by the action of mitochondrial GDH. When linked with aminotransferase reactions, GDH activity enables the synthesis of the nutritionally dispensable amino acids and the degradation of all amino acids.

Although the basic functions of GDH have long been recognized, research continues to demonstrate more diverse aspects of its characterization (Table 28.2), action and important attributes. It is sometimes assumed that GDH serves primarily to facilitate the metabolism of amino acids, whether by disposing of excess or ameliorating deficiencies through linkage with aminotransferase activity. The incidence of the novel hyperinsulinism-hyperammonaemia syndrome in hypoglycaemic children has provided the impetus for elucidating the expression (Anno et al., 2004), regulation (Herrero-Yraola et al., 2001; Fang et al., 2002) and other functional characteristics of GDH (Fujioka et al., 2001; Tanizawa et al., 2002; Choi et al., 2007; Stanley, 2009). In addition, possible interactions of GDH and glutamine synthetase in the prefrontal cortex of patients with psychiatric and neurodegenerative disorders should sustain further research (Burbaeva et al., 2003, 2005).

28.4.2 Aminotransferases (transaminases)

Aminotransferases or transaminases catalyse the transfer of an amino group from one amino acid to a keto acid to form another amino acid (Chapter 2). These enzymes require pyridoxal phosphate as cofactor to maximize catalytic efficacy. In theory, all aminotransferase reactions should be reversible. However, within mammalian tissues only a limited number of α-keto acids are readily transaminated to their respective amino acids (Table 28.4).

The initial step in the degradation of most amino acids involves a transamination reaction, which, when coupled with the action of GDH, results in the production of ammonia. The liver is the primary site for

Table 28.4. α-Keto acids readily transaminated in mammalian tissues.

α-Keto acid	Amino acid product
α-Ketoglutarate	Glutamate
Oxaloacetate	Aspartate
Pyruvate	Alanine
α-Ketoisocaproate	Leucine
α-Keto-β-methylvalerate	Isoleucine
α-Ketoisovalerate	Valine
Phenylpyruvate	Phenylalanine

coupled reactions of this type, enabling catabolism of all amino acids. The ammonia may be re-utilized or detoxified in the hepatic synthesis of urea prior to excretion via the kidneys. Skeletal muscle, however, is the major site for the transamination of the three branched-chain amino acids (BCAA), leucine, isoleucine, and valine (Harper et al., 1984). Adipose tissue may be another important site for BCAA metabolism, assuming that work with a mouse model is applicable to other mammalian systems. Herman et al. (2010) suggested that activity of catabolic enzymes in adipose tissue may be instrumental in the modulation of circulating levels of BCAA. Such a statement would imply a role for BCAA aminotransferase in this process.

The expression and metabolic significance of branched-chain aminotransferase (BCAT) in its two isoforms (Table 28.2) are reviewed in Chapter 2. The data of Sweatt et al. (2004) and Garcia-Espinosa et al. (2007) with reference to the mitochondrial isozyme ($BCAT_m$) and the cytosolic form ($BCAT_c$) in neurons (Table 28.3) are regarded as important contributions to current knowledge.

In the mammalian brain, kynurenine aminotransferase is a key enzyme in the breakdown of tryptophan, yielding the neuroactive metabolite kynurenic acid. The relationship between kynurenine aminotransferase and kynurenine 3-monooxygenase in the mammalian metabolism of tryptophan in the brain continues to attract attention (Amori et al., 2009). It is becoming increasingly clear that this pathway of tryptophan metabolism is capable of producing a number of neuroactive intermediates.

28.4.3 Glutamate decarboxylase

The conversion of glutamate into γ-aminobutyrate (GABA) typifies the physiologically-important decarboxylation reactions that lead to the synthesis of bioactive molecules such as neurotransmitters (Chapter 6). The direct reaction is catalysed by glutamic acid decarboxylase (GAD), a pyridoxal phosphate-dependent enzyme. GAD is expressed in two isoforms (Table 28.2) encoded by different genes (Korpershoek et al., 2007). GAD 65 refers to the 65 kDa form, while GAD 67 represents the 67 kDa isozyme. Based on work with the developing mouse lens, Kwakowsky et al. (2007) observed that GAD isoforms are subject to spatiotemporal expression. GAD 65 appeared in primary fibres, while GAD 67 expression predominated in the postnatal secondary fibres. More recent studies include the post-translational regulation of the functional characteristics of GAD in the brain, including protein phosphorylation and activity-dependent cleavage (Wei and Wu, 2008). Although of particular significance in neurotransmission, GAD is also expressed in the pancreas. GAD is an important auto-antigen in the development of type 1 diabetes. In non-obese diabetic mice, administration of GAD 65 isoform can prevent autoimmune degeneration of pancreatic beta-cells. The therapeutic potential of GAD in both intervention and prevention strategies for type 1 diabetic patients is currently under investigation (Ludvigsson, 2009).

28.4.4 Glutamine synthetase

The action of glutamine synthetase (GS) represents a second important mechanism of ammonia assimilation. Under the influence of GS, ammonia combines with glutamate to yield glutamine in a non-reversible reaction. Recent developments have placed GS in an enhanced perspective in terms of localization and function. Although GS is ubiquitous in mammalian tissues, its expression in the brain is predominantly within the astrocytes where it serves to modulate the glutamate–glutamine cycle (Table 28.3). This control is effected by the uptake of extracellular glutamate via specific transporters and metabolizing the amino acid to glutamine through the action of GS in the astrocytes (Lo et al., 2008).

28.4.5 Glutaminase

Glutaminase catalyses the breakdown of glutamine into glutamate and ammonia, enabling the enzyme to participate in the glutamate–glutamine cycle in the brain (Table 28.3). The synthesis of glutamate in the brain is primarily the result of the activity of glutaminase (Table 28.2), a point unequivocally underlined in Chapter 7 of this volume. The work of de la Rosa et al. (2009) and Marquez et al. (2009) have contributed to an evolving hypothesis of expression and metabolic functions. However, this synthesis of glutamate is sensitively regulated in order to avoid precipitation of excitotoxic lesions.

28.4.6 Ornithine decarboxylase

Ornithine decarboxylase (ODC) initiates the synthesis of polyamines, molecules that are essential in the regulation of cell growth and differentiation. ODC acts on ornithine to produce putrescine and CO_2. Inputs of decarboxylated 5-adenosylmethionine at two separate stages result in the synthesis of spermidine and spermine. Polyamine production appears to be an essential adjunct in all tissues that are actively synthesizing proteins. For example, polyamines act as mediators in the histological differentiation of specialized cells. Polyamine synthesis is also an important focal point for the action of antinutritional factors in legume seeds. In addition, the involvement of methionine in polyamine biosynthesis imposes competing metabolic demands, particularly when the tissue supply of cysteine may be critical.

Currently there is considerable interest in different aspects of ODC localization, regulation, and expression due to its link with carcinogenesis. Regarding intracellular localization, Schipper et al. (2004) suggested that nucleocytoplasmic shuttling might be important in the regulation and function of ODC. This process may be facilitated by its regulatory protein, antizyme 1. Regulation of ODC has been reviewed by Pegg (2006) who outlined key factors in this process at the levels of transcription, translation, and protein turnover.

28.4.7 Urea-cycle enzymes

Four enzymes participate in the urea cycle, namely ornithine transcarbamylase, argininosuccinate synthetase, argininosuccinate lyase, and arginase. The component reactions of this pathway are listed in Table 28.1. In the urea cycle the metabolism of ornithine, citrulline, argininosuccinate and arginine are linked in a pathway that allows mammals to dispose of excess N from amino acids that cannot be used for anabolic purposes. The liver is the primary site for this activity. Waste N enters the urea cycle as carbamoyl phosphate, synthesized from ammonia, carbon dioxide and ATP by the action of carbamoyl phosphate synthetase. Carbamoyl phosphate reacts with ornithine to form citrulline. However, waste N also enters the cycle directly, via aspartate which combines with citrulline to form argininosuccinate. This intermediate breaks down to arginine and fumarate. The action of arginase results in the production of urea and the regeneration of ornithine.

28.4.7.1 Arginase

The metabolic role of arginase has been given particular attention in order to reflect recent biochemical advances and clinical implications (Chapter 3). The expression of the cytosolic and mitochondrial forms (arginase I and arginase II, respectively) is a significant feature (Table 28.2). Arginase competes with nitric oxide synthase for their common substrate, arginine. Recent data suggest that arginase II is part of a system that modulates nitric oxide synthesis. Additionally, Munder (2009) claimed that arginase is a key participant in the mammalian immune system.

28.4.8 Nitric oxide synthase

Nitric oxide synthase (NOS) catalyses the synthesis of nitric oxide (NO) from arginine with the concomitant production of citrulline (Chapter 4). This reaction is facilitated by NOS isoforms expressed in specific compartments (Table 28.2). The constitutive isoform, cNOS, is always present and generates intermittent low levels of NO, whereas the inducible isozyme (iNOS) is activated by cytokines and endotoxins. Following induction, iNOS produces large and sustained quantities of NO. Barouch *et al.* (2002) referred to spatial confinement of neuronal and endothelial isoforms allowing NO signals to exert independent and even opposite effects on organ function.

There is growing evidence that NOS interacts with arginase since they share the same substrate, arginine. Thus, Topal *et al.* (2006) reported that endothelial NO synthesis depends on the activity of arginase II in the mitochondria. Subsequently, Durante *et al.* (2007) confirmed the role of arginase as a critical regulator of NO synthesis.

28.4.9 Histidine decarboxylase

Histidine decarboxylase (HDC) catalyses the synthesis of histamine from histidine with the release of carbon dioxide (Chapter 5). Histamine is credited with diverse pathophysiological functions, including the induction of allergic and other inflammatory responses, gastric acid secretion, bone loss and regulation of sleep and appetite. In addition, histamine has been attributed with transmitter and signalling functions (Haas *et al.*, 2008). A role for histamine in cognition has also been proposed (Alvarez, 2009). In other studies, neuronal histamine and its receptors have been associated with the regulation of obesity (Masaki and Yoshimatsu, 2009). Furthermore, up-regulation of HDC expression has been observed in superficial cortical nephrons during pregnancy in mice and in women (Morgan *et al.*, 2006).

28.4.10 Serine racemase

Serine, when presented as the L-isomer, is a nutritionally dispensable amino acid with unique metabolic features. It has been consistently stated that L-amino acids are utilized in mammalian systems in preference to, or in certain instances to the exclusion of, the corresponding D-isomers. In cases where the D enantiomorphs are metabolized, these must be converted to the L-isomer prior to utilization. The incorporation of L-serine during protein and peptide synthesis is totally consistent with the above principles. Uniquely, however, this doctrine is reversed for serine in its neurotransmitter/modulatory role. Relatively substantial quantities of the D-isomer occur in mammalian brain and in neuronal ganglion cells of the retina (Chapter 8). D-serine is synthesized from its L-isomer by the action of serine racemase. Aspects recently under investigation include induction of serine racemase expression (Wu et al., 2004) and feedback inhibition (Mustafa et al., 2007). Of particular interest is the neuronal expression of D-serine and serine racemase in the vertebrate retina (Dun et al., 2008).

28.4.11 Hydroxylases

Phenylalanine hydroxylase catalyses the formation of tyrosine from the indispensable amino acid, phenylalanine. A genetic deficiency of phenylalanine hydroxylase results in the well-recognized condition, phenylketonuria. Tyrosine is used in protein and in thyroxine synthesis but, critically, also contributes to the formation of 3,4-dihydroxyphenylalanine (DOPA), dopamine, noradrenaline and adrenaline. This cascade is initiated by tyrosine hydroxylase, the rate-limiting enzyme in the biosynthetic pathway. Consistent with its biochemical and physiological importance, tyrosine hydroxylase continues to be the focus of extensive research. Recent investigations include tyrosine hydroxylase gene transcription in catecholaminergic neuronal subtypes (Rusnak and Gainer, 2005); mechanisms of activation (Gelain et al., 2007); and regulation of expression in the enteric nervous system (Chevalier et al., 2008).

Tryptophan hydroxylase catalyses the rate-limiting reaction in the pathway leading to the synthesis of 5-hydroxytryptamine (serotonin) from tryptophan (Chapter 9). It is now known that tryptophan hydroxylase (TPH) exists in two forms: TPH 1, expressed in peripheral tissues and in the pineal body; and TPH 2, the neuronal isoform (Table 28.2; Winge et al., 2008). However, TPH 1 may act specifically on the development of serotonin neurons and subsequently modulate behaviour (Nakamura et al., 2006).

28.4.12 Enzymes of methionine metabolism

Key enzymes of methionine metabolism are presented in Chapter 10 and summarized in Table 28.1 of this chapter. Methionine adenosyltransferase (MAT) is expressed in three isoforms: MAT I, MAT II and MAT III (Table 28.2; Finkelstein, 2006). Other enzymes include S-adenosylhomocysteine hydrolase, methionine synthase, cystathionine β-synthase and cystathionine γ-lyase.

The mammalian metabolism of methionine proceeds along well-established routes. The principal components of these pathways include activation, transmethylation, remethylation and transsulphuration. The first three of these reactions comprises the methionine cycle, a process which serves to minimize losses of key intermediates such as S-adenosylmethionine, S-adenosylhomocysteine, homocysteine and methionine itself. The transsulphuration reaction occurs as a result of the irreversible formation of cystathionine from homocysteine, a process which leads to the synthesis of cysteine. The turnover of intermediates in the methionine cycle and, in particular, the transsulphuration of homocysteine provides the sites for metabolic regulation of methionine dynamics in different tissues and organs. In this respect, Finkelstein (2007) has considered the potential of S-adenosylmethionine and S-adenosylhomocysteine in the regulation of the methionine cycle.

Relative rates of transmethylation and transsulphuration form the basis of recent research in a variety of metabolic and physiological circumstances. For example, under normal conditions higher rates of transsulphuration occur in early gestation in humans, while higher rates of transmethylation are seen in late pregnancy (Dasarathy et al., 2010).

Rates of transmethylation in both pre-term and full-term infants were observed to be high, and transsulphuration reactions were evident even in the immediate neonatal phase (Thomas *et al.*, 2008). Polymorphisms of methionine metabolism have been implicated in meningioma formation, with the effects on transmethylation of DNA being postulated as the possible focal point (Semmler *et al.*, 2008). However, it was pointed out that methionine kinetics are not only a function of genetic factors but are also subject to dietary modulation, for example, by B-vitamin intake. In laboratory models, alterations in components of the methionine cycle may be affected by acute valproate administration (Ubeda *et al.*, 2002) or during copper accumulation (Delgado *et al.*, 2008).

Homocysteine is an independent risk factor for vascular disorders (Wagner and Koury, 2007) and other conditions such as cognitive impairment in the elderly (Kim *et al.*, 2007). The association is considered to be causal, although the pathophysiological mechanisms involved remain to be elucidated. Homocysteine status is influenced by a variety of nutritional factors, food intake, age, genetics and lifestyle (Chapter 21). A consistent relationship between plasma homocysteine levels and status of certain B vitamins is now emerging. In addition, dietary fat may be another relevant factor in determining plasma homocysteine concentrations.

Taurine is relevant here, not only by virtue of its derivation from cysteine, but also in recognition of its relationship with amino acids in human disorders. Although not a dietary essential, taurine is attributed with important physiological, modulatory and structural functions, with implications for human diseases. Thus uptake of taurine by the retinal pigment epithelium may exert consequences for the transport of small solutes between the choroid and the outer retina (Hillenkamp *et al.*, 2004). According to Hayes *et al.* (1989), taurine modulates platelet aggregation in both cats and humans. The role of taurine as a constituent of mitochondrial tRNA has been examined and new proposals have been advanced as to its function and putative relationship with the development of human mitochondrial diseases (Suzuki *et al.*, 2002). The association between plasma taurine and other amino acids in human sepsis has also been investigated (Chiarla *et al.*, 2000). The kinetics of taurine in the metabolism of healthy adult humans has been published (Rakotoambinina *et al.*, 2004).

28.5 Neurotransmitters

A number of amino acids, including glutamate, aspartate, proline, GABA, glycine, serine, β-alanine and taurine are attributed with direct neurotransmitter and/or modulatory functions; while arginine, glycine and cysteine are precursors of recognized and putative gaseous neurotransmitters including nitric oxide (NO), carbon monoxide (CO), hydrogen sulphide (H_2S) and sulphur dioxide (SO_2). In addition, tyrosine, tryptophan and histidine act as precursors of dopamine, serotonin and histamine, respectively. Several of the amino acids listed here fulfil the long-standing specific criteria required for classification as neurotransmitters. However, it is instructive to consider current evidence and, particularly, any implications for the pathophysiology of neurodegenerative and psychiatric disorders.

28.5.1 Glutamate

In nutritional classification, glutamate is identified as a dispensable amino acid, but its metabolic and neuronal roles place it in a unique category. Indeed, glutamate has been referred to as an amino acid of 'particular distinction' and detailed evidence for such a claim will be found in this volume. Of particular significance is the emergence of glutamate as the principal excitatory neurotransmitter in the mammalian central nervous system (CNS) (Chapter 25). The role of specific transporters, and ionotropic and metabotropic receptors, in the glutamatergic synapse is now well-established (Meldrum, 2000). Glutamate promotes normal synaptic transmission and long-term potentiation as well as long-term depression (Rodriguez-Moreno and Sihra, 2007). However, glutamatergic signalling in non-neuronal cells, particularly in astrocytes, is an emerging issue awaiting elucidation in terms of biochemical function and molecular mechanisms (Nedergaard et al., 2002). The conversion of glutamate into GABA typifies the physiologically-important decarboxylation reactions that result in the synthesis of key bioactive molecules. The enzyme responsible for GABA production is glutamate decarboxylase.

28.5.2 Aspartate

Although aspartate has long been associated with neurotransmitter activity, various aspects are still under investigation, particularly in relation to mechanisms of depolarization-induced release from cerebrocortical synaptosomes. The conclusions of Cavallero et al. (2009) are an appropriate representation of current views. Evidence was advanced to confirm that aspartate is released from nerve terminals by Ca-dependent exocytotic mechanisms. While the status of aspartate as an neurotransmitter is undisputed, other work emphasizes that in certain conditions, for example in the ventilatory response to hypoxia, the balance between excitatory and inhibitory amino acids may be of importance (Hehre et al., 2008).

28.5.3 Proline

The case for proline as an amino acid neurotransmitter was emphasized by Shafqat et al. (1995) who claimed that several of the classical criteria had been fulfilled for such a function. Two of these conditions included the presence of a brain-specific high-affinity L-proline transporter and the efflux of this amino acid from brain slices and synaptosomes after appropriate depolarization. Subsequently, the expression of the proline transporter in subpopulations of excitatory nerve terminals in rat forebrain indicated a role for this carrier in neurotransmission (Renick et al., 1999). The candidature of proline as a neurotransmitter was further supported by observations that L-proline (but not D-proline) induces its depressor and bradycardic activities via ionotropic excitatory amino acid receptors in the nucleus tractus solitarii of the anesthetized rat (Takemoto, 2001). In a further study, Takemoto and Semba (2006) used immunohistochemical evidence for the localization of neurons containing proline, and concluded that this amino acid may function as a neurotransmitter or neuromodulator in the brain. In the Second Proline Symposium, Phang (2008) advanced the concept of proline acting as a neurotransmitter by suppressing glutamatergic neurons.

28.5.4 γ-Aminobutyrate and glycine

It is widely acknowledged that GABA is the major inhibitory neurotransmitter in the mammalian CNS. Its *modus operandi* is primarily via the ligand-gated channel, the $GABA_A$ receptor (Wegner et al., 2008). The functioning of these receptors is determined by age, mediating excitatory effects in early development to facilitate differentiation of the brain, and inhibitory effects in more advanced stages and in adults. The physiology and function of $GABA_A$ receptors in the brain also change in subjects with epilepsy (Galanopoulou, 2008). Several anti-epileptic drugs currently in use target components of the GABAergic system, for example receptors, transport and degradation. The paper of Madsen et al. (2010) provides an insight into the potential of targeting GABA transporters in the development of anti-epileptic drugs.

The multifunctional attributes of glycine are widely recognized. It is involved in the synthesis of purines, creatine, and haem, and participates in the well-established interrelationship with serine. Glycine is also attributed with anti-inflammatory, cytoprotective and immunomodulatory properties.

Glycine is the primary inhibitory neurotransmitter in the spinal cord, brain stem and retina (Gundersen et al., 2005; Bowery and Smart, 2006). Glycine-gated chloride channels are sited in neurons of the central nervous system. Composite proposals for the extensive action of glycine have been reviewed by Gundersen et al. (2005). The localization of glycine receptors has now been accomplished with immunohistochemical techniques

(Baer et al., 2009). Furthermore, the co-release of glycine and GABA from the single synaptic terminal is an emerging issue (Katsurabayashi et al., 2004). Hernandes and Tronsone (2009) maintain that this concomitant release may be an important process to elucidate the role of glycine in forebrain neural transmission. Other studies point to the role of glycine and GABA in stimulating the release of glucagon-like peptide-1 (Gameiro et al., 2005).

28.5.5 D-Serine

Substantial quantities of D-serine occur in the brain, where it serves as an important modulator of glutamatergic neurotransmission (Chapter 8; see also Mustafa et al., 2004; Bauer et al., 2005). The case for D-serine as a neurotransmitter/modulator has been advanced by Mustafa et al. (2004) for a number of reasons:

1. synthesis of D-serine from its L-isomer occurs in astrocytic glia associated with synapses in regions of the brain that are well-endowed with NMDA receptors;
2. D-serine is more potent than glycine in the activation of certain sites at these receptors;
3. selective degradation of D-serine reduces NMDA neurotransmission;
4. glutamate initiates the release of D-serine to facilitate joint action at NMDA receptors;
5. D-serine is also implicated in neural development.

28.5.6 β-Alanine and taurine

It is widely acknowledged that β-alanine exerts a modulatory or neurotransmitter role in the mammalian CNS. β-Alanine may also act as a neurotransmitter in the visual system (Sandberg and Jacobson, 2008).

Junyent et al. (2009) attribute taurine with a number of significant properties. It is one of the most abundant free amino acids in the mammalian CNS with the capacity to reduce or prevent epileptic seizures. It is associated with neuroprotectant roles in experimental conditions, and its levels in the brain are subject to modulation by astrocytes.

Furthermore, Mori et al. (2002) proposed that β-alanine and taurine may serve as endogenous agonists at glycine receptors, and by this action may function in the maintenance of inhibitory tone in the hippocampus.

28.5.7 Gases

Important signalling gases are now known to be synthesized by both animals and humans (Li et al., 2009). Reference has already been made to NO in Chapter 4, and attention is now being directed at CO, H_2S and SO_2. The sources of these gases are, respectively, glycine (haem) and cysteine. At physiological concentrations, NO, CO and SO_2 facilitate the production of cGMP which then induces diverse reactions including vascular smooth muscle relaxation, neurotransmission and cellular metabolism. H_2S controls neurological function and also acts as a vasorelaxant (Yang et al., 2008). In addition, according to Li et al. (2009), NO, CO and H_2S impart cytoprotective and immunomodulatory functions. They further suggest that arginine, glycine, and cysteine act as both precursors and regulators of the synthesis of these gases in a cell-specific manner.

This review would be incomplete without reference to the diverse interactions involving NO, CO and sub-cellular components. There is convincing evidence that CO acts as a neurotransmitter and thus fulfils a similar function as NO (Lin et al., 2004). Furthermore, the haem-oxygenase-2 (HO2)/CO axis is thought to serve in various physiological roles including regulation of vascular tone. Lin et al. (2004) developed the concept in more detail by demonstrating interactions between CO and group II and III metabotropic glutamate receptors in central cardiovascular regulation.

Of particular relevance to this chapter is the NO–CO interaction. While the function of both neurotransmitters in the brain is well-recognized, Xue et al. (2000) concluded that they are also important in the enteric nervous system. The evidence for their claim was based first on the co-localization of their respective biosynthetic enzymes (neuronal NOS and HO2) and second on altered intestinal function of mice with genomic deletion of these enzymes. Another manifestation of the NO–CO interaction is seen in the work of Wang and Wu (2003). Their results demonstrated that NO and CO act on different amino acid residues of K_{Ca} channel proteins. It was further stated that the interactions of NO and CO determine the functional status of K_{Ca} channels in vascular smooth muscle cells.

All mammals are endowed with the capacity to produce and to salvage metabolic ammonia (NH_3). Thus NH_3 is ubiquitous, and readily takes part in key assimilation reactions catalysed by glutamate dehydrogenase, glutamine synthase and carbamoyl phosphate synthetase. Another reaction of NH_3 may be of relevance in hepatic encephalopathy, a condition with multifactorial aetiology. Jones (2002) suggested that NH_3 may act on the GABA system to enhance inhibitory neurotransmission and thus contribute to the pathogenesis of hepatic encephalopathy. Basile (2002) indicated that NH_3 is able to modulate GABAergic neurotransmission via direct and indirect mechanisms, and considered the implications for the pathogenesis of hyperammonaemic syndromes. An updated review of the role of NH_3 in the glutamate/GABA–glutamine cycle and neurotransmitter homeostasis has been published by Bak *et al.* (2006).

28.6 Molecular Interactions

Interactions comprise the very essence of amino acid metabolism with profound implications for nutrition, health, and therapeutic interventions. However, the full extent of these interrelationships is often underestimated or, in certain cases, yet to be determined. This volume contains references to several types of molecular interactions at various levels of intricacy. As stated in Chapter 13, hormonal, neuronal and nutritional factors may exert complex effects in the regulation of gene expression. Another example is illustrated by the action of mitochondrial arginase II which modulates NO synthesis in endothelial cells, with consequent implications for vascular disease (Topal *et al.*, 2006).

The interactions within the aminoacidergic and monoaminergic systems, involving intricate and coordinated activities of enzymes, neurotransmitters, transporters and receptors, exemplify a higher order of complexity. In addition, other factors may impact on such activity. For example, D-serine functions as an important modulator of glutamatergic neurotransmission. Other observations indicate that glutamate may modulate the growth rate and branching of dopaminergic axons (Schmitz *et al.*, 2009). As stated in Chapter 5, histamine interacts with other neurotransmitters including dopamine, serotonin and acetylcholine. The multifactorial nature of these interactions, although of immense scientific relevance, implies that drug development may require the targeting of multiple sites within and between aminoacidergic and monoaminergic systems. Barone (2010) concurs, advocating the development of agents that interact with several of the affected neurotransmission systems in Parkinson's disease.

28.6.1 Transport

Membrane transport of amino acids has been investigated at four principal sites: small intestine, kidney, brain and placenta. In essence, and as might be predicted, similar mechanisms operate in all mammalian systems. Typically, such mechanisms involve the interaction of transporters with the corresponding amino acids (Sengers *et al.*, 2010). The intestinal absorption and transport of amino acids (and peptides) has been exhaustively reviewed by Krehbiel and Matthews (2003). Interest in renal transport is sustained by continuing research in the inherited disorder, cystinuria, as discussed later in this chapter (Aydogdu *et al.*, 2009). Efforts are now directed towards the role of the blood–brain barrier in determining availability of amino acids to the brain for metabolism within astrocytes and neurons (Chapter 11). The practical implications of this research are now emerging. Thus, the use of large neutral amino acids (LNAA) to impede brain transport of phenylalanine has been considered for phenylketonuria (PKU) patients (Chapter 23). Competition between LNAA and tryptophan at the blood–brain barrier forms the basis for current neuropsychiatric investigations (Chapter 24). There is also increasing awareness of the potential importance of placental amino acid transport in the regulation of fetal growth (Bajoria et al., 2002), including effects in pregnancies complicated by diabetes (Jansson et al., 2002). Desforges et al. (2010) emphasized the importance of system A-mediated transport for the provision of neutral amino acids for fetal growth. An autocrine/paracrine role for leptin in regulating system A amino acid transport in the human placenta has recently been proposed (von Versen-Hoynck et al., 2009).

28.6.2 Leucine signalling

Reference to Chapter 13 will indicate the case for amino acids as signalling molecules with critical effects in the regulation of gene expression and physiological functions. It is apparent that mammals are able to modulate changes in amino acid availability by regulating expression of numerous genes.

It is worthwhile reviewing other evidence relating specifically to leucine. Studies with animal models indicate that leucine is the dominant amino acid in metabolic and nutritional antagonisms with isoleucine and valine (Chapter 19). In addition, leucine is possibly unique among the BCAA in its ability to act as a transduction molecule in the stimulation of muscle protein synthesis. This property is attributed to enhanced availability of specific eukaryotic initiation factors. It is suggested that leucine stimulates protein synthesis in skeletal muscle by enhancing both the activity and synthesis of proteins involved in mRNA translation (Anthony et al., 2001). This effect is thought to be mediated partly via the mammalian target of a rapamycin (mTOR) signalling pathway where both insulin and leucine act in concert to maximize protein synthesis. In addition, leucine may suppress protein catabolism. Leucine also regulates glucose oxidation in skeletal muscle by stimulating recycling via the glucose–alanine mechanism. Recognition of these interactions has stimulated interest in the potential use of leucine in the treatment of obesity (Layman and Walker, 2006). Studies with animal models suggest that increasing leucine intake reduces diet-induced obesity and improves glucose and cholesterol metabolism via diverse mechanisms (Zhang et al., 2007). The potential of leucine to counteract the effects of muscle-wasting manifestations of AIDS, sepsis, kidney failure and bed rest has also been considered (Drummond and Rasmussen, 2008).

28.6.3 Hormonal modulation

The anabolic effects of insulin and its relationship with leucine are well recognized, but a brief account of recent developments is appropriate here. According to Layman and Walker (2006), leucine interacts with the insulin-signalling process to enhance downstream regulation of protein synthesis. Others maintain that leucine, when consumed with glucose synergistically stimulates insulin secretion in healthy adults (Kalogeropoulou et al., 2008), while Moriyama et al. (2008) observed increased insulin and leptin secretion following amino acid infusion during off-pump coronary arterial bypass surgery. The overall efficacy of amino acids may be determined by the relative concentration of leucine (Katsanos et al., 2006; Drummond and Rasmussen, 2008). The mechanism of action of leptin may reside in its capacity to regulate amino acid transport (von Versen-Hoynck et al., 2009).

Insulin secretion may also be stimulated in patients with GDH gene defects (Anno et al., 2004; Stanley, 2009; Chapter 1). Overexpression of constitutively activated GDH induces insulin secretion by oxidizing glutamate to α-ketoglutarate, thus providing substrate for the tricarboxylic acid cycle.

Other evidence, obtained with animal models, suggests that gonadotropin and growth hormone secretion may be modulated by interactions between GABAergic and aminoacidergic pathways (Pinilla et al., 2002; Aguilar et al., 2005).

Hormonal interactions with aminoacidergic systems may operate within mutually controlled mechanisms. There is limited clinical evidence to suggest that some GABAergic neurological conditions in humans may be linked with thyroid dysfunction. Indeed,

Weins and Trudeau (2006) concluded that there is strong support for the concept of reciprocal regulation between thyroid hormone and GABA systems in vertebrates. Another view of this aspect is reflected in the observations of Leret *et al.* (2007), demonstrating the role of maternal corticosterone levels in the development and maturation of aminoacidergic systems in the rat brain.

A complex picture of amino acid–endocrine interactions is now emerging, but much more research is still required to fully elucidate the implications for human health.

28.6.4 Umami flavour

The characteristic feature of the umami flavour appears to reside in the synergy between glutamate and purinic ribonucleotides. This effect is mediated via interactions with heteromeric macromolecules of the class-C G protein-coupled receptors. The molecular mechanisms are reviewed in Chapter 20. The interaction between taste and olfactory pathways in the human brain with respect to the umami flavour has been elaborated by Rolls (2009). In addition, GABA may also act as a mediator in a taste-transduction pathway (Chapter 6).

28.6.5 Post-translational adducts

Amino acids may retain reactivity, post-translationally, to confer unique properties to proteins. Two examples are highlighted below to underline evolving implications for nutrition and health.

28.6.5.1 Advanced glycation end-products

Under particular circumstances, post-translational modification of amino acid residues of proteins may occur, resulting in the synthesis of advanced glycation end-products (AGE) (Chapter 22). The residues regularly implicated are N^ε-(carboxymethyl) lysine (CML) and N^ε-(carboxyethyl) lysine (CEL) (Hartog *et al.*, 2007). In a nutritional context, Uribarri and Tuttle (2006) indicate that there is 'compelling' evidence from experimental models and human investigations to associate excess dietary protein with the incidence of progressive kidney lesions. The effects were attributed to increased production of AGE. However, enhanced AGE synthesis has also been observed in cardiovascular disorders, diabetes and intestinal inflammation. The formation of AGE has been attributed to the accretion of reducing sugars under certain physiological conditions such as diabetes and ageing (Quintero *et al.*, 2010). The clinical and prognostic significance of recent observations are discussed later in this chapter.

28.6.5.2 Proline-rich proteins

A number of mammalian species, including humans, are endowed with the capacity to secrete salivary proteins rich in proline, as a defence mechanism against the anti-nutritional effects of dietary tannins (see Griffiths, 1991). For example, young rats fed sorghum tannins develop hypertrophy of the parotid glands, and subsequently a marked increase in the output of salivary proline-rich proteins (PRP). It is suggested that PRP may also serve to facilitate the provision of a protective milieu for the teeth by restricting bacterial adhesion to oral surfaces. The primary structures of six human salivary PRP have been elucidated by Hay *et al.* (1988) who indicated the importance of configuration on the functional properties of these proteins. The different isoforms and post-translational variants of human PRP have been further investigated by Inzitari *et al.* (2005). The abnormally high proline content of PRP confers an open type of structure with a distinctive affinity for condensed tannins. Consequently, salivary PRP are highly effective as precipitators of tannins and provide a first line of defence against such polymers (Shimada, 2006). The interaction of tannins with human salivary PRP has been investigated (Charlton *et al.*, 1996; Lu and Bennick, 1998). In particular, it has been observed that tannin interactions with full-length PRP display a higher affinity than with single proline-rich repeats (Charlton *et al.*, 1996). Furthermore, an extra-oral function of PRP has been suggested by Bennick (2007) who proposed that PRP may act as scavenger molecules preventing intestinal absorption of tannins but allowing the assimilation of other beneficial compounds such as antioxidants.

28.7 Clinical Support

28.7.1 Biochemical considerations

In common with other mammals, humans are unable to synthesize eight specific keto acids, a feature normally expressed as a dietary requirement for the corresponding amino acids. Accordingly, leucine, isoleucine, valine, phenylalanine, lysine, methionine, threonine and tryptophan are designated as nutritionally indispensable (or essential) amino acids. Dietary provision of these amino acids is therefore obligatory. On the other hand, the potential for the synthesis of other amino acids is extensive and well documented. Since α-ketoglutarate, oxaloacetate and pyruvate are ubiquitous and readily transaminated, the corresponding amino acids are considered to be nutritionally dispensable (or non-essential). However, it is important to acknowledge that although glutamate is readily synthesized in mammalian tissues and is widely distributed in foods, it exerts a critical, even unique, role in metabolic processes. Thus 'nutritional dispensability' and 'metabolic efficacy' should be recognized as distinct attributes, particularly with respect to glutamate, but also to other non-essential amino acids.

In theory, glutamine may be regarded as a nutritionally dispensable amino acid, by virtue of the action of GS. However, there is evidence that glutamine may confer benefits in particular clinical conditions, consistent with the role of a 'pharmaconutrient'. Although open to wide interpretation, this term probably encapsulates the paradoxical concept of nutritional dispensability and clinical efficacy. Normal processing within the urea cycle means that all intermediates, and arginine in particular, are nutritionally dispensable. However, Nijveldt *et al.* (2004) indicated that when degradation and/or utilization is enhanced, as for example in wound healing, trauma and sepsis, arginine assumes the role of an indispensable amino acid. The term 'conditionally indispensable' is generally used to describe the nutritional classification of arginine. Citrulline status also declines in critical illness, although levels increase spontaneously during recovery.

The transsulphuration pathway ensures that cysteine is a nutritionally dispensable amino acid as long as dietary methionine intake is adequate. However, in severe childhood undernutrition, cysteine production may be impaired due to decreased mobilization from tissue protein. This effect is exacerbated in the oedematous form of undernutrition (Jahoor *et al.*, 2006).

28.7.2 Supplements

Food constitutes the ultimate source of amino acids for all species, including humans. Systematic studies are now in progress to assess the amino acid requirements (Chapter 16) and availability in foods (Chapter 15) using modern methodology. In healthy individuals consuming a balanced diet, there is normally no need for supplements of amino acids. Indeed, there is no evidence that such supplements are more effective than high-quality food proteins in stimulating muscle protein synthesis or skeletal muscle mass (Chapter 17). Foods such as eggs, meat and milk are readily digested, inducing minimal losses of endogenous amino acids (Chapter 14). As such these foods should provide near-optimal levels of the essential and non-essential amino acids to satisfy requirements. However, there is increasing evidence (Table 28.5) that administration of particular amino acids, individually or as mixtures, may confer benefits for pre-term infants or patients with conditions such as Duchenne's dystrophy and chronic obstructive pulmonary disease (COPD). Amino acid supplements may also be of use in critical illness and in the care of the elderly.

The general strategy underlying the use of supplemental amino acids is to enhance the overall metabolic and nutritional status of vulnerable subjects. It is not intended that such measures should act as specific antidotes, but rather to contribute to well-being and management of patients.

Table 28.5. Amino acids in clinical support.

Amino acid(s)	Clinical condition	Efficacy/conclusions
Glutamine	Duchenne muscular dystrophy	Inhibition of whole-body protein degradation
	Chronic obstructive pulmonary disease	Increased plasma concentrations of citrulline and arginine
	Burn care	Favourable prospects
	Surgical patients	Attenuation of plasma interleukin-6 levels
	Infectious morbidity in critically ill surgical patients	Ineffective at dose levels used
	Major abdominal surgery for cancer	Outcome not affected
	Inflammatory bowel disease	Ineffective
Glutamate	Chronic obstructive pulmonary disease	Increased glutamate availability
Branched-chain amino acids	Chronic obstructive pulmonary disease	Enhanced whole-body protein synthesis
	Radiofrequency ablation therapy for hepatocellular carcinoma	Improved liver function
	Surgical management for hepatocellular carcinoma	Favourable prospects
	Cirrhosis and hepatocellular carcinoma	Reduced frequency of complications
	Hepatic encephalopathy; liver regeneration; hepatic cachexia	Benefits depend on type of liver disease and on the presence of inflammatory reactions
	Septic encephalopathy	Beneficial effects
Glycine	Alcoholic liver disease	Effective as a therapeutic immuno-nutrient
Arginine	Hepatic failure	Potentially harmful effects
	Transplantation	Attenuation of donor lung injury associated with haemorrhagic shock
	Post-surgical head and neck cancer	Improved local wound complications and decreased length of stay
β-alanine	Neuromuscular fatigue in elderly subjects	Improved muscle endurance
Special mixture	Sarcopenia in elderly subjects	Enhanced whole-body lean mass and insulin sensitivity

Following encouraging results with experimental models, glutamine emerged as one of the important candidate amino acids in nutritional therapy. The general rationale for the clinical use of glutamine is based on the proposal that endogenous provision may become inadequate, for example during critical illness. The insufficiency may be a consequence of declining muscle mass which is unable to maintain normal export of glutamine. The shortage may be reflected in decreased plasma concentrations of glutamine (Rutten et al., 2006a). The complexities of inter-organ fluxes of glutamine are considered in detail in Chapter 12 of this volume. It is suggested that the efficacy of glutamine administration in critical illness is due to its role as metabolic fuel and in its action in the attenuation of the inflammatory response and oxidant stress (Wischmeyer, 2007).

The effects of glutamine in children with Duchenne muscular dystrophy are reviewed in Chapter 18. However, there is currently interest in the use of glutamine and glutamate in COPD. Rutten *et al.* (2006a) observed that repeated ingestion of glutamine, but not glutamate, increased plasma concentrations of citrulline and arginine. Nevertheless, in a separate study Rutten *et al.* (2006b) concluded that glutamate supplementation might be a suitable option to increase whole-body glutamate turnover in COPD patients and in healthy elderly individuals who are likely to be dependent on dietary sources of this amino acid.

Windle (2006) reviewed the efficacy of enteral and parenteral glutamine supplementation in burn care. It was concluded that the prospects for glutamine therapy in burns are favourable. On the other hand, Gianotti *et al.* (2009) indicated that perioperative intravenous glutamine supplementation did not influence outcome in major abdominal surgery for cancer. Others question the effectiveness of enteral glutamine in reducing infectious morbidity (Schulman *et al.*, 2006) and whether the evidence supports the case for glutamine supplementation in humans (Alpers, 2006). Glutamine-enriched total parenteral nutrition conferred no biochemical or clinical advantage in patients with inflammatory bowel disease (Ockenga *et al.*, 2005), although surgical patients did benefit (Lin *et al.*, 2005). Responses to glutamine may, however, depend upon overall nutritional status of patients (Gianotti *et al.*, 2009).

The evidence for the use of BCAA supplements appears to be more consistent (Table 28.5). Thus, Engelen *et al.* (2007) concluded that BCAA supplements to soy protein enhanced whole-body protein synthesis in patients with COPD. Others observed benefits in patients under surgical management (Okabayashi *et al.*, 2008) or after radiofrequency ablation therapy (Ishikawa *et al.*, 2009) for hepatocellular carcinoma. Holecek (2010) has suggested three potential targets for BCAA use, namely hepatic encephalopathy (see also Chapter 19), liver regeneration and hepatic cachexia, although the benefits might depend upon the type of disease and on the development of inflammatory reactions. In clinical amino acid imbalance caused by liver disease and in the management of cirrhosis and hepatocellular carcinoma, BCAA supplementation may be associated with decreased frequency of complications (Charlton, 2006; Lam and Poon, 2008). Glycine may also be used for chemoprevention and treatment of hepatocellular carcinoma, according to Yamashina *et al.* (2005), who concluded that the amino acid is a potent therapeutic immunonutrient.

According to Nijveldt *et al.* (2004), the case for arginine supplementation (Table 28.5) requires careful assessment, as it is unlikely to be suitable for critically-ill patients with hepatic failure. Elevated plasma arginine concentrations occur in these patients, implying potentially harmful effects of supplementation. On the other hand, Preissler *et al.* (2009) observed that arginine attenuates donor lung injury associated with haemorrhagic shock; while De Luis *et al.* (2009) concluded that in post-surgical cancer patients, an arginine-enriched formula elicited beneficial outcomes in terms of local wound complications and duration of stay.

Recent data suggest that the elderly may also respond positively to arginine-enriched supplements of indispensable amino acids. Improvements may be seen in terms of lean body mass, strength and physical function (Borsheim *et al.*, 2008), as well as reduced plasma and liver triacylglycerols (Borsheim *et al.*, 2009). Furthermore, elderly individuals may respond positively to supplements of β-alanine (Stout *et al.*, 2008). It is suggested that enhanced tissue carnosine status improves pH regulation, thereby facilitating muscle endurance. Oral administration of an amino acid mixture enhanced whole-body lean mass and insulin sensitivity in elderly patients with sarcopenia (Solerte *et al.*, 2008). Methionine kinetics may also be altered in the elderly. Mercier *et al.* (2006) indicated that cysteine demands may increase during ageing in order to supplement host defence mechanisms against oxidative stress through the provision of glutathione.

Nutritional support is not merely a question of supplementation with amino acids. As indicated below, consumption of vegetables rich in nitrates, nitrites and antioxidants may complement the effects of arginine in ischaemic conditions. Furthermore, B-vitamin fortification may prevent incident stroke episodes and neural tube defects, presumably by reducing risks associated with elevated homocysteine levels (Chapter 21). B-vitamin deficiencies also tend to occur in PKU patients on Phe-restricted diets (Chapter 23).

28.8 Food Toxicology

28.8.1 Nitrate and nitrite

Nitrates and nitrites are widely distributed in vegetables and are also used in the production of cured meats. Epidemiological evidence of an association between high intake of cured meats and the incidence of certain forms of cancer is persuasive, but Eichholzer and Gutzwiller (2003) discounted any consistent effect of nitrates or nitrites per se. Indeed, for nitrate in vegetables, an inverse relationship was observed with the incidence of stomach cancer. Further support for the positive effects of nitrates and nitrites of plant origin is provided in Chapter 4 of this volume. The authors conclude that arginine on its own is ineffective in restoring NO bioavailability under ischaemic conditions. Provision of vegetables rich in nitrates, nitrites and antioxidants in combination with arginine may complement NO biosynthesis and homeostasis, and may thus represent a rescue or protective pathway for individuals at risk of cardiovascular disorders.

28.8.2 Plant neurotoxins

A number of neurotoxic amino acids occur in plants of economic importance (Chapter 19). β-N-oxalylamino-L-alanine (BOAA) is a common constituent of *Lathyrus sativus*, while β-cyanoalanine and α,γ-diaminobutyric acid are present in *Vicia sativa* and *Lathyrus sylvestris*, respectively. These amino acids are often referred to collectively as the neurolathyrogens. Another neurotoxic amino acid, β-N-methylamino-L-alanine (BMAA), occurs in the seed of *Cycas circinalis*.

28.8.3 Monosodium glutamate

Glutamate is arguably the most ubiquitous of all amino acids present naturally in foods (Simon and Ishiwata, 2003). In addition, the sodium form of glutamate (MSG) is routinely used in South-east Asian cuisine as a flavour-enhancing agent imparting a specific taste attribute known as 'umami' (Chapter 20). There are suggestions that dietary MSG supplementation may improve food intake in the elderly and in patients with chronic inappetence. MSG is currently regarded by the US Food and Drugs Agency as safe. Nevertheless, disquiet over its use continues, following its association with 'Chinese restaurant syndrome' (Kwok, 1968) and widespread recognition of the neuronal function of glutamate. The adverse reaction is characterized by burning sensation, headache, nausea, and chest pains. The present-day approach in the scientific community is to largely set aside safety issues and instead focus on molecular mechanisms and physiology. Thus, the 100th anniversary symposium of umami discovery published in *The American Journal of Clinical Nutrition* in 2009 included, among others, reviews on subjects such as taste receptors (Li, 2009), functional neuroimaging (Rolls, 2009), glutamate metabolism (Stanley, 2009) and the blood–brain barrier, in relation to glutamate (Hawkins, 2009). Updated versions of two of these titles appear in Chapters 11 and 20.

28.8.4 Maillard products

In the heat-processing of common foods, non-enzymatic reactions may occur between amino acid residues in proteins and the carbonyl groups of sugars (Chapter 22). The resulting Maillard products, while enhancing organoleptic properties of such foods, are also associated with deleterious effects including allergy and autoimmune diseases, and neurodegenerative and cardiovascular disorders. Two major groups of Maillard products include AGE as defined above and advanced lipoxidation end-products (ALE). The concentrations are dependent upon processing temperature as well as duration of storage at elevated temperatures. Thus AGE arises in food processing, but may also occur in body fluids and tissues with increased levels of sugars as, for example, in diabetics.

Recent investigations indicate the formation of the potential carcinogen, acrylamide, in certain plant products following cooking at relatively high temperatures as in frying, grilling and baking. Acrylamide synthesis is attributed to Maillard reactions between sugars and amino acids such as asparagine, methionine and cysteine. Highest concentrations have been found in potato crisps. In model systems, proline is highly effective in reducing acrylamide production (Koutsidis et al., 2009).

28.8.5 Lysinoalanine

The unusual amino acid, lysinoalanine, may also arise during heat processing of foods. Its occurrence is indicative of the extent of thermal damage in foods. The feeding of proteins containing lysinoalanine has been associated with reduced dietary biological values and the incidence of renal lesions in rats. However, Langhendries et al. (1992) concluded that exposure of pre-term infants to lysinoalanine and Maillard reaction products in heat-processed milk formulas did not affect kidney function.

28.9 Disorders

This volume contains numerous references to a wide range of adverse effects and specific conditions linked by complex mechanisms to the metabolism of amino acids (Tables 28.6 and 28.7). Enzyme studies have provided intriguing insights into the biochemical changes in a variety of these disorders. The hypothesis advanced here is that the metabolism of amino acids is (a) associated with, or (b) modulated by a diverse array of disorders which, in certain instances, may provide markers for risk assessment (Fig. 28.1). This model has been simplified to facilitate clarity in the presentation of the main effects, rather than the interactions of multifactorial systems. Those well-versed in disorders of amino acid metabolism will be aware of the complexities of such interactions. Thus the dopamine theory for schizophrenia, and the GABA mechanism for anxiety disorders, have not been included in Fig. 28.1. The aim here is to collate the evidence for different aspects of this model within an integrated account.

28.9.1 Clinical amino acid imbalance

The concept of clinical amino acid imbalance has been advanced to accommodate the incidence of adverse ratios of groups of amino acids in specific disease conditions of diverse aetiology (Chapter 19). In patients with septic encephalopathy or with chronic liver disease, plasma ratios of BCAA to aromatic amino acids are consistently reduced. This imbalance may be observed within 12h of the onset of septic encephalopathy. Furthermore, it has been suggested that clinical amino acid imbalance may serve as a diagnostic marker in the assessment of the severity of the septic syndrome. With regard to hepatic encephalopathy, Romero-Gomez (2005) investigated a putative role for phosphate-activated glutaminase in the pathogenesis of this condition. As stated previously, hepatic encephalopathy is a disorder of complex aetiology, with amino acid imbalance as a contributory factor (Chapter 19). Other forms of clinical amino acid imbalance have been observed in patients with chronic renal failure, Huntington's disease, and lung and breast cancer, as detailed in Chapter 19. Clinical amino acid imbalance is distinct in aetiology from the nutritional versions, as exemplified in depletion studies with humans (Chapter 24), and in contrived experiments with animal models (D'Mello, 2003). Nevertheless, nutritional interventions involving administration of BCAA-enriched supplements are beneficial in the management of septic patients or those with cirrhosis and hepatocellular carcinoma.

28.9.2 Obesity

The notion that amino acids may exert a role in the regulation of food intake and obesity is gaining support. Specifically, and not

Table 28.6. Clinical significance of enzymes involved in the metabolism of amino acids. (Disorders caused by genetic deficiencies of enzymes are presented in Table 28.7.)

Enzymes	Clinical significance
Glutamate dehydrogenase (GDH)	Linked with glutamine synthetase (see below); marker of alcohol dependence
Aminotransferases	Ornithine carbamoyltransferase to alanine aminotransferase (ALT) ratio potent indicator for hepatocellular carcinoma; obesity and elevated ALT associated with insulin resistance and cardiovascular risk in rheumatoid arthritis
Glutamate decarboxylase (GAD)	Proposed therapy with GAD 65 in diabetes; GABA and mood disorders
Glutamine synthetase (GS)	Loss of GS in human epileptogenic hippocampus proposed as possible mechanism for raised extracellular glutamate in mesial temporal epilepsy; levels of GS and GDH altered in the prefrontal cortex of patients with schizophrenia and Alzheimer's disease
Glutaminase	Co-expression of glutaminase K and L isozymes in human tumour cells; modulation of glutamine-glutamate cycle in schizophrenia; pathogenesis of hepatic encephalopathy
Ornithine decarboxylase	Over-expression in a variety of cancers
Arginase	Endothelial dysfunction; allergic asthma
Nitric oxide synthase (NOS)	Expression of inducible NOS in multiple sclerosis lesions
Histidine decarboxylase (HDC)	Histamine involved in allergy and other inflammatory responses; HDC is potential target to attenuate histamine production in certain pathological states
Tyrosine hydroxylase	Dopamine neurotransmission: implications for psychological function
Tryptophan hydroxylase	Serotonin neurotransmission: implications for psychiatric disorders
Tryptophan 2,3-dioxygenase	Key kynurenine-synthesizing enzyme: up-regulation of kynurenine pathway in patients with major psychotic disorders, including schizophrenia and bipolar disorder
Methionine adenosyltransferase	S-Adenosylmethionine synthesis and depression
S-Adenosylhomocysteine hydrolase	Homocysteine synthesis: independent risk factor for cardiovascular disease
D-Amino acid oxidase	Expression and activity increased in schizophrenia

unexpectedly, there is interest in the potential role of leucine in the treatment of obesity and the metabolic syndrome. The basis for such an expectation is the interaction of leucine with the insulin transduction pathway and regulation of glucose utilization (Layman and Walker, 2006). Studies with mice suggest that leucine reduces diet-induced obesity and improves glucose and cholesterol metabolism via multiple mechanisms (Zhang et al., 2007). In Chapter 5 of this volume, it is suggested that the histamine system in the brain might be a potential target for the treatment of eating disorders leading to obesity.

28.9.3 Neuropathologies

Derangements of aminoacidergic and/or monoaminergic neurotransmission have been implicated as predisposing or as secondary factors in the aetiology of a wide range of neurological conditions. Three major categories of CNS disorders are currently under investigation in this respect:

1. the group of neurodegenerative conditions including Alzheimer's disease, Parkinson's disease, Huntington's disease, amyotrophic lateral sclerosis, stroke and multiple sclerosis are consistently linked with glutamatergic dysfunction;

Table 28.7. Genetic disorders associated with defective enzymes of amino acid metabolism or with other aberrant mechanisms. Citation of recent references is designed to emphasize continuing research even in well-established syndromes.

Disorder	Enzyme[a] or mechanism	Clinical presentation and effects	Reference update
Hyperinsulinism/ hyperammonaemia	Glutamate dehydrogenase	Excessive insulin and ammonia synthesis	Chapter 1
Glutamine synthetase deficiency	Glutamine synthetase	Glutamine absent in physiological fluids; multi-organ failure; neonatal mortality	Haberie et al. (2006)
Carbamoyl phosphate synthetase 1 deficiency	Carbamoyl phosphate synthetase 1	Two forms: lethal-neonatal and less severe delayed-onset; brain damage; seizures	Ono et al. (2009)
Ornithine transcarbamylase deficiency	Ornithine transcarbamylase	Classical neonatal and late-onset types; acute hyperammonaemic encephalopathy; fatal outcomes	Ben-Ari et al. (2009)
Citrullinaemia	Argininosuccinate synthetase	Three clinical presentations: neonatal, infantile and late-onset; increased citrulline levels in physiological fluids; hyperammonaemic encephalopathy; mental retardation	Albayram et al. (2002)
Argininosuccinate lyase deficiency	Argininosuccinate lyase	Hyperammonaemia; accumulation of argininosuccinate; arginine depletion; systemic hypertension; seizures	Brunetti-Pierri et al. (2009)
Hyperargininaemia	Arginase	Hyperammonaemia; spastic quadriplegia; seizures; mental impairment	Hertecant et al. (2009)
Phenylketonuria	Phenylalanine hydroxylase	Vomiting; cognitive impairment	Chapter 23
Albinism	Tyrosinase	Lack of pigmentation due to reduced melanin synthesis; reduced visual acuity	Kirkwood (2009)
Tyrosinaemia			
Type 1	Fumarylacetoacetate hydrolase	Vomiting; diarrhoea; jaundice; liver failure; fatal outcomes	Croffie et al. (1999)
Type 2	Tyrosine aminotransferase	Oculocutaneous symptoms: corneal opacity, keratitis with photophobia; mental impairment	Pasternack et al. (2009)
Type 3	4-Hydroxyphenylpyruvate dioxygenase	Autism; mental impairment; neurological abnormalities	D'Eufemia et al. (2009)

Continued

Table 28.7. Continued.

Disorder	Enzyme[a] or mechanism	Clinical presentation and effects	Reference update
Alkaptonuria (defect of Tyr catabolism)	Homogentisate 1,2-dioxygenase	Dark pigmentation of urine; destruction of connective tissue; back pain; late-onset arthritis	Watts and Watts (2007)
Hypermethioninaemia	Methionine adenosyltransferase	Methionine accumulation; most affected individuals asymptomatic	Finkelstein (2006)
S-Adenosylhomocysteine hydrolase deficiency	S-Adenosylhomocysteine hydrolase	Psychomotor delay; periportal fibrosis	Finkelstein (2006)
Homocystinuria	Cystathionine β-synthase	Mental impairment	Skovby et al. (2010)
Cystinuria	Renal transport of cystine and dibasic amino acids	Urinary stones	Aydogdu et al. (2009)
Maple syrup urine disease (inborn error of branched-chain amino acid degradation)	Branched-chain α-keto acid dehydrogenase complex	Brain damage; seizures; mental impairment	Zinnanti et al. (2008); Amaral et al. (2010)
Familial hyperlysinaemia	Lysine-ketoglutarate reductase and/or saccharopine dehydrogenase	Mental impairment	Sacksteder et al. (2000)
Glutaric aciduria type 1 (inborn error of Lys and Trp degradation)	Glutaryl-coenzyme A dehydrogenase	Brain damage	Kurul et al. (2004)
Propionic acidaemia (inborn error of Met, Ileu, Thr and Val degradation)	Propionyl-CoA carboxylase	Severe neonatal-onset and late-onset presentations; vomiting, loss of appetite, heart abnormalities, stroke-like episodes; seizures, coma and possibly death	Scholl-Burgi et al. (2009)
Histidinaemia	Histidine α-deaminase	Original description: speech defects; mental impairment. Recent studies: most patients with normal intelligence	Kawai et al. (2005)
Hyperprolinaemia			
Type 1	Proline dehydrogenase	Neurological, renal and/or auditory defects; some asymptomatic individuals	Mitsubuchi et al. (2008)
Type 2	Δ-1-pyrroline-5-carboxylic acid dehydrogenase	Mental impairment; seizures	
Canavan disease (inborn error of N-acetylaspartate degradation)	Aspartoacylase	Early onset; psychomotor retardation; mental impairment	Baslow and Guilfoyle (2009)
Serine deficiency	3-Phosphoglycerate dehydrogenase	Congenital microcephaly; psychomotor retardation; seizures	de Koning (2006)
Non-ketotic hyperglycinaemia	Glycine cleavage system	Severe neonatal-onset; intractable epilepsy; convulsive seizures	Rossi et al. (2009)

[a]Defective inhibition of glutamate dehydrogenase; all other enzyme-related disorders attributed to deficiencies.

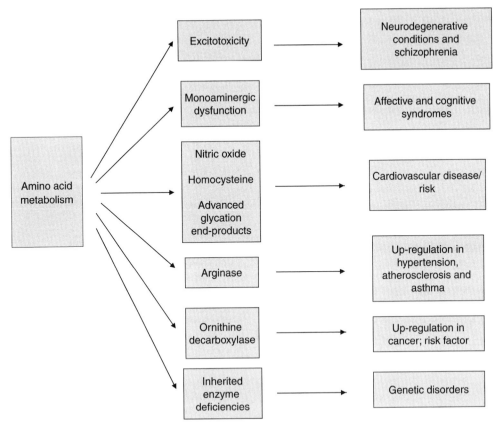

Fig. 28.1. Amino acid metabolism and disease. A provisional model to indicate that the dysfunctional metabolism of amino acids is associated with, or reflected in, a diverse array of disorders and, in certain instances, may provide markers for risk assessment. This template has been simplified to ensure clarity of presentation. Relevant details of interactions appear elsewhere in this volume.

2. among the neurochemical syndromes of relevance are affective disorders, schizophrenia and anxiety. Aggression and attention deficit/hyperactivity disorder (ADHD) are also of importance in this context; and
3. within the neurophysiological classification, epilepsy is widely regarded as a manifestation of complex aminoacidergic dysfunction.

28.9.3.1 Conditions associated with glutamate excitotoxicity

The concept of excitotoxicity is invoked almost exclusively in the context of glutamatergic dysfunction. As is well known, glutamate is the principal excitatory neurotransmitter in the CNS. The precise functioning of the glutamatergic system requires the synchronized action of the glutamine–glutamate cycle and associated enzymes (Table 28.6) and receptors. Disruption of this system has been associated with a wide range of adverse effects (Chapter 25). It is generally acknowledged that prolonged exposure to, and excess concentrations of, glutamate are toxic to neurons. According to Martel et al. (2009), during an ischaemic event, extracellular glutamate accumulates to cause excessive activation of the N-methyl D-aspartate (NMDA) subclass of glutamate receptor, which mediates Ca^{2+}-dependent cell death. The concept that glutamate excitotoxicity may prejudice health and well-being is not new. Lipton and Rosenberg (1994) proposed that glutamate and aspartate excitotoxicity represents the 'final common pathway' in the pathogenesis of neurological disorders. Glutamatergic dysfunction, mediated via excessive NMDA receptor activation, has been associated with acute neurodegenerative disorders such as stroke (Liu et al., 2007) as well as chronic forms like Parkinson's disease and Alzheimer's disease (Chapter 25). Burbaeva et al. (2005) reported perturbations in the metabolism of glutamate in the brain of patients with Alzheimer's disease, based upon data for GDH and GS. Lack of synchronization between the enzyme contributors of the glutamate–glutamine cycle may be implied. However, pathological changes in the histaminergic system have also been observed in the brain of patients with Alzheimer's disease. There is now speculation as to whether some of the cognitive symptoms of such patients might be ameliorated after treatment with histamine-related drugs (Chapter 5). In addition, neurological and psychiatric disorders may represent other manifestations of glutamate excitotoxicity (Rammes et al., 2008).

There is universal consensus now that disruption of glutamatergic neurotransmission is an underlying feature of the pathophysiology of schizophrenia (Kantrowitz and Javitt, 2010; Chapter 25), although the dopamine hypothesis is still cited in textbooks. Burbaeva et al. (2003) observed significant differences in GS and GDH levels in the prefrontal cortex of patients with schizophrenia relative to controls. It was concluded that glutamate metabolism was impaired, with the abnormal functioning of the glutamate–glutamine cycle, in the prefrontal cortex of patients with schizophrenia. A study by Maeshima et al. (2007) investigated increased plasma glutamate by antipsychotic medication and its relationship to glutaminase1 and 2 genotypes in schizophrenia. It was concluded that glutaminase genes were not risk factors for schizophrenia, although plasma glutamate status might reflect the clinical course of the condition. Gaisler-Salomon et al. (2009) confirmed the role of disturbed glutamatergic neurotransmission in the pathophysiology of schizophrenia and further suggested that modulation of glutaminase activity might provide the basis for novel therapies. Furthermore, the neurobiology of D-amino acid oxidase and its implications in schizophrenia are now emerging on the basis of genetic, biochemical, and behavioural studies (Verrall et al., 2010).

Overstimulation of glutamate receptors may also damage the myelin-producing cells of the CNS and contribute to lesions in multiple sclerosis (MS) (Pitt et al., 2000). The action of iNOS in the production of NO has been implicated in the pathogenesis of MS (Table 28.6). Liu et al. (2001) concluded that iNOS is induced in different cell types in MS lesions and that astrocyte-derived NO may influence the manifestation of inflammatory reactions, particularly at the blood–brain barrier.

Deficiency of GS in the astrocytes has been proposed as a possible molecular mechanism for elevated extracellular glutamate in seizure development in mesial temporal lobe epilepsy (Eid et al., 2004). Subsequent data with a rat model reinforced the notion that deficiency in hippocampal GS causes recurrent seizures (Eid et al., 2008). Therapeutic interventions targeting this relative deficiency of GS in the epileptogenic hippocampus are envisaged.

It follows that targeting the glutamatergic system might be part of a therapeutic strategy for conditions such as focal cerebral ischaemia (Muir and Lees, 1995), MS (Pitt et al., 2000; Sarchielli et al., 2003) and depression (Yoon et al., 2009).

Two other glutamate-related human disorders are relevant here. Both BOAA and BMAA are attributed with neurotoxic properties due to their action as potent glutamate receptor agonists (Chapter 19). BOAA is associated with neurolathyrism, a disorder characterized by muscular rigidity, paralysis of leg muscles and, in extreme cases, death. More controversially, BMAA has been implicated in Guam dementia (amyotrophic lateral sclerosis/Parkinson dementia complex).

28.9.3.2 Psychological and cognitive impairments: emerging methodology

Depletion of the amino acid precursors of monoamine neurotransmitters is emerging as a popular means of investigating psychological performance and behaviour. The technique involves the administration of amino acid mixtures devoid of the appropriate precursors.

The dopaminergic neurotransmission system has been implicated in the pathogenesis of unipolar depression and in motivated behaviour (McLean et al., 2004). Acute tyrosine and phenylalanine depletion has been employed to transiently reduce dopamine neurotransmission in both animal models and humans. Ellis et al. (2005) examined the effects of acute tyrosine depletion in healthy men, and observed that under these conditions, working memory performance was not impaired. However, stimulation of D_1/D_2 receptors during acute tyrosine depletion induced a subtle impairment in spatial working memory performance. Ellis et al. (2005) questioned the reliability of this methodology as a modulator of dopamine status and function in humans. Similarly, Lythe et al. (2005) indicated the lack of behavioural effects following acute tyrosine depletion in healthy volunteers. Thus, acute tyrosine depletion did not influence mood, while measures of memory, attention and behavioural inhibition were also unaltered. Lythe et al. (2005) were somewhat uncertain about how robust or consistent the effects of depletion were on the assessment of psychological function. The scepticism was reinforced by the paper entitled 'Acute tryptophan or tyrosine depletion test: time for reappraisal' (Badawy, 2005).

Notwithstanding these doubts, others have used the technique with interesting results. For example, Vrshek-Schallhorn et al. (2006) demonstrated that healthy individuals showed affective bias and response modulation after tyrosine depletion, in sensitivity tests to positively and negatively valenced words. Furthermore, McTavish et al. (2001) concluded that reduced tyrosine supply to the brain attenuated the pathological increases in dopamine neurotransmission after administration of the psychostimulant drug methamphetamine.

Acute tryptophan-depletion techniques have also been applied to ascertain any association between serotonin and psychiatric conditions (Chapter 24). Studies of this type have led to the conclusion that there is an inverse relationship between serotonin status and aggression in children with ADHD.

There is increasing evidence that the kynurenine pathway of tryptophan degradation may be up-regulated in patients with schizophrenia and bipolar disorder. A key enzyme in this sequence is tryptophan 2,3-dioxygenase (Miller et al., 2008; Barry et al., 2009).

Results with animal models show that histamine status affects cognitive functioning. The studies of van Ruitenbeck et al. (2009) with human subjects suggest that histidine depletion might serve as a promising technique in the assessment of histamine-based cognitive impairment. However, validation of the methodology is necessary.

28.9.4 Cardiovascular disease

Increased arginase activity is widely associated with vascular dysfunction, for example in inflammatory bowel disease (Horowitz et al., 2007) and in endothelial cell oxidative stress (Sankaralingam et al., 2010; Chapter 3). NO is a well-recognized modulator of cardiac relaxation. Hence the conclusion of Silberman et al. (2010), that uncoupled cardiac NOS mediates diastolic dysfunction, is in accordance with that concept. In infants and children with pulmonary hypertension and congenital heart disease, Hoehn et al. (2009) reported up-regulation of eNOS as well as iNOS at an early stage. It was hypothesized that such an enhancement may be a compensatory reaction to restrict the rise in pulmonary artery pressure. There is general consensus that formation of AGE is associated with the development and progression of chronic heart failure, typified by the comments of Hartog et al. (2007). Accumulation of AGE is enhanced in the cerebral vessels of diabetic patients (van Deutekom et al., 2008).

28.9.5 Diabetes

It is worth summarizing, on the basis of limited evidence, that diabetes may directly or indirectly impact on transport, metabolism and post-translational reactivity of amino acids. For example, alterations in placental activity of amino acid transporters may contribute to enhanced fetal growth rates in pregnancies complicated by diabetes, according to Jansson et al. (2002). Romero et al. (2008) indicated that diabetes-induced coronary vascular dysfunction involves enhanced arginase activity (see also Chapter 3). Experimental data imply that BCAA catabolism may be down-regulated in type 2 diabetes (Kuzuya et al., 2008). Furthermore, in type 2 diabetics with nephropathy, homocysteine metabolism is impaired, reflecting changes in the dynamics of the methionine cycle and transsulphuration reactions (Tessari et al., 2005). In addition, long-term metformin administration to patients with type 2 diabetes increases risk of vitamin B_{12} deficiency, which results in elevated homocysteine concentrations. Other studies point to the accumulation of lysine adducts (as AGE) in greater concentrations in diabetic patients. Increased levels were recorded for these subjects with renal dysfunction (Lieuw-A-Fa et al. 2004) and in the cerebral blood vessels of diabetics compared with control values (van Deutekom et al., 2008).

28.9.6 Cancer

The association between cancer and expression of amino acid-metabolizing enzymes is the subject of considerable research. In human tumour cells, Perez-Gomez et al. (2005) identified two glutaminase isoforms, namely K (kidney-type) and L (liver-type). Since glutamine is an important source of energy in neoplastic tissues, recent studies have focused on the expression and roles of glutaminases in this process (Szeliga and Obara-Michlewska, 2009).

Arginase expression and activity are enhanced in breast, colon, and prostate cancers (Chapter 3). In human prostate cancer, co-expression of both arginase II and NOS occurs in tumour cells. In lung cancer, arginase II expression neither induces immune suppression nor influences progression of the disease (Rotondo et al., 2008). The lack of effect may be attributed to the absence of NOS expression in that study.

More consistent evidence is available for ODC activity which is elevated in a variety of malignant states. Brabender et al. (2001) reported an up-regulation of ODC mRNA expression in Barrett's-associated adenocarcinoma of the oesophagus. It was suggested that high ODC mRNA expression is an early event in the initiation and progression of this condition and may be a clinically useful marker for incipient adenocarcinoma. ODC is also overexpressed in both benign prostatic hyperplasia and in neoplastic tissues, and again, Young et al. (2006) indicated that enhanced activation of the enzyme appears to be an early indicator for prostate carcinogenesis. It had previously been demonstrated that ODC was induced by androgens in human prostatic epithelial cells (Visvanathan et al., 2004). Elevated activity of ODC has been linked with other forms of cancer. Thus, Zell et al. (2009) and Brown et al. (2009) published observations on polymorphism in the ODC gene and the risk of colorectal and breast cancer, respectively. In the latter paper, increased ODC activity in breast cancer tissue, compared with benign and normal tissues, was emphasized. Work with laboratory models reinforces the above observations and conclusions. Thus susceptibility to tumour development is enhanced in transgenic mice expressing elevated levels of ODC, and diminished in those with reduced levels of this enzyme (Pegg, 2006; Young et al., 2006). Expression of non-mast cell HDC in tumour-associated microvessels might exert a regulatory role in human oesophageal squamous cell carcinoma (Li et al., 2008). The presence of HDC in neuroendocrine tumours has also been revealed using immunohistochemical and gene expression techniques (Uccella et al., 2006).

The relationship between abnormal methionine metabolism and hepatocellular cancer has been considered in Chapter 10 of this volume. S-Adenosylmethionine appears to be a key intermediate in this respect. The question now being addressed is the mechanism by which a defect or excess of hepatic S-adenosylmethionine might initiate cancer.

28.9.7 Genetic defects

Examination of Table 28.7 will confirm the wide range of genetic conditions associated with the metabolism and transport of amino acids. The disorders listed relate to virtually all the important amino acids in human metabolism. Thus, the biochemical fate of glutamate, glutamine, urea cycle intermediates, phenylalanine, tyrosine, sulphur amino acids, branched-chain amino acids, lysine, tryptophan, threonine, histidine, proline, glycine and serine may be influenced by deleterious enzyme mutations. In addition, an inherited transport disorder may affect renal function with respect to cystine and dibasic amino acids. A number of these syndromes, for example, PKU (Chapter 23), albinism, alkaptonuria and maple syrup urine disease are long-established and well-characterized. However, as shown in Table 28.7, research continues on virtually all genetic disorders, as efforts are directed at the application of modern techniques to investigate gene mutations or provide non-invasive clinical assessments of affected patients. The prospects of new products and treatment modalities, including gene therapy, provide additional impetus for ongoing investigations. The incidence of these enzyme and transport deficiencies is generally quite low, only 8 per 100,000 births for PKU, 3 per 100,000 births for albinism, and significantly lower for the remaining disorders listed in Table 28.7.

A summary of the salient features may be discerned in the light of recent advances (Table 28.7). Although the disorders relate almost exclusively to enzymes of amino acid catabolism, at least one condition, namely serine deficiency disorder, is caused by a biosynthetic enzyme. The hyperinsulinism/hyperammonaemia syndrome has been attributed to mutations that cause a loss of inhibition of GDH (Chapter 1). Anno *et al.* (2004) attributed hyperinsulinism to over-expression of constitutively activated GDH. Although considerable emphasis has been placed on neonatal screening, and justifiably so, it is salutary to note the recurring theme of late-onset presentation of disorders. Prolonged survival may be observed in the latter group, but this is not a consistent feature for all conditions. In the interests of clarity, less emphasis has been placed on metabolic changes concerning the accumulation of intermediates in tissues and physiological fluids as a result of genetic enzyme deficiencies. These observations are well documented in basic biochemistry texts. Thus, it is widely appreciated that argininosuccinate lyase deficiency is accompanied by accumulation of argininosuccinate. Similarly, in PKU, abnormally high concentrations of phenylalanine in plasma are commonly observed in affected individuals (Chapter 23). A considerable number of the congenital disorders listed in Table 28.7 are associated with a common underlying theme of brain damage, seizures and mental impairment. In many instances, gross observations are accompanied by data obtained at sub-cellular and molecular levels. As might be anticipated, hyperammonaemia occurs commonly in deficiencies of urea cycle enzymes.

Again, as might be predicted, the arginine–NO pathway has been attributed with a role in the pathophysiology of congenital urea cycle disorders, although the precise molecular mechanisms await elucidation (Brunetti-Pierri *et al.*, 2009; Nagasaka *et al.*, 2009). In addition, however, increased NO synthesis by neutrophils of a patient with tyrosinaemia type 3 has been reported (D'Eufemia *et al.*, 2009).

28.9.8 Risk factors

Recent developments highlighted in this volume indicate the potential for identifying risk factors associated with certain disorders. Elevated plasma concentrations of aminotransferases have been suggested as markers for a variety of conditions (Chapter 2; Table 28.6) including non-alcoholic fatty liver disease (Lu *et al.*, 2009), insulin resistance (Burgert *et al.*, 2006; Chen *et al.*, 2009) and hazardous alcoholic consumption (Chaudhry *et al.*, 2009). Another study indicated that serum aminotransferases are associated with insulin resistance and atherosclerosis in rheumatoid arthritis (Dessein *et al.*, 2007). Genetic factors, however, may contribute to the variation in circulating aminotransferase concentrations (Makkonen et al., 2009).

As indicated earlier in this chapter, it has been observed that high ODC mRNA expression is an early event in the initiation and progression of diverse forms of cancer. It is, therefore, logical to consider ODC up-regulation as a clinically useful risk factor in carcinogenesis (Young et al., 2006).

As stated previously, homocysteine is an independent risk factor for vascular disease and other conditions such as cognitive impairment in the elderly. The association is considered to be causal, although the pathophysiological mechanisms involved remain to be elucidated (Chapter 21).

Post-translational modification of proteins may be associated with the synthesis of advanced glycation end products (AGE) (Chapter 22). The most comprehensive set of investigations implicate AGE in vascular disease. Baidoshvili et al. (2006) indicate that CML accretion in intramyocardial blood vessels in patients with acute myocardial infarction might reflect increased risk rather than a consequence of this disorder. Hartog et al. (2007) suggested that AGE synthesis is a factor in the pathogenesis of chronic heart failure and may also reflect severity of the condition. Increased depositions of CML have also been observed in the cerebral blood vessels of diabetic patients compared with age-matched controls (van Deutekom et al., 2008). Furthermore, elevated AGE accretion has been reported in diabetic subjects with renal dysfunction (Lieuw-A-Fa, et al., 2004). In addition, the AGE burden may correlate with clinical outcomes in acute lung injury (Calfee, 2008) and there are also implications for dental implant osseointegration and stability (Quintero et al., 2010).

28.9.9 Therapeutics

As stated in Chapter 26, L-DOPA has now become the classical example of brain neurotransmitter therapy and current efforts are being directed at a more effective treatment modality for Parkinson's disease. There is much anticipation about future developments in prophylactic measures for other neurodegenerative disorders (Chapter 25). However, much work at the fundamental level remains to be accomplished.

A significant factor driving amino acid research is the quest to identify appropriate targets for therapeutic intervention. In addition to the potential use of amino acid supplements in clinical support (Table 28.5), alternative strategies are now under active consideration. The following account indicates the nature of recent work in this area and is not designed to be fully comprehensive, but as illustrative of the diversity of approaches now being considered. Furthermore, the importance of interactions should be recognized in the development of novel therapeutic agents. Thus, although aberrations in glutamatergic neurotransmission have been implicated in the aetiology of Parkinson's disease (Rodriguez-Moreno and Sihra, 2007; Chapter 25), the characteristic motor symptoms have been attributed to degeneration of dopaminergic neurons. Barone (2010) implies that agents designed to interact with several of the affected neurotransmission systems would enhance therapeutic efficacy in this disease. Nevertheless, the challenge in developing appropriate pharmaceuticals, particularly for CNS disorders, is formidable. Thus the choice of agonists as opposed to antagonists of glutamatergic neurotransmission reflects the ongoing dilemma (Chapter 25). On the other hand, tetrahydrobiopterin (BH_4) therapy may enhance outcomes in patients with PKU (Chapter 23) or with vascular conditions (Silberman, 2010). In addition, the role of BH_4 as a cofactor for tyrosine hydroxylase (Chapter 26) raises further issues regarding therapeutic potential.

28.9.10 Dietary modulation

In Chapter 1 of this volume, the case is presented for the development of alternative strategies for the treatment of GDH-mediated insulin disorders. The prevailing consensus is that the epigallocatechin gallate component of green tea might offer some therapeutic value by virtue of its specific inhibition of GDH. The authors further imply that anti-cancer treatment which combines GDH inhibitors with those that suppress glucose utilization might be effective against tumours (Chapter 1). Since elevated ODC, polyamine, and NO levels are commonly associated with tumour initiation and development, there has been some speculation as to dietary strategies to control risk. For example, Zell et al. (2007) suggested important roles for arginine and meat consumption in the control of colorectal tumours.

Recent observations suggest that arginine on its own is ineffective in restoring NO bioavailability under ischaemic conditions. Consumption of vegetables rich in nitrates, nitrites and antioxidants in combination with arginine may serve as a rescue or protective mechanism for individuals at risk to cardiovascular disorders (Chapter 4).

Dietary folate appears to be effective in reducing homocysteine concentrations in adolescents and adults. However, in clinical trials folate, vitamin B_6 and vitamin B_{12} supplementation failed to reduce the risk of recurrent coronary heart disease, stroke and venous thromboembolism. Although folic acid supplementation has been associated with reduced incidence of neural tube defects, other maternal factors should be considered in efforts to further minimize congenital risks (Chapter 21).

Gaenslen et al. (2008) point to some positive effects of nutrition on the development of Parkinson's disease, suggesting that dietary polyunsaturated fatty acids may decrease glutamate release and activate NMDA binding sites as part of the mechanism.

Reduced serotonin synthesis has been linked, in part at least, with the onset of depression (Porter et al., 2007). As a consequence of these responses, there is now interest in the use of tryptophan-rich proteins to enhance serotonin status by nutritional means (Markus et al., 2008).

28.9.11 Non-protein amino acids in cancer prevention

The potential for specific non-protein amino acids in cancer therapy (Chapter 19; D'Mello, 1991) is worth reiterating here. For example, ester derivatives of canavanine appear to be markedly more effective than the parent amino acid in suppressing the growth of cultured pancreatic carcinoma cells. The development of specific analogue inhibitors is gaining momentum (Wu et al., 2007; Bailey et al., 2010). In the latter study, for example, difluoromethylornithine was examined in skin cancer prevention in subjects with a previous history of this form of malignancy. Preclinical studies demonstrated that inhibition of ODC by this analogue decreased tissue concentrations of polyamines and prevented neoplastic growth in many tissue types. It was suggested that difluoromethylornithine therapy might form part of a preventative strategy in subjects with a previous history of skin cancer.

Se-Methylselenocysteine is most effective against mammary tumours and is also highly effective in potentiating the efficiency of anti-cancer drugs and in protecting against drug-induced toxicity. Indeed, it has been suggested that the increased therapeutic efficacy of certain anti-cancer drugs may be dependent upon the dose of the amino acid. Se-Allylselenocysteine is more effective than a number of other selenoamino acids for chemoprevention of mammary cancer in a rat methylnitrosourea model. Limited work points to the potential therapeutic use of selenomethionine, but a cautious approach is recommended to minimize cytotoxic effects. The efficacy of S-methylcysteine sulphoxide and its metabolite, methyl methane thiosulphinate, on mouse genotoxicity suggests that these two organosulphur compounds may contribute to the anti-carcinogenic properties of brassica vegetables. However, epidemiological evidence only supports the case for prevention of gastric and lung cancers through consumption of these vegetables. Finally, interest in mimosine as a potential anti-cancer agent is typified by its action in blocking cell-cycle progression, inhibiting DNA replication and inducing apoptosis.

28.9.12 Molecular targets

28.9.12.1 Enzymes

Much emphasis has been placed on the potential for the development of novel therapeutics by targeting enzymes associated with specific disorders. The following is a summary of selected examples of recent research based on evidence surveyed and referenced earlier in this chapter. Modulation of GAD in both intervention and prevention strategies for type 1 diabetes has been suggested. Deficiency of GS in the epileptogenic hippocampus may represent a new focus for treatment of seizures. Disturbed glutamatergic neurotransmission in schizophrenia may be responsive to modulation of glutaminase activity. Preclinical investigations suggest that inhibition of ODC by specific analogues may prevent neoplastic growth in diverse tissue types. Similarly, it has been suggested that tyrosine kinase blockers may provide the basis for new approaches in cancer therapy (Pytel *et al.*, 2009). Arginase inhibition may represent a mechanism for the treatment of acute and chronic asthma (Maarsingh *et al.*, 2009). As might be predicted, HDC is a potential target to attenuate histamine release in a number of pathological conditions (Table 28.6). To this end, Wu *et al.* (2008) examined inhibitory and structural properties of coenzyme–substrate analogues relative to the activity of human HDC. Employing computer-based modelling, Moya-Garcia *et al.* (2009) attempted to elucidate structural features of HDC that might provide the basis for specific inhibition. This approach represented an extension of the 'structure to function' theme proposed in an earlier paper (Moya-Garcia *et al.*, 2005).

28.9.12.2 Aminoacidergic and monoaminergic receptors

Another strategy under active investigation relates to modulation of aminoacidergic and monoaminergic receptors for therapeutic purposes. The evidence presented in Table 28.8 indicates that a wide range of receptors is currently being targeted for drug development. In summary, research has focused on receptors of the following classes and subtypes:

1. α-amino-3-hydroxy-5-methyl-4-isoxazolepropionic acid (AMPA);
2. $GABA_A$ and $GABA_C$;
3. glycine;
4. histamine H1 and H3;
5. dopamine D2 and D3;
6. serotonin; and
7. serotonin/glutamate complex.

Modulation of the NMDA and metabotropic subclasses of glutamate receptors may

Table 28.8. Aminoacidergic and monoaminergic receptors as potential targets in the development of molecular therapeutics.

Receptor	Disorder/condition	Reference
NMDA	Schizophrenia	Yang and Svensson (2008)
	Alzheimer's disease	Kotermanski and Johnson (2009)
Metabotropic (glutamate)	Schizophrenia	Conn *et al.* (2009)
Ca-permeable AMPA	L-DOPA-induced dyskinesia in Parkinson's disease	Kobylecki *et al.* (2010)
$GABA_A$	Neurons in Parkinsonian state	Xue *et al.* (2010)
$GABA_A$	Huntington's disease	Twelvetrees *et al.* (2010)
$GABA_C$	Fear and anxiety	Cunha *et al.* (2010)
Glycine	Inflammatory pain; spasticity; epilepsy	Gilbert *et al.* (2009)
Glycine	Human startle disease	Davies *et al.* (2010)
Histamine H3	Cognitive	Esbenshade *et al.* (2008)
Histamine H3	Psychosis	Ito (2009)
Histamine H1 and H3	Atypical antipsychotic weight gain	Deng *et al.* (2010)
Dopamine D2	Management of neuroendocrine tumours	Ribeiro-Oliveira *et al.* (2008)
Dopamine D3	Drug addiction	Heidbreder (2008)
Serotonin	Irritable bowel syndrome	Fayyaz and Lackner (2008)
Serotonin/glutamate complex	Psychosis	Gonzalez-Maeso *et al.* (2008)

constitute a potential mechanism for the treatment of schizophrenia and related disorders. In addition, NMDA receptor selectivity to the Alzheimer's drug memantine may be an useful model for future research. Targeting AMPA receptors might be of therapeutic value in L-DOPA-induced dyskinesia in Parkinson's disease. GABA receptors are considered as possible targets for the treatment of a variety of disorders including Parkinson's disease and Huntington's disease, as well as fear and anxiety. The glycine receptor mediates inhibitory neurotransmission and is currently emerging as a potential drug target for inflammatory pain, spasticity and epilepsy. Other defects of the glycinergic system, implicated in human startle disease, have been linked to mutations in the post-synaptic glycine receptor. The latter is a potential target for therapeutic purposes. Receptors of the histaminergic system have been proposed as potential focal points for the treatment of cognitive disorders, psychosis and atypical antipsychotic-induced weight gain. The potential role of dopamine receptors as targets in the management of neuroendocrine tumours and for drug addiction pharmacology has been suggested. In other studies, serotonin receptor modulators are being considered as prospective drugs for the treatment of irritable bowel syndrome. Of particular interest is the association of a serotonin/glutamate receptor complex with psychosis. Further studies should reveal any potential for modulating this axis by specific inhibitors.

28.9.12.3 Transporters

It is conceivable that further advances in molecular pharmacology may well emerge as a result of contemporary investigations with CNS transporters (Chapter 11). The expression of brain-specific high-affinity L-proline transporter in subpopulations of putative glutamatergic neurons implies a role in excitatory activity and a possible focus for modulation in drug development (Renick *et al.*, 1999). The work of Chen *et al.* (2003) suggesting that glycine transporter-1 blockade potentiates NMDA-mediated responses in rat prefrontal cortical neurons both *in vitro* and *in vivo* is another example of innovative approaches now being pursued. On a more definitive note, Madsen *et al.* (2010) proposed that neuronal and non-neuronal GABA transporters may serve as putative targets for anti-epileptic drugs.

28.10 Innovation

There is universal consensus that recent advances reviewed in this volume have largely been the result of developments in molecular and non-invasive techniques. The refinement and exploitation of these methodologies should contribute to further progress in the future. One example is the use of amino acid profiles in clinical diagnosis (Chapter 27). Further studies may well include measures of monoaminergic function. However, other forms of innovation are now under scrutiny.

28.10.1 Modelling

Modelling is perceived as an essential technique in a wide range of biological disciplines, including nutrition and health sciences. In general, there is widespread belief that more rapid progress might be achieved by the adoption of modelling techniques. It is suggested that only simulation processes can provide the capacity to embody complex biochemical pathways within dynamic and flexible models. In support of computational modelling, Sengers *et al.* (2010) point out that placental amino acid flux involves the interaction of 15 or more transporters for 20 amino acids. It is also claimed that the elaborate requirements of drug development demand the use of modelling methodologies (Moya-Garcia *et al.*, 2009). Nevertheless, even in such cases, validation through determination of clinical efficacy would still be necessary. Furthermore, it is argued that the identification of future research priorities is best accomplished through logic generated within simulation protocols. However, it is patently clear that virtually all the advances recorded in this volume have been the result of deliberate and arduous empirical research. On balance, it has to be conceded that a combination of approaches may be necessary in the future; in other words, the two procedures are not mutually exclusive. Indeed, the promulgation of contrived schismatic positions may well prove to be a retrogressive step in the long term.

28.11 Summary

Notable developments have recently emerged to enhance our understanding of the functional role of amino acids in human nutrition and health. The advances have unquestionably been the result of expansionary approaches adopted in diverse research programmes at a global level. The advent and innovative application of sophisticated techniques have contributed markedly to progress in virtually every aspect of this endeavour. Substantive features, ordered in a series of thematic statements with appropriate cross-referencing, are presented below.

28.11.1 Underlying theme

- Specific enzymes have been selected for review in this volume to exemplify the impact of amino acid metabolism on nutrition and health issues, including disorders, identification of risk factors and targets for development of molecular therapeutics.

28.11.2 Metabolism

- Major developments have been published on the expression, molecular characterization and regulation of key enzymes of amino acid metabolism (Chapters 1–10; Table 28.1). The localization and functional properties of isoforms of a number of these enzymes are a particular feature of recent research (Table 28.2).
- The enzymes associated with amino acid metabolism enable the synthesis of a diverse range of physiologically-important intermediates and end-products. In addition, a number of these enzymes ensure the disposal of amino acids present in excess of immediate requirements.
- A neuronal role for enzymes has now been extended to include glutamate dehydrogenase, glutamine synthetase, glutaminase, nitric oxide synthase, histidine decarboxylase, serine racemase, tyrosine hydroxylase and tryptophan hydroxylase. As such these enzymes exert a constitutive or supportive role in aminoacidergic, monoaminergic or nitrergic neurotransmission systems.
- A much more diverse range of amino acids is now attributed with neurotransmitter functions compared to a few years ago.
- The emergence of gaseous neurotransmitters and their mutual interactions is another key development indicating the need to recognize the complexity of signalling mechanisms.
- Thus, the classical view that amino acids serve merely as structural components and that associated enzymes are largely for re-distribution or disposal of surpluses has been substantially revised. For example, glutamate dehydrogenase exerts a pivotal role in insulin homeostasis and neurotransmission, in addition to ureagenesis (Chapter 1).

28.11.3 Nutrition

- A major feature of the enzymes considered in this volume is the biosynthesis of the nutritionally dispensable amino acids. As a consequence, glutamate, glutamine, aspartate, arginine, glycine, serine, tyrosine and cysteine need not be supplied in the diet, providing precursor levels are adequate. Nevertheless, glutamate, glutamine and arginine have been considered as potential supplements in particular clinical conditions.
- The distinction between nutritional dispensability and clinical efficacy of amino acids may thus need further amplification in the evaluation of interventions for vulnerable individuals.

The consensus now emerging is that the nutritional classification of glutamate, glutamine and arginine as dispensable grossly underestimates the key metabolic and clinical significance of these amino acids.
- Existing protocols derived from animal models have been applied to determinations of digestibility, availability and requirements of key indispensable amino acids (Chapters 14–16).
- The potential for nutritional interventions with amino acids (Table 28.5) will only be fully realized following further advances in fundamental issues such as transport (Chapter 11), inter-organ fluxes (Chapter 12), metabolic regulation and availability (Chapters 13, 14 and 15), and clinical imbalance and safety (Chapters 19 and 20). This effort should be enhanced by employing measurements of oxidation to quantify amino acid requirements and to assess nutritional adequacy of food proteins.
- Nevertheless, the attributes of glutamine and branched-chain amino acids in nutritional support are now emerging (Table 28.5). In addition, there may be potential in the administration of tryptophan-rich proteins and hydrolysates for the treatment of affective disorders.
- There are indications that dietary monosodium glutamate supplementation may improve food intake in the elderly and in patients with chronic inappetence.
- The dietary inclusion of vegetables rich in nitrate, nitrite and antioxidants combined with arginine may represent an optimal balance of substrates to restore and maintain nitric oxide bioavailability under conditions of ischaemia or oxidative stress (Chapter 4).
- B-vitamin fortification may reduce risks associated with elevated homocysteine levels (Chapter 21). B-vitamin deficiencies also tend to occur in PKU patients on Phe-restricted diets (Chapter 23).
- The oral administration of amino acid mixtures devoid of tryptophan (Chapter 24) or histidine or phenylalanine plus tyrosine, in order to deplete brain concentrations of the respective neurotransmitters, is emerging as a worthwhile technique in psychopharmacology.

28.11.4 Food safety

- The toxicity and safety of non-protein amino acids in food have been reviewed together with their physiological and molecular interactions (Chapters 19–20).
- There is some disquiet over the use of nitrates and nitrites in the production of cured meats. However, recent research indicates that consumption of vegetables rich in nitrates, nitrites and antioxidants may confer benefits that outweigh any perceived cancer risks (Chapter 4).
- Monosodium glutamate is currently regarded by the US Food and Drugs Agency as safe. The protective functions of the blood–brain barrier have been emphasized (Chapter 11).
- The occurrence of Maillard reaction products (Chapter 22) in processed foods is associated with adverse health effects and reductions in nutritional value.

28.11.5 Health and disease

- The structural functions of amino acids underline the requirements of these nutrients for optimal health and well-being. However, it is the neurotransmission roles in normal and, by imputation, in diseased states (Chapters 5, 7, 24, and 25) that encapsulate the modern perspective of amino acids in human health.
- Amino acid metabolism has been implicated in, or is affected by a diverse range of disorders (Fig. 28.1). In addition, metabolic dysfunction may provide markers for several clinical conditions.
- Consistent evidence is available to demonstrate that ornithine decarboxylase (ODC) activity is elevated in a variety of malignant conditions including Barrett's oesophagus and Barrett's-associated adenocarcinoma, prostate cancer, colorectal cancer and breast cancer.

- Up-regulation of the kynurenine pathway of tryptophan degradation has been observed in patients with major psychotic disorders, including schizophrenia and bipolar disorder (Table 28.6).
- Neuropsychiatric conditions and behaviour are influenced by serotonin neurotransmission as elucidated in tryptophan-depletion tests (Chapter 24).
- Dopaminergic factors appear to be involved in the pathogenesis of unipolar depression and in motivated behaviour.
- Disruption of glutamatergic function and ensuing excitotoxicity have been implicated in the pathophysiology of psychiatric and neurodegenerative disorders (Chapters 7 and 25). Detailed consideration has been given to current evidence for depression, schizophrenia, Alzheimer's disease, Parkinson's disease, Huntington's disease, amyotrophic lateral sclerosis, stroke and epilepsy, attributed principally to loss of glutamatergic transmission or to excitotoxicity (Chapter 25).
- Inducible NO synthase is expressed in different cell types in multiple sclerosis lesions, and astrocyte-derived NO may influence the manifestation of inflammatory reactions, particularly at the blood–brain barrier (Table 28.6).
- In ischaemic conditions or oxidative stress, NO homeostasis may be impaired, requiring supplementation via dietary nitrate and nitrite (Chapter 4).
- The resolution of interactions is critical for further advances in disease characterization and treatment. Thus, both glutamate excitotoxicity and NO synthesis are implicated in the pathogenesis of multiple sclerosis. Similarly, Parkinson's disease is attributed to disruption of glutamatergic neurotransmission (Chapter 25), but the characteristic motor manifestations arise with degeneration of dopaminergic neurons (Chapter 26).
- Histamine is associated with several pathological conditions including allergic reactions, inflammation, atherosclerosis, cancer and epilepsy. There is substantial evidence linking the histaminergic system in the brain with cognitive impairments observed in patients with Alzheimer's disease (Chapter 5).
- The regulation of obesity by histamine (Chapter 5) and by leucine should provide impetus for further research to elucidate the underlying mechanisms involved in this effect. The modulation of insulin signalling may represent one line of enquiry.
- Limited evidence indicates that diabetes may directly or indirectly impact on transport, metabolism and post-translational reactivity of amino acids.
- The evidence presented in Table 28.7 confirms the wide range of genetic conditions associated with the metabolism and transport of amino acids. An emerging issue is the late-onset presentation in certain disorders, permitting prolonged survival. A considerable number of the congenital disorders, including PKU (Chapter 23), are associated with a common underlying theme of brain damage, seizures and mental impairment. Novel non-invasive technologies have been employed to revisit long-established genetic disorders.
- Aminotransferases, ODC, homocysteine and post-translational lysine adducts may serve as markers or mediators of risk in a variety of disorders (Chapters 2, 21, and 22).
- The quest to identify appropriate targets for therapeutic intervention provides an important impetus for continuing research. Targets under consideration include enzymes, neurotransmitter receptors (Table 28.8) and transporters implicated in specific neurodegenerative, cognitive and psychotic disorders. However, the development of therapeutic agents that interact with several of the affected regulatory mechanisms might contribute to enhanced efficacy. A number of non-protein amino acids have been screened for anti-cancer properties (Chapter 19).

28.12 Outlook

It was always inevitable that support for the ethos of mammalian protein metabolism would decline sooner rather than later. The limitations inherent in the underlying concepts of nitrogen balance and protein turnover, for example, have long been recognized. Questions concerning protein-energy malnutrition have now been replaced by an awareness of the functional and molecular roles of individual amino acids and associated enzymes in a wide range of other disorders. *Amino Acids in Human Nutrition and Health* has been designed to formalize this transition towards a more dynamic and comprehensive approach. There is now considerable optimism that recent developments, reviewed in this volume, should provide significant impetus for continuing progress in several of the disciplines underpinning this title.

Further developments in fundamental areas of dynamics, as presented in this volume, should yield valuable data to enhance the potential of amino acids in nutritional support. Current studies designed to measure endogenous losses, requirements and availability of amino acids should ensure that nutritional support emerges as a more consistent and routine form of clinical intervention. Integral to this and other applications will be the need to evaluate the potential impact of amino acid–endocrine interactions. The role of amino acids as immune modulators should also be addressed in a more comprehensive approach.

A diverse range of disorders is now attributed to, or reflected in, the abnormal metabolism of amino acids. Disruption of the neurotransmission mechanisms has been implicated in several neurodegenerative, affective, cognitive and cardiovascular conditions, but there is clearly a need for more definitive evidence that would underpin the development of novel therapeutics. Specific components of signalling systems provide potential focal points for targeting such disorders with novel pharmaceuticals. However, the multifactorial aspects of interactions within and between these systems may well determine the efficacy of any programme of drug development. Future efforts will inevitably be directed at evaluating the clinical significance of changes in amino acid metabolism in diabetes, cancer and genetic disorders.

The role of amino acids, post-translationally modified residues and enzymes as risk factors or mediators for disease should provide the basis for future developments in diagnostic applications. There is scope for a more broad-based metabolomic approach in risk assessment.

Future advances will be critically dependent upon the refinement of existing protocols and development of innovative technologies. At the leading edge of this effort will be the application of non-invasive imaging devices and molecular methodologies. It is imperative that any strategy is not polarized or confounded by preconceptions concerning empirical and modelling approaches.

In conclusion, the prospects for enhanced use of amino acids in nutritional support should improve with further advances in kinetics and metabolic regulation. Moreover, current initiatives should establish the mechanisms whereby other nutrients and dietary constituents may complement critical properties, or mitigate adverse effects, of amino acids. It is also clear that the dysfunctional metabolism of amino acids is associated with or reflected in a diverse array of disorders and, in certain instances, may provide markers for risk assessment. In view of a more progressive agenda now emerging, there is renewed confidence that elucidation of the complex interactions underlying diverse disorders should yield the molecular basis for the development of novel therapeutics and diagnostic methodologies.

References

Aguilar, E., Tena-Sempre, M. and Pinilla, L. (2005) Role of excitatory amino acids in the control of growth hormone secretion. *Endocrine* 28, 295–302.

Albayram, S., Murphy, K.J., Gailloud, P., Moghekar, A. and Brunberg, J.A. (2002) CT findings in the infantile form of citrullinemia. *American Journal of Neuroradiology* 23, 334–336.

Alpers, D.H. (2006) Glutamine: do the data support the cause for glutamine supplementation? *Gastroenterology* 130, S106–S116.

Alvarez, E.O. (2009) The role of histamine on cognition. *Behavioural Brain Research* 199, 183–189.

Amaral, A.U., Leipnitz, G., Fernandes, C.G. and Wajner. M. (2010) Alpha-ketoisocaproic acid and leucine provoke mitochondrial bioenergetic dysfunction in rat brain. *Brain Research* 1324, 75–84.

Amori, L., Guidetti, P., Kajii, Y. and Schwarcz, R. (2009) On the relationship between the two branches of the kynurenine pathway in the rat brain *in vivo*. *Journal of Neurochemistry* 109, 316–325.

Anno, T., Uehara, S., Ohta, Y., Ueda, K., Moriyama, Y., Oka, Y. and Tanizawa, Y. (2004) Over expression of constitutively activated glutamate dehydrogenase induces insulin secretion through enhanced glutamate oxidation. *American Journal of Physiology, Endocrinology and Metabolism* 286, E280–E285.

Anthony, J.C., Anthony, T.G., Kimball, S.R. and Jefferson, L.S. (2001) Signalling pathways involved in translational control of protein synthesis in skeletal muscle by leucine. *Journal of Nutrition* 131, 856S–860S.

Aydogdu, S.D., Kirel, B., Coskun, T. and Kose, S. (2009) Prevalence of cystinuria among elementary schoolchildren in Eskisehir, Turkey. *Scandinavian Journal of Urology and Nephrology* 43, 138–141.

Badawy, A.A.-B. (2005) Acute tryptophan or tyrosine depletion test: time for reappraisal. *Journal of Psychopharmacology* 19, 429–430.

Baer, K., Waldvogel, H.J., Faull, R.L. and Rees, M.I. (2009) Localization of glycine receptors in the human forebrain, brainstem and cervical spinal cord: an immunohistochemical review. *Frontiers in Molecular Neuroscience* 2, 25–30.

Baidoshvili, A., Krijnen, P.A.J., Niessen, H.W.M. and Schalkwijk, C.G. (2006) N^ε-(carboxymethyl)lysine depositions in intramyocardial blood vessels in human and rat acute myocardial infarction. A predictor or reflection of infarction. *Arteriosclerosis, Thrombosis and Vascular Biology* 26, 2497–2503.

Bailey, H.H., Kim, K., Verma, A.K., Larson, P.O., Douglas, J., Berg, E.R. and Carbone, P.P. (2010) A randomized, double-blind placebo-controlled phase 3 skin cancer prevention study of difluoromethylornithine in subjects with previous history of skin cancer. *Cancer Prevention Research* 3, 35–47.

Bajoria, R., Sooranna, S.R., Ward, S. and Hancock, M. (2002) Placenta as a link between amino acids, insulin-IGF axis and low birth weight: evidence from twin studies. *The Journal of Clinical Endocrinology and Metabolism* 87, 308–315.

Bak, L.K., Schousboe, A. and Waagepetersen, H.S. (2006) The glutamate/GABA-glutamine cycle: aspects of transport, neurotransmitter homeostasis and ammonia transfer. *Journal of Neurochemistry* 98, 641–653.

Barone, P. (2010) Neurotransmission in Parkinson's disease: beyond dopamine. *European Journal of Neurology* 17, 364–376.

Barouch, L.A., Harrison, R.W., Skaf, M.W., Rosas, G.O., Cappola, T.P., Kobeissi, Z.A. and Hare, J.M. (2002) Nitric oxide regulates the heart by spatial confinement of nitric oxide synthase isoforms. *Nature* 416, 337–340.

Barry, S., Clarke, G., Scully, P. and Dinan, T.G. (2009) Kynurenine pathway in psychosis: evidence of increased tryptophan degradation. *Journal of Psychopharmacology* 23, 287–294.

Basile, A.S. (2002) Direct and indirect enhancement of GABAergic neurotransmission by ammonia: implications for the pathogenesis of hyperammonemic syndromes. *Neurochemistry International* 41, 115–122.

Baslow, M.H. and Guilfoyle, D.M. (2009). Are astrocytes the missing link between brain aspartoacylase activity and the spongiform leukodystrophy in Canavan disease? *Neurochemical Research* 34, 1523–1534.

Bauer, D., Broer, S., Palm, C., Zilles, K., Coenen, H. and Langen, K. (2005) Preferred stereoselective brain uptake of serine - a modulator of glutamatergic neurotransmission. *Nuclear Medicine and Biology* 32, 793–797.

Ben-Ari, Z., Dalal, A., Zinger, P., Cohen, J., Tessler, D. and Mandel, H. (2009) Adult-onset ornithine transcarbamylase (OTC) deficiency unmasked by the Atkins diet. *Journal of Hepatology* 52, 292–295.

Bennick, A. (2007) Extraoral function of salivary proteins. *Journal of Oral Bioscience* 49, 24–26.

Borsheim, E., Bui, Q.U., Tissier, S. and Wolfe, R.R. (2008) Effect of amino acid supplementation on muscle mass, strength and physical function in elderly. *Clinical Nutrition* 27, 189–195.

Borsheim, E., Bui, Q.U., Tissier, S., Ferrando, A.A., Newcomer, B.R. and Wolfe, R.R. (2009) Amino acid supplementation decreases plasma and liver triacylglycerols in elderly. *Nutrition* 25, 281–288.

Brabender, J., Dananberg, K.D., Schneider, P.H., Park, J.M., Peters, J.H. and Danenberg, P.V. (2001) Upregulation of ornithine decarboxylase mRNA expression in Barrett's oesophagus and Barrett's associated adenocarcinoma. *Journal of Gastrointestinal Surgery* 5, 174–182.

Brown, I., Halliday, S., Greig, H., Heys, S.D., Wallace, H.M. and Schofield, A.C. (2009) Genetic polymorphism in ornithine decarboxylase and risk of breast cancer. *Familial Cancer* 8, 307–311.

Brunetti-Pierri, N., Erez, A., Craigen, W. and Lee, B. (2009) Systemic hypertension in two patients with ASL deficiency: a result of nitric oxide deficiency? *Molecular Genetics and Metabolism* 98, 195–197.

Burbaeva, G.S., Boksha, I.S., Turishcheva, M.S. and Tereshkina, E.B. (2003) Glutamine synthetase and glutamate dehydrogenase in the prefrontal cortex of patients with schizophrenia. *Progress in Neuropsychopharmacology and Biological Psychiatry* 27, 675–680.

Burbaeva, G.S., Boksha, I.S., Tereshkina, E.B. and Turishcheva, M.S. (2005) Glutamate metabolizing enzymes in prefrontal cortex of Alzheimer's disease patients. *Neurochemical Research* 30, 1443–1451.

Burgert, T.S., Taksali, S.E., Goodman, T.R., Constable, R.T., Weiss, R., Savoye, M., Seyal, A.A. and Caprio, S. (2006) Alanine aminotransferase levels and fatty liver in childhood obesity: associations with insulin resistance, adiponectin and visceral fat. *Journal of Clinical Endocrinology and Metabolism* 91, 4287–4294.

Calfee, C.S. (2008) Plasma receptor for advanced glycation end products and clinical outcomes in acute lung injury. *Thorax* 63, 1080–1089.

Cavallero, A., Marte A. and Fedele, E. (2009) L-Aspartate as an amino acid neurotransmitter: mechanisms of the depolarization-induced release from cerebrocortical synaptosomes. *Journal of Neurochemistry* 110, 924–934.

Charlton, A.J., Baxter, N.J., Lilley, T.H., Haslam, E., McDonald, C.J. and Williamson, M.P. (1996) Tannin interactions with full-length human salivary proline-rich proteins display a stronger affinity than with single proline-rich repeats. *Federation of European Biochemical Societies Letters* 382, 289–292.

Charlton, M. (2006) Branched-chain amino acid enriched supplements as therapy for liver disease. *Journal of Nutrition* 136, 295S–298S.

Chaudhry, A.A., Sulkowski, M.S., Chander, G. and Moore, R.D. (2009) Hazardous drinking is associated with an elevated aspartate aminotransferase to platelet ratio index in an urban HIV-infected clinical cohort. *HIV Medicine* 10, 133–142.

Chen, L., Muhlhauser, M. and Yang, C.R. (2003) Glycine transporter-1 blockade potentiates NMDA-mediated responses in rat prefrontal cortical neurons *in vitro* and *in vivo*. *Journal of Neurophysiology* 89, 691–703.

Chen, P.H., Chen, J.D. and Lin, Y.C. (2009) A better parameter in predicting insulin resistance: obesity plus elevated alanine aminotransferase. *World Journal of Gastroenterology* 15, 5598–5603.

Chevalier, J., Derkinderen, P., Gomes, P., Thinard, R., Vanden Berghe, P. and Neunlist, M. (2008) Activity-dependent regulation of tyrosine hydroxylase expression in the enteric nervous system. *Journal of Physiology* 586, 1963–1975.

Chiarla, C., Giovannini, I., Siegel, J.H., Boldrini, G. and Castagneto, M. (2000) The relationship between plasma taurine and other amino acid levels in human sepsis. *Journal of Nutrition* 130, 2222–2227.

Choi, M.-M., Kim, E.-A., Yang, S.-J., Choi, S.Y., Cho, S.-W. and Huh, J.-W. (2007) Amino acid changes within antenna helix are responsible for different regulatory preferences of human glutamate dehydrogenase isozymes. *Journal of Biological Chemistry* 282, 19510–19517.

Conn, P.J., Lindsley, C.W. and Jones, C.K. (2009) Activation of metabotropic glutamate receptors as a novel approach for the treatment of schizophrenia. *Trends in Pharmacological Sciences* 30, 25–31.

Croffie, J.M., Gupta, S.K., Chong, S.K.F. and Fitzgerald, J.F. (1999) Tyrosinemia type I should be suspected in infants with severe coagulopathy even in the absence of other signs of liver failure. *Pediatrics* 103, 675–678.

Cunha, C., Monfils, M.H. and Ledoux, J.E. (2010) GABA (C) receptors in the lateral amygdala: a possible novel target for the treatment of fear and anxiety disorders? *Frontiers in Behavioral Neuroscience* 12, 4–6.

Dasarathy, J., Gruca, L.L., Bennett, C., Fierro, J.L. and Kalhan, S.C. (2010) Methionine metabolism in human pregnancy. *American Journal of Clinical Nutrition* 91, 357–365.

Davies, J.S., Chung, S.K., Thomas, R.H., Harvey, R.J. and Rees, M.I. (2010) The glycinergic system in human startle disease: a genetic screening approach. *Frontiers in Molecular Neuroscience* 3, 3–8.

Delgado, M., Perez-Miguelsanz, J., Garrido, F., Perez-Sala, D. and Pajares, M.A. (2008) Early effects of copper accumulation on methionine metabolism. *Cellular and Molecular Life Sciences* 65, 2080–2090.

De Luis D.A., Izaola, O., Cuellar, L., Martin, T. and Aller, R. (2009) High dose of arginine enhanced enteral nutrition in postsurgical head and neck cancer patients: a randomized clinical trial. *European Review for Medical and Pharmacological Sciences* 13, 279–283.

Deng, C., Weston-Green, K. and Huang, X.F. (2010) The role of histaminergic H1 and H3 receptors in food intake: a mechanism for atypical antipsychotic-induced weight gain. *Progress in Neuropsychopharmacology and Biological Psychiatry* 34, 1–4.

Desforges, M., Greenwood, S.L., Glazier, J.D., Westwood, M. and Sibley, C.P. (2010) The contribution of SNAT1 to system A amino acid transporter activity in human placental trophoblast. *Biochemical and Biophysical Research Communications* 398, 130–134.

Dessein, P.H., Woodiwiss, A.J., Joffe, B.I. and Norton, G.R. (2007) Aminotransferases are associated with insulin resistance and atherosclerosis in rheumatoid arthritis. *BMC Cardiovascular Disorders* 7, 31–33.

D'Eufemia, P., Finocchiaro, R., Celli, M., Raccio, I., Properzi, E. and Zicari, A. (2009) Increased nitric oxide release by neutrophils of a patient with tyrosinemia type III. *Biomedicine and Pharmacotherapy* 63, 359–361.

van Deutekom, A.W., Niessen, H.W.M., Schalkwijk, C.G., Heine, R.J. and Simsek, S. (2008) Increased N^ε-(carboxymethyl)lysine levels in cerebral blood vessels of diabetic patients and in a rat model of diabetes mellitus. *European Journal of Endocrinology* 158, 655–660.

D'Mello, J.P.F. (1991) Toxic amino acids. In: D'Mello, J.P.F., Duffus, C.M. and Duffus, J.H. (eds) *Toxic Substances in Crop Plants*. The Royal Society of Chemistry, Cambridge, pp. 21–48.

D'Mello, J.P.F. (2003) Adverse effects of amino acids. In: D'Mello, J.P.F. (ed.) *Amino Acids in Animal Nutrition*. CAB International, Wallingford, UK, pp. 125–142.

Drummond, M.J. and Rasmussen, B.B. (2008) Leucine-enriched nutrients and the regulation of mammalian target of rapamycin signaling and human skeletal muscle protein synthesis. *Current Opinion in Clinical Nutrition and Metabolic Care* 11, 222–226.

Dun, Y., Duplantier, J., Roon, P., Martin, P.M., Ganapathy, V. and Smith, S.B. (2008) Serine racemase expression and D-serine content are developmentally regulated in neuronal ganglion cells of the retina. *Journal of Neurochemistry* 104, 970–978.

Durante, W., Johnson, F.K. and Johnson, R.A. (2007) Arginase: a critical regulator of nitric oxide synthesis and vascular function. *Clinical, Experimental Pharmacology and Physiology* 34, 906–911.

Eichholzer, M. and Gutzwiller, F. (2003) Dietary nitrates, nitrites and *N*-nitroso compounds and cancer risk with special emphasis on the epidemiological evidence. In: D'Mello, J.P.F. (ed.) *Food Safety. Contaminants and Toxins*. CAB International, Wallingford, UK, pp. 217–234.

Eid, T., Thomas, M.J., Spencer, D.D., Kim, J.H. and de Lanerolle, N.C. (2004) Loss of glutamine synthetase in the human epileptogenic hippocampus: possible mechanism for raised extracellular glutamate in mesial temporal lobe epilepsy. *The Lancet* 363, 28–37.

Eid, T., Ghosh, A., Wang, Y., Lee, T.S., Lai, J.C. and de Lanerolle, N.C. (2008) Recurrent seizures and brain pathology after inhibition of glutamine synthetase in the hippocampus in rats. *Brain* 131, 2061–2070.

Ellis, K.A., Mehta, M.A., Wesnes, K.A., Armstrong, S. and Nathan, P.J. (2005) Combined D_1/D_2 receptor stimulation under conditions of dopamine depletion impairs spatial working memory performance in humans. *Psychopharmacology* 181, 771–780.

Engelen, M.P., Rutten, E.P., Wouters, E.F., Schols, A.M. and Deutz, N.E. (2007) Supplementation of soy protein with branched-chain amino acids alters protein metabolism in healthy elderly and even more in patients with chronic obstructive pulmonary disease. *American Journal of Clinical Nutrition* 85, 431–439.

Esbenshade, T.A., Bitner, R.S., Cowart, M.D. and Brioni, J.D. (2008) The histamine H3 receptor: an attractive target for the treatment of cognitive disorders. *British Journal of Pharmacology* 54, 1166–1181.

Fang, J., Hsu, B.Y.L., MacMullen, C.M., Poncz, M., Smith, T.J. and Stanley, C.A. (2002) Expression, purification and characterisation of human glutamate dehydrogenase (GDH) allosteric regulatory mutations. *The Biochemical Journal* 363, 81–87.

Fayyaz, M. and Lackner, J.M. (2008) Serotonin receptor modulators in the treatment of irritable bowel syndrome. *Therapeutics and Clinical Risk Management* 4, 41–48.

Finkelstein, J.D. (2006) Inborn errors of sulfur-containing amino acid metabolism. *Journal of Nutrition* 136, 1750S–1754S.

Finkelstein, J.D. (2007) Metabolic regulatory properties of S-adenosylmethionine and S-adenosylhomocysteine. *Clinical Chemistry and Laboratory Medicine* 45, 1694–1699.

Fujioka, H., Okano, Y., Inada, H., Asada, M., Kawamura, T., Hose, Y. and Yamano, T. (2001) Molecular characterisation of glutamate dehydrogenase gene defects in Japanese patients with congenital hyperinsulinism/hyperammonaemia. *European Journal of Human Genetics* 9, 931–937.

Gaenslen, A., Gasser, T. and Berg, D. (2008) Nutrition and the risk of Parkinson's disease: review of the literature. *Journal of Neural Transmission* 115, 703–713.

Gaisler-Salomon, I., Miller, G.M., Lee, S., Zhang, H., Wang, Y., Galloway, M.P., Moore, H.M., *et al.* (2009) Glutaminase-deficient mice display hippocampal hypoactivity to pro-psychotic drugs and potential latent inhibition: relevance to schizophrenia. *Neuropsychopharmacology* 34, 2305–2322.

Galanopoulou, A.S. (2008) GABA(A) receptors in normal development and seizures: friends or foes? *Current Neuropharmacology* 6, 1–20.

Gameiro, A., Williams, L., Simpson, A.K. and Gribble, F.M. (2005) The neurotransmitters glycine and GABA stimulate glucagon-like peptide-1 release from the GLUTag cell line. *The Journal of Physiology* 569, 761–772.

Garcia-Espinosa, M.A., Wallin, R., Hutson, S.M. and Sweatt, A.J. (2007) Widespread neuronal expression of branched-chain aminotransferase in the CNS: implications for leucine/glutamate metabolism and for signalling by amino acids. *Journal of Neurochemistry* 100, 1458–1468.

Gelain, D.P., Moreira, J.C.F., Dickson, P.W. and Dunkley, P.R. (2007) Retinol activates tyrosine hydroxylase acutely by increasing the phosphorylation of serine40 and then serine31 in bovine adrenal chromaffin cells. *Journal of Neurochemistry* 103, 2369–2379.

Gianotti, L., Braga, M. and Mariani, L. (2009) Perioperative intravenous glutamine supplementation in major surgery for cancer: a randomized multicenter trial. *Annals of Surgery* 250, 684–690.

Gilbert, D.F., Lynagh, T., Lynch, J.W. and Webb, T.I. (2009) High throughput techniques for discovering new glycine receptor modulators and their binding sites. *Frontiers in Molecular Neuroscience* 2, 17–21.

Gonzalez-Maeso, J., Yuen, T., Chan, P., Okawa, Y. and Sealfon, S.C. (2008) Identification of a serotonin/glutamate receptor complex implicated in psychosis. *Nature* 452, 93–97.

Griffiths, D.W. (1991) Condensed tannins. In: D'Mello, J.P.F., Duffus, C.M. and Duffus, J.H. (eds) *Toxic Substances in Crop Plants*. The Royal Society of Chemistry, Cambridge, pp.180–201.

Gundersen, R.Y., Vaagenes, P., Breivik, T. and Opstad, P.K. (2005) Glycine - an important neurotransmitter and cytoprotective agent. *Acta Anaesthesiologica Scandinavica* 49, 1108–1116.

Haas, H.L., Sergeeva, O.A. and Selbach, O. (2008) Histamine in the nervous system. *Physiological Reviews* 88, 1183–1241.

Haberie, J., Gorg, B., Toutain, A., Koch, H.G. and Haussinger, D. (2006) Inborn error of amino acid synthesis: human glutamine synthetase deficiency. *Journal of Inherited Metabolic Diseases* 29, 352–358.

Harper, A.E., Miller, R.H. and Block, K.P. (1984) Branched-chain amino acid metabolism. *Annual Review of Nutrition* 4, 409–454.

Hartog, J.W.L., Voors, A.A., Schalkwijk, C.G., Bakker, S.J.L., Smit, A.J. and van Veldhuisen, D.J. (2007) Clinical and prognostic value of advanced glycation end-products in chronic heart failure. *European Heart Journal* 28, 2879–2885.

Hawkins, R.A. (2009) The blood-brain barrier and glutamate. *The American Journal of Clinical Nutrition* 90, 867S–874S.

Hay, D.I., Bennick, A., Schlesinger, D.H., Minnguchi, K., Madapallimattan G. and Schluckebier, S.K. (1988) The primary structures of six human salivary acidic proline–rich proteins (PRP-1, PRP-2, PRP-3, PRP-4, PIF-s and PIF-f). *The Biochemical Journal* 255, 15–21.

Hayes, K.C., Pronczuk, A., Adessa, A.E. and Stephan, Z.F. (1989) Taurine modulates platelet aggregation in cats and humans. *American Journal of Clinical Nutrition* 49, 1211–1216.

Hehre, D.A., Devia, C.J., Bancalari, E. and Suguihara, C. (2008) Brainstem amino acid neurotransmitters and ventilatory response to hypoxia in piglets. *Pediatric Research* 63, 46–50.

Heidbreder, C. (2008) Selective antagonism of dopamine D3 receptors as a target for drug addiction pharmacology: a review of preclinical evidence. *CNS and Neurological Disorders Drug Targets* 7, 410–421.

Herman, M.A., She, P., Peroni, O.D., Lynch, C.J. and Kahn, B.B. (2010) Adipose tissue branched-chain amino acid (BCAA) metabolism modulates circulating BCAA levels. *Journal of Biological Chemistry* 285, 11348–11356.

Hernandes, M.S. and Tronsone, L.R. (2009) Glycine as a neurotransmitter in the fore-brain: a short review. *Journal of Neural Transmission* 116, 1551–1560.

Herrero-Yraola, A., Bakhit, S.M.A., Franke, P., Weise, C., Schweiger, M., Jorcke, D. and Ziegler, M. (2001) Regulation of glutamate dehydrogenase by reversible ADP-ribosylation in mitochondria. *The European Molecular Biology Organization Journal* 20, 2404–2412.

Hertecant, J.L., Al-Gazali, L.I. and Ali, B.R. (2009) A novel mutation in ARG 1 gene is responsible for arginase deficiency in an Asian family. *Saudi Medical Journal* 30, 1601–1603.

Hillenkamp, J., Hussain, A.A., Jackson, T.L., Cunningham, J.R. and Marshall, J. (2004) Taurine uptake by human retinal pigment epithelium: implications for the transport of small solutes between the choroid and the outer retina. *Investigative Ophthalmology and Visual Science* 45, 4529–4534.

Hoehn, T., Stiller, B., McPhaden, A.R. and Wadsworth, R.M. (2009) Nitric oxide synthases in infants and children with pulmonary hypertension and congenital heart disease. *Respiratory Research* 10, 110–114.

Holecek, M. (2010) Three targets of branched-chain amino acid supplementation in the treatment of liver disease. *Nutrition* 26, 482–490.

Horowitz, S., Bionion, D.G., Nelson, V.M., Kanaa, Y., Javadi, P., Lazarova, Z., Andrekopoulos, C., *et al.* (2007) Increased arginase activity and endothelial dysfunction in human inflammatory bowel disease. *American Journal of Physiology - Gastrointestinal and Liver Physiology* 292, G1323–G1336.

Inzitari, R., Cabras, T., Onnis, G., Olmi, C., Mastina, A., Sanna, M.T., Pellegrini, M.G., *et al.* (2005) Different isoforms and post-translational modifications of human salivary acidic proline-rich proteins. *Proteomics* 5, 805–815.

Ishikawa, T., Michitaka, I., Higuchi, K., Kubota, T., Ohta, H., Yoshida, T. and Kamimura, T. (2009) Oral branched-chain amino acid administration improves impaired liver dysfunction after radiofrequency ablation therapy for hepatocellular carcinoma. *Hepatogastroenterology* 56, 1491–1495.

Ito, C. (2009) Histamine H3-receptor inverse agonists as novel antipsychotics. *Central Nervous System Agents in Medicinal Chemistry* 9, 132–136.

Jahoor, F., Badaloo, A., Reid, M. and Forrester, T. (2006) Sulfur amino acid metabolism in children with severe childhood under nutrition: cysteine kinetics. *American Journal of Clinical Nutrition* 84, 1393–1399.

Jansson, T., Ekstrad, Y., Wennergren, M. and Powell, T.L. (2002) Alterations in the activity of amino acid transporters in pregnancies complicated by diabetes. *Diabetes* 51, 2214–2219.

Jones, E.A. (2002) Ammonia, the GABA neurotransmitter system, and hepatic encephalopathy. *Metabolic Brain Disease* 17, 275–281.

Junyent, F., Utrera, J., Romero, R. and Auladell, C. (2009) Synthesis, uptake and release of taurine in astrocytes treated with 8-Br-cAMP. *Neuroscience Letters* 467, 199–202.

Kalogeropoulou, D., Lafave, L., Gannon, M.C. and Nuttall, F.Q. (2008) Leucine, when ingested with glucose, synergistically stimulates insulin secretion and lowers blood glucose. *Metabolism* 57, 1747–1752.

Kantrowitz, J.T. and Javitt, D.C. (2010) Thinking glutamatergically: changing concepts of schizophrenia based upon changing neurochemical models. *Clinical Schizophrenia and Related Psychoses* 4, 189–200.

Katsanos, C.S., Kobayashi, H., Aarsland, A. and Wolfe, R.R. (2006) A high proportion of leucine is required for optimal stimulation of the rate of muscle protein synthesis by essential amino acids in the elderly. *American Journal of Physiology, Endocrinology and Metabolism* 291, E381–E387.

Katsurabayashi, S., Kubota, H., Higashi, H., Akaike, N. and Ito, Y. (2004) Distinct profiles of refilling of inhibitory neurotransmitters into presynaptic terminals projecting to spinal neurones in immature rats. *The Journal of Physiology* 560, 469–478.

Kawai, Y., Moriyama, A., Asai, K., Coleman-Campbell, C.M., Sumi, S., Morishita, H. and Suchi, M. (2005) Molecular characterization of histidinemia: identification of four missense mutations in the histidase gene. *Human Genetics* 116, 340–346.

Kim, J., Park, M.H., Kim, E., Han, C. and Jo, I. (2007) Plasma homocysteine is associated with the risk of mild cognitive impairment in an elderly Korean population. *Journal of Nutrition* 137, 2093–2097.

Kirkwood, B.J. (2009) Albinism and its implications with vision. *Insight* 34, 13–16.

Kobylecki, C., Cenci, M.A., Crossman, A.R. and Ravenscroft, P. (2010) Calcium-permeable AMPA receptors are involved in the induction and expression of L-DOPA-induced dyskinesia in Parkinson's disease. *Journal of Neurochemistry* 114, 499–511.

de Koning, T.J. (2006) Treatment with amino acids in serine deficiency disorder. *Journal of Inherited Metabolic Disease* 29, 347–351.

Korpershoek, E., Verwest, A.M., Rottier, R. and de Krijger, R.R. (2007) Expression of GAD 67 and novel GAD 67 splice variants during human fetal pancreas development: GAD 67 in fetal pancreas. *Endocrine Pathology* 18, 31–36.

Kotermanski, S.E. and Johnson, J.W. (2009) Mg^{2+} imparts NMDA receptor subtype selectivity to the Alzheimer's drug memantine. *The Journal of Neuroscience* 29, 2774–2779.

Koutsidis, G., Simons, S.P.J., Wedzicha, B.L. and Mottran, D.S. (2009) Investigations on the effect of amino acids on acrylamide, pyrazines and Michael addition products in model systems. *Journal of Agricultural and Food Chemistry* 57, 9011–9015.

Krehbiel, C.R. and Matthews, J.C. (2003) Absorption of amino acids and peptides. In: D'Mello, J.P.F. (ed.) *Amino Acids in Animal Nutrition*. CAB International, Wallingford, UK, pp. 41–70.

Kurul, S., Cakamakci, H. and Dirik, E. (2004) Glutaric aciduria type 1: proton magnetic resonance spectroscopy findings. *Pediatric Neurology* 31, 228–231.

Kuzuya, T., Katano, Y., Nakano, I. and Shimomura, Y. (2008) Regulation of branched-chain amino acid catabolism in rat models for spontaneous type 2 diabetes mellitus. *Biochemical and Biophysical Research Communications* 373, 94–98.

Kwakowsky, A., Zhang, Q., Katarova, Z.D. and Szabo, G. (2007) GAD isoforms exhibit distinct spatiotemporal expression in the developing mouse lens: correlation with Dlx 2 and Dlx 5. *Developmental Dynamics* 236, 3532–3544.

Kwok, R.H.M. (1968) Chinese restaurant syndrome. *The New England Journal of Medicine* 278, 796.

Lam, V.W. and Poon, R.T. (2008) Role of branched-chain amino acids in management of cirrhosis and hepatocellular carcinoma. *Hepatology Research* 38, S107–S115.

Langhendries, J.P., Hurrell, R.F., Finot, P.A. and Bernard, A. (1992) Maillard reaction products and lysinoalanine: urinary excretion and the effects on kidney function of preterm infants fed heat-processed milk formulas. *Journal of Paediatric Gastroenterology and Nutrition* 14, 62–70.
Layman, D.K. and Walker, D.A. (2006) Potential importance of leucine in treatment of obesity and the metabolic syndrome. *Journal of Nutrition* 136, 319S–323S.
Leret, M.L., Lecumberri, M., Garcia-Montojo, M. and Gonzalez J.C. (2007) Role of maternal corticosterone in the development of the aminoacidergic system of the rat brain. *International Journal of Developmental Neuroscience* 25, 465–471.
Li, X. (2009) T1R receptors mediate mammalian sweet and umami taste. *The American Journal of Clinical Nutrition* 90, 733S–737S.
Li, X., Bazer, F.W., Gao, H., Jobgen, W., Johnson, G.A., Li, P., McKnight, J.R., et al. (2009) Amino acids and gaseous signalling. *Amino Acids* 37, 65–78.
Li, Z., Liu, J., Tan, F., Liu, Y., Waldum, H.L. and Cui, G. (2008) Expression of non-mast cell histidine decarboxylase in tumor-associated microvessels in human oesophageal squamous cell carcinomas. *Acta Pathologica, Microbiologica et Immunologica Scandinavica* 116, 1034–1042.
Lieuw-A-Fa, M.L.M., van Hinsberg, V.W.M., Teerlink, T., Twisk, J., Stehouwer, C.D.A. and Schalkwijk, C.G. (2004) Increased levels of N^ε-(carboxymethyl)lysine and N^ε-(carboxyethyl)lysine in type 1 diabetic patients with impaired renal function: correlation with markers of endothelial dysfunction. *Nephrology, Dialysis and Transplantation* 19, 631–636.
Lin, C.-H., Lo W.-C., Hsino, M., Tung, C.-S. and Tseng, C.-J. (2004). Interactions of carbon monoxide and metabotropic glutamate receptor groups of rats. *The Journal of Pharmacology and Experimental Therapeutics* 308, 1213–1218.
Lin, M.T., Kung, S.O., Kuo, M.L., Lee, P.H. and Chen, W.J. (2005) Glutamine-supplemented total parenteral nutrition attenuates plasma interleukin-6 in surgical patients with lower disease severity. *World Journal of Gastroenterology* 11, 6197–6201.
Lipton, S.A. and Rosenberg, P.A. (1994) Excitatory amino acids as a final common pathway for neurologic disorders. *The New England Journal of Medicine* 330, 613–622.
Liu, J.S., Zhao, M.L., Brosnan, C.F. and Lee, S.C. (2001) Expression of inducible nitric oxide synthase and nitrotyrosine in multiple sclerosis lesions. *The American Journal of Pathology* 158, 2057–2066.
Liu, Y., Wong, T.P., Craig, A.M. and Wang, Y.T. (2007) NMDA receptor subunits have differential roles in mediating excitotoxic neuronal death both *in vitro* and *in vivo*. *The Journal of Neuroscience* 27, 2846–2857.
Lo, J.-C., Huang, W.-C., Chen, Y.-C., Tseng, C.-H., Lee, W.-L. and Sun, S.H. (2008) Activation of $P2X_7$ receptors decreases glutamate uptake and glutamine synthetase activity in RBA-2 astrocytes via distinct mechanisms. *Journal of Neurochemistry* 105, 151–164.
Lu, H., Zeng, L., Liang, B., Shu, X. and Xie, D. (2009) High prevalence of coronary heart disease in type 2 diabetic patients with non-alcoholic fatty liver disease. *Archives of Medical Research* 40, 571–575.
Lu, Y. and Bennick, A. (1998) Interaction of tannin with human salivary proline-rich proteins. *Archives of Oral Biology* 43, 717–728.
Ludvigsson, J. (2009) Therapy with GAD in diabetes. *Diabetes/Metabolism Research and Reviews* 25, 307–315.
Lythe, I.M., Deakin, J.F.W., Elliot, R. and Strickland, P. (2005) Lack of behavioural effects after acute tyrosine depletion in healthy volunteers. *Journal of Psychopharmacology* 19, 5–11.
Maarsingh, H., Zaagsma, J. and Meurs, H. (2009) Arginase: a key enzyme in the pathophysiology of allergic asthma opening novel therapeutic perspectives. *British Journal of Pharmacology* 158, 652–664.
Madsen, K.K., White, H.S. and Schousboe, A. (2010) Neuronal and non-neuronal GABA transporters as targets for antiepileptic drugs. *Pharmacology and Therapeutics* 125, 394–401.
Maeshima, H., Ohnuma, T., Sakai, Y., Shibata, N., Ohkubo, T., Nakano, Y., Suzuki, T., et al. (2007) Increased plasma glutamate by antipsychotic medication and its relationship to glutaminase 1 and 2 genotypes in schizophrenia - Juntendo University Schizophrenia Projects (JUSP). *Progress in Neuropsychopharmacology and Biological Psychiatry* 31, 1410–1418.
Makkonen, J., Pietilainen, K.H., Rissanen, A., Kaprio, J. and Yki-Jarvinen, H. (2009) Genetic factors contribute to variation in serum alanine aminotransferase activity independent of obesity and alcohol: a study in monozygotic and dizygotic twins. *Journal of Hepatology* 50, 1035–1042.
Markus, C.R., Firk, C., Gerhardt, C. and Smolders, G.F. (2008) Effect of different tryptophan sources on amino acid availability to the brain and mood in healthy volunteers. *Psychopharmacology* 201, 107–114.
Marquez, J., Tosina, M., de la Rosa, V., Segura, J.A., Alonso, F.J., Mates, J.M. and Campos-Sandoval, J.A. (2009) New insights into brain glutaminases: beyond their role on glutamatergic transmission. *Neurochemistry International* 55, 64–70.

Martel, M.A., Soriano, F.X., Baxter, P., Rickman, C., Duncan, R., Wyllie, D.J.A. and Hardingham, G.E. (2009) Inhibiting pro-death NMDA receptor signalling dependent on the NR2 PDZ ligand may not affect synaptic function or synaptic NMDA receptor signalling to gene expression. *Channels* 3, 12–15.

Masaki, T. and Yoshimatsu, H. (2009) Molecular mechanisms of neuronal histamine and its receptors in obesity. *Current Molecular Pharmacology* 2, 249–252.

McLean, A., Rubinsztein, J.S., Robbins, T.W. and Sahakian, B.J. (2004) The effects of tyrosine depletion in normal healthy volunteers: implications for unipolar depression. *Psychopharmacology* 171, 286–297.

McTavish, S.F.B., McPherson, M.H., Harmer, C.J., Clark, L., Sharp, T., Goodwin, G.M. and Cowen, P.J. (2001) Antidopaminergic effects of dietary tyrosine depletion in healthy subjects and patients with manic illness. *The British Journal of Psychiatry* 179, 356–360.

Meldrum, B.S. (2000) Glutamate as a neurotransmitter in the brain: review of physiology and pathology. *Journal of Nutrition* 130, 1007S–1015S.

Mercier, S., Breuille, D., Papet, I. and Obled, C. (2006) Methionine kinetics are altered in the elderly both in the basal state and after vaccination. *American Journal of Clinical Nutrition* 83, 291–298.

Miller, C.L., Llenos, I.C., Walkup, J. and Weis, S. (2008) Alterations in kynurenine precursor and product levels in schizophrenia and bipolar disorder. *Neurochemistry International* 52, 1297–1303.

Mitsubuchi, H., Nakamura, K., Matsumoto, S. and Endo, F. (2008) Inborn errors of proline metabolism. *Journal of Nutrition* 138, 2016S–2020S.

Morgan, T.K., Montgomery, K., Mason, V., Wang, L. and Higgins, J.P. (2006) Upregulation of histidine decarboxylase expression in superficial cortical nephrons during pregnancy in mice and women. *Kidney International* 70, 306–314.

Mori, M., Gahwiler, B.H. and Gerber, U. (2002) β–Alanine and taurine as endogenous agonists at glycine receptors in rat hippocampus in vitro. *The Journal of Physiology* 539, 191–200.

Moriyama, T., Tsuneyoshi, I., Takeyama, M. and Kanmura, Y. (2008) The effect of amino acid infusion during off-pump coronary arterial bypass surgery on thermogenic and hormonal regulation. *Journal of Anesthesia* 22, 354–360.

Moya-Garcia, A.A., Medina, M.A. and Sanchez-Jimenez, F. (2005) Mammalian histidine decarboxylase: from structure to function. *BioEssays* 27, 57–63.

Moya-Garcia, A.A., Pino-Angeles, A., Morreale, A. and Sanchez-Jimenez, F. (2009) Structural features of mammalian histidine decarboxylase reveal the basis for specific inhibition. *British Journal of Pharmacology* 157, 4–13.

Muir, K.W. and Lees, K.R. (1995) Clinical experience with excitatory amino acid antagonist drugs. *Stroke* 26, 503–513.

Munder, M. (2009) Arginase: an emerging key player in the mammalian immune system. *British Journal of Pharmacology* 158, 638–651.

Mustafa, A.K., Kim, P.M. and Snyder, S.H. (2004) D-serine as a putative glial neurotransmitter. *Neuron Glia Biology* 1, 275–281.

Mustafa, A.K., Kumar, M., Selvakumar, B., Ho, G.P.H., Barrow, R.K., Amzel, L.M. and Snyder S.H. (2007) Nitric oxide S-nitrosylates serine racemase, mediating feedback inhibition of D-serine formation. *Proceedings of the National Academy of Sciences* 104, 2950–2955.

Nagasaka, H., Tsukahara, H., Miida, T., Murayama, K., Kobayashi, K., Okano, Y. and Takayanagi, M. (2009) Evaluation of endogenous nitric oxide synthesis in congenital urea cycle enzyme defects. *Metabolism* 58, 278–282.

Nakamura, K., Sugawara, Y., Sawabe, K., Xiu, Y., Lin, Q.S., Hasegawa, H. and Hirose, S. (2006) Late developmental stage-specific role of tryptophan hydroxylase 1 in brain serotonin levels. *Journal of Neuroscience* 26, 530–534.

Nedergaard, M., Takano, T. and Hansen, A.J. (2002) Beyond the role of glutamate as a neurotransmitter. *Nature Reviews, Neuroscience* 3, 748–755.

Nijveldt, R.J., Siroen, M.P.C., Teerlink, T., Prins, H.A. and van Leeuwen, P.A.M. (2004) High plasma arginine concentrations in critically ill patients suffering from hepatic failure. *European Journal of Clinical Nutrition* 58, 587–593.

Ockenga, J., Borchert, K., Stuber, E., Manns, M.P. and Bischoff, S.C. (2005) Glutamine-enriched total parenteral nutrition in patients with inflammatory bowel disease. *European Journal of Clinical Nutrition* 59, 1302–1309.

Okabayashi, T., Nishimori, I., Sugimoto, T., Iwasaki, S., and Hanazaki, K. (2008) The benefit of the supplementation of perioperative branched-chain amino acids in patients with surgical management for hepatocellular carcinoma: a preliminary study. *Digestive Diseases and Sciences* 53, 204–209.

Ono, H., Suto, T., Kinoshita, Y., Sakano, T., Furue, T. and Ohta, T. (2009) A case of carbamoyl phosphate synthetase 1 deficiency presenting symptoms at one month of age. *Brain and Development* 31, 779–781.

Pasternack, S.M., Betz, R.C., Bandrup, F., Gade, E.F. and Bygum, A. (2009) Identification of two new mutations in the TAT gene in a Danish family with Tyrosinaemia type II. *British Journal of Dermatology* 160, 704–706.

Pegg, A.E. (2006) Regulation of ornithine decarboxylase. *Journal of Biological Chemistry* 281, 14529–14532.

Perez-Gomez, C., Campos-Sandoval, J.A., Alonso, F.J., Segura, J.A., Manzanares, E., Ruiz-Sanchez, P., Gonzalez, M.E., et al. (2005) Co-expression of glutaminase K and L isoenzymes in human tumour cells. *Biochemical Journal* 386, 535–542.

Phang, J.M. (2008) Introduction to Second Proline Symposium. *Amino Acids* 35, 653–654.

Pinilla, L., Gonzalez, L.C. and Aguilar, E. (2002) Interactions between GABAergic and aminoacidergic pathways in the control of gonadotropin and growth hormone secretion in pre-pubertal female rats. *Journal of Endocrinological Investigation* 25, 96–100.

Pitt, D., Werner, P. and Raine, C.S. (2000) Glutamate excitotoxicity in a model of multiple sclerosis. *Nature Medicine* 6, 67–70.

Porter, R.J., Gallagher, P. and O'Brien, J.T. (2007). Effects of rapid tryptophan depletion on salivary cortisol in older people recovered from depression, and the healthy elderly. *Journal of Psychopharmacology* 21, 71–75.

Preissler, G., Lohe, F., Huff, I., Messmer, K. and Angele, M.K. (2009) Recipient treatment with L-arginine attenuates donor lung injury associated with hemorrhagic shock. *Transplantation* 87, 1602–1608.

Pytel, D., Sliwinski, T., Poplawski, T., Ferriola, D. and Majsterek, I. (2009) Tyrosine kinase blockers: new hope for successful cancer therapy. *Anti-cancer Agents in Medicinal Chemistry* 9, 66–76.

Quintero, D.G., Winger, J.N., Khashaba, R. and Borke, J.L. (2010) Advanced glycation endproducts and rat dental implant osseointegration. *The Journal of Oral Implantology* 36, 97–103.

Rakotoambinina, B., Marks, L., Badran, A.M., Igliki, F., Thuillier, F., Crenn, P., Messing, B. and Darmaun, D. (2004) Taurine kinetics assessed using [1,2-13$_{C2}$] taurine in healthy adult humans. *American Journal of Physiology - Endocrinology and Metabolism* 287, E255–E262.

Rammes, G., Zieglgansberger, W. and Parsons, C.G. (2008) The fraction of activated N-methyl-D-aspartate receptors during synaptic transmission remains constant in the presence of the glutamate release inhibitor riluzole. *Journal of Neural Transmission* 115, 1119–1126.

Renick, S.E., Kleven, D.T., Chan, J., Stenius, K., Milner, T.A., Pickel, V.M. and Fremeau Jr, R.T. (1999) The mammalian brain high-affinity-L-proline transporter is enriched preferentially in synaptic vesicles in a subpopulation of excitatory nerve terminals in rat forebrain. *The Journal of Neuroscience* 19, 21–33.

Ribeiro-Oliveira, A., Korbonits, M. and Grossman, A.B. (2008) The potential role of D(2) dopamine receptors as a target in the management of neuroendocrine tumors. *Cancer Biology and Therapy* 7, 1979–1981.

Rodriguez-Moreno, A. and Sihra, T.S. (2007) Metabotropic actions of kainate receptors in the central nervous system. *Journal of Neurochemistry* 103, 2121–2135.

Rolls, E.T. (2009) Functional neuroimaging of umami taste: what makes umami pleasant? *The American Journal of Clinical Nutrition* 90, 804S–813S.

Romero, M.J., Platt, D.H., Tawfik, H.E., Labazi, M., El-Remessy, B., Bartoli, M., Caldwell, R.B. et al. (2008) Diabetes-induced coronary vascular dysfunction involves increased arginase activity. *Circulation Research* 102, 95–102.

Romero-Gomez, M. (2005) Role of phosphate-activated glutaminase in the pathogenesis of hepatic encephalopathy. *Metabolic Brain Disease* 20, 319–325.

de la Rosa, V., Campos-Sandoval, J.A., Martin-Rufian, M., Cardona, C., Mates, J.M., Segura, J.A., Alonso, F.J., et al. (2009) A novel glutaminase isoform in mammalian tissues. *Neurochemistry International* 55, 76–84.

Rossi, S., Daniele I., Bastrenta, P., Mastrangelo, M. and Lista, G. (2009) Early myoclonic encephalopathy and nonketotic hyperglycinemia. *Pediatric Neurology* 41, 371–374.

Rotondo, R., Mastracci, L., Piazza, T., Fabbi, M., Ratto, G.B., Ferrini, S. and Frumento, G. (2008) Arginase 2 is expressed by human lung cancer, but it neither induces immune suppression, nor affects disease progression. *International Journal of Cancer* 123, 1108–1116.

van Ruitenbeek, P., Sambeth, A., Vermeeren, A., Young, S.N. and Riedel, W.J. (2009). Effects of L-histidine depletion and L-tyrosine/L-phenylalanine depletion on sensory and motor processes in healthy volunteers. *British Journal of Pharmacology* 157, 92–103.

Rusnak, M. and Gainer, H. (2005) Differential effects of forskolin on tyrosine hydroxylase gene transcription in identified brainstem catecholaminergic neuronal subtypes in organotypic culture. *European Journal of Neuroscience* 21, 889–898.

Rutten, E.P., Engelen, M.P., Wouters, E.F. and Deutz, N.E. (2006a) Metabolic effects of glutamine and glutamate ingestion in healthy subjects and in persons with chronic obstructive pulmonary disease. *American Journal of Clinical Nutrition* 83, 115–123.

Rutten, E.P., Engelen, M.P., Wouters, E.F., Deutz, N.E. and Schols, A.M. (2006b) Effect of glutamate ingestion on whole-body glutamate turnover in healthy elderly and patients with chronic obstructive pulmonary disease. *Nutrition* 22, 496–503.

Sacksteder, K.A., Biery, B.J., Morrell, J.C., Goodman, B.K., Cox, R.P., Gould, S.J. and Geraghty, M.T. (2000) Identification of the alpha-aminoadipic semialdehyde synthase gene, which is defective in familial hyperlysinemia. *American Journal of Human Genetics* 66, 1736–1743.

Sandberg, M. and Jacobson, I. (2008) β-Alanine: a possible neurotransmitter in the visual system? *Journal of Neurochemistry* 37, 1353–1356.

Sankaralingam, S., Xu, H. and Davidge, S.T. (2010) Arginine contributes to endothelial cell oxidative stress in response to plasma from women with preeclampsia. *Cardiovascular Research* 85, 194–203.

Sarchielli, P., Greco, L., Floridi, A. and Gallai, V. (2003) Excitatory amino acids and multiple sclerosis: evidence from cerebrospinal fluid. *Archives of Neurology* 60, 1082–1088.

Schipper, R.G., de Groot, H.J.M., Thio, M. and Verhofstad, A.A.J. (2004) Intracellular localization of ornithine decarboxylase and its regulatory protein, antizyme-1. *Journal of Histochemistry and Cytochemistry* 52, 1259–1266.

Schmitz, Y., Luccarelli, J., Kim, M., Wang, M. and Sulzer, D. (2009) Glutamate controls growth rate and branching of dopaminergic axons. *The Journal of Neuroscience* 29, 11973–11981.

Scholl-Burgi, S., Gotwald, T., Albrecht, U. and Karall, D. (2009) Stroke-like episodes in propionic academia caused by central focal metabolic decompensation. *Neuropediatrics* 40, 76–81.

Schulman, A.S., Claridge, J.A., Evans, H.L. and Sawyer, R.G. (2006) Does enteral glutamine supplementation decrease infectious morbidity? *Surgical Infections* 7, 29–35.

Semmler, A., Simon, M. and Linnebank, M. (2008) Polymorphisms of methionine metabolism and susceptibility to meningioma formation. *Journal of Neurosurgery* 108, 999–1004.

Sengers, B.G., Please, C.P. and Lewis, R.M. (2010) Computational modelling of amino acid transfer interactions in the placenta. *Experimental Physiology* 95, 829–840.

Shafqat, S., Velaz-Faircloth, M., Henzi, V.A., Whitney, K.D., Yang-Feng, T.L., Seldin, M.F. and Fremeau, R.T. Jr (1995) Human brain-specific L-proline transporter: molecular cloning, functional expression and chromosomal localization of the gene in human and mouse genomes. *Molecular Pharmacology* 48, 219–229.

Shimada, T. (2006) Salivary proteins as a defence against dietary tannins. *Journal of Chemical Ecology* 32, 1149–1163.

Silberman, G.A., Fan, T.H., Liu, H., Boulden, B.M., Widder, J., Fredd, S., Harrison, D.G., et al. (2010) Uncoupled cardiac nitric oxide synthase mediates diastolic dysfunction. *Circulation* 121, 519–528.

Simon, R.A. and Ishiwata, H. (2003) Adverse reactions to food additives. In: D'Mello, J.P.F. (ed.) *Food Safety. Contaminants and Toxins*. CAB International, Wallingford, UK, pp. 235–270.

Skovby, F., Gaustadnes, M. and Mudd, S.H. (2010) A revisit to the natural history of homocystinuria due to cystathionine beta-synthase deficiency. *Molecular Genetics and Metabolism* 99, 1–3.

Solerte, S.B., Gazzaruso, C., Basso, C. and Fioravanti, M. (2008) Nutritional supplements with oral amino acid mixtures increases whole-body lean mass and insulin sensitivity in elderly subjects with sarcopenia. *The American Journal of Cardiology* 101, 69E–77E.

Stanley, C.A. (2009) Regulation of glutamate metabolism and insulin secretion by glutamate dehydrogenase in hypoglycemic children. *American Journal of Clinical Nutrition* 90, 862S–866S.

Stout, J.R., Graves, B.S., Smith, A.E., Cramer, J.T. and Harris, R.C. (2008) The effect of beta-alanine supplementation on neuromuscular fatigue in elderly (55-92 years): a double-blind randomized study. *Journal of the International Society of Sports Nutrition* 7, 5–21.

Suzuki, T., Wada, T., Saigo, K. and Watanabe, K. (2002) Taurine as a constituent of mitochondrial tRNAs: new insights into the functions of taurine and human mitochondrial diseases. *The European Molecular Biology Organization Journal* 21, 6581–6589.

Sweatt, A.J., Wood, M., Wallin, R., Willingham, M.C. and Hutson, S.M. (2004) Branched-chain amino acid catabolism: unique segregation of pathway enzymes in organ systems and peripheral nerves. *American Journal of Physiology, Endocrinology and Metabolism* 286, E64–E76.

Szeliga, M. and Obara-Michlewska, M. (2009) Glutamine in neoplastic cells: focus on the expression and roles of glutaminases. *Neurochemistry International* 55, 71–75.

Takemoto, Y. (2001) Depressor and bradycardic actions of L-proline injected into the nucleus tractus solitarii of anesthetized rats. *The Japanese Journal of Physiology* 51, 687–692.

Takemoto, Y. and Semba, R. (2006) Immunohistochemical evidence for the localization of neurons containing the putative transmitter L-proline in rat brain. *Brain Research* 1073, 311–315.

Tanizawa, Y., Nakai, K., Ohta, Y., Inoue, H., Matsuo, K., Furukawa, S. and Oka, Y. (2002) Unregulated elevation of glutamate dehydrogenase activity induces glutamine-stimulated insulin secretion: identification and characterization of a GLUD 1 gene mutation and insulin secretion studies with MIN6 cells over-expressing the mutant glutamate dehydrogenase. *Diabetes* 51, 712–717.

Tessari, P., Coracina, A., Vettore, M., Valerio, A., Zaramella, M. and Garibotto, G. (2005) Effects of insulin on methionine and homocysteine kinetics in type 2 diabetes with nephropathy. *Diabetes* 54, 2968–2976.

Thomas, B., Gruca, L.L., Bennett, C., Hanson, R.W. and Kalhan, S.C. (2008) Metabolism of methionine in the newborn infant: response to the parenteral and enteral administration of nutrients. *Pediatric Research* 64, 1–2.

Topal, G., Brunet, A., Walch, L., Boucher, J.L. and David-Dufilho, M. (2006) Mitochondrial arginase II modulates nitric oxide synthesis through nonfreely exchangeable L-arginine pools in human endothelial cells. *The Journal of Pharmacology and Experimental Therapeutics* 318, 1368–1374.

Twelvetrees, A.E., Lumb, M.J., Triller, A. and Kittler, J.T. (2010) Delivery of GABA to synapses is mediated by HAP1-K1F5 and disrupted by mutant huntingtin. *Neuron* 65, 53–65.

Ubeda, N., Alonso-Aperte, E. and Varela-Moreiras, G. (2002) Acute valproate administration impairs methionine metabolism in rats. *Journal of Nutrition* 132, 2737–2742.

Uccella, S., Cerutti, R., Vigetti, D., Furlan, D., Oldrini, R., Pelosi, G., Passi, A., *et al.* (2006) Histidine decarboxylase, DOPA decarboxylase and vesicular monoamine transporter 2 expression in neuroendocrine tumours: immunohistochemical study and gene expression analysis. *Journal of Histochemistry and Cytochemistry* 54, 863–875.

Uribarri, J. and Tuttle, K.R. (2006) Advanced glycation end products and nephrotoxicity of high-protein diets. *Clinical Journal of the American Society of Nephrology* 1, 1293–1299.

Verrall, L., Burnet, P.W., Betts, J.F. and Harrison, P.J. (2010) The neurobiology of D-amino acid oxidase. *Molecular Psychiatry* 15, 122–137.

von Versen-Hoynck, F., Rajakumar, A., Parrott, M.S. and Powers, R.W. (2009) Leptin affects system A amino acid transport in the human placenta: evidence for STAT3 dependent mechanisms. *Placenta* 30, 361–367.

Visvanathan, K., Boorman, D.W., Strickland, P.T., Hoffman, S.C., O'Brien, T.G. and Guo, Y. (2004) Association among ornithine decarboxylase polymorphism, androgen receptor gene (CAG) repeat length and prostate cancer risk. *The Journal of Urology* 171, 652–655.

Vrshek-Schallhorn, S., Wahlstrom, D., Benolkin, K., White, T. and Luciana, M. (2006) Affective bias and response modulation following tyrosine depletion in healthy adults. *Neuropsychopharmacology* 31, 2523–2536.

Wagner, C. and Koury, M.J. (2007) *S*-Adenosylhomocysteine - a better indicator of vascular disease than homocysteine? *American Journal of Clinical Nutrition* 86, 1581–1585.

Wang, R. and Wu, L. (2003) Interaction of selective amino acid residues of K_{Ca} channels with carbon monoxide. *Experimental Biology and Medicine* 228, 474–480.

Watts, R.W.E. and Watts, R.A. (2007) Alkaptonuria: a 60-year follow-up. *Rheumatology* 46, 358–359.

Wegner, F., Kraft, R., Busse, K., Hartig, W. and Hevers, W. (2008) Functional and molecular analysis of $GABA_A$ receptors in human midbrain-derived neural progenitor cells. *Journal of Neurochemistry* 107, 1056–1069.

Wei, J. and Wu, J.Y. (2008) Post-translational regulation of L-glutamic acid decarboxylase in the brain. *Neurochemical Research* 33, 1459–1465.

Wiens, S.C. and Trudeau, V.L. (2006) Thyroid hormone and γ-amino butyric acid (GABA) interactions in neuroendocrine systems. *Comparative Biochemistry and Physiology - Part A: Molecular and Integrative Physiology* 144, 332–344.

Windle, E.M. (2006) Glutamine supplementation in critical illness: evidence, recommendations and implications for clinical practice in burn care. *Journal of Burn Care Research* 27, 764–772.

Winge, I., McKinney, J.A., Ying, M., D'Santos, C.S., Kleppe, R., Knappskog, P.M. and Haavik, J. (2008) Activation and stabilization of human tryptophan hydroxylase 2 by phosphorylation and 14-3-3 binding. *Biochemical Journal* 410, 195–204.

Wischmeyer, P.E. (2007) Glutamine: mode of action in critical illness. *Critical Care Medicine* 35, S541–S544.

Wu, F., Grossenbacher, D. and Gehring, H. (2007) New transition state-based inhibitor for human ornithine decarboxylase inhibits growth of tumor cells. *Molecular Cancer Therapeutics* 6, 1831–1839.

Wu, F., Yu, J. and Gehring, H. (2008) Inhibitory and structural studies of novel coenzyme-substrate analogs of human histidine decarboxylase. *Federation of American Societies for Experimental Biology* 22, 890–897.

Wu, S.-Z., Bodles, A.M., Porter, M.M., Griffin, W.S.T., Basile, A.S. and Barger, S.W. (2004) Induction of serine racemase expression and D-serine release from microglia by amyloid β-peptide. *Journal of Neuroinflammation* 1, 2–3.

Xue, L., Farrugia, G., Miller, S.M., Ferris, C.D., Snyder, S.H. and Szurszewski, J.H. (2000) Carbon monoxide and nitric oxide as coneurotransmitters in the enteric nervous system: evidence from genomic deletion of biosynthetic enzymes. *Proceedings of the National Academy of Sciences of the USA* 97, 1851–1855.

Xue, Y., Han, X.H. and Chen, L. (2010) Effects of pharmacological block of GABA (A) receptors on pallidal neurons in normal and Parkinsonian state. *Frontiers in Cellular Neuroscience* 22, 2–4.

Yamashina, S., Ikejima, K., Enomoto, N. and Sato, N. (2005) Glycine as a therapeutic immuno-nutrient for alcoholic liver disease. *Alcoholism, Clinical and Experimental Research* 29, 162S–165S.

Yang, C.R. and Svensson, K.A. (2008) Allosteric modulation of NMDA receptor via elevation of brain glycine and D-serine: the therapeutic potentials for schizophrenia. *Pharmacology and Therapeutics* 120, 317–332.

Yang, G., Wu, L., Jiang, B., Yang, W., Qi, J., Cao, K., Meng, Q., *et al.* (2008) H_2S as a physiologic vasorelaxant: hypertension in mice with deletion of cystathionine gamma-lyase. *Science* 322, 587–590.

Yoon, S.J., Lyoo, I.K., Haws, C., Kim, T.-S., Cohen, B.M. and Renshaw, P.F. (2009) Decreased glutamate/glutamine levels may mediate cytidine efficacy in treating bipolar depression: a longitudinal proton magnetic resonance spectroscopy study. *Neuropsychopharmacology* 34, 1810–1818.

Young, L., Salomon, R., Au, W., Allan, C., Russell, P. and Dong, Q. (2006) Ornithine decarboxylase (ODC) expression pattern in human prostrate tissues and ODC transgenic mice. *Journal of Histochemistry and Cytochemistry* 54, 223–229.

Zell, J.A., Ziogas, A., Gerner, E.W. and Anton-Culver, H. (2007) Risk and risk reduction involving arginine intake and meat consumption in colorectal tumorigenesis and survival. *International Journal of Cancer* 120, 459–468.

Zell, J.A., Ziogas, A., Bobbs, A.S., Gerner, E.W. and Anton-Culver, H. (2009) Associations of a polymorphism in the ornithine decarboxylase gene with colorectal cancer survival. *Clinical Cancer Research* 15, 6208–6216.

Zhang, Y., Guo, K., LeBlanc, R.E. and Yu, Y.H. (2007) Increasing dietary leucine intake reduces diet-induced obesity and improves glucose and cholesterol metabolism in mice via multimechanisms. *Diabetes* 56, 1647–1654.

Zinnanti, W.J., Lazovic, J., Griffin, K., Paul, H.S., Bewley, M.C., Cheng, K.C. and Flanagan, J.M. (2008) Dual mechanism of brain injury and novel treatment strategy in maple syrup urine disease. *Brain* 132, 903–918.

Index

Page numbers in **bold** refer to illustrations and tables

acropathy 330
acrylamide 497
activating transcription factor (ATF) 229, 233, **234**–237
activators 61–62, 160
Acute tryptophan or tyrosine depletion test: time for reappraisal 503
adducts, post-translational 492–493
adenosine triphosphate (ATP) 61, 131, 178–180, 361, **362**, 445
adenosine diphosphate (ADP) 3, 8–11
adenosine monophosphate (AMP) 158, 159, **179**, 180, 183
S-adenosylhomocysteine hydrolase (SAH) 176, 180
S-adenosylmethionine (SAMe) 174, 177, 178–180, 181, 182–184, 185, 504
administration protocols 421–422
advanced glycation end-products (AGE)
    see AGE/ALE
advanced lipoxidation end-products (ALE)
    see AGE/ALE
adverse effects
    antagonisms 331–341
    classification 323–**324**
    excitatory amino acids 427–445
    glutamine-glutamate cycle
        disruption 501
    imbalance 323, **324**–331, 346
    homocysteine 342, 346, 369–378, **501**, 506, 507
    investigation technique 343–345
    mechanisms 326–327, 339–341

modified amino acid-based molecules
    382–397, 492, 496–497, 503, **501**,
    503, 504, 506
monosodium glutamate 496
non-protein amino acids **334**–341, **345**
phenylketonuria 406–414, **499**
potential applications 343–345
toxicity 323–**324**, 341, 342–343
see also side-effects; toxicity
age factor 261–263, 373, 388–389, 391, 431, 455
age-related macular degeneration (AMD) 390
AGE/ALE
    accumulations 384–385, 388–394, 395–396
    burden 342–343
    diabetes role 391, 504
    dietary sources 394–395, 397
    disease association 388–394, 492, **501**, 503, 504, 506
    food quality, heating effect 383–384, 496–497
    measurement methods 385
    nutrient utilization effects 328
    rich, foods 394–395
    synthesis 506
ageing 59, 292, 302–303, 373, 386, 391
aggregation 156, 164
aggression 161
agonists 146–147, 148, 430, 443–444, 445, 506
    see also glycine
akinesia 455
β-alanine 489, **494**, 495
alanine 34–35, 199, 205, 220
alanine:glyoxylate aminotransferase (AGT) 37

525

alanine aminotransferase (ALT)
    brain metabolism role 34
    cellular distribution 27–28
    diagnostic biomarker role 38–39
    elevation 39–41
    glucogenesis role 34–35
    isoforms **482**
    serum levels **40**
alanine, serine and cysteine (ASCT)
        transporters 140, 142
albumin 397
alcohol 39, 41, 505
aldose reductase 60–61
Se-allylselenocysteine 344, **345**, 507
allergenicity 388
Alzheimer's disease (AD)
    AGE/ALE accumulation 388–389
    age factor 388–389
    drug 97, 509
    enzyme alterations **498**, 502
    glutamate receptors **428**–430
    histamine system changes 98
    homocysteine status 373, 376
    memory impairment 97
    molecular therapeutics **508**
    supplementation studies 373, 376, 377
Amadori products 383
α-amino-3-hydroxy-5-methyl-4-isoxazolepropionic
        acid (AMPA) 138, 435, 436, 443, 509
α-amino-3-hydroxy-5-methyl-4-isoxazolepropionic
        acid receptor (AMPAR) **428**, 429, 436,
        441, 443
amino acid hydroxylase (AAAH) 150–164
D-amino acid oxidase (D-AAOX) 139, **498**, 502
amino acid regulatory element (AARE) 233,
        234–235
amino acid response (AAR) **234**
amino acids, *lists* **197**, 257, 263, **334**, **339**, **345**, 494
γ-aminobutyric acid (GABA)
    decreased level 434
    depression 437
    distribution 103–104
    epilepsy role 436–437, 509
    histamine co-localization 90–91
    interactions 490, 491–492
    neuropathologies, role 430, 433, 434, 435
    neurotransmission 488–489
    pathway **104**, 105, 430
    production 116, 129
    receptors 104–**105**, **428**, 434, 433, 434, 488
    storage, release and uptake 104
    thyroid dysfunction link 491–492
AminoIndex 466, 467–472, 473
aminotransferases (transaminases)
    disease biomarkers 38–41, 505
    distribution 25–28
    future directions 41–42

    inhibition 341
    isoforms 27–28, **482**
    metabolism impairment 36–38
    nitric oxide cycle **223**
    role 24, 28–36
    transamination 25, **26**, 32, 483
ammonia 54, 205–206, 216–220, 221, 490
ammonium **132**
amygdala 95, 434
β-amyloid (Aβ) 389, 429
amyloid (Aβ peptide) 428
amyotrophic lateral sclerosis (ALS) 346, **428**,
        440–442
anabolic stimuli *see* exercise
analogues, arginine 333–336, 339–340
analogues, sulphur-containing amino acids 336–337,
        340–341
analysis methods **111**, **112**, 139–140, 196, 465
angiotensin 61, 386–387
animal models 3–19, 230, 432–434
anorexia 232, 326
antagonisms **324**, 331–341
antagonists 346, 430, 444
anti-coagulants 372, 468
antibodies 107, 110, **111**–**112**, 115
antinutritional factors (ANF) 248, 249, 252
antioxidants 386, 387, 396
anxiety 95–96, 501, 509
apoptosis (cell death) 130–131, **132**, 146–147, 444,
        445, 501
appetite 93, 326, **327**, 330
arachidonic acid (ARA) 410
arginase
    activity 61–62
    L-arginine metabolism 51–**63**
    distribution 53
    expression 504
    health and disease role 54–60, **498**, **501**
    inhibitors 60, 62–63, 340, 508
    isoforms 53, **482**
    location 53–54
    metabolic role 485
    regulation 60–62
    structure 53–54
    urea cycle role 51–**52**, **74**, **219**, 223
L-arginine-nitric oxide pathway 73–76
arginine
    analogues 333–336, 339–340
    antagonism 332
    dispensable classification 493, 510, 511
    food toxicity 496
    L form 51–53, 54–55, 59, 62, 73–79
    metabolism 51–**63**, 224–225
    nitric oxide yield 323
    pathway **52**, **74**, **217**, **219**, **223**, 505
    physiology 223–224
    provision 196

role in cardiovascular disease 77–78
supplementation 224, **494**, 495
tumour control 507
argininosuccinate 52, **219**, **223**, 505
aromatic amino acid decarboxylase (AADC) 456, **457**, 458, 460
aromatic amino acids 150–164, 201, **334**, 456, 458, 460–461
see also phenylalanine hydroxylase; tryptophan hydroxylase; tyrosine hydroxylase
arousal 94
arteriosclerosis 57, 74, 369, 389–390, 505
arthritis, rheumatoid 392–393, 395
asparagine synthetase (ASNS) 229, 232, 233, **234**
aspartate 35–36, 196, 353, 357, 488
aspartate aminotransferases (AST) 27–28, **33**, 35–36, 38–41, **482**
aspartate/glutamate carrier (AGC) 35, 36
AST/ALT ratio 39
asthma 57, **501**, 508
astrocytes **128**, 129, 130, **193**, 204
asymmetrical dimethyl-arginine (ADMA) 77
atrophy 432
attention deficit/hyperactivity disorder (ADHD) 161–163, 343, 501, 503
AUF1 expression 184–185
aurintricarboxylic acid (ATA) 17
autoantibody targets 107, 110
autoimmune disease 39, 388
availability of amino acids 229–238

B$^{0,+}$ system 195, 199
Bat family proteins 195
beetroot juice, blood pressure reduction 82, 83
behaviour 93–97, 431–432, 503, 512
benchmarks, establishment 480
Best's effect 184
Bickel, Dr Horst 407, 413
binding
ligands 154–155, 164, 358–**359**, 360–**361**
order 156
sites **9**–10, 18–19, 161, 359, **362**
biochemistry 326–**327**, 480, 493
biology, modern molecular 384–385
biomarkers 38–41
see also markers
bipolar disorder 503
blood 110–113, 409
see also plasma
blood pressure 55–56, 82, 83, 180–181, 371, 373
see also hypertension
blood-brain barrier (BBB) 191–208, 419, **420**, 458, 490–491

bone 393, 410
bovine spongiform encephalopathy (BSE) 389
brain
/plasma amino acid gradients 197
amino acid concentrations **198**, 232
amino acid content regulation 194
amino acid availability 490
atrophy 432
developmental stage, tryptophan hydroxylase role 161
function, branched-chain amino acids influence 201
glutamate role 24, **29**–31, 201–202, 444–445
glutaminase expression 127–129
hippocampal slices **439**
histamine system **90**
lesions 341
metabolism 31–34, **420**, 457
neurotransmitters 93, 147–148, 487–490
regulation 124
stem, cyclic adenosine monophosphate (cAMP) effect 159
stimulatory effectors particulate preparations 126
see also blood-brain barrier; neurotransmission
branched-chain amino acids (BCAA)
antagonisms 331–333
brain function 201
brain metabolism role 31–35
brain-barrier crossing 27, 31
catabolism 504
clinical support **494**, 495
depletion 346
depressed/aromatic amino acids ratios 344
deprivation 343–344
efficacy **494**
host tissue losses replenishment 344
metabolism 31–35, 483
requirement **279**, 280
supplements 495
transamination 25, **26**, 483
see also leucine
branched-chain aminotransferase (BCAT)
brain metabolism role 31–34
cellular distribution 27
isoforms 27, **482**–483
muscle **30**
redox sensitivity 38
release 25, **26**
transamination 32
branched-chain keto-acids (BCKA) **31**, 33–34, 331
breakpoint detection **270**, 282
BSB 17
burn care **494**, 495

C/EBP homologous protein (CHOP) 232–233, **234**, 235
Ca^{2+} 434, 443–444, 445, 501
cachexia, hepatic **494**
CAG triplets 430–431
calcium 202, 456
caloric restriction (CR) 395–396
canavanine 333–**335**, **339**, 341, 344, **345**, 507
cancer
    amino acid imbalance 330, **344**
    amino acid-metabolizing enzymes association 504
    amino acids in clinical support **494**
    AminoIndex application 472–**473**
    arginase role 58–59
    drugs 344
    histidine decarboxylase expression 92
    methionine metabolism 174–178
    N-nitrosamines formation effect 83
    non-protein amino acids 507
    ornithine decarboxylase activity **501**, 504, 506, 511
    prevention 507
    RAGE role 390
    saturated and trans fatty intake association 387
    therapy 17, 344, 346, 508
    treatment 184, 506
    ZR75 human breast cancer cells 125
carbamoylphosphate synthetase (CPS) **52**, **219**
carbenoxolone (CBX) 131
carbohydrate 297, 298, 304, 387, 388
carbon dioxide (CO_2) 105, 341, 489–490
carbonyls, reactive 383
α-carboxyl group 105
carboxylation 131
carcinoma 182–185, **494**
    see also cancer
cardiovascular disease (CVD)
    AGE formation association **501**, 503
    AGE/ALE effect 389–390
    arginase role 503
    L-arginine role 77–78
    diet benefits 83, 377
    homocysteine status 372, 373, **374**–**375**, 376, 377
    modified lysine residues 343
    recurrence risk lowering **374**–**375**
    risk factors 342, 373, 376
    vegetable/arginine combined consumption 507
    see also diabetes; hypertension; obesity; vascular disease
cardiovascular function 72–84
carnitine 396
carnosine 396
cascade, biochemical **327**

casein 263, 301
Cat family proteins 195, 232
catabolism **12**, 131, 220, 504
catalysis 154, 155–156, 164, **482**
cataract 390–391
catechins **16**–17
catecholamines, inhibition role 156
catechol-O-methyltransferase (COMT) 456, **457**, 458, 460–461
cationic amino acids (CAA) transporters 195
cationic system y^+ 195–196
cells
    amino acids availability adaptation 229–238
    death (apoptosis) 130–131, **132**, 146–147, 444, 445, 501
    ganglion 144, **145**, 146
    growth switch 181
    growth synchronization 174
    Müller cell (retinal astroglia) 33, 35, 60, 138, 142, 144
    oval 183
    signalling 298–299, 303–304
    see also Müller cell
central nervous system (CNS)
    disorders 97, 161–164, 373, 388–389, 427–445, 454–461, **498**, **501**–503, 506
    entry restriction 205–206
    functioning role, glutamatergic synaptic transmission 445
    histamineric projections 90
    neurotransmitters 127, 129, 161
    regions sensitive to dietary amino acid imbalance 327
    structural components 410
    see also blood-brain barrier
cerebral ischaemia 442, 443–445, 502
    see also stroke
cerebrospinal fluid (CSF) 197, 207, 330, 442
children, growth data 409
chimeric receptor **359**
Chinese restaurant syndrome 496
cholesterol 389
p-chlorophenylalanine (PCPA) 157–158
choline 97, **174**, 428–429
CHOP gene 232–233
choreoathetosis 430, 431
chromatin immunoprecipitation 233
chromatography 116, 385, 468
chromogranin-A 422
chronic obstructive pulmonary disease (COPD) 392, **494**–495
circulation, glutamate role 202
circumvallate papillae 354
cirrhosis 39, 185, **494**
citrulline 52, 62, 73, **74**, **217**, **219**, 222–224, 225, 493
cocaine 95
Coxsackie virus 110

cognition
    deficits 410
    disorders **501**, 502–503, 509
    disturbances 430
    function 373–376, 377, 430, 503
    impairment 342, 389, **501**, 502–503, 506
    losses 431
    systems 502
Collaborative Study of Children treated for PKU 407
colorectomy 247
complexes 3–4, 35–36
conditions
    clinical *list* **494**, **508**
    medical 371–372
    pathological 35, 330, 512
conformation change 154–155
congenitalness 407, 408, 512
Consensus Conference for Phenylketonuria, National Institute for Health (NIH) 413
cooperativity, negative 4
copper-zinc superoxide dismutase 1 (SOD1) gene mutations 440
coronary artery disease (CAD) 77, 78
coronary heart disease (CHD) 372, 373, **374–375**, 376–377, 387
corticosterone, maternal levels 492
critical illness and trauma 220–221
crystal structure 154–155
crystallinity 260, 261
β-cyanoalanine **334**, 337–338, **339**, 341
cystathionine β-synthase (CBS) **175**, **177**, 370, 486
cystathioninuria 341
cysteine 108, 177, 196, **273**, 493, 495
cystinuric patients 330
cytochromes **182**
cytokines 61, 124, 388, 393

dairy products 387–388, 394
    see also milk
data, stability, influencing factors 468
death-associated protein kinase 1 (DAPK 1) 444
deficiency sensing 236–238
dementia 97, 334, 373–376, 377
Demographics and Memory Study (2002) 373
demography, characteristics 370–372
dendrites 429, 432, 434–435
dental implant osseointegration 506
deoxyribonucleic acid (DNA) fragmentation detection 146
dephosphorylation 110
depression **428**, 435–436, 503, 507, 512
deprivation 232, 237–238, 343–344
diabetes
    AGE/ALE role 391
    arginase role 55
    diagnostic tool 107–108, 116
    glutamic acid decarboxylase modulation role 508
    impact on amino acids 503–504, 512
    onset, autoantibody appearance 110
    patients 384, 393
    rats discrimination from normal 466
    renal dysfunction 506
    retinopathy 146
    ROS formation increase 60
    see also insulin
diagnosis 39, 464–473
α (γ)-diaminobutryric acid **334**, 338, **339**
diet
    amino acid sources 397
    cardiovascular benefits 83, 377
    choice 387
    constituents 513
    deficiency 237
    fibre contents 250, **251**
    homocysteine metabolism 370–372
    imbalance 231–232, 237, 324–328
    modulation 506–507
    normal **174**
    phenylalanine restricted 407, 409, 410
    preferences 326
    protein-free 247, 249
    therapy 409–411, 412
    see also food; nutrition; supplements
Dietary Approaches to Stop Hypertension (DASH) study 83
diffusion, *defined* 420
digesta 246–248, 249
digestibility 251–252, 253, 493
digestive system 113, **246**
dihydroxyphenylacetic acid (DOPAC) 456
dihydroxyphenylalanine (DOPA) 454–461
dimethylarginine dimethylaminohydrolase (DDAH) 78
dinitrogen trioxide (N_2O_3) formulation equation 82
direct amino acid balance (DAAB) 268, 272, **273**–274, 275, **281**
direct amino acid oxidation (DAAO) 272–**273**, **274**, 281
direct amino acids 268, 272–275, 280
disorders
    age-related macular degeneration (AMD) 390
    aggression 161
    allergy 388
    Alzheimer's disease (AD) 97, 98, 373, 376, 388–389, **428**–430, **498**, 502, **508**
    amyotrophic lateral sclerosis (ALS) 338, 346, **428**, 440–442
    ALS/Parkinsonism dementia complex (PDC) 338
    anorexia 232, 326
    anxiety 95–96, 501, 509

530 Index

disorders (*continued*)
  asthma 57, **501**, 508
  atherosclerosis 57–58, 389–390, **501**
  attention deficit hyperactivity disorder (ADHD) 161–163, 343, 501,503
  autoimmune disease 39, 388
  cancer 58–59, 174–178, 182–185, 330, **344**,390, **494**, 472–**473**, **501**, 504, 506, 507, 511
  cardiovascular disease (CVD) 77–78, 372–373, **374**–**375**, 389–390, **501**, 503
  cataract 390–391
  of central nervous system (CNS) 97, 161–164, 373, 388–389, 427–445, 454–461, **498**, **501**-503, 506
  Chinese restaurant syndrome 496
  chronic obstructive pulmonary disease (COPD) 392, **494**–495
  cirrhosis 39, 185, **494**
  coronary heart disease (CHD) 372–373, **374**–**375**, 376–377, 387
  of cognition, 342, 389, **501**, 502–503, 506
  dementia 97, 334, 338, 373–376, 377
  depression **428**, 435–436, 503, 507, 512
  diabetes 55, 60,107–108, 110, 116, 146, 391, 503–504, 508, 512
  Duchenne muscular dystrophy (DMD) 312–318, **494**–495
  dyskinesias 458–460, 506
  endocrine 391–392, 513
  epilepsy **428**, 436–440, **498**, **501**, 502, **508**, 509
  of the eye 390–391
  fibrosis 61, 467, 468–**470**
  genetic disorders 406–414, **499**–**501**, 505, 512
  hepatic encephalopathy 330
  hepatocellular carcinoma (HCC) 182–185
  homocysteinaemia 372–373
  homocystinuria 372
  Huntington's disease (HD) 330, **428**, 430–434, 509
  hyperhomocysteinaemia 342, 371, 372, 373, 376
  hyperinsulinism/hyperammonaemia syndrome (HHS) 11–13, 16–17, 505
  hyperlysinaemia 332–333
  hypertension 55–56, 82, 83, 180–181, 371, 373
  hypoglycaemia 341, 346
  imbecillitas phenylpyruvica 406–407
  inflammation 343, 385, 386–387, 509, 512
  ischaemia 57, 78–79, 84, 442, 443–445, 496, 502, 512
  Kawasaki disease 163
  lists **494**, 497, **498**, **499**–**501**, **508**, 512
  liver disease 39–41, 173–178, 182–185, 221, 344, 346, 467, 468–**470**, **494**, 505
  maple syrup urine disease (MSUD) 37, **500**
  metabolic syndrome (MetS) 470–**471**
  mood 419, 422, 436
  movement 430, 431, 458, 460, 512
  multiple sclerosis **498**, 502, 512
  nephropathy 58, 394
  neural tube defects (NTD) 369, 371, 376, 371, 377, 378, 496, 507
  neurodegenerative 37–38, 388–389, 427–445, 454–461, **498**, **501**, 502, 506, 512
  neurolathyrism 346, 502
  neurological 427–445
  neuropsychiatric 418–423, **501**, 502–503
  neurotoxicity 334, 337, 341, 496
  non-alcoholic fatty liver disease (NAFLD) 39, 41, 173–174, 185, 505
  obesity 373, 395–396, 497–498, 512
  osteoporosis 158, 393
  Parkinson's disease (PD) 346, 389, **428**, 429–430, 454–461, **498**, 502, 506, 509
  pellagra 332
  phenylketonuria (PKU) 156, 343, 406–414, 496, **499**, 505
  psychotic **498**, 512
  retinopathy 60
  rheumatoid arthritis 392–393, 395
  schizophrenia **428**, 434–435, **501**, 502, 503, **508**, 509
  seizures 436–437, **438**, 502, 508
  septic encephalopathy 329–330
  short bowel syndrome (SBS) 314–315
  sickle cell disease 56
  steatohepatitis 181–182
  stress **315**, 386, 397, 435
  stroke 372–373, **374**, **375**, 376, 377, **428**, 442–445, 496, 498, 502
  sudden infant death syndrome (SIDS) 163
  trauma 220–221
  tumours 92, 122, 124, 344, 346, 507, 509
  uraemia 384
  vascular disease 59, 61, 77, 78, 371, 372, 373, 376–377, 387, 506
  venous thromboembolism (VTE) 372, 373, 377
  'vomiting sickness' 338
dispensable amino acids 493, 510, 511
  see also non-essential amino acids
docosahexaenoic acid (DHA) 410
dopamine (DA)
  biosynthesis 456
  deficiency 410, 454, 455
  delivery tool 460
  distribution 156–157
  factors 512
  hypothesis 502
  hypothesis of reward 94–95
  metabolism 456, **457**
  neurons degeneration 429
  neurotransmission system 503

pools 343
receptors role 509
schizophrenia theory 434
system 95
see also levodopa
Down's syndrome 97, 389
drugs
    addiction 509
    addictive 95
    Alzheimer's disease 97, 509
    anti-cancer 344
    binding sites 18–19
    development 513
    glutaminase expression suppression 131
    rewards 94–95
    targets 107, 110, 432, 506, 507–509, 512
    tetrahydrobiopterin (BH_4) 412–413
    see also inhibitors
Duchenne muscular dystrophy 312–318, **494**–495
dyskinesias 458–460, 506
    see also movement disorders; Parkinson's disease

elderly 296, 301, 303, 304, 495
    see also age factor; ageing
electrostatic interactions, substrate orientation importance 154
emerging methods 502–503
emotional disturbances 430
encephalopathy 221, 329, 344, 346, 466, **494**
endocrine 391–392, 513
endogeny 146–147, 245–253, 513
endothelial nitric oxide synthase (eNOS) 73, **76**
endothelium 59–60, 61, 72–84, 192, **193**, 204
endurance exercise (EE) 296–298, 304
energy 250, 395–396, 481
entacapone 458
enzyme-hydrolysed protein methods 247–248
enzymes
    S-adenosylhomocysteine hydrolase (SAH) 176, 180
    D-amino acid oxidase (D-AAOX) 139, **498**, 502
    aminotransferases 24–42, **482**, 483, 505
    arginase 51–**63**, **74**, **219**, 223, **482**, 485, **498**, **501**, 504, 508
    AMP-activated protein kinase (AMPK) **179**, 180–185
    aromatic amino acid decarboxylase (AADC) 456, **457**, 458, 460
    asparagine synthetase (ASNS) 229,232–**234**
    carbamoylphosphate synthetase (CPS) **52**, **219**
    cystathionine β-synthase **175**, **177**, 370, 486
    in genetic disorders 406–414, **499**–**501**, 505
    glutamate decarboxylase (GAD) 103–116, **482**, 484, 508

glutamate dehydrogenase (GDH) 3–19, 36, **482**–483, 491, 505, 506
glutaminase (GA) 122–**132**, **223**, **482**, 484, **498**, 504
glutamine synthetase (GS) 30, **313**, 484, 502, 508
γ-glutamyl transpeptidase (GGT) 206–207
glycine N-methyltransferase (GNMT) 176–177, 181, 184–185
histidine decarboxylase (HDC) 89–98, 105–106, **481**, **482**, 485, **498**, 504, 508
kinases 62, 159, **179**–180, 183, 236–237, 508
lists **282**, **481**, **482**–487, **498**, **499**, **500**, **501**
methionine adenosyltransferase (MAT) 174, **175**–178, 180–185, **482**, 486
methylene-THF reductase(MTHFR) **175**, 177, 178, 370, 372
as molecular targets 507–508
monoamine oxidase (MAO) 151, **420**, 456, **457**
neuronal role 28–34, 36, **75**, **90**, 93, 95, 103, 104, 126–131, 142–144, 146–147, **151**, 152, 161, **482**
nitric oxide synthase (NOS) 57, 72–81, 196, 222, **223**, 408, **482**, 485, **498**
ornithine carbamoyl-transferase (OCT) **52**, 341
ornithine decarboxylase (ODC) 54, 340, 484–485, **498**, **501**, 504, 506, 507, 508, 511
phenylalanine hydroxylase 150–151, **153**, 406, 408, 413, 486
regulation 3–11, 14–15, 17–19, 60–63, 125–127, 156–161, 180–182, 233
serine racemase 137–148, 485–486
tryptophan hydroxylase (TPH) 150–164, **420**, **482**, 486
tyrosine hydroxylase (TH) 150–151, 456, 486, 506
of urea cycle 51–**52**, **219**, 341, 485
eosin-stained JB-4 plastic embedded section, C57B1/6 mouse retina **138**
epigallocatechin (EGC) **16**
epigallocatechin gallate (EGCG) **16**–17
epilepsy **428**, 436–440, **498**, **501**, 502, **508**, 509
epitopes **112**–113
erectile dysfunction 56, 60
essential amino acids (EAA)
    classification 292, 493
    ingestion 303
    lists **200**, 231
    muscle protein synthesis maximization requirement 296
    source, food 230, 292
    synthesis, gut microbes 253
    synthesis inability 230, 292
    see also indispensable amino acids
estimation methods **251**, 256–257, 258, 263–264, 267–284, 493
ethanol 95
ethanolamine 174

ethylendiamine tetracetic acid disodium salt
    (EDTA 2Na) 468
p-ethynylphenylalanine 158
Examination Committee of Criteria for Metabolic
    Syndrome 471
exaption 15
exchange, inter-organ **217**
excitatory amino acid (EAA)
    disorders 428–445
    major 437
    neurological/neurodegenerative disorders
        role 427–445
    neuropathies **428**
    principle 342
    receptors **428**–436
    retinal 138
    transport system 199
    see also aspartate; glutamate
Excitatory amino acids as a final common pathway for
    neurological disorders 342
excitotoxicity
    advanced glycation end-products 441
    adverse effect subdivision 346
    blocking 444
    concept 342
    epilepsy role 436–437
    glutamate 146, 433, 501–502
    hypothesis 202, 433
    neuropathologies role 441, 445
    see also adverse effects; toxicity
exercise 292–298, 299, 301, 302, 303, 304
exogenous amino acids, mechanism
    of action **293**
extracellular fluid (ECF) 191, 195, 197,
    203, 208
eye disorders 390–391
    see also retina

factorial prediction, requirements 281–282
fatty acids
    deficiency 410
    dietary modulation 507
    essential 410
    homeostasis regulation 237–238
    intake 387
    mobilization **182**
    oxidation 15
    supplements 377
fear 95–96, 509
fibre 250, 253
fibrosis 61, 467, 468–**470**
Fischer's ratio 466, 467, **470**
flora, intestinal 396
fluorescence measuring 385
α-fluoromethylhistidine 92, 93–94
fluxes, inter-organ 215–226, 481

folate (folic acid)
    clinical efficacy 373
        dietary 507
    cycle **175**
    deficiency 410
    homocysteine status role 371, 372, **374**–**375**,
        376, 377, 507
foliate papillae **354**
folic acid *see* folate
Følling, Asbjørn 406–407, 413
food
    additives 342, 346, 358, 496, 511
    AGE/ALE rich 394–395
    amino acids, availability 256–264, 493
    amino acids, source 257, 258, 260–261, 493
    aversion triggering 236–237
    dry matter intake **251**
    intake 93, 94, 236–237, 326
    medical, manufacturers **411**
    nitrate/nitrite source **80**, 82–83
    preparation habits changing 395
    processing
        adverse effects 511
        damage 252
        heat **260**, 261, 263, 383–384, 394,
            496–497
        industrial 382–397
        microwaving avoidance 395
        nutritional value reductions 511
    proteins 256–264
    quality 304
        reward 363
    safety 511
    toxicology 496–497
free amino acid pool 216, 230–231
fruit consumption 83
fungiform papillae **354**
Furchgott, Robert Francis 81

G protein coupled receptors (GPCR)
    modulators 359–360
galanin 91
Garrod, Archibald 407
gases 489–490
gastrointestinal system (GI) 164, 250, 386, 392
GCN2/ATF4 pathway **234**, 235–238
gel shift experiments 233
general control non-derepressive 2 (GCN2) **234**,
    235–238
Genetic Metabolic Dieticians International
    (GMDI) 413
genetics
    disorders 406–414, **499**–**501**, 505, 512
    gene
        coding 151–152
        expression 158, 229–238, 490

factors 372
GCH1/TH availability ratio 460
histidine decarboxylase 91
knock-out 92–93, 131
mutations 440
polymorphism 92
regulation, amino acid starvation 233
structure, glutamic acid decarboxylase 110
therapy 413, 459–460
transcripts 123–125, 130, 221, 232–238
viral vector-mediated transfer delivery method 460, 461
homocysteine status 372
molecular genetic techniques 92
genotypes 372
glaucoma 391
gliomas, malignant 128–129
gliosis 432
glucocorticoids 123, 158, 435–436
gluconeogenesis 34, 220, 323
glucose 34, 35, 60–61, 131, 220, 507
glucose-alanine cycle **30**, 34
glutamate
   adverse effects 496
   binding 5
   chemistry 115–116
   classification 487–488, 511
   in clinical support **494**, 495
   compartmentation 202
   concentrations 205
   cycle **29**, **32**, 34–35, **128**, 129–130, **498**
   disease contribution 146, 502
   dysfunction 498
   excitotoxicity 146, 433, 501–502
   fates 30
   formation 31–32
   inhibition 33, 126–127, 438, 445
   L form 103, 105, 138, 353, **357**
   location 436
   metabolism 35–36, 442, 493, 502
   molecular interactions 490
   near depletion 131
   neurotransmission 128, 342, 436–437
   neurotransmitter function 201–202, 487–488
   oxidation 36
   plasma 201–202
   pool maintenance 24
   recognition 359
   receptors 428–430, 434–436, 441, 443–445, **508**
   recycling 129
   regulation 434
   release 434, 438, **439**
   synthesis 33, 122, 131
   system 445, 502, 506, 508
   toxicity 37–38, 342
   transport 196, 200, 202–**204**, 205, 442
   uptake 196
   utilization 130
   see also taste; umami
glutamate decarboxylase (GAD)
   antibody reactive protein detection **111**
   characterization 107–110
   clinical significance **498**
   decarboxylation reaction 105–107
   decreased level 434
   diabetes diagnostic tool 107–108
   distribution 107–110
   expression in blood leucocytes 110–113
   gene structure 110
   genetics 107–108, 110–**113**, 114, **115**, 116
   isoforms 105–106, 107, 129, **482**, 484
   modulation 508
   post-translational modification 108
   purification 110
   review 103–116
   sequence **108–109**, 110–113
   taste signalling 113–115
   see also γ-aminobutyric acid
glutamate dehydrogenase (GDH)
   active site 5–11
   allostery 8–9, 11, 14–15
   animal 3–19
   antenna region **14**
   clinical significance **498**
   dynamics 7
   evolution **14**
   genetic defects 505
   glutamate metabolism role 36
   inhibition 7–8, **16**, 17–19, 505
   insulin disorders 11–14, 16–17, 491, 505, 506
   isoforms **482**
   neurobiological function **482**–483
   regulation 8–13
   structure 4–**5**, 6
   suppression need 15
glutaminase (GA)
   apoptosis, role 131–**132**
   clinical significance **498**
   expression 127–130
   genes and transcripts 123–125
   glutamate-glutamine cycle, role **128**–130, 484
   isoforms 125–127, **482**, 504
   nitric oxide cycle, role **223**
glutamine
   accumulation 205
   ammonia balance 205
   anatomical location 313
   catabolism 131
   clinical outcomes 317–318
   conversion 130

glutamine (*continued*)
  cycle 29, 32, 34–35, **128**, 129–130, **498**
  dispensable classification 493, 510, 511
  enhanced fluxes 220
  enteral administration 224
  genes 130
  metabolism 122, 216–**220**, 224, **313**–317
  nutritional therapy importance 494, **495**
  oxidation 30–31, 36
  pharmaconutrient role 493
  physiology 222–223
  plasma, concentration decline 220–221
  substrate 124–125
  supplementation 316–318, 495
  toxicity 131
  transcriptional factors 130
  transport 196, **204**, 206
  uptake 218, 222
  utilization 123
glutamine synthetase (GS) 30, **313**, 484, 502, 508
γ glutamyl transpeptidase (GGT) 206–207
glutathione (GSH) 206, 386, 495
glutenoids intake 387
glycation 389, 393, 492
glycine 148, 199, 488–489, 509
glycine *N*-methyltransferase (GNMT) 176, 177, 181, 184, 185
glycogen 298
glycolysis 181
glycomacropeptide 406, 412
Golgi metal impregnation method 432
gonadotropin modulation 491
gradients, brain and plasma 197
growth hormone (GH) 231
Guam dementia 334, 338, 502
guanosine triphosphate (GTP) 3, 7–**8**, **12**, 15, 456, **457**
guanosine monophosphate (GMP) 353–354
guanylyl cyclase 75
gut 158, 164, 249–250, 253
Guthrie, Robert 407, 413

haematoxylin **138**
health and disease 511–512
heart disease 372, 373, 376–377, 387, 407, 408
  see also cardiovascular disease
heat-processing, food **260**, 261, 263, 383–384, 394, 496–497
hepatic *see* liver
hepatitis 39, 41, 470
hepatocarcinogenesis 185
hepatocellular carcinoma (HCC) 182–185
hepatocytes 174–181, 184–185
hexachlorophene (HCP) 18
hibernation 81
high density lipoproteins (HDL) 389–390

high performance liquid chromatography (HPLC) 385, 468
high-fructose corn syrup (HFCS) 387, 391
histamine
  co-localization 90–91
  cognitive function role 503
  dementia, role 97
  depletion 96–98
  interactions 490
  learning and memory role 96
  metabolism 90
  neuronal 90
  neurophysiology and behaviour, role 93–97
  physiological function role 89–90
  receptors 92, 93, 502, **508**, 509
  release 508
  stress response regulation 95
  synthesis 89, **90**
  system **90**, 498
histidine 89–**90**, 383, 396, 503
histidine decarboxylase (HDC) 89–98, 105–106, **481**, **482**, **498**, 485, 504, 508
homeostasis 230–238, 386
homoarginine **334**, 335–336, **339**, 340
homocysteinaemia 372–373
homocysteine 342, 346, 369–378, **501**, 506, 507
homocystinuria 372
homology 107, **108–109**
homovanillic acid (HVA) 456, **457**
homozygotes onset, age 431
hormones 386, 388, 391, 409, 491–492
human antigen R (HuR) **179**, 180, 184–185
human startle disease 509
humoral factors 60–61, 330
huntingtin protein 430, 432, 433, 434
Huntington's disease (HD) 330, **428**, 430–434, 509
hydrogen sulphide (H_2S) 489
hydrolation mechanism 164
hydrolysate 301
hydroxyproline 467
hyperammonaemia 221, 505
hyperargininaemia 59
hyperhomocysteinaemia 342, 371, 372, 373, 376
hyperinsulinism/hyperammonaemia (HHS) 11–13, 16–17, 505
hyperlysinaemia 332–333
hyperparathyroidism 386
hypertension 55–56, 82, 83, 180–181, 371, 373
hypoglycaemia 341, 346
hypoglycin **334**, **336**, 338, **339**, 341, 346
hypothalamic-pituitary-adrenal axis 436
hypothalamus 94

ILEA Commission on Classification and Terminology 436
ileum 245–253, 261

illness, critical 220–221
imbalance
  adverse effects 323, **324**–331, 346
  clinical 328–331, 497
  clinical benefit 343–**344**
  concept 324, 497
  diet 231–232, 237, **324**–328
  disorders 327, 330, **344**, 497
  imposition 343
  nutritional 324–328
  precipitating **325**
  research titles 329
  therapeutic potential **344**
imbecillitas phenylpyruvica 406–407
imidazolamine histamine 89–90
immune modulators 513
immune system 238, 386
immunodetection **143**, **145**
immunohistochemistry **113**, 385
immunostaining **113**
index, diagnostic, algorithm 466
indicator amino acid balance (IAAB) 268, **278**, **280**, **281**, 283–284
indicator amino acid oxidation (IAAO) 258–259, 260–261, **262**, 276–280, **281**, 283
indispensable amino acids (IAA)
  conditional 230, 493
  graded intakes, metabolic responses **281**
  protein malnutrition metabolism adjustment 230–231
  requirements **271**, **273**, **279**, **280**, **282**, **284**
  see also essential amino acids
indospicine **334**, 336, **339**, 340, 341
inducible nitric oxide synthase (iNOS) 58, 502
infarct 442, 443
inflammation 343, 385, 386–387, 509, 512
ingestion timing 292, 296, 297–298, 300, 304
inheritance 431, 505
inhibition, pharmacological 92
inhibitors 17, 61, 62, 78, 164
innovation 509
inosine monophosphate (IMP) 353–354, 357, 359
institutional review board (IRB) approval 421
insulin
  antiproteolytic effects 303
  disorders 11–14, 16–17, 491, 506
  exercise insulinotropic stage **297**
  homeostasis 11, 15
  hyperstimulated secretion **12**
  regulation 11
  resistance 388, 505
  signalling process 491
  see also diabetes
insulin-like growth factors (IGF) 231
interactions 154, 490–493, 512, 513
interleukin 6 (IL-6) elevations 386
intermediates, dispensability 493

interneurons, aspiny 432
intestine, small **113**
ions, transport 193–194
irinotecan, anti-cancer drug 344
iron, reduction mechanisms 155–156
irritable bowel syndrome 509
ischaemia 57, 78–79, 84, 442–445, 496, 502, 512
isoleucine **26**
isotope dilution 248
isotopic carbon dioxide ($^{13}CO_2$) 277, 279–280, 341
isozymes **482**

kainate receptors (KAR) 138, **428**, 435, 437–440, 443
Kawasaki disease 163
ketamine 436
α-keto acids 35, **483**
keto-acids 25, **26**, 493
ketogenesis 323
kidney 123, 221, 343, 371
kidney glutaminase (KGA) **123**, **125**, 126, 127, 129, 131, 504
kinases 62, 159, **179**–180, 183, 236–237, 508
kindling 437, **438**
kinetics 126, 513
Kruskal-Wallis test 469–470
Kure, Professor Shigeo 408
Kuvan® 406, 412–413

L-1 system 195, 419
labels 129, **192**, 248, 259–260
lactate **32**, 35, 36
lactate-alanine shuttle 34
lactic acid bacteria (LAB) 396–397
large neutral amino acids (LNAA) 199, 201, 406, 412, 419, 490
learning, memory 96–97
Lenke, R 407
leptin 409
leucine
  ageing sarcopenia role 302–303
  balance 258, 268, 280, 281, **283**
  brain metabolism role 31–33
  deprivation 237–238
  glutamate dehydrogenase regulation 4, 15
  induced antagonisms 331–332
  insulin relationship 17, 491
  large neutral amino acids affinity 199
  metabolism measurement **314**
  obesity treatment role 498
  oxidation 268, 278, 296
  pellagra 332
  requirements **273**, 275, 277, 282
  signalling 491
  supplementation 303

leucine (*continued*)
 transamination 32
 utilization 258
leucine carboxyl methyltransferase-1 (LCMT1) 180
leucocytes 110–113
levodopa (L-DOPA) 158, 429, 454–461, 506, 509
Levy, Harvey 407
ligands
 binding 154–155, 164, 358–**359**, 360–**361**
 list **157**
 neurotransmission 15
lipopolysaccharide (LPS) 397
lipotropism **174**
liver
 ammonia production 219–220
 arginase 54
 catabolism increase acceleration **12**
 cirrhosis 39, 185, **494**
 disease 39–41, 173–178, 182–185, 221, 344, 346, 505
 disorders 330, 392, **494**
 dysfunction 341, 467
 fat 39, 41, 173–**174**, **182**, 185, 505
 fibrosis 467, 468–**470**
 function tests markers 39
 gluconeogenesis substrate 124–125
 glutamate production and consumption 220
 glutaminase **123**, 124, **125**, 126–127, 504
 injury markers **40**
 isozymes 123
 kinase 179–180
 methionine metabolism **175**, **177**, 180–182
 nutritional imbalance effect **327**
 regeneration 180–182, 185
 S-adenosylmethionine action spectrum **183**
 treatment 467
 urea cycle enzymes expression **219**, 485
 see also liver glutaminase
long-duration response (LDR) 458
losses determination 248
lung 343, 392, 506
lysine
 adducts 346, 504
 antagonism 332
 availability **260**, 261
 food processing effect **252**, 383
 gut-endogenous flows 250, **251**
 intake against N balance, non-linear regression **270**
 modification 387
 requirement **273**, 278, **279**, **280**, 281, 283
 residues, modified 342–343
 supplements 326
 transport 199, 340
lysinoalanine 497

Maillard, Louis-Camille 383, 384
Maillard products 252, 383, 384, 496–497
 see also AGE/ALE
malate dehydrogenase 36
malate/aspartate shuttle 35
mammalian target of rapamycin (mTOR) 291
maple syrup urine disease (MSUD) 37, **500**
markers 38–41, 162, 497, 505, 512, 513
mass spectrography 385
matrix metalloproteinases (MMP) 393
meat 394, 496, 511
mediators 460, 461, 503, 513
medical food manufacturers **411**
medication use 371–372
 see also drugs
Mediterranean diet pyramid 83
melanoids (pigments) 383
memantine 509
membranes 192, **194**, **201**, 420
memory 96–97, 431, 503
mental retardation 406
metabolic ammonia (NH_3) 490
metabolic availability (MA) determination 257, 258, **260**, 261–263, 264
metabolic syndrome (MetS) 470–**471**
metabolism
 adjustment 230–231
 after supplements post-enteral administration 224
 alterations 437
 arginine 51–63, 72–84, 219, 223, 485
 canavanine 333–**335**
 clinical disorders list **498**, **499**–**501**
 co-enzyme 422
 cost 249–252
 cycles 216
 disorders 407, 497, **498**–**501**, 511
 DOPA **457**–458
 dysfunctional **501**, 513
 efficacy 493
 enzymes lists **481**, **482**, **498**–**501**
 ethos support 512–513
 glutamate 3–19, 103–117, 313, **482**–**483**, 484
 glutamine 122–132, 484
 histidine 89–98, 485
 homocysteine 370
 imbalance consequences 464–465
 major developments 510
 major sites 481
 mammalian **481**–482
 measurement **314**
 methionine 173–185, 486–487
 ornithine 54, 484–485
 reactions list **481**
 regulation 229, 230–235, 513
 selenomethionine **336**
 summary 510

transamination 24–42, 483
tryptophan 150–164, **420**, 486
zonation **220**
metabolites 3–4, 29, 36, 465
  see also glutamate; leucine
metabotropic glutamate receptor (mGluR) 357, **428**, 434, 435, 436, 443–444
metal bridging 53–54
METAVIR scoring system 469
methamphetamine 95, 503
methionine
  auxotrophy 184
  control 185
  cycle 175, **175**
  enzymes **482**, 486–487
  hepatocytes 174–178
  inherited disorder 372
  kinetics alteration 495
  manipulation 184–185
  metabolism 173–185, 372, 486–487, 504
  regulation 180–182
  requirement estimation studies **273**, **279**, **280**
  synthase deficiency 369
  therapeutic aspects 344
  toxicity 342
methionine adenosyltransferase (MAT) 174–177, 180–181, 184, 185, **482**, 486
methodologies
  carbon balance 283
  detection 90
  emerging 502–503
  enzyme-hydrolysed protein methods 247–248
  Golgi metal impregnation 432
  IAAO/IAAB, strengths and limitations **278**
  issues 376–377
  measurement 257, 259–260, **314**, 385, 468, 513
  molecular 92, 513
  N balance 268, **270**, **271**, 283
  peptide alimentary 247–248
  tracer 271–281, 283
  transport systems 192–194
  ultrafiltration 247–248
  see also analysis; estimation methods
N-methyl D-aspartate (NMDA) 138, 139–140, 142, 147–148, 501, 508
N-methyl D-aspartate receptor (NMDAR)
  agonists 146–147, 430
  antagonist (ketamine) 436
  blocking 443
  co-agonist 139–140
  disproportionate loss 433
  preferential activation 444
  role, neuropathologies **428**, 429, 433, 436, 441, 444, 445
  signalling 435

β-methylamino-L-alanine (BMAA) **334**, 338, **339**, 346, 496, 502
methylation 180, 185
S-methylcysteine sulphoxide (SMCO) **334**, **336**, 337, **339**, **345**, 507
methylenetetrahydrofolate reductase (MTHFR) **175**, 177, 178, 370, 372
methylglyoxal (MGO) 391
Se-methylselenocysteine 344, **345**, 346
methylselenocysteine 344
Michaelis-Menten kinetics 419
microcephaly 407, 408
microflora, intestinal 397
milk 295–296, 301, 302, 304, 387–388, 393
mimosine **334**, 337, **339**, 341, **345**, 507
mitochondrial arginase II 490
mitogen-activated protein kinase (MAPK) 62
modelling approaches 509–510, 513
Moja-De protocol 422
Molecule of the Year (1992) 74–75
molecules, modified amino acid-based 382–397
monoamine oxidase (MAO) **151**, **420**, 456, **457**
monosodium glutamate (MSG) 342, 358, 496, 511
mood disorders 419, 422, 436
morbidities, off-set 302
mossy fibre (MF) terminals 438
motor function 431, 458, 460, 512
movement disorders 430, 431, 458, 460, 512
mRNA 90, 92–93, 123, 158, 293
Müller cell (retinal astroglia) 33, 35, 60, 138, 142, 144
  see also retina
multiple sclerosis **498**, 502, 512
muscle 218, 220, 291–304, 313–316, **327**, 393
  see also Duchenne muscular dystrophy
muscle protein breakdown (MPB) 292, 294, **295**
muscle protein synthesis (MPS) 292–293, 294–**295**, 296, 297, 298–299, 302, 303, 304
mutations 13–14, 36–37
Myc expression 130, 131–132
myocardial I/R 81
myofibre, maintenance and adaptation **293**
myoglobin, half-loading point 81
myosin glycation 393

Na$^+$-LNAA 199
naso-intestinal intubation 247
National PKU Collaborative Study 409
neoplasm 508
  see also cancer; tumours
nephropathy 58, 394
nerve cells *see* neurons
net postprandial protein utilization (NPPU) 257–258
net protein balance (NPB) 292–293, 294, 298, 303
neural death, excitotoxicity hypothesis 202

neural tube defects (NTD) 369, 371, 376, 377, 378, 496, 507
neurochemical disorders 501
 see also anxiety; attention deficit/hyperactivity disorder; schizophrenia
neurodegeneration
 causes 36
 disease 388–389, 498
 disorders 346, 427–445, 454–461, **498**, **501**, 502, 506, 512
 glutamate toxicity role 37–38
 see also Alzheimer's disease; Parkinson's disease; stroke
neuroimaging 362–363
neurolathyrism 346, 502
neurolathyrogens 496
neurology 427–445
neurons
 degeneration 428
 dendritic architecture long-term changes 435–436
 dopaminergic 456
 enzymes 482
 glutamate/glutamine transport role **128**, **204**
 induced damage 428
 ischaemic, death mechanisms 445
 loss 432, 434
 morphology studies 432
 plasticity 237–238
 retinal 142
 umami tuned 363
neuropathologies **428**, 498, 499–503
neurophysiology 93–97, 343
neuroprotection 55
neuropsychiatry 418–423, 491, 512
neurotoxicity **334**, 337, 341, 496
neurotransmission
 abnormalities 435
 alterations 433
 disruption 513
 dopaminergic 503
 excitatory 127, 342
 glutamate ligands role 15
 health role 511
 histamine interactions 93
 inhibitory 103, 116
 N-methyl D-aspartate, role 147–148
 new momentum emergence 487
 receptors 128, 147–148, 342, 436–437
 review 487–490
 see also receptors; signalling systems
neurotransmitters
 lists 93, 487
 see also carbon dioxide; dopamine; γ-aminobutyric acid; glutamate; nitric oxide; serotonin

neutral amino acids (NAA) 196, 199
 see also glutamine; histidine; methionine; phenylalanine; serine; threonine; tryptophan; tyrosine
neutral detergent fibre (NDF) 250, **251**
nicotinamide 185
nicotinamide adenine dinucleotide (NAD$^+$) 4, 422
nicotinamide adenine dinucleotide phosphate (reduced) (NADPH) 4, 5–11, 61
nitrate 72–84, 496
nitrate-nitrite-nitric oxide pathway 79
nitric oxide (NO)
 bioavailability 60, 77, 84
 carbon monoxide interaction 489–490
 cardiovascular role **501**
 cycle, enzymes and substrates **223**, 225, 226
 formation 78, **80**, **81**, **223**
 generation 78–79
 production 60, 62, 75, 341
 synthesis 73, **76**, 196, 490, 505
nitric oxide synthase (NOS)
 clinical significance **498**
 co-factor 408
 co-localization 222
 diastolic dysfunction mediation 503
 inhibition 78
 isoforms 74–75, 196, **482**, 485
 nitric oxide generation 78, **80**, **223**
 substrate 73–76
 uncoupling 57
nitrite 72–84, 496
nitrogen
 /leucine balances estimation 258
 balance 268–271, 292, 513
 carrier 35
 dietary, ileal digestibility estimates **251**
 endogenous 245–246, 248–**249**
 fluxes **128**, 129
 loss 220
 sources 245–**246**
 utilization efficiency 258
non-alcoholic fatty liver disease (NAFLD) 39, 41, 173–174, 185, 505
non-alcoholic steatohepatitis (NASH) 174
non-essential amino acids **200**, 201, 292, 493
 see also dispensable amino acids
non-protein amino acids 333–341, 343–344, **345**, 507
noradrenaline 386
nucleophile 54
nutrient-sensing 233
nutrients 174, 300–301, 327–328, 513
 see also food
nutrition
 amino acid imbalance **327**
 appetite control 93–94
 dispensability attributes 493

guidelines development 413–414
Parkinson's disease effect 507
signals 230
sources, post-exercise **295**
summary 510–511
support 312–318
see also diet; food; supplements

obesity 373, 395–396, 497–498, 512
obligatory amino acid oxidative loss (OAAL) 268, 281
obligatory nitrogen loss (ONL) 281
observational studies 373
oral cavity issues 393
organs **217**
ornithine 51–53
ornithine carbamoyl-transferase (OCT) **52**, 341
ornithine decarboxylase (ODC) 54, 340, 484–485, **498**, **501**, 504, 506, 507, 508, 511
ornithine transcarbamylase **219**
osteoporosis 158, 393
outlook 512–513
oxaloacetate (OAA) 35–36
β-N-oxalylamino-L-alanine (BOAA) **334**, 337, **339**, 346, 496, 502
oxidation
　AST and GDH importance 36
　characterization 127–128
　direct amino acid 268, 272–275
　energy provision 30–31, 296–297
　fatty acids 15
　indicator amino acids 258–261, **262**, 276–280, 283
　leucine 268, 278, 296
　phenylalanine 259–260
oxidative stress 84, 431
oxygen (O_2) 75, **81**, **157**, 250

palmitoylation 108, 110
pancreas **12**
papillae 113, **114**, **115**, 354
parasites 59, 282–283
Parkinson, James 454
Parkinson's disease (PD)
　brain AGE/ALE accumulations 389
　dementia 346
　excitatory amino acids, receptors and effects **428**, 512
　glutamate receptors 429–430
　glutamatergic dysfunction 498, 502
　L-DOPA therapy efficacy 454–461
　nutrition effect 507
　treatment 506, 509
pathological conditions 35, 512
pathophysiology 220–221

pathways 183, 216, 235–236, 457, 481–487, 505
　see also signalling systems
patient, history taking 39
peas **260**, 261, 263
PEGylated recombinant phenylalanine ammonia lyase (PEG-PAL) 413
pellagra 332
pentosidine 390, 393, 395
pentylenetetrazole (PTZ) model of epilepsy 437
periodontitis 393
peripheral arterial disease 372
perspectives 130
pH sensitivity 445
pharmaceuticals 396, 513
pharmacodynamics 458
pharmacokinetics, clinical 458
pharmaconutrients 493
pharmacotherapy, L-DOPA 456–458
phenylalanine
　concentrations 412
　deficiency syndrome 409
　depletion 503
　genetic disorder 343, 406–414, **499**, 505
　indicator balance measurement 277
　oxidation 259–260
　requirements **273**, **280**
　restricted diets 407, 409, 410
　toxicity 343, 346
　transport **200**, 490
phenylalanine ammonia lyase (PAL) 413
phenylalanine hydroxylase (PAH) 150–151, **153**, 406, 408, 413, 486
phenylketonuria (PKU)
　genetic disorder 343, 406–414, **499**, 505
　identification, newborn to adult 406–414
　large neutral amino acids, role 406, 490
　plasma (blood) phenylalanine concentrations 407–409, 412, 413, 505
　therapy, maternal 407–408
　treatment 156, 409–413, 506
　vitamin B deficiency link 410–411, 496
phosphoprotein phosphatase 2A (PP2A) 180
phosphorylation
　binding site 161
　protein stabilization 158, 164
　pyridoxal phosphate dependent enzymes 108, 110
　reversible 159–160
　signalling pathway 236
　stimulation 292
physiological function control 236
physostigmine 97
pigments (melanoids) 383
plants 83, 253, **333**, **334**, 396, 496

plasma
    amino acids
        AminoIndex generation **467**
        concentrations **198**
        distribution, liver fibrosis **469**
        gradients to brain 197
        levels 465
    glutamate 201–202
    glutamine concentration decline 220–221
    membrane domains 194
    nutritional imbalance effect **327**
    storage 468
plasticity 237–238, 509
polyamines 53, 484
polycystic ovary syndrome (PCOS) 391–392
polyglutamine 431
polymerase chain reaction (PCR) analysis **112**, 196
polymorphisms 162–163
polypeptide 293
polyphenols **16**
positron emission tomography (PET) studies 423
postprandial protein utilization (PPU) 257, 280–281
pre-Nitric-Oxide-era (1953) 81
prefrontal cortex (PFC) 436, **498**
prion proteins 389
probiotics 396–397
proline (Pro) 53, 294, 488, 492–493, 497, 509
protein
    consumption after exercise 297
    deficiency 231–232
    digestibility-corrected amino acid score (PDCAAS) 251, 257
    dysfunctioning 394
    endogenous, loss 246
    fast/slow 301
    foods **257**–258, 260–261, **353**
    -free diet 247
    ingestion during exercise 298
    metabolism 316–317, 512
    nutritional value measure 257
    prescription 409–410
    proline-rich 492–493
    quality 232, 257–258, 262–263
    regulation 233, 292, **293**
    requirements 294
    sources **263**, 302, 304, **325**, 412
    states 466
    synthesis **259**, 301
    translation process 293
    turnover 292–293, 301, 513
    undernutrition 231
    utilization 280–281, 328
protein digestibility-corrected amino acid score (PDCAAS) 251, 257
proteolysis, suppression 301

protocols 276, 281, 409, 421–422, 513
protosystemic shunting 221
psychiatric disorders 160, 162, 164, 343, 346, **498**, 512
psychology, impairments **501**, 502–503
psychosis **508**, 509
psychotic disorders **498**, 512
    see also schizophrenia
pulmonary hypertension (PH) 56, 180–181
purification 110, 156, 164
pyridoxal phosphate (PLP)
    -dependent enzymes, classification 25
    affinity 107
    decarboxylases 105
    deficiency 39
    histamine synthesis co-factor 89
    post-translational modification 108, 110
    Schiff **26**
pyridoxamine (PMP) 25, **26**
pyroglutamate 206–208
pyruvate 35, 131

randomised clinical trials (RCT) 373, **374–375**, 376, 377
rapid tryptophan depletion (RTD) 418–423
reabsorption 246
reactions, metabolic **481–487**
reactive astrocytosis (gliosis) 432
reactive nitrogen species (RNS) 38
reactive oxygen species (ROS)
    enhanced production 130
    formation 60–61, 81
    generation 38
    nitric oxide bioavailability role 77
    production 55, 57
receiver operator characteristic (ROC) curves **470**, **471**
receptor for advanced glycation end products (RAGE) 382, 385, 386, 389, 390–391, 392, 393, 397
receptors
    altered expression 433
    aminoacidergic **508–509**
    γ-aminobutyric acid 104–**105**, 488
    amyotrophic lateral sclerosis 441
    classes and subtypes 508–509
    dopamine role 509
    glutamatergic **428–436**
    histamine 90, 92, 93, 502, **508**, 509
    homeostasis 127
    identification 384–385
    inhibitory metabotropic 445
    list 428–429
    modulators 359–360, 509

monoaminergic **508**–509
neurological/neurodegenerative
    diseases 434–435, 436, 441,
    443–445, 509
overstimulation 502
phylogenic tree **356**
polymorphisms 431
postsynaptic membrane-associated
    receptors 436
proteins 113
T1R family 355–**358**, **360**
transport, inhibition 445
see also neurotransmission; signalling
    systems
recovery enhancement 296–298
redox sensitivity 38
Reelin signalling 429
regeneration 55, 180–182, 185
regulation
    amino acid metabolism 230–232
    enzymes 3–11, 14–15, 17–19, 60–63, 125–127,
        156–161, 180–182, 233
    gene expression 229–238
    molecular mechanisms 232–236
regulators 3, 233, 465
see also adenosine diphosphate; guanosine
    triphosphate
renal *see* kidney
renin 386–387
renin angiotensinaldosterone system (RAAS) 61
reperfusion injury 57
requirements 250–251, 256–257, 260, 263–264,
    267–284, 493, 513
research suggestions 115–116, 225
research titles, clinical amino acid imbalance **329**
residues 105–107, 154, 359
resistance exercise (RE) 292–298, 299, 301, 302,
    303, 304
retina
    artery occlusions 371
    astroglia 33, 35, 60, 138, 142, 144
    branched-chain aminotransferase
        role 32–33
    disease 391
    disorders 59, 60
    embedded section **138**
    excitatory amino acid 138
    ganglion cell death 55
    serine racemase 137–148
    D-serine role 139–142
    D-serine uptake 140–142
rewards, drugs 94–95
rheumatoid arthritis (RA) 392–393, 395
ribonucleic acid (RNA) 62–63, 90, 92–93,
    123, 158, 293
ribonucleotides, purinic 353
risk 369–378, 497, **501**, 505–506, 513

Ross Protocols 409
RT-PCR analysis 112

safety 421, 511
samples, handling standardization 468
sapid molecules (tastants) 313, 353, **362**
    see also taste
sarcopenia 292, 302–303
schizophrenia
    neurotransmission derangements
        effect **501**, 502
    potential treatment mechanism 509
    receptors 428, 434–435, **508**
    theory, dopamine 434
    tryptophan pathway degradation
        effect 503
scopolamine 96
Scrivener, Charles 413
seizures 436–437, **438**, 502, 508
selenoamino acids 336–337, **339**, 344
selenocystine **334**
selenomethionine **334**, **336**, 344–**345**, 507
sensors 178–180, 233, 236–238, 354–355
septic encephalopathy 329–330
septic patients 343
sequences 92–93, **106**, **108–109**,
    110–113, 233
D-serine 137–148, 489, 490
serine racemase 137–148, 485–486
serotonin, aromatic amino acid decarboxylase
    source 460
serotonin (5-hydroxytryptamine)
    aggression in ADHD children,
        relationship 503
    biosynthesis 150–164, **420**
    depletion 157–158, 419
    diminished uptake 420
    gut-derived 158
    neurons 459
    neurotransmission role 161,
        418–419, 512
    pathway **151**
    psychiatric investigations 343,
        418–423
    receptor modulators **508**, 509
    regulation 421
    reuptake inhibitor(s) **151**, 419
    synthesis 201, 507
short bowel syndrome (SBS), infants 314–315
short-chain 3-hydroxtacyl-CoAdehydrogenase
    (SCHAD) 13–14
short-duration response (SDR) 458
shuttles **31**, 35
sickle cell disease 56
side-effects 422–423, 458–459
    see also adverse effects

signalling systems
    cells 298–299, 303–304
    components, pharmaceutical
        targeting 513
    emergence and new momentum 491
    gases 489–490
    mechanisms 236
    molecules 221
    nutrition 230
    pathways **116**, 178–180, 183, 235–236, 361–362
    Reelin 429
    regulation 82
    responses 298–299
    sensing 178–180
    transduction mechanisms 61–62, 361–362
    transmission 115
    see also neurotransmission; receptors
silent information regulator (Sirt) 13
single nucleotide polymorphisms (SNPs) 161
Sirt4 mutations 13
sirtuins 13
skeletomuscular disorders 392–393
skin 392, 507
sleep 94
slope ratio growth assay 261
smoking 371
soy proteins 263, 301
stable isotope 248, 257–258, 268, 272–274
state of the art 130
steatohepatitis 181–182
steatosis 174, 177, 181–182
stomach **113**
storage 230–231, 456, 468
stress
    chronic 435
    control 397
    Duchenne muscular dystrophy patient **315**
    mental 386
    oxidative 84, 431
    response regulation 95
striatum structures 429, 430, 432
stroke 372, 373, **374**, **375**, 376, 377, **428**, 442–445, 496, 498, 502
substrates
    glutathione 206, 386, 495
    inhibition 156, 419
    kinetic characteristics **197**
    list **197**
    liver gluconeogenesis 124–125
    nitric oxide cycle **223**
    orientation importance 154
    putative 199, 200

    recognition mechanisms 106
    selectivity 140
    systems 199, 205
    γ-glutamyl cycle 206
    see also glutamine
subthalamic nucleus (STN) 130
sucralose enhancer 360
sudden infant death syndrome (SIDS) 163
SU.FOL.OM3 trial 377
sugar 387
sulphur amino acids 257, 263, **334**, 340–341
    see also cysteine; methionine
supplements
    acute studies 294, 301–302
    benefits 493–496
    clinical support role 493–496, 506, 507, 510–511
    disease progression slowing 316–318, 377
    enteral administration 224–225
    exercise enhancement 293–298
    imbalance rectification **325–326**
    mixtures 279, 410, 493
    muscular performance 291–304
    protection role 302–303, 396
    protein 293, 294, 295, 296–298, 303
    studies 295, 302, 373, 376, 377
support, clinical 312–318, 493–496, 506, 507, 510–511
swine, feed **263**
synbiotics 396–397
synergy 353–354
systematic inflammation 386–387

T1R2 VFT domain, molecular model **360**
tacrine 97
targets, molecular 507–509
tastants 313, 353, **362**
taste
    biology 363
    qualities 353
    receptor cells 354–356, **358**, **359**, 360, 361–**362**, 363–364
    signalling systems 113–115, 354–355, 361–362
    sweet-taste receptor **358**, 360
    umami 113, 353–364, 492, 496
taurine 396, 489
tautomerization 25
tea **16**, 506
technologies, innovative development 513
tele-methylhistamine 89, **90**
tetrahydroisoquinolines (TIQs) 158
tetrahydrobiopterin (BH_4)
    dependent enzymes, regulation 155
    DOPA synthesis role 460

drug 406, 412–413
reduction 456
therapy 506
treatment 408
Tetrahymena Genome Project 14
therapeutics 343–345, 454–461, 506, 507, **508**, 509, 512, 513
thioretinaco ozonide depletion 377
threonine 250, **251**, **262**, 263, **273**, **280**
thromboembolism, venous 372, 373, 377
thymidylate synthase (TYMS) 178
thyroid dysfunction 491–492
tongue 114, **115**, 354
  see also papillae; taste
toxicity
  amino acids elimination 201
  cured meat production, disquiet 511
  glutamate 37–38, 146, 342
  glutamine 131
  health implications 346
  Huntington's disease pathogenic mechanisms 431
  neurodegeneration role 37–38
  see also adverse effects; excitotoxicity; neurotoxicity
toxicology, food 496
tracers 271–281, 283
transamination
  branched-chain amino acids 25, **26**
  gluconeogenic amino acids 220
  α-keto acids 32, 35, **483**
  reactions **26**, 130
  see also aminotransferases
transaminases *see* aminotransferases
transcription factors 123–125, 130, 221, 232–238
transduction cascade 361, **362**
transgenics 107, 432–434
transmethylation 174
transmitters excitatory 138
  see also neurotransmission
transport systems
  active 193–194, 202, 203
  blood brain barrier 191–208
  disorders, inherited **500**, 505
  facilitative 195–**197**, 203, 205
  ions 193–194
  L-1 419
  mechanisms 140, 192, 490–491
  methodologies 192–194
  Na⁺-dependent 194, 197–**200**, **201**, 203, 205, 206–208
  organization 200–201
  passive 193–194, 420
  receptors, inhibition 445
  sites 490–491
  study methods 192–194

transporters
  facilitative 194–**197**, **198**
  inhibition 445
  innovative approaches 509
  kinetic characteristics **197**, **201**
  list **197**
  membrane barriers 192
  neurons role **128**, **204**
  studies 140–142
  see also substrates
transsulphuration pathway **175**
trauma 220–221
treatment, modalities 410
trials 373, **374**–**375**, 376, 377
tricarboxylic acid (TCA) cycle 15, 31, 34, 131
triglycerides (TGL) 173
tryptophan
  -rich proteins 507
  availability 420–421
  brain entry impairment 201
  competition 490–491
  degradation 512
  depletion 343, 418–423, 503
  imbalance, induced 346
  influx mechanisms **420**
  nicotinamide generation 323
  requirement estimation **280**
  tests 512
  transport 151
  see also aromatics
tryptophan hydroxylase (TPH)
  clinical significance **498**
  domain organization 152–154
  dysfunction 161–164
  enzyme regulation 156–161
  function **152**–**156**, **420**
  isoforms 153, **482**, 486
  kinetic parameters **157**
  knockout studies 161
  ligand binding 154–155
  properties 150–152
  structure 152–156, 158
tumours
  cell proliferation 92
  development 124
  dietary control 507
  inhibition 344, 346
  management 509
  proliferative capacity 122
  see also cancer
TUNEL assay 146
tyrosinaemia **499**, 505
tyrosine
  conversion 456, **457**
  depletion 503
  kinase blockers 508
  requirements **273**, 277, **280**

tyrosine hydroxylase (TH) 150–151, 456, 486, 506

ultrafiltration 247–248
umami 113, 353–364, 492, 496
under-nourishment 283
under-nutrition 282
uraemia 384
urea cycle
    ammonia detoxification mechanisms 218
    disorders 505
    enzymes 51–**52**, **219**, 341, 485
    primary function **74**
    substrates 124–125, **219**
    synthesis of urea 124–125, 219
ureagenesis **12**, 220
urogenital disorders 394
urolithiasis 37

valine **273**, **280**, 344
vascular disease
    AGE effect 506
    age-related changes 59
    artery 77, 78
    dysfunction 60
    heart 372, 373, 376–377, 387
    homocysteine levels 371, 373, 376, 377
    remodelling 61
    study differences 376–377
    see also cardiovascular disease; stroke
vasodilation, mediation 82
vegans 388
vegetables 83, 495–496, 507
    see also plants

vegetarians 388
vein occlusions 371
venous thromboembolism (VTE) 372, 373, 377
venus flytrap (VFT) domain 359
vesicles, storage 456
viral vector-mediated gene transfer delivery method 460, 461
vitamins
    administration method 423
    B_6 370, 373, **374–375**, 376, 377, 507
    B_{12} 373, **374–375**, 376, 377, 410, 411, 507
    deficiencies 386, 410–411, 496
    efficacy 373–376
    genetic mutations, treatment 372
    sources 396
    trials **374–375**, 376–377, 507

waking 94
Warburg effect 177, 178, 181
websites **411**
weight gain 509
    see also obesity
Western blot analysis **111**, 196
wheat germ agglutinin (WGA) 362
whey protein 301, 302, 304
white matter abnormalities 410
whole-body protein 260, **314**
whole-body responses **327**
Woo, Savio 413
wound healing 54–55, 60

yeast artificial chromosome (YAC) 433